Baumann's Cosmetic Dermatology

Baumann's Cosmetic Dermatology

THIRD EDITION

Leslie S. Baumann, MD
Dermatologist, Author and Researcher
Private practice
CEO of Skin Type Solutions.com
Miami, Florida

Evan A. Rieder, MD
Dermatologist, Psychiatrist
The Ronald O. Perelman Department of Dermatology
New York, New York

Mary D. Sun, MD, MSCR
Icahn School of Medicine at Mount Sinai
New York, New York

New York   Chicago   San Francisco   Athens   London   Madrid   Mexico City
Milan   New Delhi   Singapore   Sydney   Toronto

Baumann's Cosmetic Dermatology, Third Edition

Copyright © 2022 by McGraw Hill LLC. All rights reserved. Printed in China. Except as permitted under the United States Copyright Act of 1976, no part of this publication may be reproduced or distributed in any form or by any means, or stored in a data base or retrieval system, without the prior written permission of the publisher.

Previous edition copyright @ 2002, 2009 by the McGraw-Hill Companies, Inc.

1 2 3 4 5 6 7 8 9 DSS 27 26 25 24 23 22

ISBN 978-0-07-179419-0
MHID 0-07-179419-0

The editors were Leah Carton, Karen Edmonson, and Christina M. Thomas.
The production supervisor was Richard Ruzycka.
The cover designer was W2 Design.
Project management was provided by Anamika Singh, MPS Limited.

Library of Congress Cataloging-in-Publication Data

Names: Baumann, Leslie, editor. | Rieder, Evan A., editor. | Sun, Mary D.,
    editor. | Baumann, Leslie. Cosmetic dermatology.
Title: Baumann's cosmetic dermatology / [edited by] Leslie Baumann, Evan A.
    Rieder, Mary D. Sun.
Other titles: Cosmetic dermatology
Description: Third edition. | New York : McGraw Hill, [2022] | Preceded by
    Cosmetic dermatology / Leslie Baumann, Sogol Saghari, Edmund Weisberg.
    2nd ed. c2009. | Includes bibliographical references and index. |
    Summary: "This title covers the field of cosmetic dermatology including
    medications, cosmeceuticals, and procedures in a simple and easy way
    with clear prose and ample illustrations and figures"—Provided by
    publisher.
Identifiers: LCCN 2021045692 | ISBN 9780071794190 (hardcover) | ISBN
    9780071800907 (ebook)
Subjects: MESH: Skin Diseases—therapy | Cosmetic Techniques | Skin
    Care—methods
Classification: LCC RL71 | NLM WR 650 | DDC 616.5—dc23
LC record available at https://lccn.loc.gov/2021045692
Unsubscribe | Notification Preferences

McGraw Hill books are available at special quantity discounts to use as premiums and sales promotions, or for use in corporate training programs. To contact a representative please visit the Contact Us pages at www.mhprofessional.com.

This book is dedicated to all of the aestheticians, skincare specialists, medical providers, and doctors who take the time to learn the science of cosmetic dermatology before treating clients and patients. It takes time, energy, and passion to learn all the aspects of skincare, cosmetic treatments, and procedures.
For those of you who take this field seriously—please help keep the bar high in this field as a plethora of practitioners enter this space. It's up to you to support each other and work together to advance the science of cosmetic dermatology.

Contents

Contributors

Lisa Akintilo, MD, MPH
PGY-4 Dermatology Resident
Ronald O. Perelman Department of Dermatology
New York University Grossman School of Medicine
New York, New York

Peter B. Chansky, MD
Resident Physician
Ronald O. Perelman Department of Dermatology
New York University
New York, New York

Alina Goldenberg, MD
Director of Contact Dermatitis Clinic
Dermatologist Medical Group of North County
San Diego, California

Daniel Gutierrez, MD
Assistant Professor
The Ronald O. Perelman Department of Dermatology
NYU Grossman School of Medicine
New York, New York

Kerry Heitmiller, MD
Dermatology Associates of Concord
Concord and Cambridge, Massachusetts

Sharon E. Jacob, MD
Professor
Loma Linda University
Clinical Professor (Medicine and Pediatrics)
University of California, Riverside
Loma Linda, California

Jenny Kim, MD, PhD
Professor, Director of Micrographic Surgery and
Dermatologic Oncology and Cosmetic Dermatology
Division of Dermatology, Department of Medicine
David Geffen School of Medicine
University of California
Los Angeles, California

Elizabeth J. Kream, MD
Resident Physician
Department of Dermatology
University of Illinois College of Medicine
Chicago, Illinois

Helen Liu, BS
Medical Student
Icahn School of Medicine at Mount Sinai
New York, New York

Joseph N. Mehrabi, MD
Resident Physician
Department of Medicine
Maimonides Medical Center
Brooklyn, New York

Krystal Mitchell, MD, MBA
Dermatology Resident
Department of Dermatology
Icahn School of Medicine at Mount Sinai
New York, New York

Gabrielle Pastorek, MFA
Content Developer
Skin Type Solutions Inc
Miami, Florida

Paula Purpera, MSHS, PA-C
Physician Assistant
Baumann Cosmetic and Research Institute
Miami, Florida

Jennifer M. Rullan, MD
Consultant for Scripps Mercy Hospital
Chula Vista, California
Dermatology Institute Private Practice
Chula Vista and Coronado, California

Nazanin Saedi, MD
Dermatology Associates of Plymouth Meeting
Clinical Associate Professor
Thomas Jefferson University
Philadelphia, Pennsylvania

Rachel Sally, BA
Medical Student
NYU Langone School of Medicine
New York, New York

Lana X. Tong, MD, MPH
Dermatologist
Palo Alto Foundation Medical Group
Affiliated with Palo Alto Medical Foundation
Sutter Health
Sacramento, California

Amy R. Vandiver, MD, PhD
Resident Physician
Division of Dermatology
Department of Medicine
David Geffen School of Medicine
University of California
Los Angeles, California

Jordan V. Wang, MD, MBE, MBA
Medical Research Director
Laser & Skin Surgery Center of New York
New York, New York

Edmund M. Weisberg, MS, MBE
Senior Science Writer
Johns Hopkins University
Baltimore, Maryland

Kiyanna Williams, MD
Department of Dermatology
Section Head, Skin of Color Section
Cleveland Clinic
Cleveland, Ohio

Heather Woolery-Lloyd, MD
Director, Skin of Color Division
Dr. Phillip Frost Department of Dermatology and Cutaneous Surgery
University of Miami Miller School of Medicine
Miami, Florida

Joshua Zeichner, MD
Associate Professor
Department of Dermatology
Icahn School of Medicine at Mount Sinai
New York, New York

Preface

Before I begin, I want to make my financial disclosure clear. I am the CEO of Skin Type Solutions, a software company that automatically designs skincare regimens according to the Baumann Skin Type.® This book describes the Baumann Skin Types in Chapter 10 and mentions them in the skin type chapters. Chapter 34 includes a mention of the Skin Type Solutions software. I included it because at the time of publication, over 100 dermatologists and 240 doctors were using the system in their office.

I also need to disclose that I have done clinical trials for most of the companies that make injectable medical devices used in cosmetic dermatology practices such as AbbVie (Botox, Juvéderm, Voluma, Kybella), Galderma (Dysport and the Restylane products), Revance (Daxibotulinum Toxin A), Endo International (Qwo), Merz (Ulthera) and others.

With that said, I would love to tell you why I spent many months during COVID updating this bestselling textbook. The original *Cosmetic Dermatology* text (McGraw Hill, 2002) was the first textbook on cosmetic dermatology that I know of written in any language. Botox was approved by the FDA in 2002 and the first hyaluronic acid fillers were not approved until 2003. I was involved in those research trials, so I had the insights and experience to discuss these procedures in the 2002 edition. *Cosmetic Dermatology: Principles and Practice* (2002) was translated into many languages and was a best seller around the world. If you go back and look at Edition 1, you will see it is tiny. At that time Botox was newly approved for glabellar wrinkles, hyaluronic acid fillers were not yet FDA approved in the USA, and we were still using bovine collagen injections that did not last long, had a risk of allergic reaction, and required skin testing weeks before treatment. The field of cosmetic dermatology has grown exponentially since that time as have my children. When I dedicated the first edition to my family, I had one young child and was pregnant with my second son. I wrote the entire book myself. (It is amazing how much more time we all had before social media.)

Now it is 20 years after publication of the first edition. One of those children has graduated from college and the other is still in college—a visual reminder of how much time has passed. The field of cosmetic dermatology has blossomed. There are 20+ FDA-approved hyaluronic acid dermal fillers and at least five Type A botulinum toxins that are approved by the FDA. The laser, light, and radiofrequency fields have grown so much that most cosmetic dermatology practices have at least one of these devices. I got busier as well. Although I wrote the 2nd edition of this book mostly by myself, I could not do this Edition 3 alone. There was just so much material to cover because the field has grown so much. Karen Edmonson at McGraw Hill patiently prodded me to do Edition 3 for the last 5 years and I just did not have the time. She helped motivate me during the 2020 COVID quarantine to partner with Evan Rieder, MD, who had worked with Karen on other textbooks and proven himself to be a great writer. We also brought in a young, bright, and motivated medical student, Mary Sun, to organize us and motivate us to meet the deadlines. The three of us divided up the book, assigned chapters, and worked diligently during the days of COVID to review all of the latest research and completely rewrite this edition. I am passionate about skincare and cosmeceuticals, so I wrote most of the skincare chapters myself. We changed the name of the book to *Baumann's Cosmetic Dermatology* in anticipation of Edition 4, which I may not be a part of (I will be old by then!).

Although this book has detailed scientific explanations, it is written in an easy-to-understand manner so that practitioners who are novices in performing cosmetic dermatology procedures can learn the proper techniques and understand the science. My goal is to help all medical providers give accurate medical advice and care to their patients. At the time this book was published, physician-dispensed skincare was the most rapidly growing skincare market segment. I have included chapters on how to retail skincare in your medical practice and how to choose the best physician-dispensed skincare products.

My goal is to help medical providers look beyond the marketing claims to understand the science and to empower medical providers help patients achieve the healthiest skin possible. It is my hope that this book will help all medical professionals including cosmetic chemists, medical aestheticians, physician assistants, nurse practitioners, and doctors understand the most important scientific principles in the field.

Leslie S. Baumann, MD

Opportunities to collaborate with legends in your field of practice do not come along often. Thus, when Dr. Baumann was looking for a collaborator for an upcoming edition of her renowned text, I jumped at the opportunity. I was fortunate to have written and edited a textbook immediately prior to joining Dr. Baumann, and understood the labor of love that would be required. I was also fortunate to have been introduced to a dynamic, organized, and incredibly intelligent medical student, Mary Sun. Mary had been my instrumental collaborator and right hand in several projects over the previous few years; I knew that she would be the glue that kept us together and a motivating force pushing the project along.

The field of cosmetic dermatology has been rapidly evolving in numerous ways since the launch of Botox nearly 20 years ago; around the time of this textbook's first edition. What was initially a single neurotoxin being utilized by a small subset of doctors has expanded to numerous aesthetic injectables, devices, and topical cosmetics being employed by physicians, nurses, physician assistants, aestheticians, cosmetic chemists, and beyond. While expanded options and more practitioners have brought about numerous opportunities and challenges, what has not changed is the need for accurate, evidence-based information, and a practical approach to patient care. In a field rife with marketing schemes and cosmetic treatments promising results that often seem too good to be true, it is incumbent upon us to sort through the smoke and mirrors and help our colleagues understand and make the best decisions about their practices. True to the original concept behind this tome, *Baumann's Cosmetic Dermatology* gives readers of a variety of backgrounds the tools to grasp the science behind cosmetic dermatology and the practical information to help their patients along their aesthetic journeys.

Evan A. Rieder, MD

Acknowledgments

There are so many people to thank as expressed in the two previous editions. The wonderful mentors, family members, coworkers, staff, and friends who have helped me are too numerous to list here. A few noteworthy people must be thanked.

My husband Roger Baumann, who has been important in my life since 1989, has protected, guided, motivated, and put up with me for decades. I would never have achieved what I have without his support, patience, and collaboration. My biggest achievements—my two sons, Robert and Max Baumann, are dedicated to making the world a better place. They have been so flexible and supportive of me and my career. They have taught me as much as I have taught them. I am so proud of them!

My managing editor, Edmund Weisberg, has worked with me as an editor for over 20 years. We have both put a part of our heart and soul into the previous editions and this new edition, which I hope is evident to you when you read it. I would not have done this 3rd edition without the determination of Karen Edmonson at McGraw Hill to get this completed.

My executive assistant, Elizabeth Fernandez, helped me organize chapters, consents, all of the many phone and Zoom calls, and helped me protect my time to get this accomplished. She has been organizing my life for the last 9 years. My physician assistant Paula Purpera, who is an excellent writer, helped me with several chapters and participated in research trials at the Baumann Cosmetic and Research Institute in addition to seeing patients and building a social media following @ Paulasperfectpout. Paula and I share a love of literature, writing, art, and, of course, patient care. Amy Koberling, my other physician assistant who joined my practice in the last few years, has excelled at skincare as well as injectables, and has developed a large following on social media @the_skinenthusiast. The newest addition to my medical practice, dermatologist Dr. Chloe Goldman, is destined to be a star. I have been blessed with so many wonderful colleagues like Heather Woolery-Lloyd, MD, and Laura Scott, MD, that make my job a pleasure.

I sold my medical practice in 2019 and would like to thank Dr. Reuven Porges for all of his kindness and support in making the transition seamless and helping me keep my entire team content and productive. He is one of the gentlest souls that I have ever met.

Thanks to Evan Rieder and Mary Sun for helping me get this 3rd edition completed. I never thought we would be able to do it—but we did it! And lastly, **thanks to all the readers who have helped keep this book one of the most popular textbooks on cosmetic dermatology since its first edition in 2002. We did this new edition for you!**

Leslie S. Baumann, MD

I feel privileged to have been invited to work on this text with Dr. Baumann, one of the luminaries of the field of cosmetic dermatology. I am also indebted to Mary Sun, who has demonstrated herself to be a true dynamo and productive collaborator over the past few years. And to NYU Dermatology for seeing potential in me and taking a chance on training a psychiatrist to become a dermatologist! Finally, a special thanks to Karen Edmonson and the McGraw Hill team for their assistance in bringing this great project to fruition.

Evan A. Rieder, MD

I am deeply fortunate to have worked on this text with Drs. Baumann and Rieder, who have been so generous with their knowledge and mentorship. Thank you to Karen Edmonson for her belief in me and this project, and to Leah, Christina, and the rest of the McGraw Hill team for their excellent work. Many thanks and kudos to the brilliant authors who lent their time and expertise to this undertaking. As a medical trainee, I am grateful to the advisors and educators at Mount Sinai who have supported my extracurricular pursuits. A loving thanks to my parents Michelle and John, who made everything possible, and to my partner David—you are the best copilot I could ask for.

Mary D. Sun, MD, MSCR

Baumann's Cosmetic Dermatology

SECTION 1

Basic Concepts of Skin Science

CHAPTER 1

Basic Science of the Epidermis

Leslie S. Baumann, MD

SUMMARY POINTS

What's Important?
1. Keratinocytes have multiple receptors that give them several important functions.
2. Every skincare product placed on the skin affects the keratinocytes in some way.
3. Stem cells in cosmeceutical products have no activity.

What's New?
1. Circadian rhythms increase TEWL at night.
2. Keratinocytes focus on cell protection in the daylight and cell repair at night.
3. Cosmeceuticals can manipulate epidermal skin cells.
4. Visible light injures mitochondria and lysosomes, and ages skin.

What's Coming?
1. New research on CBD in skincare products.
2. New treatments to remove lipofuscin and rejuvenate lysosomes.
3. New modalities to protect mitochondria.
4. More studies on the effects of light on keratinocytes.

The skin is composed of three primary layers: epidermis, dermis, and subcutaneous tissue (**Fig. 1-1**). The epidermis is the outermost superficial layer of the skin. It is very important from a cosmetic standpoint because it is this layer that gives the skin its texture and moisture, contributes to color, and affects light reflection. If the surface of the epidermis is dry, the skin feels rough and poorly reflects light. When patients complain that their skin is "dull" or "not radiant," the problem lies in the epidermis. This is the layer targeted by salespeople when they urge you to "just try" their product. The product is almost always an exfoliator that removes the uppermost layer of the epidermis providing instant smoothness and light reflection. The epidermis is the layer to target when patients want instant results or radiant skin overnight. However, the changes to the epidermis are temporary as the keratinization cycle continues to produce new cells and push away old cells to the skin's surface. The best topical formulations and skincare

procedures target both the epidermis and the dermis. The epidermis is much more complex than described in this chapter, which is meant to focus on what parts of the epidermis are important to enhance the skin's beauty, appearance, and health with minimal focus on skin disease.

SKIN CELLS IN THE EPIDERMIS: THE KERATINOCYTE

Keratinocytes, also known as corneocytes, are the cells that comprise most of the epidermis. The skin cells in the epidermis are called keratinocytes because they contain keratin, a protein found in the epidermis, nails, and hair. Keratin is also found in the beaks and feathers of birds, and shells. The word "keratin" comes from the Proto-Indo-European root *ker*, which means horn. Keratin composes 30–80% of the total protein of the human epidermis.

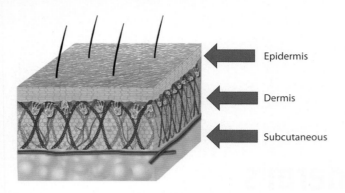

FIGURE 1-1. Human skin.

The epidermis has an abundance of the keratin filaments that make up an intermediate filament cytoskeleton. There are two classes of keratins: Type I is slightly acidic (K9–40) and Type II, more basic (K1–8 and K71–86). Both types of keratin filaments must be present for a keratin filament to develop.[1] In other words, an acidic type and a basic type form a keratin filament together. The keratin genes are found on chromosomes 12q and 17q. There are over 100 known skin, hair, and nail disorders linked to keratin genes.

Keratinocytes perform numerous functions, primarily the delivery of structural support and physical protection. Keratinocytes produce keratin filaments, which provide firmness to the skin and resilience against mechanical stress. They provide a physical barrier to prevent toxins and pathogens from entering the skin. Keratinocytes exhibit an immunomodulatory function and can secrete cytokines, activate Langerhans cells, and stimulate inflammation to protect the skin from pathogens. Keratinocytes are surrounded by bilayer lipid membranes that prevent water loss and keep hydrophilic compounds from entering the skin. They can sense peptides and function as antigen-presenting cells.

Organelles in Keratinocytes

Mitochondria

Mitochondria play a crucial role in skin health and beauty because they are responsible for energy production through a multistep process called oxidative phosphorylation or the electron transport chain. The mitochondria are the primary organelle affected by intrinsic and extrinsic aging.[2] Dysfunction of the mitochondria is a major cause of aging because energy is needed for cells to divide and differentiate, to produce the extracellular matrix (ECM) and proteins, as well as to repair themselves. Keratinocyte differentiation, for example, depends on functional mitochondria; increased Ca^{2+} causes keratinocyte differentiation based on mitochondrial calcium uptake.[2]

The mitochondria produce energy via a process called oxidative phosphorylation by converting adenosine diphosphate (ADP) to adenosine triphosphate (ATP), which occurs in the intricate inner membranes of the mitochondria. The mitochondria use oxygen as a carrier for electrons and consume oxygen in the process of oxidative phosphorylation.

The flow of electrons through the electron transport chain generates energy that is stored in ATP and results in an excess number of electrons, which become reactive oxygen species. These free radicals harm the mitochondrial membranes, as well as cause damage to and mutations in the mitochondrial DNA. Mutations of mitochondrial DNA engender disorder in the energy production process and can lead to an increased number of free radicals. The cycle is perpetuated as these free radicals create more mitochondrial DNA mutations. Mutated and damaged mitochondria do not produce ATP efficiently and represent one cause of aging.[3] At this time there are no ingredients known to repair damaged mitochondria; therefore, mitochondrial damage must be prevented in order to slow aging by using sun protection, sunscreen, and antioxidants.

Cosmeceutical ingredients and mitochondria

Secreted by the pineal gland, melatonin regulates circadian rhythm. Melatonin also exerts effects on keratinocyte proliferation, skin pigmentation, inflammation, and immune response, all of which involve the mitochondria. Melatonin and the mitochondria have a symbiotic relationship. The mitochondria are the site of melatonin biosynthesis and metabolism. Melatonin directly enhances ATP production by donating electrons and provides antioxidant protection to the mitochondria.[2]

Coenzyme Q_{10} (CoQ_{10}) is a lipophilic antioxidant that plays a role in ATP production in the mitochondria. Levels of CoQ_{10}, also known as ubiquinone, are 10-fold higher in the epidermis as compared to the dermis.[2] The statin cholesterol-lowering drugs decrease levels of CoQ_{10} and have been associated with oxidative stress and mitochondrial dysfunction leading to premature aging of skin fibroblast cells in vitro.[4] Topical application of CoQ_{10} has been shown to improve the appearance of aged skin.[5]

The vitamin A family, including retinol, influences the metabolic fitness of the mitochondria by affecting ATP production. Low levels of vitamin A are associated with minimal ATP synthesis, while increasing vitamin A results in a significantly higher energy output.[6] This may be mediated by the c-Raf and protein kinase C (PKC) families,[7] which contain high affinity retinol binding sites in their regulatory domains,[8] and play a critical role in mitochondrial function.

Cosmetic procedures and mitochondria

For the past decade, dermatologists who perform copious light and laser procedures have begun to suspect that the wavelengths of light may have effects on the skin that transcend what is presently understood. It is well known that UV light and blue light can damage mitochondria, and artificial visual light weakens mitochondrial function.[9–11] However, other studies have shown that red light and near-infrared light stimulate mitochondrial activity and ATP production by cytochrome c oxidase.[12–14] For this reason, a sunscreen that protects against visible light should be used daily. More studies are needed to understand the effects of various wavelengths of light on mitochondria.

Lysosomes

Lysosomes are the garbage disposal of the cells. Dysfunction of the lysosome allows cellular waste products to accumulate inside the cell. Genetic defects of lysosomes lead to severe disorders called lysosomal storage diseases (e.g., Tay-Sachs disease and Gaucher's disease).

Lysosomes are intracellular organelles that contain enzymes that degrade and recycle cellular waste. The enzymes require various levels of acidity (different pHs) to work properly; therefore, the lysosome membrane contains a pump that requires ATP to propel hydrogen ions into the lysosome to regulate acidity. To rid the cell of waste, the lysosome needs (1) the correct enzymes, (2) the ideal pH for that enzyme to work, and (3) energy produced by the mitochondria in the form of ATP.

Acquired lysosome dysfunction occurs with aging. When lysosomes are unable to degrade cellular waste, lipofuscin accumulates. Lipofuscin is resistant to degradation and not subject to exocytosis; therefore, it accumulates inside cells, produces free radicals, and causes other cellular disturbances. Under a microscope and with proper staining, lipofuscin appears fluorescent and is thus easily visualized. The age of cells can be ascertained by the amount of lipofuscin seen.[15,16] It is now known that mitochondria play a role in lipofuscin accumulation.[17]

Studies have shown that oxidative stress by free radicals leads to an increase in lipofuscin. Accumulation of lipofuscin hampers the ability of lysosomes to work effectively, altering acidity and disrupting the supply of enzymes.[18] Lipofuscin in keratinocytes generates singlet oxygen free radicals and causes DNA mutations upon exposure to blue light and visible light.[19,20]

Treatments to prevent aging caused by lysosomal damage or increase of lipofuscin would have to achieve one of the following: (1) preserve lysosomal function, (2) increase breakdown of lipofuscin and cellular waste, (3) reduce free radical formation, or (4) enhance lysosomal function. Medical discoveries often occur first in areas of severe disease because these advances are most needed and may receive the most attention and funding. Gaucher's disease,

which is a severe disorder caused by a lack of a lysosomal enzyme, is successfully treated with intravenous infusion of the missing enzyme.[21] Genetic treatments are being developed for Tay-Sachs disease. At this time, there are no genetic or enzyme treatments for accumulation of lipofuscin or cellular waste.

Cosmeceutical ingredients that affect lysosomes and lipofuscin

Antioxidants have been shown to slow the rate of lipofuscin accumulation. Studies have demonstrated beneficial effects from flavanols, polyphenols, catechins, and oligomeric procyanidins. Examples of ingredients that have been successful are grape seed extract, curcumin, tocopherol (vitamin E), CoQ_{10}, beta carotene, and dihydroquercetin.[22–25]

Receptors on Keratinocytes

Keratinocytes, once thought only to confer strength to the skin, play a major role in sensation, cell communication, and activation of the immune system among other functions. They contain receptors that give them several different activities. There are many more receptors on keratinocytes than discussed in this chapter, which will focus on keratinocyte receptors important in skincare.

Cannabinoid Receptors on Keratinocytes

Keratinocytes have cannabinoid receptors, both Type 1 (CB1) and Type 2 (CB2), which play a role in skin inflammation and display immunomodulatory functions (**Fig. 1-2**). Cannabidiol (CBD) regulates pathways involved in keratinocyte differentiation by inducing expression of various genes and exhibits antioxidant and anti-inflammatory properties.[26] CB1 seems to help limit topical allergic response to contact allergens by inhibiting the production of proinflammatory cytokines.[27] Activation of CB2 reduces inflammation and speeds re-epithelialization.[28] CB1 and CB2 are activated by Δ-9-tetrahydrocannabinoid (THC).[29] CB2 is also activated by eugenol, which is found in basil, cloves, and bay leaves. Although many CBD skincare products are on the market, it

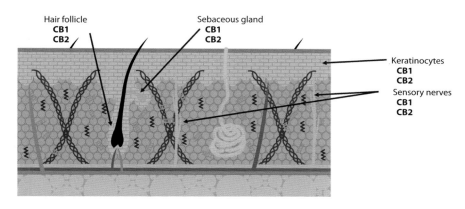

FIGURE 1-2. Cannabinoid receptors in the skin.

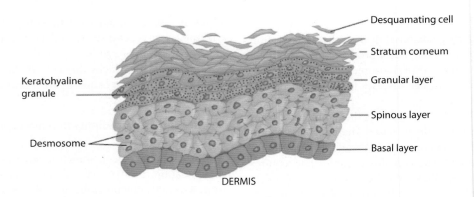

FIGURE 1-3. The layers of the epidermis.

is too early to know which are the most effective and what are the best ways to formulate them to maximize penetration.

Sensory Receptors on Keratinocytes

Keratinocytes have numerous sensory receptors such as transient receptor potential channels (TRP), which can sense temperature, pH, touch, osmolarity, pheromones, and heat. When activated, these TRP receptors release hormones, vasoactive peptides, or neurotransmitters.[29] Activation of these keratinocyte sensors can engender a cascade of effects on skin including pain, itch, activation of inflammation, or perception of heat or cooling.

Transient receptor potential vallinoid 1 (TRPV1) and TRPV4 are heat receptors and play an important role in pain and itch. TRPV1, the receptor that senses capsaicin (a component of chili peppers), gives a sensation of heat, and is activated by CBD and eugenol. TRPV3 is also triggered by eugenol. Transient receptor potential melastatin 8 (TRPM8) is a sensor of low temperatures and is activated by camphor and menthol.[30] This is why menthol, peppermint, and eucalyptus give a cooling sensation. Transient receptor potential ankyrin (TRPA) is responsible for pungent, tingling, and burning taste and feeling when bound to components of cinnamon, garlic, mustard, onion, frankincense, curcumin, and horseradish.[29]

Massage and body oils often contain these natural ingredients. They are used to deliver a sensation of cooling or heat. Knowledge of these receptors can help the practitioner choose which natural oils to include in skincare products to treat various conditions.

Keratinization

The epidermis resembles a brick wall with the bricks representing keratinocytes. It has an inner basal layer of mitotically active cells and suprabasal layers of differentiating cells. Keratinocytes are "born" at the base of the epidermis at the dermal–epidermal junction (DEJ). They are produced by stem cells, some of which reside at the base—basal layer—of the epidermis, while other stem cells are found in the hair follicle. When the stem cells divide, they create "daughter cells," which slowly migrate to the top of the epidermis.[31] This process of keratinocytes being born from stem cells, maturing, and moving to the outermost layer of the skin is called keratinization.

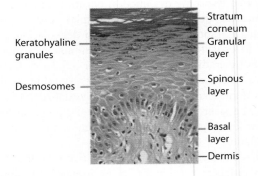

FIGURE 1-4. Histopathology of the epidermis demonstrating the four layers. (Image courtesy of George Ioannides, MD.)

After keratinization, the cells undergo apoptosis and desquamate from the skin's surface.

As keratinocyte cells migrate away from the basal layer and move outward toward the skin surface, they turn off production of proteins such as integrin and laminin and execute a terminal differentiation program. Keratinocyte cells migrate upwards in the epidermis after they loosen their attachments to each other and are pushed from below by younger keratinocytes.

As keratinocytes approach the skin's surface, they mature and develop different characteristics (known as differentiation). The layers of the epidermis are named for these characteristic traits. For example, the first (and deepest) epidermal layer is the basal layer because it is located at the base of the epidermis. The next layer is referred to as the spinous layer because the cells in this layer have prominent, spiny attachments holding the cells together. The next layer is the granular layer because these cells contain visible granules. The last, outermost layer is the stratum corneum (SC), a flattened layer of cells that have lost their nuclei and granules (**Figs. 1-3 and 1-4**). The SC is covered by a protein material called the cell envelope and bathed in lipids that protect the epidermis and help the skin remain hydrated.

As keratinocytes migrate through the layers of the epidermis, their contents and functions change according to, or depending on, the specific epidermal layer in which they are moving. Keratinocyte activity, such as the release of cytokines, can be affected by topical products administered to the skin.

THE LAYERS OF THE EPIDERMIS

The Basal Layer (Stratum Basale)

Cuboidal in shape, basal cells are found at the DEJ attached to the basement membrane that divides the epidermis and dermis. Basal cells produce the ECM components of the underlying basement membrane that separates the epidermis from the dermis.[32] Basal cells attach to the dermis below with hemidesmosomes and to neighboring basal cells and the overlying spinous cells via desmosomes. These basal keratinocytes contain keratins 5 and 14 that form a cytoskeleton allowing for cellular flexibility. This flexibility enables cells to proceed out of the basal layer to migrate superficially, thus undergoing the keratinization process. Mutations of the keratin 5 and 14 genes result in an inherited blistering disease called epidermolysis bullosa simplex.

Basal cells are responsible for maintaining the epidermis by constantly producing new keratinocytes. In the basal layer, 10% of keratinocytes are stem cells, 50% are amplifying cells, and 40% are postmitotic cells. Normally, stem cells are slowly dividing cells, but under certain conditions such as wounding or exposure to growth factors, retinoids, and defensins, they divide faster. Basal cells give rise to transient amplifying cells that are responsible for most of the cell division in the basal layer, producing more keratinocytes. Postmitotic cells undergo terminal differentiation and move superficially to become suprabasal cells that continue their upward migration to become granular cells and ultimately part of the SC (**Fig. 1-5**).

The Spinous Layer (Stratum Spinosum)

The stratum spinosum contains 8–10 layers of keratinocytes connected by spiny attachments called desmosomes that hold the cells together. These spiny desmosomes function as an adhesion point for the intermediate filaments, provide resistance against skin tearing, and play an important role in wound healing. Desmosomes are complex structures composed of adhesion molecules and other proteins that are important in cell adhesion and cell transport.

Lamellar granules, also called Odland bodies, first appear in the spinous layer of the epidermis. These lamellar granules contain lipids such as ceramides, cholesterol, and fatty acids that are produced by the cell. These lipids are packaged into granules, migrate to the surface, and extrude their contents into the space between keratinocytes, bathing the keratinocytes in protective lipids. The lamellar granules protect the contents until they are released at their target point. The lamellar granules also contain hydrolytic enzymes needed for desquamation such as proteases, acid phosphatase, lipases, and glycosidases. The antimicrobial peptide cathelicidin is also stored in the lamellar granules.[33]

Keratins 1 and 10 are first seen in this spinous layer of suprabasal keratinocytes. These keratins form a rigid cytoskeleton that confers mechanical strength to the cell.

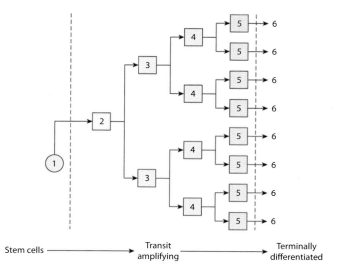

Stem cells ⟶ Transit amplifying ⟶ Terminally differentiated

FIGURE 1-5. The stem cells divide and produce amplifying cells that greatly increase the number of keratinocytes. These in turn become the mature, terminal, and differentiated cells. The numbers indicate the cell generation.

In hyperproliferative conditions such as actinic keratosis, wound healing, and psoriasis, keratins 6 and 16 are expressed in the spinous layer. The cytoplasm of the spinous layer keratinocytes contains proteins not found in the basal layers such as involucrin, keratolinin, and loricrin. These proteins become cross-linked in the SC to impart strength to the skin.

The Granular Layer (Stratum Granulosum)

The granular layer contains 3–4 layers of keratinocytes that are characterized by granular dots seen in the keratinocytes. These keratohyalin granules contain profilaggrin, the precursor to filaggrin. Filaggrin is a **fil**ament **aggr**egating prote**in** that binds to the keratin cytoskeleton and forms a protein scaffold upon which proteins and lipids can attach. The filaggrin cross-links to keratin filaments providing strength and structure. A genetic defect of the filaggrin gene predisposes an individual to the triad of atopic dermatitis (eczema), allergies, and asthma or may result in a dry skin disorder known as ichthyosis vulgaris.

The proteins of the cornified cell envelope (involucrin, keratolinin, the pancornulins, and loricrin) are cross-linked in this layer by the calcium-requiring enzyme transglutaminase (TGase) to form the cell envelope. There are four types of transglutaminases present in the epidermis: TGase 1 or keratinocyte TGase, TGase 2 or tissue TGase, TGase 3 or epidermal TGase, and TGase 5. Only TGases 1, 3, and 5 participate in the development of the corneocyte envelope. TGase 2 has other functions including a role in apoptosis (programmed cell death). TGase activity increases when Ca^{2+} levels increase,[34] and results in the formation of the cornified cell envelope.

Calcium is an inducer of keratinocyte differentiation,[35,36] and a suppressor of keratinocyte proliferation.[37,38] It has been shown that in the state of low Ca^{2+} levels keratinocytes are in a proliferative stage, while increases in Ca^{2+} levels lead to expression of differentiation markers such as keratins 1 and 10, TGase, and filaggrin.[37]

BOX 1-1

1,25-Dihydroxyvitamin D_3 [1,25(OH)$_2$D$_3$] stimulates the differentiation and prohibits the proliferation of keratinocytes. It exerts its effects via the nuclear hormone receptor known as vitamin D receptor (VDR). VDR operates with the aid of coactivator complexes. There are two known coactivator complexes: vitamin D interacting protein complex (DRIP) and the p160 steroid receptor coactivator family (SRC/p160). It has been proposed that the DRIP mediator complex is involved in proliferation and early differentiation, while the SRC/p160 complex is engaged in advanced differentiation.[11] The vitamin D receptors of undifferentiated keratinocytes bind to the DRIP complex, inducing early differentiation markers of K1 and K10.[12] The DRIP complex on the vitamin D receptor is then replaced by the SRC complex. The SRC complex induces gene transcription for advanced differentiation, which occurs with filaggrin and loricrin.[12] The replacement of the DRIP complex with the SRC complex on the vitamin D receptor is believed to be necessary for keratinocyte differentiation. It is important to realize that vitamin D levels are lower in older people and that this reduction may play a role in the slower wound healing characteristic in the elderly.

The form of vitamin D known as 1,25-dihydroxyvitamin D_3 [1,25(OH)$_2$D$_3$] plays a role in keratinocyte differentiation because it enhances the Ca^{2+} effect on the keratinocytes and increases transglutaminase activity as well as involucrin levels.[39] These combined effects induce corneocyte envelope formation.[40,41] (See **Box 1-1**.)

Granular cells exhibit anabolic properties such as synthesis of filaggrin, cornified cell envelope proteins, and high molecular weight keratins. However, they also cause catabolic events such as dissolution of the cell nucleus and organelles, which disappear prior to moving into the SC. The granular layer is the uppermost viable layer of the epidermis because the layer above it contains no organelles.

The Stratum Lucidum

This layer is 2–3 cell layers thick in most of the body and 8–10 layers thick in the palms and soles.[42] It is clear when viewed under the microscope and not easily seen in routine stains, so many skin anatomy texts contend that it does not exist other than in the palms and soles. Some consider the stratum lucidum a part of the SC. The author suggests that it is reasonable to think that most of the body has four major epidermal layers, but areas such as the palms and soles have five such layers, including the stratum lucidum.

The keratinocytes in this layer have not yet lost all their nuclei, have sparse organelles, and are filled with eleidin, which is a byproduct of keratohyalin.[42] This layer overlies the vermilion border in the lip and its lucidity allows the red blood vessels to show through, giving the vermilion border of light skin types a red appearance.

The Stratum Corneum (SC)

The most superficial layer of the epidermis is the SC or horny layer, which forms a protective layer on the skin's surface.

The keratinocytes that reside in this layer are the most mature and have completed the keratinization process. These keratinocytes contain no nuclei or organelles. Although the SC plays a very important role in skin hydration and protection, it is described as the "dead layer" of the epidermis because these cells do not exhibit protein synthesis and are unresponsive to cellular signaling.[43]

The SC is approximately 15 cell layers thick but this depends upon the location on the body.[44,45] The SC has the most cell layers on the palms and the soles. If present on the lips, the SC is only about three layers thick, which is why the lips dehydrate easily and become chapped.

The SC is composed of protein-rich corneocytes embedded in a bilayer lipid lamellar matrix assembled in a "brick and mortar" fashion. The "bricks" are composed of keratinocytes and the "mortar" is made up of the contents extruded from the lamellar granules including ceramides, cholesterol, and fatty acids (**Fig. 1-6**). These lipids form bilayer lamellar membranes known as the "skin barrier." When viewed under a cross-polarizing microscope, these lamellar lipids form a Maltese cross-pattern when the skin barrier is intact (**Fig. 1-7**). One of its protective functions is to prevent transepidermal water loss (TEWL).

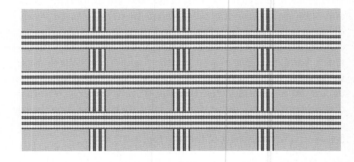

FIGURE 1-6. The keratinocytes are surrounded by multiple bilayers of lipids that form a lamellar structure. This resembles a brick and mortar structure.

FIGURE 1-7. Maltese Cross image seen under cross-polarizing microscope when bilayer lamellar membranes are intact.

Filaggrin, the structural protein synthesized in the granular layer and packaged in keratohyalin granules, is broken down into amino acids inside the keratinocyte cells. These amino acids form a substance known as natural moisturizing factor (NMF). Genetic defects of filaggrin lead to reduced levels of NMF intracellularly in the SC.[46] Cells of the midcornified layer possess the highest amino acid content and, therefore, have the greatest capability for binding to water, while the deeper layers have less water-binding capacity.[47] Intracellularly located NMF and lipids released by the lamellar granules, located extracellularly, play an important role in skin hydration, suppleness, and flexibility (see Chapter 12, Dry Skin).

THE KERATINOCYTE CELL CYCLE

Keratinization is the process of the keratinocytes beginning in the basal layer and maturing and moving to the top of the epidermis and desquamating from the skin's surface. The keratinization process of young epidermis is about 26 to 42 days but can vary due to skin thickness, age, genetics, skincare products, and other factors.[48] Most references cite 28 days as the turnover time for the cells to transition from the basal layer to the SC.[49] However, because studies differ and it is best to manage patients' expectations about when to see changes from a new skincare regimen, this text will cite that in an average person's epidermis with a thickness of 0.1 mm, the keratinization process transpires over 4–6 weeks.[50] This is significant because changes from topical skin treatments depend on keratinization time, and treating acne or pigmentation or significantly changing the epidermis takes 4–6 weeks to see results (**Fig. 1-8**).

This series of events, known also as desquamation, normally occurs invisibly with shedding of individual cells or small clumps of cells. Disturbances of this process may result in the accumulation of partially detached keratinocytes, which cause the clinical findings of dry skin. Disease states may also alter the keratinization cycle. For example, psoriasis causes a dramatic shortening of the keratinization cycle, resulting in the formation of crusty cutaneous eruptions. Keratinization lengthens in time as humans age.[51] This means that the cells at the superficial layer of the SC are older and their function

may be impaired. Results from such compromised functioning include slower wound healing and a skin appearance that is dull and lifeless.

The keratinization process is regulated by epidermal growth factor, retinoids, cytokines, and the presence of lipids such as linoleic acid and other factors.[52] Age, diet, genetics, and the use of skincare products affect keratinization duration. Using exfoliants such as scrubs, microdermabrasion, peels, and lasers can accelerate keratinization. Several cosmetic products such as retinol, growth factors, topical defensins, and alpha hydroxy acids quicken the pace of keratinization, yielding younger keratinocytes at the superficial layers of the SC, thus imparting a more youthful appearance to the skin.

Skin Stem Cells in the Epidermis

The epidermis constantly renews itself in a perpetual cycle of growth and desquamation. Epidermal stem cells (EPSCs) and hair follicles maintain this cycle and drive healing of the epidermis. EPSCs cycle between stemness, differentiation, and senescence, regulated by the p63 gene.[53] The stem cells of the epidermis are found in the hair follicle, sebaceous gland, sweat gland, and the interfollicular epidermis between the hair follicles, each with its own specialized stem cells (SCs). The interfollicular epidermal stem cells (IFE-SCs) and the sebaceous gland stem cells are constantly self-renewing, while hair follicle stem cells cycle between growth, involution, and resting stages as seen with the stages of hair growth (anagen, telogen, and catagen). IFEs are not well characterized yet. There are many stem cells in the hair follicle that are beginning to be understood (**Fig. 1-9**). LGR6+ is important in skincare science because

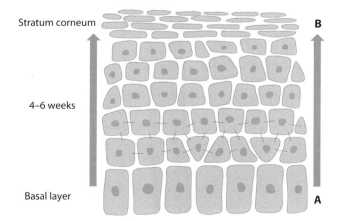

FIGURE 1-8. Movement of keratinocytes from the basal layer to the stratum corneum can take 4–6 weeks. This process is called keratinization.

Stratum corneum

4–6 weeks

Basal layer

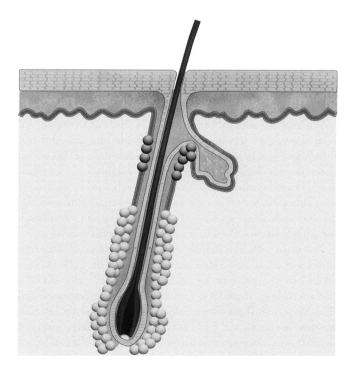

FIGURE 1-9. There are many stem cells in the hair follicle as shown in different colors along the hair follicle. The LGR6+ stem cell location is shown in green.

it is activated by defensin and can regenerate the epidermis when activated. LGR6+ is an important stem cell in wound healing.[54]

Stem cell-containing areas are divided into three niches, each with a specific microenvironment of growth factors, ECM, and various cell types. The niches are the basal layer of the epidermis, the bulge of the hair follicle, and the base of the sebaceous gland.[55] New data is emerging to reveal how stem cells interact with the ECM. For example, the stem cells interact with the ECM via integrins, and insulin-like growth factor-binding protein (IGFBP)-2 and microRNA (miR135b) have been shown to play a role in the regenerative capacity of the epidermis.[56,57] Aging, due to a multitude of reasons, results in decreases of stem cell numbers or function in these niches.[58] Stem cells are damaged from aging, exposure to UV light and free radicals, shortening of telomeres, inflammation, accumulation of senescent cells, and other factors that render them sluggish.[59–62] Reactive oxygen species, also known as free radicals, affect the proliferative ability of EPSCs and enhance their differentiation while decreasing their stemness.[63]

EPSCs are subject to the circadian clock, which affects both proliferation and differentiation.[64,65] Circadian clock disruption leads to an increase in differentiation or EPSCs that resemble the changes seen in the aging process.[66] An increased level of senescent keratinocytes in older skin causes a reduction in stem cell population.[67]

Cosmeceuticals That Act on Epidermal Stem Cells in Skincare Products

There are several benefits to manipulating the microenvironment around EPSCs to promote renewal including improvement of the skin's appearance, strength, and texture and to speed wound healing. Using over-the-counter cosmetic products that contain stem cells is not the answer. The stem cells found in these mass-market skincare products are useless and exert no activity on the epidermis. One reason is that the stem cells in skincare products are plant derived, often from apples, and deliver no activity in human skin. Even if the stem cells were active, they would need to be cultured in stringent conditions and would not survive in a skincare product on a shelf. Companies include apple stem cells in products because consumers have heard about stem cell research and skin rejuvenation. However, the stem cells used to rejuvenate skin and treat chronic wounds are grown in controlled laboratory conditions and do not sit on a shelf in uncontrolled conditions.[68]

The stem cells that display efficacy and are used in dermatology are adult associated mesenchymal stem cells (MSCs). MSCs are divided into adipose-derived stem cells (ADSCs) that are isolated from fat and bone marrow-derived stem cells (BM-MSCs).[69] These stem cells, whether from fat or bone marrow, are extracted from the patient and injected into the target tissue. They are not formulated in products sold commercially. ADSCs are used more often because they are easily available through liposuction with minimal added procedure costs.[70] Mice receiving subcutaneous injections of ADSCs have demonstrated increased procollagen Type 1, increased collagen density, angiogenesis, and increased dermal thickness.[70,71] It is unknown exactly how the ADSCs cause these effects, but it is assumed that they activate dermal fibroblasts (which affects the dermis rather than the epidermis). Human studies using amniotic membrane stem cell-conditioned media (as compared to a saline control group) applied with microneedling have shown improvement in pore size, wrinkles, and pigmentation.[72]

Another approach is using ingredients to stimulate the stem cells or improve the microenvironment in their niche in a manner that helps them renew.[73] On a cautionary note, increasing replication of skin cancer cells is not desirable, so special care must be used when tampering with these cells to avoid causing or worsening skin cancer. Although there is no evidence that the topically applied skincare ingredients discussed in this section have ever engendered or contributed to skin cancer, it is best to first ensure that the skin is free of skin cancer before using these ingredients.

Cosmeceutical ingredients affect stem cells directly or through their microenvironment. Ascorbic acid (vitamin C) has been shown to promote formation of ECM, increase integrin expression, and augment the stemness proliferation potential of EPSCs.[67] The mushroom-derived cosmeceutical ingredient *Ganoderma lucidum*, the flowering plant *Rhodiola sachalinensis*, resveratrol from grapes and berries, and the Chinese herb *Eleutherococcus senticosus* (also known as Siberian ginseng) have been demonstrated to increase integrin expression, and enhance the stemness proliferation potential of EPSCs.[67]

Alpha and beta defensins are peptides produced by the immune system during wound healing and repair. They stimulate the usually dormant LGR6+ stem cells found in the hair follicle to form EPSCs resulting in new keratinocytes. Defensins have been found to rejuvenate skin when used topically.[74,75]

Retinol plays an important role in regulating EPSCs by maintaining self-renewal and preventing differentiation of pluripotent stem cells.[6,76] Over 500 genes are influenced by retinoic acid and many of them affect EPSCs. While retinol prevents differentiation of EPSCs, retinoic acid promotes EPSC differentiation through the expression of mRNA and microRNA, as well as by increasing DNA methylation.[77]

Cellular Senescence

Cellular senescence occurs when stem cells undergo irreversible cell cycle arrest and lose the ability to divide. Cellular senescence is the way the body naturally rids itself of dysfunctional or damaged cells. Cancer occurs when cells lose the ability to become senescent and continue dividing and reproducing even when damaged. The presence of senescent cells in the skin leads to cutaneous aging and the presence of senescent cells is characteristic of aging skin.[78] Senescent cells secrete substances that affect the microenvironment around them. They take up space, make the skin stiffer, interfere with cell-to-cell communication, damage surrounding cells, and affect the functions of EPSCs.[79] Aging, reactive oxygen species, and inflammation contribute to an increase in senescent cells.[80]

CIRCADIAN RHYTHM IN THE EPIDERMIS

Keratinocytes have a circadian clock governed by a clock gene,[65] and evince endogenous rhythmicity.[81,82] Keratinocytes can directly sense light, which affects the circadian rhythm. Blue light specifically has been shown to directly influence keratinocyte clock gene expression when shined on cells at night.[83]

Studies have demonstrated that undifferentiated keratinocytes respond to differentiation cues between late night and early morning. Keratinocytes proliferate in daylight hours at the same time they turn on genes to help protect their DNA from UV light.[65] The repair of UV damaged cells occurs at night. In general, these rhythms allow the skin to focus on protection in the daytime and repair at night. Many circadian rhythm studies of the skin show that DNA repair occurs best at night and requires adequate sleep. Keratinocyte clock oscillations are affected by the stiffness of the surrounding ECM, the presence of inflammation, and aging.[84–86]

Circadian rhythm affects TEWL, which is higher in the evening than in the morning, and blood flow to the skin, which is highest in the late afternoon and night.[87] Skin penetration of topical products has been shown to be the highest at night with the peak at 4:00 A.M.[88]

Circadian rhythms should be considered when applying skincare products. Sun protection and antioxidants are recommended in the morning to protect the skin. Apply products that do not penetrate well in the evening because TEWL is higher. Follow with a barrier repair moisturizer. DNA repair enzymes should be applied at night.

Light and the Epidermis

When light hits keratinocytes, gene expression changes depending on the type of light.[9] Blue light treatments are used for acne because the light has been shown to kill *Cutibacterium acnes*. In addition, blue light is emitted from phone screens and computer screens. Blue light up to 453 nm reduces proliferation of keratinocytes in vitro by inducing differentiation.[89] Aquaporins are water channels that play an important role in skin hydration, movement of fluids between cells, and proliferation and differentiation of keratinocytes. Blue light causes lipofuscin in aged skin cells to generate aging free radicals as discussed earlier in relation to lysosomes. Red light is often used to treat skin inflammation and its use attenuates inflammatory factors.[90]

Studies have shown that keratinocytes and fibroblasts are affected by light differently.[91,92] Fibroblasts seem to be more sensitive than keratinocytes to light, especially UV, infrared, and visible light, which may be due to a higher antioxidant capacity in keratinocytes as compared to fibroblasts.[93,94] Keratinocytes also contain higher levels of ferritin than fibroblasts, allowing them to chelate iron, reducing the levels of damaging free radicals.[95] Chapter 26, Lasers and Lights, will include a more in-depth discussion on the effects of light on the skin.

GROWTH FACTORS

Growth factors can be classified into two groups: proliferative and differentiative. Proliferative factors increase DNA synthesis and result in proliferation of cells. Differentiative factors inhibit the production of DNA and suppress growth, thereby resulting in differentiation of the keratinocytes.

Epidermal growth factor (EGF) is one of the integral chemokines in the regulation of growth in human cells. It binds to the epidermal growth factor receptor (EGFR) located on the basal and suprabasal cells in the epidermis and activates tyrosine kinase activity, which ultimately results in proliferation of the cells.[96] Keratinocyte growth factor (KGF), a member of the fibroblast growth factor family, also exerts a proliferative effect via the tyrosine kinase receptor on epidermal cells.[97] It has been shown that KGF contributes to and enhances wound healing.[98] In addition, KGF has been demonstrated to promote hyaluronan synthesis in keratinocytes.[99]

Other important growth factors include the polypeptide transforming growth factors, which consist of two types: transforming growth factor alpha (TGF-α) and transforming growth factor beta (TGF-β). They differ in both configuration and function. TGF-α is a proliferative factor, similar to EGF, and works by stimulating a tyrosine kinase response. TGF-β is a cytokine that inhibits growth of epidermal keratinocytes and stimulates growth of dermal fibroblasts. TGF-β promotes differentiation and plays an important role in controlling production of the ECM.[100] TGF-β is critical for regulating collagen synthesis. In fact, the primary cause of the decrease in Type 1 procollagen after UV exposure is inhibition of a TGF-β pathway.[101] TGF-β has also been proven to contribute to scarring, and antibodies to this factor have been shown to decrease the inflammatory response in wounds and reduce scarring.[102,103] TGF-β levels are increased by calcium, phorbol esters, as well as TGF-β itself.

Insulin-like growth factor (IGF) has been shown to yield a photoprotective effect on skin. IGF signaling regulates DNA repair.[104,105] In fact, exogenous IGF added to irradiated keratinocyte cultures has been demonstrated to rescue the irradiated cells, increase keratinocyte survival, and reduce photodamage.[106]

Growth Factors in Cosmeceuticals

Various growth factors are found in cosmeceuticals although there is a paucity of research on which growth factors are best to treat the skin.[107] Skincare products containing growth factors isolated from cells cultured in conditioned media have been on the market for decades. The efficacy and safety of these growth factors is still poorly understood; however, there have not been any proven cases of skin cancer arising from their use. The concern is that these growth factors could cause undesirable skin cells to flourish. For example, TGF-β, known as a tumor growth factor, is present in the conditioned media used in some skincare products.[108,109] Multiple cancer research studies show that TGF-β is a potent trigger of cancer-related pathways,[110,111] and prepares a favorable microenvironment for cancer cells.[112,113] These issues will be examined more completely in Chapter 37, Anti-Aging Ingredients.

ANTIMICROBIAL PEPTIDES

Antimicrobial peptides (AMPs) have recently become an area of interest because of their involvement in the innate immune system of human skin. AMPs exhibit broad-spectrum activity against bacteria, viruses, and fungi.[114,115] The cationic peptide of the AMPs attracts the negatively charged bacteria, becoming pervasive in the bacterial membrane in the process, and ultimately eliminates the bacteria. Cathelicidin and defensin are the two major groups of AMPs believed to have an influence in the antimicrobial defense of the skin. Cathelicidin has been identified in the keratinocytes of human skin at the area of inflammation, as well as in eccrine and salivary glands.[116–118] In addition to antimicrobial activity, cathelicidin LL-37 demonstrates a stimulatory effect on keratinocyte proliferation in the process of wound healing.[119] Pig cathelicidin PR-39 has been shown to induce proteoglycan production (specifically, syndecan-1 and -4) in the ECM in wound repair.[120] Defensin is also expressed in the human keratinocytes[121] and mucous membranes.[122,123] β-Defensin 1 seems to promote differentiation in the keratinocytes by increasing expression of keratin 10.[124] Interestingly, UVB radiation has been shown to increase the levels of human β-defensin mRNA in the keratinocytes.[125]

AMPs have been demonstrated to be involved in several dermatologic conditions including atopic dermatitis, psoriasis, and leprosy,[115] as well as wound healing, all of which are beyond the scope of our discussion. The role of AMPs in the epidermal barrier will be discussed in Chapter 12.

MOISTURIZATION OF THE STRATUM CORNEUM

The main function of the SC is to prevent TEWL and regulate the water balance in the skin. The two major components that allow the SC to perform this role are lipids and the NMF.

Natural Moisturizing Factor

Released by the lamellar granules, NMF is composed of amino acids and their metabolites, which are byproducts formed from the breakdown of filaggrin (**Box 1-2**). NMF is found exclusively inside the cells of the SC and gives the SC its humectant (water-binding) qualities (**Fig. 1-10**).

NMF is composed of highly water-soluble chemicals; therefore, it can absorb large amounts of water, even when humidity

---

BOX 1-2

Filaggrin, named for *filament aggr*egating prote*in*, derived its name from the fact that it binds keratin filaments to form a structural matrix in the SC. Genetic defects in the filaggrin gene are known to play a role in a subset of ichthyosis vulgaris cases.[38] Interestingly, filaggrin is not present in the superficial layers of the SC. Studies have shown that it is completely degraded into amino acids within 2 to 3 days of profilaggrin formation and its constituents are further metabolized to form the NMF.[40] This is nature's way of keeping its water-binding capabilities in the top layer of the SC where they are needed while preventing the lower layers of the SC from being disrupted by having too much water present. In addition, the level of NMF is regulated by the water activity present in the SC.

---

levels are low. This allows the SC to retain substantial water content even in a dry environment. The NMF also provides an important aqueous environment for enzymes that require such conditions to function. The importance of NMF is clear when one notes that ichthyosis vulgaris patients, who have been shown to lack NMF, manifest severe dryness, and scaling of the skin.[126] It has been demonstrated that normal skin exposed to normal soap washing has significantly lower levels of NMF when compared to normal skin not washed with surfactants.[127] NMF levels have also been reported to decline with age, which may contribute to the increased incidence of dry skin in the elderly population (see Chapter 12).

Lipids

In order of abundance, the composition of skin surface lipids includes triglycerides, fatty acids, squalene, wax esters, diglycerides, cholesterol esters, and cholesterol.[128] These lipids are an integral part of the epidermis and are involved in preventing TEWL and the entry of harmful bacteria. They also help prevent the skin from absorbing water-soluble agents. For decades it has been known that the absence of lipids in the diet leads to unhealthy skin (see Chapter 12). More recently, it has been shown that inherited defects in lipid metabolism, such as the deficiency of steroid sulfatase seen in X-linked ichthyosis, will lead to abnormal skin keratinization and hydration.[129] It is now known that SC lipids are affected by age, genetics, seasonal variation, and diet. Deficiency of these lipids predisposes the individual to dry skin. This has been demonstrated in mice with essential fatty acid deficiency (EFAD): when fed a diet deficient in linoleic acid these mice developed increased TEWL.[130] Interestingly, the administration of hypocholesterolemic drugs has also been associated with dry skin changes.[131]

Skin lipids are produced in and extruded from the lamellar granules as described earlier or are synthesized in the sebaceous glands and then excreted to the skin's surface through the hair follicle. The excretion of sebum by sebaceous glands is hormonally controlled (see Chapter 11, Oily Skin). Lipids help keep the NMF inside the cells where it is needed to maintain hydration and aqueous enzyme functioning. Although this is less well characterized, lipids can themselves influence enzyme function.

Role of lipids in TEWL

The major lipids found in the SC that contribute to the water permeability barrier are ceramides, cholesterol, and fatty acids.

Since the 1940s, when the SC was first identified as the primary barrier to water loss, many hypotheses have been developed as to exactly which lipids are important in the SC. The research with the EFAD mice described earlier led to a focus on phospholipids because they contain linoleic acid. However, it was later found that phospholipids are almost completely absent from the SC.[132] In 1982, ceramide 1 was discovered. This linoleic acid-rich compound is believed to play a major role in structuring SC lipids essential for barrier function.[133] Later, five more distinct types of ceramides were discovered and

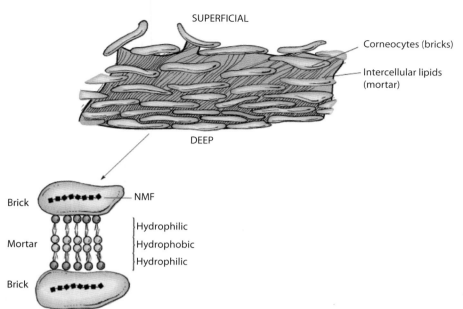

SUPERFICIAL

Corneocytes (bricks)

Intercellular lipids (mortar)

DEEP

Brick — NMF

Mortar — Hydrophilic / Hydrophobic / Hydrophilic

Brick

FIGURE 1-10. The keratinocytes are embedded in a lipid matrix that resembles bricks and mortar. Natural moisturizing factor (NMF) is present within the keratinocytes. NMF and the lipid bilayer prevent dehydration of the epidermis.

named according to the polarity of the molecule. Ceramide 1 is the most nonpolar and ceramide 6 is the most polar.

Although the ceramides were once thought to be the key to skin moisturization, studies now suggest that no particular lipid is more important than the others. It appears that the proportion of fatty acids, ceramides, and cholesterol is the most significant parameter. This was demonstrated in a study in which after altering the water barrier with acetone, the application of a combination of ceramides, fatty acids, and cholesterol resulted in normal barrier recovery.[134] Application of each of the separate entities alone resulted in delayed barrier recovery. Manufacturers now include ceramides or a mixture of ceramides, cholesterol, and fatty acids in several available products based on these findings. However, the use of these mixtures to treat atopic dermatitis and other ichthyotic disorders has been disappointing.

CONCLUSION

The epidermis is implicated in many of the skin complaints of cosmetic patients. It is the state of the epidermis that causes the skin to feel rough and appear dull. A flexible, well-hydrated epidermis is more supple and radiant than a dehydrated epidermis. The popularity of buff puffs, exfoliating scrubs, masks, moisturizers, chemical peels, and microdermabrasion attests to the obsession that cosmetic patients have with the condition of their epidermis. It is important to understand the properties of the epidermis in order to understand which cosmetic products and procedures can truly benefit patients as opposed to those that are based on myths or hype.

References

1. Chu D. Overview of biology, development, and structure of skin. In: Wolff K, Goldsmith L, Katz S, Gilchest B, Paller A, Leffell D, eds. *Fitzpatrick's Dermatology in General Medicine.* 7th ed. New York, NY: McGraw-Hill; 2008:60.

2. Sreedhar A, Aguilera-Aguirre L, Singh KK. Mitochondria in skin health, aging, and disease. *Cell Death Dis.* 2020;11(6):444.

3. Krutmann J, Schroeder P. Role of mitochondria in photoaging of human skin: the defective powerhouse model. *J Investig Dermatol Symp Proc.* 2009;14(1):44–49.

4. Marcheggiani F, Cirilli I, Orlando P, et al. Modulation of Coenzyme Q10content and oxidative status in human dermal fibroblasts using HMG-CoA reductase inhibitor over a broad range of concentrations. From mitohormesis to mitochondrial dysfunction and accelerated aging. *Aging (Albany NY).* 2019;11(9):2565–2582.

5. Blatt T, Littarru GP. Biochemical rationale and experimental data on the antiaging properties of CoQ(10) at skin level. *Biofactors.* 2011;37(5):381–385.

6. Khillan JS. Vitamin A/retinol and maintenance of pluripotency of stem cells. *Nutrients.* 2014;6(3):1209–1222.

7. Hoyos B, Imam A, Chua R, et al. The cysteine-rich regions of the regulatory domains of Raf and protein kinase C as retinoid receptors. *J Exp Med.* 2000;192(6):835–845.

8. Imam A, Hoyos B, Swenson C, et al. Retinoids as ligands and coactivators of protein kinase C alpha. *FASEB J.* 2001;15(1):28–30.

9. Sun X, Kim A, Nakatani M, Shen Y, Liu L. Distinctive molecular responses to ultraviolet radiation between keratinocytes and melanocytes. *Exp Dermatol.* 2016;25(9):708–713.

10. Nakashima Y, Ohta S, Wolf AM. Blue light-induced oxidative stress in live skin. *Free Radic Biol Med.* 2017;108:300–310.

11. Rascalou A, Lamartine J, Poydenot P, Demarne F, Bechetoille N. Mitochondrial damage and cytoskeleton reorganization in human dermal fibroblasts exposed to artificial visible light similar to screen-emitted light. *J Dermatol Sci.* 2018:S0923-1811(18)30213-30215.

12. Hu WP, Wang JJ, Yu CL, Lan CC, Chen GS, Yu HS. Helium-neon laser irradiation stimulates cell proliferation through

photostimulatory effects in mitochondria. *J Invest Dermatol.* 2007;127(8):2048–2057.

13. Hawkins DH, Abrahamse H. Time-dependent responses of wounded human skin fibroblasts following phototherapy. *J Photochem Photobiol B.* 2007;88(2-3):147–155.

14. Karu TI, Pyatibrat LV, Kalendo GS. Photobiological modulation of cell attachment via cytochrome c oxidase. *Photochem Photobiol Sci.* 2004;3(2):211–216.

15. Baumann LS. Overview of Aging. In: *Cosmeceuticals and Cosmetic Ingredients.* New York: McGraw-Hill; 2014:317–321.

16. Skoczyńska A, Budzisz E, Trznadel-Grodzka E, Rotsztejn H. Melanin and lipofuscin as hallmarks of skin aging. *Postepy Dermatol Alergol.* 2017;34(2):97–103.

17. König J, Ott C, Hugo M, et al. Mitochondrial contribution to lipofuscin formation. *Redox Biol.* 2017;11:673–681.

18. Terman A, Kurz T, Navratil M, Arriaga EA, Brunk UT. Mitochondrial turnover and aging of long-lived postmitotic cells: the mitochondrial-lysosomal axis theory of aging. *Antioxid Redox Signal.* 2010;12(4):503–535.

19. Höhn A, Jung T, Grimm S, Grune T. Lipofuscin-bound iron is a major intracellular source of oxidants: role in senescent cells. *Free Radic Biol Med.* 2010;48(8):1100–1108.

20. Tonolli PN, Martins WK, Junqueira HC, et al. Lipofuscin in keratinocytes: Production, properties, and consequences of the photosensitization with visible light. *Free Radic Biol Med.* 2020;160:277–292.

21. Barton NW, Brady RO, Dambrosia JM, et al. Replacement therapy for inherited enzyme deficiency—macrophage-targeted glucocerebrosidase for Gaucher's disease. *N Engl J Med.* 1991;324 (21):1464–1470.

22. de Freitas V, da Silva Porto P, Assunção M, Cadete-Leite A, Andrade JP, Paula-Barbosa MM. Flavonoids from grape seeds prevent increased alcohol-induced neuronal lipofuscin formation. *Alcohol Alcohol.* 2004;39(4):303–311.

23. Shen LR, Parnell LD, Ordovas JM, Lai CQ. Curcumin and aging. *Biofactors.* 2013;39(1):133–140.

24. Marzabadi MR, Sohal RS, Brunk UT. Effect of alpha-tocopherol and some metal chelators on lipofuscin accumulation in cultured neonatal rat cardiac myocytes. *Anal Cell Pathol.* 1990;2(6):333–236.

25. Vekshin NL, Frolova MS. Formation and Destruction of Thermo-Lipofuscin in Mitochondria. *Biochem Anal Biochem.* 2018;7(357).

26. Casares L, García V, Garrido-Rodríguez M, et al. Cannabidiol induces antioxidant pathways in keratinocytes by targeting BACH1. *Redox Biol.* 2020;28:101321.

27. Gaffal E, Cron M, Glodde N, et al. Cannabinoid 1 receptors in keratinocytes modulate proinflammatory chemokine secretion and attenuate contact allergic inflammation. *J Immunol.* 2013;190(10):4929–4936.

28. Wang LL, Zhao R, Li JY, et al. Pharmacological activation of cannabinoid 2 receptor attenuates inflammation, fibrogenesis, and promotes re-epithelialization during skin wound healing. *Eur J Pharmacol.* 2016;786:128–136.

29. Premkumar LS. Transient receptor potential channels as targets for phytochemicals. *ACS Chem Neurosci.* 2014;5(11):1117–1130.

30. Takaishi M, Uchida K, Suzuki Y, et al. Reciprocal effects of capsaicin and menthol on thermosensation through regulated activities of TRPV1 and TRPM8. *J Physiol Sci.* 2016;66(2):143–155.

31. Lechler T, Fuchs E. Asymmetric cell divisions promote stratification and differentiation of mammalian skin. *Nature.* 2005;437 (7056):275–280.

32. Blanpain C, Fuchs E. Epidermal stem cells of the skin. *Annu Rev Cell Dev Biol.* 2006;22:339–373.

33. Braff MH, Di Nardo A, Gallo RL. Keratinocytes store the antimicrobial peptide cathelicidin in lamellar bodies. *J Invest Dermatol.* 2005;124:394.

34. Li L, Tucker RW, Hennings H, et al. Inhibitors of the intracellular Ca(2+)-ATPase in cultured mouse keratinocytes reveal components of terminal differentiation that are regulated by distinct intracellular Ca2+ compartments. *Cell Growth Differ.* 1995;6:1171.

35. Green H. The keratinocyte as differentiated cell type. *Harvey Lect.* 1980;74:101.

36. Eckert RL, Crish JF, Robinson NA. The epidermal keratinocyte as a model for the study of gene regulation and cell differentiation. *Physiol Rev.* 1997;77:397–424.

37. Yuspa SH, Kilkenny AE, Steinert PM, et al. Expression of murine epidermal differentiation markers is tightly regulated by restricted extracellular calcium concentrations in vitro. *J Cell Biol.* 1989;109:1207.

38. Sharpe GR, Gillespie JI, Greenwell JR. An increase in intracellular free calcium is an early event during differentiation of cultured human keratinocytes. *FEBS Lett.* 1989;254:25.

39. Su MJ, Bikle DD, Mancianti ML, et al. 1,25-Dihydroxyvitamin D3 potentiates the keratinocyte response to calcium. *J Biol Chem.* 1994;269:14723.

40. Hosomi J, Hosoi J, Abe E, et al. Regulation of terminal differentiation of cultured mouse epidermal cells by 1 alpha, 25-dihydroxyvitamin D_3. *Endocrinology.* 1983;113:1950.

41. Smith EL, Walworth NC, Holick MF. Effect of 1 alpha,25-dihydroxyvitamin D3 on the morphologic and biochemical differentiation of cultured human epidermal keratinocytes grown in serum-free conditions. *J Invest Dermatol.* 1986;86:709.

42. Usui ML, Underwood RA, Fleckman P, Olerud JE. Parakeratotic corneocytes play a unique role in human skin wound healing. *J Invest Dermatol.* 2013;133(3):856–858.

43. Egelrud T. Desquamation. In: Loden M, Maibach H, eds. *Dry Skin and Moisturizers.* 1st ed. Boca Raton, FL: CRC Press; 2000:110.

44. Christophers E, Kligman AM. Visualization of the cell layers of the stratum corneum. *J Invest Dermatol.* 1964;42:407.

45. Blair C. Morphology and thickness of the human stratum corneum. *Br J Dermatol.* 1968;80:430.

46. Kezic S, Kemperman PM, Koster ES, et al. Loss-of-function mutations in the filaggrin gene lead to reduced level of natural moisturizing factor in the stratum corneum. *J Invest Dermatol.* 2008;128(8):2117–2119.

47. Proksch E, Jensen J. Skin as an organ of protection. In: Wolff K, Goldsmith L, Katz S, Gilchest B, Paller A, Leffell D, eds. *Fitzpatrick's Dermatology in General Medicine.* 7th ed. New York, NY: McGraw-Hill; 2008:383–395.

48. Proksch E, Jensen J. Skin as an organ of protection. In: Wolff K, Goldsmith L, Katz S, Gilchest B, Paller A, Leffell D, eds. *Fitzpatrick's Dermatology in General Medicine.* 7th ed. New York, NY: McGraw-Hill; 2008:87.

49. Usui ML, Mansbridge JN, Carter WG, Fujita M, Olerud JE. Keratinocyte migration, proliferation, and differentiation in chronic ulcers from patients with diabetes and normal wounds. *J Histochem Cytochem.* 2008;56(7):687–696.

50. Tortora GJ, Derrickson BH. *Principles of Anatomy and Physiology.* New York, NY: John Wiley & Sons; 2018:149.

51. Yaar M, Gilchrest B. Aging of Skin. In: Freedberg IM, Eisen A, Wolff K, Austen K, Goldmsith L, Katz S, Fitzpatrick T, eds. *Fitzpatrick's Dermatology in General Medicine.* 5th ed. New York, NY: McGraw-Hill; 1999:1697–1706.

52. Lambrechts IA, de Canha MN, Lall N. Exploiting medicinal plants as possible treatments for acne vulgaris. In *Medicinal Plants for Holistic Health and Well-Being.* San Diego, CA: Academic Press; 2018:117–143.

53. Candi E, Amelio I, Agostini M, Melino G. MicroRNAs and p63 in epithelial stemness. *Cell Death Differ.* 2015;22(1):12–21.

54. Snippert HJ, Haegebarth A, Kasper M, et al. Lgr6 marks stem cells in the hair follicle that generate all cell lineages of the skin. *Science.* 2010;327(5971):1385–1389.

55. Yang R, Liu F, Wang J, Chen X, Xie J, Xiong K. Epidermal stem cells in wound healing and their clinical applications. *Stem Cell Res Ther.* 2019;10(1):229.

56. Fernandez TL, Van Lonkhuyzen DR, Dawson RA, Kimlin MG, Upton Z. Insulin-like growth factor-I and UVB photoprotection in human keratinocytes. *Exp Dermatol.* 2015;24(3):235–238.

57. Choi HR, Nam KM, Park SJ, et al. Suppression of miR135b increases the proliferative potential of normal human keratinocytes. *J Invest Dermatol.* 2014;134(4):1161–1164.

58. Zijl S, Vasilevich AS, Viswanathan P, et al. Micro-scaled topographies direct differentiation of human epidermal stem cells. *Acta Biomater.* 2019;84:133–145.

59. Doles J, Keyes WM. Epidermal stem cells undergo age-associated changes. *Aging (Albany NY).* 2013;5(1):1–2.

60. Panich U, Sittithumcharee G, Rathviboon N, Jirawatnotai S. Ultraviolet Radiation-Induced Skin Aging: The Role of DNA Damage and Oxidative Stress in Epidermal Stem Cell Damage Mediated Skin Aging. *Stem Cells Int.* 2016;2016:7370642.

61. Liu L, Rando TA. Manifestations and mechanisms of stem cell aging. *J Cell Biol.* 2011;193(2):257–266.

62. Giangreco A, Goldie SJ, Failla V, Saintigny G, Watt FM. Human skin aging is associated with reduced expression of the stem cell markers beta1 integrin and MCSP. *J Invest Dermatol.* 2010;130(2):604–608.

63. Ji AR, Ku SY, Cho MS, et al. Reactive oxygen species enhance differentiation of human embryonic stem cells into mesendodermal lineage. *Exp Mol Med.* 2010;42(3):175–186.

64. Janich P, Pascual G, Merlos-Suárez A, et al. The circadian molecular clock creates epidermal stem cell heterogeneity. *Nature.* 2011;480(7376):209–214.

65. Janich P, Toufighi K, Solanas G, et al. Human epidermal stem cell function is regulated by circadian oscillations. *Cell Stem Cell.* 2013;13(6):745–753.

66. Welz PS, Benitah SA. Molecular Connections Between Circadian Clocks and Aging. *J Mol Biol.* 2020;432(12):3661–3679.

67. Kwon SH, Park KC. Antioxidants as an Epidermal Stem Cell Activator. *Antioxidants (Basel).* 2020;9(10):958.

68. Dabiri G, Heiner D, Falanga V. The emerging use of bone marrow-derived mesenchymal stem cells in the treatment of human chronic wounds. *Expert Opin Emerg Drugs.* 2013;18(4):405–419.

69. Wang JV, Schoenberg E, Zaya R, Rohrer T, Zachary CB, Saedi N. The rise of stem cells in skin rejuvenation: A new frontier. *Clin Dermatol.* 2020;38(4):494–496.

70. Kim JH, Jung M, Kim HS, Kim YM, Choi EH. Adipose-derived stem cells as a new therapeutic modality for ageing skin. *Exp Dermatol.* 2011;20(5):383–387.

71. Kim WS, Park BS, Park SH, Kim HK, Sung JH. Antiwrinkle effect of adipose-derived stem cell: activation of dermal fibroblast by secretory factors. *J Dermatol Sci.* 2009;53(2):96–102.

72. Prakoeswa CRS, Pratiwi FD, Herwanto N, et al. The effects of amniotic membrane stem cell-conditioned medium on photoaging. *J Dermatolog Treat.* 2019;30(5):478–482.

73. Moore KA, Lemischka IR. Stem cells and their niches. *Science.* 2006;311(5769):1880–1885.

74. Taub A, Bucay V, Keller G, Williams J, Mehregan D. Multi-Center, Double-Blind, Vehicle-Controlled Clinical Trial of an Alpha and Beta Defensin-Containing Anti-Aging Skin Care Regimen With Clinical, Histopathologic, Immunohistochemical, Photographic, and Ultrasound Evaluation. *J Drugs Dermatol.* 2018;17(4):426–441.

75. Berens AM, Ghazizadeh S. Effect of defensins-containing eye cream on periocular rhytids and skin quality. *J Cosmet Dermatol.* 2020;19(8):2000–2005.

76. Chen L, Yang M, Dawes J, Khillan JS. Suppression of ES cell differentiation by retinol (vitamin A) via the overexpression of Nanog. *Differentiation.* 2007;75(8):682–693.

77. Godoy-Parejo C, Deng C, Zhang Y, Liu W, Chen G. Roles of vitamins in stem cells. *Cell Mol Life Sci.* 2020;77(9):1771–1791.

78. Dimri GP, Lee X, Basile G, et al. A biomarker that identifies senescent human cells in culture and in aging skin in vivo. *Proc Natl Acad Sci U S A.* 1995;92(20):9363–9367.

79. Youn SW, Kim DS, Cho HJ, et al. Cellular senescence induced loss of stem cell proportion in the skin in vitro. *J Dermatol Sci.* 2004;35(2):113–123.

80. Toutfaire M, Bauwens E, Debacq-Chainiaux F. The impact of cellular senescence in skin ageing: A notion of mosaic and therapeutic strategies. *Biochem Pharmacol.* 2017;142:1–12.

81. Tanioka M, Yamada H, Doi M, et al. Molecular clocks in mouse skin. *J Invest Dermatol.* 2009;129(5):1225–1231.

82. Lyons AB, Moy L, Moy R, Tung R. Circadian Rhythm and the Skin: A Review of the Literature. *J Clin Aesthet Dermatol.* 2019;12(9):42–45.

83. Dong K, Goyarts EC, Pelle E, Trivero J, Pernodet N. Blue light disrupts the circadian rhythm and create damage in skin cells. *Int J Cosmet Sci.* 2019;41(6):558–562.

84. Williams J, Yang N, Wood A, Zindy E, Meng QJ, Streuli CH. Epithelial and stromal circadian clocks are inversely regulated by their mechano-matrix environment. *J Cell Sci.* 2018;131(5):jcs208223.

85. Greenberg EN, Marshall ME, Jin S, et al. Circadian control of interferon-sensitive gene expression in murine skin. *Proc Natl Acad Sci U S A.* 2020;117(11):5761–5771.

86. Solanas G, Peixoto FO, Perdiguero E, et al. Aged Stem Cells Reprogram Their Daily Rhythmic Functions to Adapt to Stress. *Cell.* 2017;170(4):678–692.e20.

87. Smolander J, Härmä M, Lindqvist A, Kolari P, Laitinen LA. Circadian variation in peripheral blood flow in relation to core temperature at rest. *Eur J Appl Physiol Occup Physiol.* 1993;67(2):192–196.

88. Reinberg AE, Soudant E, Koulbanis C, et al. Circadian dosing time dependency in the forearm skin penetration of methyl and hexyl nicotinate. *Life Sci.* 1995;57(16):1507–13.

89. Liebmann J, Born M, Kolb-Bachofen V. Blue-light irradiation regulates proliferation and differentiation in human skin cells. *J Invest Dermatol.* 2010;130(1):259–269.

90. Sun Q, Kim HE, Cho H, Shi S, Kim B, Kim O. Red light-emitting diode irradiation regulates oxidative stress and inflammation through SPHK1/NF-κB activation in human keratinocytes. *J Photochem Photobiol B.* 2018;186:31–40.

91. Hudson L, Rashdan E, Bonn CA, Chavan B, Rawlings D, Birch-Machin MA. Individual and combined effects of the infrared, visible, and ultraviolet light components of solar radiation on damage biomarkers in human skin cells. *FASEB J.* 2020;34(3):3874–3883.

92. D'Errico M, Lemma T, Calcagnile A, Proietti De Santis L, Dogliotti E. Cell type and DNA damage specific response of human skin cells to environmental agents. *Mutat Res.* 2007;614(1–2):37–47.

93. Oyewole AO, Birch-Machin MA. Mitochondria-targeted antioxidants. *FASEB J.* 2015;29(12):4766–4771.

94. Liebel F, Kaur S, Ruvolo E, Kollias N, Southall MD. Irradiation of skin with visible light induces reactive oxygen species and matrix-degrading enzymes. *J Invest Dermatol.* 2012;132(7):1901–1907.

95. Qian W, Van Houten B. Alterations in bioenergetics due to changes in mitochondrial DNA copy number. *Methods.* 2010;51(4):452–457.

96. Jost M, Kari C, Rodeck U. The EGF receptor—an essential regulator of multiple epidermal functions. *Eur J Dermatol.* 2000;10:505.

97. Miki T, Bottaro DP, Fleming TP, et al. Determination of ligand-binding specificity by alternative splicing: two distinct growth factor receptors encoded by a single gene. *Proc Natl Acad Sci U.S.A.* 1992;89:246.

98. Brauchle M, Fässler R, Werner S. Suppression of keratinocyte growth factor expression by glucocorticoids in vitro and during wound healing. *J Invest Dermatol.* 1995;105:579.

99. Karvinen S, Pasonen-Seppänen S, Hyttinen JM, et al. Keratinocyte growth factor stimulates migration and hyaluronan synthesis in the epidermis by activation of keratinocyte hyaluronan synthases 2 and 3. *J Biol Chem.* 2003;278:49495.

100. William I, Rich B, Kupper T. Cytokines. In: Wolff K, Goldsmith L, Katz S, Gilchest B, Paller A, Leffell D, eds. *Fitzpatrick's Dermatology in General Medicine.* 7th ed. New York, NY: McGraw-Hill; 2008:116.

101. Quan T, He T, Kang S, Voorhees JJ, Fisher GJ. Solar ultraviolet irradiation reduces collagen in photoaged human skin by blocking transforming growth factor-beta type II receptor/Smad signaling. *Am J Pathol.* 2004;165(3):741–751.

102. Shah M, Foreman DM, Ferguson MW. Neutralisation of TGF-beta 1 and TGF-beta 2 or exogenous addition of TGF-beta 3 to cutaneous rat wounds reduces scarring. *J Cell Sci.* 1995;108:985.

103. Shah M, Foreman DM, Ferguson MW. Control of scarring in adult wounds by neutralising antibody to transforming growth factor beta. *Lancet.* 1992;339:213.

104. Andrade MJ, Van Lonkhuyzen DR, Upton Z, Satyamoorthy K. Unravelling the insulin-like growth factor I-mediated photoprotection of the skin. *Cytokine Growth Factor Rev.* 2020;52:45–55.

105. Loesch MM, Collier AE, Southern DH, et al. Insulin-like growth factor-1 receptor regulates repair of ultraviolet B-induced DNA damage in human keratinocytes in vivo. *Mol Oncol.* 2016;10(8):1245–1254.

106. Andrade MJ, Satyamoorthy K, Upton Z, Van Lonkhuyzen DR. Insulin-like growth factor-I rescue of primary keratinocytes from pre- and post-ultraviolet B radiation effects. *J Photochem Photobiol B.* 2020;209:111951.

107. Baumann L. How to Use Oral and Topical Cosmeceuticals to Prevent and Treat Skin Aging. *Facial Plast Surg Clin North Am.* 2018;26(4):407–413.

108. Meirelles Lda S, Fontes AM, Covas DT, Caplan AI. Mechanisms involved in the therapeutic properties of mesenchymal stem cells. *Cytokine Growth Factor Rev.* 2009;20(5–6):419–427.

109. Falanga V, Qian SW, Danielpour D, Katz MH, Roberts AB, Sporn MB. Hypoxia upregulates the synthesis of TGF-beta 1 by human dermal fibroblasts. *J Invest Dermatol.* 1991;97(4):634–637.

110. de Gramont A, Faivre S, Raymond E. Novel TGF-β inhibitors ready for prime time in onco-immunology. *Oncoimmunology.* 2016;6(1):e1257453.

111. Neuzillet C, Tijeras-Raballand A, Cohen R, et al. Targeting the TGFβ pathway for cancer therapy. *Pharmacol Ther.* 2015;147:22–31.

112. López-Novoa JM, Nieto MA. Inflammation and EMT: an alliance towards organ fibrosis and cancer progression. *EMBO Mol Med.* 2009;1(6–7):303–314.

113. Jakowlew SB. Transforming growth factor-beta in cancer and metastasis. *Cancer Metastasis Rev.* 2006;25(3):435–457.

114. Ganz T, Lehrer RI. Defensins. *Curr Opin Immunol.* 1994;6:584.

115. Izadpanah A, Gallo RL. Antimicrobial peptides. *J Am Acad Dermatol.* 2005;52:381.

116. Frohm M, Agerberth B, Ahangari G, et al. The expression of the gene coding for the antibacterial peptide LL-37 is induced in human keratinocytes during inflammatory disorders. *J Biol Chem.* 1997;272:15258.

117. Murakami M, Ohtake T, Dorschner RA, et al. Cathelicidin anti-microbial peptide expression in sweat, an innate defense system for the skin. *J Invest Dermatol.* 2002;119:1090.

118. Murakami M, Ohtake T, Dorschner RA, et al. Cathelicidin anti-microbial peptides are expressed in salivary glands and saliva. *J Dent Res.* 2002;81:845.

119. Heilborn JD, Nilsson MF, Kratz G, et al. The cathelicidin anti-microbial peptide LL-37 is involved in re-epithelialization of human skin wounds and is lacking in chronic ulcer epithelium. *J Invest Dermatol.* 2003;120:379.

120. Gallo RL, Ono M, Povsic T, et al. Syndecans, cell surface heparan sulfate proteoglycans, are induced by a proline-rich antimicrobial peptide from wounds. *Proc Natl Acad Sci U S A.* 1994;91:11035.

121. Ali RS, Falconer A, Ikram M, et al. Expression of the peptide antibiotics human beta defensin-1 and human beta defensin-2 in normal human skin. *J Invest Dermatol.* 2001;117:106.

122. Mathews M, Jia HP, Guthmiller JM, et al. Production of beta-defensin antimicrobial peptides by the oral mucosa and salivary glands. *Infect Immun.* 1999;67:2740.

123. Dunsche A, Acil Y, Dommisch H, et al. The novel human beta-defensin-3 is widely expressed in oral tissues. *Eur J Oral Sci.* 2002;1110:121.

124. Frye M, Bargon J, Gropp R. Expression of human beta-defensin-1 promotes differentiation of keratinocytes. *J Mol Med.* 2001;79:275.

125. Seo SJ, Ahn SW, Hong CK, et al. Expressions of beta-defensins in human keratinocyte cell lines. *J Dermatol Sci.* 2001;27:183.

126. Sybert VP, Dale BA, Holbrook KA. Ichthyosis vulgaris: identification of a defect in synthesis of filaggrin correlated with an absence of keratohyaline granules. *J Invest Dermatol.* 1985;84:191.

127. Scott IR, Harding CR. Physiological effects of occlusion-filaggrin retention (abstr). *Dermatology.* 1993;2000:773.

128. Downing DT, Strauss JS, Pochi PE. Variability in the chemical composition of human skin surface lipids. *J Invest Dermatol.* 1969;53:322.

129. Webster D, France JT, Shapiro LJ, et al. X-linked ichthyosis due to steroid-sulphatase deficiency. *Lancet.* 1978;1:70.

130. Prottey C. Essential fatty acids and the skin. *Br J Dermatol.* 1976;94:579.

131. Elias PM. Epidermal lipids, barrier function, and desquamation. *J Invest Dermatol.* 1983;80:44s.

132. Rawlings AV, Scott IR, Harding CR, et al. Stratum corneum moisturization at the molecular level. *J Invest Dermatol.* 1994;103:731.

133. Swartzendruber DC, Wertz PW, Kitko DJ, et al. Molecular models of the intercellular lipid lamellae in mammalian stratum corneum. *J Invest Dermatol.* 1989;92:251.

134. Man MQ, Feingold KR, Elias PM. Exogenous lipids influence permeability barrier recovery in acetone-treated murine skin. *Arch Dermatol.* 1993;129:728.

CHAPTER 2

Basic Science of the Dermis

Leslie S. Baumann, MD

SUMMARY POINTS

What's Important?

1. Fibroblasts produce collagen, elastin precursors, and ECM constituents such as hyaluronic acid and heparan sulfate.
2. Young skin is characterized by elongated fibroblasts that are more productive (synthesize more collagen and ECM components) than those in older skin.
3. Old fibroblasts become compact and have less connection to the ECM.

What's New?

1. The tissue skeleton connects the fibroblast genomic DNA to the ECM.
2. The fibroblast connects to the ECM and exerts "mechanoforces" that affect gene expression.
3. Geometrical changes in the nucleus of the fibroblast influence gene transcription.
4. The matrisome, or microenvironment of the ECM, affects the gene expression of fibroblasts.
5. Papillary fibroblasts and reticular fibroblasts exhibit a 29% difference in gene expression[1] and different cell markers.

What's Coming?

1. Linkers of the nucleoskeleton and cytoskeleton (LINCS) are connected to genomic DNA. Research is ongoing to understand how LINCS affects DNA expression and to which signals they respond.
2. Ongoing research is assessing the tissue skeleton and modulations that occur with aging.
3. More is to be learned about epigenetics and the effects on fibroblast function.
4. More will be learned about cannabinoid receptors and fibroblasts.

The dermis lies between the epidermis and the subcutaneous fat. It is responsible for the thickness, strength, elasticity, and volume of the skin, and as a result plays a key role in the cosmetic appearance of the skin. The thickness of the dermis varies over different parts of the body and the size doubles between the ages of 3 and 7 years and again at puberty. The dermis is laden with nerves, blood vessels, melanocytes, and sweat glands surrounded by extracellular matrix, collagen, elastin, and hyaluronic acid (HA).

The dermal layer contributes most to the aged appearance of the skin. With aging, the dermal layer decreases in thickness and function. Fibroblasts become sluggish, less responsive to cell signals, and divide less frequently with age. These changes result in thinner skin with fine lines and wrinkles.

Loss of elastin in this layer leads to skin sagging, while loss of collagen yields fragility, and loss of HA engenders a decrease in moisture-holding capacity and volume. The dermis is the layer where dermal fillers are injected to increase volume and improve the skin's appearance. Although the epidermis reflects light, gives skin its texture, and regulates moisturization, changes in the epidermis affect the skin's appearance temporarily because of this layer's rapid cell turnover. Dermal changes are more durable and significant, but these less superficial changes take longer to see. Dysfunction of the dermis causes long-term issues like keloids, stretch marks, and acne scars. Protection of the dermis is critical because many problems located in this layer cannot be completely corrected.

ANATOMY OF THE DERMIS

The Dermal-Epidermal Junction

The dermal-epidermal junction (DEJ) is made up of the lower basement membrane of the basal keratinocytes and is an extremely important area of the skin (**Fig. 2-1**). It is composed of four zones that contain anchoring filaments, laminins, Type IV collagen, Type VII collagen, nidogens, and perlecan, among other structural constituents. (Note that the collagen in the basement membrane is not the same type as the Type I collagen found in the ECM of the dermis.) The components of the DEJ are synthesized by both keratinocytes and fibroblasts.[2] The DEJ junction itself functions to separate the epidermis and the dermis and, paradoxically, to attach them together. The DEJ also acts to provide a barrier to entry to the dermis that can filter large molecules, allowing some to pass. Other functions of the DEJ include anchoring the epidermis to the dermis and providing mechanical stability and tissue resilience.

When the skin blisters, the level of the split can occur in the epidermis (intra-epidermal) or below the epidermis (subepidermal). Intra-epidermal blisters arise above the DEJ and are caused by issues such as dyshidrotic eczema, friction blisters, insect bites, and herpes simplex virus. Subepidermal blistering disorders involve the DEJ and force the epidermis and dermis to separate. The subepidermal blistering diseases are severe and are caused by antibodies to structures in the DEJ, drug reactions, genetic disorders resulting in a missing DEJ structural component, or external insults such as a severe burn. Dermatitis herpetiformis is an example of a subepidermal blistering disorder caused by IgA antibodies in celiac disease. Subepidermal blisters are dangerous because they create separation of the epidermis and dermis that can lead to significant skin loss, dehydration, scarring, and other deleterious consequences. A discussion of disorders of the DEJ is beyond the scope of this chapter, but much is known about these sometimes devastating diseases.

A portion of the DEJ, known as the lamina densa, becomes duplicated in UV-exposed skin, which leads to a weakened DEJ, decreased resistance to shear force, and skin fragility.[3] In sun-exposed old patients, their skin may contain multiple layers of duplicated lamina densa.

Matrix metalloproteinases (MMPs) can break down various parts of the DEJ. Urokinase-type plasminogen activator (uPA) may degrade the basement membrane in the DEJ (see Chapter 6, Extrinsic Aging). Heparanase and other enzymes can also dissolve components in the DEJ. Perlecan, a substance composed of chains of heparan sulfate, stores and releases growth factors (GFs), acting as a GF reservoir in the DEJ. These GFs are held until needed. Heparanase, an enzyme that breaks down the HS chains in perlecan, disrupts the storage of GFs in the basement membrane, which attacks GF signaling. Heparanase levels are increased with inflammation and UV exposure resulting in a dramatic reduction in GF activity.[3] To prevent damage to the basement membrane of the DEJ, measures should be taken to reduce heparanase, free radicals, uPA, and MMPs. In other words, sun protection, sun avoidance, and sunscreen are recommended. Suffice it to say, the DEJ junction plays a critical role in skin health and skin youthfulness.

The Dermis

The dermis is divided into the upper papillary dermis and the lower reticular dermis. For years it was hard to distinguish the papillary fibroblasts (Fp) from the reticular fibroblasts (Fr), but new techniques have shown they have different markers. RNA sequencing data in healthy human skin has identified three subsets of fibroblasts (see **Table 2-1**).[4] These three fibroblast types are not spatially restricted to either the papillary or reticular dermis; rather, they are the predominant fibroblast type found in that area. Fp and Fr share some of the same gene expression, but 29% of the gene expression varies between the two types of fibroblasts. A list of expressed genes can be found in a 2019 paper by Haydont.[1] The functionality of fibroblasts is affected by their microenvironment, so when fibroblasts appear in the papillary dermis microenvironment they act like Fp and when in the reticular dermis microenvironment they act like Fr. Fibroblasts are so versatile that they can also shift to become myofibroblasts, after wounding, for example.

Papillary Dermis

The uppermost portion of the dermis, which lies beneath the epidermis, is known as the papillary dermis (**Fig. 2-2**). The papillary dermis is highly vascular with high cell density, smaller collagen bundles, and loose connective tissue. Fibroblasts in the papillary dermis give rise to the dermal sheath, papilla, and arrector pili muscle. Oxytalan fibers in the DEJ connect to fibrillin- and elastin-containing elaunin fibers in the lower papillary dermis, providing elasticity to the skin. There is a larger ratio of fibrillin to elastin in the papillary dermis.

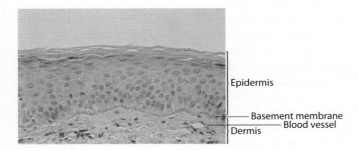

FIGURE 2-1. Histopathology of the dermal-epidermal junction. The basement membrane separates the epidermis and the dermis. (*Image courtesy of George Loannides, MD.*)

TABLE 2-1	Fibroblast Types, Actions, and Markers	
Fibroblast Location	Cell Surface Markers	Actions
Papillary	FAP+, CD90−, CD39	Proliferative
Reticular	FAP−, CD90+	Adipogenesis
Reticular	FAP+, CD90+	Adipogenesis

*Adapted from Ref. 4.

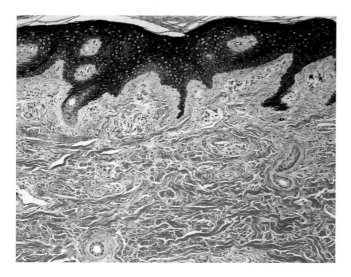

FIGURE 2-2. The dermis is divided into the papillary dermis and the reticular dermis. (Photo licensed from Shutterstock Dec 2020.)

Reticular Dermis

The lower portion of the dermis is the reticular dermis, which is characterized by low cell density surrounded by collagen and other connective tissue proteins. The reticular fibroblasts synthesize the extracellular matrix and adipocytes of the hypodermis.[5] Elastin fibers run parallel to the DEJ in the reticular dermis and there is a higher ratio of elastin to fibrillin.

Cells in the Dermis

Fibroblasts are the primary cell type in the dermis. They produce collagen, elastin, other matrix proteins, and enzymes such as collagenase and stromelysin. These structural components will be discussed individually because each exhibits significant characteristics that influence the function of the skin. Immune cells such as mast cells, polymorphonuclear leukocytes, lymphocytes, and macrophages are also present in the dermis.

Many cell types move in and out of the dermis including various types of immune cells and melanocytes. Endothelial cells and pericytes are also located in the dermis. These cells communicate with GFs, cytokines, and chemokines as well as other cells in the dermis and with the epidermis and DEJ.

Fibroblasts

Fibroblasts are the main cell type in the dermis. They can become pluripotent stem cells. The fibroblasts of the papillary dermis and reticular dermis were thought to be the same for many years, but recent evidence has shown they are distinct and respond to different signals.[4] Fibroblasts in cell culture (*in vitro*) alter the genes they express as compared to when in the dermis in humans (*in vivo*), which means they act differently in cell cultures than they do in live skin. This has made them hard to study and understand. This is also why cell culture data for cosmeceuticals cannot be relied upon to determine product efficacy.

Wounded skin. When skin is wounded, the fibroblasts change to a myofibroblastic phenotype critical for wound healing. These myofibroblasts express α smooth muscle actin and myosin II, which allows them to produce mechanical force. This change is regulated by cytokines and GFs such as the TGF-β/Smad signaling pathway. The diminished wound healing that is seen in older individuals is due partly to the decrease of HA, as well as loss of EGF and TGF-β growth factor signaling.[6]

Aged dermis. Aged dermis is characterized by less collagen, fragmented glycated elastin, fewer ECM components, and an accumulation of senescent fibroblasts that lead to reduced collagen production and an increase in MMP production.[7] Aged skin contains smaller fibroblasts than younger skin. Oder fibroblasts release an increased level of age-related MMPs and upregulate the expression of c-Jun/c-Fos and AP-1, which increases collagenases resulting in collagen breakdown.[8] (See Chapter 5, Intrinsic Aging, and Chapter 6 for more details.)

Organelles in fibroblasts

Fibroblasts contain the same type of cellular organelles as the epidermis (see Chapter 1, Basic Science of the Epidermis). The mitochondria play a critical role in energy production that fibroblasts need to synthesize the ECM components. The mitochondria in aged fibroblasts exhibit electron transport chain dysfunction, which leads to production of reactive oxygen species (ROS). Decreases in autophagy of mitochondria contribute to aging (see Chapter 5).

Receptors in the Dermis

Estrogen and Androgen Receptors in the Skin

All steroid hormones, such as estradiol and testosterone, exert their biologic action by binding to nuclear receptors, thereby initiating transcription and translation of proteins. The classic estrogen receptor (ER-α) was discovered in the 1970s; ER-β was discovered and isolated from human tissue in 1996.[9] Since then, studies have shown that ER-β is the predominant estrogen receptor in human skin and highly expressed in the epidermis, blood vessels, dermal fibroblasts, and outer root sheath of the hair follicle (the location of the bulge and stem cells). ER-α and the androgen receptor (which can bind testosterone or DHT) are expressed only in dermal papilla cells of the hair follicle.[10,11] All three receptors are also found in sebaceous glands.[10,11] In eccrine sweat glands, ER-β is highly expressed as are, to a lesser extent, androgen and progesterone receptors.[11] Recent studies of human adipose tissue found that sex hormone receptors differ by site, with ER-β being highly expressed in subcutaneous tissue.[12] With all these recent findings, it is clear that sex hormones are involved in the proliferation, differentiation, and function of the skin, adnexal structures, as well as fat, and that this regulation is far more intricate than previously thought. In addition, the recent description of the ER-β receptor (ER-β1–5) isoforms has made this subject more complex.[12]

Thyroid Receptors

Thyroid receptors are found on fibroblasts.[13] The number of thyroid receptors on fibroblasts tends to stay the same from ages 40 to 85. However, the number of overall fibroblasts declines with age, which results in a general decrease of thyroid hormone receptors in older skin.

Cannabis Receptors in the Dermis

The endocannabinoid system plays an important role in the skin. Cannabinoid receptors have been found in cutaneous nerve fibers, epidermal keratinocytes, and skin appendages. Although cannabinoid receptors have not been identified on fibroblasts, a study showed that a cannabinoid CB1 antagonist inhibited the TGF-β-induced differentiation of fibroblasts into myofibroblasts. This study found that TGF-β produced an increase in CB1 expression.[14] Another study demonstrated that fibroblasts did not have CB1 receptors, but when they transformed into pluripotent stem cells, the CB1 receptor was expressed.[15] It is still too early to know which types of fibroblasts have cannabinoid receptors and what role they play in fibroblast function.

Botulinum Toxin and Fibroblasts

BTX-A has been shown to inhibit fibroblast to myofibroblast differentiation *in vitro* and reduces the level of α-smooth muscle actin (α-SMA) and myosin II expression.[16,17] BTX-A also suppresses fibroblast proliferation and expression of TGF-β1.[18,19] It is unknown how this occurs, but it is likely due to the actions of BTX-A on the SNARE complex. TGF-β1 also significantly increases MMP-2 and MMP-9 expression, which is blocked by BTX-A.[20]

Structural Components of the Dermis

The structural components of the dermis give it the thickness, volume, strength, cushioning ability, and resiliency associated with youthful skin. The ECM of the dermis is important for many reasons that will be discussed in this chapter and Chapters 5 and 6. The ECM microenvironment affects the activity of the fibroblasts and is referred to as the matrisome.[21] The proteoglycans bind water and impart volume to the skin. Perlecan and HA reservoirs in the DEJ and ECM store and release GFs. Woven through the water-laden GAGs is an intricate cytoskeleton that makes up the "tissue skeleton" of the dermis. Intracellular actin filaments bind to the extracellular fibronectin-containing fibers via fibronexus junctions. Fibronectin molecules bind to integrin receptors on myofibroblasts and fibroblasts allowing cell signaling. The tissue skeleton connects the ECM to the genomic DNA of the fibroblast via a series of mechanical relay points: focal adhesion points, cytoskeleton, LINC complexes, and nucleoskeleton.[22] (See **Fig. 2-3**.) The fibroblast can pull against the tissue skeleton causing mechanoforces that result in cell signaling. When there are fewer GAGs and less collagen, as seen in aged skin, the fibroblast cannot adhere to the tissue skeleton as well and becomes compacted and smaller with less ability to exert mechanical forces on the tissue skeleton. Several other cellular components are involved in the tissue skeleton and dermal infrastructure.

Collagen

Collagen makes up 75% of the dry weight of the skin and provides durability, thickness, resilience, and a youthful appearance to skin. Types IV and VII collagen are found in the DEJ. Reduced levels of Types I and III collagen in the dermis have been associated with an aged skin appearance and a decrease in Type IV collagen in the basement membrane is associated with the increased fragility seen in aged skin.[23]

Increasing skin collagen has been the focus of much anti-aging research and the target of skin products and procedures for decades. Many topical cosmeceuticals increase collagen synthesis such as glycolic and ascorbic acids, as well as retinoids. Resurfacing techniques such as microneedling, chemical peels, lasers, and dermabrasion activate wound

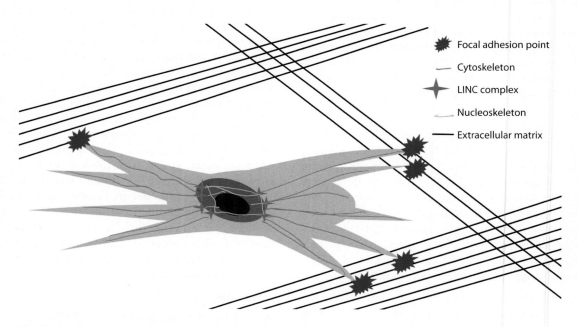

Focal adhesion point
Cytoskeleton
LINC complex
Nucleoskeleton
Extracellular matrix

FIGURE 2-3. Connection of the ECM to the genomic DNA via a series of mechanical relay points. Adapted from reference.[79]

healing mechanisms that result in increased collagen production. Skin-tightening procedures are intended to shorten collagen using heat. The efficacy of these anti-aging treatments will be discussed separately in upcoming chapters; however, it is necessary first to gain an understanding of the structure and function of collagen.

"Collagen" is actually a complex family of 18 proteins, 11 of which are present in the dermis. Collagen fibers are always seen in the dermis in the final, mature state of assembly as opposed to elastin, the immature fibers of which are seen in the superficial dermis with the more mature fibers found in the deeper layer of the dermis. Each type of collagen is composed of three chains (**Fig. 2-4**). Collagen is synthesized in the fibroblasts in a precursor form called procollagen. Proline residues on the procollagen chain are converted to hydroxyproline by the enzyme prolyl hydroxylase. This reaction requires the presence of Fe^{++}, ascorbic acid (vitamin C), and α-ketoglutarate. Lysine residues on the procollagen chain are also converted to hydroxylysine; in this case, by the enzyme lysyl hydroxylase. This reaction also requires the presence of Fe^{++}, ascorbic acid, and α-ketoglutarate. It is interesting to note that a deficiency of vitamin C, which is an essential mediating component in these reactions, leads to scurvy, a disease characterized by decreased collagen production.

The key types of collagen found in the dermis (Table 2-1)

Type I collagen comprises 80% to 85% of the collagen in the dermis, which is responsible for the tensile strength of the dermis. The amount of Type I collagen has been shown to be lower in photoaged skin, and to be increased after dermabrasion procedures.[24] Therefore, it is likely that Type I collagen is the most important collagen type pertaining to skin aging.

Type III collagen makes up 8% to 15% of the matrix of dermal collagen.[25] This collagen type has a smaller diameter than Type I and forms smaller bundles allowing for skin pliability. Type III is also known as "fetal collagen" because it predominates in embryonic life. It is concentrated around the blood vessels and beneath the epidermis and is involved in fibrosis. The production of Type III collagen increases with age, suggesting that tissue fibrosis increases with age.[26]

Type IV collagen forms a structural lattice found in the basement membrane zone. Type IV collagen levels in the basement membrane have been shown to decrease with menopause.[26] The degradation of Types I and III collagen are regulated differently than the degradation and synthesis of Type IV collagen.[26] Type V collagen, which is diffusely distributed throughout the dermis, comprises approximately 4% to 5% of the dermal matrix collagen. Type VII collagen makes

up the anchoring fibrils in the DEJ. For example, patients with the inherited blistering disease known as dominant dystrophic epidermolysis have a scarcity of Type VII collagen with resulting abnormalities in their anchoring fibrils. An acquired bullous disease, epidermolysis bullosa acquisita (EBA), is caused by antibodies to this same collagen type. Patients with chronic sun exposure have also been found to have alterations in Type VII collagen. Some investigators have postulated that a weakened bond between the dermis and epidermis caused by loss of the anchoring fibrils (Type VII collagen) may lead to wrinkle formation.[27] Type XVII collagen is located in the hemidesmosome and plays an important structural role as well. The significance of these collagens and other structural proteins is evident in genetic diseases characterized by a lack of these structures and in acquired diseases characterized by antibody formation to these crucial structures. The importance of collagen and the changes seen in aged skin will be discussed further in Chapters 5 and 6.

Elastin

Elastin stays in the skin for decades; therefore, it is susceptible to damage over time. Production of the main component of elastin decreases in adulthood and, to date, cannot be stimulated by any topically applied cosmeceutical ingredients or drugs.[28–30] Older skin is characterized by reduced elastin production and accumulation of damaged elastin, which results in sagging skin.[31–33]

Elastic fibers represent one of the essential components of the ECM in connective tissue (**Fig. 2-5**). They confer resilience and elasticity to skin as well as other organs such as the lungs and blood vessels. Elastogenesis starts during fetal life and reaches its maximum near birth and the early neonatal period. It then decreases significantly and is virtually nonexistent by adult life. Elastic fibers have two components, of which elastin, an amorphous, insoluble connective tissue protein, is the main one. The central elastin core is surrounded by peripheral microfibrils. Elastin constitutes 2% to 3% of the dry weight of skin, 3% to 7% of lung, 28% to 32% of major blood vessels, and 50% of elastic ligaments.[34]

Elastin is produced from its precursor tropoelastin in the fibroblasts as well as endothelial cells and vascular smooth

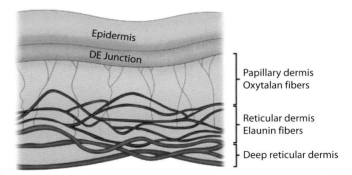

FIGURE 2-5. The elastic fiber network in the dermis consists of immature oxytalan fibers in the superficial dermis and the more mature elaunin fibers in the middle dermis. The most mature elastic fibers are unnamed and are found in the deep reticular dermis.

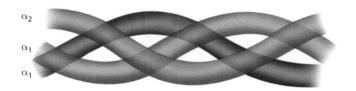

FIGURE 2-4. Collagen is formed when three chains come together to form a triple helix.

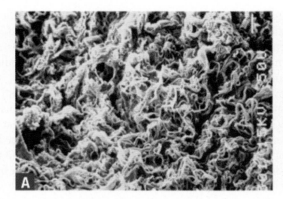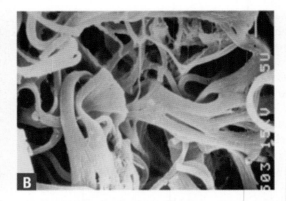

FIGURE 2-6A and B. Scanning electron micrographs of the elastic fibers in human skin. Adapted from Fitzpatrick's Dermatology in General Medicine, seventh edition (McGraw Hill), page 532, with permission.

muscle cells. In contrast to collagen fibers, elastin fibers are present in the dermis in various levels of maturity. The least mature fibers are called oxytalan. They course perpendicularly from the DEJ, through the papillary dermis to the top of the reticular dermis. More mature elastin fibers, called elaunin, then attach to a horizontal plexus of fibers found in the reticular dermis. Elaunin is more mature because it contains more elastin deposited on the fibrillin mesh. The most mature elastin fibers are unnamed and are found deeper in the reticular dermis (**Figs. 2-5 and 2-6A and B**).

Microfibrils play a critical role in elastogenesis and act as a scaffold for tropoelastin deposition and assembly.[35] Microfibrils are primarily composed of glycoproteins from the fibrillin family and microfibril-associated glycoprotein (MAGP)-1 and -2. Fibrillin-1 has been shown to be influential in elastic fiber development and wound repair.[36,37] Microfibrils are adjacent to tropoelastin-producing cells and parallel to the developing elastin fiber,[38] and form a template on which tropoelastin is deposited. The tropoelastin polypeptides are then covalently cross-linked to form elastin. Tropoelastin polypeptides contain alternating hydrophilic and hydrophobic regions. The hydrophobic domains, which are rich in proline, valine, and glycine, are believed to be responsible for the elasticity of the elastin tissue.[39] The hydrophilic domains on the other hand are rich in alanine and lysine, and interact with the enzyme lysyl oxidase in the process of cross-linking.[40] The cross-linking of elastin is a complex process necessary for its proper function and stability. This process is mediated via the copper-requiring enzyme lysyl oxidase,[41] and the subsequent formation of desmosine and isodesmosine cross-links, which result in an insoluble elastin network.[42]

Although much is known about elastin, its relevance in cosmetic dermatology is negligible at this time because there are no treatments proven to increase skin elastin content. It seems certain that collagen, hyaluronic acid (HA), and elastin bind each other covalently and create a three-dimensional structure that is impaired in aged skin. There is a commonly held belief that these three components must be increased in order to give skin a younger appearance. However, the trick is that *de novo* elastin production does not occur in adulthood. Trying to

replace elastotic elastin in adults with newer elastin is a focus of cosmetic dermatology research.

The elastic fiber's structure provides clues about its ability to interact with HA and collagen. Mature elastic fibers contain an array of proteoglycans. Versican is one of the most widely studied proteoglycans and is a member of the hyaluronan binding family that also includes aggrecan and neurocan.[43] Versican contributes to cell adhesion, proliferation, and migration and can interact with multiple ECM proteins to mediate assembly. Mature elastic fibers are found at the periphery of collagen bundles, offering a clue that elastin has significant interactions with collagen as well as with HA.

Elastic fibers are degraded by the elastolytic enzymes such as human leukocyte elastase (HLE). With significant levels of sun exposure, elastin degrades and is seen as an amorphous substance in the dermis when viewed by light microscopy. This resultant "elastosis" is a hallmark of photoaged skin. Interestingly, there are protective mechanisms in the skin preventing elastin degradation. Lysozymes are believed to play a protective role in this matter. They have been shown to increase and deposit on the elastin fibers of UV-exposed skin.[44] By binding to elastin, lysozymes prevent the proper interaction between elastase and elastin, thereby inhibiting the proteolytic activity of the elastolytic enzymes.[45,46] It is also believed that damage to the elastin fibers leads to the decreased skin elasticity seen in aged skin.[47] Defects or damage to elastin may lead to wrinkles even in the absence of sun exposure and aging. Indeed, in one case, a child with "wrinkled skin syndrome" was shown to have a deficiency of elastin fibers,[48] which demonstrates the importance of elastin in skin integrity. Defective elastic fibers can lead to multiple dermatologic diseases including cutis laxa, pseudoxanthoma elasticum (PXE), elastosis perforans serpiginosa (also known as Lutz-Miescher's syndrome), and dermatofibrosis lenticularis (also known as Buschke-Ollendorff syndrome).

Intrinsically aged skin displays fragmentation of the elastin network, while extrinsically aged skin contains clumps of elastotic material.[49] Studies have demonstrated a reduction in the elastin content in protected areas of the skin with aging. In a study performed on Egyptian subjects, the relative amount of elastin in the non-UV-exposed abdominal skin significantly decreased from 49.2% ± 0.6% in the first decade to 30.4% ± 0.8% in the ninth decade.[50] Another study on elastin content in the nonexposed buttock skin of 91 Caucasians between 20 and 80 years of age showed a reduction of 51% in elastin tissue.[46] Although UV exposure may result in elastosis and a higher content of elastin tissue, the elastic fibers are rendered structurally abnormal,[50] which is microscopically seen as thickened and twisted granular deposits of elastin in the dermis.

Elastin and stretch marks

Striae distensae, commonly known as stretch marks, are linear atrophic dermal scars in areas of volume change caused by skin stretching from weight gain or increased muscle mass. They are thought to be related to disorganization of elastin.[45] In some cases, stretch marks may be caused by impaired fibroblast function as demonstrated by reduced expression of fibronectin and Types I and III procollagen in striae.[51,52]

Increasing elastin in skin

Elastin prevents skin sagging by providing recoil and stretch. Intact elastic fiber networks are required for skin to retain elasticity, but over time elastin degrades and damaged fragments accumulate in the skin. Production of new elastin decreases with aging. For this reason, there is significant research into finding ways to increase functional elastin in the skin.

Replacing the elastin component of the ECM with new elastin has always posed a challenge in skin rejuvenation approaches. Researchers have investigated the production of recombinant and cross-linked tropoelastin in great detail.[53] Efforts to create elastin that can be applied topically and permeate human skin have failed. The remaining options include stimulating the dermis to produce elastin or injecting functional elastin into the skin. At the time of publication of this text, and despite the claims of some manufacturers, there were no topical elastin products that could increase skin elastin. There are some preliminary studies looking at the potential of elastin injections into the skin.

Elastin-derived peptides. Elastin is broken down by elastase and MMP-2, MMP-7, MMP-9, and MMP-12 into peptides. Elastin-derived peptides (EDPs) regulate MMP expression and may decrease elastase, inhibit fibroblast apoptosis, promote fibroblast proliferation, and increase hydroxyproline and water content in the skin.[54] EDPs are thought to play a role in cancer tumor progression.[55] Some cosmeceuticals contain EDPs, but these have not been proven to be safe (see Chapter 37, Anti-Aging Ingredients).

Glycoproteins

Glycoproteins (GPs) influence cell migration, adhesion, and orientation. Fibronectin and tenascin are the GPs most relevant in the dermis although vitronectin, thrombospondin, and epibolin are also present in the dermis. Fibronectin is a filamentous GP that mediates platelet binding to collagen, development of granulation tissue, and re-epithelialization. Chemotactic for monocytes, fibronectin contains six binding sites including one for collagen, two for heparin, and a region that binds fibrin. Tenascin is abundant in developing skin but found only in the papillary dermis in adult skin. These matrix components play a significant role in tissue remodeling and are important in wound healing following cosmetic procedures.

Glycosaminoglycans

Glycosaminoglycans (GAGs) are polysaccharide chains composed of repeating disaccharide units linked to a core protein. Together the GAGs and attached core protein form proteoglycans. Their cross-linking to other matrix proteins such as the collagen network results in a critical infrastructure and microenvironment that affects the function of fibroblasts. HA is the only nonsulfated GAG.

Although all the functions of GAGs are not understood, it is known that these compounds avidly bind water, contribute to the maintenance of salt and water balance, and affect fibroblast function. GAGs are found in areas with a fibrous matrix where cells are closely associated but have little space for free movement. Studies on human skin show an age-related decline in overall sulfated GAG content and HA content. Heparan sulfate (HS) and chondroitin sulfate are increased in photoaged skin, but the overall level of sulfated GAGs is decreased. The most abundant GAGs in the dermis are HA and dermatan sulfate. The other GAGs include HS, heparin, keratan sulfate, chondroitin-4, and chondroitin-6-sulfate.

Heparan sulfate

HS is an essential glycosaminoglycans that enhances cellular response to GFs by promoting the response of old, indolent fibroblasts to cellular signals. HS binds and stores GFs and protects them until they arrive at their target receptors. Once at the receptor, they present the GF or cytokine to the appropriate binding site.[56] In a way, they chaperone the cell signals until they get to their destination. As with other ECM components, HS levels are lower in aged skin.

Hyaluronic acid

HA is a vital constituent of the dermis that is responsible for attracting water and giving the dermis its volume. The name reflects its glassy appearance (the Greek word for glass is *hyalos*) and the presence of a sugar known as uronic acid. HA plays a prominent role in cell growth, membrane receptor function, and adhesion. Its structure is identical, whether it is derived from bacterial cultures, animals, or humans (**Fig. 2-7**). HA appears freely in the dermis and is more concentrated in areas where cells are less densely packed. In young skin, HA is found at the periphery of collagen and elastin fibers and at the interface of these types of fibers. These connections with

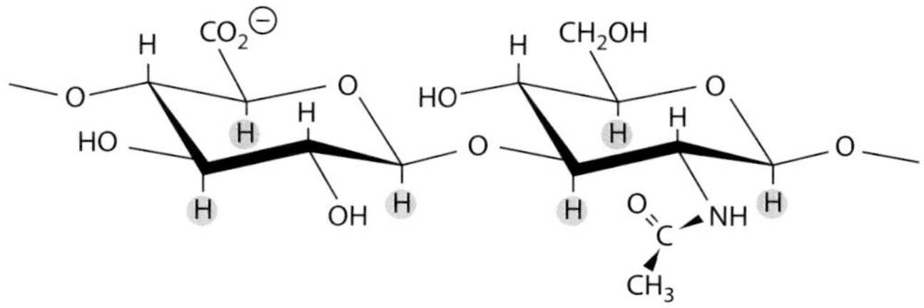

FIGURE 2-7. HA is made of repeating dimers of glucuronic acid and N-acetyl glucosamine assembled into long chains.

HA are absent in aged skin.[57] HA appears to also play a role in keratinocyte differentiation and formation of lamellar bodies via its interaction with CD44,[58] a cell surface glycoprotein receptor with HA binding sites.[59–61] HA can bind GFs and cytokines and hold them, creating gradients of these communicating factors.[62] HA is a popular ingredient in cosmetic products because it acts as a humectant (see Chapter 37). Several types are also available in an injectable dermal filler version for the treatment of wrinkles (see Chapter 23, Botulinum Toxins).

Other glycosaminoglycans

Chondroitin sulfate, dermatan sulfate, keratan sulfate, and heparin are other GAGs found in the ECM in addition to HS and HA. Intrinsically aged skin is characterized by decreased heparan sulfate and chondroitin sulfate and increased keratan sulfate and dermatan sulfate.[63,64]

Decorin

Decorin is a member of the small leucine-rich proteoglycans (SLRPs) found in the ECM protein. Its name is derived from its apparent "decorating" of collagen fibers. Decorin contains a core protein with a high content of leucine repeats and GAG chains of dermatan or chondroitin sulfate. It is shaped in a "horseshoe" pattern and binds to collagen fibrils, resulting in their proper organization.[65] Decorin-deficient mice have demonstrated clinical skin fragility and irregular collagen fibrils with increased interfibrillar space on histology.[66] In addition to collagen fibrillogenesis, decorin interacts with fibronectin and fibrinogen, thereby playing a role in wound healing and hemostasis.[67,68] Decorin also reduces the proliferation of cells in neoplasms by halting their growth in the G_1 phase of the cell cycle.[69] Carrino et al. studied the catabolic fragment of decorin in adult skin.[70] They noted a higher content of the altered decorin in adult dermis as opposed to nonmeasurable amounts in fetal skin and named it "decorunt." Decorunt was shown to have a lower affinity for collagen fibrils. This finding may explain some of the changes related to collagen disorganization in aging skin. Decorin is sparse in photoaged skin.[71]

MECHANO-SENSITIVE TRANSCRIPTION FACTORS

The interaction between the fibroblast and the ECM is intricate and communicative. The intracellular actin filaments in young, elongated fibroblasts use fibronexus junctions to bind extracellular fibronectin. This allows the fibroblast to mechanically pull the ECM. The ECM proteins bind the intracellular cytoskeleton via adhesion points that connect to the nucleoskeleton via links called "linker of neuroskeleton and cytoskeleton" (LINCS). The neuroskeleton links to the genomic DNA.[1] The fibroblast induces movements that stimulate mechano-sensible receptors that can elicit a quick or a delayed response by changing genomic DNA expression.

Growth Factors in the Dermis

Growth factors are regulatory proteins that act on the cell membrane, usually by binding tyrosine kinase receptors, to initiate biochemical pathways such as transcription of kinases in the cell nucleus. The dermal GFs play an important role in skin repair and rejuvenation. GFs are discussed in Chapter 37. Two primary GFs that affect the dermis are fibroblast GFs and transforming growth factor-β.

Fibroblast Growth Factors

Fibroblast growth factors (FGFs) are a family of GFs that increase the proliferation of fibroblasts and activate them to synthesize collagen and stimulate angiogenesis. FGF-1 induces the synthesis of collagen and elastin.

Transforming growth factor-β

TGF-β is a major profibrotic cytokine that regulates multiple cellular functions including differentiation, proliferation, and the induction of ECM protein synthesis. TGF-β promotes differentiation and plays an important role specifically in controlling production of the ECM.[38] TGF-β is critical for regulating collagen synthesis. In fact, the primary cause of the decrease in Type 1 procollagen after UV exposure is inhibition of a TGF-β pathway.[72] TGF-β has also been proven to have a role in scarring, and antibodies to this factor have been shown to mitigate the inflammatory response in wounds and reduce scarring.[39,40] TGF-β levels are increased by calcium, phorbol esters, as well as TGF-β itself.

In human skin, TGF-β inhibits the growth of epidermal keratinocytes but stimulates the growth of dermal fibroblasts. Moreover, TGF-β induces synthesis and secretion of the major ECM proteins, collagen and elastin. TGF-β also inhibits expression of certain enzymes involved in the breakdown of collagen, including MMP-1 and MMP-3. TGF-β1 significantly increases MMP-2 and MMP-9 expression.[20]

HA-containing dermal fillers stimulate collagen production by acting on the TGF-β/Smad pathway.[73] HA facilitates interaction between CD44 and EGFR, thus promoting MAPK/ERK phosphorylation and inducing TGF-β1-dependent fibroblast proliferation.

Light and the Dermis

Ultraviolet light exposure results in epidermal- and dermal-derived GF cross-talk and stimulates production of KGF and EGF. After UV exposure, FGF acts synergistically with melanin-stimulating hormone to increase melanogenesis.[74] Dermal fibroblasts are the main targets of visible light in the skin.[75] Light alters the cytoskeleton of fibroblasts, damages the mitochondria, affects the transcriptome significantly, and causes compaction of fibroblasts as seen with older fibroblasts when the ECM is altered.[76,77]

Circadian Rhythm

Fibroblasts exhibit a circadian oscillation that affects the expression of multiple genes. The fibroblasts are controlled by a light-sensitive master circadian clock in mammals known as the suprachiasmatic nucleus (SCN). The SCN is composed of multiple circadian oscillator neurons that receive input from light and a variety of intrinsic and extrinsic factors. Reduced levels of SIRT1 adversely affect clock function.[78] The circadian clock regulates many processes involved in skin aging including proteasome activity, autophagy of mitochondria, and the activity of antioxidant defense systems.[79]

Hypodermis

The hypodermis, or subcutis, located beneath the dermis, is composed mostly of fat, which is a key energy source for the body. This layer also contains collagen Types I, III, and V. As humans age, some subcutaneous fat is lost or redistributed into undesired areas. This phenomenon contributes to the aged appearance. Fat injections have been employed to move fat from undesired areas into desired ones where fat has been lost, such as the lower face (see Chapter 23).

The adipocytes secrete a hormone called leptin, a product of the obesity (*ob*) gene. Leptin exhibits a regulatory effect on human metabolism and appetite and therefore affects adipose tissue mass. Leptin has been shown to be higher in the serum of obese patients, with commensurate levels of body fat percentage.[80] It is believed that a higher percentage of body fat results in elevated leptin levels and the turning off of signals to the brain for appetite reduction. Recombinant leptin injections in mice have been associated with reduction of weight and body fat percentage.[81] However, more research is needed to ascertain the therapeutic potential of leptin in humans.

CONCLUSION

The epidermis is the target of most topical cosmetic products because these products do not penetrate to the dermis, while the dermis is the target for many of the injectable treatments for aging. The dermis is an extremely important component in skin appearance because it is responsible for imparting thickness and suppleness to the skin. A thinner dermis and an altered DEJ are hallmarks of aged skin. Loss of collagen, elastin, and GAGs located primarily in the dermis contribute significantly to cutaneous aging. Various measures intended to prevent or decelerate aging target these key constituents of the dermis.

References

1. Haydont V, Neiveyans V, Fortunel NO, Asselineau D. Transcriptome profiling of human papillary and reticular fibroblasts from adult interfollicular dermis pinpoints the 'tissue skeleton' gene network as a component of skin chrono-ageing. *Mech Ageing Dev.* 2019;179:60–77.

2. Aumailley M. Laminins and interaction partners in the architecture of the basement membrane at the dermal-epidermal junction. *Exp Dermatol.* 2021;30(1):17–24.

3. Amano S. Characterization and mechanisms of photoageing-related changes in skin. Damages of basement membrane and dermal structures. *Exp Dermatol.* 2016;25(Suppl 3):14–19.

4. Korosec A, Frech S, Gesslbauer B, et al. Lineage Identity and Location within the Dermis Determine the Function of Papillary and Reticular Fibroblasts in Human Skin. *J Invest Dermatol.* 2019;139(2):342–351.

5. Driskell RR, Lichtenberger BM, Hoste E, et al. Distinct fibroblast lineages determine dermal architecture in skin development and repair. *Nature.* 2013;504(7479):277–281.

6. Vedrenne N, Coulomb B, Danigo A, Bonté F, Desmoulière A. The complex dialogue between (myo)fibroblasts and the extracellular matrix during skin repair processes and ageing. *Pathol Biol (Paris).* 2012;60(1):20–27.

7. Mays PK, Bishop JE, Laurent GJ. Age-related changes in the proportion of types I and III collagen. *Mech Ageing Dev.* 1988;45(3):203–212.

8. Qin Z, Balimunkwe RM, Quan T. Age-related reduction of dermal fibroblast size upregulates multiple matrix metalloproteinases as observed in aged human skin in vivo. *Br J Dermatol.* 2017;177(5):1337–1348.

9. Dyer DG, Dunn JA, Thorpe SR, et al. Accumulation of Maillard reaction products in skin collagen in diabetes and aging. *J Clin Invest.* 1993;91(6):2463–2469.

10. Verzijl N, DeGroot J, Oldehinkel E, et al. Age-related accumulation of Maillard reaction products in human articular cartilage collagen. *Biochem J.* 2000;350(Pt 2):381–387.

11. Mizutari K, Ono T, Ikeda K, Kayashima K, Horiuchi S. Photo-enhanced modification of human skin elastin in actinic elastosis by N(epsilon)-(carboxymethyl)lysine, one of the gly-coxidation products of the Maillard reaction. *J Invest Dermatol.* 1997;108(5):797–802.

12. Tomasek JJ, Haaksma CJ, Eddy RJ, Vaughan MB. Fibroblast contraction occurs on release of tension in attached collagen lattices: dependency on an organized actin cytoskeleton and serum. *Anat Rec.* 1992;232(3):359–368.

13. Gunin AG, Golubtsova NN. Thyroid hormone receptors in human skin during aging. *Adv Gerontol.* 2018;31(1):82–90.

14. Correia-Sá IB, Carvalho CM, Serrão PV, et al. AM251, a cannabinoid receptor 1 antagonist, prevents human fibroblasts differentiation and collagen deposition induced by TGF-β - An in vitro study. *Eur J Pharmacol.* 2021;892:173738.

15. Bobrov MY, Bezuglov VV, Khaspekov LG, Illarioshkin SN, Novosadova EV, Grivennikov IA. Expression of Type I Cannabinoid Receptors at Different Stages of Neuronal Differentiation of Human Fibroblasts. *Bull Exp Biol Med.* 2017;163(2):272–275.

16. Zhang X, Lan D, Ning S, Jia H, Yu S. Botulinum toxin type A prevents the phenotypic transformation of fibroblasts induced by TGF-β1 via the PTEN/PI3K/Akt signaling pathway. *Int J Mol Med.* 2019;44(2):661–671.

17. Chen M, Yan T, Ma K, et al. Botulinum Toxin Type A Inhibits α-Smooth Muscle Actin and Myosin II Expression in Fibroblasts Derived From Scar Contracture. *Ann Plast Surg.* 2016;77(3):e46–e49.

18. Jeong HS, Lee BH, Sung HM, et al. Effect of Botulinum Toxin Type A on Differentiation of Fibroblasts Derived from Scar Tissue. *Plast Reconstr Surg.* 2015;136(2):171e–178e.

19. Xiao Z, Zhang F, Lin W, Zhang M, Liu Y. Effect of botulinum toxin type A on transforming growth factor beta1 in fibroblasts derived from hypertrophic scar: a preliminary report. *Aesthetic Plast Surg.* 2010;34(4):424–427.

20. Xiao Z, Zhang M, Liu Y, Ren L. Botulinum toxin type a inhibits connective tissue growth factor expression in fibroblasts derived from hypertrophic scar. *Aesthetic Plast Surg.* 2011;35(5):802–807.

21. Cole MA, Quan T, Voorhees JJ, Fisher GJ. Extracellular matrix regulation of fibroblast function: redefining our perspective on skin aging. *J Cell Commun Signal.* 2018;12(1):35–43.

22. Bouzid T, Kim E, Riehl BD, et al. The LINC complex, mechanotransduction, and mesenchymal stem cell function and fate. *J Biol Eng.* 2019;13:68.

23. Varani J, Dame MK, Rittie L, et al. Decreased collagen production in chronologically aged skin: roles of age-dependent alteration in fibroblast function and defective mechanical stimulation. *Am J Pathol.* 2006;168(6):1861–1868.

24. Nelson BR, Majmudar G, Griffiths CE, et al. Clinical improvement following dermabrasion of photoaged skin correlates with synthesis of collagen I. *Arch Dermatol.* 1994;130(9):1136–1142.

25. Oikarinen A. The aging of skin: chronoaging versus photoaging. *Photodermatol Photoimmunol Photomed.* 1990;7(1):3–4.

26. Vázquez F, Palacios S, Alemañ N, Guerrero F. Changes of the basement membrane and type IV collagen in human skin during aging. *Maturitas.* 1996;25(3):209–215.

27. Craven NM, Watson RE, Jones CJ, Shuttleworth CA, Kielty CM, Griffiths CE. Clinical features of photodamaged human skin are associated with a reduction in collagen VII. *Br J Dermatol.* 1997;137(3):344–350.

28. Monnier VM, Kohn RR, Cerami A. Accelerated age-related browning of human collagen in diabetes mellitus. *Proc Natl Acad Sci U S A.* 1984;81(2):583–587.

29. Schnider SL, Kohn RR. Effects of age and diabetes mellitus on the solubility and nonenzymatic glucosylation of human skin collagen. *J Clin Invest.* 1981;67(6):1630–1635.

30. Yamada K, Miyahara Y, Hamaguchi K, et al. Immunohistochemical study of human advanced glycosylation end-products (AGE) in chronic renal failure. *Clin Nephrol.* 1994;42(6):354–361.

31. Vitek MP, Bhattacharya K, Glendening JM, et al. Advanced glycation end products contribute to amyloidosis in Alzheimer disease. *Proc Natl Acad Sci U S A.* 1994;91(11):4766–4770.

32. Yan SD, Chen X, Schmidt AM, et al. Glycated tau protein in Alzheimer disease: a mechanism for induction of oxidant stress. *Proc Natl Acad Sci U S A.* 1994;91(16):7787–7791.

33. Takeuchi M, Kikuchi S, Sasaki N, et al. Involvement of advanced glycation end-products (AGEs) in Alzheimer's disease. *Curr Alzheimer Res.* 2004;1(1):39–46.

34. Vrhovski B, Weiss AS. Biochemistry of tropoelastin. *Eur J Biochem.* 1998;258(1):1–18.

35. Robb BW, Wachi H, Schaub T, Mecham RP, Davis EC. Characterization of an in vitro model of elastic fiber assembly. *Mol Biol Cell.* 1999;10(11):3595–3605.

36. Kielty CM, Sherratt MJ, Shuttleworth CA. Elastic fibres. *J Cell Sci.* 2002;115(Pt 14):2817–2828.

37. Amadeu TP, Braune AS, Porto LC, Desmoulière A, Costa AM. Fibrillin-1 and elastin are differentially expressed in hypertrophic scars and keloids. *Wound Repair Regen.* 2004;12(2):169–174.

38. Mithieux SM, Weiss AS. Elastin. *Adv Protein Chem.* 2005; 70:437–461.

39. Li B, Daggett V. Molecular basis for the extensibility of elastin. *J Muscle Res Cell Motil.* 2002;23(5-6):561–573.

40. Rosenbloom J, Abrams WR, Mecham R. Extracellular matrix 4: the elastic fiber. *FASEB J.* 1993;7(13):1208–1218.

41. Smith-Mungo LI, Kagan HM. Lysyl oxidase: properties, regulation and multiple functions in biology. *Matrix Biol.* 1998;16(7):387–398.

42. Starcher BC. Determination of the elastin content of tissues by measuring desmosine and isodesmosine. *Anal Biochem.* 1977;79(1-2):11–15.

43. Wight TN. Versican: a versatile extracellular matrix proteoglycan in cell biology. *Curr Opin Cell Biol.* 2002;14(5):617–623.

44. Suwabe H, Serizawa A, Kajiwara H, Ohkido M, Tsutsumi Y. Degenerative processes of elastic fibers in sun-protected and sun-exposed skin: immunoelectron microscopic observation of elastin, fibrillin-1, amyloid P component, lysozyme and alpha1-antitrypsin. *Pathol Int.* 1999;49(5):391–402.

45. Park PW, Biedermann K, Mecham L, Bissett DL, Mecham RP. Lysozyme binds to elastin and protects elastin from elastase-mediated degradation. *J Invest Dermatol.* 1996;106(5):1075–1080.

46. Seite S, Zucchi H, Septier D, Igondjo-Tchen S, Senni K, Godeau G. Elastin changes during chronological and photo-ageing: the important role of lysozyme. *J Eur Acad Dermatol Venereol.* 2006;20(8):980–987.

47. Escoffier C, de Rigal J, Rochefort A, Vasselet R, Lévêque JL, Agache PG. Age-related mechanical properties of human skin: an in vivo study. *J Invest Dermatol.* 1989;93(3):353–357.

48. Boente MC, Winik BC, Asial RA. Wrinkly skin syndrome: ultrastructural alterations of the elastic fibers. *Pediatr Dermatol.* 1999;16(2):113–117.

49. Langton AK, Sherratt MJ, Griffiths CE, Watson RE. Differential expression of elastic fibre components in intrinsically aged skin. *Biogerontology.* 2012;13(1):37–48.

50. El-Domyati M, Attia S, Saleh F, Brown D, Birk DE, Gasparro F, et al. Intrinsic aging vs. photoaging: a comparative histopathological, immunohistochemical, and ultrastructural study of skin. *Exp Dermatol.* 2002;11(5):398–405.

51. Keen MA. Striae distensae: what's new at the horizon? *Br J Med Practitioners.* 2016;9(3).

52. Lee KS, Rho YJ, Jang SI, Suh MH, Song JY. Decreased expression of collagen and fibronectin genes in striae distensae tissue. *Clin Exp Dermatol.* 1994;19(4):285–288.

53. Mithieux SM, Wise SG, Raftery MJ, Starcher B, Weiss AS. A model two-component system for studying the architecture of elastin assembly in vitro. *J Struct Biol.* 2005;149(3): 282–289.

54. Blanchevoye C, Floquet N, Scandolera A, et al. Interaction between the elastin peptide VGVAPG and human elastin binding protein. *J Biol Chem.* 2013;288(2):1317–1328.

55. Maquart FX, Bellon G, Pasco S, Monboisse JC. Matrikines in the regulation of extracellular matrix degradation. *Biochimie.* 2005;87(3-4):353–360.

56. Simon Davis DA, Parish CR. Heparan sulfate: a ubiquitous glycosaminoglycan with multiple roles in immunity. *Front Immunol.* 2013;4:470.

57. Ghersetich I, Lotti T, Campanile G, Grappone C, Dini G. Hyaluronic acid in cutaneous intrinsic aging. *Int J Dermatol.* 1994;33(2):119–122.

58. Bourguignon LY, Ramez M, Gilad E, et al. Hyaluronan-CD44 interaction stimulates keratinocyte differentiation, lamellar body formation/secretion, and permeability barrier homeostasis. *J Invest Dermatol.* 2006;126(6):1356–1365.

59. Aruffo A, Stamenkovic I, Melnick M, Underhill CB, Seed B. CD44 is the principal cell surface receptor for hyaluronate. *Cell.* 1990;61(7):1303–1313.

60. Culty M, Miyake K, Kincade PW, Sikorski E, Butcher EC, Underhill C. The hyaluronate receptor is a member of the CD44 (H-CAM) family of cell surface glycoproteins. *J Cell Biol.* 1990;111(6 Pt 1):2765–2774.

61. Underhill C. CD44: the hyaluronan receptor. *J Cell Sci.* 1992;103(Pt 2):293–298.

62. Strnadova K, Sandera V, Dvorankova B, et al. Skin aging: the dermal perspective. *Clin Dermatol.* 2019;37(4):326–335.

63. Lee DH, Oh JH, Chung JH. Glycosaminoglycan and proteoglycan in skin aging. *J Dermatol Sci.* 2016;83(3):174–181.

64. Oh JH, Kim YK, Jung JY, et al. Intrinsic aging- and photoaging-dependent level changes of glycosaminoglycans and their correlation with water content in human skin. *J Dermatol Sci.* 2011;62(3):192–201.

65. Scott JE. Proteodermatan and proteokeratan sulfate (decorin, lumican/fibromodulin) proteins are horseshoe shaped. Implications for their interactions with collagen. *Biochemistry.* 1996;35(27):8795–8799.

66. Danielson KG, Baribault H, Holmes DF, Graham H, Kadler KE, Iozzo RV. Targeted disruption of decorin leads to abnormal collagen fibril morphology and skin fragility. *J Cell Biol.* 1997;136(3):729–743.

67. Schmidt G, Robenek H, Harrach B, Glössl J, Nolte V, Hörmann H, et al. Interaction of small dermatan sulfate proteoglycan from fibroblasts with fibronectin. *J Cell Biol.* 1987;104(6):1683–1691.

68. Dugan TA, Yang VW, McQuillan DJ, Höök M. Decorin binds fibrinogen in a Zn2+-dependent interaction. *J Biol Chem.* 2003;278(16):13655–13662.

69. De Luca A, Santra M, Baldi A, Giordano A, Iozzo RV. Decorin-induced growth suppression is associated with up-regulation of p21, an inhibitor of cyclin-dependent kinases. *J Biol Chem.* 1996;271(31):18961–18965.

70. Carrino DA, Onnerfjord P, Sandy JD, et al. Age-related changes in the proteoglycans of human skin. Specific cleavage of decorin to yield a major catabolic fragment in adult skin. *J Biol Chem.* 2003;278(19):17566–17572.

71. Bernstein EF, Fisher LW, Li K, LeBaron RG, Tan EM, Uitto J. Differential expression of the versican and decorin genes in photoaged and sun-protected skin. Comparison by immunohistochemical and northern analyses. *Lab Invest.* 1995;72(6):662–669.

72. Quan T, He T, Kang S, Voorhees JJ, Fisher GJ. Solar ultraviolet irradiation reduces collagen in photoaged human skin by blocking transforming growth factor-beta type II receptor/Smad signaling. *Am J Pathol.* 2004;165(3):741–751.

73. Fan Y, Choi TH, Chung JH, Jeon YK, Kim S. Hyaluronic acid-cross-linked filler stimulates collagen type 1 and elastic fiber synthesis in skin through the TGF-β/Smad signaling pathway in a nude mouse model. *J Plast Reconstr Aesthet Surg.* 2019;72(8):1355–1362.

74. Andrade MJ, Van Lonkhuyzen DR, Upton Z, Satyamoorthy K. Unravelling the insulin-like growth factor I-mediated photoprotection of the skin. *Cytokine Growth Factor Rev.* 2020;52: 45–55.

75. Bennet D, Viswanath B, Kim S, An JH. An ultra-sensitive biophysical risk assessment of light effect on skin cells. *Oncotarget.* 2017;8(29):47861–47875.

76. Rascalou A, Lamartine J, Poydenot P, Demarne F, Bechetoille N. Mitochondrial damage and cytoskeleton reorganization in human dermal fibroblasts exposed to artificial visible light similar to screen-emitted light. *J Dermatol Sci.* 2018:S0923-1811(18) 30213–30215.

77. Opländer C, Hidding S, Werners FB, Born M, Pallua N, Suschek CV. Effects of blue light irradiation on human dermal fibroblasts. *J Photochem Photobiol B.* 2011;103(2):118–125.

78. Asher G, Gatfield D, Stratmann M, et al. SIRT1 regulates circadian clock gene expression through PER2 deacetylation. *Cell.* 2008;134(2):317–328.

79. Tigges J, Krutmann J, Fritsche E, et al. The hallmarks of fibroblast ageing. *Mech Ageing Dev.* 2014;138:26–44.

80. Considine RV, Sinha MK, Heiman ML, et al. Serum immunoreactive-leptin concentrations in normal-weight and obese humans. *N Engl J Med.* 1996;334(5):292–295.

81. Pelleymounter MA, Cullen MJ, Baker MB, et al. Effects of the obese gene product on body weight regulation in ob/ob mice. *Science.* 1995;269(5223):540–543.

CHAPTER 3

Fat and the Subcutaneous Layer

Mary D. Sun, MSCR, MS
Edmund M. Weisberg, MS, MBE
Leslie S. Baumann, MD

SUMMARY POINTS

What's Important?

1. Adipocytes, or fat cells, are a major component of the subcutaneous tissue in the human body. In addition to playing roles in thermogenesis and metabolism, these cells perform various nonmetabolic functions including antimicrobial defense, hair cycling, and wound healing.
2. Changes in the production, distribution, and degeneration of facial adipose tissue have significant aesthetic implications that can be targeted with cosmetic procedures.

What's New?

1. Collagenase clostridium histolyticum injections have been shown to improve cellulite and were approved by the FDA in 2020.
2. Emerging biomechanical studies have improved the clinical understanding of the sex- and age-related pathogenesis of cellulite and other adipose-related disease processes.
3. Newly uncovered mechanisms of adipocyte plasticity are promising avenues of research in the prevention of cutaneous disease and advancement of regenerative medicine.

What's Coming?

1. Further study is needed to characterize macro- and micro-characteristics of facial adipose tissue and their age-related changes across different anatomic compartments.
2. Large-scale, standardized, and prospective clinical studies are necessary to evaluate various harvesting, processing, and delivery methods for autologous fat transfer. The risks and benefits of supplementation strategies including platelet-rich plasma, progenitor cells, and functional growth factors should be similarly evaluated.

Subcutaneous tissue, or the hypodermis, is one of the largest tissues in the human body. The major components of this layer are adipocytes, fibrous tissue, and blood vessels. It is estimated that this layer represents 9% to 18% of body weight in normal-weight men and 14% to 20% in women of normal weight.[1] In severe obesity, fat mass can increase by up to four times and represent 60% to 70% of total body weight.[2] Though gaining fat in the body is undesirable for many, losing fat in the face has cosmetic implications as well. Adipose tissue gains and losses and volume changes contribute to the aged appearance of the face and body. This chapter will review the importance of the subcutaneous tissue and its various functions.

The subcutaneous tissue is usually not given as much attention as the dermis and epidermis because pathology at superficial layers is easier to detect or diagnose by a shave or small punch biopsy. Subcutaneous tissue usually must have an extensive defect before it is noticed, and an incision or large punch biopsy (e.g., 6 mm) is required to biopsy this area. During histologic tissue processing of biopsy tissue, the triglyceride component, which is the major component of adipocytes, is removed by alcohol and xylol. For this reason, subcutaneous tissue has long been ignored. However, with advances in diagnostic methods and new treatments, much more has been learned about the subcutaneous layer

- The largest repository of energy in the body.
- Stores fat-soluble vitamins (A, D, E, K), including their derivatives such as retinoic acids.
- Helps to shape the surface of the body, and form fat pads that act as shock absorbers.
- Helps distribute force or stress to mitigate damage to underlying organs.
- Protects against physical injury from excessive heat, cold, or mechanical factors.
- Fills up spaces between other tissues and helps to keep organs in place.
- Involved in thermoregulation by insulating the body from heat loss.
- Functions as a secretory organ that releases many cytokines.
- Plays a role in regulating androgen and estrogen levels.[3]

(Box 3-1). It is important for dermatologists and cosmetically oriented physicians to pay close attention to this tissue because it plays multiple roles in cosmetic dermatology and general appearance.

ADIPOCYTES

Adipocytes in adults were previously considered stable, nondividing cells, like other mature cells. However, recent data reveal that adipocytes in adults have the potential to increase in number or revert to stem cells. These stem cells can differentiate to other tissue, such as fibroblasts, collagen, elastic fibers, and hematopoietic stromal cells.[3] Fat cells are derived from undifferentiated fibroblast-like mesenchymal cells that have the capacity for multipotential differentiation.[4] Under certain conditions, these mesenchymal cells give rise to adipose cells. Adipose tissue is classified into two morphologic types: white and brown adipose tissue. White adipose tissue (WAT) normally appears yellow because of the accumulation of β-carotene, while brown adipose tissue (BAT) was named based on its appearance derived from its rich vascular supply.[5] Mature white adipocytes are called round unilocular fat cells. They have a copious supply of cytoplasm, which contains a single, large lipid droplet that pushes the nucleus to the border of the cell. Brown adipocytes, called polygonal multilocular fat cells, have multiple small lipid droplets.

WAT stores excess energy as fat, while BAT is responsible for energy expenditure via the thermoregulatory function of uncoupling protein 1 (UCP1). An imbalance between the two can lead to obesity and a study has shown that dietary supplementation can potentially reduce obesity by inducing BAT browning.[5] In humans, WAT is thought to be a loosened dermal compartment of functionally linked adipocytes.[6] Recent evidence suggests that there is a differentiation between the superficial and deeper parts of subcutaneous adipose tissue.[7,8] In the dermis, adipocytes are conically arranged around pilosebaceous units, with the wider aspect of the cone extending inferiorly into subcutaneous WAT.[9]

WAT is newly recognized as involved in various nonmetabolic functions as well, including antimicrobial defense, roles in hair cycling, and wound healing.[10] Adipose tissue contains nearly every immune cell type and can produce adipokines and antimicrobial peptides. It has significant innate immune antimicrobial function.[10-12] WAT surrounding hair follicles expands during anagen and regresses during telogen.[13] Specifically, anagen can trigger WAT hyperplasia and hypertrophy via Wnt signaling pathways. Adipocytes regenerate from myofibroblasts during wound healing. Myofibroblasts were previously thought to be differentiated and nonadipogenic.[14]

When observed with an electron microscope, brown adipocytes demonstrably contain much more mitochondria and smooth endoplasmic reticulum than white adipocytes. In humans, brown adipocytes play a major role in nonshivering thermogenesis. Studies in humans have demonstrated that adipose-enabled thermogenesis processes are influenced by internal temperature (suggesting a role in both heat and cold acclimation) as well as oxidative metabolism (suggesting a role in crosstalk with skeletal muscle).[15,16] In animal models, adipose-related thermogenesis can also be induced by exogenous chemical exposures such as methotrexate.[17] BAT can be found during the fetal and early neonatal phases, while the majority of adipocytes in adults are white adipocytes.

In the past, it was believed that the number of adipocytes, which develop during the 30th week of gestation, does not increase after birth. However, newer evidence has shown that adipocytes can increase in number and size in certain situations or environments. For instance, obesity and metabolic activity lead to compositional and morphological changes in adipose tissue.[18] In general, adipocytes are thought to have two periods of growth. The first period occurs from the embryonic stage to 18 months after birth, and the second period occurs during puberty. Changes in adipose tissue mass are determined by both size and number of adipocytes.[19] An increase in size (hypertrophy)[20] usually precedes an increase in the number of cells (hyperplasia).[21] Mitochondrial dysfunction affects the redistribution and lower activation of BAT during the aging process.[22] Adipose tissue (specifically WAT) has been implicated in the pathogenesis of various skin conditions including systemic sclerosis.[23]

ANATOMY

Subcutaneous tissue, also known as the superficial fascia, is divided into three layers: apical, mantle, and the deeper layer. The apical layer is located beneath the reticular dermis surrounding sweat glands and hair follicles. It contains blood vessels, lymphatic vessels, and nerves. It is also rich in carotenoids and tends to be yellow in gross appearance. Damage to this layer can lead to hematoma, seroma, paresthesia, and full-thickness skin necrosis. The mantle layer is composed of columnar-shaped adipocytes and is absent from the eyelids, nail beds, bridge of the nose, and penis. It contributes to the ability to resist trauma by distributing pressure across a large field. The deeper layer is located under the mantle layer and its shape depends on gender, genetics, anatomic area, and diet. Adipocytes in this layer are arranged in lobules between septae as well as between fibrous planes. This layer is suitable for liposuction. Vertical extrusion and/or expansion of this layer can cause cellulite (**Fig. 3-1**).

Subcutaneous tissue is found throughout the body except for the eyelids, proximal nail fold, penis, scrotum, and the entire auricle of the external ear except the lobule. In particular, subcutaneous tissue is prominent at the temples, cheeks, chin, nose, abdomen, buttocks, and thighs, as well as infraorbital areas. It is very thick at the palms and soles. Age, gender, and lifestyle choices determine the distribution and density of adipose deposits. For example, in newborns adipose tissue has a uniform thickness throughout the body, while in adults the tissue tends to disappear from some areas of the body and increase in other areas under the influence of hormones. Subcutaneous WAT is subdivided by fibrous septae into discrete areas and is classified into two types. Type 1 is present in the medial and lateral midface, parts of the periorbital region, as well as the temple, forehead, and neck.[24] The formation of nasolabial, medial, middle, lateral, and buccal subcutaneous fat compartments results from the arrangement of type 1 WAT in the midface. Type 2 occurs in the perioral and nasal regions

and around the eyebrows.[24] WAT has been further described at the microstructural level (categorized as deposit or metabolic WAT, structural WAT, and fibrous WAT, further divided into lobular and nonlobular subtypes), a thorough discussion of which is beyond the focus of this chapter.[24] All these fat types differ in adipocyte size and the collagenous composition of their extracellular matrix, which translates to mechanical properties. Most minimally invasive interventions (e.g., soft tissue fillers or fat grafting) that attempt to restore the youthful face should account for different properties in various facial fat areas.

The plasticity of WAT cells has been an important focus of research over the past two decades. Reversible adipocyte dedifferentiation into adipocyte progenitor cells (pre-adipocytes) has been demonstrated in dermal adipose tissue; adipocyte plasticity could be a major avenue of future research in regenerative cutaneous medicine.[25] Adipose tissue is distributed differently in men and women. Men tend to accumulate fat in an android or upper abdominal body distribution (apple shape). In contrast, women tend to accumulate fat in a gynoid or lower body distribution that predominantly involves the lower

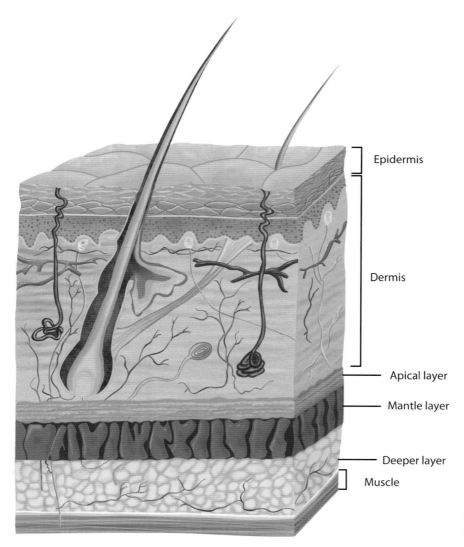

FIGURE 3-1. The three layers of the subcutaneous tissue.

abdomen, hips, and thighs (pear shape) (**Fig. 3-2**). Notably, the visceral adiposity index (VAI) is a reliable sex-specified indicator of visceral adipose distribution and function.[26] A sex-dependent VAI has been identified in pathways pertaining to primary bile acid biosynthesis, branched-chain amino acids, as well as the biosynthesis of pantothenate and coenzyme A (CoA).[27]

In the elderly, hyper- or hypoaccumulation of fat occurs in various areas. For example, infraorbital eye bags, buccal fat pad accumulation (chipmunk feature), wattle of the anterior neck, loose skin and fat accumulation in the posterior arm, increase in breast size of males, and an increase in abdomen, buttock, and thigh fat are common. Subcutaneous fat can also be lost in the malar fat pad during the aging process. This can lead to prominent flattening of the cheek/buccal area, sagging of the skin of the face, and prominent deep wrinkles, such as nasolabial folds and marionette lines or jowls. Structural cells such as keratinocytes, fibroblasts, and adipocytes contribute to barrier immunity. Age-related changes in adipose distribution result in an increased incidence of cancer and skin infections due to skin structure alterations (e.g., thinning of the epidermis and dermis, increased water loss, and fragmentation of collagen and elastin). These changes also modify skin immune composition (e.g., reduced Langerhans cells, decreased antigen-specific immunity, and increased regulatory populations such as Foxp3+ regulatory T cells), which diminishes skin barrier immunity in the elderly.[6,28] Adipocytes residing in adjacent tissue are active participants in pro-inflammatory signaling after injury. In conjunction with fibroblast cells, adipocyte-altered cellular communication can contribute to irregular inflammation associated with delayed or irregular wound healing with implications for cutaneous disease.[29]

Role of Lipids in the Human Body

Lipids can be found in different areas of the skin, not only in subcutaneous tissue. They are constituents of phospholipids in the myelin sheaths of nerve tissue and cell membranes (lipid bilayers), play an important role in the skin barrier of the epidermis, and are essential for steroid production. Lipids are water-insoluble organic molecules because they are nonpolar. However, after esterification (a condensation reaction between acid and alcohol), they are more water-soluble than their parent forms.

The most common lipids in the diet are triglycerides (triacylglycerol), which are composed of a glycerol subunit attached to three fatty acids (**Fig. 3-3**). Lipids can be saturated or unsaturated. Generally, an unsaturated fatty acid contains at least one double bond while saturated fatty acids do not. Unsaturated fatty acids provide slightly less energy during metabolism than saturated fatty acids with the same number of carbon atoms. In addition, saturated fatty acids are usually solids at room temperature and unsaturated fats are usually liquids at room temperature.

Lipid Metabolism

During digestion, fats in the food are broken down in the duodenum by pancreatic lipase into free fatty acids and glycerol. The intestinal epithelium absorbs these substances and re-esterifies them in the smooth endoplasmic reticulum into triglycerides. These triglycerides are then absorbed into the circulation and lymphatic system. When they arrive in the circulation, they are combined with apoprotein to form a lipoprotein, which is called a chylomicron. Chylomicrons are exposed to lipoprotein lipase, which is synthesized by adipocytes and stored at the surface of endothelial cells. Lipoprotein lipase cleaves the chylomicron into free fatty acids and glycerol

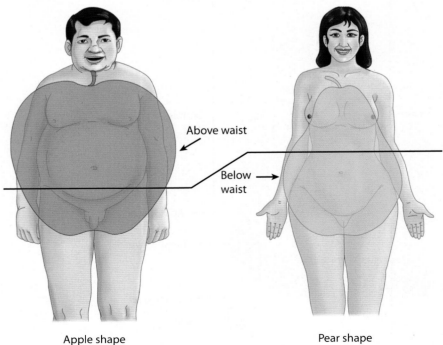

Apple shape

Pear shape

FIGURE 3-2. Android (apple) and gynoid (pear) fat distribution patterns in men and women.

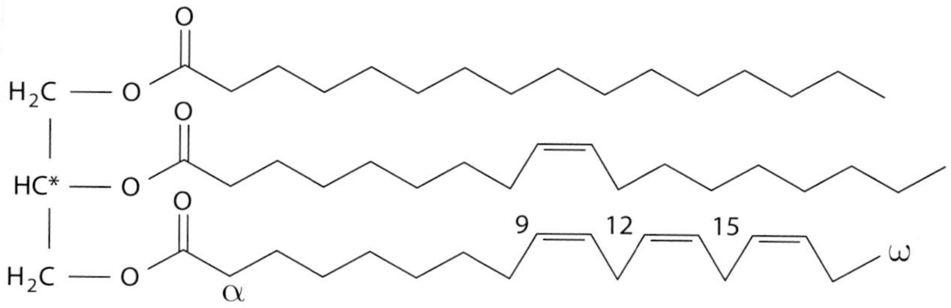

FIGURE 3-3. Triglyceride chemical structure.

again. These free fatty acids pass into adipocytes and combine with intracellular glycerol phosphate to form triglycerides and are stored for energy.

Adipose tissue can also convert excessive glucose and amino acids into fatty acids when stimulated by insulin. This explains why people who consume a low-fat diet or fat-free diet still gain weight if they do not reduce the total amount of calories they consume or have a high-carbohydrate diet. High blood glucose can stimulate insulin synthesis and insulin can increase synthesis of lipoprotein lipase from adipocytes to help absorb triglycerides into the cells. People who want to control their weight should avoid any foods that can stimulate insulin production. Individuals with Type II diabetes have high levels of insulin; therefore, they have a higher risk of becoming overweight or obese than nondiabetic individuals.

Abnormal lipid metabolism (which includes cellular synthesis, uptake, modification, degradation, and transport) is a hallmark of malignant tumors and supplies necessary substrates for rapid cell growth. It is also associated with lipid peroxidation, which plays an important role in a newly discovered type of regulated cell death termed *ferroptosis*. DNA correlates of this process have been associated with the occurrence and progression of cancer. Indeed, these correlates seem to be key regulators of abnormal lipid metabolism and ferroptosis in cancer.[30]

Lipoproteins

There are many different types of lipoproteins. Low-density lipoprotein (LDL) brings fat to the cells, while high-density lipoprotein (HDL) brings fat from the circulation to the liver for excretion in bile. High levels of LDL are associated with a high incidence of coronary artery disease and atherosclerosis. HDL, or the "good lipoprotein," can be elevated with exercise. Lipoproteins are associated with important cardiovascular and liver disease risk factors such as hypertriglyceridemia and androgen-dependent tissue factor pathways.[31–33]

Lipid Synthesis

Triglycerides are derived from foods or synthesized from excessive glucose or amino acids. In humans, triglycerides are stored mainly in adipose tissue, which constitutes the body's reserve energy source. However, excessive consumption of calories can lead to the synthesis and accumulation of more fat in subcutaneous tissues. Unfortunately, fat storage is unlimited in the subcutaneous tissue, unlike glycogen storage in the liver

and muscle. Therefore, excessive fat accumulation will not only change a person's cosmetic appearance but also increase their risk for osteoarthritis, diabetes, hypertension, as well as other diseases.

VOLUME EXCESS

Obesity

Obesity is defined as unhealthy, excessive fat mass. There are many regimens, products, and exercise programs available to fight obesity; however, there is still a rising epidemic in the United States[34] when compared to the past.[35] Obesity and hyperlipidemia are major risk factors and can lead to significant morbidity and mortality.

Pathophysiology

Obesity results from both environmental and genetic factors. Two genes that are known to exert direct effects on obesity are the leptin (*ob gene*)[36,37] and pro-opiomelanocortin (POMC) genes.[38] These genes can control eating behavior and satiety. Defects in these genes can cause severe obesity. However, almost all people gain weight when they get older because of diminished physical activity and aging-induced changes in the chemical activity of hormones. Obesity is also known to be a salient secondary cause of hypertriglyceridemia, which predisposes individuals to cardiovascular disease (CVD).[39] Further, several clinical trials have revealed an association between psoriasis and an array of cardiometabolic comorbidities, including CVDs, obesity, diabetes mellitus, and metabolic syndrome.[40]

Body mass index [BMI: body weight divided by the square of height (kg/m^2)] is a popular index used for determining body weight status. The Centers for Disease Control and Prevention (CDC) and World Health Organization (WHO) use this index to classify adults into four groups (**Table 3-1**).

TABLE 3-1	Body Mass Index (BMI) Categories
BMI	**Weight Status**
Less than 18.5	Underweight
18.5–24.9	Normal
25.0–29.9	Overweight
30.0 and greater	Obese

A normal BMI does not necessarily mean that a person has a "perfect" shape. Many people with a BMI less than 25 have fat accumulation in some areas, such as the abdomen or buttocks. Though BMI has been criticized in recent years, evidence suggests that in most populations it remains a reliable estimator of body fat percentage.[41] Other clinically validated tools to consider include the body roundness index (BRI) and a body shape index (ABSI).[42]

Impact of Obesity on the Skin

Obesity is responsible for changes in skin barrier function by significantly increasing transepidermal water loss, which can lead to dry skin and impaired barrier function.[43] Hyperfunction of sebaceous glands due to high levels of androgen-like hormone or insulin-like growth factor hormone can aggravate the severity of acne and hirsutism;[44,45] delay wound healing and collagen deposits in the wound healing process;[46] and disturb both blood and lymphatic circulation, which can cause angiopathy[47] and lymphedema, potentially precipitating chronic leg ulcers.[48] Rapid weight gain can cause striae distensae (stretch marks), which are challenging to treat.[49-52] In addition, in intertriginous areas such as the underarms, breasts, and groin, moisture accumulation can lead to candida infection (intertrigo).

It is widely known that obesity increases the risk of coronary heart disease, hypertension, hyperlipidemia, osteoarthritis, and diabetes. It is also known to be directly related to increased risk of sleep apnea; breast, endometrial, and colon cancers; gallbladder disease; musculoskeletal disorders; severe pancreatitis and diverticulitis; infertility; urinary incontinence; and idiopathic intracranial hypertension. Additionally, obesity has indirectly been linked to anxiety, impaired social interaction, and depression.

Obesity is implicated in a wide spectrum of dermatologic diseases, including acanthosis nigricans, acrochordons, keratosis pilaris, hyperandrogenism and hirsutism, striae distensae, adiposis dolorosa, fat redistribution, lymphedema, chronic venous insufficiency, plantar hyperkeratosis, cellulitis, skin infections, hidradenitis suppurativa, psoriasis, insulin resistance syndrome, and tophaceous gout.[40,53]

To determine the severity of a person's obesity, BMI can be used. In fact, the more overweight a person is the higher the mortality rate (**Table 3-2**).

Treatment

Though this is much more easily said than done, as any dieting person will avow, dietary control is very important in the treatment of obesity. In 2011, a randomized, controlled trial [the Diet, Obesity, and Genes (DiOGenes) Study] tested five different diets as a controlled dietary intervention in 932 overweight European adults who first reduced their weight on an 8-week low-calorie diet before being randomized into a 26-week diet (high or low protein or high or low glycemic index in four combinations, or control). The study's results indicated that low-glycemic-index carbohydrates and a low-protein diet, to a lesser degree, may diminish low-grade inflammation and related comorbidities in the overweight/obese adult population.[54]

Patients must understand the principle of energy intake and expenditure. Weight reduction is usually not accomplished without exercise. However, exercise alone will usually produce little long-term benefit. The combination of exercise with dietary therapy can prevent weight being regained. In addition, regular exercise (30 min daily) will improve general health. Indeed, exclusive walking has been shown to help normalize total cholesterol and LDLs in women with overweight and obesity.[55] The best results are obtained with education in well-motivated patients. Constant supervision by healthcare professionals and by family or friends can help to encourage compliance.

Prevention

Prevention of obesity is key because once fat is gained and maintained over time, it is more difficult to lose. A high-fat diet can induce an increase in the number of adipocytes.[56,57] A low-fat and complex carbohydrate diet is recommended to reduce body weight. There is an important difference between preventing weight gain and producing weight loss. To prevent weight gain, portion size and composition of food are controlled. For weight loss, restriction of calorie intake is the most effective treatment.

Liposuction

Overweight patients frequently consult plastic surgeons and dermatologists for liposuction.[58-60] Liposuction is one of the most commonly performed cosmetic surgery procedures in the United States.[61] Physicians must inform their patients that liposuction is a modality for improving body contour and not for treatment of generalized obesity. In addition, excess fatty tissue will return if regular exercise and diet control are not maintained.

Large-volume liposuction may decrease weight and fat mass; however, there has been controversy or disagreement regarding whether it significantly improves insulin resistance and other obesity-associated metabolic abnormalities.[62-64] Recent findings suggest a significant positive correlation between gastric bypass and CVD risk factor reduction in patients who are diabetic or > 50 years old, with no significant differences in non-diabetic and younger patients (in addition to significant side effects). However, a few studies show that a less invasive removal of abdominal subcutaneous adipose tissue via lipectomy consistently and significantly improved CVD risk factors.[65] Current data appear to indicate that large-volume liposuction can improve cardiovascular risk factors, metabolic balance, and insulin resistance.[66] The most common areas treated are the neck, jowls, arms, abdomen, thighs, knees, and ankles. Other conditions that can be

TABLE 3-2	Classification of Overweight and Obesity by BMI
BMI	**Weight Status**
25.0–29.9	Overweight
≥30.0	Obese
30.0–35.0	Moderate obesity (Class I)
35.0–40.0	Severe obesity (Class II)
≥40.0	Morbid obesity (Class III)

improved by liposuction include lipoma, gynecomastia, buffalo hump, and axillary hyperhidrosis.

There are strict guidelines from both the American Society of Dermatologic Surgery (ASDS) and the American Academy of Cosmetic Surgery (AACS) on the volume restrictions during liposuction. Tumescent liposuction is considered the safest method for performing the procedure. This technique relies on the infiltration of dilute anesthesia based on body weight, and the removal of limited amounts of adipose tissue during each operation. Tumescent anesthesia consists of very dilute lidocaine and epinephrine solutions ranging from 0.05% to 0.1% of lidocaine with 1:1,000,000 epinephrine and sodium bicarbonate. The total safe concentration of lidocaine that can be used in this formula is 35 to 55 mg/kg based on patient weight and any coexisting medical conditions. **Table 3-3** is a synopsis of the 2006 ASDS guidelines of care for tumescent liposuction.[59]

TABLE 3-3	Synopsis of 2006 ASDS Guidelines of Care for Tumescent Liposuction
Indications	
Aesthetic body contouring: most common regions include thighs, abdomen, hips, arms, back, buttocks, neck, breasts, and calves	
Other indications: treatment of lipomas, gynecomastia, lipodystrophy, axillary hyperhidrosis, axillary bromidrosis, and subcutaneous fat debulking during reconstructive procedures	
Pre-operative evaluation	
History: diet patterns, exercise, unwanted regions, underlying disorders such as poor wound healing, bleeding abnormalities, diabetes mellitus, keloid formation, problems with past surgical procedures, personal or family history of thrombophlebitis, pulmonary emboli, and drugs that may interfere with blood coagulation or the metabolism of lidocaine	
Explanation: procedure, risk and benefits, expected outcomes, needing a touch-up procedure	
Physical examination: assessment of both general physical health and specific sites amenable to liposuction	
Laboratory studies: may or may not be necessary for a given patient depending on the type and extent of anticipated liposuction procedure	
Some surgeons may wish to obtain CBC, PT, PTT, LFT, UA, pregnancy test, screening for HIV, hepatitis B, and hepatitis C	
Technique	
Tumescent anesthesia: consists of very dilute lidocaine and epinephrine solutions ranging from 0.05%–0.1% of lidocaine with epinephrine (around 1:1,000,000), sodium bicarbonate and +/− triamcinolone	
Volume removal	
Removal of more than 4 L of supranatant fat should be divided into more than one operative session	
Monitoring: pulse oximetry, cardiac monitoring, and intermittent monitoring of BP, HR, and RR	
Post-operative care	
Use compression garments for 1 to 4 wk	

Liposuction Complications

While there have been reports of mortality with general anesthesia, there have been no reports of death with tumescent anesthesia alone. When practitioners adhere to the AACS and ASDS guidelines, tumescent liposuction is a safe outpatient procedure. Common complications are bruising, swelling, localized paresthesia, and irritated incision sites after liposuction. Other complications include hematomas, seromas, and infection. There are serious complications that the surgeon must be aware of, however, such as the development of a fat embolus, visceral perforation (particularly of the abdomen), pneumothorax, deep vein thrombosis, congestive heart failure, lidocaine toxicity, and toxic shock syndrome.[67,68] Fortunately, these complications are very rare during tumescent liposuction. The relative skills and experience level of the operating physician represent important contributing factors to the incidence of adverse events from liposuction.

Careful patient selection is the key to a successful outcome. Younger patients, those with good skin tone, and those close to their ideal weight tend to be the best candidates. Poor patient selection may lead to the development of rippling or poor skin contraction.

VOLUME LOSS

Normal Aging

The aging face shows characteristic changes, many of which were once solely attributed to the effects of gravity on skin, muscle, and fat. It is for this reason that the main approach to the aging face was to lift and reposition "ptotic" tissue. However, we now recognize that there are complex changes occurring in which volume loss is a significant contributor. These changes include muscle atrophy, bone resorption, and fat atrophy. There are some well-designed studies that have considered the bony changes of the face and the changes in the malar fat pad with time. Results have demonstrated that the lower midfacial skeleton becomes retrusive with age relative to the upper face.[69] The study's authors speculate that the skeletal remodeling of the anterior maxillary wall allows soft tissues to be repositioned downward, thereby accentuating the nasojugal fold and malar mound. Obagi has described the increasing incidence of a "negative vector face" as one ages.[70] A "negative-vector" patient is one in whom most malar fat pads lie posterior to a line drawn straight down from the cornea to the orbital rim. With this change, the lower eyelid fat pads appear more prominent but are not truly hypertrophied.

In a magnetic resonance imaging (MRI) study by Gosain et al., the deepening appearance of the nasolabial fold with age seems to be a combination of ptosis and fat/skin hypertrophy.[71] They found a difference with age in the redistribution of fat within the malar fat pad, with older women exhibiting a relatively increased thickness of the midportion of the malar fat pad and overlying skin compared to younger females. More interestingly, they did not find an increase in the length or projection of the levator labii superioris muscle between young and old subjects.

Normal aging might also be influenced by ethnic and racial differences in the distribution of adipocity. For instance, visceral adipose tissue (VAT) and abdominal subcutaneous adipose tissue (SAT) have varying associations with cardiometabolic risk factors based, in part, on ethnic differences in populations of Inuit, Africans, and Europeans.[72] Specifically, adiposity-related population differences appear to affect risk for important health conditions such as diabetes mellitus.[73] Since 2011, obesity and adiposity measures have generally increased among US adults.[74]

In 2007, a cadaveric study considered the fat distribution of the face.[75] The authors found distinct facial fat compartments and subdivisions within these areas. The malar fat pad was composed of three separate compartments: medial, middle, and lateral temporal–cheek fat. The nasolabial fold was uniformly a discrete unit with distinct anatomic boundaries and little variation in size from one cadaver to the next. The forehead also consisted of three anatomic units: central, middle, and lateral temporal–cheek fat. Orbital fat was noted in three compartments determined by septal borders. However, the superior orbital fat did not connect to the inferior orbital fat. The jowl fat was the most inferior of the subcutaneous fat compartments and was found to be closely associated with the depressor anguli oris muscle.

One of the easiest ways for a cosmetic surgeon to begin to understand such changes in patients is by evaluating photographs of the patient both in youth and at the time of presentation for a consultation. This can be seen in the works of surgeons that have performed a great deal of volume restoration surgeries over several years.[76,77]

Autologous Fat Transplantation

Fat transplantation is the re-injection of aspirated adipocytes into an area that has lost volume due to aging, trauma, or an inflammatory process. Autologous fat transplantation (AFT) offers certain advantages over other fillers, most notably that it is an autograft with the same human leukocyte antigen; therefore, there is no allergic reaction or rejection via immune processes. In clinical settings, there are important restrictions on fat transfer procedures based on retention and reproducibility. The FDA regulates the use of human cells, tissues, and cellular or tissue-based products in humans. Title 21 of the Code of Federal Regulations Part 1271 details criteria governing the regulation of adipose therapeutics. Cell-assisted lipotransfer is categorized by the FDA as "more than minimal manipulation" due to enzymatic degradation of the tissue and isolation of cell-rich adipose fluid.[78]

Indications for AFT are volume loss anywhere in the face such as the nasolabial folds, lips, under eye hollow and tear trough deformity, submalar depressions, zygoma enhancement, chin augmentation, and malar augmentation; congenital, traumatic, and surgical defects; as well as acne scarring, idiopathic lipodystrophy, facial hemiatrophy, rejuvenation of hands, body contour defects, depressions caused by liposuction or trauma, etc.[70,79,80] A 2018 systematic review indicated that autologous fat grafting to the face was most commonly performed for cosmetic purposes (75.39%), followed by facial reconstruction in patients with lipodystrophy (8.33%), post-operative soft tissue defects (4.71%), hemifacial atrophy

(4.61%), facial trauma (1.61%), burns (1.47%), and scarring (1.13%).[81] In a 2021 study of 30 patients (aged 18 to 40), autologous injections of nanofat were histopathologically found to be effective in the treatment of scars, with increases noted in epidermal thickness, number and density of collagen and elastic fibers, and neovascularization.[82]

AFT can be divided into two processes: harvesting fat from the donor site and re-injecting it into the recipient sites. The medical literature is replete with different techniques by which fat is harvested, prepared, and infiltrated into the tissue. The variation in these techniques probably accounts for why some surgeons find success with this modality and others do not achieve long-lasting results.[83] Factors that influence survival of fat after injection include the anatomic sites of harvesting and placement, the degree of mobility in the recipient area, the vascularity of the recipient tissue, and the overall health and age of the patient.[84]

Fat aspirated from the lateral thigh has been found to last longer than fat taken from the abdomen. Even during harvesting, one will find a noticeable difference in the quality of the fat between the two areas. The fat of the upper arms, inner thighs, and abdomen tends to be softer with less connective tissue. Fat from the lateral thigh tends to be denser and more fibrous. Furthermore, placement of the fat into the tissues is critical to ensure viability. Adipocytes require a healthy and vascular bed in which to engraft. For this reason, fat must be placed in small parcels and in multiple layers, including in and under muscles. The less movement in the recipient site, the more that fat survives. Therefore, the malar and infraorbital areas do well while the nasolabial folds and lips require touch-ups to achieve the desired effect. Maximum graft regenerative zones of about 1.5 mm are acceptable before a central zone of necrosis forms.[78] The use of platelet-rich fibrin combined with autologous high-density fat transplantation significantly increases fat-retention rates and demonstrates stable long-term effects without obvious adverse reactions in clinical augmentation rhinoplasty.[85]

Complications

Reports of complications from AFT and autologous fat grafting range from 2.27% to 6%.[86] Most complications of facial autologous fat grafting occur in patients with injections in the middle third of the face. Common complications include skin irregularities, telangiectasias, erythema, and activation of skin acne.[81] Some rarer complications are swelling, ecchymosis, hematoma, infection, and subconjunctival fat infiltration.[87] Known cases of blindness and cerebral strokes resulting after fat transplantation at the glabella[88-90] and paranasal areas[91] have been noted. In these cases, a sharp needle or large syringe was used to inject the fat. By using only blunt cannulas and 1 mL syringes, this complication has not been reported in the literature.

Fat Cells as a Source for Stem Cells and Collagen Stimulation

There is evidence that supports the utility of adipocytes for a potential stem cell role as well as collagen stimulation. First, it is known that the human body can increase the number and size of fat cells even after puberty. Second, subcutaneous tissue contains not only adipocytes but also fibrous tissue and blood vessels. These tissues are active cells and can proliferate when there is an increase in the size of subcutaneous tissue.[92] In addition, there is evidence demonstrating that aspirated fluid from liposuction contains cells that can differentiate into bone, cartilage, muscle, neurons, and adipocytes.[93–96]

In contrast to harvesting stem cells from the bone marrow, harvesting adipocytes from the subcutaneous tissue is much easier and complications at the donor site can easily be visualized. In addition, adipocytes can be harvested multiple times and from many areas. Using adipose tissue grafts as a biological scaffold is advantageous for clinical translation as these grafts are readily available, easy to harvest, and present low morbidity risk.[78] Cellular components of an adipose graft can contribute to reducing inflammation as well as to both graft retention and the nonvolumetric benefits of autologous fat grafts.[78] A decellularized adipose matrix may also stimulate regeneration *in situ* without the need for an additional donor site.[78]

Although the skin of patients continues to improve and show a reduction in rhytides and aging symptoms over time after autologous fat augmentation, an improvement not seen in patients receiving synthetic fillers, the use of mesenchymal stem cells along with fat injection has been found to increase the survival rate of transferred fat.[97]

MISCELLANEOUS ADIPOSE CONDITIONS

Cellulite

Cellulite, also referred to as edematous fibrosclerotic panniculopathy (as well as gynoid lipodystrophy or orange peel syndrome), is a common cosmetic condition that affects most post-adolescent women. It is characterized by skin dimpling and nodularity that results in an inhomogeneous, irregular appearance that can be measured in stages using the photonumeric Hexsel Cellulite Severity Scale (Box 3-2).[98] Cellulite is most frequently observed in the gluteal and posterior thigh areas, though many areas of the body can be affected including the abdomen. While this condition is generally asymptomatic, severe cellulite has been associated with local temperature increases and painful nodules suggestive of inflammation in the dermis and adipose tissue.[4] Risk factors include lack of

---

BOX 3-2   Hexsel Classification of Cellulite[a]

- At Stage 0, the skin's surface is not altered.
- At Stage I, skin is smooth when the individual is standing or lying down, but some cellulite appears if the skin is pinched.
- At Stage II, skin appears dimpled without any pinching or manipulation.
- At Stage III, skin appears both dimpled and raised in some areas.

[a]Personal communication with Doris Hexsel, Porto Allegre, Brazil.

---

exercise; being female, overweight/obese, elderly; age; weight fluctuations; and having excess hormones and poor lymphatic drainage.[99–101] These skin changes can be significantly distressing and embarrassing for patients. Cellulite largely results from changes in the dermis rather than changes in the subcutaneous tissue.

A 2021 ultrasound investigation of the subcutaneous anatomy of cellulite found that the preponderance of fibrous bands characterizing cellulite demonstrated an oblique (versus perpendicular) orientation to the skin (84.4%), with the majority (90.2%) originating from the superficial fascia (versus the deep fascia). A small percentage of bands had an associated vascular structure. Overweight and obese patients, even after stratification by BMI, had a significantly higher likelihood of having an associated blood vessel visualized (P = 0.01).[102] Although cellulite is frequently found in healthy, non-obese patients, it is aggravated by obesity.[103–105]

Pathogenesis

The pathophysiology of cellulite is not completely understood, but many theories have been postulated. One of the most important factors is the anatomy of this condition. There are morphologic differences in the fat lobes between males and females, which may explain the large frequency of cellulite in females and rare occurrence in males.

A 2019 biomechanical study of 10 cellulite donors found that increased age was significantly related to decreased dermal thickness, independent of sex. The mean number of subdermal fat lobules was significantly higher in males than females, suggesting that there are more septal connections between the superficial fascia and dermis in men. Female sex and increased BMI were associated with increased height of superficial fat lobules. The force needed to cause septal breakage in males was significantly greater than in females. Therefore, cellulite can be understood as an imbalance between containment and extrusion forces at the subdermal junction. Aged women with high BMI have the greatest risk of developing cellulite.[99]

Cellulite is thought to be formed from the breakdown of collagen in the reticular dermis, which leads to weakness in the dermis and herniation of subcutaneous fat into the dermis, as well as compression of the microcirculation of the dermis. Congestion of fluid and protein in the dermis is believed to lead to formation of fibrotic bands between the subcutaneous tissue and dermis resulting in retraction, dimpling, or nodularity. The etiology of cellulite is considered multifactorial as it is influenced by genetic, hormonal, and environmental factors, with endothelial dysfunction and microcirculation disorders now believed to be significantly involved.[106] A 2021 histological study of 60 patients with cellulite found several different histological aspects present in the same patient; effectively, cellulite may be considered a degenerative disease.[107]

Treatment

This condition is considered normal in post-adolescent women and is innocuous. Many people think that it is cosmetically unappealing both visually and tactilely. Cellulite may not improve by weight reduction; however, weight control may improve the appearance of cellulite in some patients.

Several modalities have been proposed to treat this condition by stimulation of collagen production in the dermis, such as infrared, diode laser, and radiofrequency.[108] These methods are relatively new and their efficacy remains unknown at this point. The most effective method to treat cellulite is to improve blood and lymphatic circulation and drainage of waste products with massage; however, the effects are temporary. Efforts to increase exercise can stimulate lymph flow and decrease fluid accumulation. A decrease in fat mass can also occur by lipolysis, such as with exercise and diet, liposuction, ultrasound-assisted lipolysis, and mesotherapy. In severe dimpling lesions, minimally invasive procedures such as subcision can lead to improvement.[109]

Injections of collagenase received FDA approval in July 2020 for the treatment of cellulite. Collagenase clostridium histolyticum-aaes (CCH; QWO, Endo Aesthetics LLC, Malvern, PA) for injection is composed of two purified bacterial collagenases (AUX-I and AUX-II [Clostridial class I and II collagenases]) that hydrolyze collagen Types I and III. This injectable product reduces the collagen fibers in the fibrous septae that are believed to cause the dimpling seen in cellulite.[110] Reducing cellulite requires three treatments spaced 21 days apart.[111] Side effects include bruising, swelling, hyperpigmentation, and discomfort. There is a risk of anaphylaxis so the practitioner should be prepared for this. We recommend having two Epipens® and injectable Solumedrol available although the risk is very low.

Numerous topical products claim to treat cellulite. The most effective of these contain caffeine and theophylline, which dehydrate the fat cells, temporarily shrinking them. Despite the volume of cellulite treatments on the market, none have been shown to be convincingly effective for more than 24 hours. Clinical studies suggest that targeting collagen-rich fibrous septae in cellulite dimples through mechanical, surgical, or enzymatic approaches is most likely to provide sustained improvement of skin topography and the appearance of cellulite.[112]

Lipodystrophy

Lipodystrophy refers to the abnormal increase of subcutaneous fat (lipohypertrophy) or the abnormal decrease of subcutaneous fat (lipoatrophy). It can be congenital or acquired, and generalized, partial, or localized. The two most common forms of lipodystrophy include lipodystrophy due to the aging process and HIV-associated lipodystrophy. Aging skin is characterized by a loss of subcutaneous tissue and laxity of the anterior supporting dermis. A decrease in supporting bone mass and loss of muscle tone can cause patients to look older. In HIV-associated lipodystrophy, most patients are treated with highly active antiretroviral therapy (HAART). This combination therapy contains nonnucleoside reverse transcriptase inhibitors that can hinder DNA polymerase leading to adipocyte apoptosis.

Common areas affected by lipodystrophy are the cheeks and forehead, as well as the temporal, infraorbital, and jowl fat compartments. Losing fat in some areas can affect the general appearance in other areas. For example, decreasing subcutaneous fat in the malar cheeks can cause a prominent nasolabial fold, or decreasing jowl fat can cause prominent marionette lines and jowls. Treatment can be performed by using synthetic filler agents or AFT. However, many HIV patients lack adequate fat for aspiration and transplantation, or their fat is very fibrous, which renders harvesting difficult. Polylactic acid (Sculptra™, Dermik Laboratories, Berwyn, Pennsylvania), FDA-approved for the treatment of facial lipoatrophy in HIV patients, is a very useful product that works by stimulating collagen synthesis. The more recent use of higher dilutions and longer reconstitution times has led to a decrease in the formation of granulomas after injection of this agent (see Chapter 28, Sclerotherapy).

FUTURE DIRECTIONS

Understanding the biology of adipocytes is crucial to our ability to develop innovative lipolysis techniques and potentially use adipocytes as stem cells. More research is also required to characterize macro- and micro-characteristics of facial adipose tissue and their age-related changes across different anatomic compartments. In addition, various methods for fat removal are being investigated, including drugs or chemicals that can stimulate lipolysis (e.g., phosphatidylcholine, isoproterenol, theophylline, aminophylline, caffeine, carnitine, carbon dioxide, and herbal extracts) and device-assisted liposuction such as ultrasound (to burst fat cells) or 1064 nm Nd:YAG laser (to melt the fat cells). These newer methods need to be analyzed for safety and efficacy. Large-scale, standardized, and prospective clinical studies are also necessary to assess various harvesting, processing, and delivery methods for autologous fat transfer. The risks and benefits of supplementation strategies including platelet-rich plasma, progenitor cells, and functional growth factors should be similarly evaluated.

CONCLUSION

Adipocytes and subcutaneous tissue are important subjects to which the cosmetic dermatologist should pay attention. There are cosmetic concerns related to both excess and loss of fat for which the patient will seek cosmetic intervention. Advances in this field will be centered on more directed therapies of fat removal or disruption in heavy patients and on stem cell purification and injection in thinner patients. It is the role of the cosmetic dermatologist to keep abreast of these changes. Furthermore, cosmetic dermatologists and surgeons should take an active role in counseling patients on proper nutrition and weight management from both extremes (too thin or too heavy).

References

1. Hausman DB, DiGirolamo M, Bartness TJ, et al. The biology of white adipocyte proliferation. *Obes Rev*. 2001;2(4):239–254.

2. Avram MM, Avram AS, James WD. Subcutaneous fat in normal and diseased states: 1. Introduction. *J Am Acad Dermatol*. 2005;53(4):663–670.

3. Wang B, Han J, Gao Y, et al. The differentiation of rat adipose-derived stem cells into OEC-like cells on collagen scaffolds by co-culturing with OECs. *Neurosci Lett*. 2007;421(3):191–196.

4. Emanuele E. Cellulite: advances in treatment: facts and controversies. *Clin Dermatol*. 2013;31(6):725–730.

5. Sellheyer K, Krahl D. Skin mesenchymal stem cells: prospects for clinical dermatology. *J Am Acad Dermatol*. 2010;63(5):859–865.

6. Chen SX, Zhang LJ, Gallo RL. Dermal White Adipose Tissue: A Newly Recognized Layer of Skin Innate Defense. *J Invest Dermatol*. 2019;139(5):1002–1009.

7. Cappellano G, Morandi EM, Rainer J, et al. Human Macrophages Preferentially Infiltrate the Superficial Adipose Tissue. *Int J Mol Sci*. 2018;19(5):1404.

8. Kosaka K, Kubota Y, Adachi N, et al. Human adipocytes from the subcutaneous superficial layer have greater adipogenic potential and lower PPAR-γ DNA methylation levels than deep layer adipocytes. *Am J Physiol Cell Physiol*. 2016;311(2): C322–C329.

9. Kruglikov IL, Scherer PE. Dermal Adipocytes: From Irrelevance to Metabolic Targets? *Trends Endocrinol Metab*. 2016;27(1):1–10.

10. Segalla L, Chirumbolo S, Sbarbati A. Dermal white adipose tissue: Much more than a metabolic, lipid-storage organ? *Tissue Cell*. 2021;71:101583.

11. Zhang R, Kikuchi AT, Nakao T, et al. Elimination of Wnt Secretion From Stellate Cells Is Dispensable for Zonation and Development of Liver Fibrosis Following Hepatobiliary Injury. *Gene Expr*. 2019;19(2):121–136.

12. Zhang LJ, Guerrero-Juarez CF, Hata T, et al. Innate immunity. Dermal adipocytes protect against invasive Staphylococcus aureus skin infection. *Science*. 2015;347(6217):67–71.

13. Kruglikov IL, Scherer PE. Dermal adipocytes and hair cycling: is spatial heterogeneity a characteristic feature of the dermal adipose tissue depot? *Exp Dermatol*. 2016;25(4):258–262.

14. Plikus MV, Guerrero-Juarez CF, Ito M, et al. Regeneration of fat cells from myofibroblasts during wound healing. *Science*. 2017;355(6326):748–752.

15. Søberg S, Löfgren J, Philipsen FE, et al. Altered brown fat thermoregulation and enhanced cold-induced thermogenesis in young, healthy, winter-swimming men. *Cell Rep Med*. 2021;2(10):100408.

16. Pan R, Chen Y. Management of Oxidative Stress: Crosstalk Between Brown/Beige Adipose Tissues and Skeletal Muscles. *Front Physiol*. 2021;12:712372.

17. Verma N, Perie L, Corciulo C, et al. Browning of adipose tissue and increased thermogenesis induced by Methotrexate. *FASEB Bioadv*. 2021;3(11):877–887.

18. Garritson JD, Boudina S. The Effects of Exercise on White and Brown Adipose Tissue Cellularity, Metabolic Activity and Remodeling. *Front Physiol*. 2021;12:772894.

19. Prins JB, O'Rahilly S. Regulation of adipose cell number in man. *Clin Sci (Lond)*. 1997;92(1):3–11.

20. Faust IM, Miller HM Jr. Hyperplastic growth of adipose tissue in obesity. In: Angel A, Hollenberg CH, Roncari DAK, eds. *The Adipocyte and Obesity: Cellular and Molecular Mechanisms*. New York, NY: Raven Press; 1983: 41–51.

21. Spiegelman BM, Flier JS. Adipogenesis and obesity: rounding out the big picture. *Cell*. 1996;87(3):377–389.

22. Macêdo APA, da Silva ASR, Muñoz VR, et al. Mitochondrial dysfunction plays an essential role in remodeling aging adipose tissue. *Mech Ageing Dev*. 2021;200:111598.

23. Varga J, Marangoni RG. Systemic sclerosis in 2016: Dermal white adipose tissue implicated in SSc pathogenesis. *Nat Rev Rheumatol*. 2017;13(2):71–72.

24. Kruglikov I, Trujillo O, Kristen Q, et al. The Facial Adipose Tissue: A Revision. *Facial Plast Surg*. 2016;32(6):671–682.

25. Bielczyk-Maczynska E. White Adipocyte Plasticity in Physiology and Disease. *Cells*. 2019;8(12):1507.

26. Amato MC, Giordano C, Galia M, et al. Visceral Adiposity Index: a reliable indicator of visceral fat function associated with cardiometabolic risk. *Diabetes Care*. 2010;33(4):920–922.

27. Palacios-González B, León-Reyes G, Rivera-Paredez B, et al. Serum Metabolite Profile Associated with Sex-Dependent Visceral Adiposity Index and Low Bone Mineral Density in a Mexican Population. *Metabolites*. 2021;11(9):604.

28. Chambers ES, Vukmanovic-Stejic M. Skin barrier immunity and ageing. *Immunology*. 2020;160(2):116–125.

29. Cooper PO, Haas MR, Noonepalle SKR, et al. Dermal Drivers of Injury-Induced Inflammation: Contribution of Adipocytes and Fibroblasts. *Int J Mol Sci*. 2021;22(4):1933.

30. Huang J, Wang J, He H, et al. Close interactions between lncRNAs, lipid metabolism and ferroptosis in cancer. *Int J Biol Sci*. 2021;17(15):4493–4513.

31. Kee Z, Ong SM, Heng CK, et al. Androgen-dependent tissue factor pathway inhibitor regulating protein: a review of its peripheral actions and association with cardiometabolic diseases. *J Mol Med (Berl)*. 2021 Nov 19. Epub ahead of print.

32. Rezaei S, Tabrizi R, Nowrouzi-Sohrabi P, et al. The Effects of Vitamin D Supplementation on Anthropometric and Biochemical Indices in Patients With Non-alcoholic Fatty Liver Disease: A Systematic Review and Meta-analysis. *Front Pharmacol*. 2021;12:732496.

33. Rezaei S, Tabrizi R, Nowrouzi-Sohrabi P, et al. GLP-1 Receptor Agonist Effects on Lipid and Liver Profiles in Patients with Nonalcoholic Fatty Liver Disease: Systematic Review and Meta-Analysis. *Can J Gastroenterol Hepatol*. 2021;2021:8936865.

34. Manson JE, Bassuk SS. Obesity in the United States: a fresh look at its high toll. *JAMA*. 2003;289(2):229–230.

35. Kuczmarski RJ, Flegal KM, Campbell SM, et al. Increasing prevalence of overweight among US adults. The National Health and Nutrition Examination Surveys, 1960 to 1991. *JAMA*. 1994;272(3):205–211.

36. Friedman JM, Halaas JL. Leptin and the regulation of body weight in mammals. *Nature*. 1998;395(6704):763–770.

37. Montague CT, Farooqi IS, Whitehead JP, et al. Congenital leptin deficiency is associated with severe early-onset obesity in humans. *Nature*. 1997;387(6636):903–908.

38. Krude H, Biebermann H, Schnabel D, et al. Obesity due to proopiomelanocortin deficiency: three new cases and treatment

trials with thyroid hormone and ACTH4–10. *J Clin Endocrinol Metab.* 2003;88:4633.

39. Khan TZ, Schatz U, Bornstein SR, et al. Hypertriglyceridaemia: contemporary management of a neglected cardiovascular risk factor. *Glob Cardiol Sci Pract.* 2021;2021(3):e202119.

40. Cai J, Cui L, Wang Y, et al. Cardiometabolic Comorbidities in Patients With Psoriasis: Focusing on Risk, Biological Therapy, and Pathogenesis. *Front Pharmacol.* 2021;12:774808.

41. Pacheco M, de Maio Godoi Filho JR, et al. The relation between body mass index and body fat percentage in Brazilian adolescents: assessment of variability, linearity, and categorisation. *Ann Hum Biol.* 2021 Nov 7:1-6. Epub ahead of print.

42. Calderón-García JF, Roncero-Martín R, Rico-Martín S, et al. Effectiveness of Body Roundness Index (BRI) and a Body Shape Index (ABSI) in Predicting Hypertension: A Systematic Review and Meta-Analysis of Observational Studies. *Int J Environ Res Public Health.* 2021;18(21):11607.

43. Löffler H, Aramaki JU, Effendy I. The influence of body mass index on skin susceptibility to sodium lauryl sulphate. *Skin Res Technol.* 2002;8(1):19–22.

44. Deplewski D, Rosenfield RL. Growth hormone and insulin-like growth factors have different effects on sebaceous cell growth and differentiation. *Endocrinology.* 1999;140(9):4089–4094.

45. Cappel M, Mauger D, Thiboutot D. Correlation between serum levels of insulin-like growth factor 1, dehydroepiandrosterone sulfate, and dihydrotestosterone and acne lesion counts in adult women. *Arch Dermatol.* 2005;141(3):333–338.

46. Goodson WH 3rd, Hunt TK. Wound collagen accumulation in obese hyperglycemic mice. *Diabetes.* 1986;35(4):491–495.

47. de Jongh RT, Serné EH, IJzerman RG, et al. Impaired microvascular function in obesity: implications for obesity-associated microangiopathy, hypertension, and insulin resistance. *Circulation.* 2004;109(21):2529–2535.

48. García-Hidalgo L. Dermatological complications of obesity. *Am J Clin Dermatol.* 2002;3(7):497–506.

49. Pribanich S, Simpson FG, Held B, et al. Low-dose tretinoin does not improve striae distensae: a double-blind, placebo-controlled study. *Cutis.* 1994;54(2):121–124.

50. Hernández-Pérez E, Colombo-Charrier E, Valencia-Ibiett E. Intense pulsed light in the treatment of striae distensae. *Dermatol Surg.* 2002;28(12):1124–1130.

51. Jiménez GP, Flores F, Berman B, et al. Treatment of striae rubra and striae alba with the 585-nm pulsed-dye laser. *Dermatol Surg.* 2003;29(4):362–365.

52. Goldberg DJ, Sarradet D, Hussain M. 308-nm Excimer laser treatment of mature hypopigmented striae. *Dermatol Surg.* 2003;29(6):596–598.

53. Yosipovitch G, DeVore A, Dawn A. Obesity and the skin: skin physiology and skin manifestations of obesity. *J Am Acad Dermatol.* 2007;56(6):901–916.

54. Gögebakan O, Kohl A, Osterhoff MA, et al. Effects of weight loss and long-term weight maintenance with diets varying in protein and glycemic index on cardiovascular risk factors: the diet, obesity, and genes (DiOGenes) study: a randomized, controlled trial. *Circulation.* 2011;124(25):2829–2838.

55. Ballard AM, Davis A, Wong B, et al. The Effects of Exclusive Walking on Lipids and Lipoproteins in Women with Overweight and Obesity: A Systematic Review and Meta-Analysis. *Am J Health Promot.* 2021 Nov 22:8901171211048135. Online ahead of print.

56. Lemonnier D. Effect of age, sex, and sites on the cellularity of the adipose tissue in mice and rats rendered obese by a high-fat diet. *J Clin Invest.* 1972;51(11):2907–2915.

57. Faust IM, Johnson PR, Stern JS, et al. Diet-induced adipocyte number increase in adult rats: a new model of obesity. *Am J Physiol.* 1978;235(3):E279–E286.

58. Coleman WP 4th, Hendry SL 2nd. Principles of liposuction. *Semin Cutan Med Surg.* 2006;25(3):138–144.

59. Svedman KJ, Coldiron B, Coleman WP 3rd, et al. ASDS guidelines of care for tumescent liposuction. *Dermatol Surg.* 2006;32(5):709–716.

60. Coleman WP 3rd, Glogau RG, Klein JA, et al. Guidelines of care for liposuction. *J Am Acad Dermatol.* 2001;45(3):438–447.

61. Dolsky RL. State of the art in liposuction. *Dermatol Surg.* 1997;23(12):1192–1193.

62. Giese SY, Bulan EJ, Commons GW, et al. Improvements in cardiovascular risk profile with large volume liposuction: a pilot study. *Plast Reconstr Surg.* 2001;108(2):510–519.

63. Klein S, Fontana L, Young VL, et al. Absence of an effect of liposuction on insulin action and risk factors for coronary heart disease. *N Engl J Med.* 2004;350(25):2549–2557.

64. Giugliano G, Nicoletti G, Grella E, et al. Effect of liposuction on insulin resistance and vascular inflammatory markers in obese women. *Br J Plast Surg.* 2004;57(3):190–194.

65. Rocic P. Comparison of Cardiovascular Benefits of Bariatric Surgery and Abdominal Lipectomy. *Curr Hypertens Rep.* 2019;21(5):37.

66. Sailon AM, Wasserburg JR, Kling RR, et al. Influence of Large-Volume Liposuction on Metabolic and Cardiovascular Health: A Systematic Review. *Ann Plast Surg.* 2017;79(6):623–630.

67. Liu Z, Zhang W, Zhang B, et al. Toxic shock syndrome complicated with symmetrical peripheral gangrene after liposuction and fat transfer: a case report and literature review. *BMC Infect Dis.* 2021;21(1):1137.

68. Skorochod R, Fteiha B, Gronovich Y. Perforation of Abdominal Viscera Following Liposuction: A Systemic Literature Review. *Aesthetic Plast Surg.* 2021 Aug 30. Epub ahead of print.

69. Pessa JE, Zadoo VP, Mutimer KL, et al. Relative maxillary retrusion as a natural consequence of aging: combining skeletal and soft-tissue changes into an integrated model of midfacial aging. *Plast Reconstr Surg.* 1998;102(1):205–212.

70. Obagi S. Autologous fat augmentation: a perfect fit in new and emerging technologies. *Facial Plast Surg Clin North Am.* 2007;15(2):221–228, vii.

71. Gosain AK, Amarante MT, Hyde JS, et al. A dynamic analysis of changes in the nasolabial fold using magnetic resonance imaging: implications for facial rejuvenation and facial animation surgery. *Plast Reconstr Surg.* 1996;98(4):622–636.

72. Rønn PF, Andersen GS, Lauritzen T, et al. Abdominal visceral and subcutaneous adipose tissue and associations with cardiometabolic risk in Inuit, Africans and Europeans: a cross-sectional study. *BMJ Open.* 2020;10(9):e038071.

73. Maskarinec G, Raquinio P, Kristal BS, et al. Body Fat Distribution, Glucose Metabolism, and Diabetes Status among Older Adults: The Multiethnic Cohort Adiposity Phenotype Study. *J Epidemiol.* 2021 Feb 27. Epub ahead of print.

74. Liu B, Du Y, Wu Y, et al. Trends in obesity and adiposity measures by race or ethnicity among adults in the United States 2011-18: population based study. *BMJ.* 2021 Mar 16;372:n365.

75. Rohrich RJ, Pessa JE. The fat compartments of the face: anatomy and clinical implications for cosmetic surgery. *Plast Reconstr Surg.* 2007;119(7):2219–2227.

76. Donofrio LM. Fat distribution: a morphologic study of the aging face. *Dermatol Surg.* 2000;26(12):1107–1112.

77. Coleman SR. Concepts of aging: rethinking the obvious. *Structural Fat Grafting.* St. Louis, MO: Quality Medical Publishing; 2004: xvii–xxiv.

78. Hanson SE. The Future of Fat Grafting. *Aesthet Surg J.* 2021; 41(Suppl 1):S69–S74.

79. Kranendonk S, Obagi S. Autologous fat transfer for periorbital rejuvenation: indications, technique, and complications. *Dermatol Surg.* 2007;33:572.

80. Narins RS. Fat transfer with fresh and frozen fat, microlipoinjection, and lipocytic dermal augmentation. In: Klein AW, ed. *Tissue Augmentation in Clinical Practice.* 2nd ed. New York, NY: Taylor and Francis; 2006: 1–19.

81. Gornitsky J, Viezel-Mathieu A, Alnaif N, et al. A systematic review of the effectiveness and complications of fat grafting in the facial region. *JPRAS Open.* 2018;19:87–97.

82. Rageh MA, El-Khalawany M, Ibrahim SMA. Autologous nanofat injection in treatment of scars: A clinico-histopathological study. *J Cosmet Dermatol.* 2021;20(10):3198–3204.

83. Eremia S, Newman N. Long-term follow-up after autologous fat grafting: analysis of results from 116 patients followed at least 12 months after receiving the last of a minimum of two treatments. *Dermatol Surg.* 2000;26(12):1150–1158.

84. Sommer B, Sattler G. Current concepts of fat graft survival: histology of aspirated adipose tissue and review of the literature. *Dermatol Surg.* 2000;26(12):1159–1166.

85. Yan D, Li SH, Zhang AL, et al. A Clinical Study of Platelet-Rich Fibrin Combined With Autologous High-Density Fat Transplantation in Augmentation Rhinoplasty. *Ear Nose Throat J.* 2021 May 31:1455613211016902. Epub ahead of print.

86. Moak TN, Ebersole TG, Tandon D, et al. Assessing Clinical Outcomes in Autologous Fat Grafting: A Current Literature Review. *Aesthet Surg J.* 2021;41(Suppl 1):S50–S60.

87. Vatansever M, Dursun Ö, Özer Ö, et al. A Rare Ocular Complication of Autologous Fat Injection: Subconjunctival Fat Infiltration. *J Craniofac Surg.* 2021;32(7):e679–e680.

88. Egido JA, Arroyo R, Marcos A, et al. Middle cerebral artery embolism and unilateral visual loss after autologous fat injection into the glabellar area. *Stroke.* 1993;24(4):615–616.

89. Teimourian B. Blindness following fat injections. *Plast Reconstr Surg.* 1988;82(2):361.

90. Dreizen NG, Framm L. Sudden visual loss after autologous fat injection into the glabellar area. *Am J Ophthalmol.* 1989;107(1):85–87.

91. Danesh-Meyer HV, Savino PJ, Sergott RC. Case reports and small case series: ocular and cerebral ischemia following facial injection of autologous fat. *Arch Ophthalmol.* 2001;119(5):777–778.

92. Pinski KS, Coleman WP 3rd. Microlipoinjection and autologous collagen. *Dermatol Clin.* 1995;13(2):339–351.

93. Strem BM, Hicok KC, Zhu M, et al. Multipotential differentiation of adipose tissue-derived stem cells. *Keio J Med.* 2005;54(3):132–141.

94. Mizuno H, Zuk PA, Zhu M, et al. Myogenic differentiation by human processed lipoaspirate cells. *Plast Reconstr Surg.* 2002;109(1):199–209.

95. De Ugarte DA, Morizono K, Elbarbary A, et al. Comparison of multi-lineage cells from human adipose tissue and bone marrow. *Cells Tissues Organs.* 2003;174(3):101–109.

96. Kokai LE, Rubin JP, Marra KG. The potential of adipose-derived adult stem cells as a source of neuronal progenitor cells. *Plast Reconstr Surg.* 2005;116(5):1453–1460.

97. Khorasani M, Janbaz P. Clinical evaluation of autologous fat graft for facial deformity: a case series study. *J Korean Assoc Oral Maxillofac Surg.* 2021;47(4):286–290.

98. Hexsel DM, Dal'forno T, Hexsel CL. A validated photonumeric cellulite severity scale. *J Eur Acad Dermatol Venereol.* 2009;23(5):523–528.

99. Rudolph C, Hladik C, Hamade H, et al. Structural Gender Dimorphism and the Biomechanics of the Gluteal Subcutaneous Tissue: Implications for the Pathophysiology of Cellulite. *Plast Reconstr Surg.* 2019;143(4):1077–1086.

100. Emanuele E, Minoretti P, Altabas K, et al. Adiponectin expression in subcutaneous adipose tissue is reduced in women with cellulite. *Int J Dermatol.* 2011;50(4):412–416.

101. Smalls LK, Hicks M, Passeretti D, et al. Effect of weight loss on cellulite: gynoid lypodystrophy. *Plast Reconstr Surg.* 2006;118(2):510–516.

102. Whipple LA, Fournier CT, Heiman AJ, et al. The Anatomical Basis of Cellulite Dimple Formation: An Ultrasound-Based Examination. *Plast Reconstr Surg.* 2021;148(3):375e–381e.

103. Draelos ZD, Marenus KD. Cellulite. Etiology and purported treatment. *Dermatol Surg.* 1997;23(12):1177–1181.

104. Draelos ZD. The disease of cellulite. *J Cosmet Dermatol.* 2005;4(4):221–222.

105. Piérard GE, Nizet JL, Piérard-Franchimont C. Cellulite: from standing fat herniation to hypodermal stretch marks. *Am J Dermatopathol.* 2000;22(1):34–37.

106. Tokarska K, Tokarski S, Woźniacka A, et al. Cellulite: a cosmetic or systemic issue? Contemporary views on the etiopathogenesis of cellulite. *Postepy Dermatol Alergol.* 2018;35(5):442–446.

107. Scarano A, Petrini M, Sbarbati A, et al. Pilot study of histology aspect of cellulite in seventy patients who differ in BMI and cellulite grading. *J Cosmet Dermatol.* 2021 Nov 6. Epub ahead of print.

108. Alexiades-Armenakas M. Laser and light-based treatment of cellulite. *J Drugs Dermatol.* 2007;6(1):83–84.

109. Hexsel DM, Mazzuco R. Subcision: a treatment for cellulite. *Int J Dermatol.* 2000;39(7):539–544.

110. Kaufman-Janette J, Joseph JH, Kaminer MS, et al. Collagenase Clostridium Histolyticum-aaes for the Treatment of Cellulite in Women: Results From Two Phase 3 Randomized, Placebo-Controlled Trials. *Dermatol Surg.* 2021;47(5):649–656.

111. Sadick NS, Goldman MP, Liu G, et al. Collagenase Clostridium Histolyticum for the Treatment of Edematous Fibrosclerotic Panniculopathy (Cellulite): A Randomized Trial. *Dermatol Surg.* 2019;45(8):1047–1056.

112. Bass LS, Kaminer MS. Insights Into the Pathophysiology of Cellulite: A Review. *Dermatol Surg.* 2020;46(Suppl 1(1)):S77–S85.

CHAPTER 4

The Skin Microbiome

Edmund M. Weisberg, MS, MBE
Leslie S. Baumann, MD

SUMMARY POINTS

What's Important?
1. Diversity in the bacterial microbiome is the healthiest state.
2. It is too soon to recommend probiotic skincare products.
3. Diet and environment play a major role in the microbiome.

What's New?
1. The skin and gut microbiome play a role in skin inflammation.
2. The microbiome allows communication with the gut, brain, and skin.

What's Coming?
1. Understanding the effects of skin and gut microbiomes on skin disease.
2. Healthier ways to manipulate the microbiome to treat skin issues.
3. Identifying which combinations of bacteria have the best outcomes in skin disease.

INTRODUCTION

In this era of personalized or precision medicine, we have come to learn about the great deal of recent research focusing on the gut microbiome and its role in individual health. Human skin, too, hosts a copious and disparate array of bacteria, fungi, viruses, and arthropods, with as many as a billion microbes inhabiting a single square centimeter of skin.[1,2] And these microbes, too, play an important role in skin health that research is now uncovering. Human skin, the largest organ of the body, serves not only as an ecosystem but also as a protective barrier against pathogenic microorganisms and other exogenous material, and we are elucidating much more about the microbiome of the skin and its balancing act between beneficial, neutral, and harmful flora mediated by the innate and adaptive immune systems.[3]

As Dréno et al. remind us, Antoni van Leuwenhoek made the first discovery that the skin hosts a wide array of microscopic creatures in 1683.[3] Modern techniques have verified that, indeed, the human skin is colonized by an abundance of diverse microscopic communities. These microbes play an important role in skin health and disease. It should be noted that less is known about viral species than any other genera of the cutaneous microbiome.[3] The body of knowledge on microbes is most advanced on bacteria, which also are predominantly implicated in some of the skin disorders discussed here.

The skin, like the gut, plays a significant role in human health as an interface organ. As noted by O'Neill et al., the skin also expresses several co-morbidities with gut disorders.[4] Bacteria, more than other microbes, also constitute a preponderance of the gut microbiome, and the skin-gut nexus warrants exploration as these critical interface organs can impact one another in health and disease.

Dysbiosis is said to have occurred when a healthy equilibrium is disrupted by a microbial imbalance internally or externally. Infections, wounds, and microbial colonization are all regulated by the cutaneous immune system; dysregulation of this system manifests in various skin conditions.[5] The etiologies of various skin disorders, including acne, atopic dermatitis (AD), seborrheic dermatitis, hidradenitis suppurativa, and chronic wounds, have been ascribed, at least in part, to microbial sources.[5,6] Research into the dynamic role of the skin microbiome in cutaneous health and disease is essentially in its infancy, particularly in relation to the novel genomic sequencing methods now being used to elucidate the genetic and epigenetic underpinnings of health. Despite the relative dearth of data on the potential interconnections between the skin as well as gut microbiome and manifestations of skin disease, current research is pointing in many fascinating directions.

THE MICROBIOME'S ROLE IN SKIN HEALTH

Skin Surface Area

Just as humans have adapted to hostile environments through the millennia, microbial communities have adapted and continue to adapt to and navigate the nutrient-deficient, relatively cool, acidic, and dry environment of human skin—as compared to the human gut—and thrive on particular regions of the diverse topography of the expansive surface area.[5,7]

The cutaneous environment hosts microbial communities in physiologically discrete sebaceous or nonsebaceous, hairy or smooth, moist or dry, and creased or noncreased areas, with skin bacterial communities having been shown through gene sequencing as being specific to particular skin niches, with wide variations in ultraviolet (UV) exposure, pH, and temperature as well.[7-9] For example, *Propionibacterium acnes* has been found to be more prevalent in highly sebaceous sites on the head and upper torso as compared to moist skin creases or greater expanses of skin.[8] Other host factors that affect which microorganisms colonize the skin and where include hair follicle thickness, sebaceous gland density, age, sex, and diet, as well as the environmental contributors climate (including impacts from the declining biodiversity at the micro-ecological level as well as human microbial habitats), occupation, and personal hygiene.[5,10-12] The cutaneous microbiome of normal, healthy human skin is characterized by wide inter- and intra-individual variability.[13]

Insightfully, Gallo pointed out that estimates of the cutaneous microbiome's impact on human health via skin have failed to acknowledge the inner follicular surface, thus drastically undervaluing the potential of the cutaneous microbiome to influence systemic health.[14] Specifically, he suggested that the surface area of skin has been miscalculated as 2 m² based on considering it a flat surface, which ignores the plethora of hair follicles and sweat ducts that significantly broaden the epithelial surface closer to 25 m².[14] The epithelial linings of these skin appendages are in contact with microbes and represent a more expansive skin microbiome than has been previously recognized, he noted.

Progress in sequencing technologies has spurred advances in the study of the microbiome, with genomic sequencing yielding a more thorough assessment and characterization of its previously underappreciated variety while skirting the pitfalls of cultivating microbial isolates.[8,15]

The Key Residents, Where They Reside, and Changes in the Cutaneous Microbiome

Notably, as skin type can change with travel, seasons, and through a lifetime, the skin microbiome varies across individuals and is also labile, undergoing change from birth and through health and disease, even subject to influence from an adjacent skin microbiome, such as between cohabiting couples, as well as ambient air pollution.[16-18] Significantly, the cutaneous microbiome has been shown to be affected by delivery method, with the microbiota of vaginally delivered neonates manifesting vaginal bacteria and neonates delivered by cesarean evincing cutaneous bacteria.[8] The skin microbiome is also associated with alteration during puberty, with more lipophilic species such as *Propionibacteriaceae* and *Corynebacteriaceae* overcoming the earlier preponderance of *Firmicutes*, *Bacteroidetes*, and *Proteobacteria*.[8,19] Changes in the skin microbiome that may characterize later stages of the healthy life cycle remain to be ascertained. Cutaneous commensal microbial communities have been found through longitudinal studies to be stable over a two-year period, though.[7] In general, *Propionibacteriaceae* hold sway in sebaceous areas, whereas *Corynebacteriaceae* and *Staphylococcaceae* prevail in moist regions, such as the navel or axilla, with dry expanses hosting the widest diversity of microbes, including *Corynebacterium*, *Enhydrobacter*, *Micrococcus*, *Propionibacterium*, *Staphylococcus*, and *Streptococcus* species.[3,5,20]

Skin barrier stability or dysfunction, itself a function of the symbiotic or commensal relationship between host tissue and resident microbial communities on and in the skin, has been shown by research to be influenced by the volume and diversity of such microbes.[21] In a 2016 study testing the hypothesis that differences in sebum and hydration levels in specific facial areas account for inter-individual variation in facial skin microbiomes, Mukherjee et al. measured sebum and hydration from the forehead and cheeks of 30 healthy female volunteers. They found that the most significant predictor of microbiome composition was cheek sebum level, followed by forehead hydration level, while cheek hydration and forehead sebum levels were not predictive. The prevalence of *Actinobacteria*/*Propionibacterium* rose while microbiome diversity diminished with an increase in cheek sebum, with such trends reversed in relation to forehead hydration. The investigators concluded that site-specific sebum and water levels impact the nature and diversity of the facial skin microbiome.[22] Pyrosequencing assays of bacterial 16S rRNA genes have been used by investigators to distinguish and describe the wide variety of resident and transient microorganisms on the skin and elucidate their roles in skin health and disease.[3] Diversity of the microbiome seems to be very important.

Stability of the microbial community is an important contributor to skin health, as microbes interact, collaborate, and oppose one another while exerting influence on and being affected by the host. Effective communication among the innate and adaptive parts of the immune system, epithelial cells, and cutaneous microbiota is essential for optimal functioning of the skin.[5,7]

Chehoud et al. hypothesized that the complement system (a key inflammatory mediator and integral constituent of innate immunity)[23] impacts cutaneous host-microbe interactions. Culture-independent high-throughput sequencing of bacterial 16S rRNA genes from C57BL/6J mice were used to show that suppressing an important ingredient of complement diminished diversity and changed the composition of the cutaneous microbiota as skin inflammatory cell infiltration declined and skin defense and immune gene expression were downregulated. The investigators concluded that these findings, including the regulation of complement genes in the skin by cutaneous microbiota, imply interactivity of complement and the skin microbiome.[24]

In 2017, Maguire and Maguire reviewed recent studies of the gut and skin microbiomes and suggested that *Nitrobacter*, *Lactobacillus*, and *Bifidobacterium* are bacteria that can improve skin health and could be useful adjuvants in a probiotic and prebiotic strategy in homeostatic renormalization when skin health is compromised.[25] *Nitrobacter* has displayed antifungal activity against dermatophytes and *Staphylococcus*; *Lactobacillus* has exhibited anti-inflammatory effects and was shown to improve adult acne in a small study; *Bifidobacterium* combined with *Lactobacillus* lowered the incidence of atopic eczema in early childhood; and *Bifidobacterium* and the prebiotic galactooligosaccharides prevented hydration level losses in the stratum corneum among other beneficial effects in a double-blind, placebo-controlled, randomized trial.[25]

A more recent study by Holowacz et al. of oral probiotics administered to hairless SKH-1 mice with chronic skin inflammation induced by multiple applications of 12-O-tetradecanoylphorbol-13-acetate may suggest that *Lactobacillus salivarius* and *Lactobacillus rhamnosus* have potential to help maintain skin integrity and homeostasis through their actions on gut microbiota, and could help alleviate cutaneous disorders such as AD.[26]

Cosmeceutical Effects on the Skin Microbiome

The emerging body of knowledge on the cutaneous microbiome could influence how practitioners advise their patients to maintain skin health, even at the level of daily washing. In a 2016 study on the impact of acute treatment with topical skin cleansers on the cutaneous microbiome, investigators evaluated multiple common skin cleansers in the washing of human forearms. The amount of the antimicrobial peptide LL-37 and the abundance and diversity of bacterial DNA were measured, with small but significant declines in LL-37 levels noted on the skin soon after washing. No significant alterations in the bacterial community were observed. The results buttressed prior studies showing the benefits of hand washing in the health care setting, as Group A *Streptococcus* growth faltered after washing with soaps infused with antimicrobial compounds such as benzalkonium chloride or triclocarban. The researchers cautioned that much more research is necessary to ascertain the effects of chronic washing as well as the role skincare products may play in skin homeostasis or dysbiosis in some individuals.[27]

In a 2017 analysis of the effects of cosmetics on the skin microbiome of facial cheeks with high and low hydration levels over 4 weeks, Lee et al. found that bacterial diversity was higher in the low hydration group, with increases in both observed after the use of cosmetics. Common to both groups were the phyla Actinobacteria, Proteobacteria, Firmicutes, and Bacteroidetes and the genera Propionibacterium, Ralstonia, Burkholderia, Staphylococcus, Corynebacterium, Cupriavidus, and Pelomonas. The high hydration group showed a greater supply of *Propionibacterium*. Cosmetic use was found not to have caused a shift in bacterial communities in the low hydration group.[28]

Understanding the dynamic and convoluted ways in which the skin microbiome interacts with and supports healthy skin barrier function is also critical for the development of optimal skincare formulations.[21]

THE MICROBIOME'S ROLE IN SKIN DISEASE

Acne

An immune-mediated chronic inflammatory condition, acne has long been known to have a multifactorial etiologic pathway, not all of which has been completely elucidated. Of course, *Propionibacterium acnes* and *Malassezia* spp. have been long known to contribute to acne by affecting sebum secretion, comedone development, and inflammatory response.[29] It is increasingly thought that understanding the role of the skin barrier and such microbes in the microbiome in acne pathophysiology may lead to enhanced treatments.[30]

In 2017, Dréno et al. studied the skin microbiota in 26 subjects with mild to moderate acne and ascertained alterations after 28 days of treatment with erythromycin 4% or a dermocosmetic. Proteobacteria and Firmicutes were overrepresented at baseline and Actinobacteria were underrepresented. While Staphylococci were present in greater numbers on lesional as opposed to non-lesional skin, Propionibacteria was found in less than 2% of cutaneous bacteria. Upon conclusion of the study, Actinobacteria and Staphylococci were reduced in the dermocosmetic group while only Actinobacteria numbers were lowered in the erythromycin group.[31]

Early in 2018, Kelhälä et al. provided the first-time report on the influence of systemic acne treatment (isotretinoin and lymecycline) on cutaneous microbiota in the cheeks, back, and axillae of mild to moderate acne patients using gene sequencing. In the sebaceous regions of healthy control skin and untreated acne skin, *P. acnes* was the most prevalent species at baseline, and acne severity positively correlated with *P. acnes* levels. There were significant variations in microbiota, including a Streptococcus taxon, in the cheek skin of acne patients and the controls. Clinical acne grades and *P. acnes* levels were decreased by both treatments. Other species were found in significantly greater abundance in treated cheeks compared with untreated ones, and microbiota diversity was greatly enhanced on the cheek and back after systemic acne treatments.[32]

New gene sequencing technologies, particularly those based on *recA* and *tly* loci, are teaching us more about the Gram-positive, anaerobic bacterium *P. acnes*, which is a commensal member of the cutaneous microbiome and well known as a pathogen in the emergence of acne, that may eventually lead to treatment advances.[33]

Atopic Dermatitis

The chronic inflammatory disorder atopic dermatitis (AD) is observed in 15–20% of children and 2–5% of adults in the developed world,[34] with prevalence estimated as 10–20% of the general population.[35] AD is associated with dysbiosis of cutaneous microbiota that renders diminished diversity in microbial communities.[10,36] There is also a robust epidemiologic relationship between the cutaneous and gut microbiomes and AD.[37,38]

Although the role of *Staphylococcus aureus* in AD has not been ascertained, it is known that the bacterium selectively colonizes the lesional skin of AD patients but is notably lacking on the skin of most healthy people.[34] Evidence suggests that reduced microbiome diversity in patients with AD is associated with greater disease severity and elevated intrusion of harmful bacteria such as *S. aureus*.[39]

In a 2017 literature review, Bjerre et al. found that while the data were not extensive, AD-affected skin was characterized by low bacterial diversity—with *S. aureus* and *S. epidermidis* more abundant and other genera, including *P. acnes*, more scarce—and a mouse study suggested an etiologic role of dysbiosis in eczema.[36] Also that year, Williams and Gallo reported on a prospective clinical trial in children that colonization by *S. aureus* occurred before the emergence of AD symptoms, suggesting that this microbe may engender AD in some people.[40] Since then, Lunjani et al. have noted that *S. aureus* overgrowth with diminished *S. epidermidis* is characteristic of AD, though is not limited to such cutaneous disorders.[41]

In 2018, Clausen et al. reported on an observational case-control study of 45 adult healthy controls and 56 adult patients with AD between January and June 2015 to evaluate skin and nasal microbiome diversity and composition and to elucidate the relationship between disease severity and filaggrin gene mutations in AD patients. Next-generation sequencing targeting 16S ribosomal RNA was used to show that microbiome diversity was lower in the lesional skin, nonlesional skin, and nose in AD patients compared with controls. Such diversity was also found to be inversely correlated with disease severity, and microbiome composition in nonlesional AD skin was found to be associated with filaggrin gene mutations. The authors concluded that host genetics and skin microbiome may be connected in AD.[42] Kong et al. previously observed in a study on children with AD that microbial diversity during AD flares hinged on the administration of recent treatments, with enhanced bacterial diversity seen with even spotty treatment as opposed to no recent treatment.[43]

Marrs and Flohr observed that the eradication of *S. aureus* does not appear to account for improvement in AD and the rise in bacterial diversity after the use of antimicrobial and anti-inflammatory therapy to treat a flare.[44]

While treatment strategies for these conditions vary, Egert et al. have contended that because alterations in cutaneous microbiota are associated with disorders such as acne, rosacea, and atopic dermatitis, the use of pre- and probiotics, including transplantation therapies, in addition to antibiotics, warrants consideration for such conditions.[45] Paller et al. pointed out that various early clinical studies support the topical application of commensal organisms (such as *Staphylococcus hominis* or *Roseomonas mucosa*) to allay AD symptoms and reduce *S. aureus* colonization.[39]

Rosacea

Rosacea is a chronic inflammatory skin condition long associated with Demodex mites (*Demodex folliculorum* and *Demodex brevis*), which are believed to be included among the commensal cutaneous microbiome, with significant prevalence rates in healthy skin.[46] In rosacea-affected skin, Demodex mites are found to occur in greater density than in unaffected skin.[47] Notably, microbiota-linked alterations have been detected on the skin and in the small intestines in cases of rosacea.[45] In addition, Picardo and Ottaviani have observed that an irregular activation of the innate immune system has been linked to rosacea pathophysiology, and that both the skin and gut microbiomes appear to play a role.[48]

Seborrheic Dermatitis

In 2017, Park et al. studied the relationship between scalp microbiota and dandruff/seborrheic dermatitis, analyzing the bacterial and fungal species on the scalps of 102 subjects. They found that the microbiome composition varied significantly between normal and diseased scalps.[49] Paulino has suggested that advances in sequencing technology and bioinformatics have been critical in uncovering data that should broaden our perspective to the involvement in dandruff and seborrheic dermatitis of microbial communities beyond the long-implicated Malassezia yeasts.[50]

Psoriasis

The chronic inflammatory skin disease psoriasis, which affects about 2% of the world's population and is linked to heart disease,[51,52] can be triggered or aggravated by various microbes, including viruses (human papillomavirus and endogenous retroviruses), fungi (*Malassezia* and *Candida albicans*), and especially bacteria (*Staphylococcus aureus* and *Streptococcus pyogenes*).[53] Psoriatic plaques have been found to host copious amounts of *Corynebacteria*, *Propionibacteria*, *Staphylococci*, and *Streptococci*, though studies have revealed reduced diversity of species,[54] with *Streptococci* more abundant in normal and psoriatic skin, while *Staphylococci* and *Propionibacteria* are more sparse in psoriasis compared to normal limb skin in some studies.[51,55–58] Wang and Jin have cautioned that much more research is necessary to ascertain direct connections in the cutaneous microbiome and psoriasis though extant evidence shows that the microbiome in healthy controls is distinct from that in individuals with psoriasis.[55] Langan et al. added that a more accurate way to understand or depict the floral landscape of the skin is to realize that there is no "single microbiome," but various microbiomes based on site- and skin microenvironment-dependent cutaneous microbial populations.[54] Paetzold et al., who have successfully used living bacteria to alter the balance of the cutaneous microbiome, have speculated that modulating the composition of the skin microbiome may be a viable approach to treating disorders such as psoriasis and acne.[59]

Skin Cancer, the Environment, and the Skin Microbiome

There is a dearth of knowledge on the relationship of the skin microbiome and skin cancers, particularly on the topic of chemoprevention, but several studies are underway to better understand skin cancer risk and to explore the potential of using the skin microbiome to prevent, achieve earlier diagnosis, and treat skin cancers.[60] Patra et al. advised that because UV radiation, a primary environmental factor affecting the skin, can modulate the innate and adaptive immune systems in favorable and pernicious ways, it is important to consider the potential impact of UV-induced changes to the cutaneous microbiome, which itself interacts with and shares control of the immune system.[46]

Further, Prescott et al. made the compelling case on the interconnected nature of the larger ecosystem and its waning biodiversity as well as the diversity in human skin and mucosal communities. Specifically, in acknowledging the role of stratum corneum disruptions in various cutaneous conditions (e.g., acne, psoriasis, rosacea, allergic disorders such as eczema and food allergy, as well as skin aging), they reminded us that advancing climate change, the built environment and accelerated urbanization, global losses in biodiversity, and human disconnection from nature are integral factors in the decline of biodiversity at the micro-ecological as well as human microbial levels, which reinforces the notion that dysbiosis and the risk of inflammatory diseases across the life course in humans is inextricably linked to the wider ecosystem dysbiosis.[12,61] Humans are not separate from nature.

CONCLUSION

The skin microbiome is a fertile area for a plethora of microbes as well as for research, and we are certain to hear of many new developments in the discovery of cutaneous microbiome-related data and the application of such information into the therapeutic realm. In order to better understand the characteristics of cutaneous microbiota in dermatologic disorders, the emerging research in establishing a baseline for healthy skin is most welcome. We are in the early stages as we strive to learn more about the microbiome to leverage such knowledge to enhance skin health.

It is increasingly clear, though, that recent findings reveal that the cutaneous microbiome is a factor in various skin disorders. Research, particularly using advanced gene sequencing, is focused on and instrumental in ascertaining which species contribute to the etiologic pathway of skin conditions. Such investigations are pointing us toward more expansive therapeutic approaches to tackling some of the most vexing chronic dermatologic issues. This is an exciting area of scientific inquiry that holds much promise in enhancing the armamentarium against conditions such as acne, atopic dermatitis, seborrheic dermatitis, psoriasis, and rosacea, among the most prominent skin problems.

References

1. Weyrich LS, Dixit S, Farrer AG, Cooper AJ, Cooper AJ. The skin microbiome: Associations between altered microbial communities and disease. *Australas J Dermatol.* 2015;56(4):268–274.

2. Grice EA. The skin microbiome: potential for novel diagnostic and therapeutic approaches to cutaneous disease. *Semin Cutan Med Surg.* 2014;33(2):98–103.

3. Dréno B, Araviiskaia E, Berardesca E, et al. Microbiome in healthy skin, update for dermatologists. *J Eur Acad Dermatol Venereol.* 2016;30(12):2038–2047.

4. O'Neill CA, Monteleone G, McLaughlin JT, Paus R. The gut-skin axis in health and disease: A paradigm with therapeutic implications. *Bioessays.* 2016;38(11):1167–1176.

5. Grice EA, Segre JA. The skin microbiome. *Nat Rev Microbiol.* 2011;9(4):244–253.

6. Ring HC, Thorsen J, Saunte DM, et al. The Follicular Skin Microbiome in Patients With Hidradenitis Suppurativa and Healthy Controls. *JAMA Dermatol.* 2017;153(9):897–905.

7. Byrd AL, Belkaid Y, Segre JA. The human skin microbiome. *Nat Rev Microbiol.* 2018;16(3):143–155.

8. Kong HH, Segre JA. The molecular revolution in cutaneous biology: investigating the skin microbiome. *J Invest Dermatol.* 2017;137(5):e119–e122.

9. Costello EK, Lauber CL, Hamady M, et al. Bacterial community variation in human body habitats across space and time. *Science.* 2009;326(5960):1694–1697.

10. Rodrigues Hoffmann A. The cutaneous ecosystem: the roles of the skin microbiome in health and its association with inflammatory skin conditions in humans and animals. *Vet Dermatol.* 2017;28(1):60–e15.

11. Moestrup KS, Chen Y, Schepeler T, et al. Dietary control of skin lipid composition and microbiome. *J Invest Dermatol.* 2018;138(5):1225–1228.

12. Prescott SL, Larcombe DL, Logan AC, et al. The skin microbiome: impact of modern environments on skin ecology, barrier integrity, and systemic immune programming. *World Allergy Organ J.* 2017;10(1):29.

13. Zeeuwen PL, Kleerebezem M, Timmerman HM, Schalkwijk J. Microbiome and skin diseases. *Curr Opin Allergy Clin Immunol.* 2013;13(5):514–520.

14. Gallo RL. Human skin is the largest epithelial surface for interaction with microbes. *J Invest Dermatol.* 2017;137(6):1213–1214.

15. Kong HH. Skin microbiome: genomics-based insights into the diversity and role of skin microbes. *Trends Mol Med.* 2011;17(6):320–328.

16. Ross AA, Doxey AC, Neufeld JD. The skin microbiome of cohabiting couples. *mSystems.* 2017 Jul 20;2(4).

17. Mancebo SE, Wang SQ. Recognizing the impact of ambient air pollution on skin health. *J Eur Acad Dermatol Venereol.* 2015;29(12):2236–32.

18. He QC, Tavakkol A, Wietecha K, Begum-Gafur R, Ansari SA, Polefka T. Effects of environmentally realistic levels of ozone on stratum corneum function. *Int J Cosmet Sci.* 2006;28(5):349–357.

19. Oh J, Conlan S, Polley EC, et al. Shifts in human skin and nares microbiota of healthy children and adults. *Genome Med.* 2012;4(10):77.

20. Zeeuwen PL, Boekhorst J, van den Bogaard EH, et al. Microbiome dynamics of human epidermis following skin barrier disruption. *Genome Biol.* 2012;13(11):R101.

21. Baldwin HE, Bhatia ND, Friedman A, et al. The role of cutaneous microbiota harmony in maintaining a functional skin barrier. *J Drugs Dermatol.* 2017;16(1):12–18.

22. Mukherjee S, Mitra R, Maitra A, et al. Sebum and hydration levels in specific regions of human face significantly predict the nature and diversity of facial skin microbiome. *Sci Rep.* 2016;6:36062.

23. Ricklin D, Hajishengallis G, Yang K, Lambris JD. Complement: a key system for immune surveillance and homeostasis. *Nat Immunol.* 2010;11(9):785–797.

24. Chehoud C, Rafail S, Tyldsley AS, Seykora JT, Lambris JD, Grice EA. Complement modulates the cutaneous microbiome and inflammatory milieu. *Proc Natl Acad Sci U S A.* 2013;110(37):15061–15066.

25. Maguire M, Maguire G. The role of microbiota, and probiotics and prebiotics in skin health. *Arch Dermatol Res.* 2017;309(6):411–421.

26. Holowacz S, Blondeau C, Guinobert I, Guilbot A, Hidalgo S, Bisson JF. Lactobacillus salivarius LA307 and Lactobacillus rhamnosus LA305 attenuate skin inflammation in mice. *Benef Microbes.* 2018;9(2):299–309.

27. Two AM, Nakatsuji T, Kotol PF, et al. The cutaneous microbiome and aspects of skin antimicrobial defense system resist acute treatment with topical skin cleansers. *J Invest Dermatol.* 2016;136(10):1950–1954.

28. Lee HJ, Jeong SE, Lee S, et al. Effects of cosmetics on the skin microbiome of facial cheeks with different hydration levels. *Microbiologyopen.* 2018;7(2):e00557.

29. Xu H, Li H. Acne, the Skin Microbiome, and Antibiotic Treatment. *Am J Clin Dermatol.* 2019;20(3):335–344.

30. Rocha MA, Bagatin E. Skin barrier and microbiome in acne. *Arch Dermatol Res.* 2018;310(3):181–185.

31. Dreno B, Martin R, Moyal D, et al. Skin microbiome and acne vulgaris: Staphylococcus, a new actor in acne. *Exp Dermatol.* 2017;26(9):798–803.

32. Kelhälä HL, Aho VTE, Fyhrquist N, et al. Isotretinoin and lymecycline treatments modify the skin microbiota in acne. *Exp Dermatol.* 2018;27(1):30–36.

33. McDowell A. Over a decade of recA and tly gene sequence typing of the skin bacterium Propionibacterium acnes: What have we learnt? *Microorganisms.* 2017;6(1).

34. Yamazaki Y, Nakamura Y, Núñez G. Role of the microbiota in skin immunity and atopic dermatitis. *Allergol Int.* 2017;66(4):539–544.

35. Wollina U. Microbiome in atopic dermatitis. *Clin Cosmet Investig Dermatol.* 2017;10:51–56.

36. Bjerre RD, Bandier J, Skov L, et al. The role of the skin microbiome in atopic dermatitis: a systematic review. *Br J Dermatol.* 2017;177(5):1272–1278.

37. Knaysi G, Smith AR, Wilson JM, et al. The skin as a route of allergen exposure: Part II. Allergens and role of the microbiome and environmental exposures. *Curr Allergy Asthma Rep.* 2017;17(1):7.

38. Thomas CL, Fernández-Peñas P. The microbiome and atopic eczema: More than skin deep. *Australas J Dermatol.* 2017;58(1):18–24.

39. Paller AS, Kong HH, Seed P, et al. The microbiome in patients with atopic dermatitis. *J Allergy Clin Immunol.* 2019;143(1):26–35.

40. Williams MR, Gallo RL. Evidence that human skin microbiome dysbiosis promotes atopic dermatitis. *J Invest Dermatol.* 2017;137(12):2460–2461.

41. Lunjani N, Hlela C, O'Mahony L. Microbiome and skin biology. *Curr Opin Allergy Clin Immunol.* 2019;19(4):328–333.

42. Clausen ML, Agner T, Lilje B, Edsley SM, Johannesen TB, Andersen PS. Association of disease severity with skin microbiome and filaggrin gene mutations in adult atopic dermatitis. *JAMA Dermatol.* 2018;154(3):293–300.

43. Kong HH, Oh J, Deming C, Conlan S, Grice EA, Beatson MA, et al. Temporal shifts in the skin microbiome associated with disease flares and treatment in children with atopic dermatitis. *Genome Res.* 2012;22(5):850–859.

44. Marrs T, Flohr C. The role of skin and gut microbiota in the development of atopic eczema. *Br J Dermatol.* 2016;175(Suppl 2):13–18.

45. Egert M, Simmering R, Riedel CU. The association of the skin microbiota with health, immunity, and disease. *Clin Pharmacol Ther.* 2017;102(1):62–69.

46. Patra V, Byrne SN, Wolf P. The skin microbiome: is it affected by UV-induced immune suppression? *Front Microbiol.* 2016;7:1235.

47. Igawa S, Di Nardo A. Skin microbiome and mast cells. *Transl Res.* 2017;184:68–76.

48. Picardo M, Ottaviani M. Skin microbiome and skin disease: the example of rosacea. *J Clin Gastroenterol.* 2014;48(Suppl 1):S85–S86.

49. Park T, Kim HJ, Myeong NR, et al. Collapse of human scalp microbiome network in dandruff and seborrhoeic dermatitis. *Exp Dermatol.* 2017;26(9):835–838.

50. Paulino LC. New perspectives on dandruff and seborrheic dermatitis: lessons we learned from bacterial and fungal skin microbiota. *Eur J Dermatol.* 2017;27(S1):4–7.

51. Thio HB. The Microbiome in Psoriasis and Psoriatic Arthritis: The Skin Perspective. *J Rheumatol Suppl.* 2018;94:30–31.

52. Takeshita J, Grewal S, Langan SM, et al. Psoriasis and comorbid diseases: Implications for management. *J Am Acad Dermatol.* 2017;76(3):393–403.

53. Fry L, Baker BS. Triggering psoriasis: the role of infections and medications. *Clin Dermatol.* 2007;25(6):606–615.

54. Langan EA, Griffiths CEM, Solbach W, et al. The role of the microbiome in psoriasis: moving from disease description to treatment prediction? *Br J Dermatol.* 2018;178(5):1020–1027.

55. Wang WM, Jin HZ. Skin microbiome: an actor in the pathogenesis of psoriasis. *Chin Med J (Engl).* 2018;131(1):95–98.

56. Gao Z, Tseng CH, Strober BE, et al. Substantial alterations of the cutaneous bacterial biota in psoriatic lesions. *PLoS One.* 2008;3(7):e2719.

57. Alekseyenko AV, Perez-Perez GI, De Souza A, et al. Community differentiation of the cutaneous microbiota in psoriasis. *Microbiome.* 2013;1(1):31.

58. Fahlén A, Engstrand L, Baker BS, et al. Comparison of bacterial microbiota in skin biopsies from normal and psoriatic skin. *Arch Dermatol Res.* 2012;304(1):15–22.

59. Paetzold B, Willis JR, Pereira de Lima J, et al. Skin microbiome modulation induced by probiotic solutions. *Microbiome.* 2019;7(1):95.

60. Sherwani MA, Tufail S, Muzaffar AF, et al. The skin microbiome and immune system: Potential target for chemoprevention? *Photodermatol Photoimmunol Photomed.* 2018;34(1):25–34.

61. Prescott SL, Logan AC. Transforming life: a broad view of the developmental origins of health and disease concept from an ecological justice perspective. *Int J Environ Res Public Health.* 2016;13(11). pii: E1075.

CHAPTER 5

Intrinsic Aging

Leslie S. Baumann, MD

SUMMARY POINTS

What's Important?
1. There is much overlap between intrinsic and extrinsic aging.
2. Keratinocyte and fibroblast functions change with aging.
3. Senescent cells develop a secretory phenotype that accelerates aging.

What's New?
1. Emerging research is demonstrating the importance of the "tissue skeleton," consisting of fibroblasts and their attachments to the ECM molecules.
2. Lipofuscin contributes to skin aging by reducing the activity of the proteasome.
3. Autophagy decreases the rate of aging. Mitochondrial autophagy is especially important.

What's Coming?
1. Research evaluating the effects of mechanoforces between fibroblasts and the ECM and ascertaining how these change with age.
2. Understanding the changes in mechanoforces and how they affect genetic expression and fibroblast function.
3. Identifying epigenetic methylation patterns of aged skin.
4. Controlling macroautophagy of mitochondria may be an anti-aging strategy in the future.
5. Timely clearance of senescent cells before they create too much damage may be an approach to prevent skin aging.

There are two main causes of skin aging, intrinsic and extrinsic. The extrinsic causes can be decreased by changing lifestyle habits (see Chapter 6, Extrinsic Aging). Intrinsic aging is caused by internal cellular processes that occur due to daily metabolism and normal cellular processes. The etiology of intrinsic aging can be influenced with diet, exercise, oral supplements, topical treatments, and lifestyle habits but cannot be completely eliminated. There is much overlap between intrinsic and extrinsic aging. This chapter will discuss cellular processes and hormonal changes that affect the skin in the absence of sun and pollution exposure.[1] However, for a more complete explanation of aging, please consider this material and Chapter 6 in tandem, because some of the issues discussed in the extrinsic aging chapter apply here as well.

CHANGES TO SKIN STRUCTURE IN INTRINSIC AGING

Intrinsically aged skin is smooth, finely wrinkled, thinner, more fragile, and less elastic than younger skin. Intrinsically aged skin is seen in body areas not exposed to the sun and does not exhibit solar lentigos and other pigmentation changes associated with sun exposure. Although studies compare data from sun-exposed areas to those not exposed to the sun to elucidate the effects of intrinsic and extrinsic aging, there is much overlap because all skin withstands some sort of environmental exposure. However, there are characteristics unique to sun-protected aged skin.

Changes to the Epidermis

Keratinocytes are dynamic and change between phenotypes that display stemness, proliferation, differentiation, and senescence. The epidermis is a self-renewing tissue that relies upon the keratinocytes that exhibit stemness (i.e., that function as stem cells) to repopulate the epidermal layers. As aged keratinocytes display less stemness, the epidermis becomes thinner and develops flattening of the rete pattern. Young keratinocytes that have a high self-renewal capacity *in vitro* exhibit a high level of the epidermal stem cell marker β1 integrin, while older keratinocytes express much less of this stem cell marker. Keratinocytes that demonstrate stemness do not divide infinitely and do not remain as stem cells forever. At some point they lose the ability to divide, undergo cell division arrest known as replicative senescence, and become senescent cells.[2] Aged skin manifests an increased number of senescent keratinocytes. Senescent keratinocytes assume the senescent-associated secretory phenotype (SASP) that realizes inflammatory factors and degrading enzymes that are now believed to be the major cause of skin aging.

Changes to the Stratum Corneum

The stratum corneum (SC) normally has an acidic pH in younger skin and is referred to as the "acid mantle." The low pH is important for barrier homeostasis, SC integrity and cohesion, antimicrobial defense, cytokine activation, and proper functioning of enzymes and proteases. Under normal conditions the pH gradient in the upper SC ranges from 4.5 to 5.0 and the lower SC 6.5 to 7.0. Studies on older skin have consistently shown an increased pH on the skin's surface as compared to younger skin.

Changes to the Skin Barrier

The aged skin barrier is disrupted more easily and repaired more slowly than in younger skin due to a deficiency in lipids such as cholesterol, ceramides, and fatty acids.[3] It has been estimated that aged skin has one-third less lipid weight percentage than younger skin.[4] The activity of enzymes involved in lipid biosynthesis such as acid sphingomyelinase and ceramide synthase are decreased in aged skin. This matches the fact that the genes that play a role in lipid biosynthesis are downregulated in aged skin. Older skin also demonstrates a decrease in the intercellular lamella of the bilayer membrane of the SC and diminished lamellar body secretion.[4]

In younger skin, there is a calcium gradient with lower levels of calcium in the basal and spinous layers of the epidermis and higher levels at the granular layer. Calcium guides the terminal differentiation of keratinocytes as they approach the skin's surface. This epidermal calcium gradient is believed to guide the secretion of lamellar bodies. In aged skin, the calcium gradient disappears with equal amounts of calcium throughout the epidermis, which affects differentiation, lamellar body secretion, and the integrity of the skin barrier.

Changes to the Dermal-Epidermal Junction

The dermal-epidermal junction (DEJ) provides structural support between the epidermis and dermis and provides a highly dynamic microenvironment that changes with aging. The DEJ flattens in intrinsically aged skin; the rete ridge height declines and the number of papillae decreases. A flattened DEJ leads to a diminished surface area for nutrients, cells, and signaling molecules to traverse. Reduced adhesion of the epidermal basal keratinocytes to the underlying dermis results in less resistance to mechanical shearing forces. The DEJ is also a place where growth factors are held in reservoir by a perlecan/heparan sulfate (HS) structure that breaks down with aging and the presence of heparanase. Aging in the DEJ yields skin fragility, decreased transport between the epidermis and dermis, and impeded cellular communication.[5]

Changes to the Dermis

The loss of all types of collagen occurs with intrinsic aging, and leads to thinner, fragile skin with fine lines. Many studies have shown that levels of Type I collagen in the dermis correspond to the skin's appearance. Most cosmeceutical products and procedures aim to increase skin collagen.

Aged dermis demonstrates decreased recoil and elasticity. The changes in elastin tissue vary in intrinsically aged skin as compared to extrinsically aged skin, which displays elastosis. In intrinsic aging, the fibrillin-rich microfibrils in the papillary dermis that impart skin elasticity are degraded in a process that involves fibulin-5. In addition, aged skin has decreased levels of the lysyl oxidase enzyme required to produce elastin precursors.[6]

The role of the extracellular matrix (ECM) in aging is becoming clearer with recent studies. It is now known that the matrisome, or microenvironment of the ECM, plays a critical role in skin aging. The glycosaminoglycans of the ECM are involved in cell-to-cell communication, water retention, and the tissue skeleton infrastructure. Loss of hyaluronic acid (HA) is usually seen in extrinsically aged skin but is mentioned here because old fibroblasts produce fewer of all ECM components, including HA. When ECM components such as HA, HS, and collagen levels are decreased, fibroblasts become compacted, lose the ability to synthesize proteins and other ECM components, and act like senescent cells. Gene expression in the fibroblasts changes.[7] Emerging research is demonstrating the importance of the "tissue skeleton," consisting of fibroblasts and their attachments to the ECM molecules (see Fig. 2–3 in Chapter 2, Basic Science of the Dermis). The linkages of the fibroblasts to the ECM are intricate.[7] When the tissue skeleton is diminished, there is less contact area between fibroblasts and the ECM and the fibroblasts' ability to generate a mechanical force on the tissue skeleton is impaired. The lack of mechanical force on the tissue skeleton results in changes in chromatin expression and histone deacetylation activity. Glycosaminoglycans such as HA and HS play an important role in the tissue skeleton.

HS is a proteoglycan found in the ECM that facilitates cell-to-cell communication by helping growth factors find and bind receptors. Chains of HS form perlecan, a component of the basement membrane. Perlecan is a reservoir that stores and regulates the release of growth factors such as fibroblast growth factors as well as vascular endothelial growth factor-A (VEGF-A). When perlecan is broken down by heparanase, its ability to hold growth factors falters. Heparanase levels increase with sun exposure; however, it can also be stimulated by inflammatory cytokines in the absence of UV exposure.[8]

MOLECULAR MECHANISMS IN SKIN AGING

While discrete phenomena, the causes of intrinsic and extrinsic aging can be inextricably linked, and there are notably similar mechanisms within each type of aging that provoke the cutaneous changes characteristic of aged skin. The mainstay of anti-aging skincare is to increase production of proteins, saccharides, and glycoproteins and prevent the processes that break them down. The most common proteins discussed in skin aging science are collagen and elastin while the most common saccharides are HA and HS; however, there are several components in the ECM that decrease or lose function with aging. **Fig. 5-1** shows an overview of how time and reactive oxygen species (ROS) lead to a decrease in skin collagen and elastin.

There are various cellular and molecular processes and pathways that play a role in skin aging and much overlap among them as they may upregulate and downregulate each other. These processes involved in skin aging are discussed in alphabetical order to facilitate cross-referencing.

Advanced Glycation End Products (AGEs)

When sugar binds to protein in a process called the Maillard reaction, advanced glycation end products (AGEs) are formed. The nonenzymatic glycosylation aging theory is used to explain why people with diabetes tend to manifest signs of aged skin as compared to those who do not have diabetes.[9] AGEs accumulate in aging skin, damage collagen and elastin, and promote skin aging.[10,11] AGEs can be produced in the absence of sugar when the dicarbonyl compounds glyoxal (GO) and methylglyoxal (MG) react with proteins.[12] The enzyme glyoxalase detoxifies GO and MG and becomes less efficient with age allowing the accumulation of AGEs.

Collagen Glycation

Glycation of collagen and other proteins plays an important role in aging. (This is not to be confused with glycosylation of collagen, which is an enzyme-mediated process in the intracellular step of collagen biosynthesis.) Glycation is a nonenzymatic series of biologic events that involves adding a reducing sugar molecule (such as glucose or fructose) to proteins. This cascade of events is known as the Maillard reaction, which is the same reaction that occurs when onions are caramelized or bread is toasted. It is well known to chefs because it imparts flavor to foods. However, in skin, the Maillard reaction resulting in glycation of skin proteins is undesirable and leads to cutaneous aging. In glycation, a sugar molecule reacts with the amino group side chains of lysine and arginine in collagen and other proteins. Subsequently, the product of this process undergoes oxidative reactions resulting in the formation of AGEs (**Fig. 5-2**). AGEs have been implicated in the aging process and age-related diseases such as diabetes mellitus,[13–15] chronic renal failure,[16,17] and Alzheimer's disease.[18–20] It is believed that with time, AGEs increase, accumulate on human collagen and elastin fibers, and contribute to aging of the skin.[21–23]

As a result of glycation, collagen networks lose their ability to contract, and they become stiffer and resistant to remodeling. Fibroblasts apply contracture force on the collagen lattice

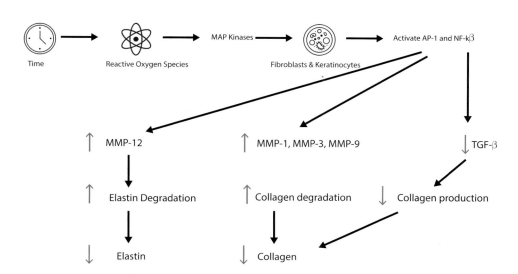

FIGURE 5-1. Normal metabolism results in the creation of ROS. With time, the buildup of ROS leads to losses of ECM proteins such as collagen and elastin. Green arrows = activation, red arrows = inhibition.

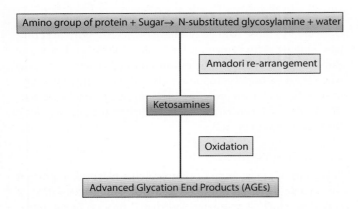

FIGURE 5-2. Glycation of proteins results in advanced glycation end products (AGEs).

via their actin cytoskeleton, which turns on gene expression.[24] Glycated collagen modifies the actin cytoskeleton of the fibroblasts, thereby diminishing their collagen contraction capacity.[25] In cell cultures, glycation of collagen used to prepare the dermal compartment has resulted in an increase in matrix metalloproteinase (MMP)-1, MMP-2, and MMP-9, thickening of the basement membrane zone, and modification of α6 and β1 integrin patterns in the epidermis.[26]

Elastin Glycation

Several AGEs can be seen when elastin is exposed to sugar. AGEs accumulate on elastin fibers and render them resistant to elastase degradation. AGE modification of elastin decreases skin elasticity by modifying the elastin sheet structure. Studies have shown that UV exposure contributes to the production of AGEs, which causes a decrease in elastin degradation resulting in the accumulation of elastotic fibers called elastosis characteristic of extrinsically aged skin. Ne-(carboxymethyl)lysine (CML) seems to be the predominant form that accumulates on elastin fibers and makes them resistant to elastase degradation.[11] CML is higher in sun-exposed skin as compared to sun-protected skin.[23] AGE-modified proteins act as endogenous photosensitizers in human skin via oxidative stress mechanisms induced by UVA light.[27,28]

Metformin

Metformin is an oral medication widely used to treat diabetes by lowering blood glucose levels. Its topical absorption is limited. In an *in vitro* fibroblast model, addition of metformin to cell cultures led to decreased apoptosis, increased production of collagen Types I and II, and decreased levels of NF-κβ. When metformin was placed in solid liponanoparticles to increase topical penetration, it attenuated fibroblast senescence.[29] Another study on human dermal fibroblasts showed that addition of metformin to cultures prior to UVA exposure decreased the production of free radicals as well as MMP-1 and MMP-3, and decreased expression of collagen Type 1 mRNA that is usually seen with UVA exposure.[30]

Autophagy

Autophagy is the process of cellular self-digestion that involves delivering cytoplasmic material into lysosomes for degradation.[31,32] It serves the purpose of eliminating damaged organelles, proteins, and pathogens, as well as regulating apoptosis, cell differentiation, immunity, and inflammation. Therefore, autophagy slows the rate of aging by maintaining cellular homeostasis and removing substances that stimulate or cause aging. It diminishes with age, thus contributing to an aged phenotype.[33,34] Autophagy regulates ECM metabolism by modulating MMPs. Blocking autophagy leads to an increase in MMPs and an increase in collagen breakdown. TGF-β is involved in the regulation of autophagy.[34] Maintenance of the ability for mitochondria to practice autophagy is particularly important in preventing aging.

Autophagy is subject to circadian rhythms and is induced by nutrient starvation, oxidative stress, infection, and two protein kinases (unc-51-like kinase complex and the phosphatidylinositol 3-kinase complex).[35,36] There are three forms of autophagy: microautophagy, chaperone-assisted autophagy, and macroautophagy. Microautophagy occurs with invagination of the endosomal membrane that traps and degrades material. Chaperone-mediated autophagy requires a chaperone molecule that binds the material, unfolds it, and binds it to the lysosomal lumen via a lysosome-associated membrane protein (LAMP). Macroautophagy is controlled by autophagy-related proteins and involved in packaging the unwanted material in double-membraned autophagosomes in the cytoplasm.[37] Macroautophagy is the process that removes dysfunctional mitochondria.

Autophagy is seen in both proliferating and differentiating keratinocytes and supports the maintenance of keratinocyte stem cells. It promotes the removal of oxidized molecules, improves nucleotide excision repair, and removes lipofuscin.[38,39] Autophagy levels in aged human dermal fibroblasts are significantly lower than those of young fibroblasts. Loss of autophagy and the capacity to remove oxidized or misfolded proteins leads to the induction of cellular senescence. (Cellular senescence leads to aging as discussed below.) Upregulation of autophagy is thought to contribute to the prolongation of lifespan seen with caloric restriction.

Increasing autophagy, especially in mitochondria, is an anti-aging strategy. Genetically increasing autophagy delays aging in flies, worms, and mice.[40] Substances that induce autophagy such as lithium and trehalose have been shown in nematodes and mice to improve mitochondrial function, reduce senescence, and expand the lifespan.

Sirtuin-1 (SIRT-1) mediates the effects of caloric restriction on health and longevity. SIRT-1 is activated by resveratrol. Activation of SIRT-1 induces autophagy as do resveratrol and melatonin.[41,42]

DNA Damage

Age-related increases in DNA damage and structural chromosomal mutations are seen in aged senescent fibroblasts. Accumulation of oxidative damage is one reason for this. UV radiation causes DNA mutations (see Chapter 6). The capacity for DNA repair decreases with age.

Extracellular Vesicles

Extracellular vesicles (EVs) are lipid bilayer bound vesicles secreted by cells. There are numerous EV subtypes of which exosomes are the smallest and most studied. DNA damage results in a p53-dependent increase in EV secretion.[43] EVs can cross from the dermis to epidermis and function as a conduit of communication between keratinocytes, melanocytes, and fibroblasts.[44]

EVs can carry multiple types of cargo between cells such as proteases (MMPs), inflammatory cytokines, growth factors, and functional RNA. EVs can deliver miRNA from SASPs to surrounding cells. They have even been found to carry mitochondrial DNA and genomic DNA.

EV production can occur in multiple cell types after senescence-inducing stimuli. Senescent cells (SCs) are deleterious because they secrete MMPs and other factors that age skin. SCs turn into a dynamic SASP that is currently believed to be the primary cause of aging. The SASPs release EVs, which is how the SASPs mainly affect cells around them, leading to aging. Circulating EVs have been shown to be increased in older individuals as compared to younger people.[45]

Fibroblast Interactions

In young skin, fibroblasts adhere to the ECM, containing Type I collagen, and use this infrastructure to spread itself in an elongated shape and exert mechanical forces on the surrounding ECM (see Chapter 2). With time and sun exposure, the ECM is degraded, collagen I levels decrease, and the ability of the fibroblasts to adhere declines. This results in compacted fibroblasts with a collapsed morphology that are less able to synthesize ECM components. This self-perpetuating cycle has other consequences such as increased ROS production by mitochondria, activation of activator protein-1 (AP-1), and elevation of MMPs. When the ECM components are renewed, the fibroblasts regain their elongated appearance. This illustrates the importance of the entire ECM on skin aging.[46]

Growth Factors

There are multiple growth factors involved in aging but transforming growth factor-β (TGF-β) is one of the prominent ones because it controls collagen production and degradation via the Smad pathway. Activation of the TGF-β/Smad signaling pathway turns on the genes involved in the synthesis of collagens, fibronectin, decorin, and versican. The TGF-β/Smad signaling network also upregulates the tissue inhibitor of metalloproteinases (TIMPs) and downregulates MMPs. Impairment of the TGF-β/Smad signaling pathway leads to skin aging. In skin, ROS upregulate AP-1 expression, which directly inhibits the TGF-β/Smad pathway (see **Fig. 5-3**). This is one of several mechanisms by which ROS cause cutaneous aging.[46] Growth factors are discussed in Chapter 37, Anti-Aging Ingredients.

Inflammation

There are myriad causes of inflammation. The presence of ROS has long been known to lead to inflammation. UV exposure, the immune system, cytokines such as TNF, and other endogenous mediators like IL-1 all contribute to inflammation. This is such a significant cause of aging that it is referred to as "inflammaging," characterized by elevated levels of blood inflammatory markers that carry a high susceptibility to inflammation-related disorders such as heart disease and diabetes. Causes of inflammaging include a genetic predilection, central obesity, increased gut permeability, dysfunctional mitochondria, immune cell dysregulation, and chronic infections.[47] Senescent cells contribute significantly to aging because they develop the detrimental SASP phenotype (see the senescent cells section of this chapter).[48] Inflammation will

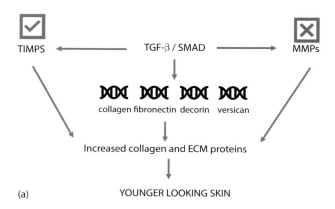

FIGURE 5-3A. Activation of the TGF-β/Smad signaling pathway turns on the genes involved in the synthesis of collagens, fibronectin, decorin, and versican. The TGF-β/Smad signaling network upregulates TIMPs and downregulates MMPs resulting in increased collagen production and decreased collagen breakdown. This results in younger-looking skin.

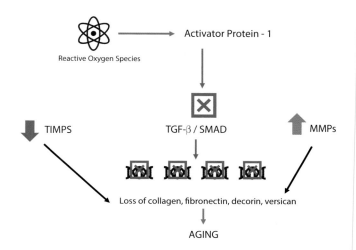

FIGURE 5-3B. ROS increase the expression of AP-1. This inhibits the TGF-β/Smad signaling pathway leading to loss of ECM proteins including collagen. This results in aged skin.

be discussed more in depth in Chapters 13, Sensitive Skin, and 37, Anti-Aging Ingredients.

Lipofuscin

The word "lipofuscin" is derived from the Greek work *lipo* (lipids) and the Latin word *fuscus* (dark). Lipofuscin is a waste material of intracellular structures that has been broken down into proteins, lipids, and carbohydrates. For years, before epigenetics and telomeres were discovered, lipofuscin staining was the method used to determine the age of cells. Studies are showing that lipofuscin production is related to the presence of ROS generated by autophagocytosis of mitochondria. Lipofuscin accumulation in fibroblasts renders them more susceptible to free radical damage with less lysosomal degradation of waste.[49] Lipofuscin is not degradable and accrues in the lysosomes of older cells. Fibroblast autophagy is required for the removal of lipofuscin.[39] It is believed that lipofuscin contributes to skin aging by reducing the activity of the proteasome.

Lysosomes

Lysosomes are the garbage disposals/recycle bins of the cell; their role is to eliminate dysfunctional cell parts. There are three major autophagy pathways that deliver substrate to lysosomes (see the autophagy section): macroautophagy, chaperone-mediated autophagy, and microautophagy.

Aging causes decreased function of lysosomes and their enzymes. One reason for this is that aged skin manifests an increased number of senescent cells, and senescent cells exhibit significant changes in their lysosomes: they increase in number and size due to indigestible material such as lipofuscin. Senescent cells display dysfunctional lysosomal activity, which is related to an increase in lipofuscin and production of EVs.

Reduced function of lysosomes decreases mitochondrial autophagy, which disrupts mitochondrial turnover.[40] Non-autophagocytosed mitochondria produce ROS. The accumulation of ROS forms lipofuscin. Diminished lysosomal activity promotes further oxidation of lipids and proteins, thereby increasing lipofuscin production. This self-perpetuating cycle is known as the lysosomal-mitochondrial axis.[40] (See **Fig. 5-4**.)

Lysosomes contain many enzymes that depend on a low pH (4.5–5). Changes in pH of the lysosome affect function. A raised pH (6.0) results in decreased activity of several lysosomal enzymes and diminished autophagy. Raising the pH results in an increase in EV production, while lowering lysosomal pH results in decreased EV formation. EVs are one of the major communication systems used by SASPs (see the senescent cell section) to transport messages to other cells that are believed to increase aging. A reduced pH in the lysosome (6.0) lowers the activity of senescence-associated β-galactosidase (SA-β-gal). Overexpression of β-galactosidase is used as a surrogate marker for an increase in lysosome number and size associated with senescence.[50]

MicroRNA

Ninety-eight percent of the human genome contains instructions for noncoding RNA that was once thought of as nonfunctional. We now know these are important. There are several

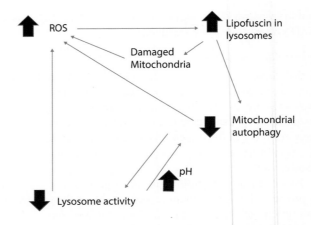

FIGURE 5-4. Lysosomes and mitochondria affect each other. When one is damaged, the other is impaired, leading to aging. Young looking skin requires healthy lysosomes and mitochondria.

categories of noncoding RNAs, one of which is microRNA (miRNA). miRNAs are small single-stranded RNA molecules that are post-transcriptional negative regulators of gene expression. They block translation and cleave mRNA targets. miRNAs are involved in all cellular processes including aging. Some examples are seen in the list in **Table 5-1**.

As seen in **Table 5-1**, many miRNA pathways have been identified that factor into human keratinocyte and fibroblast senescence. Long-term UVB exposure, pollution, and other exposures alter the expression of miRNAs, as does intrinsic aging.[56] One example is the miR-34 family: miR-34 in human dermal fibroblast (HDF) cells regulates cell function and expression of MMP-1, the Type 1 collagen (COL1A1) gene, and elastin production. miRNA 378b inhibits mRNA expression of COL1A1 by interfering with Sirtuin-6 (SIRT-6) in human dermal fibroblasts, while miRNA 217 regulates the senescence of human skin fibroblasts by directly targeting DNA methyltransferase. miR-23a-3p controls cellular senescence by targeting enzymes to control HA synthesis. Some miRNAs have been shown to be associated with longer life spans such as lin-4, let-7, miR-17, and miR-34: these are known as longevity-related miRNAs.[57] Many studies thus show that microRNAs regulate the skin aging process.[1,58]

MicroRNA is one of the ways that SASP cells communicate with surrounding cells. EVs can carry microRNA to other cells resulting in a paracrine senescence effect on surrounding cells. The most often secreted miRNAs from SASP cells target pro-apoptotic transcription factors, suggesting a role for EV-packaged miRNAs as anti-apoptotic members of the SASP.[44]

Mitochondrial Function

Mitochondria can be thought of as the powerhouses and fuel tanks of cells because these double-membraned organelles synthesize the ATP used by cells as chemical energy. Mitochondria produce energy through oxygen-dependent mitochondrial respiration (also called oxidative phosphorylation) that results

TABLE 5-1	miRNAs Involved in Cellular Aging		
miRNA[51–55]	Action	Skin Section	Genes Affected
miR-203	Promotes differentiation by restricting proliferation	Epidermis	P63, Skp2, Msi2
miR-720	Epidermal differentiation	Suprabasal epidermis	P63, iASPP
miR-574-3p	Epidermal differentiation	Suprabasal epidermis	P63, iASPP
miR-34a, miR-34c	Inhibit keratinocyte proliferation	Epidermis	
miR-205	Keratinocyte survival, cell migration, and cytoskeletal reorganization	Epidermis	
miR-194	Inhibits TGF-β/Smad pathway	Dermis	
miR-302b-3p	Accelerates fibroblast senescence, suppresses SIRT-1	Dermis	JNK2
miR-152	Induces senescence	Dermal fibroblasts	
miR-181a	Induces senescence, increases collagen XVI synthesis	Dermal fibroblasts	
miR-34	Activates MMPs (collagenase)	Dermis	
miR-137	Increases senescence-associated β-galactosidase activity	Epidermal keratinocytes	p53, ERK
miR-668	Increases senescence-associated β-galactosidase activity	Epidermal keratinocytes	p53

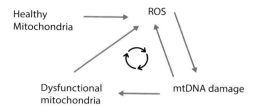

FIGURE 5-5. Mutations of mitochondrial DNA (mtDNA) result in an increase in ROS and dysfunction of mitochondria that engenders production of more ROS causing a destructive feedback loop.

respiration depends upon Ca^{2+}. Increasing Ca^{2+} also increases keratinocyte differentiation, which illustrates the relationship of the mitochondria to keratinocyte differentiation. Terminal differentiation of keratinocytes is associated with activation of the mitochondrial caspase-dependent apoptotic pathway.[60]

A melatonin-mitochondrial axis exists in the skin in which a symbiotic relationship manifests. Cutaneous melatonin biosynthesis and metabolism occur in cutaneous mitochondria. At the same time, melatonin increases the electron flux through the mitochondrial respiratory chain and enhances ATP production by donating electrons. A lysosome-mitochondrial axis also exists in which they both affect the function of the other (see the lysosome and senescence sections for further discussion).

Mitochondrial dysfunction is a hallmark of aging and results in oxidative stress, decreased ATP levels, increased lipofuscin in lysosomes, and calcium imbalances. Aged cells contain mitochondria with increased mass and size caused by a functional decline due to increased ROS. This large mitochondrial size may be one reason decreased macroautophagy is seen in older mitochondria (see the autophagy section).

Mitochondria generate ROS during their normal functions. Aged fibroblast mitochondria demonstrate decreased activity in Complex II of the electron transport chain (this is not seen in keratinocytes),[61] which causes an increase in ROS. These free radicals damage the mitochondrial membranes and leak out of the mitochondria to attack nearby structures. In other words, normal cellular function causes damage to mitochondria and surrounding structures (such as lysosomes) via ROS. This oxidative damage plays a role in both aging and cancer.

Mitochondria have their own DNA called mitochondrial DNA (mtDNA) that is derived from the mother. These mtDNA are highly susceptible to mutations from exposure to UV or ROS. Aged mitochondria are characterized by mutations and deletions in mtDNA, the most common of which is a 4977 base pair deletion known as the "common deletion."[59] The common deletion, increased in extrinsically aged (sunexposed) cells, leads to increased production of ROS. Once these mutations occur, mitochondrial function is hampered. The production of ROS causes a negative feedback loop that generates more ROS (**Fig. 5-5**).

The lysosomal-mitochondrial axis plays a critical role in aging and generation of senescent cells. Decreased lysosomal function reduces mitochondrial function, which further reduces lysosomal function.

in the production of ATP from ADP. ATP is produced in the electron transport chain located in the inner membrane of the mitochondria. Mitochondria are critical for microbial defense, glycolysis, and energy production and are involved in fatty acid oxidation, heme and steroid biosynthesis, apoptosis, and calcium signaling.

Mitochondria play a regulatory role in differentiation of cell lineages and are essential to skin homeostasis. The epidermis is a self-renewing layer that constantly utilizes energy to produce more keratinocytes and to differentiate and migrate. Mitochondrial respiration is necessary for keratinocyte differentiation and results in the formation of ROS.[59] Mitochondrial

Coenzyme Q_{10} is part of the electron transport chain of the mitochondria and plays an important role in shuttling electrons between different complexes of the mitochondria. CoQ_{10} levels are much higher in the epidermis compared to the dermis. Reduced CoQ_{10} levels in the skin occur with age and are associated with lower activity of the mitochondrial complexes I/III and increased generation of ROS.[62] This is reversed by exogenous CoQ_{10}, either oral supplements or topical cosmeceuticals.

Damaged mitochondria are cleared away in a pathway called macroautophagy. Controlling macroautophagy may be an anti-aging strategy in the future. A groundbreaking study in mice showed that mitochondrial dysfunction resulted in wrinkled skin that became unwrinkled when mitochondrial function was restored.[63] Revitalizing the lysosomal-mitochondrial axis is required to revert cells from senescence back to a more youthful cell type. This can be achieved by decreasing the pH of the lysosome, which increases the decomposition of mitochondrial fragments, restores autophagy, and decreases the number of senescent cells (see **Fig. 5-6**).[40] Supplementation with the oxidized form of cellular nicotinamide adenine dinucleotide (NAD+) in mice stem cells leads to mitochondrial functional recovery and prevents senescence of stem cells.[64]

Matrix Metalloproteinases

The MMPs, which include a large family of zinc-dependent endopeptidases, are crucial to the turnover of ECM components. MMPs can be produced by endothelial cells as well as immune cells and, more commonly, by keratinocytes and fibroblasts.

Collagenases

Interstitial collagenase, or MMP-1, was the first enzyme discovered in this group. MMP-1 is secreted from fibroblasts and is mainly involved in the degradation of collagen Types I, II, III, and VII. It is the most important enzyme that degrades collagen. Once collagen is cleaved by MMP-1 it is further broken down by MMP-3 and MMP-9.[65]

Human neutrophil collagenase (MMP-8), another type of collagenase, is engaged in cleaving collagen Types I and III. Collagenase-3 (MMP-13) is the third member of this group of enzymes, and it is known to fragment fibrillar collagens. It is also believed to have a role in scarless wound healing by enhancing fibroblast proliferation and survival.[65]

Gelatinases

Gelatinases consist of two types of enzymes, gelatinase A (MMP-2) and gelatinase B (MMP-9), which are responsible for attacking gelatin and collagen Type IV in the basement membrane.

Stromelysins

Stromelysins include MMP-3, MMP-10, and MMP-11. These are mainly involved in degradation of proteoglycans, laminins, and collagen Type IV.

Matrilysins

Matrilysins are MMP-7 and MMP-26, which are expressed on stromal tissue, fetal skin, and in the setting of carcinomas.[66]

Membrane Type MMPs

Membrane type (MT) MMPs include MMP-14, MMP-15, and MMP-16.

Tissue Inhibitor of Metalloproteinases

The activity of MMPs is regulated by endogenous TIMPs. TIMPs are naturally produced proteins that specifically inhibit the MMPs. There are four such protease inhibitors: TIMP-1, TIMP-2, TIMP-3, and TIMP-4. TIMPs help control MMPs and keep the balance between synthesis and degradation; however, in skin aging this balance is lost and MMPs outnumber TIMPs.[66]

The balance between MMPs and their inhibition by TIMPs leads to proper tissue remodeling. TIMPs are regulated via expression of cytokines (such as IL-1), growth factors, and even retinoids.[66] Retinoids have been shown to provoke a two- to threefold increase in the biosynthesis of human fibroblast-derived TIMPs *in vitro*.[66] Increased production of MMPs and decreased production of TIMPs have a role in the metastatic behavior of tumors. Synthetic inhibitors of MMPs are of interest to investigators especially in cancer research. These inhibitors, such as hydroxamates, contain a zinc-chelating group that binds to the active site of MMPs leading to its

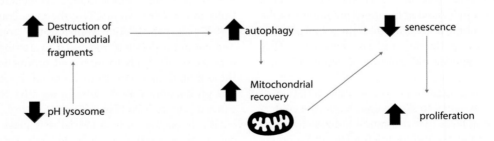

FIGURE 5-6. Decreasing the pH of the lysosome increases the destruction of mitochondrial fragments, restores autophagy, and decreases the number of senescent cells. This results in mitochondrial recovery and an increase in cell proliferation, thus returning to a healthier state.

inhibition. Currently, their use is mostly limited to research studies because of their side-effect profile. Certain medications such as doxycycline are also known for their inhibitory effect on MMPs and have been studied in myriad MMP-related conditions such as periodontal and atherosclerotic diseases.

Oxidative Stress and Reactive Oxygen Species (Free Radicals)

Oxidative stress contributes significantly to cutaneous aging. It is caused by ROS, also known as free radicals, which are reactive molecules that contain an oxygen atom. Free radicals are a vital part of metabolism and are generated by normal cellular functions. Examples of free radicals include hydroxyl (OH•), superoxide (O_2-), nitric oxide (NO•), thyl (RS•), and peroxyl (RO•). Peroxynitrite (ONOO−), hypochlorous acid (HOCl), hydrogen peroxide (H_2O_2), singlet oxygen ($1O_2$), and ozone (O_3) can easily become free radicals.[67]

External and internal factors such as the mitochondria's oxidative metabolism, UV exposure, and other insults lead to the production of ROS. The accumulation of ROS engenders DNA damage, induces inflammation, reduces antioxidant enzymes, and activates nuclear factor-kappa B (NF-κB) and AP-1, all of which inhibit collagen production and increase MMPs that break down proteins in the dermis.[68] Antioxidants, both endogenous and exogenous, combat ROS, but these are easily exhausted, thus requiring continuous replacement. Oxidative stress and antioxidants are discussed in Chapter 39, Antioxidants.

p53

The TP53 gene (also known as p53) is a tumor suppressor gene that is also an important inducer of organismal aging. The TP53 gene modulates cellular senescence, apoptosis, and DNA repair. Increased activity of p53 has been directly tied to skin changes with aging; increased expression of p53-mediated skin aging increases the loss of subdermal fat and decreases sebaceous gland activity; p53 is commonly discussed in the epigenetic literature.[69] One study found that methylation of the p53 promoter was controlled by the miR-377–DNMT1 axis (see epigenetic discussion below).[70] DNMT1 causes methylation of CnG islands resulting in reduced expression of p53. Inhibition of DNMT1 augments p53 expression and cellular senescence in human skin fibroblasts, resulting in skin aging.[71]

Proteostasis

The quality control of protein synthesis is known as proteome homeostasis or proteostasis. Loss of proteostasis results in accumulation of oxidized proteins or glycated proteins and is seen in aged fibroblasts.[72,73] Oxidation of proteins occurs when they are exposed to ROS. Glycated proteins arise in the presence of glucose and ROS (see the AGEs section). Unless the oxidized proteins or AGEs are removed or repaired by the proteosome or autophagy, they amass in cells causing deleterious effects such as skin aging. Modified proteins are found in the mitochondria of senescent fibroblasts and affect energy metabolism, quality control stress response, and

cytoskeletal organization. The accrual of oxidized proteins in aged fibroblasts is related to an impaired function of the 20S proteasome.[74] Impaired proteosomes cause dysfunction of mitochondria and inhibition of mitochondrial function, which in turn impairs the proteosome.[75] Autophagy plays an important role in proteostasis. Proteosome activity is controlled by circadian rhythm.

Senescent Cells

Fibroblast and keratinocyte cells can be found in five different phases: stem, proliferation, differentiation, senescence, and apoptosis. Senescent cells have gone into cell cycle arrest, stay viable and functional, and are not eliminated from the skin as are apoptotic cells. Senescent cells have lost the ability to proliferate but have not undergone apoptosis. Senescent cells are known to be the main drivers of the age-related phenotype.[76]

Senescent human skin fibroblasts lose the youthful spindle-like shape and become enlarged as well as flattened in cell cultures, with pronounced changes in their lysosomes and mitochondria, both of which lose functionality.[77,78] Senescent cells collect in older skin due to age-related decline of senescent cell removal systems such as the immune system and the autophagy-lysosomal pathway.[79,80]

Senescent cells affect each other and the cells around them when they assume the SASP. The SASP creates havoc and is believed to be one of the major causes of aging. When senescent cells become the SASP, they communicate with nearby cells using proinflammatory cytokines, catabolic modulators such as MMPs, and EVs. EVs are lipid bilayer-lined vesicles that move cargo between cells, allowing cross-talk between keratinocytes, fibroblasts, and melanocytes.[81] EVs can even transport functional RNA and microRNA between cells. EVs have been shown to be able to cross over from the dermis, through the DEJ into the epidermis. EVs are partially accountable for the communication abilities of the SASP human dermal fibroblasts.[81] For example, senescent melanocytes induce telomere dysfunction and limit proliferation of surrounding basal keratinocytes,[82] while senescent fibroblasts alter melanocyte differentiation by upregulating the expression of the melanogenesis regulators MITF and tyrosinase in melanocytes.[76]

The SASP phenotype is dynamic and evolves during the stages of cellular senescence based on the influence of transcription factors such as NF-κβ. One beneficial effect of the SASP is that it increases the removal of senescent cells via immune cell recruitment.[44,83] The SASP is likely a natural tumor-suppressive mode by cells to prevent cells with cancerous mutations from undergoing replication.[84] However, the deleterious effects seem to surpass the beneficial effects when it comes to aging. SASP is the major contributor to a prolonged state of inflammation, known as "inflammaging,"[48] which is detrimental to the skin's appearance.

Senescent cells that have developed into the SASP modulate their environment via gene expression that is distinctive compared to differentiating or proliferating cells.[85] SASP cells are known to release growth factors, cytokines, chemokines, matrix-modeling enzymes, lipids, and EVs.[81] Human fibroblasts that have assumed the SASP secrete pro-inflammatory cytokines, MMPs and release ROS resulting in degradation of the surrounding ECM.[86,87] Loss of the ECM leads to fibroblast compaction and reduced DNA synthesis, all caused by SASPs (**Fig. 5-7**).

Several factors can induce cellular senescence. NRF2 is a key regulator of the skin's antioxidant defense system, which controls the transcription of genes encoding ROS-detoxifying enzymes and various other antioxidant proteins.[88] Activation of NRF2 induces cellular senescence via direct targeting of certain ECM genes. Loss of mitochondrial autophagy induces senescence as does activation of the TP53 gene, inactivity of SIRT-1, and short telomeres (**Fig. 5-8**).

Evidence shows that decreasing the number of senescent cells exerts an anti-aging effect; therefore, the goal should be to prevent senescence or turn senescent cells back to a more juvenile form (proliferating or differentiating). Removal of senescent cells postpones the onset and severity of age-related diseases and extends the life span of mice.[81,89] Timely clearance of senescent cells before they create too much damage is an approach to prevent skin aging.[90] Restoration of the lysosomal-mitochondrial axis has been shown to revert SASP back to a juvenile status. Normalization of the lysosomal-mitochondrial axis is a prerequisite to reverse senescence.[40]

Sirtuins

Silent information regulator-1 (SIRT-1) was first described as a conserved, energy-sensitive anti-aging protein that mediated the beneficial effects of calorie restriction.[91] SIRT-1 is one of seven members of the sirtuin family of nicotinamide adenine dinucleotide (NAD)-dependent deacetylases.[92] SIRT-1, a NAD-dependent histone deacetylase, is known to affect gene expression involved in modulating cellular differentiation, metabolism, immunity and stress response, as well as replicative senescence.[54]

Activation of SIRT-1 extends the lifespan in mammals, while its inactivity induces cellular senescence. SIRT-1 galvanizes the "longevity gene" FOX01, which stimulates autophagy. Macroautophagy mediates the downregulation of SIRT-1 in aging (see the earlier discussion of autophagy).[93]

SIRT-1 acts as a regulator in circadian clock genes by modulating deactylation. It is believed that SIRT-1 plays a positive role in regulating circadian rhythm and that when SIRT-1 expression is decreased, dysfunction of the circadian clock occurs. There is still more to learn about SIRT-1 and its effects on the circadian clock; however, the circadian clock plays a role in aging and its dysfunction could be one of the ways that SIRT-1 activation prevents aging.[94]

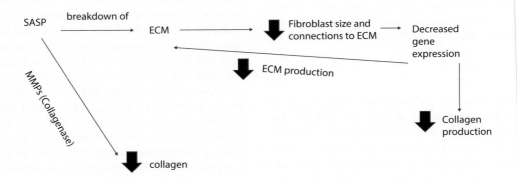

FIGURE 5-7. SASP cells secrete pro-inflammatory cytokines, MMPs, and release of ROS causing degradation of the surrounding ECM including loss of collagen.

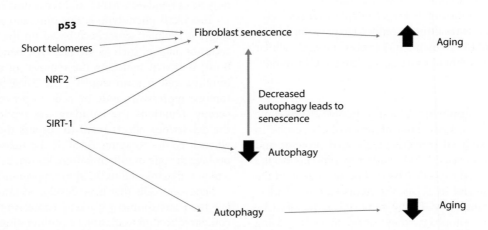

FIGURE 5-8. Cellular senescence leads to aging. Activation of SITR-1 inhibits senescence and promotes autophagy leading to more youthful cellular function and decreased aging. Loss of mitochondrial autophagy induces senescence as does activation of the p53 gene, activation of NRF2, inactivity of SIRT-1, and short telomeres. Green arrows = activation, red arrows = inhibition.

Anti-aging therapies are aimed at increasing SIRT-1 expression, which can also be accomplished by caloric restriction and exercise.[95] Resveratrol and Aquatide (a molecule based on resveratrol and pyrrolidone carboxylic acid, a natural moisturizing factor) have both been shown to activate SIRT-1.[36,41]

Decreasing or inhibiting SIRT-1 has consequences (see discussion of sirtuins). Aging is associated with a reduction in SIRT-1 levels and their protective effects, leading to numerous age-related diseases.[54,96] Prolonged insulin-like growth factor exposure inhibits SIRT-1, increases p53 acetylation, and promotes cellular senescence.[97] One major goal of anti-aging therapies is to increase SIRT-1 expression.

Stem Cells

Epidermal stem cells are found in the basal keratinocytes, appendages such as sebaceous glands, and cells present in the hair follicle such as LGR6+ cells (see Chapter 1, Basic Science of the Epidermis). In the dermis, the fibroblast can assume a stem cell phenotype and exert "stemness" behavior (see Chapter 2). Keratinocytes and fibroblasts have five modes: stem, proliferation, differentiation, senescence, or apoptosis. The microenvironment, ECM, cytokines, and growth factors around them determine the mode for these cells. Aged skin is characterized by a decline in the activity and number of cells exhibiting stemness and an increased number of senescent cells.

Telomere Shortening

Telomeres are composed of repetitive TTAGGG sequences at the ends of chromosomes. These small pieces of DNA-protein control the cell cycle. Telomeres are regulated by telomerase reverse transcriptase (TERRA) and telomerase. TERRAs provide telomere stability while telomerase is an enzyme that elongates the telomeres. The circadian clock controls TERRA and telomerase and therefore plays an important role in telomere length. Each cell division shortens the telomere, and shortened telomeres seem to cause cellular senescence. Several studies in cell cultures suggest that fibroblasts can acquire senescence when telomeres are shortened. Keratinocyte stem cells with short telomeres have been shown in some studies to have a poor proliferative capacity, which can be corrected by introducing telomerase. However, the role of telomere shortening in replicative senescence is unclear as illustrated by an observation that keratinocytes cultured for at least 100 doublings never reached replicative senescence. Most studies of telomeres in keratinocytes and fibroblasts have been conducted on cells in culture, so they may not translate to *in vivo* findings. At this time, it is believed but not certain that telomere shortening causes intrinsic aging in keratinocytes and fibroblasts.[98] There is evidence to suggest that telomeres are shortened by ROS, physiologic stress, inflammation, and other factors.

GENETICS AND AGING SKIN

In the last two decades much excitement about the role of genetics and how genes affect skin appearance has prompted several companies to make exaggerated claims about skincare products. The problem was that the science was just not there yet. We did not know which genes were important in aging and skin appearance. Studies over the last few years are pushing progress but the knowledge about epigenetics and its effects on gene expression have complicated the picture even more. Fortunately, new methods of research are beginning to shed light on which genes are important in skin appearance and function. It is still many years too early to develop skincare products targeted to "genetic deficiencies," but some trends in genetic expression changes with age are becoming clear.

Multiple studies have established that mutations in the melanocortin 1 receptor gene (MC1R) that regulates skin pigmentation, imparts red hair, and predisposes to melanoma formation also play a role in intrinsic aging. Studies show that research subjects with decreased function of the MC1R gene are perceived as an average of 2 years older when compared to those with a normally functioning MCR1 gene.[99] This is believed to be due to the fact that the MC1R gene is required to produce eumelanin, which confers antioxidant activity as opposed to the pro-oxidant pigment pheomelanin.[100] Genes involved in cellular metabolism, DNA transcription, signal transduction, and cell cycle regulation have been implicated in intrinsic aging.

In 2009, cRNA samples from sun-exposed and unexposed areas from young women (aged 19–20) and photodamaged women (aged 63–65) were compared.[101] The older skin from both groups, whether exposed to the sun or not exhibited downregulation of lipid synthesis genes, especially those involved in cholesterol and fatty acid synthesis (see **Table 5-2**). Genes associated with epidermal differentiation, keratin filaments, and cornified envelope proteins were downregulated in older skin. Both intrinsically aged and extrinsically aged skin displayed increased expression of inflammation-related genes, cytokine activity, and protease genes.

In 2013, Glass et al. looked at gene expression changes and remarked that the changes observed were tissue specific.[102] In other words, gene studies on aging must be performed in human skin to elucidate the mechanisms of skin aging. In 2018, a study demonstrated that aged skin was linked to the downregulation of genes associated with lipid biosynthesis, skin barrier integrity, mitochondrial function, cytokine production, and immune response.[103,104]

In 2018, Kimball et al. evaluated gene expression in sun-exposed and non-sun-exposed areas from 158 women who were divided into categories based on whether they looked younger, equal to, or older than their age.[103] Findings revealed that 2,100 epidermal genes were associated with younger-looking skin. Most of these genes were involved in DNA repair, cell replication, response to oxidative stress, autophagy, mitochondrial function, and protein metabolism. All aging processes accelerated in subjects in their 60s and 70s and co-occurred with menopause. Results revealed that older women with younger-looking skin exhibited gene expression patterns that matched those with chronologically younger skin, illustrating the strong effect of genetic expression on skin aging. The epidermal structure, skin barrier, and dermal structure were better maintained in younger-looking skin with preserved genetic

TABLE 5-2	Biological Processes That Have Genetic Changes Associated with Aging		
Biologic Process	**Intrinsic Aging**	**Extrinsic Aging**	**References**
Epidermal differentiation	+	+	(100,104)
Epidermal structure	++		(103)
Lipid biosynthesis	+++	+	(100,104)
Steroid biosynthesis	+++		(100)
Keratin filaments	+++		(100)
Keratinocyte differentiation	+++		(100)
Cornified envelope	++		(100)
ECM organization and biosynthesis		+++	(100)
Cell adhesion	+++	+++	(100)
ECM components	++	+++	(100,103,104)
Elastin genes		+++	(100,104)
Collagen genes		+	(104)
Inflammation		+	(104,105)
Cell senescence		+++	(103)
Mitochondria structure and metabolism		+++	(103)
Barrier function		++	(103)

+ some change in expression, ++ moderate amount of change in expression, +++ very significant change in expression. This table is adapted from multiple sources. For exact data please refer to the original source as noted.

TABLE 5-3	Genes Thought to Influence Cutaneous Aging
Gene	**Associated Activity**
MFAP4	Organization of elastin fibers in the ECM[107]
IRF4	Tanning response, pigmentation[107]
NEK6	Cell cycle, prevents senescence[107]
MMPs 2, 3, 8, 10, and 13	Breakdown of collagen and ECM[108]
Epidermal differentiation complex (EDC)	Skin barrier function[108]
FGF2	Growth factor, angiogenesis[108]
TGFBR1, TGFBR2, TGHBR3	Growth factor, angiogenesis[108]
VEGF	Growth factor, angiogenesis[108]
CDKN2A	Cell senescence[103]
COX7A2L	Cytochrome C oxidase in mitochondria[103]
GLUD1	Glutamate dehydrogenase 1 in mitochondria[103]
NMRK1	Nicotinamide riboside kinase, involved in NAD and coenzyme A in mitochondria[103]
PANK4	Pantothenate kinase involved in NAD and Coenzyme A in mitochondria[103]
CDH1	Cadherin 1, adherens junctions, cell-cell adhesion [103]
LAMA 5	Laminin subunit α5, attachment of keratinocyte to basement membrane[103]
DSC3	Desmocollin-3, desmosome, cell-cell adhesion [103]

function relating to maintenance of those structures. Notably, cyclin-dependent kinase inhibitor (CDKN2A) was three-fold higher in older-appearing women in sun-exposed areas and two-fold higher in non-sun-exposed areas as compared to younger and younger-appearing women. CDKN2A indicates cell senescence and codes for multiple proteins including p16[INK4A], which induces cellular senescence. This illustrates the role of both intrinsic and extrinsic aging in cellular senescence and skin aging.

In 2019, human dermal fibroblasts were cultured and the gene expression was evaluated in the absence of UV exposure to ascertain which genes were expressed as the cells aged.[106] This *in vitro* model on intrinsic aging showed decreased expression of the following genes with intrinsic aging (mostly due to shortened telomeres): COL1A1, COL1A2, COL4A1, MMP-1, MMP-2, MMP-7, MMP-8, MMP-9, TIMP-1, TIMP-2, TIMP-3, and TIMP-4. This contrasted with the findings in the extrinsic aging model that demonstrated that UV irradiation of the fibroblasts led to an increase in MMP-1, MMP-3, MMP-9, MMP-10, MMP-12, MMP-13, MMP-14, TIMP-1, TIMP-2, and TIMP-4. It is easier to distinguish the etiology between intrinsic and extrinsic aging in cell cultures and animal studies. Human studies are more difficult because there

is no standardized objective measurement for aged skin, so subjective measurements are used. For example, in 2020, researchers looked at genetic expression associated with subjective measures of perceived age.[107] A genome-wide association study (GWAS) was performed using the following question: "Do people say you look: 1. Older than you are, 2. About your age, 3. Younger than you are, or 4. Do not know or prefer not to say?" Those that reported "do not know or prefer not to say" were excluded leaving 423,992 adult participants. Approximately 9.6 million single nucleotide variants (SNVs) were tested for association. The results supported the fact that there are multiple biologic processes involved in maintaining a youthful appearance. MFAp4, IRF4, and NEK6 were cited as having a correlation with perception of skin age. There have been several studies that considered genes and skin aging. **Table 5-3** lists some of the genes thought to play a role in skin aging.

In summary, genes involved in fundamental cellular repair, protection from oxidation, metabolic processes, mitochondrial function, and barrier repair all play a role in skin aging. The link of CDKN2A expression to aged skin provides support for the hypothesis that cells with the SASP may hasten skin aging. There is still much to be learned about the genetics of aging and the effects of epigenetics.

Epigenetics

DNA methylation (DNAm) is an enzyme-induced modification of gene expression that does not change the DNA sequence and is reversible. Areas with a cytosine followed by a guanine are called CpG islands. CpG islands are frequently methylated sites. When the cytosine nucleotide acid residue in the CpG island of genes is methylated, gene expression changes (usually expression is downregulated). Analysis of DNA methylation patterns obtained in epidermal suction blisters and whole skin punch biopsies from sun-protected areas of skin from young and old individuals has shown that intrinsic aging was associated with hypermethylation of CpG islands (while sun-exposed areas demonstrated hypomethylation).[98] DNA methylation is closely correlated with chronological age and CpG islands have been used as an "epigenetic clock" indicating biologic age.

DNA methylation is regulated by DNA methyltransferases (DNMTs) while demethylation is regulated by ten-eleven translocation (TET) enzymes.[109] The expression of these enzymes declines with age. DNA methylation functions to maintain correct gene expression. Dysregulation of DNMT1 has been associated with various diseases.[110] One study showed that DNMT1 expression was markedly higher in young human skin fibroblasts and knock out of the DNMT1 caused cellular senescence. In mice, knock out of the DNMT1 resulted in premature aging signs such as alopecia and deep wrinkles. Epigenetics is an exciting area of study and will likely provide myriad insights into aging over the next decade.

HORMONES AND AGING SKIN

Hormones are known to play a role in skin aging, especially in women. Studies on hormones and aging show that menopausal women have decreased estrogen, which correlates with lower levels of collagen Types I and IV in skin.[111] While it has long been known that the skin contains hormone receptors, the role of hormones in cutaneous aging is still being deciphered. The aim of this section is to review the actions of hormones on the skin and to examine the roles of these hormones in skin aging.

Synthesis of Hormones and Their Decline During Aging

Gonads and Sex Hormones

Sex hormones are mainly synthesized in the ovaries, testicles, and adrenal glands of humans. Testosterone and estrogen are no longer considered male or female hormones, although most females have more estrogen than males and most males have more testosterone than women. The way society views gender has evolved and is no longer considered binary; in other words, it is more complicated than discussing males vs. females. The vast majority of research trials have been conducted with the classic binary definitions of male and female, however. Consequently, although the author understands and appreciates the complexities of gender variation and fluidity, for scientific clarity this section will refer to females as those individuals who have more endogenous and exogenous estrogen than testosterone and males as individuals who have more endogenous and exogenous testosterone as compared to estrogen. The reader should understand that the scientific data described here is based on binary gender definitions and should be interpreted as such.

In females, the ovaries synthesize two groups of sex hormones, progesterone and estrogen, There are three forms of estrogen: estradiol, estrone, and estriol. Estrone is the predominant estrogen after menopause, and estriol is synthesized by the placenta during pregnancy (**Table 5-4**).

In males, the testes produce 20% of circulating estrogens. The remaining estrogen is produced by fat cells, the brain, skin, and bone, which convert testosterone to estrogen via the enzyme aromatase. Estradiol E_2 is important for bone health and sexual desire in men and falls in parallel with the decline of serum testosterone levels.[112]

During puberty, both the male and female gonads begin to secrete testosterone. In females, most of the testosterone produced by the ovaries is converted into estradiol (17β-estradiol), the physiologically active and most abundant estrogen during this stage of life. In males, the prostate and hair follicles can convert testosterone into the more potent dihydrotestosterone (DHT), which has an affinity five times as strong as testosterone for the androgen receptor. DHT is the hormone responsible for male pattern baldness and medications to block the conversion of testosterone to DHT are used to prevent both prostatic hypertrophy and hair loss.

Sex Hormones and Skin Aging

Collagen loss increases dramatically and skin becomes thinner when women reach menopause.[113] Collagen Types I and III decline by as much as 30% in the first 5 years after estrogen levels drop. Lowered estrogen levels decrease the skin's defense against oxidative stress.

Sex Hormones and Wound Healing

Sex hormones also influence wound healing. Estrogen can regulate the production of dermal components, namely collagen and HA, by increasing the production of TGF-β.[114]

TABLE 5-4	Types of Estrogen, Their Origin, and When Each Type Prevails		
Estrogen Type	Stage Of Production/ Prevalence	Synthesized By	Relative Potency
Estradiol (E2)	Reproductive years	Ovaries	Most potent
Estriol (E3)	Pregnancy	Placenta	Least potent
Estrone (E1)	Post-reproductive years	Fat cells, adrenal glands	

A randomized, double-blind study by Ashcroft et al. examined the effects of topical estrogen on cutaneous wound healing in healthy elderly men and women after receiving punch biopsies and related these effects to the inflammatory response and local elastase levels (an MMP known to be upregulated in chronic wounds); it was found that compared to placebo treatment, estrogen treatment increased the extent of wound healing in both elderly males and females.[25] These authors further determined that estrogen treatment was associated with a decrease in wound elastase levels secondary to reduced neutrophil numbers and decreased fibronectin degradation. Similarly, an observational study showed that HRT recipients are approximately 30% to 40% less likely to develop a venous leg ulcer or a pressure ulcer than nonrecipients.[115] In contrast, androgens appear to prolong inflammation and inhibit wound healing.[116–118] Estrogen also promotes wound healing by increasing tissue expression of vascular endothelial growth factor (VEGF), an effect that is antagonized by androgens; therefore, estrogen can promote neovascularization that is necessary for wound healing while androgens inhibit it.[116]

As estrogen has a direct stimulatory influence on dermal fibroblasts, it also affects scarring. Aged skin is associated with a reduced rate of cutaneous wound healing and improved quality of scarring, while young skin heals quickly but often with thick, visible scars. Keloids and hypertrophic scars are generally conditions of youth, owing to an increase in TGF-β production by dermal fibroblasts, while scarless wound healing is a characteristic of fetal skin that, like aged skin, has lower levels of TGF-β.[119] As estrogen is known to increase TGF-β, and is therefore profibrotic, anti-estrogens such as tamoxifen have been shown to decrease TGF-β levels,[120,121] and are antifibrotic. Therefore, tamoxifen or other estrogen receptor modulators may be useful in improving scar cosmesis.

Pituitary Hormones

Production of pituitary hormones diminishes with age, with the exception of thyrotropin hormone (TSH), which increases with age. The pituitary gland produces the growth hormone (GH) prolactin, insulin-like growth factor-1 (IGF-1), luteinizing hormone (LH), follicle-stimulating hormone (FSH), melanocyte-stimulating hormone, and thyroid-stimulating hormone. The pituitary also synthesizes stress hormones in the adrenocorticotropic family such as cortisol.

Adrenal Glands and Hormones

In the adrenal gland, the precursor to both estrogens and androgens is dehydroepiandrosterone (DHEA), a derivative of cholesterol. DHEA is converted into androstenedione in the adrenal gland. Both androstenedione and DHEA, which by themselves display weak androgenic activity, can enter the systemic circulation and be converted into testosterone or estrogen by peripheral target cells. The enzyme responsible for this conversion is aromatase. Testosterone can be converted into estradiol via this enzyme in men and women. Besides the gonads, other tissues containing aromatase, and hence the ability to produce estradiol or testosterone from DHEA, are bone, brain, vascular tissue, fetal liver, placenta, adipose tissue, and the skin (**Table 5-5**).[15,16]

Hormone Replacement Therapy

Hormones are well known to play a role in skin aging in both men and women. Hormone replacement therapy (HRT) is believed to prevent some of the signs of aging. A complete discussion of hormones and aging skin is beyond the scope of this chapter, which will conclude with a high-level review of the hormones used to prevent skin aging.

Estrogen

Menopause is the cessation of menses that occurs in females as ovarian follicles diminish over time, with a subsequent decline in serum estradiol levels. In the fourth and fifth decades of life, many women begin to notice alterations in their skin that are associated with changes seen in menopause, such as skin thinning, dryness, an increase in wrinkles, and decreased elasticity. In fact, studies have shown that as much as 30% of skin collagen (both Type I, which confers strength to the skin, and Type III, which contributes to the elasticity of skin) is lost in the first 5 years after menopause,[122] and total collagen levels are estimated to decline on an average of 2% per postmenopausal year over 15 years.[123]

These skin changes can be reversed by estrogen replacement therapy. Estrogen replacement increases keratinocyte proliferation and collagen production by increasing expression of TGF-β, upregulating the expression of TIMPs, and downregulating the expression of MMPs.[124–126] Estrogen increases production of ECM components by triggering the release of epidermal growth factor from keratinocytes that stimulates production of versican and HA by fibroblasts.[98] Reports of increased skin elasticity after estrogen therapy may be due to the fact that estrogen increases levels of tropoelastin and fibrillin, but these are unlikely to form mature elastic fibers after puberty.

In a study that evaluated the effects of aging and postmenopausal hypoestrogenism on Types I and III collagen content in the skin of premenopausal and postmenopausal women, a decrease in skin collagen was more closely related to years of postmenopause than to chronologic age.[122] While collagen content seems to quickly diminish with increased postmenopausal years, several studies demonstrate that postmenopausal women who start receiving HRT with estrogen have an increase in skin collagen content,[123,127–129] with as much as a 6.5% increase in skin collagen content after 6 months of estrogen replacement.[128] In a study by Brincat et al. examining

TABLE 5-5	Tissues That Contain Aromatase
Gonads	
Bone	
Brain	
Vascular tissue	
Fetal liver	
Placenta	
Adipose tissue	
Skin	

different regimens of estrogen replacement therapy in post-menopausal women, the authors found that all regimens of estrogen therapy under consideration increased skin collagen content and that estrogen replacement therapy was prophylactic in women who had higher skin collagen levels and both prophylactic and therapeutic in women with lower skin collagen levels.[123] Similarly, a study by Castelo-Branco et al. examining skin collagen changes and HRT in postmenopausal women at 0 and 12 months of treatment showed that various forms of HRT with estrogen induced increases in skin collagen content in postmenopausal women, whereas the postmenopausal control group had experienced significant decreases when assessed at the same time points (**Box 5–1**).[129] In another study by Brincat et al. examining skin collagen changes in postmenopausal women receiving topical estradiol applied to the abdomen and thigh, the authors noted a strong correlation between the change in skin collagen content and the original skin collagen content, indicating that the change in response to estrogen therapy is dependent on the original collagen level, and that there is no further increase in collagen production once an "optimum" skin collagen level is reached.[130] This study is particularly noteworthy insofar as it suggests that there is

BOX 5-1

Hormone replacement therapy (HRT), already in widespread use primarily to reduce the risk of osteoporosis, gained much attention, and some notoriety, when one of the studies in the Women's Health Initiative (WHI) was halted in 2002. The National Institutes of Health (NIH) National Heart, Lung, and Blood Institute (NHLBI) halted the Prempro phase (HRT phase) of the WHI during the summer of 2002 because of a higher-than-expected rise in breast cancer, heart attacks, strokes, and blood clots in the legs among this cohort as well as the failure of the expected benefits to materialize. The two studies consisted of an HRT phase, estrogen plus progestin in women with a uterus, and an estrogen replacement therapy (ERT) phase in women without a uterus. HRT is sometimes recommended for women who have undergone natural menopause; ERT is more appropriate for women whose menopause is surgically induced. The ERT phase of the WHI ended in 2006. Follow-up of the women in both studies concluded in 2010. Over 16,000 women were randomized in the HRT phase to estrogen + progestin or placebo and approximately 10,000 women in the ERT phase were likewise randomized to estrogen or placebo. Few of the participants were taking HRT (13% in the HRT cohort and 6% in the ERT cohort), though the numbers that had ever used HRT were three-fold higher. It has been suggested that the results of these studies are not generalizable to premenopausal/perimenopausal women, who are more likely to be experiencing menopausal symptoms, because many of the women in the study may not have been experiencing menopausal symptoms any longer.

Women should decide on the appropriateness of HRT or ERT therapy in medical consultation based on the individual's specific risk factors and medical profile. See the NIH Web site (http://www.nhlbi.nih.gov/health/women/pht_facts.pdf) for more information.

a therapeutic window in which estrogen exerts its maximal effect in stimulating collagen production.

Estrogen can also combat skin dryness by decreasing transepidermal water loss (TEWL). In a study by Piérard-Franchimont et al. that examined TEWL in menopausal women, the authors found that women receiving transdermal hormone replacement with estrogen exhibited a significantly increased water-holding capacity of the SC as compared with menopausal women not receiving hormone replacement.[131] In addition, in a study examining changes in TEWL and cutaneous blood flow during the menstrual cycle, Harvell et al. found that TEWL was higher on the day of minimal estrogen/progesterone secretion as compared with the day of maximal estrogen secretion on both back ($P = 0.037$) and forearm ($P = 0.021$) skin in normal women.[132] The use of topical estrogen has been shown to increase epidermal thickness in postmenopausal women.[133,134] However, whether the beneficial effects of estrogen on skin dryness are attributable to its influence on the fibroblast and an increase in HA content, with the concomitant increase in water-retaining capacity of the dermis, or a direct effect of estrogen on the epidermis remain unclear.

While the number of sebaceous glands remains the same during life, as androgen levels decline with advanced age, sebum levels tend to decrease.[135] Although the level of surface lipids falls with age owing to diminished sebaceous gland function, paradoxically the sebaceous glands become larger, rather than smaller, as a result of slower cellular turnover.[135]

Subcutaneous fat is also important in maintaining the appearance of youth, and fat distribution is another area where sex hormones play a vital role. In postmenopausal women, the reduction in estrogen and the unmasking effects of systemic androgens lead to central fat accumulation. In a study by Dieudonne et al. examining androgen receptors in mature human adipocytes, androgen binding sites were found to differ by location, with twice as many androgen binding sites in intra-abdominal fat than in subcutaneous fat.[136] This finding was the same for fat deposits in men and women.[136] Another study by Dieudonne et al. investigating the location of estrogen receptors in mature human adipocytes of both men and women found that the predominant estrogen receptor was ER-α and that its level of expression was the same regardless of origin (intra-abdominal or subcutaneous fat).[137] These results suggest that the deposition of subcutaneous fat is mainly influenced by estrogen, while the deposition of abdominal fat depends more on androgen.

While many postmenopausal women would derive great cutaneous benefits from estrogen therapy, as estrogens are known to affect several organ systems, this subject is best addressed on a case-by-case basis and as part of a team approach with other physicians so that all risks and benefits are weighed. The primary risks associated with HRT are related to breast cancer and cardiovascular health; the primary benefits include relief of menopausal symptoms (such as vasomotor instability, sexual dysfunction, mood fluctuation, and skin atrophy) and reduced fracture risk. Current recommendations specify that HRT should only be used short term, for moderate to severe vasomotor symptoms, and primarily in younger women who are close to menopause (early menopause or first 5 years after menopause). It is important to note that estrogen-containing creams are contraindicated for women who have been diagnosed with estrogen-responsive cancers. Regarding the use of topical versus oral estrogens, topical estrogens are easily absorbed (hence the popularity of estrogen replacement in patch or gel form), but the cutaneous route avoids hepatic first-pass metabolism and high plasma levels of estrogen metabolites are associated with oral administration.

Progesterone

Studies have shown that women who take HRT that contains both estrogen and progesterone display an increase in skin surface lipids that is not seen in patients that take estrogen alone.[138] Progesterones are known to stimulate sebaceous gland activity.[139]

Testosterone

Men experience an age-associated decline in gonadal secretion of testosterone, termed "*andro*pause" for the drop in androgen levels, and it is associated with various symptoms, such as sexual dysfunction, hypogonadism, and psychologic changes.[19] In men, serum total testosterone falls 1–2% per year after age 30 so that by the age of 75, men have about 30% of the amount of serum testosterone as they did at age 25.[112] Obesity, metabolic syndrome, frailty, and other abnormalities are associated with lower serum testosterone levels. The reason(s) for this steady androgen decline in men are not as well understood as menopause in women, but the decline is attributed to decreased secretion of GnRH (gonadotropin-releasing hormone, secreted by the hypothalamus).[20]

Women also are treated with testosterone replacement therapy. Studies demonstrate that women on both estrogen and testosterone have a 48% higher collagen content of the skin as compared to women treated with estrogen alone.[140] Estrogen and testosterone increase Type II collagen.[141]

DHEA

As both men and women age, the levels of DHEA and DHEAS (its sulfate ester that can be measured in serum) produced by the adrenal glands begin to decline, so that by 70 to 80 years of age peak concentrations are only 10% to 20% of those found in young adults.[17] This steady decline in DHEA and DHEAS has been termed "*adreno*pause," for the associated decline in the adrenal secretion of DHEA/DHEAS,[17] although the levels of glucocorticoids and mineralocorticoids (other adrenal hormones) stay relatively constant throughout life (**Table 5-6**).

TABLE 5-6	Menopause, Andropause, and Adrenopause. These age-related conditions are characterized by a decline in the hormones listed.
Condition	Hormone That Decreases
Menopause	Estrogen (Estradiol)
Adrenopause	DHEA/DHEAS
Andropause	Androgens

Since many age-related disturbances have been reported to begin with the decline of this hormone, there has been much interest in the use of DHEA as a replacement therapy in aging.

In one randomized, double-blind, controlled trial examining men and women aged 60 to 88 years with low serum DHEAS levels, DHEA replacement therapy for 1 year improved hip bone mineral density;[18] however, most other studies examining the effects of DHEA administration in the elderly have displayed mixed results.

Oral supplementation of 50 mg of DHEA improved skin hydration, sebum production, epidermal thickness, and skin pigmentation in one study.[142] Topical DHEA has also been shown to augment sebum production, skin thickness, and collagen production.[143]

Human Growth Hormone

Low levels of human growth hormone (HGH) seen in older individuals correlates with skin thinning. After 18 months on HGH, elderly men were measured to have an increase of 4% in skin thickness compared to a decrease in 96% of patients not treated with HGH.[144] Another study on men over 60 years of age showed that HGH for 6 months increased skin thickness by 7%.[145]

Thyroid Hormone

Thyrotropin-releasing hormone (TRH) binds to the TRH receptor and stimulates the production and secretion of thyroid-stimulating hormone (TSH). TSH binds to the TSH receptor (TSHR) and induces TH production resulting in the release of triiodothyronine (T3) and tetraiodothyronine (T4), also known as thyroxine. T3 and T4 increase mitochondrial activity in fibroblasts.[146] Both T3 and T4 increase gene expression of mitochondrial cytochrome c oxidase. They have also been shown to increase ATP production,[147] reduce ROS, and increase antioxidant enzymes in cultured human keratinocytes. T3 increases SIRT-1 expression by an unknown mechanism and increases synthesis of Types I and III collagen, helping to thicken skin. T3 increases fibrillin-1, but it is unknown if this results in an increase of mature functional elastin, which is unlikely. Paus et al. have suggested that topical thyroid hormone might be an approach to treat aging skin.[146]

Summary

Hormonal influences on the health and function of skin are an important topic in dermatology that warrant due consideration by the cosmetic practitioner in assessing the health or prescreening of patients' skin prior to performing corrective procedures. The beneficial effect of estrogen on collagen production and in the promotion of wound healing is clear. Future investigations into the effects of other hormones on the skin remain unproven but promising.

CONCLUSION

Intrinsic aging occurs in everyone due to normal cellular metabolism. Investigations into aging and longevity from basic science research have yielded insights and clues as to the causes of intrinsic aging that will result in anti-aging strategies. Although the fountain of youth has not yet been discovered, it is certain that one major goal is to prevent cellular senescence without promoting tumor growth. The balance between the five phases of cells (stem, differentiating, proliferating, senescent, and apoptosis) is the key to safe anti-aging strategies. One important target to achieve this is normalizing mitochondrial and lysosomal function. As more is learned about the processes described in this chapter, new anti-aging therapies will emerge.

References

1. Cao C, Xiao Z, Wu Y, Ge C. Diet and Skin Aging-From the Perspective of Food Nutrition. *Nutrients*. 2020;12(3):870.

2. Strnadova K, Sandera V, Dvorankova B, et al. Skin aging: the dermal perspective. *Clin Dermatol*. 2019;37(4):326–335.

3. Elias PM, Ghadially R. The aged epidermal permeability barrier: basis for functional abnormalities. *Clin Geriatr Med*. 2002;18(1):103–120, vii.

4. Choi EH. Aging of the skin barrier. *Clin Dermatol*. 2019;37(4):336–345.

5. Roig-Rosello E, Rousselle P. The Human Epidermal Basement Membrane: A Shaped and Cell Instructive Platform That Aging Slowly Alters. *Biomolecules*. 2020;10(12):1607.

6. Langton AK, Sherratt MJ, Griffiths CE, Watson RE. Differential expression of elastic fibre components in intrinsically aged skin. *Biogerontology*. 2012;13(1):37–48.

7. Haydont V, Neiveyans V, Fortunel NO, Asselineau D. Transcriptome profiling of human papillary and reticular fibroblasts from adult interfollicular dermis pinpoints the 'tissue skeleton' gene network as a component of skin chrono-ageing. *Mech Ageing Dev*. 2019;179:60–77.

8. Chen G, Wang D, Vikramadithyan R, et al. Inflammatory cytokines and fatty acids regulate endothelial cell heparanase expression. *Biochemistry*. 2004;43(17):4971–4977.

9. Dyer DG, Dunn JA, Thorpe SR, et al. Accumulation of Maillard reaction products in skin collagen in diabetes and aging. *J Clin Invest*. 1993;91(6):2463–2469.

10. Farrar MD. Advanced glycation end products in skin ageing and photoageing: what are the implications for epidermal function? *Exp Dermatol*. 2016;25(12):947–948.

11. Yoshinaga E, Kawada A, Ono K, et al. N(ε)-(carboxymethyl)lysine modification of elastin alters its biological properties: implications for the accumulation of abnormal elastic fibers in actinic elastosis. *J Invest Dermatol*. 2012;132(2):315–323.

12. Radjei S, Gareil M, Moreau M, et al. The glyoxalase enzymes are differentially localized in epidermis and regulated during ageing and photoageing. *Exp Dermatol*. 2016;25(6):492–494.

13. Liskowski L, Rose DP. Experience with a simple method for estrogen receptor assay in breast cancer. *Clin Chim Acta*. 1976;67(2):175–182.

14. Bassas E. Experimental studies on seborheic alopecia. III. Localization of testosterone receptors in human hairy follicles. *Med Cutan Ibero Lat Am*. 1975;3(1):77–79.

15. Bulun SE, Takayama K, Suzuki T, Sasano H, Yilmaz B, Sebastian S. Organization of the human aromatase p450 (CYP19) gene. *Semin Reprod Med*. 2004;22(1):5–9.

16. Simpson ER. Aromatase: biologic relevance of tissue-specific expression. *Semin Reprod Med*. 2004;22(1):11–23.

17. Genazzani AD, Lanzoni C, Genazzani AR. Might DHEA be considered a beneficial replacement therapy in the elderly? *Drugs Aging*. 2007;24(3):173–185.

18. Jankowski CM, Gozansky WS, Schwartz RS, et al. Effects of dehydroepiandrosterone replacement therapy on bone mineral density in older adults: a randomized, controlled trial. *J Clin Endocrinol Metab*. 2006;91(8):2986–2993.

19. Mooradian AD, Korenman SG. Management of the cardinal features of andropause. *Am J Ther*. 2006;13(2):145–160.

20. Keenan DM, Takahashi PY, Liu PY, et al. An ensemble model of the male gonadal axis: illustrative application in aging men. *Endocrinology*. 2006;147(6):2817–2828.

21. Mosselman S, Polman J, Dijkema R. ERβ: identification and characterization of a novel human estrogen receptor. *FEBS Lett*. 1996;392(1):49–53.

22. Thornton MJ, Taylor AH, Mulligan K, et al. Oestrogen receptor beta is the predominant oestrogen receptor in human scalp skin. *Exp Dermatol*. 2003;12(2):181–190.

23. Pelletier G, Ren L. Localization of sex steroid receptors in human skin. *Histol Histopathol*. 2004;19(2):629–636.

24. Pedersen SB, Bruun JM, Hube F, Kristensen K, Hauner H, Richelsen B. Demonstration of estrogen receptor subtypes alpha and beta in human adipose tissue: influences of adipose cell differentiation and fat depot localization. *Mol Cell Endocrinol*. 2001;182(1):27–37.

25. Ashcroft GS, Greenwell-Wild T, Horan MA, Wahl SM, Ferguson MW. Topical estrogen accelerates cutaneous wound healing in aged humans associated with an altered inflammatory response. *Am J Pathol*. 1999;155(4):1137–1146.

26. Pageon H, Bakala H, Monnier VM, Asselineau D. Collagen glycation triggers the formation of aged skin in vitro. *Eur J Dermatol*. 2007;17(1):12–20.

27. Dekkers OM, Thio BH, Romijn JA, Smit JW. Acne vulgaris: endocriene aspecten [Acne vulgaris: endocrine aspects]. *Ned Tijdschr Geneeskd*. 2006;150(23):1281–1285. Dutch.

28. Wondrak GT, Roberts MJ, Cervantes-Laurean D, Jacobson MK, Jacobson EL. Proteins of the extracellular matrix are sensitizers of photo-oxidative stress in human skin cells. *J Invest Dermatol*. 2003;121(3):578–586.

29. Nayeri Rad A, Shams G, Safdarian M, Khorsandi L, Grillari J, Sharif Makhmalzadeh B. Metformin loaded cholesterol-lysine conjugate nanoparticles: A novel approach for protecting HDFs against UVB-induced senescence. *Int J Pharm*. 2020;586:119603.

30. Cui B, Liu Q, Tong L, Feng X. The effects of the metformin on inhibition of UVA-induced expression of MMPs and COL-I in human skin fibroblasts. *Eur J Inflamm*. 2019;17:2058739219876423.

31. Levine B, Kroemer G. Biological Functions of Autophagy Genes: A Disease Perspective. *Cell*. 2019;176(1-2):11–42.

32. Mizushima N, Levine B, Cuervo AM, Klionsky DJ. Autophagy fights disease through cellular self-digestion. *Nature*. 2008;451(7182):1069–1075.

33. Rubinsztein DC, Mariño G, Kroemer G. Autophagy and aging. *Cell*. 2011;146(5):682–695.

34. Jeong D, Qomaladewi NP, Lee J, Park SH, Cho JY. The Role of Autophagy in Skin Fibroblasts, Keratinocytes, Melanocytes, and Epidermal Stem Cells. *J Invest Dermatol*. 2020;140(9):1691–1697.

35. Solanas G, Peixoto FO, Perdiguero E, et al. Aged Stem Cells Reprogram Their Daily Rhythmic Functions to Adapt to Stress. *Cell*. 2017;170(4):678–692.e20.

36. Lim CJ, Lee YM, Kang SG, et al. Aquatide Activation of SIRT1 Reduces Cellular Senescence through a SIRT1-FOXO1-Autophagy Axis. *Biomol Ther (Seoul)*. 2017;25(5):511–518.

37. Eckhart L, Tschachler E, Gruber F. Autophagic Control of Skin Aging. *Front Cell Dev Biol*. 2019;7:143.

38. Qiang L, Zhao B, Shah P, Sample A, Yang S, He YY. Autophagy positively regulates DNA damage recognition by nucleotide excision repair. *Autophagy*. 2016;12(2):357–368.

39. Höhn A, Sittig A, Jung T, Grimm S, Grune T. Lipofuscin is formed independently of macroautophagy and lysosomal activity in stress-induced prematurely senescent human fibroblasts. *Free Radic Biol Med*. 2012;53(9):1760–1769.

40. Park JT, Lee YS, Cho KA, Park SC. Adjustment of the lysosomal-mitochondrial axis for control of cellular senescence. *Ageing Res Rev*. 2018;47:176–182.

41. Morselli E, Maiuri MC, Markaki M, et al. Caloric restriction and resveratrol promote longevity through the Sirtuin-1-dependent induction of autophagy. *Cell Death Dis*. 2010;1(1):e10.

42. Lee JH, Moon JH, Nazim UM, et al. Melatonin protects skin keratinocyte from hydrogen peroxide-mediated cell death via the SIRT1 pathway. *Oncotarget*. 2016;7(11):12075–12088.

43. Lespagnol A, Duflaut D, Beekman C, et al. Exosome secretion, including the DNA damage-induced p53-dependent secretory pathway, is severely compromised in TSAP6/Steap3-null mice. *Cell Death Differ*. 2008;15(11):1723–1733.

44. Wallis R, Mizen H, Bishop CL. The bright and dark side of extracellular vesicles in the senescence-associated secretory phenotype. *Mech Ageing Dev*. 2020;189:111263.

45. Im K, Baek J, Kwon WS, et al. The comparison of exosome and exosomal cytokines between young and old individuals with or without gastric cancer. *Int J Gerontol*. 2018;12(3):233–238.

46. Shin JW, Kwon SH, Choi JY, et al. Molecular Mechanisms of Dermal Aging and Antiaging Approaches. *Int J Mol Sci*. 2019;20(9):2126.

47. Ferrucci L, Fabbri E. Inflammageing: chronic inflammation in ageing, cardiovascular disease, and frailty. *Nat Rev Cardiol*. 2018;15(9):505–522.

48. Franceschi C, Campisi J. Chronic inflammation (inflammaging) and its potential contribution to age-associated diseases. *J Gerontol A Biol Sci Med Sci*. 2014;69(Suppl 1):S4–S9.

49. Skoczyńska A, Budzisz E, Trznadel-Grodzka E, Rotsztejn H. Melanin and lipofuscin as hallmarks of skin aging. *Postepy Dermatol Alergol*. 2017;34(2):97–103.

50. Hwang ES, Yoon G, Kang HT. A comparative analysis of the cell biology of senescence and aging. *Cell Mol Life Sci*. 2009;66(15):2503–2524.

51. Botchkareva NV. The Molecular Revolution in Cutaneous Biology: Noncoding RNAs: New Molecular Players in Dermatology and Cutaneous Biology. *J Invest Dermatol*. 2017;137(5):e105–e111.

52. Qu S, Yang L, Liu Z. MicroRNA-194 reduces inflammatory response and human dermal microvascular endothelial cells permeability through suppression of TGF-β/SMAD pathway by inhibiting THBS1 in chronic idiopathic urticaria. *J Cell Biochem*. 2020;121(1):111–124.

53. Tan J, Hu L, Yang X, et al. miRNA expression profiling uncovers a role of miR-302b-3p in regulating skin fibroblasts senescence. *J Cell Biochem*. 2020;121(1):70–80.

54. Gerasymchuk M, Cherkasova V, Kovalchuk O, Kovalchuk I. The Role of microRNAs in Organismal and Skin Aging. *Int J Mol Sci*. 2020;21(15):5281.

55. Shin KH, Pucar A, Kim RH, et al. Identification of senescence-inducing microRNAs in normal human keratinocytes. *Int J Oncol*. 2011 Nov;39(5):1205–1211.

56. Shin CH, Byun J, Lee K, et al. Exosomal miRNA-19a and miRNA-614 Induced by Air Pollutants Promote Proinflammatory M1 Macrophage Polarization via Regulation of RORα Expression in Human Respiratory Mucosal Microenvironment. *J Immunol*. 2020;205(11):3179–3190.

57. Kinser HE, Pincus Z. MicroRNAs as modulators of longevity and the aging process. *Hum Genet*. 2020;139(3):291–308.

58. Joo D, An S, Choi BG, et al. MicroRNA-378b regulates α-1-type 1 collagen expression via sirtuin 6 interference. *Mol Med Rep*. 2017;16(6):8520–8524.

59. Sreedhar A, Aguilera-Aguirre L, Singh KK. Mitochondria in skin health, aging, and disease. *Cell Death Dis*. 2020;11(6):444.

60. Allombert-Blaise C, Tamiji S, Mortier L, et al. Terminal differentiation of human epidermal keratinocytes involves mitochondria- and caspase-dependent cell death pathway. *Cell Death Differ*. 2003;10(7):850–852.

61. Bowman A, Birch-Machin MA. Age-Dependent Decrease of Mitochondrial Complex II Activity in Human Skin Fibroblasts. *J Invest Dermatol*. 2016;136(5):912–919.

62. Hoppe U, Bergemann J, Diembeck W, et al. Coenzyme Q10, a cutaneous antioxidant and energizer. *Biofactors*. 1999;9(2-4):371–378.

63. Singh B, Schoeb TR, Bajpai P, Slominski A, Singh KK. Reversing wrinkled skin and hair loss in mice by restoring mitochondrial function. *Cell Death Dis*. 2018;9(7):735.

64. Zhang H, Ryu D, Wu Y, et al. NAD$^+$ repletion improves mitochondrial and stem cell function and enhances life span in mice. *Science*. 2016;352(6292):1436–1443.

65. Fisher GJ, Datta SC, Talwar HS, et al. Molecular basis of sun-induced premature skin ageing and retinoid antagonism. *Nature*. 1996;379(6563):335–339.

66. Quan T, Little E, Quan H, Qin Z, Voorhees JJ, Fisher GJ. Elevated matrix metalloproteinases and collagen fragmentation in photodamaged human skin: impact of altered extracellular matrix microenvironment on dermal fibroblast function. *J Invest Dermatol*. 2013;133(5):1362–1366.

67. Poljšak B, Dahmane RG, Godić A. Intrinsic skin aging: the role of oxidative stress. *Acta Dermatovenerol Alp Pannonica Adriat*. 2012;21(2):33–36.

68. Kammeyer A, Luiten RM. Oxidation events and skin aging. *Ageing Res Rev*. 2015;21:16–29.

69. Kim J, Nakasaki M, Todorova D, et al. p53 Induces skin aging by depleting Blimp1+ sebaceous gland cells. *Cell Death Dis*. 2014;5(3):e1141.

70. Xie HF, Liu YZ, Du R, et al. miR-377 induces senescence in human skin fibroblasts by targeting DNA methyltransferase 1. *Cell Death Dis*. 2017;8(3):e2663.

71. Stadtman ER. Protein oxidation and aging. *Free Radic Res*. 2006;40(12):1250–1258.

72. Waldera-Lupa DM, Kalfalah F, Florea AM, et al. Proteome-wide analysis reveals an age-associated cellular phenotype of in situ aged human fibroblasts. *Aging (Albany NY)*. 2014;6(10):856–878.

73. Hamon MP, Ahmed EK, Baraibar MA, Friguet B. Proteome Oxidative Modifications and Impairment of Specific Metabolic Pathways During Cellular Senescence and Aging. *Proteomics.* 2020;20(5-6):e1800421.

74. Chondrogianni N, Petropoulos I, Franceschi C, Friguet B, Gonos ES. Fibroblast cultures from healthy centenarians have an active proteasome. *Exp Gerontol.* 2000;35(6-7):721–728.

75. Kozieł R, Greussing R, Maier AB, Declercq L, Jansen-Dürr P. Functional interplay between mitochondrial and proteasome activity in skin aging. *J Invest Dermatol.* 2011;131(3):594–603.

76. Yoon JE, Kim Y, Kwon S, et al. Senescent fibroblasts drive ageing pigmentation: A potential therapeutic target for senile lentigo. *Theranostics.* 2018;8(17):4620–4632.

77. Papadopoulou A, Kanioura A, Petrou PS, Argitis P, Kakabakos SE, Kletsas D. Reacquisition of a spindle cell shape does not lead to the restoration of a youthful state in senescent human skin fibroblasts. *Biogerontology.* 2020;21(6):695–708.

78. López-Otín C, Blasco MA, Partridge L, Serrano M, Kroemer G. The hallmarks of aging. *Cell.* 2013;153(6):1194–1217.

79. Rodier F, Campisi J. Four faces of cellular senescence. *J Cell Biol.* 2011;192(4):547–556.

80. Dutta D, Calvani R, Bernabei R, Leeuwenburgh C, Marzetti E. Contribution of impaired mitochondrial autophagy to cardiac aging: mechanisms and therapeutic opportunities. *Circ Res.* 2012;110(8):1125–1138.

81. Terlecki-Zaniewicz L, Pils V, Bobbili MR, et al. Extracellular Vesicles in Human Skin: Cross-Talk from Senescent Fibroblasts to Keratinocytes by miRNAs. *J Invest Dermatol.* 2019;139(12):2425–2436.e5.

82. Victorelli S, Lagnado A, Halim J, et al. Senescent human melanocytes drive skin ageing via paracrine telomere dysfunction. *EMBO J.* 2019;38(23):e101982.

83. Yun MH, Davaapil H, Brockes JP. Recurrent turnover of senescent cells during regeneration of a complex structure. *Elife.* 2015;4:e05505.

84. Campisi J, d'Adda di Fagagna F. Cellular senescence: when bad things happen to good cells. *Nat Rev Mol Cell Biol.* 2007;8(9):729–740.

85. Coppé JP, Desprez PY, Krtolica A, Campisi J. The senescence-associated secretory phenotype: the dark side of tumor suppression. *Annu Rev Pathol.* 2010;5:99–118.

86. Nelson G, Wordsworth J, Wang C, et al. A senescent cell bystander effect: senescence-induced senescence. *Aging Cell.* 2012;11(2):345–349.

87. Passos JF, Saretzki G, Ahmed S, et al. Mitochondrial dysfunction accounts for the stochastic heterogeneity in telomere-dependent senescence. *PLoS Biol.* 2007;5(5):e110.

88. Hiebert P, Wietecha MS, Cangkrama M, et al. Nrf2-Mediated Fibroblast Reprogramming Drives Cellular Senescence by Targeting the Matrisome. *Dev Cell.* 2018;46(2):145–161.e10.

89. Baker DJ, Childs BG, Durik M, et al. Naturally occurring p16(Ink4a)-positive cells shorten healthy lifespan. *Nature.* 2016;530(7589):184–189.

90. Mavrogonatou E, Pratsinis H, Papadopoulou A, Karamanos NK, Kletsas D. Extracellular matrix alterations in senescent cells and their significance in tissue homeostasis. *Matrix Biol.* 2019;75-76:27–42.

91. Guarente L, Picard F. Calorie restriction—the SIR2 connection. *Cell.* 2005;120(4):473–482.

92. Hall JA, Dominy JE, Lee Y, Puigserver P. The sirtuin family's role in aging and age-associated pathologies. *J Clin Invest.* 2013;123(3):973–979.

93. Xu C, Wang L, Fozouni P, et al. SIRT1 is downregulated by autophagy in senescence and ageing. *Nat Cell Biol.* 2020;22(10):1170–1179.

94. Osum M, Serakinci N. Impact of circadian disruption on health; SIRT1 and Telomeres. *DNA Repair (Amst).* 2020;96:102993.

95. Koo JH, Kang EB, Oh YS, Yang DS, Cho JY. Treadmill exercise decreases amyloid-β burden possibly via activation of SIRT-1 signaling in a mouse model of Alzheimer's disease. *Exp Neurol.* 2017;288:142–152.

96. Korman B. Evolving insights into the cellular and molecular pathogenesis of fibrosis in systemic sclerosis. *Transl Res.* 2019;209:77–89.

97. Tran D, Bergholz J, Zhang H, et al. Insulin-like growth factor-1 regulates the SIRT1-p53 pathway in cellular senescence. *Aging Cell.* 2014;13(4):669–678.

98. Tigges J, Krutmann J, Fritsche E, et al. The hallmarks of fibroblast ageing. *Mech Ageing Dev.* 2014;138:26–44.

99. Liu F, Hamer MA, Deelen J, et al. The MC1R Gene and Youthful Looks. *Curr Biol.* 2016;26(9):1213–1220.

100. Stout R, Birch-Machin M. Mitochondria's Role in Skin Ageing. *Biology (Basel).* 2019;8(2):29.

101. Robinson MK, Binder RL, Griffiths CE. Genomic-driven insights into changes in aging skin. *J Drugs Dermatol.* 2009;8(7 Suppl):s8–s11.

102. Glass D, Viñuela A, Davies MN, et al. Gene expression changes with age in skin, adipose tissue, blood and brain. *Genome Biol.* 2013;14(7):R75.

103. Kimball AB, Alora-Palli MB, Tamura M, et al. Age-induced and photoinduced changes in gene expression profiles in facial skin of Caucasian females across 6 decades of age. *J Am Acad Dermatol.* 2018;78(1):29–39.e7.

104. McGrath JA, Robinson MK, Binder RL. Skin differences based on age and chronicity of ultraviolet exposure: results from a gene expression profiling study. *Br J Dermatol.* 2012;166(Suppl 2):9–15.

105. Lener T, Moll PR, Rinnerthaler M, Bauer J, Aberger F, Richter K. Expression profiling of aging in the human skin. *Exp Gerontol.* 2006;41(4):387–397.

106. Lago JC, Puzzi MB. The effect of aging in primary human dermal fibroblasts. *PLoS One.* 2019;14(7):e0219165.

107. Roberts V, Main B, Timpson NJ, Haworth S. Genome-Wide Association Study Identifies Genetic Associations with Perceived Age. *J Invest Dermatol.* 2020;140(12):2380–2385.

108. Cho BA, Yoo SK, Seo JS. Signatures of photo-aging and intrinsic aging in skin were revealed by transcriptome network analysis. *Aging (Albany NY).* 2018;10(7):1609–1626.

109. Qian H, Xu X. Reduction in DNA methyltransferases and alteration of DNA methylation pattern associate with mouse skin ageing. *Exp Dermatol.* 2014;23(5):357–359.

110. Johnson AA, Akman K, Calimport SR, Wuttke D, Stolzing A, de Magalhães JP. The role of DNA methylation in aging, rejuvenation, and age-related disease. *Rejuvenation Res.* 2012;15(5):483–494.

111. Vázquez F, Palacios S, Alemañ N, Guerrero F. Changes of the basement membrane and type IV collagen in human skin during aging. *Maturitas.* 1996;25(3):209–215.

112. Decaroli MC, Rochira V. Aging and sex hormones in males. *Virulence.* 2017;8(5):545–570.

113. Brincat M, Moniz CJ, Studd JW, et al. Long-term effects of the menopause and sex hormones on skin thickness. *Br J Obstet Gynaecol.* 1985;92(3):256–259.

114. Ashcroft GS, Dodsworth J, van Boxtel E, et al. Estrogen accelerates cutaneous wound healing associated with an increase in TGF-beta1 levels. *Nat Med.* 1997;3(11):1209–1215.

115. Margolis DJ, Knauss J, Bilker W. Hormone replacement therapy and prevention of pressure ulcers and venous leg ulcers. *Lancet.* 2002;359(9307):675–677.

116. Kanda N, Watanabe S. Regulatory roles of sex hormones in cutaneou biology and immunology. *J Dermatol Sci.* 2005;38(1):1–7.

117. Gilliver SC, Wu F, Ashcroft GS. Regulatory roles of androgens in cutaneous wound healing. *Thromb Haemost.* 2003;90(6):978–985.

118. Fimmel S, Zouboulis CC. Influence of physiological androgen levels on wound healing and immune status in men. *Aging Male.* 2005;8(3-4):166–174.

119. Adzick NS, Lorenz HP. Cells, matrix, growth factors, and the surgeon. The biology of scarless fetal wound repair. *Ann Surg.* 1994;220(1):10–18.

120. Chau D, Mancoll JS, Lee S, et al. Tamoxifen downregulates TGF-beta production in keloid fibroblasts. *Ann Plast Surg.* 1998;40(5):490–493.

121. Mikulec AA, Hanasono MM, Lum J, Kadleck JM, Kita M, Koch RJ. Effect of tamoxifen on transforming growth factor beta1 production by keloid and fetal fibroblasts. *Arch Facial Plast Surg.* 2001;3(2):111–114.

122. Affinito P, Palomba S, Sorrentino C, et al. Effects of postmenopausal hypoestrogenism on skin collagen. *Maturitas.* 1999;33(3):239–247.

123. Brincat M, Versi E, Moniz CF, Magos A, de Trafford J, Studd JW. Skin collagen changes in postmenopausal women receiving different regimens of estrogen therapy. *Obstet Gynecol.* 1987;70(1):123–127.

124. Liu T, Li N, Yan YQ, et al. Recent advances in the anti-aging effects of phytoestrogens on collagen, water content, and oxidative stress. *Phytother Res.* 2020;34(3):435–447.

125. Thornton MJ. Estrogens and aging skin. *Dermatoendocrinol.* 2013;5(2):264–270.

126. Kassira N, Glassberg MK, Jones C, et al. Estrogen deficiency and tobacco smoke exposure promote matrix metalloproteinase-13 activation in skin of aging B6 mice. *Ann Plast Surg.* 2009;63(3):318–322.

127. Patriarca MT, Goldman KZ, Dos Santos JM, et al. Effects of topical estradiol on the facial skin collagen of postmenopausal women under oral hormone therapy: a pilot study. *Eur J Obstet Gynecol Reprod Biol.* 2007;130(2):202–205.

128. Sauerbronn AV, Fonseca AM, Bagnoli VR, Saldiva PH, Pinotti JA. The effects of systemic hormonal replacement therapy on the skin of postmenopausal women. *Int J Gynaecol Obstet.* 2000;68(1):35–41.

129. Castelo-Branco C, Duran M, González-Merlo J. Skin collagen changes related to age and hormone replacement therapy. *Maturitas.* 1992;15(2):113–119.

130. Brincat M, Versi E, O'Dowd T, et al. Skin collagen changes in post-menopausal women receiving oestradiol gel. *Maturitas.* 1987;9(1):1–5.

131. Piérard-Franchimont C, Letawe C, Goffin V, Piérard GE. Skin water-holding capacity and transdermal estrogen therapy for menopause: a pilot study. *Maturitas.* 1995;22(2):151–154.

132. Harvell J, Hussona-Saeed I, Maibach HI. Changes in transepidermal water loss and cutaneous blood flow during the menstrual cycle. *Contact Dermatitis.* 1992;27(5):294–301.

133. Creidi P, Faivre B, Agache P, Richard E, Haudiquet V, Sauvanet JP. Effect of a conjugated oestrogen (Premarin) cream on ageing facial skin. A comparative study with a placebo cream. *Maturitas.* 1994;19(3):211–223.

134. Fuchs KO, Solis O, Tapawan R, Paranjpe J. The effects of an estrogen and glycolic acid cream on the facial skin of postmenopausal women: a randomized histologic study. *Cutis.* 2003;71(6):481–488.

135. Zouboulis CC, Boschnakow A. Chronological aging and photoaging of the human sebaceous gland. *Clin Exp Dermatol.* 2001;26(7):600–607.

136. Dieudonne MN, Pecquery R, Boumediene A, Leneveu MC, Giudicelli Y. Androgen receptors in human preadipocytes and adipocytes: regional specificities and regulation by sex steroids. *Am J Physiol.* 1998;274(6):C1645–C1652.

137. Dieudonné MN, Leneveu MC, Giudicelli Y, Pecquery R. Evidence for functional estrogen receptors alpha and beta in human adipose cells: regional specificities and regulation by estrogens. *Am J Physiol Cell Physiol.* 2004;286(3):C655–C661.

138. Rosenthal A, Jacoby T, Israilevich R, Moy R. The role of bioidentical hormone replacement therapy in anti-aging medicine: a review of the literature. *Int J Dermatol.* 2019 Oct 11.

139. Sator PG, Schmidt JB, Sator MO, Huber JC, Hönigsmann H. The influence of hormone replacement therapy on skin ageing: a pilot study. *Maturitas.* 2001;39(1):43–55.

140. Brincat M, Moniz CF, Studd JW, Darby AJ, Magos A, Cooper D. Sex hormones and skin collagen content in postmenopausal women. *Br Med J (Clin Res Ed).* 1983;287(6402):1337–1338.

141. Savvas M, Bishop J, Laurent G, Watson N, Studd J. Type III collagen content in the skin of postmenopausal women receiving oestradiol and testosterone implants. *Br J Obstet Gynaecol.* 1993;100(2):154–156.

142. Baulieu EE, Thomas G, Legrain S, et al. Dehydroepiandrosterone (DHEA), DHEA sulfate, and aging: contribution of the DHEAge Study to a sociobiomedical issue. *Proc Natl Acad Sci USA.* 2000;97(8):4279–4284.

143. Nouveau S, Bastien P, Baldo F, de Lacharriere O. Effects of topical DHEA on aging skin: a pilot study. *Maturitas.* 2008;59(2):174–181.

144. Rudman D, Feller AG, Cohn L, Shetty KR, Rudman IW, Draper MW. Effects of human growth hormone on body composition in elderly men. *Horm Res.* 1991;36(Suppl 1):73–81.

145. Rudman D, Feller AG, Nagraj HS, et al. Effects of human growth hormone in men over 60 years old. *N Engl J Med.* 1990;323(1):1–6.

146. Paus R, Ramot Y, Kirsner RS, Tomic-Canic M. Topical L-thyroxine: The Cinderella among hormones waiting to dance on the floor of dermatological therapy? *Exp Dermatol.* 2020;29(9):910–923.

147. Vidali S, Knuever J, Lerchner J, et al. Hypothalamic-pituitary-thyroid axis hormones stimulate mitochondrial function and biogenesis in human hair follicles. *J Invest Dermatol.* 2014;134(1):33–42.

CHAPTER 6

Extrinsic Aging

Leslie S. Baumann, MD
Edmund M. Weisberg, MS, MBE

SUMMARY POINTS

What's Important?

1. The AhR signaling pathway is turned on by ozone and other pollutants and results in increased production of MMPs.
2. The common deletion in mitochondria occurs in photoaged skin and is associated with decreased mitochondrial function.
3. There is much overlap with intrinsic aging; therefore, reading Chapter 5 will provide useful supplemental information.

What's New?

1. The ECM components are broken down with sun exposure and other extrinsic insults resulting in changes in fibroblast activity.
2. Pollution from traffic is a major cause of skin aging.
3. Infrared and visible light can age skin.

What's Coming?

1. Knowledge on genetic expression and epigenetic methylation changes in sun-exposed vs. non-sun-exposed skin will increase.
2. Studies on mitochondria and how to improve autophagy and mitochondrial function in aged skin are ongoing.
3. It is still not possible to upregulate elastin levels in the skin by any means. Studies are ongoing to try and find ways to increase the quantity of mature elastin fibers that are bound to a microfibrillar backbone in the skin.

Since the end of the 19th century, dermatologists have discussed the notion that sunlight contributes to premature aging.[1] However, tanning beds remain popular and the majority of people continue to avoid consistent daily sun protection. In addition, in the last 15 years, studies have shown that environmental influences such as pollution also play an important role in skin aging. The rise in popularity of vaping will likely impart deleterious effects to the skin of some individuals, also, but it is too early to know if the effects of this new technology will engender cutaneous aging as does traditional smoking of tobacco products.

The consequences to the skin from sun and environmental exposure are readily apparent when one compares the exposed skin of the face, hands, or neck to the unexposed skin of the buttocks, inner thighs, or inner arms (**Fig. 6-1**). This damage can be highlighted by using a Wood's lamp, blue light, or an ultraviolet (UV) camera system, rendering the epidermal pigment component more noticeable (**Figs. 6-2**, **6-3**, and **6-4**). Showing such results to patients can prove useful in convincing them of the havoc that environmental exposures have wreaked on their skin.

Although the sun is not the sole source or cause of skin aging, it is the major external cause among several components, both endogenous and exogenous. This chapter will concentrate on the role of the sun in the extrinsic aging process of the skin, also known as photoaging.

SKIN AGING

There are two main processes of skin aging, intrinsic and extrinsic. Intrinsic aging reflects the genetic background of an individual and results from the passage of time. It is inevitable

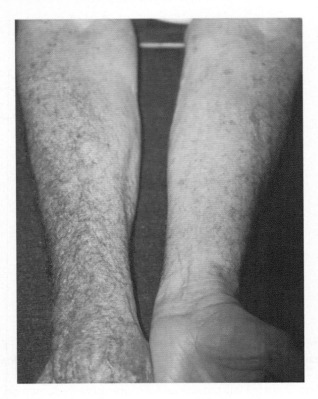

FIGURE 6-1. Comparing the sun-exposed surface of the forearm to the non-sun-exposed surface demonstrates the sun's ability to cause skin changes.

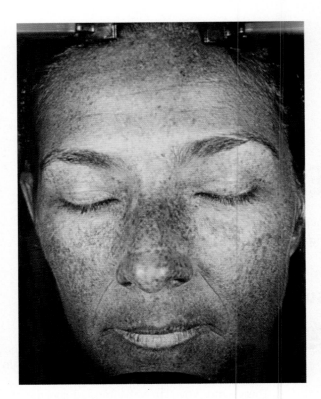

FIGURE 6-3. Photoaging is accentuated by using UV light.

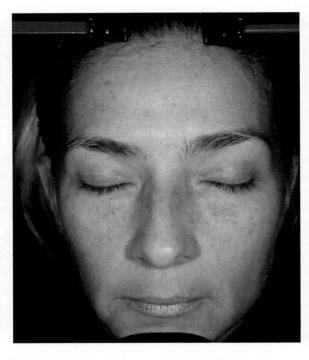

FIGURE 6-2. Facial skin of 25-year-old with normal lens. Sun damage is barely visible.

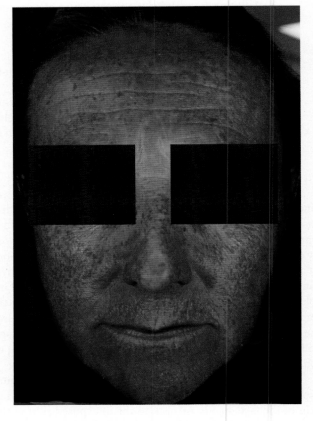

FIGURE 6-4. Photoaging as seen under blue light.

and, thus, beyond voluntary control. Extrinsic aging is engendered by external factors such as smoking, excessive use of alcohol, poor nutrition, and sun exposure, which in many cases can be reduced with effort. This process, then, is not inevitable and, by definition, refers to premature skin aging. It is believed that as much as 80% of facial aging can be ascribed to sun exposure.[2]

INTRINSIC VERSUS EXTRINSIC AGING

Intrinsically aged skin is smooth and unblemished, with exaggerated expression lines but preservation of the normal geometric patterns of the skin. Under the microscope, such skin demonstrates epidermal atrophy, flattening of the epidermal rete ridges, and dermal atrophy.[3] Collagen fibrils are not thickened but are elevated in number with an increase in the collagen III to collagen I ratio.[4]

Extrinsically aged skin appears predominantly in exposed areas such as the face, chest, and extensor surfaces of the arms. It is a result of the total effects of a lifetime of exposure to UV radiation (UVR). Clinical findings of photoaged skin include wrinkles and pigmented lesions such as freckles, lentigines, and patchy hyperpigmentation, and depigmented lesions such as guttate hypomelanosis (**Fig. 6-5**). Interestingly, a study in the *Journal of the American Medical Association* reported that children with the tendency to freckle developed 30% to 40% fewer freckles when treated with an SPF 30 sunscreen daily as compared to children not treated with a sunscreen.[5] This study illustrates the importance of sun protection in the prevention of these pigmented lesions that render an older appearance to the skin and are associated with an increased risk of melanoma. Other signs of skin aging include a loss of tone and elasticity, increased skin fragility, areas of purpura owing to blood vessel weakness, and benign lesions such as keratoses, telangiectasias, and skin tags (**Fig. 6-6**).

The histopathologic alterations in photoaged skin are easily distinguished and characterized by elastosis (**Fig. 6-7**). Photoaged skin is also marked by epidermal atrophy and

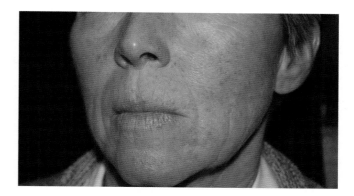

FIGURE 6-6. Photoaged skin shows telangiectasias, solar lentigos, and wrinkles.

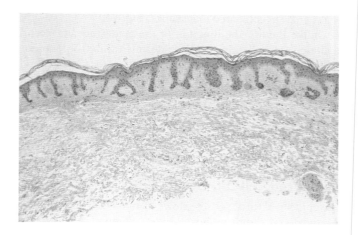

FIGURE 6-7. Hematoxylin and eosin (H and E) stain of sun-damaged skin demonstrates significant elastosis in the dermis and multiple solar lentigos. *(Image courtesy of George Ioannides, MD.)*

discrete changes in collagen and elastic fibers. In severely photoaged skin, collagen fibers are fragmented, thickened, and more soluble.[6] Elastic fibers also appear fragmented and may exhibit progressive cross-linkage and calcification.[7] These alterations in collagen and elastic fibers have been demonstrated to worsen with continued UV exposure.

Molecular Causes of Extrinsic Aging

Several different reactions occur when the skin is exposed to various insults such as UV radiation. Matrix metalloproteinases (MMPs) are enzymes that break down multiple cellular components. MMPs 1, 2, 3, and 9 are increased when skin is exposed to UV radiation. Free radicals, advanced glycation end products, microRNA, heparinase and many other enzymes, cytokines, and growth factors are increased or decreased by external insults. These are also seen in intrinsic aging and are discussed in Chapter 5, Intrinsic Aging.

CHARACTERISTICS OF AGED SKIN

Regardless of the etiology of skin aging, there are important characteristics of aged skin that must be considered.

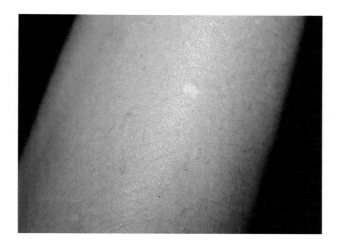

FIGURE 6-5. Photograph of idiopathic guttate hypomelanosis.

These changes occur throughout the epidermis, dermis, and subcutaneous tissue and can result in wide-ranging alterations in the topography of the skin.

Epidermis

Although age-related changes in the dermis are more pronounced than those in the epidermis, the epidermis does exhibit such alterations. Some studies suggest that aged skin displays a thinner epidermis,[6,8] but other studies do not support such findings.[9,10] Most studies are in agreement, though, that the thickness of the stratum corneum (SC) is unchanged with aging. The authors of one report did demonstrate that the spinous layer of a wrinkle was thinner at the bottom or valley of the wrinkle than the spinous layer at the wrinkle's flanks.[11] This study also showed that fewer keratohyaline granules are present in the base of a wrinkle as compared to its flanks (**Fig. 6-8**).

Unlike the SC, the junction of the epidermis and dermis is altered in aged skin. Aged epidermis exhibits a flattening of the dermal-epidermal junction (DEJ) with a correspondingly smaller connecting surface area. One study of abdominal skin showed that the surface area of the DEJ decreased from 2.64 mm^2 in subjects aged 21 to 40 years to 1.90 mm^2 in subjects aged 61 to 80 years.[12] This loss of DEJ surface area may lead to increased skin fragility and may also result in less nutrient transfer between the dermis and epidermis.

Decreased Cell Turnover in Epidermis

The epidermal turnover rate slows from 30% to 50% between the third and eighth decades of life.[7] Kligman demonstrated that SC transit time was 20 days in young adults and 30 or more days in older adults.[13] This lengthening of the cell cycle corresponds to a prolonged SC replacement rate and decelerated wound healing. In fact, it has been shown that older patients take twice as long to re-epithelialize after dermabrasion resurfacing procedures when compared with younger patients.[14] The slow cell cycle is combined with less effective desquamation in many elderly individuals. Heaps of corneocytes result, rendering the skin surface dull and rough in appearance. Consequently, many cosmetic dermatologists employ products such as hydroxy acids or retinoids to "speed up" the cell cycle with the belief that a faster turnover rate will ameliorate skin appearance and accelerate wound healing after cosmetic procedures.

Dermal-Epidermal Junction

The dermal-epidermal junction plays an important role in the skin (see Chapter 2, Basic Science of the Dermis). It becomes damaged when exposed to UV light, which leads to fragility due to decreased resistance to shear force caused by a weakened DE junction. The DE junction is discussed in Chapters 2 and 5.

Dermis

Elderly individuals exhibit a loss of approximately 20% of dermal thickness.[14] Examination of the structure of aged dermis reveals that it is relatively acellular and avascular.[3] Aged dermis is further characterized by changes in collagen production and the development of fragmented elastic fibers. The dermis that has been exposed to UV light also manifests disorganized collagen fibrils and the accumulation of abnormal elastin-containing material (Fig. 6-7).[15] The three components of the dermis that have received the most attention in anti-aging research are collagen, elastin, and glycosaminoglycans. Among the glycosaminoglycans, hyaluronic acid (HA) and heparan sulfate (HS) are the substances most often investigated.

COLLAGEN

Awareness of the importance of collagen in the aging process has led to the manufacture of many skincare products, supplements, and injectable treatments the aim of which is to augment skin collagen. There are even collagen beverages that are touted to render skin smoother and younger. Cosmeceutical ingredients in skincare products, such as vitamin C, retinol, and glycolic acid, owe some of their popularity to the studies revealing that these agents can increase collagen synthesis. Such products are usually labeled as "antiwrinkle creams." Although wrinkles are common, it is interesting that little is really known about their pathogenesis.[16] This is because neither an animal model nor an in vitro model of wrinkling has been developed. It is well established, however, that alterations in collagen seem to be important in the aging process, which accounts for the popularity of anti-aging products designed to increase collagen production.

What Is Skin Collagen?

Collagen constitutes 70% of dry skin mass.[17] The collagen in aged skin is characterized by thickened fibrils organized in rope-like bundles, which are in disarray as compared to the organized pattern seen in younger skin.[3] Type I collagen comprises 80% and type III collagen comprises approximately 15% of the total skin collagen of young skin. However, as the skin ages, the ratio of type III to type I collagen has been shown to increase (meaning that there is less type I collagen with aging).[18] Collagen type I levels have been shown to decrease by 59% in irradiated skin;[15] this reduction was found to correlate with the extent of photodamage.[19] It is known that the

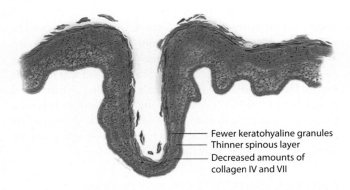

FewerKeratohyaline granules
Thinner spinous layer
Decreased amounts of collagen IV and VII

FIGURE 6-8. The spinous layer is thinner and there are fewer keratohyaline granules in the valley of the wrinkle. Levels of collagens IV and VII are also decreased in the valley of a wrinkle when compared to the flanks.

overall collagen content per unit area of skin surface decreases by approximately 1% per year.[20] Although type I collagen is the most abundant in the skin, the other types of collagen in the dermis may also be affected by aging.

Collagen IV, a key component in the DEJ, provides a framework for other molecules and is important in the maintenance of mechanical stability. Although studies have shown no difference in collagen IV levels in sun-exposed skin in comparison to nonexposed skin, a significant diminution of collagen IV was found in the bottom of wrinkles when compared to the flanks of wrinkles (Fig. 6-8). This loss of collagen IV may affect the mechanical stability of the DEJ and contribute to wrinkle formation.[11]

Anchoring fibrils, made of collagen VII, are important because they attach the basement membrane zone to the underlying papillary dermis. Patients with chronically sun-exposed skin have been characterized as having a significantly lower number of anchoring fibrils when compared to normal controls. The investigators who made this observation postulated that a weakened bond between the dermis and epidermis owing to loss of anchoring fibrils leads to wrinkle formation.[21] Interestingly, a more recent study demonstrated that this loss of collagen VII was more pronounced at the base of the wrinkle (similar to that seen with collagen IV in the same study).[11]

The mechanism of action of how UVR induces collagen damage has been well characterized in the last 15 years. It is now known that UVR exposure dramatically upregulates the production of several types of collagen-degrading enzymes known as MMPs. This occurs by the following mechanism: UV exposure causes an increase in the amount of the transcription factor c-Jun (c-Fos is abundant without UV exposure). These two transcription factors, c-Jun and c-Fos, combine to produce activator protein-1 (AP-1), which activates the MMP genes resulting in production of collagenase, gelatinase, and stromelysin. It has been demonstrated in humans that MMPs, specifically collagenase and gelatinase, are induced within hours of UVB exposure.[22] Fisher et al. showed that multiple exposures to UVB yield a sustained induction of MMPs.[15] Because collagenase degrades collagen, long-term elevations in collagenase and other MMPs likely result in the disorganized and clumped collagen seen in photoaged skin. These MMPs may represent the mechanism through which collagen I levels are reduced following UV exposure.

Mitogen-Activated Protein Kinases and Aging

Mitogen-activated protein kinases (MAPKs) are serine–threonine protein kinases, meaning they phosphorylate the OH side chain of serine and threonine. Significantly, they are involved in signal transduction pathways for cell proliferation, differentiation, and apoptosis. Thus far, four groups of MAPKs have been identified: extracellular signal-regulated kinases (ERKs), c-Jun amino-terminal kinases (JNKs), also known as stress-activated protein kinases (SAPKs), p38 kinase, and ERK5. ERKs are activated via growth factors and play a role in cell proliferation and differentiation. JNKs, on the other hand, respond to stressful stimuli such as UV light, osmotic

shock, or cytokines,[23] and are involved in cellular apoptosis.[24] In addition, p38 kinase is activated via stress-induced stimuli. It has been demonstrated that a synchronized inhibition of ERKs and activation of JNK/p38 must be present for cellular apoptosis, suggesting that a "balance" among these groups influences cell survival versus death.[25] The MAPKs have been implicated in both intrinsic and extrinsic aging of skin. Chung et al. demonstrated that JNK activity is higher and ERK activity lower in intrinsically aged skin.[26] As previously mentioned, the combination of UV-induced c-Jun (through the JNK pathway), and naturally expressed c-Fos produces AP-1, which promotes the degrading of collagen and the extracellular matrix by increasing MMPs.[27] AP-1 has an additional impact in collagen loss by decreasing collagen I gene expression.[28] Therefore, some collagen reduction in photoaged skin may be explained by the role of AP-1 in both increasing MMPs and decreasing collagen synthesis.

ELASTIN

Changes in elastic fibers are so characteristic in photoaged skin that "elastosis," an accumulation of amorphous elastin material, is considered a hallmark of photoaged skin. Thickening and coiling of elastic fibers in the papillary dermis distinguish the alterations induced by UV exposure. Continued UV exposure leads to these same changes in the reticular dermis.[29] Electron microscopy examination of the elastic fibers reveals an increase in the complexity of the shape and arrangement of the fibers, a decrease in the number of microfibrils, a higher number of electron-dense inclusions, and more interfibrillar areas.[30] Elastin extracted from the skin of elderly patients has been demonstrated to contain small amounts of sugar and lipids and an abnormally high level of polar amino acids.[3] The mechanism of these changes is not as well understood as it is in collagen; however, MMPs likely play a role because MMP-2 has been shown to degrade elastin.[31]

Elastin and Sun Exposure

Fibrillin, fibulin, and other microfibrillar components of elastin fibers are sensitive to UV light,[32] while tropoelastin is not.[33] The initial response of elastic fibers to UV light is hyperplastic, resulting in increased elastic tissue. The magnitude of this response depends on the degree of sun exposure. The second phase of response, seen in aged elastic fibers, is degenerative, resulting in reduced elasticity and resiliency of the skin.[34,35] Aged skin that has suffered this degenerative response manifests an alteration in the normal pattern of immature elastic fibers, called oxytalan, which is found in the papillary dermis. In young skin, these fibers form a network that ascends perpendicularly from the uppermost portion of the papillary dermis to just below the basement membrane (Fig. 2–5 in Chapter 2). As skin ages, this network gradually disappears.[36] In fact, a loss of skin elasticity has been shown to incrementally increase with age.[37] This loss of elasticity accounts for much of the sagging often seen in the skin of elderly individuals. In darker, melanized skin of color, skin sagging also occurs from sun exposure. However, darker skin types exhibit less solar elastosis, which implies that sagging is due to more than just elastotic elastin and seems to be due to remodeling of fibrillin-rich microfibrils.[38]

GLYCOSAMINOGLYCANS

Glycosaminoglycans (GAGs) are important molecules because they can bind water up to 1,000 times their volume. The GAG family includes HA, chondroitin sulfate, HS, and dermatan sulfate, among many other constituents. Numerous studies report that GAGs, especially HA, are decreased in amount in photoaged skin and HS is lowered in aged skin.[39] However, some conflicting studies report no change in the amount of GAGs in aged skin.[40]

A study by Uitto demonstrated that photoaged skin exhibits a reduction in HA and an increase in chondroitin sulfate proteoglycans,[41] which, interestingly, is a pattern also seen in scars. In young skin, the HA is found at the periphery of collagen and elastin fibers and at the interface of these types of fibers. Such connections with HA are absent in aged skin.[39] Decreases in the amount of HA, leading to its lack of association with collagen and elastin and decreased water binding, may play a role in the changes seen in aged skin including decreased turgidity, diminished capacity to support the microvasculature, wrinkling, and altered elasticity.

MELANOCYTES

The number of melanocytes decreases from 8% to 20% per decade. This is displayed clinically by a reduction in the number of melanocytic nevi in older individuals.[3] Because melanin absorbs carcinogenic UV light, the skin of older patients is less able to protect itself from the sun and, consequently, is at greater risk for developing sun-induced cancers. It is for this reason that sun protection is important even for patients who feel it is "too late" to begin adding a sunscreen to their skincare regimens.

Vasculature

Many studies have shown that aged skin is relatively avascular. One investigation demonstrated a 35% reduction in the venous cross-sectional area in aged skin as compared to young skin.[42] This reduction in the vascular network is particularly obvious in the papillary dermis with loss of the vertical capillary loops. Such a reduction of vascularity results in decreased blood flow, diminished nutrient exchange, impaired thermoregulation, lower skin surface temperature, and skin pallor.

Subcutaneous Tissue

Elderly skin displays both a loss and a gain of subcutaneous tissue that is site specific. Subcutaneous fat is decreased in the face, as well as the dorsal aspects of the hands and the shins. Other areas, however, such as the waist in women and the abdomen in men, accumulate fat with aging (see Chapter 3, Fat and Subcutaneous Layer).[3]

UV IRRADIATION AND UROCANIC ACID ISOMERS

The cutaneous barrier is the initial line of bodily defense, protecting other organs from external antigens, bacteria, and viruses, as well as UV light. UV irradiation is well understood as an exogenous factor that can diminish cutaneous immunity, leading to impaired recognition of abnormal cells that may eventually develop into skin cancers. *Trans*-urocanic acid (*trans*-UCA), a metabolite of histidine, is commonly present in the epidermal skin layers. As discussed in Chapter 12, Dry Skin, histidine is mostly derived from filaggrin in the epidermis and gets converted to *trans*-UCA, which plays an integral role in epidermal hydration. Following UV exposure, *trans*-UCA is photoisomerized into *cis*-urocanic acid (*cis*-UCA), a known photoreceptor for UV light (**Fig. 6-9**). *cis*-UCA is a well-recognized immunosuppressant in the skin. Impaired delayed hypersensitivity reaction and decreased function of epidermal antigen-presenting cells (Langerhans cells) occur following exposure to *cis*-UCA through TNF-α release.[43,44] Interestingly, the effect of *cis*-UCA is dose dependent.[45] In addition to UV irradiation dose, skin pigmentation is an important factor. Fair-skinned subjects have been shown to produce more *cis*-UCA with lower doses of UV light when compared to darker-skinned individuals.[46] It has been suggested that *cis*-UCA decreases the ability of APCs to present the abnormal cells and antigens to the immune system, thereby contributing to UV carcinogenesis.[47] However, the exact role of *cis*-UCA in skin cancers is not well understood and the few studies performed on this subject have not revealed a direct association between the total UCA levels and skin cancer. In a study by de Fine Olivarius et al. of the total UCA and percentage of *cis*-UCA in sun-exposed and sun-protected areas of skin in patients with a history of basal cell carcinoma (BCC), patients with malignant melanoma, and healthy subjects, the total UCA and *cis*-UCA levels did not differ among the three groups, while

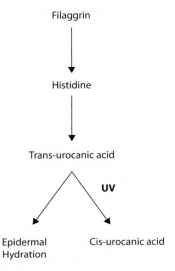

FIGURE 6-9. Filaggrin breaks down into *cis*-urocanic acid through the pathway shown.

the percentage of *cis*-UCA was found to be higher in patients with a history of BCC and melanoma as compared to healthy individuals.[48] Another study conducted by Snellman et al. also failed to demonstrate a statistically significant increase of UCA with UV exposure in subjects with a history of BCC and melanoma.[49]

FREE RADICALS AND LIGHT EXPOSURE

Free radicals, also known as reactive oxygen species, are composed of oxygen with an unpaired electron and are created by UV exposure, blue light, pollution, stress, smoking, and normal metabolic processes. They are suspected to be the cause, or at least a major contributor, to the aging process. There is evidence to suggest that free radicals induce changes in gene expression pathways that lead to the degradation of collagen and accumulation of elastin characteristic of photoaged skin (**Fig. 6-10**).[31] Antioxidants neutralize these reactive oxygen species by providing another electron, which gives the oxygen ion an electron pair, thereby stabilizing it (see Chapter 39, Antioxidants).

It has been demonstrated that following a single dose of UV irradiation there is an initial decrease in expression and activity of antioxidant enzymes in the cultured fibroblasts of skin.[50] In this study, the antioxidant enzymes increased even to higher than pre-exposure levels in a few days, probably as a defense mechanism in preparation for more potential UV exposure.

UV radiation is not the only kind of light that can cause free radicals in the skin. Blue-violet light (380–495 nm) has been clearly shown to utilize skin carotenoids demonstrating free radical generation by blue-violet light on the skin.[51] Infrared radiation (IR) induces expression of MMP-1 resulting in collagen breakdown.[52]

SKIN LIPIDS AND LIGHT EXPOSURE

Skin lipids are critical for proper barrier function. UV exposure has long been known to cause dry skin. In 2016, a study showed that UV light affects the ceramide lipid subclasses and squalene levels in the skin, which may account for some of the dryness seen in sun-exposed skin.[53] In the same study, visible and infrared light exerted different effects on these same ceramide subclasses, suggesting that the type of light is important.

EFFECTS OF LIGHT ON MITOCHONDRIA

Large-scale deletions of mitochondrial DNA are seen in photoaged skin.[54,55] The "common deletion," a 4,977b deletion, is 10 times more common in photoaged skin compared to sun-exposed skin of the same subject.[56] This DNA mutation leads to oxidative stress and altered gene expression, which impacts surrounding structural components in the fibroblast and the extracellular matrix resulting in cutaneous aging.

IR also affects mitochondria but seems to spur deleterious effects even faster than UV light because a single exposure to IR has been shown to cause reactive oxygen species inside the mitochondria of human skin fibroblasts.[57] IR may be more damaging because it reacts with constituents of the mitochondrial electron transport chain such as copper. This disturbs the electron flow and results in generation of free radicals and

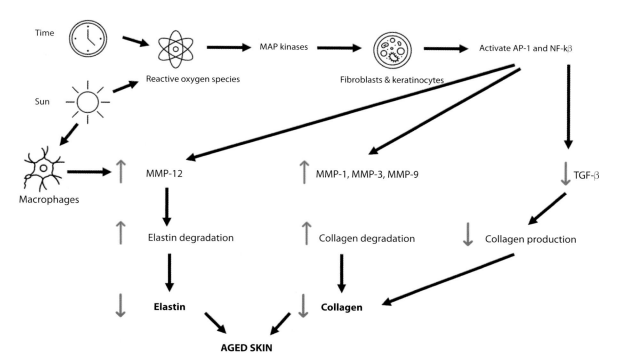

FIGURE 6-10. The sun and other pollutants activate matrix metalloproteinases that turn on the aging process that overlaps with intrinsic aging.

damage to mitochondrial DNA. This effect is blocked by anti-oxidants added to the fibroblast cultures.

TANNING AND ITS EFFECTS ON THE SKIN

UV light stimulates the production of melanin by causing α-melanocyte-stimulating hormone (α-MSH) to be secreted by keratinocytes. Redheads have a defect in the proopiomelanocortin (POMC) gene that prevents this tanning response from occurring. Data published in *Cell* showed that the tumor suppressor protein p53, when "stressed" by UV, activates the POMC gene, which leads to both tanning and an increase in β-endorphin.[58] This may explain why some people state that they feel good after tanning. Of course, many companies are looking at ways to safely stimulate p53 to create a "protective" tan but much more research is necessary.

Tanning beds are especially pernicious to skin because they utilize UVA, which penetrates deeper into the dermis than UVB and does not immediately induce erythema to warn of impending harm. For this reason, tanning beds are dangerous. Several studies describe the damage to skin that tanning beds cause. One reason they are so harmful is that UVA exposure causes a 40% increase in the levels of the common deletion in the dermal mitochondria.[59] These DNA mutations lead to an increase of reactive oxygen species, inflammation, and skin aging.

AIR POLLUTION AND SKIN AGING

Pollution is divided several into categories by the US Environmental Protection Agency (EPA). Of these, the following have proven effects on skin: (1) ground level ozone, (2) particulate matter, (3) persistent organic pollutants like dioxin and pesticides, and (4) gaseous pollutants. Traffic-related pollution is a mixture of various types of pollutants.

Tropospheric ozone (increased levels of ozone that make it to the earth) engenders an oxidative stress response resulting in free radicals. Long-term exposure to tropospheric ozone has been associated with premature skin aging.[60,61] Ozone has also been shown to affect the aryl hydrocarbon receptor (AhR), which is another mechanism that accounts for the aging effects of ozone on the skin. Activation of AhR induces the expression of xenobiotic metabolizing enzymes like cytochrome P450. The AhR is involved in hypoxia signaling, circadian rhythms, and the induction of MMP-1 expression.[62] We know that AhR directly affects MMP-1 synthesis in fibroblasts because treating fibroblasts with AhR inhibitors blocks MMP-1 production.[63]

Ambient particulate matter in air has deleterious effects on the skin, mainly by causing oxidative stress through free radical generation. Traffic-related pollution is a mixture of pollutants that includes polycyclic aromatic hydrocarbons (PAHs), formaldehyde, and benzene. To evaluate the effects of pollution on cutaneous aging, 400 Caucasian women aged 70–80 were followed to see the effects of pollution on the skin. This well-designed study showed that air pollution exposure caused an increase in dark spots on the skin and, to a lesser degree, wrinkles.[64] Other studies have demonstrated that

traffic pollution increases skin aging.[65] The mechanisms by which pollution leads to signs of skin aging are not completely understood but hydrocarbons such as dioxin have been shown to stimulate melanocyte pigmentation in mice.[66]

There are several mechanisms by which pollutants can affect skin aging including generation of free radicals, induction of inflammation, activation of the AhR receptor, and alterations to the skin microbiome.

SMOKING, VAPING, AND SKIN AGING

Numerous studies since 1971 have demonstrated that smoking tobacco increases skin wrinkles because tobacco induces MMP-1 leading to collagen breakdown.[67–70] Tobacco smoke contains several PAHs, which are generated from the incomplete combustion of organic compounds and found in burning wood, cigarettes, and electronic-cigarettes (e-cigarettes). PAHs are often toxic or carcinogenic and are known to trigger the AhR signaling pathway. All PAHs can contribute to collagen loss in the skin through this mechanism. E-cigarettes have far fewer PAHs than cigarettes; therefore, tobacco vaping may cause less skin aging than tobacco cigarettes.

Already widespread, cannabis use has gained even greater popularity over the last few years with increasing legalization but there is a paucity of research on the effects of cannabis on the skin. The delivery method of cannabis is important to consider when researching the cutaneous effects of cannabis. It is very likely that combusted cannabis imparts aging effects on the skin because of the presence of PAHs. Ingested and vaporized cannabis may not adversely affect the skin. For example, cannabis vapor from a volcano device contained no PAHs while combusted cannabis did have PAHs.[71]

CHANGES IN SKIN APPEARANCE

Dry Skin and Dull Skin

Elderly people often display dry, dull, scaled skin. It loses radiance due to a decrease in light reflection caused by an uneven surface. Dry, dull skin arises in part because of the barrier function decline and skin dehydration that occur with increasing age (see Chapter 12). Aged skin exhibits increased transepidermal water loss; therefore, it is susceptible to becoming dry in low-humidity environments. The recovery of damaged barrier function has been shown to be slower in aged skin leading to an increased susceptibility to dryness. This is caused by a combination of factors including lower lipid levels in lamellar bodies and a reduction in epidermal filaggrin (see Chapter 12).[72,73] Roughness, wrinkling, skin pallor, and the appearance of dark and light spots also affect the appearance and texture of aged skin. In addition, aged skin is typically characterized by laxity, fragility, easy bruising, and benign neoplasms.

Benign Neoplasms in Aging Skin

The surface texture and appearance of skin can change dramatically through age with the emergence of acrochordons (skin tags), cherry angiomas, seborrheic keratoses, lentigos (sun spots), and sebaceous hyperplasias. It is not uncommon for cosmetic patients to request removal of these benign neoplasms. There are several different destructive treatment modalities available, such as hyfrecation, curettage, and laser.

Wrinkles and Sagging Skin

Aged skin is more fragile and thinner than young skin as well as less elastic. Loss of collagen leads to loss of strength, while decreased HA decreases skin volume. Alterations in elastin cause skin sagging. All of these changes contribute to skin wrinkling.

TREATMENT

Several different topical agents and in-office procedures are used to treat photoaged skin. Most of these remedies function by "resurfacing" the epidermis. The goal is to remove the damaged epidermis and, in some instances, dermis, and allow them to be replaced with remodeled skin layers. There is some evidence that resurfacing procedures can induce the formation of new collagen with a normal staining pattern in contrast to the basophilic elastotic masses of collagen present in photoaged skin.[74] Although there are multiple treatments available for aged skin, prevention is still paramount and should be emphasized to all patients.

PREVENTION

Vitamin D Protects Skin from Sun Exposure

The importance of vitamin D in health is becoming better understood. The $1\alpha,25$-dihydroxyvitamin D_3 form of vitamin D, known as $1,25(OH)_2D_3$, has been shown to protect skin against the DNA mutation known as thymine dimers.[75] Vitamin D has also evinced protection from reactive nitrogen species that are formed by excess levels of nitric oxide arising from increased production due to UV upregulation and enhanced release. The form of vitamin D known as $1,25(OH)_2D_3$ is not an antioxidant but has been demonstrated to protect *ex vivo* human skin from various types of DNA mutations after UV exposure.[76]

Estrogen and Sun Damage

Dermal fibroblasts contain numerous estrogen receptors and estrogen plays a role in stimulating fibroblasts to produce collagen through transforming growth factor β.[77] Estrogen also increases levels of HA. Hormone replacement therapy has been shown to decrease skin aging and increase collagen levels.[78,79] This appears to be achieved by increasing collagen synthesis. UV exposure raises levels of MMP-1, which breaks down collagen. One study looked at topical estradiol 0.05% applied behind the ear in postmenopausal women not on hormone replacement therapy. Topical estradiol did not alter MMP levels after UV exposure, nor increase procollagen I and III messenger RNA levels in sun-exposed photodamaged skin,[80] but did increase procollagen in sun-protected skin on the hip. Currently, there is evidence that estrogen can improve

the skin's appearance but does not seem to protect skin from sun-induced damage.

Sunscreen and Sun Avoidance

It is well established that sun avoidance and sunscreen use are important adjuvants to anti-aging regimens. Obviously, sun avoidance is not always possible and hardly a popular behavioral adjustment for many patients. However, patients should be discouraged from engaging in unnecessary sun exposure, particularly between 10 AM and 4 PM, and any exposure to tanning beds. Sunscreen should be recommended for use on a daily basis, even when the patient remains indoors. Patients should be reminded that UVA rays have the capacity to pass through glass, thus individuals are at risk of solar exposure even in their cars and homes as well as at work. UVA shields can be placed on windows, providing some protection. Sun-protective clothing, such as a broad-brimmed hat and SPF 45 clothing, should be encouraged for patients planning any protracted exposure to the sun. Many patients believe that their sun exposure is minimal and does not warrant daily use of sunscreen. Use of a Wood's or a UV light to reveal solar damage is a helpful way to convince patients of the necessity of sun avoidance. Such a demonstration will also make them more likely to employ preventive measures, such as sunscreens, antioxidants, and retinoids, when sun avoidance is impractical. Sunscreens, antioxidants, and retinoids are discussed in upcoming chapters.

CONCLUSION

Extrinsic and intrinsic aging often coincide and it may be difficult to separate out the effects of each. For this reason, many of the mechanisms that lead to extrinsic aging are also discussed in Chapter 5. Figure 6-10 shows how these overlap from a molecular point of view. Rough, dry skin, mottled pigmentation, and wrinkling epitomize the clinical appearance of extrinsic aging, particularly photoaging. Extensive or severe photodamage can also be a precursor to skin cancer. Despite increasing awareness of the risks of prolonged sun exposure, too many people remain unaware that the proverbial "healthy tan" is, in fact, evidence of photodamage and indicative of premature aging. It is incumbent upon the dermatologist to educate patients on the ravages of the sun, the importance of sun avoidance and sun-protective behavior, and, as always, tailor treatments to individual patient needs.

References

1. Unna PG. *Histopathologie der Hautkrankheiten*. Berlin, Germany: A. Herschwald; 1894.
2. Uitto J. Understanding premature skin aging. *N Engl J Med*. 1997;337:1463.
3. Fenske NA, Lober CW. Structural and functional changes of normal aging skin. *J Am Acad Dermatol*. 1986;15:571.
4. Lovell CR, Smolenski KA, Duance VC, et al. Type I and III collagen content and fibre distribution in normal human skin during ageing. *Br J Dermatol*. 1987;117:419.

5. Gallagher RP, Rivers JK, Lee TK, et al. Broad-spectrum sunscreen use and the development of new nevi in white children: a randomized controlled trial. *JAMA.* 2000;283:2955.

6. Lavker RM. Structural alterations in exposed and unexposed aged skin. *J Invest Dermatol.* 1979;73:59.

7. Yaar M, Gilchrest B. Aging of skin. In: Freeberg I, Eisen A. Wolff K, et al. eds. *Fitzpatrick's Dermatology in General Medicine.* 5th ed. New York, NY: McGraw-Hill; 1999:1697.

8. Lock-Andersen J, Therkildsen P, de Fine Olivarius, et al. Epidermal thickness, skin pigmentation and constitutive photosensitivity. *Photodermatol Photoimmunol Photomed.* 1997;13:153.

9. Whitton JT, Everall JD. The thickness of the epidermis. *Br J Dermatol.* 1973;89:467.

10. Sandby-Moller J, Poulsen T, Wulf HC. Epidermal thickness at different body sites: relationship to age, gender, pigmentation, blood content, skin type and smoking habits. *Acta Derm Venereol.* 2003;83:410.

11. Contet-Audonneau JL, Jeanmaire C, Pauly G. A histological study of human wrinkle structures: comparison between sun-exposed areas of the face, with or without wrinkles, and sun-protected areas. *Br J Dermatol.* 1999;140:1038.

12. Katzberg AA. The area of the dermo-epidermal junction in human skin. *Anat Rec.* 1985;131:717.

13. Kligman AM. Perspectives and problems in cutaneous gerontology. *J Invest Dermatol.* 1979;73:39.

14. Orentreich N, Selmanowitz VJ. Levels of biological functions with aging. *Trans NY Acad Sci.* 1969;31:992.

15. Fisher GJ, Wang ZQ, Datta SC, et al. Pathophysiology of premature skin aging induced by ultraviolet light. *N Engl J Med.* 1997;337:1419.

16. Kligman AM, Zheng P, Lavker RM. The anatomy and pathogenesis of wrinkles. *Br J Dermatol.* 1985;113:37.

17. Gniadecka M, Nielsen OF, Wessel S, et al. Water and protein structure in photoaged and chronically aged skin. *J Invest Dermatol.* 1998;111:1129.

18. Oikarinen A. The aging of skin: chronoaging versus photoaging. *Photo-dermatol Photoimmunol Photomed.* 1990;7:3.

19. Griffiths CE, Russman AN, Majmudar G, et al. Restoration of collagen formation in photodamaged human skin by tretinoin (retinoic acid). *New Engl J Med.* 1993;329:530.

20. Shuster S, Black MM, McVitie E. The influence of age and sex on skin thickness, skin collagen and density. *Br J Dermatol.* 1975;93:639.

21. Craven NM, Watson RE, Jones CJ, et al. Clinical features of photodamaged human skin are associated with a reduction in collagen VII. *Br J Dermatol.* 1997;137:344.

22. Fisher GJ, Datta SC, Talwar HS, et al. Molecular basis of sun-induced premature skin ageing and retinoid antagonism. *Nature.* 1996;379:335.

23. Rosette C, Karin M. Ultraviolet light and osmotic stress: activation of the JNK cascade through multiple growth factor and cytokine receptors. *Science.* 1996;274:1194.

24. Ham J, Babij C, Whitfield J, et al. A c-Jun dominant negative mutant protects sympathetic neurons against programmed cell death. *Neuron.* 1995;14:927.

25. Xia Z, Dickens M, Raingeaud J, et al. Opposing effects of ERK and JNK-p38 MAP kinases on apoptosis. *Science.* 1995; 270:1326.

26. Chung JH, Kang S, Varani J, et al. Decreased extracellular-signal-regulated kinase and increased stress-activated MAP kinase activities in aged human skin in vivo. *J Invest Dermatol.* 2000;115:177.

27. Fisher GJ, Voorhees JJ. Molecular mechanisms of retinoid actions in skin. *FASEB J.* 1996;10:1002.

28. Chung KY, Agarwal A, Uitto J, et al. An AP-1 binding sequence is essential for regulation of the human alpha2(I) collagen (COL1A2) promoter activity by transforming growth factor-beta. *J Biol Chem.* 1996;271:3272.

29. Mitchell RE. Chronic solar dermatosis: a light and electron microscopic study of the dermis. *J Invest Dermatol.* 1967;48:203.

30. Tsuji T, Hamada T. Age-related changes in human dermal elastic fibers. *Br J Dermatol.* 1981;105:57.

31. Scharffetter-Kochanek K, Brenneisen P, Wenk J, et al. Photoaging of the skin from phenotype to mechanisms. *Exp Gerontol.* 2000;35:307.

32. Naylor EC, Watson RE, Sherratt MJ. Molecular aspects of skin ageing. *Maturitas.* 2011;69(3):249–256.

33. Hibbert SA, Watson REB, Gibbs NK, et al. A potential role for endogenous proteins as sacrificial sunscreens and antioxidants in human tissues. *Redox Biol.* 2015;5:101–113.

34. Matsuoka L, Uitto J. Alterations in the elastic fibers in cutaneous aging and solar elastosis. In: Balin A, Kligman AM, eds. *Aging and the Skin.* New York, NY: Raven Press; 1989:141.

35. Lavker RM. Cutaneous aging: chronologic versus photoaging. In: Gilchrest BA. *Photodamage.* 1st ed. Cambridge, MA: Blackwell Science; 1995:128.

36. Montagna W, Carlisle K. Structural changes in aging human skin. *J Invest Dermatol.* 1979;73:47.

37. Escoffier C, de Rigal J, Rochefort A, et al. Age-related mechanical properties of human skin: an in vivo study. *J Invest Dermatol.* 1989;93:353.

38. Langton AK, Alessi S, Hann M, et al. Aging in skin of color: disruption to elastic fiber organization is detrimental to skin's biomechanical function. *J Invest Dermatol.* 2019;139(4):779–788.

39. Ghersetich I, Lotti T, Campanile G, et al. Hyaluronic acid in cutaneous intrinsic aging. *Int J Dermatol.* 1994;33:119.

40. Pearce RH, Grimmer BJ. Age and the chemical constitution of normal human dermis. *J Invest Dermatol.* 1972;58:347.

41. Bernstein EF, Underhill CB, Hahn PJ, et al. Chronic sun exposure alters both the content and distribution of dermal glycosaminoglycans. *Br J Dermatol.* 1996;135:255.

42. Gilchrest BA, Stoff JS, Soter NA. Chronologic aging alters the response to ultraviolet-induced inflammation in human skin. *J Invest Dermatol.* 1982;79:11.

43. Kurimoto I, Streilein JW. cis-urocanic acid suppression of contact hypersensitivity induction is mediated via tumor necrosis factor-alpha. *J Immunol.* 1992;148:3072.

44. Kurimoto I, Streilein JW. Deleterious effects of cis-urocanic acid and UVB radiation on Langerhans cells and on induction of contact hypersensitivity are mediated by tumor necrosis factor-alpha. *J Invest Dermatol.* 1992;99:69S.

45. Ross JA, Howie SEM, Norval M, et al. Ultraviolet-irradiated urocanic acid suppresses delayed-type hypersensitivity to herpes simplex virus in mice. *J Invest Dermatol.* 1986;87:630.

46. de Fine Olivarius F, Wulf HC, Crosby J, et al. Isomerization of urocanic acid after ultraviolet radiation is influenced by skin pigmentation. *J Photochem Photobiol B.* 1999;48:42.

47. Beissert S, Mohammad T, Torri H, et al. Regulation of tumor antigen presentation by urocanic acid. *J Immunol.* 1997;159:92.

48. de Fine Olivarius F, Lock-Andersen J, Larsen FG, et al. Urocanic acid isomers in patients with basal cell carcinoma and cutaneous malignant melanoma. *Br J Dermatol.* 1998;138:986.

49. Snellman E, Jansen CT, Rantanen T, et al. Epidermal urocanic acid concentration and photoisomerization reactivity in patients with cutaneous malignant melanoma or basal cell carcinoma. *Acta Derm Venereol.* 1999;79:200.

50. Leccia MT, Yaar M, Allen N, et al. Solar simulated irradiation modulates gene expression and activity of antioxidant enzymes in cultured human dermal fibroblasts. *Exp Dermatol.* 2001;10:272.

51. Vandersee S, Beyer M, Lademann J, Darvin ME. Blue-violet light irradiation dose dependently decreases carotenoids in human skin, which indicates the generation of free radicals. *Oxid Med Cell Longev.* 2015;2015:579675.

52. Yoon HS, Kim YK, Matsui M, Chung JH. Possible role of infrared or heat in sun-induced changes of dermis of human skin in vivo. *J Dermatol Sci.* 2012;66(1):76–78.

53. Lohan SB, Müller R, Albrecht S, et al. Free radicals induced by sunlight in different spectral regions–in vivo versus ex vivo study. *Exp Dermatol.* 2016;25(5):380–385.

54. Yang JH, Lee HC, Wei YH Photoageing-associated mitochondrial DNA length mutations in human skin. *Arch Dermatol Res.* 1995;287:641–648.

55. Yang JH, Lee HC, Lin KJ, Wei YH. A specific 4977-bp deletion of mitochondrial DNA in human ageing skin. *Arch Dermatol Res.* 1994;286:386–390.

56. Berneburg M, Gattermann N, Stege H, et al. Chronically ultraviolet-exposed human skin shows a higher mutation frequency of mitochondrial DNA as compared to unexposed skin and the hematopoietic system. *Photochem Photobiol.* 1997;66:271–275.

57. Krutmann J, Schroeder P. Role of mitochondria in photoaging of human skin: the defective powerhouse model. *J Investig Dermatol Symp Proc.* 2009;14(1):44–49.

58. Cui R, Widlund HR, Feige E, et al. Central role of p53 in the suntan response and pathologic hyperpigmentation. *Cell.* 2007;128:853.

59. Berneburg M, Plettenberg H, Medve-Konig K, et al. Induction of the photoaging-associated mitochondrial common deletion in vivo in normal human skin. *J Invest Dermatol.* 2004;122:1277–1283.

60. Hüls A, Schikowski T, Krämer U, et al. Ozone exposure and extrinsic skin aging: Results from the SALIA cohort. *J Invest Dermatol.* 2015;135:S49.

61. Fuks KB, Hüls A, Sugiri D, et al. Tropospheric ozone and skin aging: Results from two German cohort studies. *Environ Int.* 2019;124:139–144.

62. Morita A, Torii K, Maeda A, Yamaguchi Y. Molecular basis of tobacco smoke-induced premature skin aging. *J Investig Dermatol Symp Proc.* 2009;14(1):53–55.

63. Ono Y, Torii K, Fritsche E, et al. Role of the aryl hydrocarbon receptor in tobacco smoke extract-induced matrix metalloproteinase-1 expression. *Exp Dermatol.* 2013;22(5):349–353.

64. Vierkötter A, Schikowski T, Ranft U, et al. Airborne particle exposure and extrinsic skin aging. *J Invest Dermatol.* 2010;130(12):2719–2726.

65. Schikowski T, Hüls A. Air Pollution and Skin Aging. *Curr Environ Health Rep.* 2020;7(1):58–64.

66. Krutmann I, Lux B, Luecke S, et al. Involvement of arylhydrocarbon receptor (AhR-) signaling in skin melanogenesis. *J Invest Dermatol.* 2008;128:S220.

67. Daniell HW. Smoker's wrinkles. A study in the epidemiology of "crow's feet." *Ann Intern Med.* 1971;75(6):873–880.

68. Kadunce DP, Burr R, Gress R, Kanner R, Lyon JL, Zone JJ. Cigarette smoking: risk factor for premature facial wrinkling. *Ann Intern Med.* 1991;114(10):840–844.

69. Ernster VL, Grady D, Miike R, Black D, Selby J, Kerlikowske K. Facial wrinkling in men and women, by smoking status. *Am J Public Health.* 1995;85(1):78–82.

70. Francès C, Boisnic S, Hartmann DJ, et al. Changes in the elastic tissue of the non-sun-exposed skin of cigarette smokers. *Br J Dermatol.* 1991;125(1):43–47.

71. Gieringer D, St. Laurent J, Goodrich S. Cannabis vaporizer combines efficient delivery of THC with effective suppression of pyrolytic compounds. *J Cannabis Ther.* 2004;4(1):7–27.

72. Ghadially R, Brown BE, Sequeira-Martin SM, et al. The aged epidermal permeability barrier. Structural, functional, and lipid biochemical abnormalities in humans and a senescent murine model. *J Clin Invest.* 1995;95:2281.

73. Tezuka T, Qing J, Saheki M, et al. Terminal differentiation of facial epidermis of the aged: immunohistochemical studies. *Dermatology.* 1994;188:21.

74. Nelson BR, Majmudar G, Griffiths CE, et al. Clinical improvement following dermabrasion of photoaged skin correlates with synthesis of collagen I. *Arch Dermatol.* 1994;130:1136.

75. Song EJ, Gordon-Thomson C, Cole L, et al. 1α,25-Dihydroxyvitamin D3 reduces several types of UV-induced DNA damage and contributes to photoprotection. *J Steroid Biochem Mol Biol.* 2013;136:131–138.

76. Gordon-Thomson C, Gupta R, Tongkao-on W, et al. 1α,25 dihydroxyvitamin D3 enhances cellular defences against UV-induced oxidative and other forms of DNA damage in skin. *Photochem Photobiol Sci.* 2012;11(12):1837–1847.

77. Ashcroft GS, Dodsworth J, van Boxtel E, et al. Estrogen accelerates cutaneous wound healing associated with an increase in TGF-beta1 levels. *Nat Med.* 1997;3(11):1209–1215.

78. Baumann L. A dermatologist's opinion on hormone therapy and skin aging. *Fertil Steril.* 2005;84(2):289–290; discussion 295.

79. Piérard GE, Letawe C, Dowlati A, Piérard-Franchimont C. Effect of hormone replacement therapy for menopause on the mechanical properties of skin. *J Am Geriatr Soc.* 1995;43(6):662–665.

80. Rittié L, Kang S, Voorhees JJ, Fisher GJ. Induction of collagen by estradiol: difference between sun-protected and photodamaged human skin in vivo. *Arch Dermatol.* 2008;144(9):1129–1140.

CHAPTER 7

Facial Anatomy and Aging

Leslie S. Baumann, MD

SUMMARY POINTS

What's Important?
1. The various ethnicities age differently.
2. Women's faces are more often curved while men more often have angular faces and these are considered aesthetic ideals.
3. Terminology helps patients communicate their aesthetic goals.

What's New?
1. Bone loss, rather than gravity, is the main cause of facial shape changes with aging.
2. HA fillers prevent aging by increasing collagen production and improving the ECM.
3. Botulinum toxins prevent the development of fine lines.
4. Lengthening of the lip occurs with aging rather than volume loss.

What's Coming?
1. Medications and supplements may be developed to reduce bone loss in the face.
2. The exact effects of hormone status and facial bone loss are unknown, but may be elucidated with ongoing research.
3. Use of injectables to "prejuvenate" the face and prevent aging.

Faces differ according to gender, ethnicity, genetics, and aging. In general, faces can be classified by shapes. Square and rectangular facial shapes are perceived as more masculine while round and heart-shaped faces are seen as more feminine. With aging, the face becomes more square-shaped as the brows lower, cheeks flatten, and jowling occurs. Overuse and improper placement of dermal fillers can result in an exaggerated heart shape. It is important to consider face shape when deciding placement of dermal fillers (**Fig. 7-1**).

THE AGING FACE

The face is composed of skin, fat, muscles, cartilage, and bone: each of these changes with age. The skin thins, sags, and develops an uneven tone. Although the skin becomes thinner with loss of collagen, hyaluronic acid (HA), and other components, it is the loss of fat, muscle, and bone that causes the shape and volume alterations characteristic of facial aging. An understanding of the changes in facial shape and volume with aging is important when approaching the patient who desires facial rejuvenation. Skin aging is discussed in Chapters 5 (Intrinsic Aging) and 6 (Extrinsic Aging). This chapter focuses on the changes in the other layers of the face that lead to an aged appearance.

The main changes seen in an aged face are (**Fig. 7-2**):

- Decreased forehead fullness
- Concavity of the temple
- Lowered brows
- Increased size of the orbits
- Increased length and width of the nose
- Hollowing of the cheeks
- Loss of distinctive arches and curves on the face
- Lowering and widening of the chin

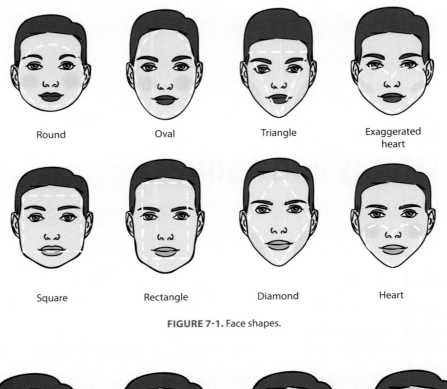

| Round | Oval | Triangle | Exaggerated heart |

| Square | Rectangle | Diamond | Heart |

FIGURE 7-1. Face shapes.

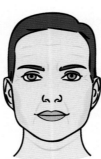 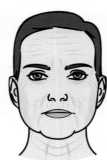 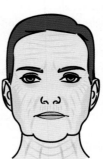

FIGURE 7-2. Face shape changes with aging.

- Loss of jaw definition
- Squaring of the face

CAUSES OF FACIAL AGING CHANGES

There are two main theories of why aging occurs in the face: the gravitational theory and the volumetric theory.[1] Both theories have credence and are not mutually exclusive. The gravitational theory focuses on the gravitational pull on the ligaments that causes them to change position and affect the facial structures, most notably the fat pads. The volumetric theory of facial aging is currently believed to be the more important of the two because changes in volume can affect the positions of the ligaments. Several studies have demonstrated alterations in volume of facial compartments.[2-4] This chapter provides an overview of the volumetric changes in various parts of the face that lead to an aged appearance.

BONE AND FACIAL AGING

Facial bone undergoes selective resorption, with certain regions resorbing faster than others.[5] Changes in bone lead to a reduction in facial height and an increase in width, which results in a squaring of the facial shape. Notable bone resorption occurs around the nasal, maxillary, and frontal bones, yielding linear and angular alterations followed by rotation and posterior displacement of the midface as well as increased aperture of the orbital rim.[6] The maxillary bone decreases in size.[7] The shape and size of the mandible are affected by resorption of bone in the alveolar ridge and loss or changes in the teeth. The orbits increase in size and the supraorbital ridges expand. The lateral cheek projection flattens with loss of the ogee curve of the cheekbone. (The "ogee curve" is an architectural term used to describe a double curve.) The projection of the chin also changes with age.

In Caucasians, the glabellar, orbital, maxillary, and pyriform angles decrease with age and the maxillary pyriform angles as well as infraorbital rim regress with age.[8,9] As compared with Caucasians, Asians have been shown to undergo fewer changes in the orbital and maxillary angles but experience more prominent changes in the pyriform angle with aging.[8,10] African Americans have decreased rates of bone resorption compared with Caucasians.[11] One study showed a significant decrease in frontozygomatic junction diameter and a significant widening of the pyriform aperture in the black population over a 10-year period. This study concluded that less bone loss was seen in subjects with black skin as compared with those with light skin.[6]

Bone loss widens the orbits and affects the position of the ligaments and fat pads, leading to numerous signs of facial aging. There are also significant changes found in the fat pads themselves.

FAT AND FACIAL AGING

Fat in the face is divided into superficial and deep compartments separated by the superficial musculoaponeurotic system (SMAS). The adipose of the face is contained in fat pads held in place by surrounding structures (**Fig. 7-3**). The superficial fat pads are adjacent to the facial muscles, while the deep fat pads lie atop the facial bones. Rohrich and Pessa, in particular, have conducted several studies to delineate these fat pads.[2,3,12–14] Their results have been confirmed by others.[1]

Fat pads are important because they change size and position in the aging face due to alterations in bone mass and movement of the ligaments (**Fig. 7-4**). For example, a decrease in the size of the bony structures of the maxilla leads to anterior movement of the malar fat pad. This results in increased depth of the nasolabial fold.[7,15] Identification of which fat pad has moved or changed in size is an excellent approach to determining where to inject facial fillers.

FACIAL MUSCLES AND AGING

Facial muscles lengthen with age and become stiffer.[16] It is unknown how much of this is due to sarcopenia and how much is due to shifting facial ligaments. Many people have proposed that facial muscle exercises can mitigate facial aging and increase facial volume; however, aged muscles exhibit increased tone, so this does not make sense scientifically. A review of publications investigating facial exercise-induced changes in profiles of facial soft tissues showed that 8- to 12-week interventions of facial muscle contractions or

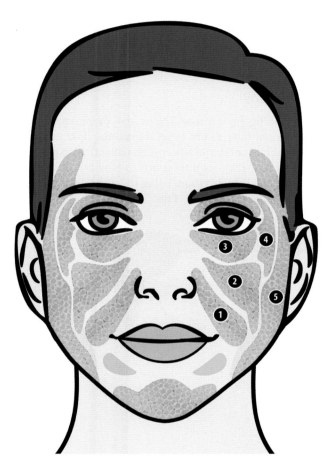

FIGURE 7-3. Fat pads in the face.

Aging of facial fat pads

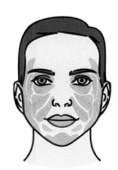 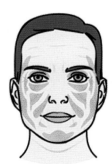 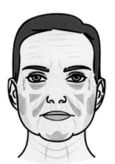 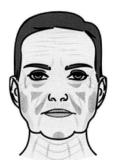

FIGURE 7-4. Changes in facial fat pads with aging.

oscillatory movement devices may increase facial muscle size in middle-aged women.[17] It was unclear if the exercises in the reviewed studies resulted in muscle hypertrophy or a change in the resting length of the muscle.

Further, it is unknown whether the increase in facial muscle size reported after facial exercises is due to increased muscle size, a change in the resting length of muscle, changes to muscle tone, or changes to associated ligaments.[17] Although studies have demonstrated an augmentation in facial muscle size, they have not definitively shown an improvement in facial appearance.

A small controlled study of 18 participants evaluated the efficacy of four isometric exercises targeting five facial areas for 7 weeks (9 subjects used facial exercises, while 9 did not). This study did not demonstrate a significant difference between groups.[18] A literature search that reviewed nine studies concluded that the evidence as of 2014 was insufficient to conclude that facial exercises are an effective way to achieve facial rejuvenation.[19] At this time it is concluded that facial exercises do not improve the appearance of the aging face. In fact, the increased movement could increase, deepen, or lengthen wrinkles based on the fact that botulinum toxins reduce wrinkles by decreasing movement.

JAWLINE AND AGING

A youthful male jawline is typically broad with a sharp right angle that approximates 90 degrees, while young women usually have a less angular jawline. The decrease in bone volume of the mandible and chin combined with forward movement of the fat pads result in loss of definition of the jawline and development of jowls (**Fig. 7-5**).

THE LIP

Lip Anatomy

Understanding lip anatomy helps the practitioner choose which dermal filler to use to rejuvenate the lips. Anatomical terms facilitate communication with patients who often have an idea of how they want their lips to look but do not know how to articulate their vision. Using these charts to communicate with patients may help (**Figs. 7-6–7-8**).

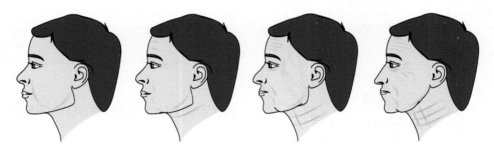

FIGURE 7-5. Changes in jawline with facial aging.

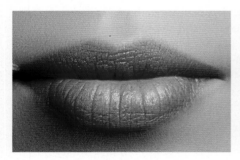

Perfect lip

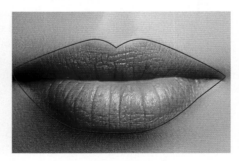

Vermillion border

Philtral column   Philtral dimple   Philtral column

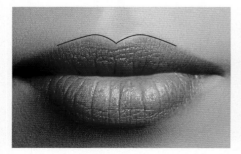

Cupid's bow

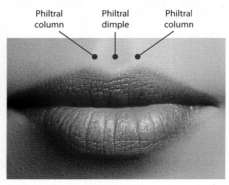

Philtrum

FIGURE 7-6. Basic lip anatomy.

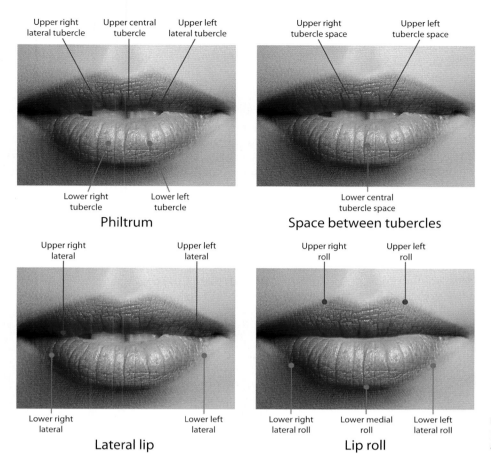

FIGURE 7-7. Lip anatomy vocabulary that patients can use to show where they want augmentation.

Lip styles

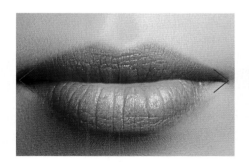

Oral commissures

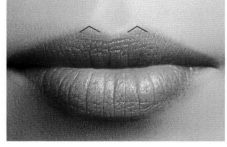

G-K points

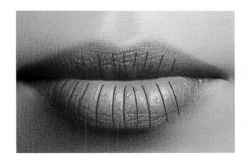

Vertical lip body lines

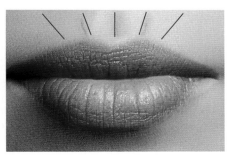

Bar code lines

FIGURE 7-8. Areas where aging of the lip is most obvious.

The Lip and Aging

The decrease in size of the maxilla bone and thinning of the orbicularis oculi muscle lead to less support for the upper lip.[7] Although fillers are often used to increase the size of lips in an effort to make them look younger, many believe that the appearance of aging lips is not due to loss of volume, but rather to ptosis of the upper lip.[20] One study examined 182 photographs of the upper lip that were measured and correlated with age.[21] A significant lengthening of the upper lip with aging was shown.

Aging lips reveal flattening of the cupid's bow, philtrum columns, and vermilion border with lowering and loss of the GK points. Aging lips display an increased distance between the oral commissures, bar code lines, and vertical lip body lines.

PREJUVENATION OF THE FACE

"Prejuvenation" is a term gaining popularity to describe efforts to prevent aging, especially facial aging. Most prejuvenation treatments are in the form of topical skin care, supplements, or injectables.

Prevention of Facial Bone Loss

There have been no studies on the effects of estradiol replacement on bone loss in the face of postmenopausal women; however, many studies have shown that estrogen replacement slows skeletal bone loss. New studies suggest that increased levels of follicle stimulating hormone may play a role in bone loss in women.[22] Men also experience facial bone loss with aging, but there is a paucity of data on the role testosterone may play in preventing facial aging bone loss. New purported mechanisms of bone loss in men are being evaluated.[23] In the future, we may have more data on anabolic hormones and other medications to prevent bone loss in the face.

Injectables to Prevent Facial Aging

Hyaluronic acid dermal fillers prevent facial aging by changing the ECM

Early use of HA fillers may prevent skin aging by preserving facial volume and increasing collagen production.[24] Filler injections stimulate localized proliferation of fibroblasts. Fibroblasts, when stretched, tend to upregulate collagen production.[25] Restylane and Juvéderm injections are known to increase collagen production, but this result has not yet been proven with other HA fillers.[26–28] The increase in collagen that occurs may be due to direct effects of the HA on the fibroblast or a result of stretching of the fibroblasts.[29]

Aged skin is characterized by altered fibroblast attachments to the extracellular matrix (ECM) resulting in decreased mechanical forces on the fibroblasts.[30] Accumulation of fragmented collagen and elastin in the dermis alters the physical properties of the dermal microenvironment and reduces ECM binding by fibroblasts, which in turn lessens mechanical force. Diminished mechanical forces render a collapsed shape to fibroblasts,[31] which then produce less Type I collagen[32] and more matrix metalloproteinases. When HA is injected into the dermis, fibroblast spreading is induced. This fibroblast elongation upregulates the TGF-β signaling pathway and its downstream targets CTGF/CCN2, stimulating Type I collagen synthesis.[27]

Botulinum toxin injections to prevent facial aging

Botulinum toxin injections prevent muscle movement, stiffness, and hypertrophy. Long-term consistent use of botulinum toxin has been associated with the development of fewer facial wrinkles. An examination of two identical twin females aged 38 years demonstrated the protective role against aging that botulinum toxins impart. One twin had received regular Botox injections for 14 years, while the other twin had only been injected twice in that same 14-year period. The twin who had received regular injections had fewer facial wrinkles than the twin who had not.[33] The same results were observed at 19 years.[34] A case study that followed two subjects over a 7-year period showed improved skin quality and fewer wrinkles over time.[35]

CONCLUSION

The aging face evinces distinctive characteristics due to bone loss, lengthening of ligaments, and movement of fat pads. Skin aging, as discussed in Chapter 6, Extrinsic Aging, also contributes to an aged appearance. Facial rejuvenation treatments may include fillers, botulinum toxins, lights, lasers, peels, microneedling, and, of course, topical skin care. The use of HA fillers to elongate fibroblasts and stimulate them to increase collagen production as well as botulinum toxin to prevent fine lines can be enhanced by the combined topical use of ascorbic acid and retinoids.

References

1. Wan D, Amirlak B, Rohrich R, Davis K. The clinical importance of the fat compartments in midfacial aging. *Plast Reconstr Surg Glob Open.* 2014;1(9):e92.
2. Rohrich RJ, Pessa JE. The fat compartments of the face: anatomy and clinical implications for cosmetic surgery. *Plast Reconstr Surg.* 2007;119:2219–2227.
3. Rohrich RJ, Pessa JE. The anatomy and clinical implications of perioral submuscular fat. *Plast Reconstr Surg.* 2009;124:266–271.
4. Gosain AK, Klein MH, Sudhakar PV, et al. A volumetric analysis of soft-tissue changes in the aging midface using high-resolution MRI: implications for facial rejuvenation. *Plast Reconstr Surg.* 2005;115:1143–1152. Discussion 1153–1155.
5. Mendelson B, Wong CH. Changes in the facial skeleton with aging: implications and clinical applications in facial rejuvenation. *Aesthetic Plast Surg.* 2012;36(4):753–760.
6. Buziashvili D, Tower JI, Sangal NR, et al. Long-term Patterns of Age-Related Facial Bone Loss in Black Individuals. *JAMA Facial Plast Surg.* 2019;21(4):292–297.
7. Coleman SR, Grover R. The anatomy of the aging face: volume loss and changes in 3-dimensional topography. *Aesthet Surg J.* 2006;26(1S):S4–9.

8. Cotofana S, Fratila AA, Schenck TL, Redka-Swoboda W, Zilinsky I, Pavicic T. The Anatomy of the Aging Face: A Review. *Facial Plast Surg.* 2016;32(3):253–260.

9. Richard MJ, Morris C, Deen BF, Gray L, Woodward JA. Analysis of the anatomic changes of the aging facial skeleton using computer-assisted tomography. *Ophthal Plast Reconstr Surg.* 2009;25(5):382–386.

10. Kim SJ, Kim SJ, Park JS, Byun SW, Bae JH. Analysis of age-related changes in Asian facial skeletons using 3D vector mathematics on picture archiving and communication system computed tomography. *Yonsei Med J.* 2015;56(5):1395–1400.

11. Henry YM, Eastell R. Ethnic and gender differences in bone mineral density and bone turnover in young adults: effect of bone size. *Osteoporos Int.* 2000;11(6):512–517.

12. Rohrich RJ, Pessa JE, Ristow B. The youthful cheek and the deep medial fat compartment. *Plast Reconstr Surg.* 2008;121:2107–2112.

13. Rohrich RJ, Pessa JE. The retaining system of the face: histologic evaluation of the septal boundaries of the subcutaneous fat compartments. *Plast Reconstr Surg.* 2008;121:1804–1809.

14. Rohrich RJ, Arbique GM, Wong C, et al. The anatomy of suborbicularis fat: implications for periorbital rejuvenation. *Plast Reconstr Surg.* 2009;124:946–951.

15. Owsley JQ. Elevation of the malar fat pad superficial to the orbicularis oculi muscle for correction of prominent nasolabial folds. *Clin Plast Surg.* 1995;22(2):279–293.

16. Le Louarn C, Buthiau D, Buis J. Structural aging: the facial recurve concept. *Aesthetic Plast Surg.* 2007;31(3):213–218.

17. Abe T, Loenneke JP. The influence of facial muscle training on the facial soft tissue profile: A brief review. *Cosmetics.* 2019;6(3):50.

18. De Vos MC, Van den Brande H, Boone B, Van Borsel J. Facial exercises for facial rejuvenation: a control group study. *Folia Phoniatr Logop.* 2013;65(3):117–122.

19. Van Borsel J, De Vos MC, Bastiaansen K, Welvaert J, Lambert J. The effectiveness of facial exercises for facial rejuvenation: a systematic review. *Aesthet Surg J.* 2014;34(1):22–27.

20. Penna V, Stark GB, Eisenhardt SU, Bannasch H, Iblher N. The aging lip: a comparative histological analysis of age-related changes in the upper lip complex. *Plast Reconstr Surg.* 2009;124(2):624–628.

21. Iblher N, Kloepper J, Penna V, Bartholomae JP, Stark GB. Changes in the aging upper lip—a photomorphometric and MRI-based study (on a quest to find the right rejuvenation approach). *J Plast Reconstr Aesthet Surg.* 2008;61(10):1170–1176.

22. Khosla S. Estrogen Versus FSH Effects on Bone Metabolism: Evidence From Interventional Human Studies. *Endocrinology.* 2020;161(8):bqaa111.

23. Laurent MR, Dedeyne L, Dupont J, Mellaerts B, Dejaeger M, Gielen E. Age-related bone loss and sarcopenia in men. *Maturitas.* 2019;122:51–56.

24. Kerscher M, Bayrhammer J, Reuther T. Rejuvenating influence of a stabilized hyaluronic acid-based gel of nonanimal origin on facial skin aging. *Dermatol Surg.* 2008;34(5):720–726.

25. Kessler D, Dethlefsen S, et al. Fibroblasts in mechanically stressed collagen lattices assume a "synthetic" phenotype. *J Biol Chem.* 2001;276(39):36575–36585.

26. Wang F, Garza LA, Kang S, et al. In vivo stimulation of de novo collagen production caused by cross-linked hyaluronic acid dermal filler injections in photodamaged human skin. *Arch Dermatol.* 2007;143(2):155–163.

27. Quan T, Wang F, Shao Y, et al. Enhancing structural support of the dermal microenvironment activates fibroblasts, endothelial cells, and keratinocytes in aged human skin in vivo. *J Invest Dermatol.* 2013;133(3):658–667.

28. Paliwal S, Fagien S, Sun X, et al. Skin extracellular matrix stimulation following injection of a hyaluronic acid-based dermal filler in a rat model. *Plast Reconstr Surg.* 2014;134(6):1224–1233.

29. Skutek M, van Griensven M, Zeichen J, Brauer N, Bosch U. Cyclic mechanical stretching modulates secretion pattern of growth factors in human tendon fibroblasts. *Eur J Appl Physiol.* 2001;86(1):48–52.

30. Varani J, Schuger L, Dame MK, et al. Reduced fibroblast interaction with intact collagen as a mechanism for depressed collagen synthesis in photodamaged skin. *J Invest Dermatol.* 2004;122(6):1471–1479.

31. Fisher GJ, Varani J, Voorhees JJ. Looking older: fibroblast collapse and therapeutic implications. *Arch Dermatol.* 2008;144(5):666–672.

32. Varani J, Dame MK, Rittie L, et al. Decreased collagen production in chronologically aged skin: roles of age-dependent alteration in fibroblast function and defective mechanical stimulation. *Am J Pathol.* 2006;168(6):1861–1868.

33. Binder WJ. Long-term effects of botulinum toxin type A (Botox) on facial lines: a comparison in identical twins. *Arch Facial Plast Surg.* 2006;8(6):426–431.

34. Rivkin A, Binder WJ. Long-term effects of onabotulinumtoxinA on facial lines: a 19-year experience of identical twins. *Dermatol Surg.* 2015;41(Suppl 1):S64–S66.

35. Bowler PJ. Dermal and epidermal remodeling using botulinum toxin type A for facial, non reducible, hyperkinetic lines: two case studies. *J Cosmet Dermatol.* 2008;7(3):241–244.

Immunology of Skin Aging

Amy R. Vandiver, MD, PhD
Jenny Kim, MD, PhD

SUMMARY POINTS

What's Important

- The skin provides the first line of defense against external pathogens through a physical, chemical, and antimicrobial barrier maintained by the epidermis and the cutaneous microbiome.
- In addition to barrier function, the skin acts as an innate immune sentinel, with Toll-like receptors responding to external pathogens and cellular damage to activate the local immune response.
- Cytokines and growth factors released upon activation of innate immune signaling regulate local inflammation and function of resident skin cells. Growth factors specifically play an important role in regulating epidermal proliferation and synthesis of the dermal matrix.
- Aging of the skin is associated with a decline in barrier function and increased activation of the innate immune system. These changes contribute to altered growth factor and MMP signaling which impair maintenance of the dermal matrix.

What's New

- Advances in sequencing technology have allowed increased insight into the diversity of the cutaneous microbiome. The balance of bacterial species and strains in each body site plays a role in regulating immune function.
- Induction of innate immune signaling through activation of Toll-like receptors as part of a damage response plays an important role in regeneration and wound healing.
- Anti-aging treatments targeted at modulating innate immune signaling have shown benefit for improving photoaging phenotypes.

What's Coming

- Therapy aimed at restoration of the skin barrier will clarify the role of skin barrier changes in initiating skin and systemic aging changes.
- Better characterization of the cutaneous microbiome will facilitate understanding of shifts associated with aging to offer more targeted probiotic therapy for cutaneous aging.
- Increased understanding of the role of the innate immune system in injury-mediated regeneration will offer new targets for promoting rejuvenation.

Little is known about the relationship between immunology and skin appearance; however, it is certain that the immune system plays an important role in the health of the skin and evidence is accumulating to indicate that the immune response plays a role in skin aging phenotypes. Work is ongoing to elucidate how this vital system interacts with the largest organ of the body. It is very likely that this segment of research, as it pertains to cosmetic dermatology, will offer significant potential for discovery of new therapeutics and procedures. This chapter will serve as a brief introduction to the skin as an immune organ and how the immune response plays a role in cutaneous aging.

In the past, the skin was viewed primarily as a physical barrier to prevent invading pathogens and other environmental toxins, including UV radiation, from penetrating into internal organs. However, we now know that the skin acts as an immense and integral immune organ and first point of contact with the environment, capable of initiating an intricate series of events leading to host defense. A basic review of skin immunology, including the role of antimicrobial peptides and lipids, the microbiome, cytokines and growth factors, will be provided as an important part of this discussion. Mechanisms of various immune responses found in skin disease, the interplay between innate immunity and extracellular matrix synthesis and the relevance of the local immune system to skin aging, particularly photoaging, will be emphasized. Finally, emerging immune-targeted anti-aging treatments will be highlighted.

SKIN—AN INNATE IMMUNE ORGAN

The immune response can be divided into innate and adaptive immunity. The innate immune response occurs rapidly and without specificity after exposure to a danger trigger. The cells of the innate immune system use pattern recognition receptors (PRRs) to recognize potential threats and respond by secreting soluble factors that can lead to both inflammation and host defense including antimicrobial response. The adaptive immune response is specific to individual encountered microbes but occurs more slowly as activation of adaptive immune cells, such as B and T cells, requires stimulation from antigen-presenting cells and receptor gene rearrangement. The adaptive immune system can mount either humoral immunity (B cells, which make antibodies) or cell-mediated immunity (T cells). Furthermore, the adaptive immune system is responsible for immune memory, which confers long-term protection to the host. Although the two systems appear distinct, they are not separate, and in fact can act synergistically, insofar as the innate immune system instructs the adaptive immune response and the adaptive immune system instructs the innate system.

As the skin is constantly interfacing with the environment, its function as a rapidly responding innate immune organ is particularly prominent. Prior to encountering an environmental trigger, the epidermis plays a prominent role in promoting immunity through maintenance of an antimicrobial barrier through synthesis of a physical barrier and antimicrobial peptides (AMPs) and function of the cutaneous microbiome. In the epidermis, keratinocytes, sebocytes, Langerhans cells and likely melanocytes act as innate immune cells. In addition, neutrophils, macrophages, and dendritic cells present within the dermis play a role in innate immunity. When a foreign substance is encountered, activation of innate cells occurs through PRRs, including the Toll-like receptors (TLRs), which are reviewed below. Upon activation, the skin resident innate immune cells become capable of inducing a direct antimicrobial response by producing factors that can help protect the host from external insults. These factors include reactive oxygen and nitrogen intermediates (also known as "free radicals") and antimicrobial peptides. In addition, activated innate immune cells produce cytokines and other inflammatory mediators that can instruct adaptive immunity. Paradoxically, this same protective innate immune response can induce pro-inflammatory cytokine production that can lead to inflammation and tissue injury. Accumulating evidence suggests that this proinflammatory environment contributes to aging and particularly photoaging changes. Below, details of these levels of innate immune function and evidence for their involvement in aging will be reviewed.

Epidermal Barrier Function

The first line of defense is the epidermal barrier. The primary barrier function of the epidermis comes from the topmost layer, the stratum corneum, which is made up of anucleate corneocyte cells attached by corneodesmosomes and surrounded by a dense network of proteins and lipids to form a semipermeable barrier. This barrier serves the dual function of preventing pathogens from entering the body and preventing water loss through the skin. In addition to the physical barrier function, the stratum corneum also acts as a chemical barrier through maintenance of an acidic pH as well as the production of protective lipids. Disruption of barrier function is most classically seen in atopic dermatitis. In this setting, impaired barrier function is associated with immune dysregulation in which both the immune system is activated and increased inflammatory cytokines are seen, but the ability to clear common pathogens is decreased.

SKIN LIPIDS

The lipids present in the epidermis were classically thought to function primarily in forming a physical barrier, however there is growing evidence that they play a broader role in innate immunity. Lipids accumulate in keratinocytes beginning in the stratum granulosum, in which keratinocytes store glucosylceramides, sphingomyelin, and phospholipids in lamellar bodies. As keratinocytes differentiate to form the stratum corneum, these are enzymatically modified to ceramides and free fatty acids, as well as sphingosines. Free fatty acids and ceramides lipid envelope of the stratum corneum together with cholesterol and alterations in the content of these lipids are associated with impaired barrier function.[1,2]

In addition to their structural role, lipids and their metabolism function in the antimicrobial barrier through other means. Production of free fatty acids plays an important role in acidification of the stratum corneum.[2] Further, multiple lipid metabolites have been demonstrated to have bactericidal activity. The sphingosines have been shown to have broad activity against gram positive and negative bacteria in vitro.[3] Free fatty acids, in particular the medium to long chain forms, have bactericidal activity against gram positive bacteria,[4] a defense which is partly mediated by increased activation of the innate immune system.[5]

ANTIMICROBIAL PEPTIDES

In addition to their role in forming a physical barrier, keratinocytes create an antimicrobial barrier through secretion of antimicrobial peptides (AMPS). AMPs are a diverse family of secreted peptides that are typically small, positively charged and hydrophobic, and function to prevent local pathogen growth. They are produced by all organisms. Those produced by eukaryotic organisms typically target bacteria, fungi, and enveloped viruses through disruption of membranes. In addition to their antimicrobial action, many AMPs regulate the innate immune system. There is evidence of AMPs acting both to amplify local inflammatory responses through chemotactic signaling and to decrease inflammatory response through modulation of TLR signaling. Whether AMPs play a pro-inflammatory or modulatory role has been demonstrated to depend on the type and context of pathogen encounter, suggesting a complex relationship in which AMPs help fine tune the inflammatory response.

Multiple AMPs have been identified in the skin. Keratinocytes constitutively excrete andrenomedullin, ß-defensin-1, and the ribonuclease RNase 7.[6,7] In the setting of inflammation challenge, RNase7 and ß-defensin-2 and 4 are upregulated.[8–10] In addition, keratinocytes produce the antimicrobial peptide cathelicidin/LL-37, which is stored in the cytoplasm and released upon stimulation.[11,12] These have broad action against many of the common cutaneous pathogens: Adrenomedullin demonstrating activity against gram negative and positive bacteria, while the ß-defensins, RNase7, and cathelicidin show efficacy against bacteria, enveloped viruses and candida species. Sebocytes also produce ß-defensin-2 and cathelicidin as well as dermcidin, a peptide with antibacterial activity first characterized in eccrine glands.[13–15]

Research in psoriasis and atopic dermatitis suggest AMP expression is intimately linked to keratinocyte function and pathology. AMPs are upregulated and abundant in psoriatic lesions, but decreased in atopic dermatitis, consistent with impaired immunity seen in atopic dermatitis.[16] Low dose UVB exposure upregulates keratinocyte expression of antimicrobial peptides in mice, however the effects of chronic exposure and aging on this system are not well understood.[17] Deeper in the skin, there is increasing evidence that dermal fat cells play an antimicrobial role through secretion of cathelicidin in response to pathogens.[18] Intriguingly, this capacity is reduced in aged mice, possibly due to increased TGF-ß signaling.[19]

The Skin Microbiome

With advances in sequencing technology, we have recently gained insight into the diverse array of microorganisms that live on the skin surface and make up the cutaneous microbiome. As the ability to characterize these populations increases, we are rapidly learning about their regulation of cutaneous immunity and their role in skin pathology. The skin microbiome consists of bacteria, fungi and viruses. Among bacteria, most found on the skin are part of four phyla: Actinobacteria, Firmicutes, Bacteriodetes and Proteobacteria. The composition of individuals' skin microbiome is first established in the neonatal period. The composition shifts during puberty and then is thought to remain relatively stable throughout adulthood. While the composition is relatively stable within an individual throughout their lifetime, it varies within an individual based on region of the body. Across all sites,

staphylococcus epidermidis is the most frequently isolated organism. Sebaceous rich regions such as the face are dominated by cutibacterium and staphylococcus species, while moist areas such as the antecubital fossa are dominated by corynebacterium, staphylococcus and beta-proteobacteria species.[20] Within each species, variation in strains is observed. For some bacteria such as cutibacterium acnes, the identified strains vary more between individuals than between body sites of a single individual, while for others such as staph epidermidis, there is more variation between body sites within an individual than between individuals.[21] Between individuals, the composition of the microbiome is seen to vary with immune status, genetic background and lifestyle factors. Settings of systemic and local inflammation have been shown to acutely alter the microbiome composition within specific body sites.

Under steady state conditions, the majority of microbes found on the skin function as commensal organisms, they do not cause pathology but may contribute positively to immune function. The immune system learns to tolerate colonizing bacteria when bacteria are encountered in the absence of inflammatory signals through action of T-regulatory cells in the neonatal period.[22,23] There is growing evidence that once established as commensals, at least some components of the skin microbiome function in innate immunity. Cutibacterium and staph epidermidis specifically have been shown to both produce antimicrobial peptides and to stimulate production of antimicrobial peptides within the epidermis. Staph epidermidis and other commensals have also been shown to interact with tissue resident dendritic cells to stimulate migration of populations of protective T cells to skin when introduced to the skin of germ free mice.[24] In wound healing models, staph epidermidis components binding to epidermal TLR2 is shown to decrease inflammation and promote improved healing.[25]

While methods are rapidly evolving to study the microbiome, initial work has indicated that the microbiome is altered in multiple settings of skin disease and that targeting this population may be beneficial. In atopic dermatitis, the microbiome has been observed to shift to become less diverse, with increased staphylococcus and corynebacterium and reduced streptococcus, propionibacterium and acinetobacter during flares. This shift improves when eczema activity is reduced.[26] More severe AD has been associated with higher proportions of staph aureus versus staph epidermidis.[27] In diabetic wounds, the specific species and strains in the wound microbiome are associated with clinical course and illicit responses in mice that correspond to patient wound course.[28]

Cytokines and Growth Factors

Cytokines are soluble mediators of the immune system secreted by particular cell types in response to a variety of stimuli. They differ in molecular weight, structure, and mechanism of action. In general, secreted cytokines act locally in either an autocrine (effect on the producing cell itself) or paracrine (effect on adjacent cells) fashion. While there have been numerous cytokines identified to date, this section will focus on the common cytokines present in the skin and the changes that occur in expression profiles with aging.

TABLE 8-1	Summary of Cytokines and Growth Factors Within the Skin and the Cells That Produce Them
	Cell Type
Cytokines	
Pro-inflammatory	
IL-1 (α, β)	Keratinocytes (IL-1α), Langerhans cells, melanocytes, fibroblasts, T cells, B cells, macrophages, neutrophils
TNF-α	Keratinocytes, Langerhans cells, melanocytes, fibroblasts, T cells, B cells, macrophages, neutrophils, eosinophils, basophils
IL-2	T cells
IL-4	T cells, mast cells, basophils, eosinophils
IL-5	Mast cells, T cells, eosinophils
IL-6	Keratinocytes, Langerhans cells, melanocytes, fibroblasts, T cells, B cells
IL-8	Keratinocytes, Langerhans cells, melanocytes, fibroblasts, T cells, B cells, macrophages, neutrophils, eosinophils, basophils
IL-12	Keratinocytes, Langerhans cells, macrophages, mast cells, B cells
Anti-inflammatory	
IL-10	T cells, mast cells, macrophages, B cells
Growth factors	
TGF-α	Keratinocytes, macrophages, eosinophils
TGF-β	Keratinocytes, melanocytes, fibroblasts, T cells, B cells, macrophages
EGF	Keratinocytes, eccrine ducts

In the epidermis, cytokines are primarily produced by keratinocytes, melanocytes, and Langerhans cells, while fibroblasts, endothelial cells, mast cells, macrophages, dendritic cells, lymphocytes, and other inflammatory cells are responsible for cytokine production within the dermis (**Table 8-1** summarizes cytokines present in the skin and the cells that produce them).

PRO-INFLAMMATORY CYTOKINES

Activation of the immune system is an important step in protecting the skin from pathogens and other environmental toxins; however, paradoxically, activation of the immune mechanism can also lead to inflammation, thus promoting disease and aging. Interleukin (IL)-1, a cytokine expressed by keratinocytes and most other cell types, exhibits a broad spectrum of biologic activity. Whereas IL-1β is predominantly expressed in most cells, IL-1α is expressed by keratinocytes.[29] IL-1 induces keratinocyte proliferation, promotes differentiation of B cells, activates neutrophils and macrophages, and

initiates the expression of other pro-inflammatory cytokines. In addition, IL-1 is capable of enhancing the activation of T cells and is involved in aspects of both humoral (B cells) and cellular immunity (T cells). IL-1 is continuously expressed at low levels in normal epidermis but is markedly enhanced when the skin barrier is disrupted. Furthermore, upon UV radiation, keratinocytes can secrete IL-1, which then initiates a cytokine cascade, and the biologic sequelae may accelerate changes seen in photoaging.

Tumor necrosis factor (TNF-α), although structurally unrelated to IL-1, shares similar biologic spectra. TNF-α is a potent inducer of inflammation and also induces prostaglandin synthesis in macrophages, further contributing to its pro-inflammatory nature. Within the skin, both IL-1 and TNF-α are expressed by keratinocytes and Langerhans cells. IL-6, produced by keratinocytes, Langerhans cells, and resident immune cells within the skin, synergizes with other cytokines, mainly potentiating the effects of TNF-α and IL-1.

Other members of the interleukin family are expressed by various cells within the skin and contribute to local innate and adaptive immunity. IL-2 is secreted by activated T cells within the skin and promotes clonal T cell proliferation as well as cytokine production and is critical for activation of the adaptive immune response. IL-4, expressed by activated T cells, mast cells, and eosinophils, is important in allergic disease processes and has been shown to promote IgE production and the maturation of mast cells and eosinophils. IL-5, expressed by monocytes and eosinophils, serves mainly as an eosinophil growth and differentiation factor. IL-8, produced by keratinocytes and resident immune cells within the skin, is a potent chemoattractant for neutrophils. IL-12, produced by antigen presenting cells, is a critical regulator of innate and adaptive immunity, and serves to potentiate cell-mediated immunity. It is also expressed by keratinocytes and Langerhans cells.

ANTI-INFLAMMATORY CYTOKINES

Not all members of the interleukin family are pro-inflammatory. IL-10 inhibits the inflammatory immune response through various mechanisms. Specifically, it lowers the activity of antigen presenting cell function by downregulating major histocompatibility complex (MHC) class II expression. Along with T cells, macrophages, and B cells, keratinocytes express IL-10. Moreover, IL-10 disrupts cytokine production by immune effector cells and inhibits the generation of reactive oxygen species (via oxidative burst) and nitric oxide production. UVB radiation is established to induce local immunosuppression partially through increased IL-10 production in keratinocytes.[30] In addition, the production of IL-10 by nonmelanoma skin cancer can inhibit the function of tumor infiltrating lymphocytes and promote tumor growth.[31] Interestingly, the immune cells of older individuals have been shown to produce high levels of IL-10 in comparison to younger adults, suggesting that IL-10 is in part responsible for the immunosuppression observed in the elderly.[32]

GROWTH FACTORS

Growth factors are proteins that have an effect on cellular proliferation and differentiation. While some cytokines can also be classified as growth factors, not all cytokines are considered growth factors (see **Table 8-2** for a summary of the functions of cytokines and growth factors). There are numerous families of growth factors. The epidermal growth factor (EGF) family and the transforming growth factor (TGF)-β superfamilies will be discussed further.

TGF-α is a member of the EGF family of growth factors, which also consists of EGF, amphiregulin (AR), epiregulin, and neuregulin 1, 2, and 3. These growth factors are secreted by keratinocytes and bind to the EGF receptor in an autocrine manner to induce keratinocyte proliferation.[33] In addition to increasing epidermal thickness and contributing in a complex chain of events to the regulation of keratinocyte differentiation, EGF is important in wound healing.[34] Notably, EGF and TGF-α enhance migration of normal keratinocytes.[35] EGF accelerates wound healing in mice and enhances lateral migration of keratinocytes, wound closure, and subsequent re-epithelialization.[36] Moreover, EGF stimulates fibroblast migration and proliferation and is critical for wound repair and dermal regeneration.[37,38]

The TGF-β superfamily has a broad spectrum of functions dependent on the dosage and the target cell type. In the wound healing process, TGF-β is responsible for recruiting monocytes, neutrophils, and fibroblasts to the wound site. Higher concentrations of TGF-β activate monocytes to release numerous growth factors and stimulate fibroblasts to increase matrix synthesis and decrease matrix degradation. The effects of TGF-β on keratinocytes are inconclusive with some studies showing an inhibitory role in growth, while others favor keratinocyte chemoattraction and activation. This apparent discrepancy is perhaps linked to the temporal kinetics, dose of TGF-β administered, and also the dual activity TGF-β exerts on keratinocytes.

TGF-β is best known in cosmetic dermatology for its ability to promote the production of the extracellular matrix, notably the synthesis of procollagen.[39] TGF-β also serves as a growth factor for fibroblasts, the cells that produce collagen and play an important role in wound healing. The subcutaneous injection of TGF-β into unwounded skin results in increased collagen deposition at the injection site.[40] Moreover, collagen synthesis is enhanced in animal models when TGF-β is administered locally or systemically.[41,42] Despite the encouraging results of TGF-β on collagen synthesis, its effects on re-epithelialization are less predictable. *In vivo* studies have shown both accelerated and impaired re-epithelialization in animal wound models,[43,44] echoing the contradictory effects of TGF-β on keratinocytes.

Toll-like Receptors

The discovery of TLRs has created a new paradigm for how we view the innate immune system. TLRs appear to play important roles in acne and other inflammatory skin diseases. Considering the partial pro-inflammatory nature of UV exposure, it is possible that TLRs factor into the aging process. Because TLRs are often activated early in the innate immune response resulting in cytokine production, part of the age-related cytokine aberration may be linked to changes in TLR expression and function. The background of TLRs and their known roles in skin disease and photoaging will be discussed in this chapter. In addition, the effect of retinoids on TLR expression and function will be explored.

The importance of innate immunity became clear with the discovery of TLRs a decade ago. The toll receptor, initially described in relation to drosophila, was shown to be crucial in preventing fungal infection in flies. Subsequently, it was demonstrated that TLRs play a role in human host defense.[45] To date, 10 human TLRs have been described and their role in innate immunity has greatly influenced our view of the immune system. TLRs are PRRs capable of recognizing a variety of conserved microbial motifs collectively referred to as pathogen-associated molecular patterns. Each TLR recognizes a unique microbial motif, such as bacterial cell wall components, fungal elements, viral RNA, and bacterial DNA. Moreover, individual TLRs can form dimers in

TABLE 8-2	Summary of Function of Cytokines and Growth Factors
	Function
Cytokines	
Pro-inflammatory	
IL-1 (α, β)	Keratinocyte differentiation, B cell differentiation, activates neutrophils and macrophages
TNF-α	Similar to IL-1, prostaglandin synthesis in macrophages
IL-2	T-cell proliferation, cytokine production
IL-4	IgE production, mast cell and eosinophil maturation
IL-5	Eosinophil growth and differentiation
IL-6	Potentiates effects of TNF-α and IL-1
IL-8	Neutrophil chemoattractant
IL-12	Potentiates cell-mediated immunity
Anti-inflammatory	
IL-10	Downregulates MHC class II, disrupts cytokine production, inhibits production of reactive oxygen species and NO
Growth Factors	
TGF-α	Enhances keratinocyte migration and keratinocyte differentiation
TGF-β	Recruits monocytes, neutrophils, and fibroblasts, decreases matrix degradation
EGF	Enhances keratinocyte migration and keratinocyte differentiation, accelerates wound healing, stimulates fibroblast migration and proliferation

order to increase specificity. A summary of TLRs and their respective ligands can be found in **Fig. 8-1**. Although their extracellular domains vary in specificity for their respective microbial ligands, the intracellular domains of TLRs are conserved and converge onto a common pathway. TLR signaling is thought to occur primarily in a MyD88-dependent pathway that ultimately leads to nuclear translocation of the transcription factor NF-κB. This in turn results in the transcription of immunomodulatory genes, including those that encode for various cytokines and chemokines.[46] In addition to a MyD88-dependent pathway, certain TLR activation can lead to MyD88-independent signaling resulting in an immune response.[47]

TLRs are expressed by various cells of the innate immune system such as keratinocytes, sebocytes, melanocytes, neutrophils, monocytes, macrophages, dendritic cells, and mast cells. Moreover, as TLRs are key players in the innate response to pathogens, the expression and function of TLRs at sites of host-pathogen interaction are critical for host defense. It is therefore of little surprise that the skin, which is the first point of contact with cutaneous pathogens, exhibits functionally significant TLR expression. It is now known that keratinocytes express TLRs 1, 2, and 5, with TLR2 and 5 showing preferential staining in the basal keratinocytes.[48] In addition, other studies have identified expression of TLR4 in cultured human keratinocytes.[49] TLR9 has been shown to be preferentially expressed in keratinocytes found in the granular layer.[50] A more recent study has found that cultured keratinocytes constitutively express TLR1, 2, 3, 4, 5, 6, 9, and 10 mRNA, but not TLR7 or 8.[51,52] It has also been suggested that keratinocyte expression of TLR can be influenced by cytokines and growth factors, such as TGF-α.[50] Furthermore, TLR expression within the epidermis may correlate with keratinocyte maturation; as cells progress from the basal layer to the surface of the skin, patterns of TLR expression may change. TLRs are also expressed on sebocytes, melanocytes, and fibroblasts, though the *in vivo* function remains less characterized. Cultured sebocytes constitutively express TLR2 and 4.[53,54] Cultured melanocytes express TLRs 2–5, 7, 9 and 10, *in vitro* stimulation of which increases IL-8 and IL-6 as well as melanin content.[55–57] Cultured dermal fibroblasts express all 10 TLRs at higher levels than cultured keratinocytes, with *in vitro* stimulation increasing IL-6, IL-8 and MMP-1 expression.[58]

The importance of TLRs in skin has been gleaned through the study of various inflammatory skin diseases. For example, TLR2 has been implicated in the pathogenesis of acne vulgaris. *Cutibacterium acnes*, a Gram positive anaerobe that plays a *sine qua non* role in the pathogenesis of acne, induces the production of pro-inflammatory cytokines, such as IL-6 and IL-12, by binding TLR2.[59] Furthermore, TLR2 plays an important role in the production of key host defense components, such as antimicrobial peptides, which have been demonstrated to increase in culture systems when keratinocytes are stimulated with *C. acnes*.[60] Subtle variability in the expression of TLR1, 2, 5, and 9 has been described in psoriatic lesions when compared to normal skin, although these variances in TLR expression have not been linked to the etiology or pathogenesis of the disease.[48,61] Nevertheless, TLR2 is thought to be a key factor in host response to *Mycobacteria leprae*, the organism implicated in leprosy. The expression of TLR2 and TLR1 is markedly increased in tuberculoid leprosy (resistant form of leprosy) when compared to lepromatous leprosy (susceptible form of leprosy), suggesting that TLR2/1 is important for activating cell-mediated immunity.[62]

Accumulating evidence suggests a role for keratinocyte TLRs in UV-induced damage. Activation of TLR3 by RNA released from damaged keratinocytes has been shown to be essential for induction of UVB-mediated inflammatory response.[25] Intriguingly, recent evidence has implicated keratinocyte TLR3 activation and signaling in damage response and regeneration in wound healing. Studies of mouse wounding have demonstrated that dsRNA released upon tissue damage activates TLR3 signaling and that this signaling alters keratinocyte regeneration to promote a progenitor cell phenotype

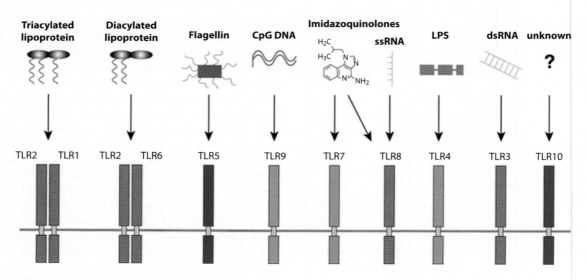

FIGURE 8-1. Toll-like receptors and their respective ligands.

through IL-6, STAT3, and retinoic acid signaling.[63–65] TLR4 has also been implicated in response to acute UVB, with mice lacking TLR4 showing reduced UV-induced immunosuppression and improved nucleotide excision repair following UV-induced damage.[66,67]

Since TLR expression and function appear to play a role in the pathogenesis of various inflammatory and infectious skin conditions, modulation of the expression and function of these PRRs with pharmacologic agents appears to be a potential mechanism for altering damage and regenerative responses which are central to skin aging phenotypes.

Matrix Metalloproteinases

Recently, TLRs have been directly linked to collagen synthesis or breakdown by mediating the expression of various

TABLE 8-3	Types and Function of Select MMPs		
Group	Enzyme	ECM Substrate	Other Select Substrates
Collagenases	MMP-1 (Collagenase-1)	Collagen I, II, III, VII, X	Pro-TNF, IL-1β, MMP-2, MMP-9
	MMP-8 (Collagenase-2)	Collagen I, II, III	
	MMP-13 (Collagenase-3)	Collagen I, II, III, IV, X	MMP-9
Gelatinases	MMP-2 (Gelatinase-A)	Gelatin I	IL-1β, MMP-1, MMP-9, MMP-13
		Collagen IV, V, VII, X	
		Fibronectin	
		Elastin	
	MMP-9 (Gelatinase-B)	Gelatin I, V	IL-1β
		Collagen IV, V	
		Fibronectin	
		Elastin	
Stromelysins	MMP-3 (Stromelysin-1)	Proteoglycans	IL-1β
		Fibronectin	
		Laminin	
		Gelatin I, III, IV, V	
	MMP-10 (Stromelysin-2)	Fibronectin Gelatin I, III, IV, V	MMP-1, MMP-8
	MMP-11 (Stromelysin-3)	Fibronectin	IGF binding protein
		Gelatin	
		Laminin	
		Collagen IV	

metalloproteinases. Matrix metalloproteinases (MMPs) are a group of enzymes responsible for the breakdown of collagen and can be classified into four subfamilies: (1) Collagenases, (2) gelatinases, (3) stromelysins, and (4) membrane-type MMPs (**Table 8-3** for a summary of the functions of the first three types). Initial breakdown of collagen depends on members of the collagenase family that are capable of cleaving native triple helical collagen. After the initial cleavage of collagen, the resultant fragments are further degraded by gelatinases and stromelysins.[68] The expression of MMPs is tightly regulated and regulation of the extracellular matrix involves a balance between synthesis of structural components and MMPs. MMPs are expressed primarily by fibroblasts, but also by macrophages and keratinocytes and the expression of MMPs is modulated by cytokines. For example, MMP-1 production from fibroblasts is stimulated by IL-1, IL-6, and TNF-α.[69–71] Moreover, other cytokines such as IL-4 inhibit MMP expression and are chemoattractant for fibroblasts, favoring collagen and fibronectin synthesis and matrix preservation.[72]

In addition to regulation at the transcriptional level, MMP activity is regulated by tissue inhibitors of metalloproteinase (TIMP). TIMPs, low molecular weight glycoproteins, are synthesized mainly in fibroblasts and macrophages,[73] and inhibit MMP activity by forming heat-stable 1:1 stoichiometric complexes. The expression of TIMPs is also regulated by cytokines and growth factors. For example, TIMP-1 is induced by IL-1, IL-6, and EGF.[39,70] Although both MMPs and TIMPs can be induced by similar stimuli, the expression can be regulated in both a coordinated and reciprocal manner. The critical balance between MMP and TIMP expression determines the balance between matrix degradation and matrix preservation. During periods of extracellular matrix homeostasis, the expression of MMP and TIMP is tightly coordinated providing for appropriate remodeling without excessive tissue breakdown. However, if the amount of MMP expression is increased relative to TIMP expression, excessive matrix degradation is thought to occur.

In addition to their ability to induce cytokines and chemokines, TLRs have been implicated in the induction of MMPs. Several preliminary studies have shown that microbial agents are capable of inducing MMP expression through a TLR-dependent pathway. For example, in Lyme disease the causative agent *Borrelia burgdorferi* is capable of inducing MMP-9 through a TLR2-dependent mechanism.[74] Moreover, mycobacterial cell wall components are also thought to increase MMP-9 through TLR2.[75] More recently, CpG oligodeoxynucleotide, the ligand for TLR9, exhibited the capacity to induce MMP-9 expression in macrophages via a TLR9/NF-κB-dependent signaling pathway.[76]

ALTERED IMMUNE FUNCTION IN CUTANEOUS AGING

Aging of the skin is typically studied as two distinct processes—photoaging refers to the changes seen over time in skin exposed to the sun, while intrinsic or chronological aging refers to changes seen in photo-protected skin. Photoaging and chronological aging have both common and unique clinical manifestations and underlying mechanisms, more completely addressed in Chapter 6. Chronological aging is associated with fine lines, increased skin laxity, loss of volume and xerosis. Photoaging is associated with deeper wrinkles, volume loss, dyspigmentation and increased incidence of malignancy. Histologically, both are associated with epidermal thinning and loss of the dermal extracellular matrix, with photoaging having more prominent loss of dermal extracellular matrix and increased dermal inflammation. The molecular mechanisms underlying these changes are complex and remain incompletely understood. In photoaging, there is a prominent role for UV-induced signaling alterations and oxidative damage in initiating a series of changes including epigenetic alterations, metabolic dysfunction and cellular senescence, all of which amplify impaired epidermal maintenance and degradation of the dermal extracellular matrix.

While cutaneous aging was not originally thought to be an immunologic process, there is increasing evidence that the innate immune system plays an important role in initiating these changes as part of the response to UV exposure. The most prominent evidence indicating a role for immune regulation in aging is the repeatedly observed increase in NF-κB signaling in aged tissue and particularly in photoaged skin. NF-κB is a family of transcription factors which regulate the expression of many genes activated in acute and chronic inflammation. NF-κB is a target of TLR signaling and known as a master regulator of the innate immune system. Intriguingly NF-κB signaling has also been identified as a key regulator of aging phenotypes across multiple tissues including skin[89] and inhibition of NF-κB signaling was shown to be sufficient to reverse aging phenotypes in mouse skin.[77] While the mechanisms underlying these changes remain unclear, the current data indicates a role for impaired barrier function, altered growth factor signaling, increased MMP expression and altered cytokine signaling in initiating and propagating changes in chronological aging and photoaging.

BARRIER FUNCTION IN SKIN AGING

The physical, chemical, and antimicrobial barriers maintained by the epidermis and cutaneous microbiome provide the first line of defense against external pathogens. Alterations in this function are seen as both a trigger and consequence of age-associated inflammation. Consistent with the observed thinning of the epidermis, both chronological aging and UV induced photoaging have also been associated with decreased barrier function as well as diminished capacity to recover a functional barrier after injury.[78] This decrease in barrier function predisposes older patients to multiple skin conditions including xerosis, pruritus, contact dermatitis and cutaneous infections. Once present, recent work suggests that disruptions of the epidermal permeability barrier as seen in aging can increase systemic inflammatory markers, possibly predisposing to systemic aging linked pathology.[79]

The processes underlying the decline in epidermal barrier function are likely multifactorial. Increased NF-kB signaling likely plays a role in decreased keratinocyte regenerative

capacity, suggesting that immune system activation may amplify this defect. Alterations in the cutaneous microbiome may also initiate or perpetuate this process. Multiple studies have demonstrated that the microbiome of facial skin from aged individuals is distinct from younger individuals, however the nature and functional consequences of these differences remain to be elucidated.[80–82] Multiple small studies have demonstrated change in both the cutaneous and gastrointestinal microbiome with acute UV radiation, suggesting a possible role for chronic UV exposure in these changes.[83,84]

MMP AND GROWTH FACTOR SIGNALING IN SKIN AGING

There is also significant evidence that the degradation of the dermal extracellular matrix which is so central to skin aging phenotypes is at least partially a consequence of immune signaling. Both *in vivo* and *in vitro* work have established central roles for MMPs and growth factor signaling in aging of the extracellular matrix. Both photoaging and intrinsic aging are associated with increased activation of AP-1, a transcription factor which increases expression of MMP-1, 3, and 9 and decreases expression of TGF-β and pro-collagen. These MMPs, particularly MMP-1, degrade dermal collagen, which alters the environment for dermal fibroblasts and amplifies AP-1 activation within these cells to further promote matrix degradation. This signaling is directly induced with UV exposure, indicating that chronic UV exposure may induce the increased MMP expression seen in photoaged skin.[85,86] Further, UV exposure has been shown to decrease TGF-β function through downregulation of both the TGF-β type II receptor (TGF-β RII) and TGF-β, and upregulation of Smad7, a negative regulator of TGF-β,[87,88] further decreasing collagen synthesis in the dermis.

Alterations in growth factor signaling are also linked to aged-related deficits in wound healing. Decreased responsiveness of EGF receptors is also seen with increasing age, possibly because of a lower number and density of receptors, as well as reduced ligand binding, receptor autophosphorylation, and internalization.[89] In addition, amphiregulin expression is downregulated in aged epidermis.[90] Diminished EGF activity and amphiregulin expression lead to a subsequent decrease in fibroblast migration and proliferation at the site of wound healing. These events contribute to the impaired wound healing that is observed in aged skin.

TOLL-LIKE RECEPTORS AND AGING

The Toll-like receptors (TLRs) are pattern recognition receptors which respond to both exogenous pathogens and internal damage signals to activate the innate immune system. Given that the Toll-like receptors (TLRs) activate NF-kB signaling and are directly linked to MMP regulation in multiple cutaneous diseases, it is likely TLRs play a role in both the altered barrier function and extracellular matrix changes seen in cutaneous aging. While the specific details of this relationship in skin remain to be clarified, TLR expression and function have been demonstrated to change with aging in other systems. Studies evaluating the levels of TLR expression in murine macrophages in aged mice have shown significantly lower levels of expression of TLRs. Moreover, when stimulated with known ligands to TLR2/1, 2/6, 3, 4, 5, and 9, significantly lower levels of IL-6 and TNF-α were produced, indicating a decline in function.[91] This supports the observation that increased susceptibility to pathogens and altered immunity in elderly individuals may be caused by a decline in TLR expression and function. A more recent study characterized TLR2/1 function in humans. TNF-α and IL-6 production from peripheral blood-derived monocytes were significantly reduced in those older than 65 years when compared to the cohort aged 21 to 30 years. Moreover, surface expression of TLR1 was decreased but TLR2 was unchanged as a function of aging.[92] While these studies have shown decreased TLR expression in monocytes, the effects of aging on cutaneous TLR expression have not been thoroughly examined. A small study indicated decreased TLR 1–5 in adult skin as compared to prenatal and infant skin, however the changes have not been examined throughout aging.[93]

CYTOKINES AND PHOTOAGING

Cytokines are soluble signaling molecules secreted by many cell types within the skin to modulate immune function (**Table 8-1**). They serve as an intermediary between different types of immune cells to coordinate the local response as well as modulate the function of surrounding cells. Specific cytokines can either promote or decrease local inflammation. An altered cytokine balance is implicated in systemic aging in which chronic elevations in IL-6 and TNF-α are linked to age related frailty and morbidity.[94,95] In cutaneous aging, the relationship between specific cytokines and specific aging phenotypes remains to be clarified; however, there is a clear relationship between UV exposure and cytokine signaling, suggesting cytokines may play an important role in photoaging.

At this time, the effects of acute UVB exposure on inflammatory signaling have been most extensively characterized. Acute UVB exposure, linked to sunburn, is associated with increased pro-inflammatory cytokines by resident skin cells, including IL-1, TNF-α, IL-6, and IL-8. These cytokines cause inflammation, but also initiate activation of macrophages, and other immune cells that generate reactive oxygen species, resulting in cellular damage. In addition, these reactive oxygen species initiate the production of activator protein (AP)-1 and the formation of destructive enzymes such as collagenases that contribute to skin aging (see Chapter 6).[86] UV exposure also increases the production of TGF-α from keratinocytes.[96] However, the effect of acute UVB is not completely pro-inflammatory as acute UVB is also linked to increased IL-10 which has immunosuppressive effects as discussed above.

While the effects of acute UVB exposure on cytokine production have been well characterized, the effects of UVA and more chronic UVB exposure are less well understood. The current data suggests a complex relationship. The changes in chronically sun exposed skin are less clear. Elevated IL-1 and TNF-α mRNA are seen in mice exposed to chronic UVB.[97] However, samples of stratum corneum from aged individuals suggest that in chronically photo-exposed tissue the ratio of IL-1 α to its antagonist, IL-1r α is dramatically decreased compared to sun protected aged tissue, indicating there may be less active IL-1 α.[98]

The consequences of these alterations for aging phenotypes are also unclear. Interestingly, UVB-induced cytokines display opposing functions with regard to keratinocyte proliferation. Specifically, IL-1, IL-6, and TGF-α, which are known to augment keratinocyte proliferation, while TNF-α is known to suppress keratinocyte growth. Further, mice lacking IL-1 receptor demonstrate epidermal barrier deficits similar to those seen in aging, further suggesting a possible beneficial role for inflammatory signaling in epidermal function.[90]

Keratinocyte- and dermal-derived cytokines that result from UV exposure may also partially account for the dyspigmentation seen with photoaging. An experimental model has demonstrated that UVA-induced granulocyte-monocyte colony-stimulating factor (GM-CSF) from keratinocytes may play a role in melanocyte proliferation and thus result in UVA-induced pigmentation in the epidermis.[99] However, other studies have shown that IL-1 and TNF-α can inhibit melanogenesis, suggesting that the relationship is complex.[100] Further studies are needed to clarify the role of UV-induced cytokines on melanocyte growth and function.

SKIN RESIDENT IMMUNE CELLS AND AGING

In addition to the prominent role of keratinocytes and lesser role of fibroblasts in orchestrating the primary immune response within the skin, multiple immune cell populations are present in the skin that coordinate the immune response and are altered with aging and photoaging. In the epidermis, Langerhans cells, a population of tissue-resident macrophages, act as a critical bridge between the innate immune system and the adaptive immune system. Similar to keratinocytes, they express Toll-like receptors, specifically TLR1, 2 and 6, which facilitate maturation in response to foreign stimuli.[101] Once activated, they produce cytokines and antimicrobial peptides as part of the innate immune response and also act as antigen presenting cells and migrate to lymph nodes to initiate an adaptive immune response. Intrinsic aging of skin is associated with decreased numbers of Langerhans cells within the epidermis. This effect is exacerbated in photoaged tissue. In addition, remaining Langerhans cells have decreased migratory and secretory function, which has been linked to decreased IL-1 β expression in aged skin.[102–104] In the photoaging model, UV inhibits the antigen presenting function of Langerhans cells and its ability to activate T cells via IL-10 dependent mechanism.[105]

A more mixed immune cell population is present in the dermis. Dermal dendritic cells and macrophages act as phagocytic antigen presenting cells to coordinate the innate and adaptive immune responses, with macrophages also playing an important role in wound healing. Mast cells are present in the dermis that contain granules of histamine and other components, these contribute to a local inflammatory response in allergic and other conditions. The role of these populations in aging and photoaging is less well defined than epidermal Langerhans cells. While dermal dendritic cell counts are stable with aging and photoaging, mouse studies suggest they may have decreased migratory and stimulatory function with chronological aging.[106] By contrast, dermal macrophages and mast cells are increased in number with UV exposure and in photoaging, with no clear change in their functional capacity.

Skin resident T memory cells facilitate a more rapid adaptive immune response to repeat infections. This population has been demonstrated to play an important role in responding to skin infections and controlling melanoma and is implicated in vitiligo and other cutaneous autoimmune diseases. With age there are no clear changes in the number of skin resident T cells; however, multiple groups have noted decreased T cell mediated response to recall antigens in aged cells, suggesting this population may have functional impairments. Multiple pathways have been implicated in this functional decline. Increased expression of the inhibitory receptor PD-1 was noted on CD4 T cells isolated from skin of aged individuals.[107] Further, an increased proportion of immunomodulating regulatory T cells has been noted in skin from aged individuals and linked to the age- and UV-associated increase in IL-10.[107–109]

IMMUNE TARGETED ANTI-AGING TREATMENTS

As evidence accumulates that innate immune function is altered in skin aging, interest has grown in developing therapies to mitigate or reverse these changes in order to counteract the effects of photoaging. These include topical products meant to supplement the reduced growth factor signaling seen in aged skin, alter the skin microbiome or directly activate TLR signaling. Intriguingly, recent research has also suggested multiple well established anti-aging treatments, retinoids and laser resurfacing may act in part through modulations of the innate immune system and that other candidate anti-aging compounds may work through decreasing inflammatory signaling.

TOPICAL GROWTH FACTORS

Given the alterations in growth factors and growth factor response associated with aging and photoaging, many cosmeceuticals now contain various growth factors including EGF and TGF-β. Although these growth factors can theoretically induce keratinocyte differentiation and dermal remodeling, whether any of the products available to consumers demonstrate significant clinical effectiveness in preventing or reversing photoaging has not yet been established. Since cosmeceuticals are not subject to the same FDA regulatory requirements as drugs, well-controlled clinical studies that support the efficacy of cosmeceuticals are generally not available. Multiple small studies have shown clinical improvement in aging phenotypes with growth factors and cytokines, including EGF, TGF-β, platelet-derived growth factor (PDGF), FGF, IL-1 and TNF-α. However, the mechanistic role of topical growth factors remains unclear. Many growth factors and cytokines are large, hydrophilic molecules with greater than 15,000 Da molecular weight, and it has previously been shown that hydrophilic molecules greater than 500 Da have low penetration past the stratum corneum.[110] Companies have developed shorter peptides that contain active properties derived from the larger growth factors and advanced delivery systems have been developed for better delivery of peptides; however, more evidence and larger clinical trials are needed to demonstrate the effectiveness of peptide therapy in skin aging.

PROBIOTICS

With the growing understanding that the cutaneous microbiome plays a role in regulating skin function, there is increasing interest in developing therapies to manipulate the microbiome through addition of specific live bacteria in the form of probiotics, or prebiotics compounds that are meant to induce growth of beneficial bacteria. While prebiotics are commonly added to topical products, there have been minimal studies characterizing the effect on the microbiome after application. There is accumulating evidence to support the use of topical probiotics in multiple skin conditions including acne, rosacea and atopic dermatitis.[111] One small study of 20 women over age 65 demonstrated that addition of cream containing *Streptococcus thermophilus* increased ceramide levels and barrier function, suggesting probiotics may be beneficial for treatment of aging phenotypes as well.[112] Intriguingly, small studies in mice and humans demonstrate that supplementation with oral probiotics may mitigate acute UV-induced changes,[113,114] emphasizing the interaction between the cutaneous and gastrointestinal microbiome.

IMIQUIMOD

The increasing evidence for TLR signaling in skin aging suggests that modulating specific TLRs may have a role in anti-aging treatment. Imiquimod, a TLR7 and 8 ligand with approved anti-viral and anti-neoplastic indications, has been shown to downregulate production of MMP-9 while simultaneously upregulating TIMP expression.[115] Clinical evidence to support a broader role in reversal of photoaging has been supported by multiple small studies which demonstrate histological reversal of solar elastosis and restoration of epidermal thickness with use of topical imiquimod.[116,117] In this regard, imiquimod appears to have potential as a novel therapy for reversal of photoaging as well as the prevention of cutaneous neoplasms. The exact role imiquimod exerts in regulating the expression of MMP *in vivo* has not been determined and further studies are warranted in this area.

RETINOIDS

Retinoids, a class of vitamin A-derived compounds that bind various members of the retinoic acid receptor family, have long been used for the treatment of numerous inflammatory and hyperproliferative skin diseases and are well established to improve photoaging phenotypes. Many studies have demonstrated a benefit of topical bioactive retinoid, tretinoin, for use on photoaged skin. Topical tretinoin is shown to improve epidermal thickness, dermal ECM content, and reduce wrinkles and skin laxity in photoaged skin, with both short term and longer term benefit seen,[118,119] and evidence suggesting that higher strength formulations have more prominent clinical improvement.[120] *In vitro* work has established that retinoids work to increase synthesis of collagen, increase TIMP expression and decrease MMP-1 expression through decreased activity of AP-1 signaling,[121] and has suggested retinoids may act through regulation of innate immune signaling as well. Topical retinoids have been seen to specifically downregulate TLR2 expression in the epidermis of skin explants from acne patients, suggesting that modulation of the innate immune system may be central to this role.[122] Intriguingly, stimulation of TLR3 has also been demonstrated to induce retinoic acid signaling, suggesting retinoid therapy may modulate downstream inflammatory signaling as well.[65]

INJURY-MEDIATED REGENERATION

Many of the well-established therapies with clinical benefit for photoaging, including chemical peels, micro-needling, micro-dermabrasion and fractional lasers have been demonstrated to induce improved collagen synthesis through induction of local skin injury to stimulate a repair response. The increasing evidence for the innate immune system and particularly TLR signaling in mediating the damage response in wound healing and regeneration suggests that this system may also play a prominent role in these anti-aging procedures. This is supported by a gene expression study comparing facial skin before and after non-ablative laser treatment which showed enrichment for dsRNA-induced signaling.[65] This intriguing overlap supports the idea that modulation of the innate immune system may offer a novel mechanism for treating skin aging.

RESVERATROL

Resveratrol (3,5,4'-trihydroxystilbene) is a natural polyphenol found as a major constituent of red wine that has drawn attention as an anti-aging compound across many systems. The best understood anti-aging roles of resveratrol are in regulation of cellular metabolism through activation of sirtuins and promotion of mitochondrial function and anti-oxidant function.[123] However, there is also evidence that resveratrol may play an anti-inflammatory role through modulation of NF-kB signaling. Resveratrol has been shown to decrease NF-kB activation in multiple systems *in vivo*,[124,125] and blocks UV-induced activation of NF-kB in cultured keratinocytes.[126] Topical application has been shown to block irritant-stimulated NF-kB activation in mouse epidermis.[127] However, despite the strong potential for resveratrol as a topical anti-aging agent, currently only small clinical trials of topical formulations have been performed which have unclear evidence of benefit, possibly due to questionable bioavailability.[123]

NICOTINAMIDE

Nicotinamide is the amide form of vitamin B3 and the precursor of nicotinamide adenine dinucleotide (NAD), which functions as an essential cofactor for multiple cellular processes. Oral and topical nicotinamide supplementation have recently been shown to have benefit for multiple cutaneous diseases including bullous pemphigoid, acne, rosacea and nonmelanoma skin cancer.[128] Two randomized controlled trials have evaluated the use of nicotinamide for photoaging of the face: one study used 4% nicotinamide for 8 weeks in 30 Japanese females[129] and one used 5% nicotinamide for 12 weeks in 50 Caucasian females.[130] The mechanism of nicotinamide is likely multifactorial as NAD serves as a co-factor for multiple enzymes and plays an important role in regulating cellular metabolism. Nicotinamide has been seen to decrease inflammatory cytokine induction *in vitro*.[131] Evidence for the anti-inflammatory role of nicotinamide comes from its role as a co-factor and inhibitor of the enzyme PARP, a nuclear repair protein which regulates NF-kB activation.

SUMMARY

We are beginning to see evidence that the immune system plays a role in skin appearance, including the phenomena of aging and photoaging. While various hypotheses for aging exist, persistent inflammation via NF-kB signaling has received much attention as one of the critical factors influencing aging across many systems. Immune cells within the skin appear to respond to pathogens, UV radiation, and other environmental toxins to engender an immune response to protect the host. Yet the same mechanisms through the activation of various receptors including the TLRs can lead to cytokine alterations and have important implications in cellular apoptosis, inflammation, and tissue injury. For example, the loss of TGF-β or decreased responsiveness to EGF leads to a decrease in collagen production, as well as the increased breakdown of collagen and hyaluronic acid, accounting for the dermal alterations characteristic of photoaging.

A better understanding of the mechanisms of skin aging, and photoaging in particular, from an immunologic perspective will likely lead to the development of improved novel therapies. Although currently there are no FDA-approved cytokine and growth factor therapies for photoaging, numerous cosmeceutical treatments containing these factors have been developed. It is important to note that for those who practice evidence-based medicine, not enough data are available to know if these products reverse or prevent photoaging and further studies are warranted. With the discovery of TLRs and their relationship to cytokine production as well as their indirect and direct links to collagen synthesis, it may be possible that TLRs could prove to be realistic targets for the prevention of photoaging. Furthermore, therapeutics that directly target downstream events of TLR activation such as modulators of MMPs and TIMPs may be of use. More research into the role of local immune response in skin aging should help provide physicians with tools to better treat and educate our patients.

References

1. Meguro S, et al. Relationship between covalently bound ceramides and transepidermal water loss (TEWL). *Arch Dermatol Res*. 2000;292(9):463–468.

2. Fluhr JW, et al. Generation of free fatty acids from phospholipids regulates stratum corneum acidification and integrity. *J Invest Dermatol*. 2001;117(1):44–51.

3. Bibel DJ, Aly R, Shinefield HR. Antimicrobial activity of sphingosines. *J Invest Dermatol*. 1992;98(3):269–273.

4. Drake DR, et al. Thematic review series: skin lipids. Antimicrobial lipids at the skin surface. *J Lipid Res*. 2008;49(1):4–11.

5. Nguyen MT, et al. Skin-Specific Unsaturated Fatty Acids Boost the Staphylococcus aureus Innate Immune Response. *Infect Immun*. 2016;84(1):205–215.

6. Martinez A, et al. Expression of adrenomedullin and its receptor in normal and malignant human skin: a potential pluripotent role in the integument. *Endocrinology*. 1997;138(12):5597–5604.

7. Fulton C, et al. Expression of natural peptide antibiotics in human skin. *Lancet*. 1997;350(9093):1750–1751.

8. Liu AY, et al. Human beta-defensin-2 production in keratinocytes is regulated by interleukin-1, bacteria, and the state of differentiation. *J. Invest Dermatol*. 2002;118(2):275–281.

9. Harder J, et al. Differential gene induction of human beta-defensins (hBD-1, -2, -3, and -4) in keratinocytes is inhibited by retinoic acid. *J Invest Dermatol*. 2004;123(3):522–529.

10. Harder J, Schroder JM. RNase 7, a novel innate immune defense antimicrobial protein of healthy human skin. *J Biol Chem*. 2002;277(48):46779–46784.

11. Sorensen OE, et al. Wound healing and expression of antimicrobial peptides/polypeptides in human keratinocytes, a consequence of common growth factors. *J Immunol*. 2003;170(11):5583–5589.

12. Braff MH, Di Nardo A, Gallo RL. Keratinocytes store the antimicrobial peptide cathelicidin in lamellar bodies. *J Invest Dermatol*. 2005;124(2):394–400.

13. Georgel P, et al. A Toll-like receptor 2-responsive lipid effector pathway protects mammals against skin infections with gram-positive bacteria. *Infect Immun*. 2005;73(8):4512–4521.

14. Nagy I, et al. Propionibacterium acnes and lipopolysaccharide induce the expression of antimicrobial peptides and pro-inflammatory cytokines/chemokines in human sebocytes. *Microbes Infect*. 2006;8(8):2195–2205.

15. Dahlhoff M, Zouboulis CC, Schneider MR. Expression of dermcidin in sebocytes supports a role for sebum in the constitutive innate defense of human skin. *J Dermatol Sci*. 2016;81(2):124–126.

16. Ong PY, et al. Endogenous antimicrobial peptides and skin infections in atopic dermatitis. *N Engl J Med*. 2002;347(15):1151–1160.

17. Hong SP, et al. Biopositive effects of low-dose UVB on epidermis: coordinate upregulation of antimicrobial peptides and permeability barrier reinforcement. *J Invest Dermatol*. 2008;128(12):2880–2887.

18. Zhang LJ, et al. Innate immunity. Dermal adipocytes protect against invasive Staphylococcus aureus skin infection. *Science*. 2015;347(6217):67–71.

19. Zhang LJ, et al. Age-Related Loss of Innate Immune Antimicrobial Function of Dermal Fat Is Mediated by Transforming Growth Factor Beta. *Immunity*. 2019;50(1):121–136 e5.

20. Grice EA, et al. Topographical and temporal diversity of the human skin microbiome. *Science*. 2009;324(5931):1190–1192.

21. Oh J, et al. Biogeography and individuality shape function in the human skin metagenome. *Nature*. 2014;514(7520):59–64.

22. Naik S, et al. Commensal-dendritic-cell interaction specifies a unique protective skin immune signature. *Nature*. 2015;520(7545):104–108.

23. Scharschmidt TC, et al. A Wave of Regulatory T Cells into Neonatal Skin Mediates Tolerance to Commensal Microbes. *Immunity*. 2015;43(5):1011–1021.

24. Naik S, et al. Compartmentalized control of skin immunity by resident commensals. *Science*. 2012;337(6098):1115–1119.

25. Lai Y, et al. Commensal bacteria regulate Toll-like receptor 3-dependent inflammation after skin injury. *Nat Med*. 2009;15(12):1377–1382.

26. Kong HH, et al. Temporal shifts in the skin microbiome associated with disease flares and treatment in children with atopic dermatitis. *Genome Res*. 2012;22(5):850–859.

27. Byrd AL, et al. Staphylococcus aureus and Staphylococcus epidermidis strain diversity underlying pediatric atopic dermatitis. *Sci Transl Med*. 2017;9(397).

28. Kalan LR, et al. Strain- and Species-Level Variation in the Microbiome of Diabetic Wounds Is Associated with Clinical Outcomes and Therapeutic Efficacy. *Cell Host Microbe*. 2019;25(5):641–655 e5.

29. Bell TV, et al. Expression of mRNA homologous to interleukin 1 in human epidermal cells. *J Invest Dermatol*. 1987;88(4):375–379.

30. O'Connor A, et al. DNA double strand breaks in epidermal cells cause immune suppression in vivo and cytokine production in vitro. *J Immunol*. 1996;157(1):271–278.

31. Kim J, et al. IL-10 production in cutaneous basal and squamous cell carcinomas. A mechanism for evading the local T cell immune response. *J Immunol*. 1995;155(4):2240–2247.

32. Uyemura K, Castle SC, Makinodan T. The frail elderly: role of dendritic cells in the susceptibility of infection. *Mech Ageing Dev*. 2002;123(8):955–962.

33. Cohen S. The stimulation of epidermal proliferation by a specific protein (EGF). *Dev Biol*. 1965;12(3):394–407.

34. Schultz GS, et al. Epithelial wound healing enhanced by transforming growth factor-alpha and vaccinia growth factor. *Science*. 1987;235(4786):350–352.

35. Barrandon Y, Green H. Cell migration is essential for sustained growth of keratinocyte colonies: the roles of transforming growth factor-alpha and epidermal growth factor. *Cell*. 1987;50(7):1131–1137.

36. Ando Y, Jensen PJ. Epidermal growth factor and insulin-like growth factor I enhance keratinocyte migration. *J Invest Dermatol*. 1993;100(5):633–639.

37. Blay J, Brown KD. Epidermal growth factor promotes the chemotactic migration of cultured rat intestinal epithelial cells. *J Cell Physiol*. 1985;124(1):107–112.

38. Carpenter G, Cohen S. Human epidermal growth factor and the proliferation of human fibroblasts. *J Cell Physiol*. 1976;88(2):227–237.

39. Edwards DR, et al. Transforming growth factor beta modulates the expression of collagenase and metalloproteinase inhibitor. *EMBO J*. 1987;6(7):1899–1904.

40. Roberts AB, et al. Transforming growth factor type beta: rapid induction of fibrosis and angiogenesis in vivo and stimulation of collagen formation in vitro. *Proc Natl Acad Sci U S A.* 1986;83(12):4167–4171.

41. Beck LS, et al. One systemic administration of transforming growth factor-beta 1 reverses age- or glucocorticoid-impaired wound healing. *J Clin Invest.* 1993;92(6):2841–2849.

42. Mustoe TA, et al. Accelerated healing of incisional wounds in rats induced by transforming growth factor-beta. *Science.* 1987;237(4820):1333–1336.

43. Quaglino DJr. et al. Transforming growth factor-beta stimulates wound healing and modulates extracellular matrix gene expression in pig skin. I. Excisional wound model. *Lab Invest.* 1990;63(3):307–319.

44. Hebda PA. Stimulatory effects of transforming growth factor-beta and epidermal growth factor on epidermal cell outgrowth from porcine skin explant cultures. *J Invest Dermatol.* 1988;91(5):440–445.

45. Medzhitov R, Preston-Hurlburt P, Janeway CAJr. A human homologue of the Drosophila Toll protein signals activation of adaptive immunity. *Nature.* 1997;388(6640):394–397.

46. Takeda K, Kaisho T, Akira S. Toll-like receptors. *Annu Rev Immunol.* 2003;21:335–376.

47. Doyle SE, et al. Toll-like receptors induce a phagocytic gene program through p38. *J Exp Med.* 2004;199(1):81–90.

48. Baker BS, et al. Normal keratinocytes express Toll-like receptors (TLRs) 1, 2 and 5: modulation of TLR expression in chronic plaque psoriasis. *Br J Dermatol.* 2003;148(4):670–679.

49. Pivarcsi A, et al. Expression and function of Toll-like receptors 2 and 4 in human keratinocytes. *Int Immunol.* 2003;15(6):721–730.

50. Miller LS, et al. TGF-alpha regulates TLR expression and function on epidermal keratinocytes. *J Immunol.* 2005;174(10):6137–6143.

51. Mempel M, et al. Toll-like receptor expression in human keratinocytes: nuclear factor kappaB controlled gene activation by Staphylococcus aureus is Toll-like receptor 2 but not Toll-like receptor 4 or platelet activating factor receptor dependent. *J Invest Dermatol.* 2003;121(6):1389–1396.

52. Lebre MC, et al. Human keratinocytes express functional Toll-like receptor 3, 4, 5, and 9. *J Invest Dermatol.* 2007;127(2):331–341.

53. Oeff MK, et al. Differential regulation of Toll-like receptor and CD14 pathways by retinoids and corticosteroids in human sebocytes. *Dermatology.* 2006;213(3):266.

54. Torocsik D, et al. Genome wide analysis of TLR1/2- and TLR4-activated SZ95 sebocytes reveals a complex immune-competence and identifies serum amyloid A as a marker for activated sebaceous glands. *PLoS One.* 2018;13(6):e0198323.

55. Ahn JH, et al. Human melanocytes express functional Toll-like receptor 4. *Exp Dermatol.* 2008;17(5):412–417.

56. Yu N, et al. Cultured human melanocytes express functional toll-like receptors 2-4, 7 and 9. *J Dermatol Sci.* 2009;56(2):113–120.

57. Jin SH, Kang HY. Activation of Toll-like Receptors 1, 2, 4, 5, and 7 on Human Melanocytes Modulate Pigmentation. *Ann Dermatol.* 2010;22(4):486–489.

58. Yao C, et al. Toll-like receptor family members in skin fibroblasts are functional and have a higher expression compared to skin keratinocytes. *Int J Mol Med.* 2015;35(5):1443–1450.

59. Kim J, et al. Activation of Toll-like receptor 2 in acne triggers inflammatory cytokine responses. *J Immunol.* 2002;169(3):1535–1541.

60. Nagy I, et al. Distinct strains of Propionibacterium acnes induce selective human beta-defensin-2 and interleukin-8 expression in human keratinocytes through Toll-like receptors. *J Invest Dermatol.* 2005;124(5):931–938.

61. Curry JL, et al. Innate immune-related receptors in normal and psoriatic skin. *Arch Pathol Lab Med.* 2003;127(2):178–186.

62. Krutzik SR, et al. Activation and regulation of Toll-like receptors 2 and 1 in human leprosy. *Nat Med.* 2003;9(5):525–532.

63. Lin Q, et al. Toll-like receptor 3 ligand polyinosinic:polycytidylic acid promotes wound healing in human and murine skin. *J Invest Dermatol.* 2012;132(8):2085–2092.

64. Nelson AM, et al. dsRNA Released by Tissue Damage Activates TLR3 to Drive Skin Regeneration. *Cell Stem Cell.* 2015;17(2):139–151.

65. Kim D, et al. Noncoding dsRNA induces retinoic acid synthesis to stimulate hair follicle regeneration via TLR3. *Nat Commun.* 2019;10(1):2811.

66. Lewis W, et al. Regulation of ultraviolet radiation induced cutaneous photoimmunosuppression by Toll-like receptor-4. *Arch Biochem Biophys.* 2011;508(2):171–177.

67. Ahmad I, et al. Toll-like receptor-4 deficiency enhances repair of UVR-induced cutaneous DNA damage by nucleotide excision repair mechanism. *J Invest Dermatol.* 2014;134(6):1710–1717.

68. Birkedal-Hansen H. Matrix metalloproteinases. *Adv Dent Res.* 1995;9(3 Suppl):16.

69. Dayer JM, Beutler B, Cerami A. Cachectin/tumor necrosis factor stimulates collagenase and prostaglandin E2 production by human synovial cells and dermal fibroblasts. *J Exp Med.* 1985;162(6):2163–2168.

70. Postlethwaite AE, et al. Modulation of fibroblast functions by interleukin 1: increased steady-state accumulation of type I procollagen messenger RNAs and stimulation of other functions but not chemotaxis by human recombinant interleukin 1 alpha and beta. *J Cell Biol.* 1988;106(2):311–318.

71. Wlaschek M, et al. UVA-induced autocrine stimulation of fibroblast-derived collagenase/MMP-1 by interrelated loops of interleukin-1 and interleukin-6. *Photochem Photobiol.* 1994;59(5):550–556.

72. Zhang Y, et al. Differential regulation of monocyte matrix metalloproteinase and TIMP-1 production by TNF-alpha, granulocyte-macrophage CSF, and IL-1 beta through prostaglandin-dependent and -independent mechanisms. *J Immunol.* 1998;161(6):3071–3076.

73. Stricklin GP, Welgus HG. Human skin fibroblast collagenase inhibitor. Purification and biochemical characterization. *J Biol Chem.* 1983;258(20):12252–12258.

74. Gebbia JA, Coleman JL, Benach JL. Selective induction of matrix metalloproteinases by Borrelia burgdorferi via Toll-like receptor 2 in monocytes. *J Infect Dis.* 2004;189(1):113–119.

75. Elass E, et al. Mycobacterial lipomannan induces matrix metalloproteinase-9 expression in human macrophagic cells through a Toll-like receptor 1 (TLR1)/TLR2- and CD14-dependent mechanism. *Infect Immun.* 2005;73(10):7064–7068.

76. Lee S, et al. CpG oligodeoxynucleotides induce expression of pro-inflammatory cytokines and chemokines in astrocytes: the role of c-Jun N-terminal kinase in CpG ODN-mediated NF-kappaB activation. *J Neuroimmunol.* 2004;153(1-2):50–63.

77. Adler AS, et al. Reversal of aging by NFkappaB blockade. *Cell Cycle*. 2008;7(5):556–559.

78. Reed JT, Elias PM, Ghadially R. Integrity and permeability barrier function of photoaged human epidermis. *Arch Dermatol*. 1997;133(3):395–396.

79. Hu L, et al. Epidermal Dysfunction Leads to an Age-Associated Increase in Levels of Serum Inflammatory Cytokines. *J Invest Dermatol*. 2017;137(6):1277–1285.

80. Kim HJ, et al. Segregation of age-related skin microbiome characteristics by functionality. *Sci Rep*. 2019;9(1):16748.

81. Dimitriu PA, et al. New Insights into the Intrinsic and Extrinsic Factors That Shape the Human Skin Microbiome. *mBio*. 2019;10(4).

82. Shibagaki N, et al. Aging-related changes in the diversity of women's skin microbiomes associated with oral bacteria. *Sci Rep*. 2017;7(1):10567.

83. Burns EM, et al. Ultraviolet radiation, both UVA and UVB, influences the composition of the skin microbiome. *Exp Dermatol*. 2019;28(2):136–141.

84. Bosman ES, et al. Skin Exposure to Narrow Band Ultraviolet (UVB) Light Modulates the Human Intestinal Microbiome. *Front Microbiol*. 2019;10:2410.

85. Herrlich P, et al. The mammalian UV response: mechanism of DNA damage induced gene expression. *Adv Enzyme Regul*. 1994;34:381–395.

86. Fisher GJ, et al. Pathophysiology of premature skin aging induced by ultraviolet light. *N Engl J Med*. 1997;337(20):1419–1428.

87. Quan T, et al. Solar ultraviolet irradiation reduces collagen in photoaged human skin by blocking transforming growth factor-beta type II receptor/Smad signaling. *Am J Pathol*. 2004;165(3):741–751.

88. Quan T, et al. Ultraviolet irradiation induces Smad7 via induction of transcription factor AP-1 in human skin fibroblasts. *J Biol Chem*. 2005;280(9):8079–8085.

89. Reenstra WR, Yaar M, Gilchrest BA. Effect of donor age on epidermal growth factor processing in man. *Exp Cell Res*. 1993;209(1):118–122.

90. Ye J, et al. Alterations in cytokine regulation in aged epidermis: implications for permeability barrier homeostasis and inflammation. I. IL-1 gene family. *Exp Dermatol*. 2002;11(3):209–216.

91. Renshaw M, et al. Cutting edge: impaired Toll-like receptor expression and function in aging. *J Immunol*. 2002;169(9):4697–4701.

92. van Duin D, et al. Age-associated defect in human TLR-1/2 function. *J Immunol*. 2007;178(2):970–975.

93. Iram N, et al. Age-related changes in expression and function of Toll-like receptors in human skin. *Development*. 2012;139(22):4210–4219.

94. Saum KU, et al. Association between Oxidative Stress and Frailty in an Elderly German Population: Results from the ESTHER Cohort Study. *Gerontology*. 2015;61(5):407–415.

95. Leng SX, et al. IL-6-independent association of elevated serum neopterin levels with prevalent frailty in community-dwelling older adults. *Age Ageing*. 2011;40(4):475–481.

96. James LC, et al. Transforming growth factor alpha: in vivo release by normal human skin following UV irradiation and abrasion. *Skin Pharmacol*. 1991;4(2):61–64.

97. Schwartz E, Sapadin AN, Kligman LH. Ultraviolet B radiation increases steady-state mRNA levels for cytokines and integrins in hairless mouse skin: modulation by topical tretinoin. *Arch Dermatol Res*. 1998;290(3):137–144.

98. Hirao T, et al. Elevation of interleukin 1 receptor antagonist in the stratum corneum of sun-exposed and ultraviolet B-irradiated human skin. *J Invest Dermatol*. 1996;106(5):1102–1107.

99. Imokawa G, et al. Granulocyte/macrophage colony-stimulating factor is an intrinsic keratinocyte-derived growth factor for human melanocytes in UVA-induced melanosis. *Biochem J*. 1996;313(Pt 2):625–631.

100. Swope VB, et al. Interleukins 1 alpha and 6 and tumor necrosis factor-alpha are paracrine inhibitors of human melanocyte proliferation and melanogenesis. *J Invest Dermatol*. 1991;96(2):180–185.

101. Flacher V, et al. Human Langerhans cells express a specific TLR profile and differentially respond to viruses and Gram-positive bacteria. *J Immunol*. 2006;177(11):7959–7967.

102. Cumberbatch M, Dearman RJ, Kimber I. Influence of ageing on Langerhans cell migration in mice: identification of a putative deficiency of epidermal interleukin-1beta. *Immunology*. 2002;105(4):466–477.

103. Pilkington SM, et al. Langerhans cells express human beta-defensin 3: relevance for immunity during skin ageing. *Br J Dermatol*. 2018;179(5):1170–1171.

104. Pilkington SM, et al. Lower levels of interleukin-1beta gene expression are associated with impaired Langerhans' cell migration in aged human skin. *Immunology*. 2018;153(1):60–70.

105. Aubin F, Mechanisms involved in ultraviolet light-induced immunosuppression. *Eur J Dermatol*. 2003;13(6):515–523.

106. Grolleau-Julius A, et al. Impaired dendritic cell function in aging leads to defective antitumor immunity. *Cancer Res*. 2008;68(15):6341–6349.

107. Vukmanovic-Stejic M, et al. The Characterization of Varicella Zoster Virus-Specific T Cells in Skin and Blood during Aging. *J Invest Dermatol*. 2015;135(7):1752–1762.

108. Yamazaki S, et al. Homeostasis of thymus-derived Foxp3+ regulatory T cells is controlled by ultraviolet B exposure in the skin. *J Immunol*. 2014;193(11):5488–5497.

109. Schwarz A, et al. In vivo reprogramming of UV radiation-induced regulatory T-cell migration to inhibit the elicitation of contact hypersensitivity. *J Allergy Clin Immunol*. 2011;128(4):826–833.

110. Bos JD, Meinardi MM. The 500 Dalton rule for the skin penetration of chemical compounds and drugs. *Exp Dermatol*. 2000;9(3):165–169.

111. Knackstedt R, Knackstedt T, Gatherwright J. The role of topical probiotics in skin conditions: A systematic review of animal and human studies and implications for future therapies. *Exp Dermatol*. 2020;29(1):15–21.

112. Di Marzio L, et al. Increase of skin-ceramide levels in aged subjects following a short-term topical application of bacterial sphingomyelinase from Streptococcus thermophilus. *Int J Immunopathol Pharmacol*. 2008;21(1):137–143.

113. Bouilly-Gauthier D, et al. Clinical evidence of benefits of a dietary supplement containing probiotic and carotenoids on ultraviolet-induced skin damage. *Br J Dermatol*. 2010;163(3):536–543.

114. Sugimoto S, et al. Photoprotective effects of Bifidobacterium breve supplementation against skin damage induced by

ultraviolet irradiation in hairless mice. *Photodermatol Photoimmunol Photomed.* 2012;28(6):312–319.

115. Li VW, et al. Imiquimod as an antiangiogenic agent. *J Drugs Dermatol.* 2005;4(6):708–717.

116. Metcalf S, et al. Imiquimod as an antiaging agent. *J Am Acad Dermatol.* 2007;56(3):422–425.

117. Smith K, et al. Does imiquimod histologically rejuvenate ultraviolet radiation-damaged skin? *Dermatol Surg.* 2007;33(12):1419–1428; discussion 1428–9.

118. Ellis CN, et al. Sustained improvement with prolonged topical tretinoin (retinoic acid) for photoaged skin. *J Am Acad Dermatol.* 1990;23(4 Pt 1):629–637.

119. Bhawan J, et al. Histologic evaluation of the long term effects of tretinoin on photodamaged skin. *J Dermatol Sci.* 1996;11(3):177–182.

120. Kligman DE, Draelos ZD. High-strength tretinoin for rapid retinization of photoaged facial skin. *Dermatol Surg.* 2004;30(6):864–866.

121. Fisher GJ, et al. Molecular basis of sun-induced premature skin ageing and retinoid antagonism. *Nature.* 1996;379(6563):335–339.

122. Tenaud I, Khammari A, Dreno B. In vitro modulation of TLR-2, CD1d and IL-10 by adapalene on normal human skin and acne inflammatory lesions. *Exp Dermatol.* 2007;16(6):500–506.

123. Farris P, et al. Resveratrol: a unique antioxidant offering a multi-mechanistic approach for treating aging skin. *J Drugs Dermatol.* 2013;12(12):1389–1394.

124. Donnelly LE, et al. Anti-inflammatory effects of resveratrol in lung epithelial cells: molecular mechanisms. *Am J Physiol Lung Cell Mol Physiol.* 2004;287(4):L774–L783.

125. Ren Z, et al. Resveratrol inhibits NF-kB signaling through suppression of p65 and IkappaB kinase activities. *Pharmazie.* 2013;68(8):689–94.

126. Adhami VM, Afaq F, Ahmad N. Suppression of ultraviolet B exposure-mediated activation of NF-kappaB in normal human keratinocytes by resveratrol. *Neoplasia.* 2003;5(1):74–82.

127. Kundu JK, et al. Resveratrol inhibits phorbol ester-induced expression of COX-2 and activation of NF-kappaB in mouse skin by blocking IkappaB kinase activity. *Carcinogenesis.* 2006;27(7):1465–74.

128. Chen AC, et al. A Phase 3 Randomized Trial of Nicotinamide for Skin-Cancer Chemoprevention. *N Engl J Med.* 2015;373(17):1618–26.

129. Kawada A, et al. Evaluation of anti-wrinkle effects of a novel cosmetic containing niacinamide. *J Dermatol.* 2008;35(10):637–42.

130. Bissett DL, Oblong JE, Berge CA. Niacinamide: A B vitamin that improves aging facial skin appearance. *Dermatol Surg.* 2005;31(7 Pt 2):860–5; discussion 865.

131. Ungerstedt JS, Blomback M, Soderstrom T. Nicotinamide is a potent inhibitor of pro-inflammatory cytokines. *Clin Exp Immunol.* 2003;131(1):48–52.

CHAPTER 9

Nutrition and the Skin

Mary D. Sun, MSCR, MA
Edmund M. Weisberg, MS, MBE
Leslie S. Baumann, MD

SUMMARY POINTS

What's Important?

1. Dietary interventions affect skin health and appearance by participating in metabolic processes, mitigating oxidative damage, and/or regulating the expression of cellular components that influence the integrity of skin structure.
2. General recommendations for nutritional therapy include appropriate nutrient supplementation, calorie restriction, limitation of dairy products, and adequate protein intake in older adults. In certain situations, strategies such as intermittent fasting and epigenetic diets can confer benefits to overall health.

What's New?

1. Increases in the activation of mammalian target of rapamycin (mTOR)-1 signaling are significantly associated with acne occurrence and pro-inflammatory states.
2. Acid-rich diets can induce protein catabolism that leads to protein derangement, sometimes described as hypercatabolic protein disarrangement (HPD) syndrome. HPD can manifest with muscle wasting, inflammation, and other symptoms that accelerate aging.

What's Coming?

1. Further research is needed to understand the limitations of foodborne supplements (e.g., storage, bioavailability, solubility) and to develop effective mitigation techniques.
2. Large-scale controlled trials of non-soybean-related isoflavones are warranted in the continued study of nutrition and skin health.

Food is the only medicine that the average healthy individual requires on a daily basis. Indeed, more than 2,000 years ago, Hippocrates is said to have offered: "Let food be your medicine, and let medicine be your food."[1] It is from such a perspective—that good nutrition is a fundamental building block of good general health and healthy skin—that this discussion proceeds. Specifically, this chapter will focus on some of the key chemical components of a healthy diet that have been shown to impart benefits to the skin. In the process, cutaneous effects will be discussed in the context of vegetarianism, as well as the skin types of the Baumann Skin Typing System (BSTS). Attention will first be focused on the effects of diet on acne—the most common dermatologic condition—and, finally, on oral supplementation.

There is copious research underway now on the direct effects on health from the consumption or supplementation of various nutrients. A significant proportion of such work focuses specifically on the potential benefits delivered to the skin through the intake of certain foods or supplements. For instance, in 2003, a cross-sectional study of 302 healthy men and women collected data on serum concentrations of nutrients, dietary consumption of nutrients, as well as various cutaneous measurements (including hydration, sebum content, and surface pH). Results revealed statistically significant relationships between serum vitamin A, cutaneous sebum content, and surface pH as well as between skin hydration and dietary consumption of total fat, saturated fat, and monosaturated fat. The investigators concluded that such findings are evidence that the condition of the skin can be influenced by alterations in baseline nutritional status.[2]

In general, the ingestion of anti-aging ingredients combats skin aging in three ways. First, the peptides, essential fatty acids, and other metabolites contained in food enter the skin after absorption through the gastrointestinal system, where they participate in skin metabolism. Second, certain ingredients can reduce oxidative damage by eliminating cellular reactive oxygen species (ROS) and increasing antioxidation activity. Third, bioactive anti-aging compounds can help regulate the expression of enzymes involved in degrading, maintaining, and improving the structural integrity of skin.[3] In this way, a variety of nutrients, diet-based metabolic precursors, and diet strategies can impact skin health and aesthetic appearance.

DIET AND ACNE

Acne vulgaris is one of the most common conditions that prompt visits to a dermatologist. It is believed that acne affects as many as 40 to 50 million people in the United States alone each year.[4] Recent estimates of acne prevalence and incidence worldwide suggest that 9.4% of the global population is affected by what is the eighth most prevalent disease among humans (see Chapter 16, Acne).[5] Interestingly, epidemiologic studies in non-Westernized populations (e.g., Inuit, Okinawan Islanders, Ache hunter-gatherers, and Kitavan Islanders) in which acne is rare, indicate that dietary factors, including glycemic load, may play a role in the development of this condition, particularly since incidence of acne has risen in these communities in association with the adoption of Western lifestyles.[6–9]

Accordingly, Cordain, has argued persuasively for abandoning the traditional belief espoused in the dermatology community since the early 1970s that diet does not contribute to the pathophysiology of acne. In particular, he asserted that the dogma claiming that diet and acne are unrelated was based on two fundamentally flawed studies from 1969 by Fulton et al. and 1971 by Anderson that lacked control groups, statistical data treatment, as well as blinding and/or placebos and were characterized by inadequate sample sizes and insufficient or absent baseline diet data, among other deficiencies.[6,10,11] Furthermore, Cordain contended that substantial evidence has been amassed since these two influential studies revealing that alterations in hormonal and cytokine homeostasis engendered by diet have emerged as the leading candidates for exogenous influences on acne development. Among such data is a study suggesting that the regular, long-term consumption of high-glycemic meals, which raise insulin concentrations, may induce chronic hyperinsulinemia and insulin resistance, increasing levels of insulin-like growth factor 1 (IGF-1) and decreasing levels of insulin-like growth factor binding protein 3 (IGFBP-3), fostering keratinocyte proliferation and corneocyte apoptosis.[6,12,13] Other proximate causes of acne, such as androgen-mediated sebum production levels as well as inflammation, are also affected by diet. Cordain noted that insulin and IGF-1 incite the synthesis of androgens as well as sebum

and inhibit the hepatic production of sex hormone-binding globulin, resulting in higher levels of circulating androgens.[6]

In 2007, Smith et al. investigated the effects of a low-glycemic-load diet on acne lesion counts in 43 males between the ages of 15 and 25 years. The experimental diet, over the 12-week, parallel design study with investigator-blinded skin evaluations, included 25% energy from protein and 45% from low-glycemic-index carbohydrates and the control group diet focused on carbohydrate-rich foods without regard to the glycemic index. The low-glycemic-load participants experienced larger reductions in the number of acne lesions, weight, and body mass index and a greater improvement in insulin sensitivity than the subjects consuming the control diet.[14] In the same cohort of patients, Smith et al. also compared the impacts from an experimental low-glycemic-load diet with those from a conventional high-glycemic-load diet on acne. Subjects following the intervention diet, which included recommendations to eat more fish, exhibited lower lesion counts than the high-glycemic control group after 12 weeks, and experienced greater reductions in weight and free androgen index in addition to elevated IGFBP-1 as compared to controls. While calling for additional research, the investigators concluded that these findings reflect an active role in acne etiology of nutritional choices.[15] While accepting this overarching argument by Smith and colleagues, Logan suggested in response that aspects other than a low-glycemic index in the experimental diet, particularly its status as being lower in saturated fats as well as much higher in polyunsaturated fats and fiber, may account for hormonal alterations and inflammation that affect acne.[16] He added that greater consumption of fish, which contains anti-inflammatory ω-3 fatty acids, may have rendered the intervention diet higher in polyunsaturated fats and had a mitigating effect on acne. To further this work by Smith et al., Logan recommended research using high-fiber, high-ω-3 fatty acid, and low saturated-fat diets.

Such concerns were at least partially answered by a more recent report by Smith et al. An investigation using data on the same patients revealed a correlation between an elevated ratio of saturated to monounsaturated fatty acids of skin surface triglycerides and decreased acne lesion counts in the low-glycemic-load diet group as compared to controls after 12 weeks. An increase in monounsaturated fatty acids in sebum was also associated with greater sebum secretions. The authors concluded that desaturase enzymes may influence sebaceous lipogenesis and the emergence of acne, but suggest that more research is necessary on the interplay of sebum gland physiology and diet.[17] While additional research, particularly well controlled dietary intervention trials, is warranted and may prove revelatory in clarifying the contributory roles of specific foods in the etiologic pathway of acne, Cordain identified increased consumption of foods high in ω-3 polyunsaturated fatty acids (PUFAs), thus reducing the ratio of ω-6 to ω-3 fatty acids, as important in attacking the inflammatory aspect of acne.[6]

In recent years, an increasing number of studies demonstrate that Western "milk and sugar" diets contribute to the pathogenesis of acne vulgaris by altering metabolomic signaling pathways. Changes in these pathways induced by dietary exposures such as dairy products lead to the increased production of sebum triglycerides, monounsaturated fatty acids, and sebaceous lipids found in acne lesions. Immunohistochemical studies find that specific metabolites such as transcription factor FoxO1 and the growth factor sensitive mechanistic target of rapamycin complex 1 (mTORC1) are elevated in the skin of acne patients.[18,19] mTORC1 activation appears to stimulate leptin expression, which has been implicated in pro-inflammatory acne-related signaling. Also, mTORC1 is activated by glutaminolysis and glycolysis, metabolic processes necessary for the biochemical function of human sebaceous glands. Medical therapies shown to be effective in reducing acne are thought to attenuate mTORC1 signaling and thus reduce the inflammatory skin state characteristic of acne vulgaris.[20] Overall, these findings suggest that decreased intake of hyperglycemic carbohydrates, insulinotropic dairy proteins, and leucine-rich meat and dairy products can be effective interventions for acne patients.[21]

Acne and Milk

The possibility of an association between dietary consumption of dairy products and acne has been long considered, though it has largely been overwhelmed by the dogma of the last few decades denying a connection between diet and acne eruptions.

In an assessment of Nurses Health Study II data of 47, 355 women who completed questionnaires on high school diet in 1998 and teenage acne diagnosed by a physician as severe in 1989, Adebamowo et al. identified a positive relation between acne and consumption of total milk and skim milk, which they speculated might be attributed to the hormones and bioactive molecules present in milk.[22] In a critical response to this article, Bershad questioned the retrospective nature of the study, namely the accuracy of distantly recalled dietary habits. In addition, she suggested that the authors failed to control for the subjects' heredity, nationality, and socioeconomic status, and erred in ascribing a correlation to causation. Finally, she concluded that the most notable result of this study was not the purported link between milk consumption and acne, but the finding that acne is not caused by pizza, French fries, and sweets.[23] In a rebuttal, Adebamowo countered that the study population was similar socioeconomically by dint of job similarity. Furthermore, the study population comprised nurses of which 91.6% were non-Hispanic white women residing in the 14 most populous US states in 1989. While stipulating that socioeconomic status is a risk factor for acne development,[7] he noted that accounting for race and socioeconomic status in the study models did not significantly alter the study results. Adebamowo added that the methods of his team were well validated,[24] and that their findings of a positive relationship between milk consumption and acne and no observed association between certain foods and acne warrant further investigation.[23]

In 2006, Adebamowo et al. reported results of a prospective cohort study demonstrating a link between milk intake and acne in 6,094 girls. The subjects were 9 to 15 years old in 1996, when they reported milk consumption on as many as three food frequency questionnaires from 1996 to 1998. In 1999, questionnaires were used to evaluate the presence and severity of acne. Again, they discerned a positive relationship between milk consumption and acne development, ascribing such cutaneous results to the metabolic effects of milk.[25] In subsequent studies, Adebamowo et al., following a prospective cohort study of 4,273 boys who also responded to dietary intake questionnaires from 1996 to 1998 and a teenaged acne questionnaire in 1999, reported a positive association between the consumption of skim milk and acne. The authors attributed these findings to hormonal components in skim milk, or factors that affect endogenous hormones.[26] A more recent meta-analysis of 14 observational studies designed to evaluate the relationship between dairy products and acne development found that low-fat, skim, and total milk intake were significantly associated with acne disease states. Furthermore, there was a linear dose-response relationship between the amount of milk consumed and the occurrence of acne. Notably, no significant relationship was observed between yogurt or cheese consumption and acne.[27]

Danby, a coauthor with Adebamowo on the prospective studies above, while acknowledging the unnatural aspect of humans (particularly in post-weaned years) consuming copious amounts of another species' milk, has suggested that qualitative and quantitative research is necessary to ascertain the influence on acne pathogenesis of steroid hormones in all dairy products.[28] He also noted that Perricone's acne prescription diet is nearly devoid of dairy products,[28] and, in fact, focuses heavily on anti-inflammatory food ingredients and maintaining a low-glycemic load.[29] This may explain the success of Perricone's diet for the skin.

Acne and Iodine

In 1961, Hitch and Greenburg disproved the notion of a direct causal connection between acne and iodine intake as the largest quantities of fish and other seafood were consumed by adolescents who exhibited the lowest acne rates in their study.[30] However, in 1967, Hitch did establish that iodine consumption can aggravate acne.[31] In response to the Adebamowo et al. study on an association between dairy intake during high school and teenaged acne cited above, Arbesman indicated that the iodine content of milk may have also contributed to acne development in addition to the hormonal explanation proffered by the investigators.[32] He added that significant levels of iodine have been identified in milk in Denmark, Italy, Norway, the United Kingdom, and the United States, because of the use of iodine and iodophor at various stages of the production process, with variable levels of iodine in milk based on geography and season.[33-39]

In a reply to Arbesman, Danby countered that iodine deficiency poses a greater health risk than overdosage, and that iodine levels in milk appear to be comparable to those found in human mother's milk. Furthermore, he suggested that there are no data to uphold the notion that comedonal acne is caused by the ingestion of iodides.[40] The author had not observed an association between acne and iodine, either causally or as an exacerbating factor, but noted that Fulton, primary author of the 1969 study criticized by Cordain, argued that in individuals prone to acne, iodine excreted through the sebaceous glands may in the process irritate the pilosebaceous unit and contribute to a flare-up.

Acne and Chocolate

While Cordain and others[1] have exposed the flaws in the methodologies of the studies that denied a significant link between nutrition and acne, particularly the study by Fulton et al. that refuted a connection between chocolate and acne, such debunking has not undermined the basic truth happened upon in 1969 regarding acne and chocolate. Cordain pointed out that the actual treatment variable in the Fulton study was an ingredient of the tested bittersweet chocolate candy bar, cacao solids, which were replaced with partially hydrogenated vegetable fat in the control bar. While suggesting that the only logical conclusion of this study was that cacao solids may not contribute to the causal pathway of acne, he also noted, among other criticisms, that because subjects also consumed their normal diets in addition to the 112-g test or control bar daily for 4 weeks with no baseline measurements, there was no way of determining the quantity of cacao solids consumed in either arm of the study.[6] Indeed, it is likely that the sugar added to various chocolate delicacies is responsible for engendering multiple deleterious health effects if consumed with regularity and over time, not the cacao or chocolate ingredient. Evidence suggests that sugar and sugar products may promote such cutaneous effects through the glycosylation of proteins in the skin,[41,42] ultimately leading to skin wrinkling and photoaging (see Chapters 2, Basic Science of the Dermis, and 21, Wrinkled Skin). Interestingly, rather than serving as a culprit in acne pathogenesis, chocolate has a history dating back at least since the 1500s as a component in the medical practices of the Olmec, Maya, and Aztec peoples.[43]

Not only does chocolate per se not directly cause acne (though a steady diet of highly-sugared chocolate products can certainly contribute to it), the Borba product line now includes a Clarifying Chocolate Bar made with Swiss dark chocolate that is touted for its patented formula that is said to have the opposite effect on skin—actually clearing skin or preventing breakouts. Of course, a healthy dose of skepticism regarding the potential contributory effects of a particular food toward acne is just as appropriate toward the notion of consuming a supposedly healthier item to exert the opposite effect. A consistent pattern of good nutrition is likely the optimal choice for overall health, total cutaneous health, and reducing the risk of developing acne. It has long been known that a diet rich in fruits and vegetables is ideal. Much has been learned in recent decades, though, regarding the chemical constituents in such foods that may play direct roles in health, including the health of the skin. The beneficial activities exhibited by certain chemical ingredients in foods have, in turn, been harnessed in various medications to exert more direct effects. For instance, retinoids are a form of vitamin A, which has long been known to play a role in acne. Notably, carotenoids are one of the best dietary sources of vitamin A.

CAROTENOIDS

Certain plant constituents have been established as exerting photoprotective effects as antioxidants, including carotenoids, flavonoids and other polyphenols, tocopherols, and vitamin C. Stahl et al. demonstrated that consumption of lycopene, which is the primary carotenoid in tomatoes and also present in apricots, papaya, pink grapefruit, guava, and watermelon, was effective in preventing or curbing sensitivity to ultraviolet (UV)-induced erythema formation in volunteers consuming lycopene-rich products over 10 to 12 weeks.[44]

Stahl et al. previously investigated whether the use of dietary tomato paste, a rich source of lycopene, could deliver a protective effect against UV-induced erythema in humans. A solar simulator was used to induce erythema in the scapular area at the outset of the study and after Weeks 4 and 10. For a period of 10 weeks, 9 volunteers ingested 40 g of tomato paste with 10 g of olive oil while 10 controls ingested olive oil only. Carotenoid levels were equivalent between the two groups at the beginning of the study and there were no significant differences between the groups at Week 4. There was no change in serum carotenoids in the control group by Week 10 nor in other carotenoids but lycopene in the experimental group, but those consuming tomato paste exhibited higher serum levels of lycopene accompanied by scapular erythema development 40% less than controls.[45] In subsequent experiments that involved daily ingestion of tomato paste (16 mg/d) for 10 weeks, Stahl and Sies demonstrated similar results, with increases measured in serum levels of lycopene and total carotenoids in skin and significantly less erythema formation after 10 weeks. They also determined that there is an optimal level of protection associated with each carotenoid micronutrient.[46]

In a placebo-controlled, parallel study involving some of the same investigators, the protective effects against erythema of β-carotene (24 mg/d) were compared to those of the same dose of a carotenoid combination of β-carotene, lutein, and lycopene (8 mg/d each) or placebo for 12 weeks. Erythema intensity before and 24 hours after irradiation with a solar light simulator was recorded at baseline and following 6 and 12 weeks of supplementation. Researchers noted diminished intensity in erythema 24 hours after exposure (at Weeks 6 and 12) in both experimental groups, with substantially less erythema formation after 12 weeks in comparison to baseline. While there were no observed changes in the control group, serum carotenoid levels increased significantly also, three- to four-fold in the β-carotene group and one- to three-fold in the mixed carotenoid group.[47] Several of the same investigators later compared the photoprotective effects of synthetic lycopene to the effects of a tomato extract (Lyc-o-Mato) and a beverage containing solubilized Lyc-o-Mato (Lyc-o-Guard-Drink) after 12 weeks of supplementation. Significant increases were observed in all groups in terms of serum levels of lycopene and total skin carotenoids and a protective effect against erythema formation was seen in all groups as well, but it was substantially larger in the Lyco-o-Mato and Lyc-o-Guard groups. The researchers speculated that the carotenoid phytofluene and carotenoid precursor phytoene may have assisted in providing this additional photoprotection.[48]

Finally, lutein and zeaxanthin, found in leafy green vegetables, were supplemented for 2 weeks in the diets of female hairless Skh-1 mice to determine the cutaneous response to UVB. Investigators observed significant reductions in the edematous cutaneous response as well as decreases in the UVB-induced elevation in hyperproliferative markers.[49]

POLYPHENOLS

Comprising a broad range of more than 8,000 naturally occurring compounds, polyphenols are secondary plant metabolites that exert varying degrees of antioxidant activity. All of these diverse substances share a definitive structural component, a phenol or an aromatic ring with at least one hydroxyl group. Polyphenols are an exceedingly important part of, and the most copious antioxidants in, the human diet, and found in a vast spectrum of vegetables, fruits, herbs, grains, tea, coffee beans, propolis, and red wine (**Table 9-1**).[50,51] Flavonoids are the most abundant polyphenols in the human diet as well as the most studied polyphenols, and can be further divided into several categories. These subclasses include flavones (e.g., apigenin, luteolin); flavonols (e.g., quercetin, kaempferol, myricetin, and fisetin); flavanones (e.g., naringenin, hesperidin, eriodictyol); isoflavones (e.g., genistein, daidzein); flavanols or catechins (e.g., epicatechin, epicatechin 3-gallate, epigallocatechin, epigallocatechin 3-gallate, catechin, gallocatechin); anthocyanins (e.g., cyanidin, pelargonidin); and proanthocyanidins (e.g., pycnogenol, leucocyanidin, leucoanthocyanin) (**Table 9-2**).[51–53] Among the many other polyphenols there are stilbenes (e.g., resveratrol, found in red wine), lignans (e.g., enterodiol, found in flaxseed and flaxseed oil), tannins (e.g., ellagic acid, found in pomegranates, raspberries, strawberries, cranberries, and walnuts), hydroxycinnamic acids, and phenolic acids, among which caffeic and ferulic acids are frequently found in foods.

TABLE 9-1	Foods with Significant Polyphenol Levels[50,51]	
Vegetables	**Fruits**	**Miscellaneous**
Artichokes	Apples/pears	Cocoa
Broccoli	Apricots	Coffee beans
Cabbage	Berries (various)	Flaxseed/flaxseed oil
Eggplant	Cherries	Grains (e.g., wild rice)
Lettuce	Citrus fruits	Nuts
Olives	Currants (red and black)	Propolis
Onions	Grapes	Red wine
Soybeans	Peaches	Tea (green and black)
Spinach	Plums	

A survey of the research associated with many of these compounds and their sources is beyond the scope of this chapter, as such a discussion could fill volumes. Some of the most widely disseminated results involving polyphenols pertain to the identified efficacy of various topical applications of green tea catechins, ferulic acid, resveratrol, and other ingredients, which are discussed elsewhere in this textbook.

Polyphenols have diverse chemical structures that can be difficult to quantify in foods. In 2010, a public research institute in France created the Phenol-Explorer database (www.phenol-explorer.eu) to aggregate information about dietary polyphenol content across hundreds of studies.[54] A study that year utilized this database and comparative Folin assay methods to identify the 100 richest sources of polyphenols. Spices, dried herbs, cocoa products, berries, various seeds and nuts (e.g., flaxseed, chestnuts, hazelnuts), and some vegetables such as olives and artichoke heads provided the highest levels of polyphenols. Across dietary sources, polyphenol content appears to range from 15,000 mg/100 g in cloves to 10 mg/100 mg in some wines. Fewer than 100 food sources were found to provide more than 1 milligram of total polyphenols per serving.[55] To date, over 400 polyphenols and nearly 20,000 foods are listed in the database.[56]

TABLE 9-2	Subclasses of the Most Abundant Polyphenols, Flavonoids, and Food Sources of Each Class[51–53]					
Flavones	**Flavonols**	**Flavanones**	**Isoflavones**	**Flavanols (Catechins)**	**Anthocyanins**	**Proanthocyanidins**
Celery	Apples	Oranges	Soy	Apples	Blackberries	Apples
Fresh parsley	Broccoli	Grapefruit		Cocoa	Cherries	Dark chocolate
Sweet red pepper	Olives			Dark chocolate	Currants (black and red)	Grapes
	Onions			Tea (black and green)	Grapes	Pears
	Tea (black and green)				Plums	Red wine
					Raspberries	Tea (black and green)
					Strawberries	

A 2006 experimental success with the oral ingestion of a polyphenolic compound resulting in benefits to the skin involved a currently unmentioned food source. In an investigation of the anti-aging effects of red clover isoflavones, which in high levels in diets have already been shown to contribute to low incidence of menopausal symptoms as well as osteoporosis, researchers orally administered red clover extract containing 11% isoflavones to ovariectomized rats for 14 weeks. Their findings revealed that collagen levels increased significantly in the treatment group as compared to the control group and epidermal thickness and keratinization was normal in the treated group but diminished in the control group. The researchers concluded that skin aging engendered by estrogen depletion can be mitigated by regular dietary consumption of red clover isoflavones.[57] (See the Pigmented vs. Nonpigmented section below for additional studies on the cutaneous effects of orally administered polyphenols found in pomegranates and grapes.)

PROTEINS AND AGING

Sarcopenia, or the loss of muscle mass also known as age-related muscle wasting, is a normal part of the aging process. However, poor nutrition can predispose and even accelerate sarcopenia. A comprehensive literature review identified a range of nutritional factors affecting muscle health including protein, acid–base balance, vitamin D/calcium, and minor nutrients such as vitamin B. Protein intake appears to play the most important role, with an intake of approximately 1.0–1.2 g/kg of body weight per day generally recommended for older adults.[58] Adequate ingestion of amino acids and their precursors is also necessary for protein synthesis and muscle function; deficient intake of nutrients such as vitamin B_{12} and folic acid increases homocysteine levels, which has been correlated with advanced aging and cancerous states. Appropriate, high-quality supplementation can help stimulate protein synthesis by acting on muscle-derived growth factors that inhibit pro-inflammatory cell death and therefore muscular atrophy.[59,60]

Long-term ingestion of acid-producing foods and beverages has also been found to adversely affect muscle performance. Acidic body environments can trigger protein catabolism, where muscle wasting is an adaptive response to acidosis. Diets high in alkali-producing foods and low in net acid-producing compounds, which includes many fruits and vegetables, have been shown to help preserve lean tissue mass.[59] In 2018, researchers linked hypercatabolic states to hypercatabolic protein disarrangement (HPD) syndrome, which can manifest clinically with sarcopenia, anemia, and altered fluid compartmentation, among other symptoms. HPD is correlated with additional increases in mortality, hospitalization, and morbidity, and is a negative prognostic indicator for patients with chronic and/or inflammatory disease.[61] Especially in older individuals, calorie-restricted and nutrient-rich diets are considered the most effective nutritional intervention for preventing age-related disease. Emerging evidence suggests that strategies such as intermittent fasting, epigenetic diets, and in some cases protein restriction may be effective in helping patients achieve their nutritional goals.[62]

ESSENTIAL FATTY ACIDS AND VEGETARIAN/VEGAN DIETS

In 1984, investigators measured the ω-6 and ω-3 fatty acids (also known as n-6 and n-3 fatty acids, respectively) in the plasma phospholipids of 41 adults with atopic eczema and 50 normal controls and found the ω-6 linoleic acid (LA) to be significantly elevated, with all of its metabolites likewise reduced, and the ω-3 α-linolenic acid (ALA) elevated, but not significantly, with all of its metabolites substantially decreased. The researchers identified a link between eczema and abnormal metabolism. Oral evening primrose oil (EPO) treatment partly rectified the abnormal metabolism of ω-6, but did not alter ω-3 levels.[63] Subsequently, Galland noted data indicating an association between poor desaturation of linoleic and linolenic acids by Δ-6 dehydrogenase and eczema and other allergic conditions, as well as the alleviation of atopic eczema symptoms through dietary supplementation with essential fatty acids.[64] In 1987, investigators conducting a 12-week, double-blind study of the effects of dietary supplementation with n-3 fatty acids in patients with atopic dermatitis (AD) found that the experimental group taking eicosapentaenoic acid (EPA) experienced overall less subjective severity and pruritus than the control group taking a placebo.[65] Supplementation with n-3 fatty acids may have ameliorated symptoms of eczema in the short term. Notably, levels of n-3 fatty acids are depressed in vegetarians and vegans. Not all physicians embrace the utility of dietary modifications in the treatment of eczema. Of course, patient recommendations should include advice on bathing and skin moisturization (see Chapters 12, Dry Skin, and 43, Moisturizers) as well as dietary recommendations.

The dietary research in the 1980s helped form the theoretical framework that undergirds current studies of suitable sources for adjunct or alternative therapies for atopic eczema, such as hemp seed oil (which is rich in ω-6 and ω-3 fatty acids), EPO, and borage oil, as well as the significance of varying levels of essential fatty acids for individuals with vegetarian or vegan diets as compared to omnivores.[66–68]

A 1996 examination of lipid metabolism in 81 healthy lacto-ovovegetarians and 62 nonvegetarians buttressed previous studies that revealed higher total serum polyunsaturated acid concentrations, particularly linoleic and linolenic acids, in vegetarians compared to nonvegetarians. Significantly higher plasma levels of vitamin C, β-carotene, and selenium as well as vitamin E-to-cholesterol and vitamin E-to-triacylglycerol ratios (indicators of LDL and fatty acid protection, respectively) were observed.[69] (See **Table 9-3** for a summary of potential nutritional deficits according to diet style.)

In an interesting matched-pair study in 1987, Melchert et al. compared serum fatty acid content in 108 vegetarians (62 females, 40 males) and 108 nonvegetarians (70 females, 38 males). Palmitoleic (ω-7), vaccenic (ω-7), and docosahexaenoic (ω-3) acids were higher in nonvegetarians, and very low in vegetarians, and vegetarians exhibited higher levels of

TABLE 9-3	Potential Nutritional Deficiencies Based on Diet			
	Vitamin D	Omega-3 Fatty Acids	Polyphenols	Cholesterol[a]
Vegetarian		X		X
Vegan	X	XX		X
Lactoveg-etarian		XX		X
Lacto-ovo-vegetarian	X	XX		X
Typical Western diet			X	
Atkins diet followers			XX	
South Beach diet followers			X (in first 2 wk)	

[a]Low levels of cholesterol lead to dry skin. Topical, but not oral, supplementation is suggested (see Chapters 11, Oily Skin, and 32, Cosmetics and Drug Regulations).
X, likely deficient; XX, must supplement.

LA.[70] More supportive evidence was established in a study of essential fatty acids and lipoprotein lipids in female Australian vegetarians and omnivores, as investigators found that the vegetarians had significantly lower levels of n-6 and n-3 PUFAs and a lower ratio of n-3 to n-6 PUFAs.[71] It is also important to note, PUFAs are known to inhibit the synthesis of eicosanoids derived from arachidonic acid, and are thus effective against allergic diseases.[72]

More recently, Davis and Kris-Etherton have indicated that vegetarian, particularly vegan, diets have been shown to deliver lower levels of ALA than LA, and especially low, if any, levels of EPA and docosahexaenoic acid (DHA), resulting in lower tissue levels of long-chain n-3 fatty acids. Given such low EPA and DHA levels as well as the inefficient conversion of ALA to the more active longer-chain metabolites EPA and DHA, they suggest that vegetarians may exhibit a greater dependence on ALA conversion to its metabolites and a corresponding greater need for n-3 acids than nonvegetarians.[73] In 2005, investigators conducted a cross-sectional study of 196 omnivore, 231 vegetarian, and 232 vegan men in the United Kingdom to compare plasma fatty acid concentrations in order to ascertain if the proportions of EPA, docosapentaenoic acid (DPA), and DHA relied on strict dietary adherence (data on which was obtained through a questionnaire) or to the proportions of LA and ALA in plasma. While only minor differences were observed in DPA levels, investigators noted reduced EPA and DHA levels in vegetarians and vegans, whose DHA levels were inversely correlated with plasma LA. Interestingly, they found that duration of adherence to dietary regimens was not significantly related to plasma n-3 levels. The researchers suggested that the endogenous synthesis of EPA

and DHA is low but yields stable n-3 plasma levels in individuals whose diets exclude animal foods.[74] Such findings support the notion of vegetarian/vegan diets providing sufficient n-3 fatty acid concentration for survival. To optimize cutaneous health and appearance, though, vegetarians and vegans may benefit from adding supplemental EPA and DHA. It is worth noting that topically applied EPA has also been found to exert photoprotective and anti-aging effects to the skin.[75]

Vegetarians Versus Nonvegetarians

As stated previously, vegetarians exhibit lower levels of serum cholesterol, ALA, EPA, and DHA and higher levels of antioxidants than nonvegetarians. For example, one study estimated lipid parameters in four different groups of vegetarians, and noted higher levels of vitamin C in the blood of all four groups.[76] Furthermore, individuals on a vegan diet for an extended period may have little to no serum cholesterol. Vegans also tend to have drier skin than vegetarians.

The main dietary fat should be derived from foods and oils rich in monounsaturated fat. When monounsaturated fats predominate, saturated fats, *trans*-fatty acids, and n-6 fatty acids are counterbalanced, and the ratio of n-6 to n-3 fatty acids improves as the proportion of ω-3 acids increases. Nuts (except for walnuts and butternuts), peanuts (a legume), olive oil, olives, avocados, canola oil, high-oleic sunflower oil, and high-oleic safflower oil all contain appreciable levels of monounsaturated fats. (See **Table 9-4** for a summary of foods that may have an impact in ameliorating dry skin.) Monounsaturated fats are better to consume through whole foods as compared to oils, or supplements, because whole foods deliver several other nutrients to the diet. Certain seeds, nuts, and legumes (flaxseed, hempseed, canola, walnuts, and soy) as well as the green leaves of plants, including

TABLE 9-4	Foods That May Mitigate or Improve Dry Skin[66-69,73]
Avocados	
Borage seed oil	
Canola oil	
Evening primrose oil	
Fish (particularly albacore tuna, lake trout, mackerel, menhaden, and salmon)	
Flaxseed oil	
Hempseed	
Nuts	
Olive oil	
Olives	
Peanuts	
Safflower oil (high-oleic)	
Soy	
Sunflower oil (high-oleic)	
Walnuts	

phytoplankton and algae, are the primary sources of dietary ALA. Legumes are rich sources of anti-photoaging and anti-cancer compounds such as selenium, various vitamins, polyunsaturated fatty acids, phytic acid, and flavonoids that exert direct effects of several mitogen-activated protein kinase (MAPK)-regulated pathways. Soybeans, which contain the phenolic phytochemicals genistein and daidzein, are specifically classified by the US National Cancer Institute as a plant-based food with protective effects against cancer. Recent studies suggest that these isoflavones have potential roles in optimizing skin health, especially in preventative regimens.[77]

Although vegetarian diets are generally lower in total fat, saturated fat, and cholesterol compared to nonvegetarian diets, they deliver comparable levels of essential fatty acids. Clinical studies have shown that tissue levels of long-chain n-3 fatty acids are typically depressed in vegetarians, particularly so in vegans. However, vegetarians consume approximately one-third less saturated fat (vegans approximately one-half) and approximately one-half as much cholesterol (vegans consume none) as omnivores.[73] As stated above, fish, fish oil, and seafood are the best sources of dietary EPA and DHA. For lacto-ovovegetarians, eggs provide an adequate amount of DHA ($\leq$50 mg/egg) but minimal EPA. Microalgae and seaweed are the only plant sources of long-chain n-3 fatty acids.

EPA/DHA, Immunoresponse, and Psoriasis

DHA has been shown to inhibit inflammation and immunoresponses in the contact hypersensitivity reaction in mice. Investigators fed dietary DHA as well as EPA to mice sensitized with 2, 4-dinitro-1-fluorobenzene. They found that 24 hours after the contact hypersensitivity challenge, ear swelling was reduced by DHA ethyl ester, but not EPA ethyl ester. DHA also diminished the infiltration of CD4+ T lymphocytes into the ears, and minimized the expression of interferon-γ, interleukin (IL)-6, IL-1β, and IL-2 mRNA in the ears. The researchers concluded that the immunosuppressive activity associated with fish oil should be ascribed primarily to DHA and not its fellow n-3 PUFA.[78] However, in clinical trials, EPA and DHA in fish oils have, combined with medication, been shown to ameliorate the skin lesions and reduce the hyperlipidemia caused by etretinates (which were removed from the Canadian market in 1996 and the US market in 1998 because of elevated risks of birth defects), as well as lower cyclosporin toxicity in patients with psoriasis.[79] Furthermore, in a 14-day double-blind, randomized, parallel group multicenter study in which 83 patients hospitalized for chronic plaque-type psoriasis (with a Psoriasis Area and Severity Index [PASI] score of at least 15) were randomized to receive daily intravenous administration of either an ω-3 fatty acid-based lipid emulsion or an ω-6 emulsion, investigators observed greater improvements in the ω-3 group in terms of diminished psoriasis severity, which was echoed by patient self-assessment. The researchers concluded that chronic plaque-type psoriasis could be effectively treated with intravenous ω-3 fatty acids.[80]

MATCHING DIETARY NEEDS WITH SKIN TYPE

The BSTS, introduced in *The Skin Type Solution* (Bantam 2005), is a modern approach to classifying skin type (see Chapter 10, The Baumann Skin Typing System). The BSTS score, derived from a self-administered questionnaire, is based on the understanding that skin can be assessed according to four major parameters: oily versus dry (O/D), sensitive versus resistant (S/R), pigmented versus nonpigmented (P/N), and wrinkled versus tight (W/T). Sixteen different skin type permutations are possible. The discussion of dietary needs based on skin type proceeds according to the four major parameters. The center of the spectrum is ideal for both the O/D and S/R parameters. Dietary interventions appear to be possible to render skin less oily or dry, as well as less sensitive, but not less resistant. Sensitive skin will be discussed briefly in "the OSNW Skin Type" section below, but primarily in the context of comparing vegetarian and nonvegetarian diets and nutritional approaches to curbing inflammation, which is a fundamental presentation of all sensitive skin subtypes. Regarding the P/N and W/T parameters, the N and T poles are the ideals. While various photoprotective behaviors are recommended to achieve these ends, particularly regarding the W/T spectrum, there appear to be dietary interventions that will promote or support these skin types.

Dry Skin

In 1992, investigators studied 79 vegetarians (51 females, 28 males) and 79 age- and sex-matched nonvegetarians to assess the relative antioxidant/atherogenic risks. Plasma α-tocopherol and corresponding cholesterol values were found to be significantly lower in the vegetarians as was their risk for atherosclerosis, but their tocopherol-to-cholesterol molar ratio was significantly increased.[81] Such results explain the higher incidence of dry skin in vegetarians. Cholesterol is an important substance in maintaining a balance in the oily–dry continuum. With more vitamin E and less cholesterol, vegetarians are more likely to experience dry skin (see Chapters 12 and 43).

In a 6-week study of the mechanisms and efficacy of n-3 PUFA for the treatment of AD, investigators administered various formulas of ALA in NC/Nga mice with AD, and found that concentrations of n-3 fatty acids increased and n-6 fatty acids decreased in the red blood cell membranes, prostaglandin E_2 production was decreased, and skin blood flow was altered, increasing in the ears of mice treated with the highest dose of ALA. The researchers noted, however, that AD development was not prevented.[72]

Oily Skin Types

In the adjusted models of the cross-sectional study of 302 healthy men and women cited above, serum vitamin A acted as a predictor of sebum content and surface pH, with a higher level of vitamin A associated with a lower sebum level.[2] Such findings suggest that individuals with oily skin would benefit from eating foods rich in vitamin A. Indeed, dietary consumption of plants and fish oil, high in PUFAs, is thought to be useful in treating inflammatory skin conditions because PUFAs are known to inhibit lipid inflammatory mediators.[82] (See Chapter 11.)

The OSNW Skin Type

Each of the Baumann Skin Types has specific dietary needs. Because of space constraints, each of the diets for the 16 Baumann Skin Types cannot be discussed here. However, as an example of the utility in knowing a patient's Baumann Skin Type, the oily, sensitive, nonpigmented, wrinkled (OSNW) skin type will be briefly discussed. Individuals with OSNW skin are at an increased risk of developing nonmelanoma skin cancer (basal cell or squamous cell carcinoma). The dietary guidelines that Dr. Baumann suggests for such patients to help them reduce cutaneous inflammation as well as the proclivity to wrinkle may also help decrease their risk for skin cancer, though.[83] Generally, the diet for individuals with OSNW skin should be focused on inhibiting oil secretion, decreasing inflammation, and preventing photodamage and skin cancer.

Dietary vitamin A has been demonstrated to exhibit an association with reduced oil gland secretion.[2] Therefore, a diet rich in foods that contain vitamin A, such as cantaloupe, carrots, dried apricots, egg yolks, liver, mangoes, spinach, and sweet potatoes, is recommended. Several foods have also long been fortified with vitamin A, including milk, some margarine, instant oats, breakfast cereals, and meal replacement bars. In addition, carotenoids, which can be converted into vitamin A, have been demonstrated to display inhibitory activity against skin cancer.[84] Two of the most protective carotenoids are lycopene, found abundantly in tomatoes, and lutein, found especially in spinach, kale, and broccoli.[85,86] A diet rich in other antioxidants, in addition to carotenoids, is also recommended, including a wide variety of fruits, vegetables, and green tea. Antioxidants have been demonstrated to help reduce the production of free radicals and destructive enzymes that promote skin aging.[87] In addition, olive oil has been shown to exhibit protective properties, especially imported extra virgin olive oil.[88]

A diet rich in fish and fish oils is also recommended for OSNWs, due to the high level of ω-3 fatty acids found in such food sources. As stated previously, ω-3 fatty acids appear to confer some anticancer and anti-inflammatory effects.[78,83] Because vegetarians, particularly vegans, have been shown to manifest low levels of serum ω-3 fatty acids,[73] vegetarian or vegan OSNWs should try to add seaweed, one of the best plant sources of ω-3 fatty acids, to their diet. (As stated previously, though, vegetarians and, particularly vegans, are more likely to tend toward dry skin.) Individuals with OSNW skin who suffer from rosacea, particularly facial flushing, are advised to abstain from alcohol, hot (in temperature) foods, and spicy food. In addition, such patients should be counseled to keep a record or diary of foods that exacerbate their condition, so that they have a clear idea of specific dietary triggers to avoid.

Pigmented Versus Nonpigmented Skin Types

One focus of altering susceptibility to develop pigmentary changes (melasma, solar lentigos) is the study of endogenous agents that have the potential to impart whitening or lightening activity. For example, vitamins C and E have been reported to suppress the spread of UV-induced hyperpigmentation in the skin of hairless mice.[89] (See Chapter 41, Depigmenting Ingredients, for more information on these agents.)

In a 2006 double-blind, placebo-controlled trial, investigators examined the various effects of dietary ellagic acid-rich pomegranate extract on skin pigmentation after UV irradiation in 13 women in their 20s to 40s. Volunteers were randomly assigned to one of three groups (high dose [200 mg/d ellagic acid], low dose [100 mg/d], or placebo [0 mg/d]) for the 4-week study. Subjects completed questionnaires regarding the condition of their skin prior to and after completing the dietary intervention. Based on the minimum erythema dose (MED) value recorded the previous day, a 1.5 MED dose of UV was administered to each participant on the inner right upper arm. Based on baseline recordings and assessments at Weeks 1, 2, 3, and 4, investigators found that in the high ellagic acid dose group and the low-dose group in comparison to the control group declining luminance rates were inhibited by 1.73% and 1.35%, respectively. Questionnaire results indicated that the subjects observed improvements such as greater brightness and diminished pigmentation. The investigators concluded that the oral consumption of ellagic acid-rich pomegranate extract exerts inhibitory activity against moderate pigmentation engendered by UV exposure.[90] Previously, several of the same investigators reported that an ellagic acid-rich pomegranate extract displayed inhibitory properties against mushroom tyrosinase in vitro, comparable to the known skin-whitening agent arbutin. In addition, they demonstrated that oral administration of the pomegranate extract inhibited UV-induced skin pigmentation in brownish guinea pigs, comparable in skin-whitening effect to the use of L-ascorbic acid, although the number of DOPA-positive epidermal melanocytes was reduced by the ellagic-rich pomegranate extract but not by vitamin C. The investigators concluded that oral pomegranate extract may be a suitable skin-whitening agent, likely by dint of suppressing melanocyte proliferation and melanin production by tyrosinase in melanocytes.[91]

To determine the lightening activity of orally administered grape seed extract, which is laden with the potent polyphenolic antioxidant proanthocyanidin, Yamakoshi et al. fed diets containing 1% grape seed extract or 1% vitamin C for 8 weeks to guinea pigs with UV-induced pigmentation. No changes were seen in the vitamin C or control groups, but a lightening effect presented in the pigmented skin of the guinea pigs in the grape seed extract group, with a reduction in the number of DOPA-positive melanocytes, among other key parameters. In addition, grape seed extract was reported to have disrupted mushroom tyrosinase activity and melanogenesis without suppressing cultured B16 mouse melanoma cell growth. The researchers concluded that orally administered grape seed extract has the capacity to lighten pigmentation in guinea pig skin engendered by UV exposure, possibly through the inhibition of melanin production by tyrosinase in melanocytes as well as free radical-fueled melanocyte proliferation.[89] In a 1-year open design study, Yamakoshi et al. also evaluated the effectiveness of proanthocyanidin for the treatment of melasma. Between August 2001 and January 2002, proanthocyanidin-rich grape seed extract was orally administered to 12 Japanese female melasma patients and to 11 of these 12 subjects between March and July 2002. Improvements in the melasma of 10 of the 12 women were noted during the first period of the study and in 6 of the 11 patients during the second period, with lightening values increasing and the melanin index significantly decreasing. The investigators concluded that the polyphenolic grape seed extract is effective in diminishing the hyperpigmentation associated with melasma, with optimal results seen after 6 months of oral administration and additional supplementation perhaps helping to prevent exacerbation of the condition during the summer.[92] As is often the case, more research is necessary, but these preliminary study results support the notion of pomegranate and grape seed consumption or supplementation for combating the pigmentation tendency.

Pycnogenol® is a standardized pine bark extract containing strong polyphenolic constituents with established antioxidant activity. Research has suggested that this patented botanical extract formulation is more potent than vitamins C and E and has the capacity to recycle vitamin C, regenerate vitamin E (as does vitamin C), and promote the activity of endogenous antioxidant enzymes.[93] The efficacy of Pycnogenol in protecting against UV radiation inspired a 30-day clinical trial of 30 women with melasma in which patients took one 25 mg tablet of Pycnogenol at each meal, 3 times daily. Researchers noted that the average surface area of melasma significantly decreased, suggesting that Pycnogenol is an effective and safe treatment for this condition.[93]

Wrinkled Skin Types

In 1995, investigators estimated the levels of certain vitamins (i.e., A, C, E, and β-carotene) and trace elements (i.e., copper, selenium, and zinc) in the blood of 67 vegetarian nonsmokers and 75 nonvegetarians (all between the ages of 34 and 60 years) living in the same geographical region. The average length of vegetarianism (lacto-or lacto-ovovegetarianism) was 6.2 years. The investigators found that vegetarians had higher plasma levels of all the tested vitamins and minerals, all of which play important roles as antioxidants or in activating antioxidant enzymes.[94] In turn, such compounds are associated with various salubrious effects, including photoprotection against aging, exemplified most frequently by wrinkles.

In a 2007 double-blind, placebo-controlled trial assessing the effects of soy isoflavone aglycone on the skin, particularly the extent of linear and fine wrinkles at the lateral angle of the eyes, of 26 women in their late 30s and early 40s, the volunteers were randomly assigned to incorporate into their daily diets for 12 weeks either the experimental food containing soy (40 mg daily) or a placebo. Investigators observed statistically significant improvements of malar skin elasticity at Week 8 and fine wrinkles at Week 12 in the soy group, as compared with the control group, and concluded that the daily dietary consumption of 40 mg of soy isoflavone aglycones contributes to the amelioration of cutaneous signs of aging in middle-aged women.[95]

In an especially intriguing study of a possible association between dietary intake and skin wrinkling in sun-exposed areas, Purba et al. used questionnaires and cutaneous microtopographic measurements to evaluate diet and skin wrinkling in 177 Greek-born individuals living in Melbourne, Australia, 69 Greek subjects residing in rural Greece, 48 Anglo-Celtic Australian elderly individuals living in Melbourne, Australia, and 159 Swedish elderly participants living in Sweden. Investigators identified the Swedish elderly as exhibiting the least wrinkling in sun-exposed areas, followed by the Greek-born in Melbourne, rural Greek elderly, and then Anglo-Celtic Australians. Correlation and regression analyses revealed significant data that led the investigators to conclude that diet may very well influence skin wrinkling. Generally, they found that individuals that consumed more vegetables (especially green leafy vegetables, spinach specifically, as well as asparagus, celery, eggplant, garlic, and onions/leeks), olive oil, monounsaturated fat, and legumes as well as lower levels of milk and milk products, butter, margarine, and sugar products manifested fewer wrinkles in sun-exposed skin (**Table 9-5**). Significantly, the authors suggested that diets high in monounsaturated acids may raise the monounsaturated fatty acid levels in the epidermis, which resist oxidative damage, whereas the PUFAs are more susceptible to oxidation. They speculated that this might explain the correlation of monounsaturated olive oil and less wrinkling as well as the higher level of wrinkling associated with the consumption of polyunsaturated margarine. Specifically, the investigators identified positive associations between photodamage and dietary intake of full-fat milk (but not skim milk, cheese, or yogurt), red meat, potatoes, soft drinks/cordials, and cakes/pastries. Conversely, less actinic damage was associated with vegetables and legumes,

TABLE 9-5	Foods to Consume and Avoid to Help Keep Wrinkles at Bay[96]	
Eat	**Avoid**	
Asparagus	Butter	
Celery	Margarine	
Eggplant	Milk and milk products	
Garlic		
Legumes	Red meat	
Leeks/onions	Sugar products	
Monounsaturated fat		
Olive oil		
Spinach (and other green leafy vegetables)		

as mentioned above, as well as apples/pears, cherries, dried fruits/prunes, jam, eggs, melon, multigrain bread, nuts, olives, tea, water, and yogurt. Finally, they noted that less photodamage was correlated with a higher intake of the following nutrients: total fat, especially monounsaturated fat, vitamins A and C, calcium, phosphorus, magnesium, iron, and zinc.[96]

LIMITS TO ENDOGENOUS PHOTOPROTECTION

It is worth noting that in a review of the literature regarding the relationship of nutrient intake and the skin, particularly the photoprotective effects of nutrients, the influences of nutrients on cutaneous immune responses, and therapeutic actions of nutrients in skin disorders, investigators found that supplementation with the nutrients of focus (i.e., vitamins, carotenoids, and PUFAs) rendered protection against UV light, but not as much as topical sunscreens.[82] Oral supplements should be combined with sunscreen use (Chapter 46, Sunscreens) and sun avoidance.

ORAL SUPPLEMENTS AND THE SKIN: FROM A TO Z

The following is a brief guide to some of the most common nutritional supplements currently used or under study in the beauty and skincare realm. The focus here is on the effects that such products confer on the skin. Several of these compounds provide broad systemic effects. Of course, it is incumbent upon practitioners to remind patients that they should always discuss the use of new supplements with their physician, particularly when pregnant, breast-feeding, or undergoing treatment for any medical conditions.

Alpha-Lipoic Acid

Alpha-lipoic acid is produced naturally by the human body in small quantities, but when present in excess (as a result of

a supplement, for example), it may help prevent various diseases. It is also said to help smooth skin and combat the cutaneous signs of aging. Significantly, perhaps, α-lipoic acid was once considered an antioxidant but a 2004 report has called such a designation into question.[97] While α-lipoic acid seems to exert a positive impact on energy, and on several health conditions, Dr. Baumann does not recommend it for skin-related concerns. More research is required to better understand the protective role of α-lipoic acid and its potential applications for the skin.

Antioxidants

Several of the supplements in this list qualify as antioxidants (see Chapter 39, Antioxidants). This entry, though, refers to products that contain a blend or combination of antioxidants. For example, Imedeen Time Perfection tablets include antioxidants such as vitamin C and grape seed extract. Antioxidants are substances that protect cells from oxidative damage caused by exogenous factors such as UV light, air pollution, ozone, cigarette smoke, and even oxygen itself. In addition, antioxidants protect cells from endogenously generated oxidative stress, a natural by-product of cellular energy production. Oxidative stress, whether its origin is external or internal, contributes to inflammatory pathways mediated by the formation of free radicals, which are molecules with an uneven number of electrons and are thus highly reactive. Left unchecked, free radicals can cause damage to cell membranes, lipids, proteins, and DNA, thus contributing to skin aging, among a cascade of other deleterious effects on health. Indeed, the cumulative effects of free radicals over time form the basis of "The Damage Accumulation Theory of Aging."[98] Antioxidants scavenge and eliminate free radicals and are crucial to the success of a skincare regimen. The convenience of antioxidant products also renders them easy to use on a regular basis. Good dietary sources of antioxidants include berries; larger fruits;

TABLE 9-6	Dietary Sources of Antioxidants[99]					
Berries	Larger Fruits	Vegetables	Beans	Roots and Tubers	Cereals (Wholemeal Flours Of)	Nuts, Seeds, Dried Fruits
Black currant	Clementine	Artichoke	Broad beans	Ginger	Barley	Dried apricots
Blackberry	Date	Brussels sprouts	Groundnut	Red beets	Buckwheat	Dried prunes
Blueberry	Grape	Chili pepper	Pinto beans		Common millet	Sunflower seeds
Cloudberry	Grapefruit	Kale	Soybeans		Oats	Walnuts
Cowberry/cranberry	Kiwi	Parsley				
	Lemon	Pepper				
Crowberry	Pineapple	Red cabbage				
Dog rose	Plum	Spinach				
Rowanberry	Pomegranate					
Sour cherry	Orange					
Strawberry						

vegetables; beans; roots and tubers; cereals; as well as nuts, seeds, and dried fruits.[99] (See **Table 9-6** for specific foods high in antioxidants.)

In 2007, investigators conducted a prospective study among 1,001 randomly chosen Australian adults to evaluate the relationship between consumption of antioxidants and risk of basal cell carcinomas (BCCs) and squamous cell carcinomas (SCCs). Histologically verified cases of skin cancer were recorded between 1996 and 2004 after antioxidant intake was estimated in 1996. In individuals with a baseline skin cancer history, dietary consumption of the carotenoids lutein and zeaxanthin was correlated with a lower incidence of SCC. However, a positive association was seen with various antioxidants and BCC development in those with and without a history of skin cancer, including individuals with a specific history of BCC. The researchers concluded that their findings supported prior evidence of divergent etiologic pathways for these types of skin cancer.[100] It is important to note that such results do not undermine the efficacy of antioxidants; rather, these findings reinforce the notion that evidence trumps hype. Antioxidants are not panaceas for all health problems. They offer significant benefits, but much additional research is required to grasp the full range of their capacities. While several antioxidants impart wide-ranging ameliorative effects, it appears likely that greater benefits are bestowed by the synergistic activity of several antioxidants. For example, the oral supplement DermaVite™ consists of a combination of (in descending order of concentration) a marine protein complex, α-lipoic acid, vitamin C, red clover extract, tomato extract, pine bark extract, vitamins E and B_3, soya extract, zinc, vitamin B_5, and copper, which has demonstrated clinical efficacy in the treatment of cutaneous aging symptoms (e.g., fine and coarse wrinkles, roughness, and telangiectasia) in a randomized, double-blind, placebo-controlled study.[101]

Arnica

The use of the *Arnica montana* plant has been promoted by homeopathic practitioners for hundreds of years. Arnica is used as a supplement for its anti-inflammatory properties, which have been attributed to its constituent sesquiterpene lactones.[102] Its primary skincare application is in the treatment and prevention of bruises (see Chapter 36, Pre- and Post-Procedure Skincare). While taking arnica regularly offers little benefit to the skin, the senior author suggests it to patients before cosmetic procedures such as soft tissue augmentation. Four homeopathic arnica pills labeled with 30x dilution taken 4 to 6 hours before a cosmetic procedure is recommended. In a double-blind study of 29 patients given perioperative homeopathic *A. montana* or placebo after undergoing rhytidectomy, smaller areas of ecchymosis were measured on the 4 postprocedural observation days, with statistically significant reductions identified on 2 of the 4 days.[103] It is important to caution patients that high doses of oral arnica can be harmful, so this dose and potency should not be exceeded. If a mild rash develops, the patient is likely sensitive to the compound helenalin, a key constituent found in arnica. In this case, arnica use

should be halted. While not falling into the category of nutritional supplements, topical creams with arnica, like Donell Super Skin K-Derm Gel and Boiron Arnica Cream, are used in the primary author's practice to accelerate the pace of bruise healing.

Beta-Carotene

Beta-carotene is a member of the carotenoid family, highly pigmented (red, orange, yellow), lipid-soluble substances naturally present in several fruits, grains, oils, and vegetables (such as apricots, carrots, green peppers, spinach, squash, and sweet potatoes). Notably, in a systematic study of antioxidants in dietary plants, carrots were found to have the lowest content of antioxidants of the array of roots and tubers screened.[99] Because it can be converted into active vitamin A (retinol), β-carotene is a provitamin, as are α- and γ-carotene. Beta-carotene has received substantially more attention than the other carotenoid compounds because it has been shown to contribute much more to human nutrition as compared to its related substances.[82]

In 2006, Stahl and Krutmann reported that the systemic use of β-carotene in dosages of 15 to 30 mg/d for 10 to 12 weeks had been shown to impart protection against UV-induced erythema, but was insufficient in terms of offering full protection against UVR.[104] Subsequently, investigators reviewed the literature up to June 2007 in PubMed, ISI Web of Science, and the epidermolysis bullosa acquisita Cochrane Library in conducting a meta-analysis of supplementation studies of dietary β-carotene as protection against sunburn. Meta-analysis of the seven studies identified revealed that β-carotene supplementation did indeed confer protection against sunburn in a time-dependent fashion, with a minimum of 10 weeks of supplementation necessary.[105] Indeed, in September 2007, Stahl and Sies clarified that dietary carotenoids such as β-carotene and lycopene, as well as flavonoids, contribute to the prevention of UV-induced erythema formation after ingestion and dispersal to light-exposed areas, including the skin and eyes. Specifically, these micronutrients reduced sensitivity to UV-induced erythema in volunteers after 10 to 12 weeks of dietary intervention.[106] Clearly, there are limits to the protection afforded by β-carotene. In a large-scale randomized, double-blind, placebo-controlled 12-year primary-prevention trial of β-carotene supplementation with follow-up, investigators found that supplementing with 50 mg of β-carotene on alternate days in apparently healthy male physicians from 40 to 84 years of age in 1982 ($n = 22,071$) did not influence the development of a first BCC or SCC.[107] It is worth noting that β-carotene supplementation has been demonstrated to contribute to elevating the risk of developing lung cancer in smokers and those exposed to asbestos.[108]

There are minor risks inherent in taking too much β-carotene and other provitamin A compounds. Superficially, the tint of one's skin can be rendered more yellow by consuming excess carotenoids. Because of the inefficiency in the conversion of β-carotene into retinol, there is less risk posed by β-carotene supplementation in comparison to vitamin A supplementation. Dr. Baumann prefers to see patients derive the benefits of β-carotene primarily from diet, but it can be a useful supplement for those living in warm climates where frequent sun exposure is more likely and whose diets do not include enough of this carotenoid.

Biotin

Also known as vitamin B_7, biotin has been shown to increase nail thickness by up to 25% in patients with brittle nails while minimizing nail breakage or flaking.[109] Nail strength can also be augmented through supplementation with biotin.[110] Dr. Baumann recommends a 2.5-mg daily dose of biotin to all patients whose nails are especially susceptible to breaking or splitting with little provocation. Indeed, brittle nail syndrome has been demonstrated to improve with this dosage.[111]

Borage Seed Oil

Borage seed oil is an ω-6 fatty acid rich in γ-linolenic acid (GLA), which cannot be synthesized by human skin from the precursor LA. GLA is thought to assist in hydrating the skin. As an oral supplement, borage seed oil is thought to be effective for soothing skin inflammation and redness. It is also touted as an ingredient for moisturizing and strengthening the skin barrier. In a study of the effects of dietary supplementation with borage seed oil, 29 healthy elderly people, with an average age of nearly 69, were given daily doses of 360 or 720 mg for 2 months. A statistically significant improvement in the barrier function of the skin was observed, with reductions in transepidermal water loss and dry skin complaints. Investigators also noted decreases in saturated and monounsaturated fats, concluding that fatty acid metabolism alterations and skin function amelioration resulted from borage seed oil consumption.[112]

Bromelain

The stem of the pineapple plant, *Ananas comosus*, is the source of bromelain, a term used to designate its constituent family of sulfhydryl-containing proteolytic enzymes.[113] It is indicated for cutaneous purposes because of its anti-inflammatory properties, although it is usually administered orally to aid digestion. In one study, patients with long bone fractures who received systemic bromelain evinced significantly less postoperative edema than the placebo group.[114] In addition to its use as a digestive aid, bromelain is commonly employed to treat inflammation and soft tissue injuries. The proteolytic enzymes of bromelain have imparted various wound-healing benefits, such as alleviating bruising, edema, and pain.[115] In fact, the presurgical administration of bromelain is associated with accelerated healing after surgical procedures and other trauma,[116] especially given its ability to potentiate antibiotics.[117] However, anecdotal reports suggest that using bromelain prior to a procedure will increase bruising. For this reason, Dr. Baumann recommends 500 mg of bromelain twice daily for 3 days to all patients *after* procedures such as dermal filling, to minimize bruising (see Chapter 36). In addition, it is worth suggesting the use of bromelain to patients that bruise easily. Bromelain is contraindicated in patients using anticoagulant

agents such as warfarin. Other contraindications include children, individuals with allergies to pineapple or bee stings, and people with a history of heart palpitations.

Caffeine

The best-known ingredient of coffee, caffeine is found naturally in the leaves, seeds, or fruits in several plants, and is present in tea, chocolate, soda, and other products. Consumed in popular beverages such as coffee and tea, caffeine or its metabolites are thought to confer significant anticarcinogenic and antioxidant properties.[118-121] For example, a 23-week period of oral administration of green tea or black tea to SKH-1 mice at high risk of developing skin cancer because of twice weekly exposure to UVB (30 mJ/cm^2) yielded a lower incidence of tumors/mouse, decreased parametrial fat pad size, and decreased thickness of the dermal fat layer away from and directly under tumors. Decaffeinated teas exhibited little or no effect, but the restoration of caffeine restored the inhibitory effects.[122] Significant anticarcinogenic activity has also been displayed through the topical application of caffeine to SKH-1 hairless, tumor-free mice pretreated with UVB twice weekly for 20 weeks.[123] In topical products (e.g., La Roche-Posay Rosaliac and Replenix Cream CF), caffeine is an effective anti-inflammatory and constricts veins to reduce facial flushing. The anti-inflammatory and anticarcinogenic benefits of orally administered caffeine are compelling. Caffeine is also dehydrating and should be enjoyed with moderation, ideally along with water but without unhealthy condiments such as cream and sugar. The dehydrating effects of caffeine make it a popular additive in cellulite creams, where its effects can last around 24 hours.[124] Patients that are predisposed to facial flushing should be advised to consider iced beverages, as hot ones may exacerbate facial redness.

Coenzyme Q$_{10}$

Ubiquinone, more familiarly referred to as coenzyme Q_{10} (CoQ_{10}), is a potent antioxidant found in all human cells that assists with energy production. Good dietary sources of CoQ_{10} include fish, shellfish, spinach, and nuts. CoQ_{10}, which is a fat-soluble compound, is thought to prevent oxidative stress-induced apoptosis by inhibiting lipid peroxidation in plasma membranes, thereby suppressing free radical development. In the mitochondria of each cell of the body, CoQ_{10} plays a significant role in the energy-producing adenosine triphosphate pathways. Energy production is an important aspect of cellular metabolism, the efficiency of which is thought to decrease with age. CoQ_{10} levels also coincidentally decline with age.[125] Supplementation with ubiquinone is believed to decelerate the reduction in energy production associated with senescence and illness. In 2005, Ashida et al. found that CoQ_{10} intake augmented the epidermal CoQ_{10} level in 43-week-old hairless male mice, which, coupled with their previous finding that extended CoQ_{10} supplementation in humans lowered the wrinkle area rate and wrinkle volume per unit area around the corner of the eye, led them to conclude that CoQ_{10} supplementation may have the potential to reduce wrinkles and confer additional cutaneous benefits.[126] It is also worth noting that topical CoQ_{10} has been demonstrated to penetrate the viable layers of the epidermis and decrease the level of oxidation measured by weak photon emission, and reduce wrinkle depth. In the same study, CoQ_{10} inhibited collagenase expression in human fibroblasts after UVA irradiation. The investigators concluded that topical CoQ_{10} may be effective in preventing the deleterious effects of UV radiation exposure.[127] CoQ_{10} supplements impart a caffeine-like stimulatory effect. Therefore, the senior author recommends daily use in the morning, typically 200 mg. Individuals taking cholesterol-lowering statin drugs should be counseled to consider this supplement, as statins reduce natural CoQ_{10} levels. Low CoQ_{10} levels are associated with fatigue and muscle cramping. Those on cholesterol-lowering drugs should consider taking 400 mg every morning.

Evening Primrose Oil

Derived from the seeds of evening primrose (*Oenothera biennis*), a hardy biennial member of the Onagraceae family noted for its fragrant flowers that open at dusk during the summer, EPO is an ω-6 fatty acid that contains both LA and GLA. In fact, it is one of the best sources of GLA, a polyunsaturated essential *cis*-fatty acid important in the production of prostaglandins, which play a role in the functioning of most bodily systems. LA is used by the body to synthesize GLA. In addition, LA imparts significant benefits to the skin, maintaining stratum corneum cohesion and reducing transepidermal water loss.[128] (See Chapter 12.) Overall, though, the health benefits of EPO are attributed to GLA. In a double-blind trial assessing the effects of oral EPO on atopic eczema, researchers found a statistically significant improvement among the EPO patients in overall severity of symptoms, including reductions in percentage of body surface involvement, inflammation, xerosis, and pruritus. While patients receiving placebo experienced less inflammation, EPO patients demonstrated a significantly greater reduction and a significant increase in plasma levels of dihomo-γ-linolenic acid.[129] Consequently, some authors have speculated that supplementing with products high in GLA, such as EPO, may be effective for patients with atopic eczema.[130] EPO taken as an oral supplement has been deemed a valuable source of essential fatty acids. It is approved in Germany for eczema and PMS and other uses. In 2004, it was found in a survey of more than 21,000 adults to be the most commonly used oral supplement.[131] In addition, EPO combined with zinc has been used to soothe dry eyes, ameliorate brittle nails, and to treat acne and sunburn. Overall, this supplement may be effective in helping to hydrate the skin as well as easing inflammation and irritation. Dr. Baumann particularly recommends EPO to patients who experience frequent skin irritation.

Glucosamine

Typically derived from the shells of shellfish (although synthetic versions are also available), glucosamine and its derivative N-acetyl glucosamine are amino-monosaccharides that serve several significant biological roles, particularly in the production of cartilage. Both act as substrate precursors for hyaluronic acid (HA) as well as proteoglycans synthesis. Given its role in HA production, it is not surprising that glucosamine has been demonstrated to confer various cutaneous benefits, such as enhancing hydration, reducing wrinkles, and accelerating wound healing.[132] In addition to anti-inflammatory and chondroprotective properties, glucosamine has been shown to be effective in treating hyperpigmentation because it inhibits tyrosinase activation thereby suppressing melanin synthesis.[132] In a randomized, controlled, single-blind 5-week study with 53 female volunteers who were given an oral supplement containing glucosamine, amino acids, minerals, and various antioxidant compounds, investigators found a statistically significant reduction (34%) in the number of visible wrinkles and a reduction (34%) in the number of fine lines in the treatment group as compared to the 12-person control group.[133] Oral glucosamine supplementation has also been demonstrated to ameliorate symptoms and decelerate the development of osteoarthritis in animals as well as in clinical trials in humans, and its list of indications is expanding.[132] In a retrospective survey of the nonvitamin, nonmineral dietary supplements used among an elderly cohort between 1994 and 1999, glucosamine emerged as the most frequently used supplement.[134] Dr. Baumann recommends 1,500 mg/d, particularly to patients older than 35 years. Glucosamine supplements have been demonstrated to assist in rebuilding cartilage, in which HA is an important component. Evidence suggests that the effects of glucosamine supplementation, namely increased skin fullness and decreased wrinkles, can be seen in as little as 4 to 6 weeks.

Horse Chestnut Seed Extract

Of the various species of horse chestnuts, trees as well as bushes, the European horse chestnut (*Aesculus hippocastanum*) is the one used most often for medicinal purposes. In its oral form, horse chestnut seed extract (HCSE) has been shown to effectively enhance circulatory problems such as varicose veins and leg cramping. Indeed, researchers conducting a thorough literature review of double-blind, randomized controlled trials of oral HCSE for patients with chronic venous insufficiency in Medline, EMBASE, BIOSIS, CISCOM, and the Cochrane Library (until December 1996) found that HCSE was superior to placebo in all cases.[135] In addition, they noted reductions in lower-leg volume, leg circumference at the calf and ankle, and improvement in symptoms including leg pain, pruritus, fatigue, and tension, with only rare mild adverse reactions. The same investigators, along with a third, subsequently conducted a broad database search of Medline, EMBASE, the Cochrane Library, CISCOM, and AMED (until October 2000) on complementary and alternative medicine and found additional cogent evidence for the effectiveness of oral HCSE for the treatment of chronic venous insufficiency.[136] HCSE has been proven to improve inflammation and circulatory discomfort in its oral form. Patients taking anticoagulant drugs should be advised not to supplement with HCSE.

Hyaluronic Acid

One of the three primary constituents of the dermis, HA, also known as hyaluronan, is the most abundant glycosaminoglycan in the human dermis. HA, which has the capacity to bind water up to 1,000 times its volume, plays an important role in cell growth, adhesion, and membrane receptor function. Its main biologic function in the intercellular matrix is to stabilize intercellular structures and form the elastoviscous fluid matrix in which collagen and elastin fibers are firmly enveloped.[137,138] HA holds onto moisture, as well, and helps provide fullness and radiance to the skin. While HA is the main component of several effective and popular dermal filling agents, and has also demonstrated efficacy as an intra-articular injection agent for knee osteoarthritis,[139] oral HA supplements are also available. These products are touted for combating the decline of HA, which occurs with age. However, HA is metabolized in the stomach; therefore, the primary author does not believe there is any evidence demonstrating the effectiveness of these supplements.

Iron

Found in every cell of the body, iron is an important mineral for all-around good health and is essential in the production of hemoglobin, the blood component that distributes oxygen throughout the body. Low iron levels have been associated with hair loss. Supplementation could help control or resolve this condition. Iron deficiency may also manifest in the fingernails, as white spots or vertical ridges. Physicians should check a patient's ferritin levels prior to recommending an iron supplement. Excess iron can generate free radicals, which attack vital skin constituents, such as collagen and elastin, and accelerate cutaneous aging. Iron supplements should be recommended to patients only if it is determined that they have low iron levels. Good dietary sources of iron include dried beans, dried fruits, egg yolks, salmon, tuna, whole grains, and other foods.

Lycopene

Naturally present in human blood and tissues, lycopene is a non-provitamin A carotenoid best known as the pigment mainly responsible for the characteristic red color of tomatoes. During the last two decades, lycopene has garnered much attention for its potent antioxidant activity.[140,141] Lycopene may play a role in reducing oxidative damage to tissues, as suggested by a placebo-controlled study that examined the effects on plasma and skin concentrations of β-carotene and lycopene from ingesting a single 120-mg dose of β-carotene. The effects from UV light exposure were also examined. Lycopene levels in plasma and skin, which are comparable or greater than those of β-carotene, were unaffected by β-carotene ingestion, but β-carotene levels increased. Furthermore, a single intense exposure (three times the MED) of solar-simulated light on a small area of the volar arm resulted in a 31% to 46% decrease in skin lycopene concentration, but no significant changes in skin β-carotene, which led the investigators to conclude that lycopene may contribute to absorbing or mitigating the effects of UV radiation and other forms of oxidative insult.[142] Protection against erythema development after UV exposure has also been demonstrated as a result of increasing lycopene intake by daily consumption of tomato paste for a 10-week period.[140] Consequently, Sies and Stahl, who conducted the study, have deemed lycopene an effective oral sun protectant that can play an important role in maintaining the health of the skin. In work published by these and additional investigators in the same year, supplementation for 12 weeks with 24 mg/d of a carotenoid formulation including β-carotene, lutein, and lycopene was found in a placebo-controlled, parallel study design to exert a comparable improvement in mitigating UV-induced erythema in humans as 24 mg of β-carotene alone.[47] More recent work by some of the same investigators has further buttressed the evidence showing the photoprotective effects of lycopene supplementation, with significant increases measured in lycopene serum levels and total skin carotenoids; erythema was also demonstrably prevented after UV irradiation.[44,48] More research is necessary, but lycopene, through oral supplementation or topical administration, is also considered a potential chemopreventive agent to address nonmelanoma skin cancer.[141]

Niacin

Also known as vitamin B_3 or nicotinic acid, niacin has long been known to be essential for the healthy functioning of the skin and nervous system. Niacinamide (also called nicotinamide) is the amide form of niacin. The terms nicotinic acid and nicotinamide are used less frequently because they sound similar, though unrelated, to nicotine. Neither niacin nor niacinamide are synthesized in the human body; therefore, they must be supplied through the diet, topical application, or oral supplementation. Peanuts, brewer's yeast, fish, and meat are the best dietary sources of niacin. The deficiency of niacin and niacinamide appears to play a role in the development of several types of cancer, including skin cancer. Mice given oral niacin or topical niacinamide exhibited a 70% decrease in UV-induced skin cancers and near-complete prevention of photoimmunosuppression.[142]

For several years, niacinamide has been used both topically and orally to treat inflammatory diseases. For example, Berk et al. described the use of oral niacinamide plus tetracycline for the treatment of bullous pemphigoid.[143] Rosacea is among the indications for niacinamide treatment.[144] Niacin deficiency is also associated with pellagra, a disease characterized by diarrhea, dermatitis, and dementia. However, a 2017 study of oral niacin intake in women found no evidence of protection against the development of AD, as well as an inverse relationship between supplementary B complex and multivitamin intake and AD.[145]

The use of oral or intravenous niacin has been described for the treatment of migraines and tension-type headaches, though randomized controlled trials are lacking.[146] Indeed, niacin is well known for exhibiting vasodilatory activity.[146]

Patients who take oral niacin long-term to control hypertension tend to develop bothersome flushing. Because of this, topical products may be more desirable, though the relatively new extended-release 1,000 mg niacin ER tablet has been shown to reduce the frequency, duration, and intensity of niacin-induced flushing.[147] Although niacin supplements may be prescribed for various conditions, there is no skin-related reason to take more than what would be derived from a typical multivitamin. Niacinamide, in contrast, imparts no cutaneous side effects and is a very effective ingredient in topical formulations for treating photodamage, inflammation, hyperpigmentation, and dry skin. Niacinamide is found in the Olay brand products such as Total Effects, Regenerist, and Definity. The brand Nia24 contains an ingredient very similar to niacinamide.

Omega-3 Fatty Acids

Although they are not synthesized naturally in the body, ω-3 fatty acids are a family of polyunsaturated fatty acids (also referred to as n-3 PUFAs or PUFAs) that are crucial components of cell membranes and key constituents in the skin barrier. ALA, EPA, and DHA are the primary essential ω-3 fatty acids. The anti-inflammatory activities of these compounds are well established, as several studies have demonstrated their efficacy in combating erythema and irritation associated with cutaneous conditions such as psoriasis and rosacea. Significant anti-inflammatory activity displayed by EPA and DHA, from oily extracts of three Mediterranean fish species, against UVB-induced erythema has been revealed *in vivo* in human volunteers.[148] The hydrating qualities of ω-3 fatty acids also serve to add volume to the skin, minimizing the appearance of fine lines. Good dietary sources of the ω-3 fatty acid ALA include canola oil, walnuts, and "ω-3 eggs" (which provide much more than the typical level of ω-3 as a result of the special diet fed to the hens); for the ω-3 fatty acids EPA and DHA, fish and other seafood, as well as "ω-3 eggs" are good dietary sources.[149] The fish that contain significant levels of ω-3 fatty acids are fatty predatory fish, including albacore tuna, lake trout, mackerel, menhaden, and salmon[82] (**Table 9-7**). It is important to note that such fish do not synthesize these acids but accumulate them through their diet, which may also include toxic substances. For this reason, particularly in the case of mercury toxicity in albacore tuna, the FDA recommends limiting consumption of selected predatory fish species. Supplementing with fish oil has become an increasingly popular alternative. Cod liver oil and other fish oils are also good sources of n-3 PUFAs.[82] While noting the natural dietary sources of such nutrients, particularly fish, it is important to make dietary choices with environmental sensitivity. In particular, fish should be selected with this in mind, as several species may be endangered (e.g., cod) or approaching such status.

Sies and Stahl have contended that ω-3 fatty acids are among the various micronutrients that exhibit the capacity to deliver systemic photoprotection against UV-induced damage.[150] In addition, Black and Rhodes have suggested that there is a wide array of experimental and clinical studies indicating an important role for ω-3 fatty acids in preventing nonmelanoma

TABLE 9-7	Good Dietary Sources of Omega-3 Fatty Acids[73,82,149]	
Albacore tuna		
Canola oil		
Fish (and other seafood)		
Flaxseed/flaxseed oil		
Hempseed		
Lake trout		
Mackerel		
Menhaden		
"Omega-3 eggs"		
Salmon		
Seaweed		
Walnuts		

skin cancer, as manifested in evidence of increasing tumor latency periods, decreasing tumor number, increasing the UV radiation-mediated erythema threshold in humans, and significantly reducing pro-inflammatory and immunosuppressive prostaglandin E synthase type 2 (PGE_2) levels in human skin exposed to UVB.[151] A recent Cochrane systematic review of 11 randomized placebo-controlled trials, totaling nearly 600 participants, found that of oral zinc sulphate, selenium and selenium plus vitamin E, vitamin D and vitamin D plus vitamin E, pyridoxine, sea buckthorn oil, hempseed oil, sunflower oil (linoleic acid), DHA versus control (saturated fatty acids of the same energy value), and olive oil versus corn oil versus fish oil, only two studies of fish oil showed a small positive effect on existing atopic eczema/dermatitis.[152]

In a 2006 report in the *Journal of the American Medical Association*, MacLean et al. conducted a literature review, and consulted experts in the neutraceutical field regarding unpublished studies, to sift through mixed results on the capacity of ω-3 fatty acids to lower the risk of developing cancer. Thirty-eight articles were ultimately considered in their evaluation, yielding the conclusion that dietary supplementation with ω-3 fatty acids does not likely prevent cancer.[153] However, Chen et al. countered that none of the 38 studies reviewed considered the measurement of fatty acid composition in patients. They suggested that in reviewing dietary data, it is important to note that some fish (particularly farm-raised fish) are inadequate sources of ω-3 fatty acids. Chen et al. suggested that it remains uncertain, but is not unlikely, as to whether ω-3 fatty acids confer a preventive effect against cancer.[154] While more research is clearly needed regarding the diverse effects of dietary ω-3 fatty acids, several benefits have been patently established. The senior author recommends incorporating as many sources of ω-3 fatty acids into one's diet as desired and supplementing with 1,000 mg/d.

Polypodium Leucotomos

Derived from the fern family, the extract of *Polypodium leucotomos* has been used to treat inflammatory conditions and shown, *in vitro* and *in vivo*, to display inmunomodulating effects.[155] It is also thought to exhibit potent antioxidant activity and is considered a viable oral photoprotectant.[156,157]

In 2004, Middelkamp-Hup et al. assessed whether oral *Polypodium leucotomos* extract (PLE) could diminish the clinical and histologic phototoxic damage to human skin caused by psoralen with ultraviolet A (PUVA) treatment. Ten healthy patients with Fitzpatrick skin types II to III were exposed to PUVA alone and PUVA accompanied by 7.5 mg/kg of oral PLE. After 48 to 72 hours, clinical results revealed consistently lower phototoxicity in PLE-treated skin, with pigmentation reduced 4 months after treatment. Histologic examination indicated significantly fewer sunburn cells, and reductions in vasodilatation and the tryptase-positive mast cell infiltration, in addition to preservation of Langerhans cells in PLE-treated skin. The authors found that PLE effectively protected the skin against the known deleterious effects of PUVA.[158] Although this was a small study, the results spurred the team to additional study of PLE. In research reported later in 2004 by the same group, nine healthy individuals with Fitzpatrick skin types II to III were exposed to various doses of artificial UVR radiation without or following oral administration of 7.5 mg/kg PLE. Investigators assessed erythematous reactions 24 hours after exposure and obtained paired biopsy specimens from PLE-treated skin and untreated skin. Significantly less erythema was noted in the PLE-treated skin. In the biopsy specimens, researchers recorded fewer sunburn cells, cyclobutane pyrimidine dimers, and proliferating epidermal cells as well as less mast cell infiltration. Preservation of Langerhans cells was also achieved. The team's previous findings were supported by this study, which prompted them to conclude that oral PLE effectively protects the skin against UV insult.[159]

In a study by Middelkamp-Hup et al. of the potential of oral PLE in the treatment of vitiligo vulgaris, 50 patients were randomly administered 250 mg of oral PLE or placebo 3 times daily, combined with the first-line therapy (narrow-band UVB) twice weekly for 25 or 26 weeks. Investigators identified a definite trend in repigmentation in the head and neck area, particularly in light skin types, with the combined narrow-band UVB and oral PLE therapy.[160] PLE is most widely available in a capsule supplement known as Heliocare. It is expensive, but it helps protect the skin against UV damage, and reduces erythema caused by sun exposure. The primary author recommends one capsule taken in the morning when sun exposure is anticipated, two capsules if the exposure is expected to be prolonged.

Selenium

An important antioxidant, selenium is a trace mineral found naturally in the body and various foods, particularly Brazil nuts. Some seafood, meat, cereals, and dairy products contain selenium as do several plant foods, depending on the selenium content of the soil in which they are grown. Selenium is essential to good health, but required in only small amounts.[161] A properly functioning thyroid is also dependent on selenium. In addition, the protective activity characteristic of the immune cells is supported by the synergistic cooperation of various vitamins and minerals, including selenium.[162] Although a capacity to protect against skin cancer has been recently disproved, selenium remains among the list of potential oral or topical chemopreventive agents against other forms of cancer,[141] and it is considered an important contributor to antioxidant defense.[150,163] However, in a prospective case-cohort study of the link between arsenic-related premalignant skin lesions and prediagnostic blood selenium levels in 303 cases newly diagnosed from November 2002 to April 2004 and 849 subcohort members randomly selected from the 8,092 subjects in the Health Effects of Arsenic Longitudinal Study, investigators found that dietary selenium intake may lower the incidence of arsenic-related premalignant skin lesions among susceptible populations (those exposed to arsenic from drinking water).[164] In addition, it is thought to exhibit potent anti-inflammatory and anti-aging properties and, in oral form, appears to mitigate UV-induced skin damage. Indeed, animal studies suggest that selenium deficiency sensitizes the skin for UVB-induced oxidative damage and inflammation through the activation of p38 MAPK signaling pathways.[165]

Although more research is necessary, selenium in both oral and topical form appears to impart several benefits to the skin. It is used as a topical water to treat psoriasis, eczema, and other inflammatory skin conditions in the La Roche-Posay spa in France dedicated to the treatment of these skin conditions. Most multivitamins typically contain a sufficient amount of selenium. The recommended daily allowance of selenium for adults is 55 µg, and overdose can be harmful (generally, more than 400 µg/d). In fact, excessive amounts of selenium can lead to hair loss.

Vitamin A

Retinol, also known as vitamin A, has such status because it is not synthesized in the human body. The term "retinoids" refers to vitamin A and all its natural and synthetic derivatives including retinol. Carotenoids such as carrots, cantaloupes, sweet potatoes, and spinach are among the best dietary sources of vitamin A.[166] Milk, margarine, eggs, beef liver, and fortified breakfast cereals are also important dietary contributors of vitamin A.[167] Retinoids exhibit several important biologic functions, such as regulating growth and differentiation of epithelial cells, inhibiting tumor promotion during experimental carcinogenesis, diminishing malignant cell growth, decreasing inflammation, and enhancing the immune system[168] (see Chapter 45, Retinoids). In addition, retinoids have been shown to improve the appearance of striae as well as skin discoloration.[169] Vitamin A is also particularly beneficial for individuals with acne, as it helps diminish oil levels in the skin. In addition, retinoic acid, or tretinoin, is known to reverse the signs of photoaging by diminishing wrinkles, actinic keratoses, and lentigines as well as smoothing skin texture.[170] In cooperation with several other vitamins and minerals, including vitamins C and E, as well as zinc, vitamin A contributes to enhancing skin barrier function as well as immune cell protective activity.[162]

Vitamin A is an important part of any diet, but consuming or taking excessive amounts poses risks, including a greater susceptibility to bone fracture. There is rarely a reason to take more than what is found in a good multivitamin. It is healthier, however, to derive one's necessary vitamin A through diet, particularly by eating leafy greens, carrots, cantaloupes, sweet potatoes, spinach, broccoli, squash, and mangoes.

Vitamin C

Known historically for its role in the prevention of scurvy, vitamin C is abundantly available in citrus fruits. In fact, by the 18th century, sailors knew that eating citrus fruits prevented this condition associated with dental abnormalities, bleeding disorders, characteristic purpuric skin lesions, and mental deterioration. In the 1930s, researchers confirmed that vitamin C is the key ingredient in citrus fruit that fends off scurvy and dubbed it ascorbic acid (*scorbutus* is Latin for *scurvy*). Currently, vitamin C is considered a potent antioxidant and is used effectively as an anti-aging and anti-inflammatory agent.

In the skin, vitamin C plays an integral role in the metabolism of collagen, where it is essential for the hydroxylation of lysine and proline in procollagen (see Chapter 2). Vitamin C has also been demonstrated to augment collagen synthesis in both neonatal and adult fibroblasts when added to culture medium.[171] Aging skin is characterized by decreased collagen production (see Chapters 5, Intrinsic Aging, and 6, Extrinsic Aging). Consequently, it is thought that increasing collagen production in the skin with vitamin C should theoretically contribute to preventing or even reversing some of the signs of cutaneous aging.[172] The stimulatory effects of vitamin C on collagen synthesis are believed to be effective in preventing and treating striae alba (stretch marks). This important role in collagen synthesis indicates the relevance of vitamin C in wrinkle prevention.

In a literature review of the photoprotective effects of vitamins C and E, investigators found that topical applications of each individual antioxidant performed significantly better than their orally administered counterparts. The photoprotective effects of vitamin C and E combinations, along with other antioxidants, proved to be markedly more effective than monotherapies in delivering cutaneous protection against UVB.[173]

In a 3-month study of the effects of oral administration of a combination of vitamins C and E, investigators found significant decreases in the sunburn response to UVB exposure, with substantially fewer thymine dimers induced by UV radiation, implying a protective effect against DNA damage conferred by the antioxidant combination.[174] In a study of the effects of the oral administration of a mixture combining the antioxidants vitamins C and E, Pycnogenol, and EPO on UVB-induced wrinkle formation, female SKH-1 hairless mice received the test mixture or control vehicle for 10 weeks along with UVB irradiation 3 times weekly, with graduated increases in UVB intensity. Investigators found that UVB-induced wrinkle formation was significantly inhibited, with substantial reductions

also seen in epidermal thickness as well as UVB-engendered acanthosis, hyperplasia, and hyperkeratosis.[175]

Many physicians, including the senior author, recommend that patients take oral vitamin C 500 mg twice daily. This way they enjoy the benefits of vitamin C without the irritation and expense of topical formulations, which are difficult to stabilize. Other than an upset stomach, there is no risk of taking too much vitamin C.

Vitamin D

Perhaps best known as the vitamin skin produces when exposed to UV light, vitamin D_3, often shortened to vitamin D, is actually a hormone, and a potent antioxidant. Besides sun exposure, vitamin D can be obtained through the diet, especially by consumption of fatty fish.[176] Through the metabolic process, vitamin D is converted into 25-hydroxyvitamin D (25(OH)D) by the liver and 1,25-dihydroxyvitamin D (1,25(OH)$_2$D) by the kidneys.[176] It has been known for several years that UVB exposure induces epidermal keratinocytes to convert 7-dehydrocholesterol into vitamin D_3. Further, the metabolites of vitamin D_3, particularly calcitriol, are known to confer significant benefits, such as antiproliferative and prodifferentiating activity as well as regulating cellular activity in keratinocytes and immunocompetent cells.[177]

In addition to imparting benefits to most bodily organ systems, vitamin D plays a significant role in psoriasis treatments, including the drug Dovonex. Like all antioxidants, vitamin D exhibits the capacity to decelerate aspects of cutaneous aging. Cutaneous vitamin D_3 synthesis declines with age. Consequently, vitamin D deficiency is not uncommon in the elderly, the demographic group most in need of taking oral vitamin D supplements. Low vitamin D status is a factor in the development of osteoporosis. Vitamin D insufficiency is also associated with rickets, certain types of cancer, and various other diseases.[178]

Vitamin D deficiency can lead to an elevation in serum parathyroid hormone, contributing to bone resorption, osteoporosis, and fractures. Supplementation with vitamin D has been shown to inhibit serum parathyroid hormone, increase bone mineral density, and may reduce the incidence of fractures, particularly in the elderly.[176] In a 12-week randomized clinical study in a psychogeriatric nursing home comparing the effects of UV radiation and oral vitamin D_3 on the vitamin D status and parathyroid hormone concentration in elderly nursing home patients, investigators found UVB to be as effective as oral vitamin D_3 in raising serum 25(OH)D and serum calcium as well as inhibiting secondary hyperparathyroidism.[179]

Research has also shown that vitamin D analogs may have a role to play in the medical therapy of melanoma, even though avoiding exposure to UV remains the best protection against melanoma and nonmelanoma skin cancers.[180] In addition, research has shown that obesity-related vitamin D insufficiency likely results from the diminished bioavailability of vitamin D_3 from cutaneous and dietary sources due to deposition in body fat.[181]

In the mid-1990s, vitamin D became the subject of controversy when claims emerged that the use of sunscreen led to vitamin D deficiency.[182] Despite mounting evidence to the contrary, this remains a controversial topic. Interestingly, Gilchrest cited evolutionary changes in countering the argument for controlled exposure to UV to obtain sufficient vitamin D levels. Specifically, she suggested that when the human capacity to photosynthesize vitamin D emerged, the lifespan for human beings was considerably shorter than it is today, and the effects of long-term photodamage, or the modern option of purchasing oral vitamin D, could not be part of the equation.[183]

Currently, the tolerable upper intake level (UL) for vitamin D_3 stands at 50 µg/d (2,000 IU/d) in North Americans and Europeans, but several studies suggest that metabolic utilization of vitamin D_3 would be optimized at a UL as high as twice this level, particularly to ameliorate vitamin D status in the elderly.[178,184,185] The challenge with vitamin D is balancing the mounting evidence that cutaneous vitamin D production helps prevent various diseases, including some cancers, with the understanding that prolonged sun exposure greatly increases the risk of skin cancer and other photodamage. Oral vitamin D supplementation in place of UV exposure appears to be the safest approach and may be particularly appropriate for certain populations. For instance, individuals at high risk for skin cancer (e.g., those who have red hair and freckles, or a family history of skin cancer) should be advised to avoid unprotected sun exposure and to obtain vitamin D in oral supplement form and diet. Mushrooms have been found to be a good source of vitamin D. Blood levels of vitamin D should be checked in all patients. If levels are low, vitamin D supplementation and the addition of mushrooms to the diet should be recommended along with *limited* sun exposure. It takes only a few minutes of solar exposure each day to stimulate vitamin D synthesis. Patients should be reminded of this and advised that there is never a good reason to bake in the sun all day.

Vitamin E

Vitamin E includes the tocopherols and the tocotrienols. It is the most significant lipid-soluble antioxidant, and it is found naturally in many vegetables, especially spinach, avocados, corn, vegetable oils, sunflower seeds, soy, whole grains, nuts, and margarine. Usually referred to as α-tocopherol, its most biologically active form, vitamin E is also found in some meat and dairy products. In humans, vitamin E naturally occurs in the membranes of cells and organelles. It protects cell membranes from peroxidation and scavenges free radicals. Consequently, vitamin E is thought to help prevent cardiovascular disease and the "aging" of the arteries. It is effective in mitigating skin dryness, particularly in those taking oral retinoids.

Vitamin E has also been shown to exert anti-inflammatory effects on the skin through the inhibition of chemical mediator synthesis and release. In addition to stabilizing lysosomes, vitamin E influences prostaglandin E_2 production (decreasing it) as well as well as IL-2 production (increasing

it). Anti-inflammatory and immunostimulatory effects are the result.[168] An important component of sebum, vitamin E is found in greater supply in individuals with oily skin. This may correlate with less skin aging and less skin cancer. The lips, which have no oil glands and are thus devoid of vitamin E, are more susceptible to skin cancer than many other areas of the skin surface. Antitumorigenic, photoprotective, and skin barrier-stabilizing activities have been associated with topical and oral vitamin E.[186]

In a hairless mouse model of photocarcinogenesis induced by UVB expression, investigators showed that oral administration of α-tocopherol resulted in significant inhibitory effects on tumor incidence and number.[187] However, in a study assessing the capacity of orally administered vitamin E and β-carotene to diminish markers of oxidative stress and erythema in response to UV exposure in 16 healthy participants who took either of the lipid-soluble antioxidants for 8 weeks, results revealed that such supplementation had no effect on skin sensitivity, though the vitamin E group experienced significant decreases in cutaneous malondialdehyde. No other measures of oxidative stress in basal or UV-exposed skin were influenced by the supplementation, suggesting that neither bestowed photoprotection.[188]

While results remain conflicting over the relative photoprotective effects of oral vitamin E, the evidence strongly indicates significant photoprotective effects from the orally administered combination of vitamins C and E. In a single-blind controlled clinical trial examining the photoprotective effects of vitamins C and E, 45 healthy volunteers were divided into three groups, one receiving oral vitamin C, one receiving oral vitamin E, and one receiving an oral mixture of the two antioxidants. Daily treatments lasted 1 week. The MED was ascertained before and after treatment, with the median MED increasing the most in the combination group, suggesting that d-α-tocopherol combined with ascorbic acid yielded better photoprotective effects than either of the antioxidants alone.[189] For more information on just a few of the several reports on the success of this combination, see the "vitamin C" section above. This combination of antioxidants currently represents one of the skin's best defenses against photodamage, including photocarcinogenesis and photoaging.

Vitamin E is an important part of any diet, but there is a risk from taking too much. The senior author recommends 400 IU, in gel cap form, per day. Vitamin E can increase the likelihood of bruising if taken in large doses. Indeed, doses greater than 3,000 mg daily when taken over a long period may cause such side effects. Patients undergoing surgical procedures should avoid doses of vitamin E greater than 4,000 IU.[168] In addition, vitamin E should be discontinued 10 days prior to surgical procedures, soft tissue augmentation, or Botox injections in order to minimize the risk of bruising.

Vitamin-fortified Beverages

Various "enhanced water" products have been introduced onto the market in the last several years. As an occasional treat, they represent a much better choice than soda, which offers no health benefits. At least these products provide a few vitamins. Ersatz water products are not a substitute for a good multivitamin, however, and do not include common supplements such as glucosamine or biotin. In addition, these products often contain high levels of sugar, which can contribute to various health outcomes and, in the cutaneous realm, foster wrinkling caused by glycation as well as acne eruptions.

The appeal of this market has resulted in the emergence of sugar-free and nutrient-added formulations. For example, Coca-Cola launched a product called Enviga, a sugar-free beverage that contains green tea, one of the most potent and best-researched antioxidants available. In addition, the Borba product line features nutrient-fortified waters specifically formulated for the skin. (These have no added sugar and zero calories.) Not surprisingly, only proprietary in-house studies are available on such products. While it remains to be seen whether these products confer any health benefits, there is no reason to think that they would be harmful or unhealthy. Another way to derive cutaneous benefits from liquid nutrients, other than red wine and green and other teas, is a "water booster." These formulations, packaged in dropper-style bottles, can be added to any beverage. The senior author recommends Dr. Brandt Anti-Oxidant Water Booster/Pure Green Tea. Liquid supplements to be placed on the tongue, such as Dr. Andrew Weil for Origins™ Plantidote™ Mega-Mushroom Supplement, are also popular but unproven. These products should be combined, more importantly, with a well-rounded diet, exercise, and a good multivitamin. Finally, pomegranate juice does not require any vitamin fortification. As long as no sugar is added, pomegranate juice packs a potent antioxidant punch.

Zinc

Zinc is an essential trace element found in, but not produced by, the human body. It is present in various foods, particularly high-protein meats such as lean beef, chicken, and fish. A vegetarian diet often contains less zinc than a meat-based diet. Good vegetarian sources of zinc include beans, dairy products, lentils, nuts, seeds, particularly pumpkin seeds, whole grain cereals, and yeast.[190,191] Known as an essential dietary factor for the last half century, zinc is now also thought to exhibit antioxidant and anti-inflammatory activity.[192] In addition, zinc assists other micronutrients in bolstering the function of the skin barrier as well as the protective actions of immune cells.[162] Zinc is also necessary for synthesizing retinol-binding protein, which transmits vitamin A. Although there are no areas in the body where zinc is stored, the essential mineral is found in muscle (60%), bone (30%), skin (5%), and other organs.[190,193]

The beneficial effects on immunity are typically cited as the reason for the inclusion of zinc in various cold and flu over-the-counter remedies. Indeed, antiviral effects are now being considered. In a placebo-controlled trial reported on in 2002, investigators found oral zinc sulfate at a dose of 10 mg/kg daily to be successful for the treatment of recalcitrant viral warts after a follow-up of 2 to 3 months.[194] The overlapping,

protective roles of the skin and the immunity system appear to be reflected in the activity of zinc. In a study of the effects on the allergic response of zinc deficiency in a DS-Nh mouse model of AD, investigators fed male mice a zinc-deficient diet for 4 weeks and found that zinc deficiency affected the skin barrier and immune systems, and aggravated AD.[195]

With age, zinc absorption declines and zinc deficiency is not uncommon in the elderly, particularly individuals older than 75 years.[193] Zinc supplementation has been shown to reverse the plasma zinc reductions, plasma oxidative stress marker increases, and elevated production of inflammatory cytokines seen in the elderly.[192] The adult recommended daily amount (RDA), now referred to as the reference nutrient intake (RNI), for zinc is 15 mg/d for men and 12 mg/d for women, though pregnant women require more zinc. It is important to note that only 20% of the zinc present in the diet is actually absorbed by the body. In addition, zinc absorption is often impaired in patients with chronic GI inflammation. For oral mineral supplements, the amounts of zinc and iron should be equivalent so that they do not interfere with absorption. Zinc is lost primarily through feces, urine, hair, skin, sweat, semen, and menstrual blood.

DIET AND THE SKIN

Diet plays a crucial role in the appearance of the skin, factoring into everything from skin hydration, redness, and acne to cutaneous aging. Even broken blood vessels on the face can be caused by diet. Based on the studies reviewed above, certain dietary principles can be gleaned and formulated into suggestions for patients regarding general cutaneous health as well as specific concerns such as which foods to eat or avoid in an anti-aging or acne treatment regimen. The following discussion provides some general dietary guidelines for healthy skin (Box 9-1) as well as some specific recommendations that depend on skin type (Box 9-2). The following dietary recommendations are long-term interventions intended for good overall health and the prevention of future wrinkles, not as treatment for already extant wrinkles.

Fish and Omega-3 Fatty Acids

As stated above, predatory fish such as albacore tuna, lake trout, mackerel, menhaden, and salmon are high in ω-3 fatty acids. Salmon, in particular, is highly regarded and readily available, as is tuna. Salmon contains ω-3 and ω-6 fatty acids that help human skin hold onto water, inhibiting transepidermal water loss. The numerous ω-3 fatty acids in salmon (particularly EPA and DHA) are also anti-inflammatory; therefore, eating salmon may help curb acne and facial redness. Patients should be advised to select wild salmon because it may have a greater abundance of ω-3 fatty acids and fewer contaminants, such as PCB, as compared to farmed salmon. The senior author recommends eating salmon at least 3 times a week.

Omega-3 fatty acids as well as ω-6 fatty acids are essential for healthy human growth and development. The typical Western diet had a typical ratio of ω-6 to ω-3 fatty acids of

BOX 9-1 — General Dietary Recommendations in Brief

1. Eat salmon at least three times per week.
2. Add flaxseeds to your diet or use flaxseed oil as a salad dressing.
3. Eat foods high in antioxidants, such as a wide variety of berries and pomegranates.
4. Eat a wide variety of fruits, vegetables, and legumes—what nutritionists have been advising for decades. In particular, eating fruits and vegetables that are in season is more nutritious.
5. Use spices such as oregano, ginger, and basil, all of which exhibit antioxidant properties.
6. Drink 2 to 4 cups of green tea per day.
7. Drink plenty of water (1 to 2 L a day, depending on level of exertion, humidity conditions, and individual need).
8. Supplement with CoQ_{10}, at least one 200 mg gel cap in the AM.
9. Drink a moderate amount of red wine, which contains the polyphenolic antioxidants resveratrol and grape seed extract, both of which confer significant anti-aging benefits. Consumption of too much alcohol leads to free radical formation, which ages the skin.
10. Limit or avoid calorie-dense refined sugars, saturated fats, and processed foods. Sugar can contribute to acne and accelerate aging by causing the glycosylation of necessary proteins.
11. Following the premise that what is good for the digestion is good for the skin, eat smaller portions (the typical American diet, particularly as evidenced by restaurant portions, overdoes this considerably), and chew slowly (ideally not while reading, watching TV, or otherwise distracted).

It is important to note that these are general guidelines. Individual dietary needs may vary. In fact, the BSTS system is founded on the notion that skincare needs vary according to skin type. (See Table 9-8 for oral supplementation guidelines by BSTS.) Accordingly, some dietary needs or restrictions can be categorized by skin type. It is worth noting that ancient medical systems that continue in the present day—traditional Chinese medicine and Ayurveda, from the Indian sub-continent—base nutritional advice on evaluations of an individual's constitution and their relative deficits upon examination. Ultimately, as we are learning in the West, one healthy diet plan does not fit all—individual tailoring is necessary.

For Vegetarians: To achieve the optimal level of essential fatty acid intake, vegetarians should follow these practical guidelines: (1) Make a wide variety of whole plant foods the foundation of the diet. (2) Derive the majority of fat from whole foods—nuts, seeds, olives, avocados, and soy foods. (3) If using concentrated fats and oils, select those rich in monounsaturated fats, such as olive, canola, or nut oils. Oils rich in ω-3 fatty acids can also be used but should not be heated. Moderate use of oils rich in ω-6 fatty acids is advised. (4) Limit or avoid intake of processed foods and deep-fried foods rich in ω-6 and trans-fatty acids. (5) Reduce intake of foods rich in saturated fat. (6) Include foods rich in ω-3 fatty acids in the daily diet (ideally consuming 2–4 g ALA/d). (7) Consider using a direct source of DHA, ideally 100 to 300 mg/d.

BOX 9-2 — Dietary Quick Fixes

Alterations to one's lifestyle to ensure long-term improvements are not easy to implement. Patients are often in the market for short-term solutions for longer-term problems. Dietary guidelines for overall health as well as cutaneous health and enhancement are geared toward long-range benefits, and can withstand or blunt the effects of occasional lapses. For the patient who seeks to see a relatively quick change in the appearance of the skin through nutrition alone, however, a few immediate steps can be taken, with the understanding that the skin's individual needs must also be taken into account. The following suggestions, based on skin type or dietary restrictions, may be helpful:

For *dry skin,* increase ω-3 fatty acids, such as those in salmon, and other fatty acids and a small amount of cholesterol to remain hydrated, and increase water consumption.

For *oily skin,* increase consumption of green leafy vegetables (e.g., kale and spinach), butternut squash, cantaloupe, carrots, mangoes, pumpkins, and sweet potatoes, which are high in vitamin A and will help decrease oil production.

For *sensitive skin,* as manifested through redness and facial flushing, add ω-3 fatty acids, fish in particular, as discussed above and antioxidants, which have anti-inflammatory effects.

For *sensitive skin with the acne subtype,* attention should be paid to concentrating on eating a diet with a low glycemic load. In addition to consuming the foods just cited, foods high in vitamin A are particularly beneficial. Fruits and vegetables have lower glycemic loads than most foods. Interestingly, given the reports and studies linking milk consumption and acne, dairy foods have lower glycemic loads than fruits and vegetables.[6] (The potential role of milk in the etiologic pathways of acne appears to involve other factors, however.) Grain products, and processed foods in general, are to be avoided.

For *sensitive skin with the rosacea subtype,* add ω-3 fatty acids, particularly through fish, but also cut out hot (temperature) foods, spicy foods, alcohol, and caffeine.

For *vegans:* Add flaxseed oil to the diet. This will help hydrate the skin, reduce redness, and puff out fine lines, restoring skin radiance. Skin radiance results from reflection of light off of a smooth surface.

10:1 during the mid-1990s,[196] which has now increased to a range of approximately 15:1 to 16.7:1.[197] A healthy ratio is thought to be closer to 4:1.[196] A high ratio of ω-6 to ω-3 fatty acids has been associated with a greater risk for depression and various inflammatory diseases.[198] Omega-3 fatty acids exhibit significant anti-inflammatory activity. Good sources of ω-3 fatty acids, in addition to the fish mentioned above, are cod liver oil, fish oil, flaxseeds, and flaxseed oil. Crushed or ground flaxseeds can make a healthy complement to yogurt or oatmeal. Using flaxseed oil as a salad dressing is a great approach to keeping a healthy dish healthy—many standard salad dressings are high in sugar. Omega-3 fatty acids may also assist in skin hydration, as these compounds have been shown to contribute to improving eczema.

TABLE 9-8	Oral Supplement Recommendations by BSTS Parameter
Skin Type Parameter	**Supplement**
Dry	Borage seed oil
	Cholesterol
	Evening primrose oil
	Glucosamine
	Omega-3 fatty acids
Oily	Vitamin A
Sensitive	Fish oils, marine oils (ω-3 fatty acids, particularly eicosapentaenoic acid and docosahexaenoic acid)
Resistant	NA
Pigmented	Pycnogenol
	Vitamin C
	Soy
Nonpigmented	NA
Wrinkled	Coenzyme Q_{10}
	Green tea
	Pomegranate
	Pycnogenol
	Vitamin C
	Vitamin E
Tight	NA

Antioxidants

Antioxidants impart protection to cells from oxidative damage caused by exogenous factors such as UV light, air pollution, ozone, cigarette smoke, and even oxygen itself, as well as from endogenous insult. The expression "antioxidant" is more of a reflection of the activity exhibited by the substance rather than its chemical family or constituency. Antioxidants include carotenoids, polyphenols, vitamins, and other classes of compounds. A diet rich in various antioxidants is strongly advised.

Skin Hydration

Skin hydration is a very important factor in achieving and maintaining healthy skin. The enzymes in the skin that perform various functions require water to work. Without water skin ages more quickly and is more likely to itch and get red. EPO, black currant oil, and borage oil are all good sources of the ω-6 fatty acid GLA, which helps prevent water evaporation from the skin. Humans tend to lose approximately 2.5 L of water per day. This is partly replenished through food intake. The level of water consumption varies by individual, one's level of activity, and climate, but 1 to 2 L is probably a reasonable estimate. One must drink water to prevent becoming dehydrated. However, as far as skin is concerned it is not how much water you drink but how well the skin holds onto the water and keeps it from evaporating. Skin needs adequate

levels of fatty acids, ceramides, and cholesterol to hold onto water (see Chapter 12). This explains why vegans and people on low-cholesterol diets or cholesterol-lowering drugs often have dry skin. Any liquid can provide skin hydration; however, water consumption should be increased when drinking caffeine and alcohol, which can cause dehydration.

Caloric Restriction

During the last several years, one focus of anti-aging research has included examinations oriented toward determining whether the lifespan and healthspan of human beings can be increased. In the process, caloric restriction (CR) has been shown to prolong the mean and maximum lifespan in various species.[199] It is not yet known whether CR can extend the average and maximum lifespan or the healthspan of human beings. However, available epidemiologic evidence appears to suggest that CR has already contributed to increased life span, average, and maximum, in one human population—in Okinawa, Japan.[200] It is important to note that restricting caloric intakes to the extremes (as high as 60%) as performed in animal studies is not recommended for human beings.[200] But CR at an 8% level has been demonstrated to confer benefits on some biochemical and inflammatory biomarkers.[201]

While much more research is necessary on the viability of expanding the life- and healthspan of humans, one of the cultural practices on Okinawa—to "...eat until you are 80% full" (or *hara hachi-bu*)[200]—is sound advice alone to help stem the obesity epidemic that is afflicting an increasing proportion of the global population, particularly in the West. Such a practice would also likely benefit the skin if the individual consumes a healthy diet.

CONCLUSION

Nutrition has long been ignored or given short shrift in the Western medical community, particularly in medical school education. This has also filtered into the practice of dermatology, perhaps most saliently in the treatment of acne as manifested by dermatologists' decades-long attempts to debunk popular myths regarding certain foods and the eruption of acne. While the two seminal, and admittedly flawed, studies that Cordain cited played an influential role in dermatologists' approaches to disabusing patients and/or their parents of the myths linking certain foods to acne, the myth itself has often been misinterpreted by the public and physicians have still offered sound basic nutritional advice (i.e., recommending generous portions of fruits and vegetables) even while trying to refute misinformation. That is, in the public mind, the myth took on an all-or-none implication that either chocolate, greasy foods, or other culprits directly caused acne. We know now that the correlation between diet and the skin is more convoluted. One chocolate bar will not lead to acne eruptions, but unhealthy eating patterns can certainly contribute to the etiologic pathway of acne.

Cosmetic dermatologists, while on the front lines in terms of treating the most conspicuous disorders and, in many cases, diagnosing systemic conditions with cutaneous manifestations, are increasingly expected to help patients endogenously and exogenously maintain the appearance, and health, of the skin and forestall the cutaneous symptoms of aging. With ever-evolving technology, practitioners are increasingly better equipped to offer procedures as well as oral and topical products that meet patients' health needs and cosmetic desires. But to further carry the banner of Hippocrates, and to take a broader look at cutaneous health and anti-aging approaches, we must consider food, the only "medicine" that all individuals require on a daily basis. While the official or curricular attitudes toward nutrition are slowly changing, more rapidly accruing evidence suggests that nutrition has a varied and complex role to play in overall health as well as the health of the skin. Of course, much more research is necessary, but enough data exist to suggest that the old saw "you are what you eat" has been venerated for a reason. The food that we consume does exert far-reaching systemic influences that have the potential to result in cutaneous manifestations.

References

1. Wolf R, Matz H, Orion E. Acne and diet. *Clin Dermatol.* 2004;22(5):387–393.

2. Boelsma E, van de Vijver LP, Goldbohm RA, Klöpping-Ketelaars IA, Hendriks HF, Roza L. Human skin condition and its associations with nutrient concentrations in serum and diet. *Am J Clin Nutr.* 2003;77(2):348–355.

3. Cao C, Xiao Z, Wu Y, Ge C. Diet and Skin Aging-From the Perspective of Food Nutrition. *Nutrients.* 2020;12(3):870.

4. American Academy of Dermatology. Skin Conditions by the Numbers. https://www.aad.org/media/stats-numbers. Accessed September 30, 2021.

5. Tan JK, Bhate K. A global perspective on the epidemiology of acne. *Br J Dermatol.* 2015;172(Suppl 1):3–12.

6. Cordain L. Implications for the role of diet in acne. *Semin Cutan Med Surg.* 2005;24(2):84–91.

7. Cordain L, Lindeberg S, Hurtado M, Hill K, Eaton SB, Brand-Miller J. Acne vulgaris: a disease of Western civilization. *Arch Dermatol.* 2002;138(12):1584–1590.

8. Schaefer O. When the Eskimo comes to town. *Nutr Today.* 1971;6(6):8–16.

9. Steiner PE. Necropsies on Okinawans; anatomic and pathologic observations. *Arch Pathol (Chic).* 1946;42(4):359–380.

10. Fulton JE Jr, Plewig G, Kligman AM. Effect of chocolate on acne vulgaris. *JAMA.* 1969;210(11):2071–2074.

11. Anderson PC. Foods as the cause of acne. *Am Fam Physician.* 1971;3(3):102–103.

12. Edmondson SR, Thumiger SP, Werther GA, Wraight CJ. Epidermal homeostasis: the role of the growth hormone and insulin-like growth factor systems. *Endocr Rev.* 2003;24(6):737–764.

13. Nam SY, Lee EJ, Kim KR, et al. Effect of obesity on total and free insulin-like growth factor (IGF)-1, and their relationship to IGF-binding protein (BP)-1, IGFBP-2, IGFBP-3, insulin, and growth hormone. *Int J Obes Relat Metab Disord.* 1997;21(5):355–359.

14. Smith RN, Mann NJ, Braue A, Mäkeläinen H, Varigos GA. A low-glycemic-load diet improves symptoms in acne vulgaris patients: a randomized controlled trial. *Am J Clin Nutr.* 2007;86(1):107–115.

15. Smith RN, Mann NJ, Braue A, Mäkeläinen H, Varigos GA. The effect of a high-protein, low glycemic-load diet versus a conventional, high glycemic-load diet on biochemical parameters associated with acne vulgaris: a randomized, investigator-masked, controlled trial. *J Am Acad Dermatol.* 2007;57(2):247–256.

16. Logan AC. Dietary fat, fiber, and acne vulgaris. *J Am Acad Dermatol.* 2007;57(6):1092–1093.

17. Smith RN, Braue A, Varigos GA, Mann NJ. The effect of a low glycemic load diet on acne vulgaris and the fatty acid composition of skin surface triglycerides. *J Dermatol Sci.* 2008;50(1):41–52.

18. Monfrecola G, Lembo S, Caiazzo G, et al. Mechanistic target of rapamycin (mTOR) expression is increased in acne patients' skin. *Exp Dermatol.* 2016;25(2):153–155.

19. Agamia NF, Abdallah DM, Sorour O, Mourad B, Younan DN. Skin expression of mammalian target of rapamycin and forkhead box transcription factor O1, and serum insulin-like growth factor-1 in patients with acne vulgaris and their relationship with diet. *Br J Dermatol.* 2016;174(6):1299–1307.

20. Aghasi M, Golzarand M, Shab-Bidar S, Aminianfar A, Omidian M, Taheri F. Dairy intake and acne development: A meta-analysis of observational studies. *Clin Nutr.* 2019;38(3):1067–1075.

21. Melnik B. Dietary intervention in acne: Attenuation of increased mTORC1 signaling promoted by Western diet. *Dermatoendocrinol.* 2012;4(1):20–32.

22. Adebamowo CA, Spiegelman D, Danby FW, Frazier AL, Willett WC, Holmes MD. High school dietary dairy intake and teenage acne. *J Am Acad Dermatol.* 2005;52(2):207–214.

23. Bershad SV. Diet and acne—slim evidence, again. *J Am Acad Dermatol.* 2005;53(6):1102; author reply 1103.

24. Spiegelman D, McDermott A, Rosner B. Regression calibration method for correcting measurement-error bias in nutritional epidemiology. *Am J Clin Nutr.* 1997;65(4 Suppl):1179S–1186S.

25. Adebamowo CA, Spiegelman D, Berkey CS, et al. Milk consumption and acne in adolescent girls. *Dermatol Online J.* 2006;12(4):1.

26. Adebamowo CA, Spiegelman D, Berkey CS, et al. Milk consumption and acne in teenaged boys. *J Am Acad Dermatol.* 2008;58(5):787–793.

27. Melnik BC. Western diet-induced imbalances of FoxO1 and mTORC1 signalling promote the sebofollicular inflammasomopathy acne vulgaris. *Exp Dermatol.* 2016;25(2):103–104.

28. Danby FW. Acne and milk, the diet myth, and beyond. *J Am Acad Dermatol.* 2005;52(2):360–362.

29. Perricone N. *The Acne Prescription: The Perricone Program for Clear and Healthy Skin at Every Age.* New York, NY: Harper Collins; 2003.

30. Hitch JM, Greenburg BG. Adolescent acne and dietary iodine. *Arch Dermatol.* 1961;84:898–911.

31. Hitch JM. Acneform eruptions induced by drugs and chemicals. *JAMA.* 1967;200(10):879–880.

32. Arbesman H. Dairy and acne—the iodine connection. *J Am Acad Dermatol.* 2005;53(6):1102.

33. Rasmussen LB, Larsen EH, Ovesen L. Iodine content in drinking water and other beverages in Denmark. *Eur J Clin Nutr.* 2000;54(1):57–60.

34. Girelli ME, Coin P, Mian C, et al. Milk represents an important source of iodine in schoolchildren of the Veneto region, Italy. *J Endocrinol Invest.* 2004;27(8):709–713.

35. Dahl L, Opsahl JA, Meltzer HM, Julshamn K. Iodine concentration in Norwegian milk and dairy products. *Br J Nutr.* 2003;90(3):679–685.

36. Dahl L, Johansson L, Julshamn K, Meltzer HM. The iodine content of Norwegian foods and diets. *Public Health Nutr.* 2004;7(4):569–576.

37. Brantsæter AL, Haugen M, Julshamn K, Alexander J, Meltzer HM. Evaluation of urinary iodine excretion as a biomarker for intake of milk and dairy products in pregnant women in the Norwegian Mother and Child Cohort Study (MoBa). *Eur J Clin Nutr.* 2009;63(3):347–354.

38. Lee SM, Lewis J, Buss DH, Holcombe GD, Lawrance PR. Iodine in British foods and diets. *Br J Nutr.* 1994;72(3):435–446.

39. Pearce EN, Pino S, He X, Bazrafshan HR, Lee SL, Braverman LE. Sources of dietary iodine: bread, cow's milk, and infant formula in the Boston area. *J Clin Endocrinol Metab.* 2004;89(7):3421–3424.

40. Danby FW. Acne and iodine: reply. *J Am Acad Dermatol.* 2007;56(1):164–165.

41. Vliegenthart JF, Casset F. Novel forms of protein glycosylation. *Curr Opin Struct Biol.* 1998;8(5):565–571.

42. Freitas JP, Filipe P, Guerra Rodrigo F. Glycosylation and lipid peroxidation in skin and in plasma in diabetic patients. *C R Seances Soc Biol Fil.* 1997;191(5-6):837–843.

43. Dillinger TL, Barriga P, Escárcega S, Jimenez M, Salazar Lowe D, Grivetti LE. Food of the gods: cure for humanity? A cultural history of the medicinal and ritual use of chocolate. *J Nutr.* 2000;130:2057S.

44. Stahl W, Heinrich U, Aust O, Tronnier H, Sies H. Lycopene-rich products and dietary photoprotection. *Photochem Photobiol Sci.* 2006;5(2):238–242.

45. Stahl W, Heinrich U, Wiseman S, Eichler O, Sies H, Tronnier H. Dietary tomato paste protects against ultraviolet light-induced erythema in humans. *J Nutr.* 2001;131(5):1449–1451.

46. Stahl W, Sies H. Carotenoids and protection against solar UV radiation. *Skin Pharmacol Appl Skin Physiol.* 2002;15(5):291–296.

47. Heinrich U, Gärtner C, Wiebusch M, et al. Supplementation with beta-carotene or a similar amount of mixed carotenoids protects humans from UV-induced erythema. *J Nutr.* 2003;133(1):98–101.

48. Aust O, Stahl W, Sies H, Tronnier H, Heinrich U. Supplementation with tomato-based products increases lycopene, phytofluene, and phytoene levels in human serum and protects against UV-light-induced erythema. *Int J Vitam Nutr Res.* 2005;75(1):54–60.

49. González S, Astner S, An W, Goukassian D, Pathak MA. Dietary lutein/zeaxanthin decreases ultraviolet B-induced epidermal hyper-proliferation and acute inflammation in hairless mice. *J Invest Dermatol.* 2003;121(2):399–405.

50. Svobodová A, Psotová J, Walterová D. Natural phenolics in the prevention of UV-induced skin damage. A review. *Biomed Pap Med Fac Univ Palacky Olomouc Czech Repub.* 2003;147(2):137–145.

51. Scalbert A, Williamson G. Dietary intake and bioavailability of polyphenols. *J Nutr.* 2000;130(8S Suppl):2073S–2085SS.

52. Ross JA, Kasum CM. Dietary flavonoids: bioavailability, metabolic effects, and safety. *Annu Rev Nutr.* 2002;22:19–34.

53. Lyons-Wall P, Autenzio P, Lee E, Moss R, Samman S. Catechins are the major source of flavonoids in a group of Australian women. *Asia Pac J Clin Nutr.* 2004;13(suppl):S72.

54. Neveu V, Perez-Jiménez J, Vos F, et al. Phenol-Explorer: an online comprehensive database on polyphenol contents in foods. *Database (Oxford).* 2010;2010:bap024.

55. Pérez-Jiménez J, Neveu V, Vos F, Scalbert A. Identification of the 100 richest dietary sources of polyphenols: an application of the Phenol-Explorer database. *Eur J Clin Nutr.* 2010;64(Suppl 3):S112–S120.

56. Knaze V, Rothwell JA, Zamora-Ros R, et al. A new food-composition database for 437 polyphenols in 19,899 raw and prepared foods used to estimate polyphenol intakes in adults from 10 European countries. *Am J Clin Nutr.* 2018;108(3):517–524.

57. Circosta C, De Pasquale R, Palumbo DR, Samperi S, Occhiuto F. Effects of isoflavones from red clover (Trifolium pretense) on skin changes induced by ovariectomy in rats. *Phytother Res.* 2006;20(12):1096–1099.

58. Soenen S, Martens EA, Hochstenbach-Waelen A, Lemmens SG, Westerterp-Plantenga MS. Normal protein intake is required for body weight loss and weight maintenance, and elevated protein intake for additional preservation of resting energy expenditure and fat free mass. *J Nutr.* 2013;143(5):591–596.

59. Mithal A, Bonjour JP, Boonen S, Burckhardt P, Degens H, El Hajj Fuleihan G, et al. Impact of nutrition on muscle mass, strength, and performance in older adults. *Osteoporos Int.* 2013;24(5):1555–1566.

60. Strasser B, Volaklis K, Fuchs D, Burtscher M. Role of Dietary Protein and Muscular Fitness on Longevity and Aging. *Aging Dis.* 2018;9(1):119–132.

61. Pasini E, Corsetti G, Aquilani R, Romano C, Picca A, Calvani R, et al. Protein-Amino Acid Metabolism Disarrangements: The Hidden Enemy of Chronic Age-Related Conditions. *Nutrients.* 2018;10(4):391.

62. Hanjani NA, Vafa M. Protein Restriction, Epigenetic Diet, Intermittent Fasting as New Approaches for Preventing Age-associated Diseases. *Int J Prev Med.* 2018;9:58.

63. Manku MS, Horrobin DF, Morse NL, Wright S, Burton JL. Essential fatty acids in the plasma phospholipids of patients with atopic eczema. *Br J Dermatol.* 1984;110(6):643–648.

64. Galland L. Increased requirements for essential fatty acids in atopic individuals: a review with clinical descriptions. *J Am Coll Nutr.* 1986;5(2):213–228.

65. Bjørneboe A, Søyland E, Bjørneboe GE, Rajka G, Drevon CA. Effect of dietary supplementation with eicosapentaenoic acid in the treatment of atopic dermatitis. *Br J Dermatol.* 1987;117(4):463–469.

66. Callaway J, Schwab U, Harvima I, Halonen P, Mykkänen O, Hyvönen P. Efficacy of dietary hempseed oil in patients with atopic dermatitis. *J Dermatolog Treat.* 2005;16(2):87–94.

67. Morse NL, Clough PM. A meta-analysis of randomized, placebo-controlled clinical trials of Efamol evening primrose oil in atopic eczema. Where do we go from here in light of more recent discoveries? *Curr Pharm Biotechnol.* 2006;7(6):503–524.

68. Kanehara S, Ohtani T, Uede K, Furukawa F. Undershirts coated with borage oil alleviate the symptoms of atopic dermatitis in children. *Eur J Dermatol.* 2007;17(5):448–449.

69. Krajcovicová-Kudláčková M, Simoncic R, Béderová A, Klvanová J, Brtková A, Grancicová E. Lipid and antioxidant blood levels in vegetarians. *Nahrung.* 1996;40(1):17–20.

70. Melchert HU, Limsathayourat N, Mihajlović H, Eichberg J, Thefeld W, Rottka H. Fatty acid patterns in triglycerides,

diglycerides, free fatty acids, cholesteryl esters and phosphatidylcholine in serum from vegetarians and non-vegetarians. *Atherosclerosis.* 1987;65(1-2):159–166.

71. Li D, Ball M, Bartlett M, Sinclair A. Lipoprotein(a), essential fatty acid status and lipoprotein lipids in female Australian vegetarians. *Clin Sci (Lond).* 1999;97(2):175–181.

72. Suzuki R, Shimizu T, Kudo T, Ohtsuka Y, Yamashiro Y, Oshida K. Effects of n-3 polyunsaturated fatty acids on dermatitis in NC/Nga mice. *Prostaglandins Leukot Essent Fatty Acids.* 2002;66(4):435–440.

73. Davis BC, Kris-Etherton PM. Achieving optimal essential fatty acid status in vegetarians: current knowledge and practical implications. *Am J Clin Nutr.* 2003;78(3 Suppl):640S–646S.

74. Rosell MS, Lloyd-Wright Z, Appleby PN, Sanders TA, Allen NE, Key TJ. Long-chain n-3 polyunsaturated fatty acids in plasma in British meat-eating, vegetarian, and vegan men. *Am J Clin Nutr.* 2005;82(2):327–334.

75. Kim HH, Cho S, Lee S, Kim KH, Cho KH, Eun HC, et al. Photoprotective and anti-skin-aging effects of eicosapentaenoic acid in human skin in vivo. *J Lipid Res.* 2006;47(5):921–930.

76. Krajcovicová-Kudláčková M, Simoncic R, Babinská K, Béderová A. Lipid parameters in blood of vegetarians. *Cor Vasa.* 1993;35(6):224–229.

77. Porres JM, Cheng W. Legumes and Preventive Dermatology. In: Watson R, Zibadi S, eds. *Bioactive Dietary Factors and Plant Extracts in Dermatology.* Totowa, NJ: Humana Press; 2013:421–431.

78. Tomobe YI, Morizawa K, Tsuchida M, Hibino H, Nakano Y, Tanaka Y. Dietary docosahexaenoic acid suppresses inflammation and immunoresponses in contact hypersensitivity reaction in mice. *Lipids.* 2000;35(1):61–69.

79. Simopoulos AP. Omega-3 fatty acids in health and disease and in growth and development. *Am J Clin Nutr.* 1991;54(3):438–463.

80. Mayser P, Mrowietz U, Arengerger P, et al. Omega-3 fatty acid-based lipid infusion in patients with chronic plaque psoriasis: results of a double-blind, randomized, placebo-controlled, multicenter trial. *J Am Acad Dermatol.* 1998;38(4):539–547.

81. Pronczuk A, Kipervarg Y, Hayes KC. Vegetarians have higher plasma alpha-tocopherol relative to cholesterol than do nonvegetarians. *J Am Coll Nutr.* 1992;11(1):50–55.

82. Boelsma E, Hendriks HF, Roza L. Nutritional skincare: health effects of micronutrients and fatty acids. *Am J Clin Nutr.* 2001;73(5):853–864.

83. Liu G, Bibus DM, Bode AM, Ma WY, Holman RT, Dong Z. Omega 3 but not omega 6 fatty acids inhibit AP-1 activity and cell transformation in JB6 cells. *Proc Natl Acad Sci U S A.* 2001;98(13):7510–7515.

84. Hata TR, Scholz TA, Ermakov IV, et al. Non-invasive Raman spectroscopic detection of carotenoids in human skin. *J Invest Dermatol.* 2000;115(3):441–448.

85. Conn PF, Schaleh W, Truscott TG. The singlet oxygen and carotenoid interaction. *J Photochem Photobiol B.* 1991;11(1):41–47.

86. Lee EH, Faulhaber D, Hanson KM, et al. Dietary lutein reduces ultraviolet radiation-induced inflammation and immunosuppression. *J Invest Dermatol.* 2004;122(2):510–517.

87. Vranesić-Bender D. The role of nutraceuticals in anti-aging medicine. *Acta Clin Croat.* 2010;49(4):537–544.

88. Fielding JM, Sinclair AJ, DiGregorio G, Joveski M, Stockmann R. Relationship between colour and aroma of olive oil and nutritional content. *Asia Pac J Clin Nutr.* 2003;12(suppl):S36.

89. Yamakoshi J, Otsuka F, Sano A, et al. Lightening effect on ultraviolet-induced pigmentation of guinea pig skin by oral administration of a proanthocyanidin-rich extract from grape seeds. *Pigment Cell Res.* 2003;16(6):629–638.

90. Kasai K, Yoshimura M, Koga T, Arii M, Kawasaki S. Effects of oral administration of ellagic acid-rich pomegranate extract on ultra-violet-induced pigmentation in the human skin. *J Nutr Sci Vitaminol (Tokyo).* 2006;52(5):383–388.

91. Yoshimura M, Watanabe Y, Kasai K, Yamakoshi J, Koga T. Inhibitory effect of an ellagic acid-rich pomegranate extract on tyrosinase activity and ultraviolet-induced pigmentation. *Biosci Biotechnol Biochem.* 2005;69(12):2368–2373.

92. Yamakoshi J, Sano A, Tokutake S, et al. Oral intake of proanthocyanidin-rich extract from grape seeds improves chloasma. *Phytother Res.* 2004;18(11):895–899.

93. Ni Z, Mu Y, Gulati O. Treatment of melasma with Pycnogenol. *Phytother Res.* 2002;16(6):567–571.

94. Krajcovicová-Kudláčková M, Simoncic R, Babinská K, et al. Selected vitamins and trace elements in blood of vegetarians. *Ann Nutr Metab.* 1995;39(6):334–339.

95. Izumi T, Saito M, Obata A, Arii M, Yamaguchi H, Matsuyama A. Oral intake of soy isoflavone aglycone improves the aged skin of adult women. *J Nutr Sci Vitaminol (Tokyo).* 2007;53(1):57–62.

96. Purba MB, Kouris-Blazos A, Wattanapenpaiboon N, et al. Skin wrinkling: can food make a difference? *J Am Coll Nutr.* 2001;20(1):71–80.

97. Lin JY, Lin FH, Burch JA, et al. Alpha-lipoic acid is ineffective as a topical antioxidant for photoprotection of skin. *J Invest Dermatol.* 2004;123(5):996–998.

98. Rattan SI. Theories of biological aging: genes, proteins, and free radicals. *Free Radic Res.* 2006;40(12):1230–1238.

99. Halvorsen BL, Holte K, Myhrstad MC, et al. A systematic screening of total antioxidants in dietary plants. *J Nutr.* 2002;132(3):461–471.

100. Heinen MM, Hughes MC, Ibiebele TI, Marks GC, Green AC, van der Pols JC. Intake of antioxidant nutrients and the risk of skin cancer. *Eur J Cancer.* 2007;43(18):2707–2716.

101. Thom E. A randomized, double-blind, placebo-controlled study on the clinical efficacy of oral treatment with DermaVite on ageing symptoms of the skin. *J Int Med Res.* 2005;33(3):267–272.

102. Wagner S, Suter A, Merfort I. Skin penetration studies of Arnica preparations and of their sesquiterpene lactones. *Planta Med.* 2004;70(10):897–903.

103. Seeley BM, Denton AB, Ahn MS, Maas CS. Effect of homeopathic Arnica montana on bruising in face-lifts: results of a randomized, double-blind, placebo-controlled clinical trial. *Arch Facial Plast Surg.* 2006;8(1):54–59.

104. Stahl W, Krutmann J. Systemic photo-protection through carotenoids. *Hautarzt.* 2006;57(4):281–285.

105. Köpcke W, Krutmann J. Protection from sunburn with beta-carotene—a meta-analysis. *Photochem Photobiol.* 2008;84(2):284–288.

106. Stahl W, Sies H. Carotenoids and flavonoids contribute to nutritional protection against skin damage from sunlight. *Mol Biotechnol.* 2007;37(1):26–30.

107. Frieling UM, Schaumberg DA, Kupper TS, Muntwyler J, Hennekens CH. A randomized, 12-year primary-prevention trial of beta carotene supplementation for nonmelanoma skin cancer in the physicians' health study. *Arch Dermatol.* 2000;136(2):179–184.

108. Huang HY, Caballero B, Chang S, et al. Multivitamin/mineral supplements and prevention of chronic disease. *Evid Rep Technol Assess (Full Rep).* 2006;139:1–117.

109. Hochman LG, Scher RK, Meyerson MS. Brittle nails: response to daily biotin supplementation. *Cutis.* 1993;51(4):303–305.

110. Iorizzo M, Pazzaglia M, Piraccini BM, Tullo S, Tosti A. Brittle nails. *J Cosmet Dermatol.* 2004;3(3):138–144.

111. Scheinfeld N, Dahdah MJ, Scher R. Vitamins and minerals: their role in nail health and disease. *J Drugs Dermatol.* 2007;6(8):782–787.

112. Brosche T, Platt D. Effect of borage oil consumption on fatty acid metabolism, transepidermal water loss and skin parameters in elderly people. *Arch Gerontol Geriatr.* 2000;30(2):139–150.

113. MacKay D, Miller AL. Nutritional support for wound healing. *Altern Med Rev.* 2003;8(4):359–377.

114. Kamenícek V, Holán P, Franěk P. Systemic enzyme therapy in the treatment and prevention of post-traumatic and postoperative swelling. *Acta Chir Orthop Traumatol Cech.* 2001;68(1):45–49.

115. Maurer HR. Bromelain: biochemistry, pharmacology and medical use. *Cell Mol Life Sci.* 2001;58(9):1234–1245.

116. Rico MJ. Rising drug costs: the impact on dermatology. *Skin Therapy Lett.* 2000;5(4):1–2, 5.

117. Orsini RA; Plastic Surgery Educational Foundation Technology Assessment Committee. Bromelain. *Plast Reconstr Surg.* 2006;118(7):1640–1644.

118. Lu YP, Lou YR, Li XH, et al. Stimulatory effect of oral administration of green tea or caffeine on ultraviolet light-induced increases in epidermal wild-type p53, p21(WAF1/CIP1), and apoptotic sunburn cells in SKH-1 mice. *Cancer Res.* 2000;60(17):4785–4791.

119. Huang MT, Xie JG, Wang ZY, et al. Effects of tea, decaffeinated tea, and caffeine on UVB light-induced complete carcinogenesis in SKH-1 mice: demonstration of caffeine as a biologically important constituent of tea. *Cancer Res.* 1997;57(13):2623–2629.

120. Gómez-Ruiz JA, Leake DS, Ames JM. In vitro antioxidant activity of coffee compounds and their metabolites. *J Agric Food Chem.* 2007;55(17):6962–6969.

121. Devasagayam TP, Kamat JP, Mohan H, Kesavan PC. Caffeine as an antioxidant: inhibition of lipid peroxidation induced by reactive oxygen species. *Biochim Biophys Acta.* 1996;1282(1):63–70.

122. Lu YP, Lou YR, Lin Y, Shih WJ, Huang MT, Yang CS,. Inhibitory effects of orally administered green tea, black tea, and caffeine on skin carcinogenesis in mice previously treated with ultraviolet B light (high-risk mice): relationship to decreased tissue fat. *Cancer Res.* 2001;61(13):5002–5009.

123. Lu XP, Lou YR, Xie JG, et al. Topical applications of caffeine or (—)-epigallocatechin gallate (EGCG) inhibit carcinogenesis and selectively increase apoptosis in UVB-induced skin tumors in mice. *Proc Natl Acad Sci USA.* 2002;99(19):12455–12460.

124. Velasco MV, Tano CT, Machado-Santelli GM, Consiglieri VO, Kaneko TM, Baby AR. Effects of caffeine and siloxanetriol alginate caffeine, as anticellulite agents, on fatty tissue: histological evaluation. *J Cosmet Dermatol.* 2008;7(1):23–29.

125. Willis R, Anthony M, Sun L, Honse Y, Qiao G. Clinical implications of the correlation between coenzyme Q10 and vitamin B6 status. *Biofactors.* 1999;9(2-4):359–363.

126. Ashida Y, Yamanish H, Terada T, Oota N, Sekine K, Watabe K. CoQ10 supplementation elevates the epidermal CoQ10 level in adult hairless mice. *Biofactors.* 2005;25(1-4):175–178.

127. Hoppe U, Bergemann J, Diembeck W, et al. Coenzyme Q10, a cutaneous antioxidant and energizer. *Biofactors.* 1999;9(2-4):371–378.

128. Berbis P, Hesse S, Privat Y. Essential fatty acids and the skin. *Allerg Immunol (Paris).* 1990;22(6):225–231.

129. Schalin-Karrila M, Mattila L, Jansen CT, Uotila P. Evening primrose oil in the treatment of atopic eczema: effect on clinical status, plasma phospholipid fatty acids and circulating blood prostaglandins. *Br J Dermatol.* 1987;117(1):11–19.

130. Levin C, Maibach H. Exploration of "alternative" and "natural" drugs in dermatology. *Arch Dermatol.* 2002;138(2):207–211.

131. Harrison RA, Holt D, Pattison DJ, Elton PJ. Who and how many people are taking herbal supplements? A survey of 21923 adults. *Int J Vitam Nutr Res.* 2004;74(3):183–186.

132. Bissett DL. Glucosamine: an ingredient with skin and other benefits. *J Cosmet Dermatol.* 2006;5(4):309–315.

133. Murad H, Tabibian MP. The effect of an oral supplement containing glucosamine, amino acids, minerals, and antioxidants on cutaneous aging: a preliminary study. *J Dermatolog Treat.* 2001;12(1):47–51.

134. Wold RS, Lopez ST, Yau CL, et al. Increasing trends in elderly persons' use of nonvitamin, nonmineral dietary supplements and concurrent use of medications. *J Am Diet Assoc.* 2005;105(1):54–63.

135. Pittler MH, Ernst E. Horse-chestnut seed extract for chronic venous insufficiency. A criteria-based systematic review. *Arch Dermatol.* 1998;134(11):1356–1360.

136. Ernst E, Pittler MH, Stevinson C. Complementary/alternative medicine in dermatology: evidence-assessed efficacy of two diseases and two treatments. *Am J Clin Dermatol.* 2002;3(5):341–348.

137. Piacquadio D, Jarcho M, Goltz R. Evaluation of hylan b gel as a soft-tissue augmentation implant material. *J Am Acad Dermatol.* 1997;36(4):544–549.

138. Comper WD, Laurent TC. Physiological function of connective tissue polysaccharides. *Physiol Rev.* 1978;58(1):255–315.

139. Petrella RJ. Hyaluronic acid for the treatment of knee osteoarthritis: long-term outcomes from a naturalistic primary care experience. *Am J Phys Med Rehabil.* 2005;84(4):278–283; quiz 284, 293.

140. Sies H, Stahl W. Non-nutritive bioactive constituents of plants: lycopene, lutein and zeaxanthin. *Int J Vitam Nutr Res.* 2003;73(2):95–100.

141. Wright TI, Spencer JM, Flowers FP. Chemoprevention of nonmelanoma skin cancer. *J Am Acad Dermatol.* 2006;54(6):933–946; quiz 947–50.

142. Gensler HL, Williams T, Huang AC, Jacobson EL. Oral niacin prevents photocarcinogenesis and photoimmunosuppression in mice. *Nutr Cancer.* 1999;34(1):36–41.

143. Berk MA, Lorincz AL. The treatment of bullous pemphigoid with tetracycline and niacinamide. A preliminary report. *Arch Dermatol.* 1986;122(6):670–674.

144. Kademian M, Bechtel M, Zirwas M. Case reports: new onset flushing due to unauthorized substitution of niacin for nicotinamide. *J Drugs Dermatol*. 2007;6(12):1220–1221.

145. Drucker AM, Li WQ, Park MK, Li T, Qureshi AA, Cho E. Niacin intake and incident adult-onset atopic dermatitis in women. *J Allergy Clin Immunol*. 2017;139(6):2020–2022.e2.

146. Prousky J, Seely D. The treatment of migraines and tension-type headaches with intravenous and oral niacin (nicotinic acid): systematic review of the literature. *Nutr J*. 2005;4:3.

147. Cefali EA, Simmons PD, Stanek EJ, Shamp TR. Improved control of niacin-induced flushing using an optimized once-daily, extended-release niacin formulation. *Int J Clin Pharmacol Ther*. 2006;44(12):633–640.

148. Puglia C, Tropea S, Rizza L, Santagati NA, Bonina F. In vitro percutaneous absorption studies and in vivo evaluation of anti-inflammatory activity of essential fatty acids (EFA) from fish oil extracts. *Int J Pharm*. 2005;299(1-2):41–48.

149. Bourre JM. Dietary omega-3 fatty acids for women. *Biomed Pharmacother*. 2007;61(2-3):105–112.

150. Sies H, Stahl W. Nutritional protection against skin damage from sunlight. *Annu Rev Nutr*. 2004;24:173–200.

151. Black HS, Rhodes LE. The potential of omega-3 fatty acids in the prevention of non-melanoma skin cancer. *Cancer Detect Prev*. 2006;30(3):224–232.

152. Bath-Hextall FJ, Jenkinson C, Humphreys R, Williams HC. Dietary supplements for established atopic eczema. *Cochrane Database Syst Rev*. 2012;(2):CD005205.

153. MacLean CH, Newberry SJ, Mojica WA, et al. Effects of omega-3 fatty acids on cancer risk: a systematic review. *JAMA*. 2006;295(4):403–415.

154. Chen YQ, Berquin IM, Daniel LW, et al. Omega-3 fatty acids and cancer risk. *JAMA*. 2006;296(3):282.

155. González S, Pathak MA, Cuevas J, Villarrubia VG, Fitzpatrick TB. Topical or oral administration with an extract of Polypodium leucotomos prevents acute sunburn and psoralen-induced phototoxic reactions as well as depletion of Langerhans cells in human skin. *Photodermatol Photoimmunol Photomed*. 1997;13(1-2):50–60.

156. Gombau L, García F, Lahoz A, t al. Polypodium leucotomos extract: antioxidant activity and disposition. *Toxicol In Vitro*. 2006;20(4):464–471.

157. Gonzalez S, Alonso-Lebrero JL, Del Rio R, Jaen P. Polypodium leucotomos extract: a nutraceutical with photoprotective properties. *Drugs Today (Barc)*. 2007;43(7):475–485.

158. Middelkamp-Hup MA, Pathak MA, Parrado C, et al. Orally administered Polypodium leucotomos extract decreases psoralen-UVA-induced phototoxicity, pigmentation, and damage of human skin. *J Am Acad Dermatol*. 2004;50(1):41–49.

159. Middelkamp-Hup MA, Pathak MA, Parrado C, et al. Oral Polypodium leucotomos extract decreases ultraviolet-induced damage of human skin. *J Am Acad Dermatol*. 2004;51(6):910–918.

160. Middelkamp-Hup MA, Bos JD, Rius-Diaz F, Gonzalez S, Westerhof W. Treatment of vitiligo vulgaris with narrow-band UVB and oral Polypodium leucotomos extract: a randomized double-blind placebo-controlled study. *J Eur Acad Dermatol Venereol*. 2007;21(7):942–950.

161. Thomson CD. Assessment of requirements for selenium and adequacy of selenium status: a review. *Eur J Clin Nutr*. 2004;58(3):391–402.

162. Maggini S, Wintergerst ES, Beveridge S, Hornig DH. Selected vitamins and trace elements support immune function by strengthening epithelial barriers and cellular and humoral immune responses. *Br J Nutr*. 2007;98(Suppl 1):S29–S35.

163. Klotz LO, Kröncke KD, Buchczyk DP, Sies H. Role of copper, zinc, selenium and tellurium in the cellular defense against oxidative and nitrosative stress. *J Nutr*. 2003;133(5 Suppl 1):1448S–1451S.

164. Chen Y, Hall M, Graziano JH, Slavkovich V, van Geen A, Parvez F. A prospective study of blood selenium levels and the risk of arsenic-related pre-malignant skin lesions. *Cancer Epidemiol Biomarkers Prev*. 2007;16(2):207–213.

165. Zhu X, Jiang M, Song E, Jiang X, Song Y. Selenium deficiency sensitizes the skin for UVB-induced oxidative damage and inflammation which involved the activation of p38 MAPK signaling. *Food Chem Toxicol*. 2015;75:139–145.

166. Harrison EH. Mechanisms of digestion and absorption of dietary vitamin A. *Annu Rev Nutr*. 2005;25:87–103.

167. U.S. Department of Health and Human Services. Advance Data from Vital and Health Statistics. Dietary Intake of Selected Vitamins for the United States Population: 1999–2000. Centers for Disease Control and Prevention. National Center for Health Statistics. Number 339, 2004.

168. Keller KL, Fenske NA. Uses of vitamins A, C, and E and related compounds in dermatology: a review. *J Am Acad Dermatol*. 1998;39(4 Pt 1):611–625.

169. The Evolving Role of Retinoids in the Management of Cutaneous Conditions. New York, New York, USA. May 2–4, 1997. Conference proceedings. *J Am Acad Dermatol*. 1998;39 (2 Pt 3):S1–122.

170. Kligman AM. Cosmetics. A dermatologist looks to the future: promises and problems. *Dermatol Clin*. 2000;18(4):699–709; x.

171. Geesin JC, Darr D, Kaufman R, Murad S, Pinnell SR. Ascorbic acid specifically increases type I and type III procollagen messenger RNA levels in human skin fibroblast. *J Invest Dermatol*. 1988;90(4):420–424.

172. Phillips CL, Combs SB, Pinnell SR. Effects of ascorbic acid on proliferation and collagen synthesis in relation to the donor age of human dermal fibroblasts. *J Invest Dermatol*. 1994;103(2):228–232.

173. Eberlein-König B, Ring J. Relevance of vitamins C and E in cutaneous photoprotection. *J Cosmet Dermatol*. 2005;4(1):4–9.

174. Placzek M, Gaube S, Kerkmann U, et al. Ultraviolet B-induced DNA damage in human epidermis is modified by the antioxidants ascorbic acid and D-alpha-tocopherol. *J Invest Dermatol*. 2005;124(2):304–307.

175. Cho HS, Lee MH, Lee JW, et al. Anti-wrinkling effects of the mixture of vitamin C, vitamin E, pycnogenol and evening primrose oil, and molecular mechanisms on hairless mouse skin caused by chronic ultraviolet B irradiation. *Photodermatol Photoimmunol Photomed*. 2007;23(5):155–162.

176. Lips P. Vitamin D physiology. *Prog Biophys Mol Biol*. 2006;92(1):4–8.

177. Lehmann B, Querings K, Reichrath J. Vitamin D and skin: new aspects for dermatology. *Exp Dermatol*. 2004;13(Suppl 4):11–15.

178. Zitterman A. Vitamin D in preventive medicine: are we ignoring the evidence? *Br J Nutr*. 2003;89(5):552–572.

179. Chel VG, Ooms ME, Popp-Snijders C, et al. Ultraviolet irradiation corrects vitamin D deficiency and suppresses

secondary hyperparathyroidism in the elderly. *J Bone Miner Res.* 1998;13(8):1238–1242.

180. Bialy TL, Rothe MJ, Grant-Kels JM. Dietary factors in the prevention and treatment of nonmelanoma skin cancer and melanoma. *Dermatol Surg.* 2002;28(12):1143–1152.

181. Wortsman J, Matsuoka LY, Chen TC, Lu Z, Holick MF. Decreased bioavailability of vitamin D in obesity. *Am J Clin Nutr.* 2000;72(3):690–693.

182. Marks R, Foley A, Jolley D, Knight KR, Harrison J, Thompson SC. The effect of regular sunscreen use on vitamin D levels in an Australian population. Results of a randomized controlled trial. *Arch Dermatol.* 1995;131(4):415–421.

183. Gilchrest BA. Sun protection and vitamin D: three dimensions of obfuscation. *J Steroid Biochem Mol Biol.* 2007;103(3-5):655–663.

184. Vieth R. Critique of the considerations for establishing the tolerable upper intake level for vitamin D: critical need for revision upwards. *J Nutr.* 2006;136(4):1117–1122.

185. Heaney RP. Barriers to optimizing vitamin D3 intake for the elderly. *J Nutr.* 2006;136(4):1123–1125.

186. Thiele JJ, Ekanayake-Mudiyanselage S. Vitamin E in human skin: organ-specific physiology and considerations for its use in dermatology. *Mol Aspects Med.* 2007;28(5-6):646–667.

187. Kuchide M, Tokuda H, Takayasu J, et al. Cancer chemopreventive effects of oral feeding alpha-tocopherol on ultraviolet light B induced photocarcinogenesis of hairless mouse. *Cancer Lett.* 2003;196(2):169–177.

188. McArdle F, Rhodes LE, Parslew RA, et al. Effects of oral vitamin E and beta-carotene supplementation on ultraviolet radiation-induced oxidative stress in human skin. *Am J Clin Nutr.* 2004;80(5):1270–1275.

189. Mireles-Rocha H, Galindo I, Huerta M, Trujillo-Hernández B, Elizalde A, Cortés-Franco R. UVB photoprotection with antioxidants: effects of oral therapy with d-alpha-tocopherol and ascorbic acid on the minimal erythema dose. *Acta Derm Venereol.* 2002;82(1):21–24.

190. Vegetarian Information Sheet. https://vegsoc.org/info-hub/health-and-nutrition/zinc/. Accessed September 10, 2021.

191. Agnoli C, Baroni L, Bertini I, et al. Position paper on vegetarian diets from the working group of the Italian Society of Human Nutrition. *Nutr Metab Cardiovasc Dis.* 2017;27(12):1037–1052.

192. Prasad AS. Clinical, immunological, anti-inflammatory and antioxidant roles of zinc. *Exp Gerontol.* 2008;43(5):370–377.

193. Miyata S. Zinc deficiency in the elderly. *Nihon Ronen Igakkai Zasshi.* 2007;44(6):677–689.

194. Al-Gurairi FT, Al-Waiz M, Sharquie KE. Oral zinc sulphate in the treatment of recalcitrant viral warts: randomized placebo-controlled clinical trial. *Br J Dermatol.* 2002;146(3):423–431.

195. Takahashi H, Nakazawa M, Takahashi K, et al. Effects of zinc deficient diet on development of atopic dermatitis-like eruptions in DS-Nh mice. *J Dermatol Sci.* 2008;50(1):31–39.

196. Sugano M. Characteristics of fats in Japanese diets and current recommendations. *Lipids.* 1996;31(Suppl):S283–S286.

197. Simopoulos AP. Evolutionary aspects of diet, the omega-6/omega-3 ratio and genetic variation: nutritional implications for chronic diseases. *Biomed Pharmacother.* 2006;60(9):502–507.

198. Kiecolt-Glaser JK, Belury MA, Porter K, Beversdorf DQ, Lemeshow S, Glaser R. Depressive symptoms, omega-6:omega-3 fatty acids, and inflammation in older adults. *Psychosom Med.* 2007;69(3):217–224.

199. Carter CS, Hofer T, Seo AY, Leeuwenburgh C. Molecular mechanisms of life- and health-span extension: role of calorie restriction and exercise intervention. *Appl Physiol Nutr Metab.* 2007;32(5):954–966.

200. Willcox DC, Willcox BJ, Todoriki H, Curb JD, Suzuki M. Caloric restriction and human longevity: what can we learn from the Okinawans? *Biogerontology.* 2006;7(3):173–177.

201. Dirks AJ, Leeuwenburgh C. Calorie restriction in humans: potential pitfalls and health concerns. *Mech Ageing Dev.* 2006;127(1):1–7.

Skin Types

CHAPTER 10

The Baumann Skin Typing System

Leslie S. Baumann, MD
Edmund M. Weisberg, MS, MBE

SUMMARY POINTS

What's Important?

1. The Fitzpatrick Skin Typing System was never intended to be used to make skincare recommendations.
2. The Baumann Skin Typing System was designed as a scientific way to prescribe facial skincare routines.
3. There are four barriers to skin health: dehydration, inflammation, dyspigmentation, and aging.
4. The goal of any skincare routine is to eliminate the barriers to skin health.
5. Using a standardized skin typing taxonomy improves communication and aids research efforts.

What's New?

1. Combination skin is not a true skin type.
2. The definition of oily skin is skin with an adequate or excessive amount of sebum production.
3. An oilier skin type is healthier than a dry skin type.
4. The definition of pigmented skin is not based on ethnicity or overall skin color; rather, it is based on unevenness of skin tone with pigmented skin being uneven and nonpigmented skin being even skin toned.
5. Skin type changes over time.
6. Oily, resistant, nonpigmented, tight skin (Skin Type 10) is the healthiest skin type and can be considered "the normal skin type."

What's Coming?

1. Cosmeceutical research trials will begin to enroll subjects by Baumann Skin Type to improve standardization of results.
2. Long-term outcome research on skincare routines and skin type will be conducted.
3. Genetic studies on the Baumann Skin Types and their responses to various skincare routines are planned.
4. The effects of the microbiome on the 16 Baumann Skin Types will be studied.

A standardized, scientifically validated approach to diagnose skin type is important to ensure that skin type is correctly identified in all genders, ages, and ethnicities. Diagnosing skin type properly is a necessary step to recommending the best skincare routine to protect and improve skin health. Assigning patients to a skin type phenotype and tracking skin type improvement is beneficial because it helps the medical provider choose which skincare products to retail to match their patients' demographics and skin types (see Chapter 33, Choosing Skincare Products), prepare skincare advice and regimens ahead of time (see Chapter 35, Skincare Regimen Design), track results more effectively, communicate clearly with colleagues using the same nomenclature, and predict inventory needs by skin type prevalence in the medical practice.

SKIN TYPING SYSTEMS USED IN DERMATOLOGY

Skin typing classification systems are used to personalize and customize skincare routines. For skincare routines to precisely target the underlying barriers to skin health, the entire skincare routine, not just the individual products, should be tested on the various skin types in a controlled manner. Each product affects the efficacy of the entire regimen (see Chapter 35) and this can vary by skin type. If cosmetic chemists, cosmetic companies, dermatologists, medical providers, aestheticians, and cosmetics salespeople are not using the same nomenclature, it is impossible to standardize skincare using a scientific approach. In addition, they must all be trained to use the nomenclature properly. A good example is sensitive skin. The meaning of the expression "sensitive skin" can vary from person to person (see Chapter 13, Sensitive Skin). Another example is the misuse of the expression "combination skin," which will be discussed later in this chapter.

Many skin typing systems are available, but for a skin typing system to be considered scientifically valid and to provide reproducible results, the skin typing classification system should meet the following criteria:

- Diagnosis of skin type is made with a scientifically validated measurement instrument.
- The instrument must be shown to deliver the same results when used by different dermatologists.
- If self-administered, the instrument must be shown to give the same results when self-administered as compared to when given by a dermatologist.
- The instrument should be tested on various ages, genders, and ethnicities, as well as in different geographic locations.

Ideally, the best skin typing system would also display these traits:

- The skin typing system is preferred by dermatologists and used in their medical practices.
- The skin typing system is independent from a skincare brand or pharmaceutical company to prevent bias.

- The skin typing system is used by many different brands, doctors, researchers, chemists, aestheticians, and medical providers so that data can be accurately compared.
- The skin typing system can and should be updated by dermatologists specializing in skin typing as new scientific discoveries are made.
- Updates to the skin typing system can and should be validated scientifically.
- The skin typing system should remain unadulterated and unaltered from user to user so that the results remain consistent, updates can be adopted by all users at the same time, and the vocabulary will remain consistent among users.

There are two main skin typing systems used by dermatologists, aestheticians, and medical providers to discuss skin type: the Fitzpatrick Skin Type and the Baumann Skin Type®. These skin typing systems are not mutually exclusive because they measure different skin parameters.

Fitzpatrick Skin Type

The Fitzpatrick Skin Type corresponds with the skin tanning response to UV and light exposure (**Fig. 10-1**). It was developed by Dr. Thomas B. Fitzpatrick at Harvard to determine the proper dose of UV light to treat psoriasis.[1] The initial version included only lighter skin types and was later updated to include darker skin types. It is now used to choose laser settings. The current skin color of the patient may not correspond to the Fitzpatrick Skin Type. For example, a Fitzpatrick III Skin Type who avoids sun exposure and always wears sun-protective clothing and sunscreen may appear to be a Fitzpatrick II. Using the questionnaire in the Fitzpatrick Skin Typing Questionnaire about how the skin responds to sun exposure is a more effective method of choosing laser settings

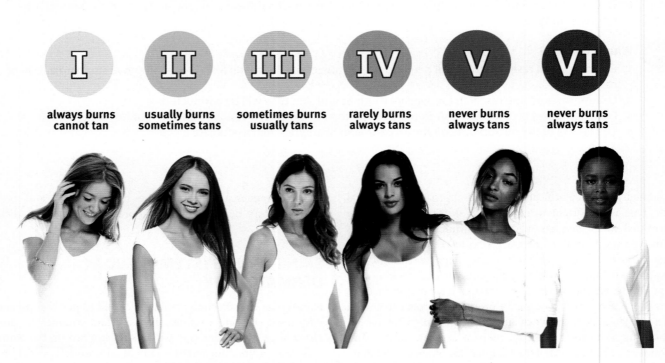

FIGURE 10-1. The Fitzpatrick Skin Type is based on how the skin reacts to UV exposure.

than looking at the skin color alone. The Fitzpatrick skin typing system is often incorrectly used to prescribe skincare, but it was never intended for this purpose; it only gives information about melanocyte response to light and not about the underlying barriers to skin health such as inflammation and dehydration. The higher the Fitzpatrick Skin Type number is, the more robust the melanin production response to light. A higher Fitzpatrick Skin Type suggests an increased risk of post-inflammatory hyperpigmentation and a lower risk of skin cancer due to sun exposure. The Fitzpatrick Skin Typing Questionnaire is more accurate when administered by a dermatologist as compared to self-administered.[2] This skin typing system may not be accurate in Asians,[3] and has been found to be unreliable in Korean skin.[4] The Fitzpatrick Skin Type is genetically determined and does not change with time unless the patient is exposed to photosensitizers.

The Fitzpatrick Skin Type

1. Measures the skin's ability to produce melanin pigment in response to UV exposure.
2. It must be assessed by a trained provider rather than self-administered.
3. Is not accurate in many Asian ethnicities.
4. Corresponds to the dose of UV or light that should be used to treat skin disorders.
5. Helps determine which laser setting to use when treating hair or pigment.
6. Helps predict post-inflammatory pigment alteration (PIPA) after lasers, lights, and other cosmetic procedures.
7. May help predict skin cancer risk.
8. Must be assessed by a trained medical provider.
9. Does not correspond to skincare routine or skincare product needs.
10. Does not change with time.
11. Applies to all the skin on the body.

Baumann Skin Type®

The Baumann Skin Type is used to prescribe facial skincare.[5] It specifies the presence or absence of four barriers to skin health: dehydration, inflammation, dyspigmentation, and aging lifestyle factors. These four parameters are combined in different permutations into 16 distinct Baumann Skin Types.[6,7] (See **Fig. 10-2A** and **B.**) The Baumann Skin Type is identified using a four-letter designation, a distinctive color, and a number to help patients remember their particular skin type. These are further divided into four sensitive skin subtypes: acne, facial redness (rosacea), skin stinging, and allergic (**Fig. 10-3**). The Baumann Skin Type reveals the underlying issues that must be addressed in the skincare routine to improve skin health.

The Baumann Skin Type

1. Identifies the four main barriers to skin health: dehydration, inflammation, dyspigmentation, and lifestyle factors that speed aging.
2. Diagnosed via a scientifically validated questionnaire.
3. Diagnostic questionnaire can be self-administered.

4. Validated for all genders and ethnicities.
5. Gives specific recommendations on what ingredients to use.
6. Gives specific recommendations on what ingredients to avoid.
7. Used to develop personalized and customized skincare regimens.
8. Changes with aging, stress, diet, hormones, geographic location, season, and skincare routine.
9. May help predict skin cancer risk by identifying unhealthy lifestyle habits.
10. Applies to facial skin only.

FOUR BARRIERS TO SKIN HEALTH

The Baumann Skin Typing System uses a questionnaire to determine if the skin suffers from one or more of the four barriers to skin health[8]: dehydration, inflammation, dyspigmentation, and aging lifestyle factors (**Fig. 10-4**). The presence of any of the four barriers to skin health provides an opportunity to improve the skin's health and appearance. The goal is to change these barriers to the corresponding attributes of healthy skin (**Fig. 10-5**). For example, skin that has underlying inflammation is designated as sensitive. The goal is to shut down the inflammatory pathways and change the skin to a resistant skin type less susceptible to inflammation. Each of the barriers to skin health has a corresponding chapter in this text that explains the underlying cause(s) and treatments.

The Baumann Skin Types are named in a way that reflects whether the skin exhibits the barrier to skin health or its corresponding attribute of healthy skin using the following taxonomy[9]:

1. oily vs. dry (O vs. D)
2. sensitive vs. resistant (S vs. R)

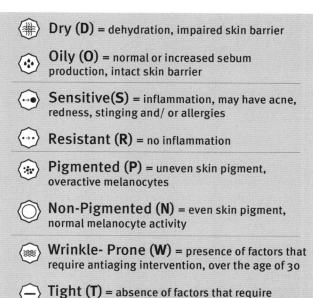

Dry (D) = dehydration, impaired skin barrier

Oily (O) = normal or increased sebum production, intact skin barrier

Sensitive (S) = inflammation, may have acne, redness, stinging and/ or allergies

Resistant (R) = no inflammation

Pigmented (P) = uneven skin pigment, overactive melanocytes

Non-Pigmented (N) = even skin pigment, normal melanocyte activity

Wrinkle- Prone (W) = presence of factors that require antiaging intervention, over the age of 30

Tight (T) = absence of factors that require antiaging intervention, under the age of 30

FIGURE 10-2A. Each skin characteristic is assigned a letter.

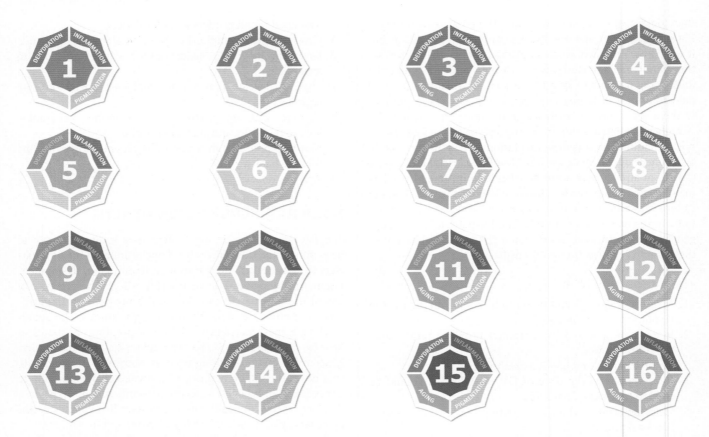

FIGURE 10-2B. The 16 Baumann Phenotypes. Each skin type exhibits barriers to skin health except 10, which is the healthiest skin type.

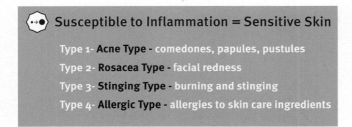

FIGURE 10-3. The sensitive skin types are further subdivided into sensitive skin subtypes. Every skin type that contains an "S" for sensitive has these 4 subtypes.

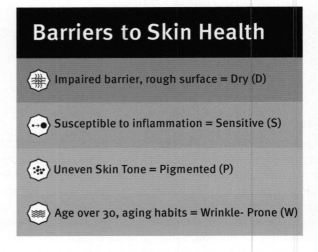

FIGURE 10-4. The four barriers to skin health.

3. uneven pigment, referred to as "pigmented skin," vs. no uneven pigment, referred to as "nonpigmented skin" (P vs. N)
4. wrinkle-prone vs. unwrinkled, referred to as "tight skin" (W vs. T)

Skin that displays only the attributes of skin health and has no underlying barriers to skin health is known as the ideal skin type and is labeled as Baumann Skin Type 10. Achieving this "Perfect 10 Skin Type," also known as normal skin, is the goal of any skincare routine and cosmetic treatment plan (**Fig. 10-6**).

Diagnosing the Baumann Skin Type

Software employing a validated self-administered questionnaire known as the Baumann Skin Type Indicator (BSTI) has been tested in all genders, multiple ethnicities, and many climates.[10–15] This system is used by hundreds of dermatologists inside and outside of the US to diagnose a patient's Baumann Skin Type,[9,16] prescribe a skincare regimen,[17–19] educate patients, and perform research.[20,21]

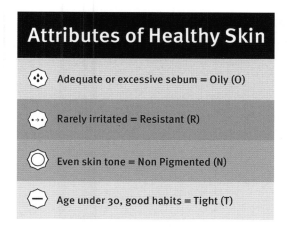

FIGURE 10-5. Attributes of healthy skin.

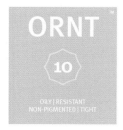

FIGURE 10-6. The ideal skin type, also known as normal skin.

The validated BSTI questionnaire identifies skin phenotype based on the presence or absence of the four barriers and four attributes of skin health.[10,15] A series of questions is asked to gather historical information to ascertain skin type. The questionnaire is even more helpful than seeing a patient's skin in person because a physical exam of facial skin only gives information about the skin's condition at that moment, while a historically based questionnaire yields information about how the skin has reacted in various situations in the past. Ideally, the patient should be evaluated in person and given the questionnaire; however, with the availability of telemedicine, the medical provider can feel confident that the questionnaire itself can provide the correct information needed to design an effective skincare routine targeted at the underlying skin concerns, even if they are unable to see the patient in person.

The Baumann Skin Types

The 16 different Baumann Skin Types are represented by a four-letter designation as well as color and number designations to help patients remember their Baumann Skin Type. For example, an individual with dry skin, facial redness, even skin tone, and fine lines would be assigned as a DRNW (Dry, Resistant, Non-pigmented, Wrinkle-prone type) (**Fig. 10-7**), which corresponds to Baumann Skin Type #16 and the color lilac.

The letters, color, and number are all used together because studies have demonstrated that some patients remember the number of their skin type, while others remember the color or

the four-letter designation. This skin-typing system facilitates communication between physicians, their staff, and patients as well as the process of prescribing the optimal products for a patient's skin type.[17] The interactivity of the questionnaire, the skin type colors, the skin type information, skincare routine steps, and follow-up communication contributes to increasing patient compliance (see Chapter 34, Skincare Retail in a Medical Setting).

There are 16 main Baumann Skin Types. However, when the sensitive skin subtypes are considered, there are actually 40 distinct skin type possibilities (**Fig. 10-8**). Using the STS software automatically assigns the skin type and corresponding regimen and obviates the need to understand all the different possible skin type variations. For the sake of simplicity, the system should be thought of as having 16 primary skin types. The sensitive skin subtypes will be discussed in corresponding chapters (see Chapters 11–19). Each of the barriers to skin health will be discussed below but first this issue of combination skin requires attention.

What Is Combination Skin?

The Baumann Skin Typing System does not have a designation for combination skin. Consumers often use the words "combination skin type," "dry combination skin," or "oily combination skin." These are misnomers. There is no scientific designation as combination skin; rather, there are two situations that patients could mean when they say they have combination skin.

1. Changing Skin Type: The skin is dry in low-humidity and cold environments and the skin is oily in hot, humid environments. In this situation, the Baumann Skin Type changes seasonally—dry skin type in the winter and oily skin type in the summer. This can be referred to as a seasonally changing skin type or a changing skin type and occurs because in dry environments the skin barrier is unable to hold up to the dry environment and loses water. Cold air holds less water, which leads to drying of the skin. Skin that produces enough sebum to compensate will not change seasonally nor will skin with an intact skin barrier unless something perturbs the barrier. Patients with a changing skin type will need a different skincare regimen seasonally as their Baumann Skin Type changes between oily and dry.
2. Oiliness in the T-zone: Some patients who state that they have combination skin have oily and dry facial skin at the same time. In all skin types, there are more sebaceous glands in the T-zone of the face than on the sides of the face. This discrepancy is obvious when the oil glands are producing an excess amount of oil. A T-zone with excessive sebum production and dryness on the cheeks may be characterized as an oily skin type or a dry skin type in the Baumann Skin Typing System depending upon the status of the skin barrier and the amount of sebum produced in the T-zone. If enough sebum is produced to cause occlusion on the skin to compensate for a compromised skin barrier, the skin is categorized as an oily Baumann Skin Type. If the T-zone does not make enough sebum to moisturize the cheeks, then the diagnosis is a Dry Baumann Skin Type.

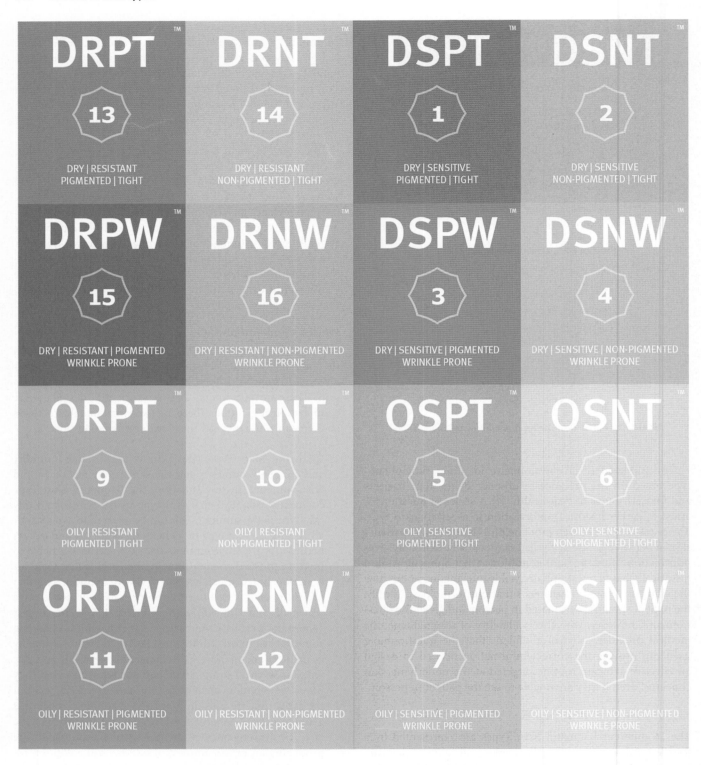

FIGURE 10-7. These are combined to form the 16 distinct Baumann Skin Types.

How Often Should the Skin Be Typed?

The Baumann Skin Type should be diagnosed at least once a year because skin type can change based on numerous factors, such as climate, lifestyle habits, diet, microbiome, hormone status, pregnancy, medication use, sun exposure, smoking, and other factors. At each visit the patient's skin type and regimen should be evaluated and updated according to the presence or absence of the four barriers to skin health. The diagnostic questionnaire can be retaken at any time that the patient or medical provider feels the skincare regimen is not working.

4 Possible Sensitive Subtypes

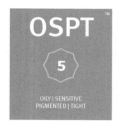

OSPT- Acne Type
OSPT- Rosacea Type
OSPT- Stinging Type
OSPT- Allergic Type

FIGURE 10-8. Each sensitive skin type has four subtypes. This example shows that a patient with adequate or increased sebum production, inflammation, uneven pigmentation, age 30 or under with healthy lifestyle habits but suffers from acne would be known as an OSPT Acne Type or OSPT1.

A CLOSER LOOK AT THE BAUMANN SKIN TYPES

This section will briefly discuss the underlying thought process behind the taxonomic classifications of the Baumann Skin Typing System. The types of questions used in the validated questionnaire to determine skin type are also focused on here. The reader is directed to the corresponding chapters later in this text to learn more about what causes dry, oily, sensitive, dyspigmented, and aged skin and how to treat these issues.

Skin Hydration: Oily (O) vs. Dry (D)

Determining whether the skin is oily or dry using a questionnaire is challenging. Studies have shown that when asked if one's skin is oily or dry, the responses do not match objective measurements.[22] Developing a scientifically validated questionnaire to measure skin oiliness took years of research and testing of questions versus sebumeter (sebum production) and tewameter (skin hydration) measurements to sort out which questions would accurately diagnose skin type.[10] Interestingly, many people, including dermatologists, have disagreed with their oily/dry diagnosis until objective measurements proved to them that their perceptions about their sebum secretion rates were incorrect. This self-misperception leads over 50% of people to use inappropriate cleansers and moisturizers for their skin type.[23,24] The Baumann Skin Type Questionnaire diagnoses skin type correctly in almost all cases. In rare situations (less than 1%), the skin type questionnaire will yield an incorrect diagnosis for the oily/dry spectrum. This occurs in patients who do not use skincare products on their face at all except water, which leads to outlying answers on a few questions that invalidate the results. An explanation for this phenomenon and how to handle it is discussed below.

In some cases, patients are confused because of their past use of or familiarity with the imprecise expressions "combination skin type" and "normal skin type," which are not skin type designations in the Baumann Skin Typing System. In the Baumann Skin Typing System, "normal skin types" are classified as oily as discussed below. Combination skin types have already been discussed. If patients are confused, explain that the Baumann Skin Typing System is based on measurable sebum secretion rates and tewameter skin hydration measurements, and the terminology is consistent with the science. Eventually they will learn the correct terminology.

Dry Skin

Dry skin is dehydrated due to an impaired skin barrier that allows excess evaporation of water from the skin's surface. It can be exacerbated by a lack of natural moisturizing factor and decreased sebum production. The skin needs water to function properly because multiple enzymes and other substances necessary for normal skin function require water. Dry skin feels rough, manifests a build-up of dead keratinocytes on the surface of the stratum corneum (SC), and reflects light poorly. Patients with dry skin complain of "dull skin" or a lack of radiance. Fine lines on the skin's surface may be noticeable. Darker skin types develop a flaking ashiness due to the accumulation of translucent skin cells on top of pigmented keratinocytes that renders a gray ashy appearance. Dehydration leads to several problems including increased susceptibility to irritant reactions, inflammation, and aging (see Chapter 12, Dry Skin). Dehydration is considered one of the four barriers to skin health.

Patients with dry skin tend to make the following statements about their skin or offer such answers to the Baumann Skin Type Questionnaire that can provide clues about the severity of dry skin. The lead author offers insights after these statements.

- "I apply a moisturizer to my facial skin once a day." This usually means they only have mildly dry skin.
- "I apply a moisturizer to my facial skin twice a day." This is the most common comment by those with moderate to severe dry skin. Those with very oily skin never choose this answer.
- "Soap dries out my skin." Very dry skin types cannot tolerate anionic and other detergent-laden foaming cleansers (see Chapter 40, Cleansing Agents).
- "My face is rough." Moderate to severe dry skin types report skin roughness.
- "My face is uncomfortable if I do not use a moisturizer." This is an important clue that the patient has dry skin. Oily skin types do not make such complaints.
- "My face feels tight and dry after washing it with a cleanser." Unless the patient used a lipid-filled creamy cleanser, all skin types (except very oily skin types) report dryness and tightness after cleansing. This does not provide much actionable information. However, if they do not feel dry right after cleansing, they are more likely to be an oily type than a dry type.
- "My face feels tight and dry for 10 to 20 minutes after washing it with a cleanser." This is more instructive because most skin types feel dry for 20 minutes after washing the face because it takes about 20 minutes for the sebaceous glands to replace the skin surface lipids removed with foaming cleansers. Dry types will continue to feel dry and uncomfortable even after 20 minutes have passed.

• "I like the feel of heavy creams and/or oil on my skin." This indicates that the patient has dry or very dry skin. In some cases, normal oily skin types who love skincare products will state that they like the feel of these heavy products. In this situation, use the Baumann Skin Type as diagnosed by the quiz but at the follow-up visit ascertain if a lighter moisturizer should be used and the patient changed to an oily skin type. Very oily skin types would never make this statement.

Oily Skin

Oily skin is hydrated due to sebum-derived lipids that coat the skin with an occlusive layer and help the skin barrier retain water. Even if a patient has a genetically or environmentally impaired skin barrier, if enough sebum is present, the skin will remain hydrated due to the actions of sebum as a hydrating and occlusive ingredient. In the Baumann Skin Typing System, "oily skin" is the healthiest and most desirable state because sebum exerts antioxidant and moisturizing activities that protect the skin from the ravages of the environment. Aging skin is characterized by lower levels of skin lipids and sebum secretion rates decline increasingly after age 30. Therefore, it is desirable to have sebum on the skin, especially in older individuals.

Oily skin in the Baumann Skin Typing System has two subtypes: very oily skin and normal oily skin (the ideal skin hydration state). Very oily skin is characterized by an excessive amount of sebum production, shininess, dislike of the feel of heavy moisturizers and sunscreens, and frequent comedones. Very oily skin is what patients commonly refer to as "oily skin." The second subtype, normal oily skin, is the skin type that patients call "normal skin." It is considered an oily skin type because in order to have healthy hydrated skin an adequate level of sebum-derived lipids is necessary for skin health. An oily skin type is a hydrated skin type.

Patients with oily skin tend to offer the following statements or questionnaire answers about their skin that can provide clues as to whether they have normal oily or very oily skin.

• "I can use any soap to wash my face without developing dryness." This statement practically guarantees that the patient has oily skin and likely has very oily skin. However, in some cases, men (and sometimes women) with dry skin who are uneducated about skincare will provide this answer.
• "I never or only occasionally apply a moisturizer." In most cases, this is diagnostic of normal oily or very oily skin. However, men and women who use no facial skincare products at all may choose this answer, which can result in an incorrect Baumann Skin Type diagnosis. If the patient is diagnosed as an oily type but they appear dry on exam or the other questions are consistent with dry skin, keep in mind that this question can yield an incorrect result. If that occurs, change the skin type diagnosis from oily to dry skin.
• "I do not apply any products to my face after cleansing." This statement is almost diagnostic of normal oily or very oily skin. However, men and women who use no facial skin-care products at all may choose this answer, contributing to an incorrect Baumann Skin Type diagnosis. If the patient is diagnosed as an oily type but they appear dry on exam or the other questions are consistent with dry skin, keep in mind that this question can give an incorrect result. If that occurs, change the skin type diagnosis from oily to dry skin.
• "My face is oily in some areas." This is the answer given by people with a changing dry to oily skin type that varies seasonally or normal oily skin types. It reflects increased sebum secretion in the T-zone.
• "My face is very oily." Several studies show that people are often wrong about how much oil they produce, and that this description alone does not correlate with sebum secretion. However, one such study suggested that people usually underestimate the amount of sebum they produce.[22] If a patient says their face is very oily, they are almost always a very oily skin type.

The ideal skin type is a normal oily skin type that makes an adequate, not excessive, amount of sebum. They are referred to as "oily skin types" in the Baumann Skin Typing System. Cleanser and moisturizer choices are linked to whether the skin is considered a dry or oily type.

Skincare for the O to D Parameter

Dry Skincare

When developing a skincare regimen for any of the eight skin types that exhibit dry skin, Phase 1 is to combat dehydration, build the skin barrier, and moisturize. The goal is to get the skin as close to a normal oily skin type as possible, meaning that the surface has protective lipids. Dehydrated skin engenders the other barriers to skin health, so it must be corrected before treating pigmentation and aging. Also, many depigmenting and anti-aging ingredients can irritate dry skin, spark inflammation, and leave the skin less healthy than when the treatments began. Addressing skin hydration in Phase 1 will speed skin recovery in the long run (**Fig. 10-9**). The choice of cleansers, water to rinse the face, and moisturizers is critical to treat dehydrated skin (see Chapters 12, 40, and 43, Moisturizers).

Oily Skincare

Oily skin types start out with an advantage because dehydration is not an issue. The main goal of using a moisturizer for oily skin is to provide any needed hydration without causing comedones. Normal oily types can use a

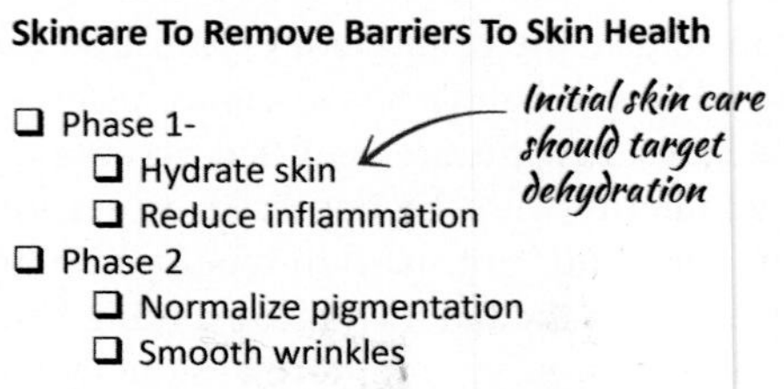

Skincare To Remove Barriers To Skin Health

☐ Phase 1-
   ☐ Hydrate skin ← *Initial skin care should target dehydration*
   ☐ Reduce inflammation
☐ Phase 2
   ☐ Normalize pigmentation
   ☐ Smooth wrinkles

FIGURE 10-9. In a phased skincare plan, hydration and inflammation should be addressed first.

light noncomedogenic moisturizer such as a hyaluronic acid (HA)-containing serum that will help facilitate penetration of the other skincare products in the regimen. Sebum can impede penetration of important ingredients, so the boost provided by HA is significant. Oily skin types with oiliness in the T-zone can only use a light moisturizer on the sides of the face, skipping the sebaceous gland-heavy T-zone. Very oily skin types can eliminate the AM and PM moisturizer. It is often difficult to get very oily skin types to wear a sunscreen; omitting a moisturizer may boost sunscreen compliance. Layering a powder over sunscreen may help reduce the greasiness that occurs in oily patients with sunscreen use. Very oily skin types will benefit from a course of low-dose isotretinoin. How to treat oily skin will be discussed in Chapter 11, Oily Skin, and Chapter 40.

Skincare for the Changing Skin Type

Skin that changes from dry in the winter or dry climates to oily in the summer and warm climates needs two completely different skincare routines. Follow the guidance for dry skin in cold, dry climates and oily guidance in the warm humid climates. The skin can easily switch from an oily type to a dry type with changes of geographic location, climate, and season.

Cosmetic Procedures for the O to D Parameter

There are not many cosmetic procedures that will treat dehydration and oiliness. Dry skin types benefit from mechanical exfoliation such as dermaplaning, microdermabrasion, and facial scrubs. Chemical exfoliation can also help smooth the SC, leaving the skin more radiant so chemical peels may be a good option for dry skin types. Oily skin types often have comedones and benefit from facial extractions, salicylic acid chemical peels, and hydrafacials®. Using lights and lasers to shrink oil glands is currently being investigated to determine if they provide a solution for oily skin.

Skin Sensitivity: Sensitive (S) vs. Resistant (R)

Sensitive skin is characterized by inflammation and manifests as acne, rosacea, burning and stinging, or skin rashes (see Chapter 12). Resistant skin is characterized by calm skin that is not easily agitated to an inflammatory state. Acne, facial redness, facial stinging, and rashes occur infrequently. While all skin types can develop an occasional pimple, flush with excitement, or develop a rash when exposed to an allergen or irritant, this occurs often in sensitive skin types and rarely in resistant skin types.

Sensitive Skin

Sensitive skin is caused by inflammation. There are numerous causes of inflammation and pathways that communicate with each other to incite inflammation. Which pathways engender inflammation depends on the sensitive skin subtype. Skin dryness can also lead to inflammation. An impaired skin barrier predisposes to sensitive skin but is not required for sensitive skin. The causes of inflammation are discussed in Chapters 13 and 16–19. Short-term inflammation is a necessary protective response that the skin uses to defend against microbes,

allergens, and irritants. However, long-term inflammation is deleterious and is being increasingly recognized as a major cause of disease and aging leading to the term "inflammaging."[25] Inflammation activates melanocytes causing uneven skin pigmentation and breakdown of collagen, HA, and elastin, resulting in sagging skin with fine lines and wrinkles. For these reasons, every effort should be made to avoid, calm, and control inflammation.

Eight of the Baumann Skin Types have sensitive skin that exhibit inflammation. These are further divided into four sensitive skin subtypes (**Fig. 10-3**). Sensitive skin types can manifest more than one sensitive skin subtype. For example, a sensitive skin type can have acne, facial redness (rosacea), and skin stinging (Chapter 13).

Resistant Skin

Individuals with resistant skin rarely experience acne, erythema, stinging, or rashes. In general, they can be treated with stronger skincare products than can those with sensitive skin. For example, resistant skin types can usually begin a retinoid faster than a sensitive skin type with fewer side effects of redness and peeling. Using the wrong skincare, increased stress, poor diet, microbiome changes, disease, new medications, and using incorrect skincare products can change a resistant skin type to a sensitive skin type.

Skincare for the S to R Parameter

Sensitive Skincare

All sensitive skin subtypes benefit from anti-inflammatory ingredients (see Chapter 38, Anti-Inflammatory Ingredients). Inflammation is important to target in Phase 1 of the skincare treatment plan because inflammation exacerbates the other barriers to skin health: pigmentation and aging. When recommending a skincare routine for sensitive skin, the products should be chosen based on which sensitive subtype is present. In the case where a patient has more than one sensitive subtype, the most damaging and severe subtypes are treated first. For example, if a patient is an allergic skin type and has an allergy to formaldehyde, then the first step is to begin formaldehyde-free skincare products; otherwise, the inflammation will never get under control. If the patient has both pimples and facial redness, the medical practitioner must decide if the patient's diagnosis is acne or rosacea and focus the skincare routine to treat the corresponding underlying cause (**Fig. 10-10**). In many cases, pimples are seen in rosacea and facial redness is seen in acne, but one pathology will be the main cause of the findings and that pathology should be targeted with skincare. Stinging skin often occurs in rosacea, so treating the underlying rosacea will often resolve the stinging. If stinging is found without facial redness, avoiding products with a low pH and fragrances as well as certain preservatives will usually resolve the stinging issues. In the case of rashes after shaving as seen in many men, it is important to delve deeper into the underlying cause because the type of razor and method of shaving can play a role. For a more in-depth discussion of skincare for sensitive skin, see Chapter 13 (**Box 10-1**).

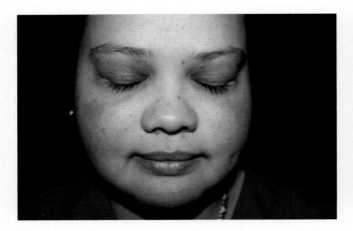

FIGURE 10-10. A patient who exhibits both Type 1 (Acne) and Type 2 (Rosacea) sensitive skin (papules, pustules, and redness), should be treated for the more severe of the two. In this image, the patient's rosacea is the cause of the papules; therefore, she would be treated with skincare targeted to rosacea. Acne medications would irritate her skin and increase her facial redness.

BOX 10-1	Ingredient Considerations for Sensitive Skin Subtypes

Ingredients to use if acne subtype:

- Glycolic acid
- Retinoids
- Salicylic acid
- Silver
- Topical antibiotics

Ingredients to avoid if stinging and burning subtype:

- Ascorbic acid
- Avobenzone
- Benzoic acid
- Foaming cleansers
- Hydroxy acids
- Menthol
- Peppermint oil
- Scrubs
- Witch hazel

Resistant Skincare

Individuals with resistant "R" skin can use most skincare products with less risk of incurring adverse reactions (e.g., acne, rashes, or a stinging response). Stronger ingredients and products can be started sooner, with less preparation, than in sensitive skin types. In the case of oily resistant types (OR types), many products are ineffective because these patients exhibit an exceedingly high threshold for product ingredient penetration. Their skin barrier is intact and their skin is coated with a protective layer of sebum; both of these conditions impede penetration of ingredients. In this situation, use of penetration-enhancing ingredients such as HA is beneficial. Salicylic acid cleansers can also help penetration in oily resistant skin (see Chapter 40).

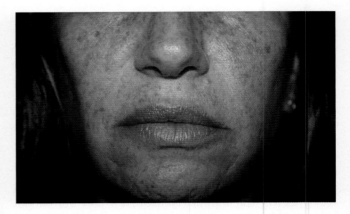

FIGURE 10-11. The diagnosis of a pigmented skin type is based upon unevenness of skin tone rather than ethnicity or Fitzpatrick Skin Type. This image is of a pigmented skin type.

Resistant types often report that products they have tried in the past "did not work." This is likely because such products were not strong enough for resistant skin. Resistant skin type patients are the ones who can be treated with higher levels of hydroxy acids and retinoids. They are less likely to develop allergic reactions to skincare products that sensitive types cannot tolerate.

Cosmetic Procedures for the S to R Parameter

Sensitive skin types that have acne and rosacea may benefit from skincare procedures. Acne types may need facial extractions or hydrafacials to remove comedones, corticosteroid injections for acne cysts, blue light to reduce bacteria, and red light or laser treatments to reduce inflammation. Chemical peels are another option to treat acne. Rosacea skin types will benefit from vascular laser treatments, red light, and possibly botulinum toxin injections, which have been reported to improve rosacea.[24,26,27] At this time, there are no cosmetic procedures to treat burning/stinging skin or allergic skin.

Sensitive skin types may also benefit from dietary alterations and lifestyle changes. Acne has been shown to worsen with dairy and sugar. Stress increases the amount of acne lesions by augmenting inflammation and sebum production. Rosacea skin types often have dietary triggers such as spicy or hot food and alcohol. Stress also affects rosacea. New research shows a correlation between the microbiome and rosacea.[28]

Skin Pigmentation: Pigmented (P) vs. Nonpigmented (N)

Ethnicity is not the focus here. Although darker skin types are more likely to exhibit the "P" (pigmented) skin type, this parameter does not refer to overall skin color; rather, it describes the evenness or unevenness of skin tone (**Fig. 10-11**). The P/N parameter measures the tendency to develop dyspigmentation due to activation of melanocytes as seen in solar lentigos, melasma, and post-inflammatory hyperpigmentation as sequelae of acne lesions.

Baumann Skin Type P/N Parameter	Fitzpatrick Skin Type
How skin looks today	How skin reacts with initial UV exposure
Independent from ethnicity	Linked to ethnicity
Determines skincare needs	Determines UV dose needed for treatments
Determines need for skin lightening	Determines laser settings
If P, then increased risk for PIPA	Predicts risk of PIPA
Defined by patient's desire to treat	Independent of patient's opinion
Changes with treatment	Consistent throughout lifetime
Not directly associated with skin cancer risk	Associated with skin cancer risk

TABLE 10-1 Comparison of the Baumann Skin Type P/N Parameter and Fitzpatrick Skin Type

The question that determines whether the patient has a P or N skin type asks patients if they have discolored marks and uneven skin pigmentation on the face. If they answer yes, they have the option of wanting to treat the uneven skin tone or leaving them alone. In many cases, the dark spots are freckles that patients want to keep. This allows for three possibilities:

- Uneven skin tone with darker areas that the patient wants to lighten = P skin type
- Uneven skin tone that the patient wants to leave as is = N skin type
- Even skin tone = N skin type

An easy way to think of this skin type is P = pigment-reducing ingredients in the regimen and N = no skin-lightening ingredients in the regimen.

The P/N parameter most closely resembles the Fitzpatrick Skin Type that assesses the skin's ability to form pigment. The difference is that the P/N parameter in the Baumann Skin Type evaluates how the skin looks at the set point in time in which the questionnaire is taken or the skin is examined. The Fitzpatrick Skin Type looks at propensity to pigmentation over a lifetime. This subtle distinction is important (see **Table 10-1**).

Skincare for the P to N Parameter

Individuals with N type skin do not require any special skincare products. However, the P skin types benefit from skin-lightening ingredients such as tyrosinase inhibitors, antioxidants, anti-inflammatories, retinoids, protease activated receptor 2 (PAR-2) blockers, and exfoliants. These ingredients are discussed at length in Chapter 41, Depigmenting Ingredients. The science of melanogenesis is discussed in Chapter 14, Skin Pigmentation, while skin disorders that cause skin pigmentation are discussed in Chapter 20, Pigmentation Disorders.

Ingredients that target pigmentation, such as retinoids and tyrosinase inhibitors, can be irritating to the skin and lead to inflammation. Inflammation, in turn, increases pigmentation and aging. For this reason, if the skin type has dryness or sensitivity, it is best to treat those barriers to skin health first in Phase 1. Then in 4 weeks, if the dryness and/or inflammation are improved, add the ingredients to target pigmentation (and aging, if applicable). Treated pigmented skin types require two different skincare regimens: one with tyrosinase inhibitors and exfoliants, and a maintenance regimen with antioxidants, PAR-2 blockers, and retinoids. Most medical providers prescribe a treatment regimen for 4 months and switch to a maintenance regimen for 1 month. After 1 month, if the skin remains a P skin type, the treatment regimen is restarted. Once the skin reaches N skin type status the maintenance regimen is used (see Chapter 14 for more details).

Cosmetic Procedures for the P to N Parameter

Individuals with N type skin do not require any cosmetic treatments. The goal for them is to keep the skin even toned. P types benefit from treatments that remove dark spots. These should be chosen based on the underlying cause of the altered pigmentation (see Chapter 20). Options include lasers, IPL, and chemical peels. In the author's experience, melasma patients do best with skincare alone because they often experience rebound effects from lasers and IPL 3 to 6 months after treatment.

Patient education is particularly critical for P skin types. Exposure to UV light, blue light from cell phones and computer screens, infrared light (heat), and stress all influence skin pigmentation. Compliance with daily sunscreen, sun protection, and sun and heat avoidance is required for successful conversion of a P skin type to an N skin type.

Skin Aging: Wrinkled (W) vs. Tight (T)

This portion of the Baumann Skin Typing System identifies habits that increase the risk of skin aging and skin cancer. The philosophy is that anyone over the age of 30 or under the age of 30 with at least three risky behaviors needs to begin using skin-protective ingredients such as antioxidants and retinoids. Patients age 30 or younger with fewer than three risky behaviors have a T skin type meaning that they do not need anti-aging and skin-protecting ingredients in their skincare routine beyond daily sunscreen. Once the patient is over 30, they will be skin typed as a W "wrinkle-prone" skin type even if they have no visible wrinkles. This is because the Baumann Skin Typing System is geared to determine the need for protective ingredients rather than labeling someone as having wrinkles or not. Wrinkle-prone types need protective ingredients, and in some cases lifestyle changes, to protect skin health.

The questionnaire asks about habits such as sun exposure, smoking, tanning bed use, stress, diet, and exercise. In addition, it asks questions about the skin of the patient's parents to ascertain the genetic influence on wrinkled skin. Patients who have three or more habits or genetic predisposition for wrinkles are considered a W skin type.

Skincare for the W to T Parameter

T skin types need daily sunscreen to keep their skin healthy. W skin types can benefit from a plethora of anti-aging ingredients discussed at length in Chapter 37, Anti-Aging Ingredients. These ingredients should be chosen based on the presence or absence of other barriers to skin health. For example, a sensitive pigmented (SP) skin type needs anti-aging ingredients that also decrease inflammation and pigmentation such as ascorbic acid.

Cosmetic Procedures for the W to T Parameter

Cosmetic treatments play an important role in the treatment of W skin types and the prevention and treatment of wrinkles. Botulinum toxins, dermal fillers, microneedling with or without PRP, skin tightening, lasers, lights, and chemical peels are some treatment options for W skin types. Combining procedures with skincare will improve results (see Chapter 36, Pre- and Post-Procedure Skincare).

PHASES OF SKINCARE TO TREAT THE FOUR BARRIERS TO SKIN HEALTH

When customizing skincare regimens by skin type, it is important to keep in mind that compliance is a concern (see the compliance section in Chapter 34). Patients should understand that the first regimen they are given is the first of at least two phases and follow-up is needed to remain on the correct path to healthy skin. If a patient is prescribed too many different products at the first visit, compliance will be compromised by budget, time, and side effects. Also, if strong depigmenting and anti-aging ingredients are used on dry or sensitive skin types, inflammation can be triggered thus attenuating all the barriers to skin health. For this reason, a phased approach is suggested. In Phase 1, the preliminary focus is dehydration and inflammation. For patients who are OR skin types, they can move directly to Phase 2 (**Fig. 10-12**). Phase 2 includes depigmenting and anti-aging ingredients (in addition to any needed hydrating, anti-inflammatory, and anti-acne ingredients from Phase 1). Patients should be given the Phase 1 plan at the baseline visit and then, in 4 weeks at the follow-up visit, be re-evaluated. In most cases at visit 2 (Day 30), the patients can be moved to Phase 2. The recommendation is to see the patients every 30 days for 3 months. If at 3 months the skin is tolerating the skincare regimen and all barriers to skin health are being addressed, patients can be seen every 6 months to assess skin type again and adjust the skincare regimen.

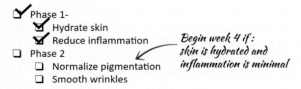

FIGURE 10-12. Phase 2 of the skincare plan focuses on regulating pigmentation and decreasing molecular events that lead to aging.

Pigmented skin types will require at least 6 months of monthly follow-ups. After 4 months of the P skin type treatment regimen, the patient should be switched to a 1-month maintenance regimen to give a "tyrosinase inhibitor holiday" as discussed in Chapter 41. After the month ends, if the altered pigmentation is still present, restart the treatment regimen. These cycles will continue until the patient achieves N skin type status.

MANAGING PATIENT EXPECTATIONS

Patients can be misled by false marketing claims that skin will improve overnight or in a few days. This is not the case. The cell cycle is 30 or more days, so it takes at least 30 days to replace the epidermis with new cells and longer for the dermis to thicken and improve. Below are some timelines that patients should be given on expectations as to when to see improvements. This timeline assumes: (1) the correct skincare regimen is prescribed, (2) patient compliance, (3) the correct amount of each product (as listed in Fig. 35–2) is applied, and (4) use of the phased skincare plan.

- Acne: results will begin to be seen at 8 weeks with clearing at 12 weeks in most cases.
- Melasma: improvement beginning at 12 weeks and more apparent at 16 weeks. Severe melasma may take longer. Lasers and IPL are not suggested. They clear up melasma faster than topical products do but it tends to recur with use of lasers and IPL.
- Rosacea: improvement at 12 weeks or sooner if combined with a vascular laser.
- Solar lentigos: improvement at 12 weeks or sooner with a pigment laser.
- Fine lines: those due to dehydration will improve in days. Those due to changes in the dermis will take 6 months or more to improve.

Explaining to a patient on the first visit that there is a phased approach to skincare will help them realize the importance of compliance and routine follow-up. They need to understand that the regimen must be adjusted monthly until they can tolerate all the products needed to target the underlying barriers to skin health.

HOW TO CHANGE THE BAUMANN SKIN TYPE

The goal of skincare regimens and cosmetic treatment plans is to change the skin type as close as possible to the healthiest, ideal skin type ORNT (number 10). This is achieved in the following order: eliminate dehydration, soothe inflammation, suppress pigmentation, and target aging.

DESCRIPTIONS OF BAUMANN SKIN TYPES

Each skin phenotype has specific characteristics and a personality. Listed below are a few of the characteristics and some of the ingredients to use and avoid. This is not a comprehensive list but gives an idea of what each skin type needs.

Baumann Skin Type ① DSPT
Dry, Sensitive, Pigmented, Tight

DSPT skin types are under the age of 30. These individuals are usually acne patients who have difficulty tolerating retinoids and benzoyl peroxide. Once their papules and pustules clear, they are left with pigmented spots. The side effects of acne medications often have interfered with their treatment plans. Using a hydrating creamy cleanser and a barrier repair moisturizer will improve tolerance and compliance to retinoid-containing acne medications.

DSPT has three barriers to skin health. Dehydration is caused by an impaired skin barrier that renders DSPT skin less able to retain water and protect against irritants and allergens. Inflammation speeds skin aging and increases the risk for pigmentation. Dyspigmentation causes an uneven skin tone. Ingredient advice for the sensitive subtypes is described in a previous section. Here is general ingredient advice for DSPTs of all sensitive subtypes.

Product Advice for DSPT

Dry skin types should not use foaming cleansers because they strip lipids from the skin. If the skin suffers from the triad of stinging, scaling, and redness, consider using filtered water to rinse off the cleanser. Treatment products may include skin lighteners, anti-inflammatories, and antioxidants. DSPTs should use barrier repair moisturizers twice a day. Avoid HA-containing moisturizers that increase penetration of retinoids until the skin has adapted to the retinoids. Retinoids can be used to treat acne if started slowly (every third night) and applied on top of a barrier repair moisturizer. A moisturizing physical sunscreen should be used daily (**Box 10-2**).

Procedure Advice for DSPT

Acne subtypes can use glycolic acid-containing chemical peels with skin-lightening ingredients. Rosacea types will benefit from vascular lasers and red light. Blue light should be avoided in DSPTs because it increases the risk for pigmentation.

Baumann Skin Type ② : DSNT
Dry, Sensitive, Non-Pigmented, Tight

DSNT has two barriers to skin health. Dehydration is caused by an impaired skin barrier that renders DSNT skin less able to retain water and protect against irritants and allergens. Inflammation speeds skin aging. Here is general ingredient advice for DSNTs of all sensitive subtypes.

Product Advice for DSNT

Dry skin types should avoid foaming cleansers because they strip lipids from the skin. Cleansers should be rinsed off using soft water with a low calcium content such as filtered water. Treatment products may include anti-inflammatories, antioxidants, and retinoids. DSNTs should use barrier repair moisturizers twice daily. Avoid HA-containing moisturizers that increase penetration of retinoids until the skin has adapted to the retinoids. Retinoids can be used to treat acne if started slowly (every third night) and applied on top of a barrier repair moisturizer. A moisturizing physical sunscreen should be used daily (**Box 10-3**).

Procedure Advice for DSNT

Acne subtypes can use glycolic acid-containing chemical peels and blue light treatments. Rosacea types will benefit from vascular lasers and red light.

Baumann Skin Type ③ : DSPW
Dry, Sensitive, Pigmented, Wrinkle-Prone

DSPW skin types usually fit one of three profiles: 1) over the age of 30 with rosacea and signs of photoaging, 2) young acne sufferers with poor lifestyle habits or increased sun exposure due to sports, or 3) adult women with acne.

DSPW skin types have four barriers to skin health. Dehydration is caused by an impaired skin barrier that renders DSPW skin less able to retain water and protect against irritants and allergens. Inflammation speeds skin aging and increases the risk for pigmentation. The uneven pigmentation gives skin an uneven skin tone. Age over 30 years or lifestyle factors that increase aging such as spending time in the sun without sunscreen make DSPW skin more prone to wrinkles and skin cancer.

BOX 10-2

Ingredients for DSPT to use:

- Aloe vera
- Argan oil
- Borage seed oil
- Ceramide
- Cholesterol
- Cucumber extract
- Defensins
- Dexpanthenol (pro-vitamin B_5)
- Feverfew
- Glycerin
- Hydroquinone
- Licorice extract
- Macadamia oil
- Methyl dihydroxybenzoate
- Myristoyl/palmitoyl oxostearamide/arachamide mea
- Niacinamide
- Pycnogenol
- Retinol
- Stearic acid
- Tetrahexyldecyl ascorbate

Ingredients for DSPT to avoid:

- Anionic surfactants
- Anything causing allergy
- Benzoyl peroxide
- Dimethyl dodecyl amido betaine
- Hard water (increased calcium)
- Isopropyl myristate
- Lauryl sulfates
- Mechanical exfoliants
- Sodium dodecyl sulfate
- Sodium laurel sulfate

BOX 10-3

Ingredients for DSNT to use:

- Allantoin
- Argan oil
- Benzoyl peroxide
- Borage seed oil
- Ceramides
- Chamomile
- Cholesterol
- Cucumber
- Dexpanthenol (pro-vitamin B_5)
- Macadamia oil
- Myristoyl/palmitoyl oxostearamide/arachamide mea
- Niacinamide
- Panthenol
- Stearic acid
- Tamanu oil
- Tea tree oil
- Willow bark

Ingredients for DSNT to avoid:

- Anionic surfactants
- Anything causing allergy
- Benzoyl peroxide
- Dimethyl dodecyl amido betaine
- Hard water (increased calcium)
- Isopropyl myristate
- Lauryl sulfates
- Mechanical exfoliants
- Sodium dodecyl sulfate
- Sodium laurel sulfate

BOX 10-4

Ingredients for DSPW to use:

- Arbutin
- Argan oil
- Ceramide
- Cholesterol
- Coenzyme Q_{10} (Ubiquinone)
- Feverfew
- Grape seed extract
- Green tea
- Hexylresorcinol
- Licorice extract
- Macadamia oil
- Methyl dihydroxybenzoate
- Mulberry extract
- Myristoyl/palmitoyl oxostearamide/arachamide mea
- Niacinamide
- Phloretin
- Resveratrol
- Retinol
- Tetrahexyldecyl ascorbate

Ingredients for DSPW to avoid:

- Alcohol
- Anionic surfactants
- Avocado oil
- Coconut oil
- Foaming cleanser
- Hard water (increased calcium)
- Isopropyl myristate
- Lanolin
- Mechanical exfoliants (scrubs)
- Myristyl propionate
- Peppermint oil
- Propylene glycol-2 (PPG-2)

Product Advice for DSPW

Dry skin types should avoid foaming cleansers with anionic surfactants that strip lipids from the skin. Instead, choose creamy lipid-filled barrier-protecting cleansers. If the skin suffers from the triad of stinging, scaling, and redness, consider using filtered water to rinse off the cleanser. Treatment products may include skin lighteners, anti-inflammatories, and antioxidants. All DSPWs should begin retinoids in Phase 1 or 2. Retinoids should be started slowly (every third night) and applied on top of a barrier repair moisturizer. Barrier repair moisturizers should be used twice daily. Sunscreen should be used daily (**Box 10-4**).

Procedure Advice for DSPW

DSPWs with acne will benefit from chemical peels containing glycolic acid and skin lighteners. These peels can be used to accelerate correction of any post-inflammatory pigment alteration (PIPA) that occurs from the acne. Blue light should be avoided due to risk of pigmentation. DSPWs with rosacea will benefit from red light or vascular laser. DSPWs with visible wrinkles and volume loss may benefit from botulinum toxin, dermal fillers, and skin tightening. Microneedling should be used in conjunction with skin lighteners, sunscreen, and sun avoidance to reduce the risk of PIPA.

Baumann Skin Type : DSNW

Dry, Sensitive, Non-Pigmented, Wrinkle-Prone

DSNW skin usually fits one of the following profiles: 1) adult with rosacea and photoaging, or 2) adult woman with acne. These require a different approach. For the acne type, retinoids are the mainstay of treatment. For the rosacea type, anti-inflammatory ingredients provide the most value.

DSNW has three barriers to skin health. Dehydration is caused by an impaired skin barrier that renders DSNW skin less able to retain water and protect against irritants and allergens. Inflammation speeds skin aging. Age over 30 years or lifestyle factors that increase aging such as spending time in the sun without sunscreen make your skin more prone to wrinkles and skin cancer.

Product Advice for DSNW

Dry skin types should avoid foaming cleansers, especially those with anionic detergents, that strip lipids from the skin. If the skin suffers from the triad of stinging, scaling, and redness, consider using filtered water to rinse off the cleanser. Treatment products may include anti-inflammatories, antioxidants, and other anti-aging products. Retinoids should be started slowly and applied over a barrier repair moisturizer. Avoid moisturizers with HA while adapting to retinoids. DSNWs should use barrier repair moisturizers twice daily. Sunscreen should be used daily.

Procedure Advice for DSNW

DSNWs with acne will benefit from chemical peels containing glycolic acid. Blue light should be avoided because it can increase skin aging. DSNWs with rosacea will benefit from red light, IPL, or vascular laser. DSNWs with visible wrinkles and volume loss may benefit from botulinum toxin, dermal fillers, microneedling, and skin tightening (**Box 10-5**).

Baumann Skin Type 5 : OSPT
Oily, Sensitive, Pigmented, Tight

OSPT skin types almost always fit this profile: younger people with a Fitzpatrick Skin Type of III or higher with acne and dark areas of PIPA on the skin where an acne lesion had been. They are often frustrated with acne treatments because they are left with months of red and brown marks on the skin. Just when the lesions clear, these individuals develop new lesions and the cycle begins again. The most important lesson for this group is

to teach them to be proactive and use their skincare to prevent acne, not to wait and use the products after the acne occurs.

OSPTs have two barriers to skin health and these are inter-related: inflammation spurs on pigmentation. The main goal is to prevent acne and pigmentation with consistent use of the proper skincare products.

Product Advice for OSPT

Oily skin types should use foaming cleansers and salicylic acid cleansers. Treatment products may include skin lighteners, anti-inflammatories, antioxidants, and retinoids. A noncomedogenic sunscreen should be used daily (**Box 10-6**).

Procedure Advice for OSPT

This skin type can benefit from salicylic acid peels that contain skin-lightening ingredients. Blue light, laser, and IPL should be avoided because these can worsen pigmentation. Facial extractions and hydrafacials are a good option.

Baumann Skin Type 6 : OSNT
Oily, Sensitive, Non-Pigmented, Tight

OSNTs are usually young patients with acne. OSNTs have one barrier to skin health: inflammation. The inflammation is usually caused by *C. acnes* bacteria on the skin or hormones leading to acne.

Product Advice for OSNT

Oily skin types should use foaming cleansers or those containing salicylic acid. Treatment products may include anti-acne and anti-inflammatory products. A light noncomedogenic moisturizer should be used. Very oily types can skip the AM moisturizer and use a sunscreen instead (**Box 10-7**).

BOX 10-5

Ingredients for DSNW to use:

- Argan oil
- Borage seed oil
- Caffeine
- Ceramide
- Chamomile
- Cholesterol
- Coenzyme Q_{10} (Ubiquinone)
- Cucumber
- Dexpanthenol (pro-vitamin B_5)
- Ferulic acid
- Feverfew
- Glycerin
- Grape seed extract
- Green tea
- Macadamia oil
- Myristoyl/palmitoyl oxostearamide/arachamide mea
- Resveratrol
- Retinol
- Stearic acid
- Tamanu oil

Ingredients for DSNW to avoid:

- Anionic surfactants
- Anything causing allergy
- Cinnamon oil
- Coconut oil
- Hard water (increased calcium)
- Isopropyl myristate

BOX 10-6

Ingredients for OSPT to use:

- Ascorbic acid
- Benzoyl peroxide
- *Glycyrrhiza glabra* (licorice)
- Hexylresorcinol
- Hydroquinone
- Kojic acid
- Methyl dihydroxybenzoate
- Niacinamide
- Resorcinol
- Retinol
- Salicylic acid
- Tetrahexyldecyl ascorbate
- Tranexamic acid

Ingredients for OSPT to avoid:

- Isopropyl myristate
- Myristyl myristate
- Myristyl propionate
- Octyl palmitate
- Octyl stearate

BOX 10-7

Ingredients for OSNT to use:

- Allantoin
- Benzoyl peroxide
- Caffeine
- *Citrus sinensis* (orange fruit)
- Feverfew
- *Glycyrrhiza glabra* (licorice)
- Hexylresorcinol
- Hyaluronic acid
- Panthenol
- Resorcinol
- Retinol
- Salicylic acid
- Tea tree oil
- Tranexamic acid
- Zinc

Ingredients for OSNT to avoid:

- Avocado oil
- Cetyl acetate
- Cocoa butter
- *Cocos nucifera* (coconut oil)
- Isopropyl myristate
- Jojoba oil
- Octyl stearate
- Squalene

BOX 10-8

Ingredients for OSPW to use:

- Ascorbic acid
- Azelaic acid
- Benzoyl peroxide
- Coenzyme Q_{10} (Ubiquinone)
- Defensins
- Feverfew
- Green tea
- Heparan sulfate
- Hexylresorcinol
- Hyaluronic acid
- Licorice extract
- Methyl dihydroxybenzoate
- Niacinamide
- Phloretin
- Retinol
- Salicylic acid
- Silver
- Tetrahexyldecyl ascorbate
- Tranexamic acid

Ingredients for OSPW to avoid:

- Bergamot oil
- Coconut oil
- Isopropyl myristate

Procedure Advice for OSNT

This skin type can benefit from salicylic acid peels. Blue light, red light, and laser can be used to treat acne lesions. Facial extractions and hydrafacials are a good option. Rosacea subtypes can be treated with IPL or the vascular laser.

Baumann Skin Type : OSPW
Oily, Sensitive, Pigmented, Wrinkle-Prone

OSPW skin types can present with several different phenotypes but most commonly fall into one of the following profiles: 1) a young person with acne who has increased sun exposure (e.g., from outdoor sports), 2) an adult with acne and photoaging, 3) an adult with facial redness and melasma, 4) an adult with acne resulting in PIPA, or 5) an adult with rosacea and photoaging. Each profile needs different skincare advice. All need daily sunscreen.

The OSPW skin type has three barriers to skin health: inflammation, which accelerates skin aging and increases the risk for pigmentation, and pigmentation itself, which can be due to acne, melasma, or sun exposure. OSPWs are over 30 years of age or have lifestyle factors that make the skin more prone to wrinkles and skin cancer.

Product Advice for OSPW

Oily skin types should use foaming cleansers or those with salicylic acid. Treatment products may include anti-acne ingredients, skin lighteners, anti-inflammatories, and anti-aging ingredients. Retinoids are a great option because they target

acne, wrinkles, and pigmentation but should be started slowly in rosacea subtypes. Sunscreen should be used daily. The moisturizer can be omitted in the AM so that the patient will be more compliant with sunscreen. (Sometimes using both feels too heavy or sticky, especially in very oily skin types) (**Box 10-8**).

Procedure Advice for OSPW

This skin type can benefit from salicylic acid peels. Blue light should be avoided because it can worsen pigmentation. Red light and laser can be used to treat rosacea. Facial extractions and hydrafacials are a good option. Botulinum toxins, dermal fillers, and skin-tightening procedures can improve wrinkles and sagging skin. Microneedling should be used with caution in Fitzpatrick Skin Type III or higher due to the risk of PIPA.

Baumann Skin Type : OSNW
Oily, Sensitive, Non-Pigmented, Wrinkle-Prone

OSNW skin types usually are either 1) a young person with acne who has significant sun exposure (e.g., from outdoor sports), 2) an older person with rosacea and photoaging, or 3) an older person with acne. The OSNW skin type has two barriers to skin health: inflammation and age or lifestyle factors that predispose to skin aging. Those with significant sun exposure are at an increased risk for skin cancer, especially if they have a Fitzpatrick Skin Type of I or II.

Product Advice for OSNW

Oily skin types should use foaming cleansers or those with salicylic acid. Treatment products may include anti-inflammatories, antioxidants, and other anti-aging ingredients. Use of

BOX 10-9

Ingredients for OSNW to use:

- Allantoin
- Argan oil
- Caffeine
- Coenzyme Q_{10} (Ubiquinone)
- Defensins
- Feverfew
- Green tea
- Heparan sulfate
- Hyaluronic acid
- Licorice extract
- Niacinamide
- Panthenol
- Resveratrol
- Retinol
- Salicylic acid
- Sulfur

Ingredients for OSNW to avoid:

- Glycolic acid
- Isopropyl myristate
- Octyl palmitate
- Octyl stearate

BOX 10-10

Ingredients for ORPT to use:

- Ascorbic acid
- Glycolic acid
- Hexylresorcinol
- Hydroquinone
- Kojic acid
- Methyl dihydroxybenzoate
- Mulberry extract
- Niacinamide
- Retinol
- Salicylic acid
- Tetrahexyldecyl ascorbate
- Tranexamic acid

Ingredients for ORPT to avoid:

- Bergamot oil
- Estrogen
- Extracts of celery, lemon, lime, parsley, fig, and carrot
- Genistein
- Melatonin

retinoids is highly recommended. If rosacea is present, begin retinoids slowly. Very oily skin types do not need a moisturizer. Normal oily skin types may choose to omit the moisturizer in the AM so that they are more likely to use a daily SPF. A non-comedogenic sunscreen should be used daily (**Box 10-9**).

Procedure Advice for OSNW

This skin type can benefit from salicylic acid peels. Blue light, red light, and lasers can be used to treat acne lesions. Red light, IPL, and lasers can be used to treat rosacea. Facial extractions and hydrafacials are a good option. Botulinum toxins, dermal fillers, microneedling with PRP, and skin-tightening procedures can improve wrinkles and sagging skin.

Baumann Skin Type 9: ORPT
Oily, Resistant, Pigmented, Tight

This is an uncommon skin type. Patients that present with this skin type are young and have uneven skin pigmentation, usually due to an excess of sun exposure. In some cases, a young woman with melasma will be an ORPT. In this case, cessation of oral contraceptives should be considered. In other cases, patients will display phytophotodermatitis that has been provoked by limes, figs, or celery juice touching the skin that is then exposed to sunlight. ORPT has one barrier to skin health: pigmentation that causes an uneven skin tone. This skin type is very close to being ideal. The focus should be on cleansing the skin and protecting it with sunscreen at a minimum. Skin-lightening and exfoliating ingredients can be used.

Product Advice for ORPT

Oily skin types should use foaming cleansers or those with salicylic acid if there are many comedones. Treatment products

may include skin lighteners. It is critical to wear sunscreen every day to improve this skin type (**Box 10-10**).

Procedure Advice for ORPT

Salicylic acid peels with skin-lightening ingredients can clear pores, speed exfoliation, and even skin tone. Microdermabrasion is an option but is not as effective as chemical peels in this skin type. Avoid blue light and microneedling to prevent worsening of pigmentation.

Baumann Skin Type 10: ORNT
Oily, Resistant, Non-Pigmented, Tight

ORNTs are 30 years of age or younger with no skin dryness. Skin is even toned, unblemished, and easily managed. ORNTs are uncommonly seen in a dermatology practice. This skin type is what some call "normal skin." ORNT has no barriers to skin health and is, therefore, the ideal skin type. It is referred to as "Perfect 10 Skin." ORNTs can be very oily, which requires salicylic acid to prevent comedones. However, in most cases ORNTs are the normal oily skin type, which produces exactly enough sebum to hydrate and protect the skin without becoming shiny. Normal oily ORNTs have one goal—to keep the skin the way it is. A salicylic acid cleanser to clear pores and daily sunscreen use are the most important products for this ideal skin type (**Box 10-11**).

Product Advice for ORNT

Oily skin types should use foaming cleansers or those that contain salicylic acid. Sunscreen should be used daily. Talc, acrysorb, and dimethicone can be used to help absorb oil and prevent streaking of makeup. Layering a powdered sunscreen over a light noncomedogenic sunscreen can help reduce shininess.

BOX 10-11

Ingredients for ORNT to use:

- Acrysorb
- Dimethicone
- Retinol
- Salicylic acid
- Talc
- Zinc oxide

Ingredients for ORNT to avoid:

- Borage seed oil
- Coconut oil
- Mineral oil
- Olive oil
- Petrolatum
- Safflower oil

BOX 10-12

Ingredients for ORPW to use:

- Ascorbic acid
- Azelaic acid
- Caffeine
- Coenzyme Q_{10} (Ubiquinone)
- Defensins
- Glycolic acid
- Green tea
- Hexylresorcinol
- Hydroquinone
- Kojic acid
- Linoleic acid
- Methyl dihydroxybenzoate
- Niacinamide
- Oleic acid
- Phloretin
- Resorcinol
- Resveratrol
- Retinol
- Salicylic acid
- Tranexamic acid

Ingredients for ORPW to avoid:

- Borage seed oil
- Coconut oil
- Mineral oil
- Olive oil
- Palmitic acid
- Petrolatum
- Safflower oil

Procedure Advice for ORNT

The only challenge for ORNTs is comedones, so facial extractions, hydrafacials, dermaplaning, and microdermabrasion are the only procedures suggested for this skin type. Avoid microneedling, chemical peels, skin tightening, blue light, red light, IPL, and other treatments that are unnecessary because they pose the risk of causing pigmentation, and would serve no purpose as this skin type is already ideal. Laser hair removal is a good option for this skin type.

Baumann Skin Type : ORPW

Oily, Resistant, Pigmented, Wrinkle-Prone

ORPWs are most likely to have one of three presentations: 1) a young person with significant sun exposure (e.g., from outdoor sports) who usually dislikes the feel of sunscreen and often displays poor sunscreen compliance due to their skin oiliness, 2) a female with melasma that may be due to pregnancy or hormone use, or 3) someone over 30 who did not use much sunscreen in the past. They have trouble finding a sunscreen that does not feel sticky to them. Very oily types have the most difficulty tolerating sunscreen. This skin type often has comedones.

ORPW has two barriers to skin health: pigmentation and risk of aging. Lighter skin types have an increased risk for skin cancer if they have a history of significant sun exposure. Improving lifestyle habits such as sunscreen use, diet, and exercise can help reduce the risk of aging (**Box 10-12**).

Product Advice for ORPW

Oily skin types should use foaming cleansers to remove oil or those with salicylic acid to clear pores. Treatment products may include skin lighteners and antioxidants, as well as other anti-aging products. The most important treatment product to begin is retinoids, which may help reduce sebum production and will target pigmentation and fine lines. Skincare ingredients have difficulty penetrating into this skin type because it has an intact barrier and is protected by a coat of sebum. Many depigmenting and anti-aging ingredients will have trouble penetrating. Use of a salicylic acid cleanser will help loosen SC attachments. Cleansing with warm water may also help penetration. Choose a moisturizer with HA to increase penetration of the treatment products. Avoid moisturizers with saturated fatty acids like palmitic acid because they augment tyrosinase activity.[29] Instead, choose moisturizers with α-linoleic acid or linoleic acid.[30] Another option is oleic acid, which inhibits tyrosinase in addition to increasing penetration of other ingredients.[31] Sunscreen should be used daily. In very oily skin types, omit the AM moisturizer to increase sunscreen compliance.

Procedure Advice for ORPW

ORPWs can benefit from salicylic acid peels with skin-lightening ingredients to clear pores, even skin tone, and give the skin radiance. Hydrafacials, dermaplaning, and microdermabrasion all help increase penetration of cosmeceutical ingredients. Pigmented lesion lasers and IPL can be used to remove solar lentigos. Botulinum toxins, dermal fillers, and skin-tightening devices will help improve sagging and fine lines. If the patient has melasma, blue light and lasers can worsen pigmentation. Microneedling is a good option if the pigmentation is due to solar lentigos rather than melasma.

Baumann Skin Type 12 : ORNW

Oily, Resistant, Non-Pigmented, Wrinkle-Prone

If a patient is over 30 years of age, this is the best of the achievable skin types. (By definition, the ideal skin type, ORNT, occurs only in ages 30 or lower, because skin over the age of 30 is more likely to age due to accumulated sun as well as mitochondrial damage, and other issues discussed in Chapters 5, Intrinsic Aging, and 6, Extrinsic Aging.) The ORNW skin type usually is one of two profiles: 1) a young person who has increased sun exposure due to outdoor sports (this skin type can be improved to ORNT with the addition of sun-protective measures such as sunscreen), or 2) an individual over 30 who has never really had any skin issues in the past. The goal is to add anti-aging skincare.

ORNW has only one barrier to skin health, which is aging (either age above 30 or deleterious lifestyle habits that can be corrected). Addition of protective ingredients such as antioxidants, retinoids, and, of course, sunscreen, are the mainstay of skincare for this coveted skin type.

Product Advice for ORNW

Oily skin types should use foaming cleansers to remove oil and salicylic acid to clear pores and increase penetration of ascorbic acid and other ingredients that follow it in the regimen. Light moisturizers containing HA and heparan sulfate provide light hydration while replacing lost components of the ECM (see Chapter 5). Retinoids are highly recommended. Antioxidants and other anti-aging products are often easily tolerated by this skin type. Sunscreen should be used daily. This skin type can use facial scrubs and brushes to help increase penetration of skincare ingredients (**Box 10-13**).

BOX 10-13

Ingredients for ORNW to use:

- Ascorbic acid
- Caffeine
- Coenzyme Q_{10} (Ubiquinone)
- Ferulic acid
- Glycolic acid
- Green tea
- Heparan sulfate
- Hyaluronic acid
- Idebenone
- Resveratrol
- Retinol
- Salicylic acid
- TGF-β
- Vitamin E

Ingredients for ORNW to avoid:

- Mineral oil
- Petrolatum
- Safflower oil

Procedure Advice for ORNW

ORNWs can benefit from salicylic acid peels to clear pores and give the skin radiance. Hydrafacials, dermaplaning, and microdermabrasion all help increase penetration of cosmeceutical ingredients and impart an instant glow. Microneedling is a great option for this skin type.

Baumann Skin Type 13 : DRPT

Dry, Resistant, Pigmented, Tight

DRPT skin types are young with dry skin and pigmentation. They often have eczema and have turned dark in areas of dryness or scratching. In other cases, this skin type may have melasma caused by use of oral contraceptives or pregnancy. This skin type is usually Fitzpatrick Skin Type III or higher and is very uncommon. DRPT has two barriers to skin health. Dehydration is caused by an impaired skin barrier that renders DRPT skin less able to retain water and protect against irritants and allergens. Pigmentation usually occurs from dryness and scratching of an affected area. In some cases, pigmentation can be due to phytophotodermatitis that occurs when this skin type is exposed to celery, lime, or figs on the skin in the presence of UV light. This can cause pigmentation.

Product Advice for DRPT

Dry skin types should avoid foaming cleansers, especially those with anionic surfactants that strip lipids from the skin (see Chapter 40). Treatment products may include skin lighteners. They should use barrier repair moisturizers twice daily with ingredients such as myristoyl/palmitoyl oxostearamide/arachamide mea. Sunscreen should be used daily (**Box 10-14**).

Procedure Advice for DRPT

DRPTs can get procedures to even the skin tone such as chemical peels, dermaplaning, microdermabrasion, and hydrafacials. Avoid blue light exposure, which can increase pigmentation. If melasma is a concern, avoid IPL, lasers, and light.

Baumann Skin Type 14 : DRNT

Dry, Resistant, Non-Pigmented, Tight

DRNTs are uncommonly seen in a dermatology practice because they only have one barrier to skin health. Their main complaints are dull skin, roughness, and occasionally itching. Dehydration allows the SC to accumulate on the skin's surface in hills and valleys, decreasing the skin's ability to reflect light. Dehydration is caused by an impaired skin barrier that renders DRNT skin less able to retain water and protect against irritants and allergens. This is an easy skin type to treat.

Product Advice for DRNT

Dry skin types should avoid foaming cleansers and instead choose a creamy nonfoaming cleanser or cleansing oil. Facial scrubs will improve skin texture and increase radiance, but excessive exfoliation can worsen dehydration. They should use barrier repair moisturizers twice daily, preferably over damp skin. If dryness continues, consider a water filter in the shower to remove

BOX 10-14

Ingredients for DRPT to use:

- Ascorbic acid
- Borage seed oil
- Ceramide
- Cholesterol
- Defensin
- Dexpanthenol (pro-vitamin B$_5$)
- Dimethicone
- Evening primrose oil
- Glycerin
- Hexylresorcinol
- Hydroquinone
- Hydroxy acids
- Jojoba oil
- Kojic acid
- Linoleic acid
- Myristoyl/palmitoyl oxostearamide/arachamide mea
- Niacinamide
- Retinol
- Safflower oil
- Shea butter
- Stearic acid
- Tranexamic acid

Ingredients for DRPT to avoid:

- Alcohol listed among first seven ingredients
- Anionic surfactants
- Bergamot oil
- Hard water (increased calcium)
- Topical estrogens

BOX 10-15

Ingredients for DRNT to use:

- Alpha hydroxy acids
- Borage seed oil
- Ceramide
- Cholesterol
- Cocoa butter
- Dimethicone
- Evening primrose oil
- Glycerin
- Grape seed oil
- Hyaluronic acid
- Jojoba oil
- Myristoyl/palmitoyl oxostearamide/arachamide mea
- Safflower oil
- Shea butter
- Stearic acid

Ingredients for DRNT to avoid:

- Acetone
- Benzyl alcohol
- Ethyl alcohol
- Isopropyl alcohol
- Olive oil
- SD alcohol

BOX 10-16

Ingredients for DRPW to use:

- Ascorbic acid
- Borage seed oil
- Glycerin
- Glycolic acid
- Grape seed extract
- Hexylresorcinol
- Hydroquinone
- Kojic acid
- Lactic acid
- Macadamia oil
- Methyl dihydroxybenzoate
- Myristoyl/palmitoyl oxostearamide/arachamide mea
- Niacinamide
- Phloretin
- Retinol
- Shea butter
- Tetrahexyldecyl ascorbate
- Tranexamic acid

Ingredients for DRPW to avoid:

- Alcohol
- Anionic detergents
- Hard water (increased calcium)

calcium. Another option is to rinse the face with filtered water. A moisturizing sunscreen should be used daily (**Box 10-15**).

Procedure Advice for DRNT

This skin type does not need any procedures, but in case they complain of decreased radiance, facials, hydrafacials, microdermabrasion, and dermaplaning will smooth the skin's surface and help it reflect light. Avoid unnecessary procedures such as microneedling, which can cause harm. Laser hair removal is safe.

Baumann Skin Type 15: DRPW
Dry, Resistant, Pigmented, Wrinkle-Prone

This very common skin type has several profiles including: (1) a person less than 30 years of age with dry skin who is often in the sun (e.g., playing outdoor sports) and does not wear SPF, (2) a person over 30 with photoaging, and (3) a person with dry skin and melasma, usually female.

DRPW has three barriers to skin health: dehydration (caused by an impaired skin barrier), pigmentation (caused by increased melanin production by melanocytes), and age over 30 or lifestyle factors that age skin (**Box 10-16**).

Product Advice for DRPW

Dry skin types should use non-foaming cleansers, such as a creamy cleanser or a cleansing oil, that deposit lipids on the skin. Hydroxy acid cleansers can be used to smooth the skin's surface. Facial scrubs can improve dull skin but should only be used two to three times a week because excessive exfoliation can injure the skin barrier leading to more dehydration.

Treatment products may include skin lighteners, retinoids, antioxidants, and other anti-aging products and should be applied before a moisturizer. A barrier repair moisturizer such as one with an equal ratio of ceramides, fatty acids, and cholesterol or with myristoyl/palmitoyl oxostearamide/arachamide mea should be used twice daily, preferably over damp skin. Sunscreen should be used daily.

Procedure Advice for DRPW

Procedures should target the pigmentation and any fine lines or sagging skin and can include skin tightening, chemical peels, botulinum toxin, and dermal fillers. Facials, dermaplaning, microdermabrasion, and chemical peels are options. Pigmented lesion lasers, resurfacing lasers, and IPL can be used when the pigmentation was caused by photoaging. However, DRPWs with melasma should avoid blue light, IPL, and lasers, which can worsen skin pigmentation.

Baumann Skin Type 16 : DRNW

Dry, Resistant, Non-Pigmented, Wrinkle-Prone

DRNW is a common skin type that has two barriers to skin health: dehydration and aging risk. The aging risk may be due to age over 30 or lifestyle habits such as sun exposure. Most DRNW skin types are either 1) older than 30 or 2) younger than 30 with deleterious lifestyle habits.

Product Advice for DRNW

Dry skin types should avoid foaming cleansers, especially those with anionic detergents (see Chapter 40). They should use barrier repair moisturizers twice daily, preferably over damp skin. Moisturizers using heparan sulfate and HA without lipids or oils are not sufficient to improve the skin barrier. Use retinoids, antioxidants, and other anti-aging products. Sunscreen should be used daily. Facial scrubs can be used two to three times a week. Avoid excessive exfoliation, which can change this skin type to a DSNW (**Box 10-17**).

Procedure Advice for DRNW

The lack of pigmentation problems makes the incidence of side effects from lasers, lights, and chemical peels lower in this skin type, so these are all good choices. Botulinum toxins, dermal fillers, microneedling with PRP, and skin tightening are ideal options for this skin type. Other choices are facials, hydrafacials, microdermabrasion, and dermaplaning, which provide a temporary benefit by smoothing the SC and increasing the skin's ability to reflect light.

USING SKIN TYPING RESEARCH

When skincare products are tested on skin, the studies should divide subjects by Baumann Skin Type. The skin types included in the study and the methods used to identify the skin type are found in the materials and methods section of the study. For example, a study that demonstrates that an anti-aging moisturizer improves fine lines without causing any side effects is less significant when sensitive skin types are excluded. Skin typing patients prior to inclusion in a study yields more robust, meaningful data.

BOX 10-17

Ingredients for DRNW to use:

- Borage seed oil
- Ceramide
- Cholesterol
- Coenzyme Q_{10} (Ubiquinone)
- Copper peptide
- Defensin
- Genistein
- Glycerin
- Glycolic acid
- Grape seed extract
- Green tea
- Idebenone
- Jojoba oil
- Lactic acid
- Lutein
- Lycopene
- Macadamia oil
- Myristoyl/palmitoyl oxostearamide/arachamide mea
- Retinol
- Safflower oil
- Shea butter
- Silymarin
- Stearic acid

Ingredients for DRNW to avoid:

- Alcohol listed among first seven ingredients
- Anionic surfactants
- Hard water (increased calcium)

CONCLUSION

The Baumann Skin Typing System has been tested on over 300,000 patients and is used by hundreds of dermatologists around the world to prescribe facial skincare routines. It requires use of the validated questionnaire to ensure that the proper diagnoses are reached. Using this taxonomy allows dermatologists, medical providers, aestheticians, cosmetic chemists, researchers, consumers, salespeople, marketers, and patients to speak a common skin type language. Standardization of skin typing using this scientifically based taxonomy allows for genetic, epigenetic, and microbiome research comparing the effectiveness of various skincare products on the Baumann Skin Types.

References

1. Fitzpatrick TB. The validity and practicality of sun-reactive skin types I through VI. *Arch Dermatol.* 1988;124(6):869–871.
2. Eilers S, Bach DQ, Gaber R, et al. Accuracy of self-report in assessing Fitzpatrick skin phototypes I through VI. *JAMA Dermatol.* 2013; 149(11):1289–1294.
3. Stanford DG, Georgouras KE, Sullivan EA, Greenoak GE. Skin phototyping in Asian Australians. *Australas J Dermatol.* 1996;37(Suppl 1):S36–S38.

4. Park SB, Suh DH, Youn JI. Reliability of self-assessment in determining skin phototype for Korean brown skin. *Photodermatol Photoimmunol Photomed*. 1998;14(5-6):160–163.

5. Baumann L. Understanding and treating various skin types: the Baumann Skin Type Indicator. *Dermatol Clin*. 2008;26(3): 359–373, vi.

6. Baumann LS. The Baumann Skin Typing System. In: Farage MA, et al. ed. *Textbook of Aging Skin*. Berlin Heidelberg: Springer-Verlag; 2017: 1579–1594.

7. Baumann L. Cosmetics and skin care in dermatology. In: *Fitzpatrick's Dermatology in General Medicine*, 7th ed. New York: McGraw Hill; 2008: 1357–2363.

8. Baumann LS. The Baumann Skin Typing System. In: Farage M, Miller K, Maibach H. eds. *Textbook of Aging Skin*. Berlin, Heidelberg: Springer; 2015: 1–19.

9. Baumann L. The Baumann skin-type indicator: A novel approach to understanding skin type. In: *Handbook of Cosmetic Science and Technology*. 3rd ed.. New York: Informa Healthcare: 2009: 29–40.

10. Baumann LS, Penfield RD, Clarke JL, Duque DK. A validated questionnaire for quantifying skin oiliness. *J Cosmet Dermatol Sci App*. 2014;4:78–84.

11. Lee YB, Ahn SK, Ahn GY, et al. Baumann skin type in the Korean male population. *Ann Dermatol*. 2019;31(6):621–630.

12. Ahn SK, Jun M, Bak H, et al. Baumann skin type in the Korean female population. *Ann Dermatol*. 2017;29(5):586–596.

13. Choi JY, Choi YJ, Nam JH, Jung HJ, Lee GY, Kim WS. Identifying skin type using the Baumann skin type questionnaire in Korean women who visited a dermatologic clinic. *Kor J Dermatol*. 2016;54(6): 422–437.

14. Baumann L. Cosmeceuticals in skin of color. *Semin Cutan Med Surg*. 2016;35(4):233–237.

15. Baumann L. Validation of a questionnaire to diagnose the Baumann skin type in all ethnicities and in various geographic locations. *J Cosmet Dermatol Sci App*. 2016;6(1):34–40.

16. Lee YB, Park SM, Bae JM, Yu DS, Kim HJ, Kim JW. Which skin type is prevalent in Korean post-adolescent acne patients?: A pilot study using the Baumann skin type indicator. *Ann Dermatol*. 2017;29(6):817–819.

17. Baumann L. 14. A scientific approach to cosmeceuticals. In: Nahai F, Nahai F, eds. *The Art of Aesthetic Surgery, Three Volume Set: Principles and Techniques*. 3rd Edition. New York: Thieme; 2020.

18. Baumann L. How to use oral and topical cosmeceuticals to prevent and treat skin aging. *Facial Plast Surg Clin North Am*. 2018;26(4):407–413.

19. Baumann L, Weisberg E. Skincare and nonsurgical skin rejuvenation, In: Neligan PC, Rubin JP. eds. *Plastic Surgery: Aesthetic*. 4th edition, vol. 2, New York: Elsevier; 2017.

20. Roberts WE. Skin type classification systems old and new. *Dermatol Clin*. 2009;27(4):529–533, viii.

21. Park JW, Park SJ, Park KY, Ahn GY, Seo SJ, Kim MN. P062: A study on the correlation of skin types with genetic factors and environmental factors in Koreans. 프로그램북 (구 초록집). 2019;71(2):354.

22. Youn SW, Kim SJ, Hwang IA, Park KC. Evaluation of facial skin type by sebum secretion: discrepancies between subjective descriptions and sebum secretion. *Skin Res Technol*. 2002;8(3): 168–172.

23. Data unpublished by author. Estimate is based on author's clinical experience and research.

24. Al-Niaimi F, Glagoleva E, Araviiskaia E. Pulsed dye laser followed by intradermal botulinum toxin type-A in the treatment of rosacea-associated erythema and flushing. *Dermatol Ther*. 2020;33(6):e13976.

25. Pilkington SM, Bulfone-Paus S, Griffiths CEM, Watson REB. Inflammaging and the Skin. *J Invest Dermatol*. 2020: S0022-202X(20)32294-6.

26. Choi JE, Werbel T, Wang Z, Wu CC, Yaksh TL, Di Nardo A. Botulinum toxin blocks mast cells and prevents rosacea like inflammation. *J Dermatol Sci*. 2019;93(1):58–64.

27. Kim MJ, Kim JH, Cheon HI, et al. Assessment of Skin Physiology Change and Safety After Intradermal Injections With Botulinum Toxin: A Randomized, Double-Blind, Placebo-Controlled, Split-Face Pilot Study in Rosacea Patients With Facial Erythema. *Dermatol Surg*. 2019;45(9):1155–1162.

28. Daou H, Paradiso M, Hennessy K, Seminario-Vidal L. Rosacea and the Microbiome: A Systematic Review. *Dermatol Ther (Heidelb)*. 2020 Nov 10.

29. Ando H, Watabe H, Valencia JC, et al. Fatty acids regulate pigmentation via proteasomal degradation of tyrosinase: a new aspect of ubiquitin-proteasome function. *J Biol Chem*. 2004;279(15): 15427–15433.

30. Ando H, Ryu A, Hashimoto A, Oka M, Ichihashi M. Linoleic acid and alpha-linolenic acid lightens ultraviolet-induced hyperpigmentation of the skin. *Arch Dermatol Res*. 1998;290(7): 375–381.

31. Naik A, Pechtold LA, Potts RO, Guy RH. Mechanism of oleic acid-induced skin penetration enhancement in vivo in humans. *J Control Release*. 1995;37(3):299–306.

CHAPTER 11

Oily Skin

Leslie S. Baumann, MD

SUMMARY POINTS

What's Important?
1. Oxidation of squalene in sebum leads to comedones and milia.
2. Oxidized squalene (squalene peroxides) has deleterious effects on skin including aging.
3. The Baumann Skin Type Indicator Questionnaire can accurately predict sebum secretion rates.
4. The average sebum production rate is 1 mg/10 cm^2 every 3 hours.

What's New?
1. Oily skin is divided into normal oily skin and very oily skin.
2. Normal oily skin has normal sebum secretion rates.
3. Botulinum toxin Type A reduces sebum production.
4. Various cannabinoids affect sebum production differently.

What's Coming?
1. PPAR and retinoid X receptor agonists and antagonists may be developed topically to control sebum production.
2. The effect of diabetes medications and insulin-like growth factor-1 (IGF-1) on sebum secretion is yet to be established.
3. Autophagy regulates sebum production and is suppressed by testosterone as well as IGF-1 and increased by vitamin D. Development of products that increase autophagy in sebocytes may lead to agents to decrease skin oiliness.
4. More data are needed to compare differences in sebum secretion rates among different ethnicities.

Sebum is a substance produced by the sebaceous gland (SG) that may follow the idiom "too much of a good thing can hurt you." Healthy skin requires a normal amount of sebum production. The average rate of sebum production in adults is approximately 1 mg/10 cm^2 every 3 hours.[1] Production of less than 0.5 mg/10 cm^2 every 3 hours results in dry skin while production of over 1.5 mg/10 cm^2 every 3 hours results in very oily skin. Neither dry nor very oily skin is desirable. Therefore, the goal is a sebum production rate between 0.6 mg and 1.4 mg/ 10 cm^2 every 3 hours.

Sebum production plays an important role in skin hydration by producing lipids, glycerol, and other components necessary for skin hydration and protection. Sebum supplies lipids to the surface of the epidermis that aid in fortifying the skin barrier and preventing transepidermal water loss (TEWL). Sebum contains the lipophilic antioxidants vitamin E and coenzyme Q_{10}, which protect the skin from free radicals.[2]

Excess sebum production produces very oily skin and contributes to the formation of comedones. With continuing advances in understanding the physiology and molecular biochemistry of SGs and lipid metabolism, scientists may soon be able to manipulate sebum secretion and oily skin. This chapter will focus on the various known causes of oily skin and their implications, a dermatologist-developed taxonomy for oily skin types, and the available treatments for oily skin.

NOMENCLATURE OF OILY SKIN TYPES

The Baumann Skin Typing System (BSTS) uses the expression "oily skin" differently than the classic skin type system of dry, normal, oily, and combination skin (see Chapter 10, The Baumann Skin Typing System). "Oily skin" in the BSTS denotes the skin produces *an adequate or excessive* amount of sebum. Oily skin in this classification has two subtypes: normal oily skin and very oily skin. Normal oily skin is healthier and equates to what consumers would describe as "normal skin." Normal oily skin synthesizes approximately 1 mg/10 cm² of sebum every 3 hours. This is the average sebum secretion rate. Skin that makes the average amount of sebum is considered an oily skin type in the BSTS; in order to have healthy hydrated skin an adequate amount of sebum-derived lipids is necessary. An oily skin type is a hydrated skin type because of the effects of sebum and its ability to slow TEWL. Very oily skin is characterized by an excessive amount of sebum production, over 1.5 mg/10 cm² every 3 hours. Very oily skin is what patients commonly refer to as "oily skin."

Is Combination Skin Oily Skin?

The BSTS does not have a designation for combination skin. Instead, there are two situations that encompass what patients might mean when they say they have combination skin.

Changing Skin Type

Many patients self-report seasonal variability in self-perceived oily skin. Strauss surmised that sebum secretion rates do not actually change but the skin is perceived as oilier in hot weather because of changes in the viscosity of skin surface lipids (SSLs) with increasing temperatures.[3] However, sebum excretion rates have been shown to be increased in higher temperatures.[4] Regional and seasonal variations in sebum secretion lead to changes of skin type from dry to oily as demonstrated in a study that tracked sebum secretion in 46 patients over an entire year.[5] Summer was the only season in which a significant increase in sebum secretion was seen. The author has also seen and evaluated several patients in which the Baumann Skin Type (BST) changes between dry and oily. In this situation, the skin is oily in hot, humid environments when there is a higher humidity index. Even if these patients have an impaired barrier, the humidity and layer of sebum on the skin can prevent dehydration, resulting in a normal oily skin type. However, there is not enough sebum production to protect them when humidity levels drop such as in an airplane, or a cold and dry environment. In this situation, the increased TEWL leads to dry skin. Skin that exhibits this behavior *alternates between a dry skin type and a normal oily skin type* seasonally. In other words, the BST changes due to environmental effects.

Oiliness in the T-Zone Type

In all skin types, there are more SGs in the T-zone of the face than on the sides of the face. In the case of a T-zone with excessive sebum production and dryness on the cheeks, this is considered an oily skin type in the BSTS. During the day, the sebum is moved around to the cheeks, which hydrates them. This is considered a *normal oily skin type* because the skin should be treated with a skincare regimen targeted at oily skin to minimize comedones and with the proper cleansers and moisturizer for this skin type.

COSMETIC IMPLICATIONS OF VERY OILY SKIN

Very oily skin is a common complaint in the adolescent age group.[6-12] Those with very oily skin may need to wash their face several times a day to prevent looking shiny during the middle of the day. Individuals with very oily skin who wear makeup report streaking of facial foundation, and an inability to find a sunscreen that does not feel greasy and sticky. These features of very oily skin are disturbing to women and men alike and are perceived to be a serious cosmetic problem leading to a negative self-perception. The shine from the flash in photos is particularly distressing in the age of social media (**Fig. 11-1**). Excessive oiliness is most apparent in the T-zone area (forehead, nose, and chin) (**Fig. 11-2**).[9] Sebum can become trapped inside the hair follicle along with desquamated keratinocytes and form comedones. Oxidation of the squalene in the sebum yields a yellow solid material that leads to the formation of comedones and milia. Oily skin types have

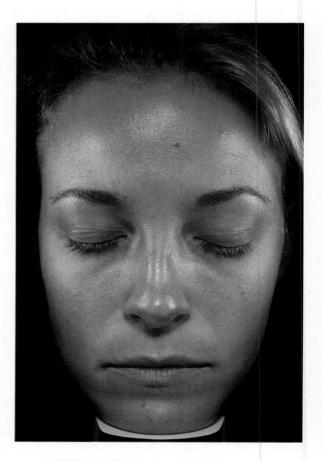

FIGURE 11-1. Oily skin shines in flash photography.

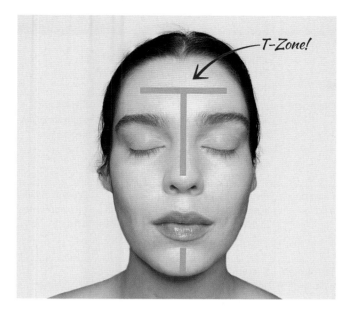

FIGURE 11-2. Sebaceous glands are more prominent in the T-zone.

Patients can be recognized by the following statements:

"I can use any soap to wash my face without developing dryness."
"I never or only occasionally apply a moisturizer."
"I do not apply any products to my face after cleansing."
"My face is oily in some areas."
"My face is very oily."
"I have trouble finding a sunscreen that is not greasy."
"My face is shiny in photographs."
"I wash my face around lunchtime due to shininess."

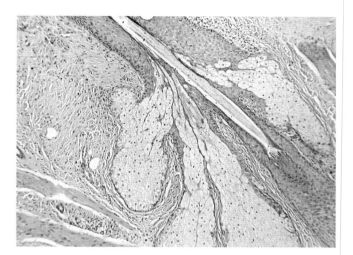

FIGURE 11-4. The pilosebaceous unit. Sebaceous glands are seen to insert into the hair follicle. (From Wikicommons. Image by Kilbad.)

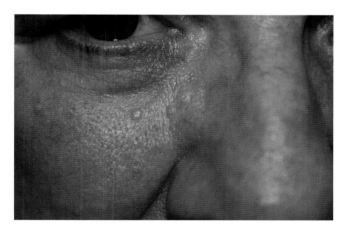

FIGURE 11-3. Sebaceous hyperplasia presents as umblicated papules in sebaceous areas.

SEBACEOUS GLANDS

SGs are uni- or multilobular and found inside hair follicles (**Fig. 11-4**). The hair follicle and SG are known collectively as the pilosebaceous unit. The number of SGs remains approximately the same throughout life, whereas their size tends to increase with age. SGs vary in size and are located throughout the body except the palms and soles. The highest concentration of SGs is found on the face and scalp, but few are found on the lips. (The lips have lower vitamin E and coenzyme Q_{10} levels than the rest of the face because of the lack of sebum.) Although SGs are most frequently associated with hair follicles, SGs are found in some non-hair-bearing or glabrous areas such as the eyelids, where they are called "meibomian glands" (**Table 11-1**).

Components of Sebum

Sebum is a mixture of mostly triglycerides, wax esters, and squalene, but may contain small amounts of cholesterol, cholesterol esters, and diglycerides (**Table 11-2**).

Sebum and the lipids produced by keratinocytes are the source of skin surface lipids that play an important role in skin protection and cell signaling. When sebum is excreted by the

larger pores than dry skin types and sebum output has been shown to correlate with pore size.[13]

SGs that become enlarged are prime for a condition known as sebaceous hyperplasia, which is characterized by 0.5 to 1.5 mm umbilicated papules (**Fig. 11-3**). These umbilicated papules are often scattered in the T-zone area.

Everyone, regardless of skin type, feels dry and sometimes tight after face washing, particularly when using anionic surfactants or hard water (see Chapter 40, Cleansing Agents). It can take SGs 20 minutes to repopulate the skin surface with sebum; therefore, any Sebumeter measurements, photographs, or skin assessments of oiliness should be conducted 30 minutes after washing. **Box 11-1** presents comments often made by individuals with very oily skin that can aid in diagnosis.

TABLE 11-1	Sebaceous Glands Found in Nonhairy Areas of the Skin
Location	Name
Eyelids	Meibomian glands
Nipples	Montgomery's glands
Genitals	Tyson's glands
Oral epithelium	Fordyce's spots

TABLE 11-2	Average Sebum Content[14,15]
Triglycerides and fatty acids	~57.5%
Wax esters	~26%
Squalene	~12%
Cholesterol	~4.5%

TABLE 11-3	Fatty Acids That Affect Sebum Production		
Lauric acid	Bactericidal activity against Gram-positive bacteria[17]	Induces expression of β-defensin 2 in sebocytes[17]	
Oleic acid	Bactericidal activity but also may increase growth of *C. acnes* in low-pH situations[17]	Induces expression of β-defensin 2 in sebocytes[17]	Strong anti-inflammatory properties[15]
Palmitic acid	Bactericidal against *C. acnes*	Induces expression of β-defensin 2 in sebocytes[23]	Broken down into sapienic acid
Palmitoleic acid	Bactericidal activity against Gram-positive bacteria[17]	Induces expression of β-defensin 2 in sebocytes[17]	
Sapienic acid	Bactericidal activity against Gram-positive bacteria[24]	Increased amounts correlate with increased sebum	Found in higher amounts in females with acne[17]
Stearic acid			Found in lower amounts in females with acne[25]

SG, it is immediately acted upon by lipotropic skin microbes, mainly bacteria and yeast, and broken down into substances such as free fatty acids (FFAs) that affect the skin's function.[16] In the case of acne, *Cutibacterium acnes* acts upon the sebum-derived lipids to produce inflammatory FFAs that cause acneiform lesions due to inflammation of the hair follicle.

Triglycerides

Triglycerides (TGs) are split into FFAs by acne-causing bacteria *C. acnes*-derived lipases.[17] Various FFAs exhibit skin activity (**Table 11-3**). FFAs, especially monounsaturated ones, play a role in keratinization, an effect at least partially due to changes in calcium dynamics.[18] Studies looking at the effects of various FFAs on acne have been contradictory and, therefore, their role is uncertain. One study showed that the fatty acid compositions of FFAs and TGs depend upon the total amount of TGs present.[17] The authors found that in females, but not males, higher levels of sapienic acid and lower levels of stearic acid were present. Sapienic acid, which is produced from palmitic acid via the Δ-6-desaturase (D6D) enzyme, is unique to human sebum. The expression of the D6D enzyme is increased when sebum production increases.[19] Low glycemic diets have been shown to change the FFA composition of sebum in males with acne.[20]

Fatty Acids

Linoleic acid and α-linolenic acid are essential fatty acids. Linoleic acid acts on peroxisome proliferator-activated receptors (PPARs). Both linoleic acid and α-linolenic acid are rapidly oxidized and degraded by fatty acid desaturases like stearoyl-CoA D6D.[21] Stearoyl-CoA D6D also converts palmitic acid into sapienic acid, a fatty acid exclusive to sebum. Sapienic acid displays bactericidal and antifungal activities and is found in increased amounts in sebum when sebum secretion rates are higher. Palmitic acid confers direct antibacterial acidity against *C. acnes*. Dietary palmitic acid has been shown to activate Toll-like receptor 2 (TLR-2).[22] TLR-2 plays a major role in acne (see Chapter 16, Acne).

Wax Esters

Wax esters play a role in skin barrier function. They are thought to vary by ethnicity.[26] The fatty acids found in wax esters may be controlled by a genetic component and are known to change with aging.[19,27] The production of wax esters is low in prepubertal children, then spikes at puberty, and slowly declines over the lifetime.[27] C_{16} fatty acids are the main components in wax esters with straight chain fatty acids more predominant than branched chain fatty acids.

Squalene

Squalene is found in large amounts in shark liver (Squalida family), which is where "squalene" derives its name. In humans, squalene is only found in sebum. It is also present in vegetable oils such as olive oil. Squalene is a triterpene with the formula $C_{30}H_{50}$. Its saturated derivate is squalane ($C_{30}H_{62}$), which appears in many cosmetic products. An average of 6–15 mg of squalene is spread on the human face daily.

Oxidation of squalene increases its ability to bind oxygen; in fact, oxidized squalene can bind 25% of its weight in oxygen. This regulates oxygen tension and affects the microbiome microenvironment in the hair follicle. The oxidization of squalene yields squalene peroxides that lead to the formation of comedones, milia, and inflammatory acne lesions.[14] Squalene peroxides are highly comedogenic as shown in an animal model.[28] Oxidized squalene also affects the sunburn process and UV-induced immunological effects.[29] These oxidized squalene peroxides have the same effects on the skin as chronic UV radiation and have been demonstrated to engender fine wrinkles in mice and hyperpigmentation in guinea pigs.[29–31] Most UVB-blocking chemical sunscreens prevent oxidation of squalene but UVA-blocking sunscreens like avobenzone and PABA enhance squalene peroxide formation.[16,29,32]

Functions of Sebum

The biologic roles of SGs are listed in **Table 11-4**. The main function of the SG is to produce sebum. Sebum significantly contributes to providing the skin surface lipids and glycerol necessary for skin hydration. Sebum functions as an occlusive moisturizing agent. It also protects against oxidative stress because it contains vitamin E and coenzyme Q_{10}, powerful antioxidants.[24] Sebum and its components affect the microbiome because resident microbes feed on triglycerides. Sebum also exhibits innate antimicrobial activity because it contains IgG, which is thought to help prevent infection.[33] Similarly, the active cells of the SG, sebocytes, express both pro- and anti-inflammatory properties, are able to utilize cholesterol as a substrate for complete steroidogenesis, present a regulatory program for neuropeptides, and selectively control the actions of hormones and xenobiotics on the skin. The importance of both the SG and sebum production in skin homeostasis is further evidenced by the numerous skin disorders associated with their aberrant activity.[25–40] Of course, the most common of such disorders is acne.

DECREASED SEBUM LEVELS

Skin surface lipids play an important role in skin hydration and communication between the outside world and the skin. Atopic dermatitis and seborrheic dermatitis have been associated with fewer skin surface lipids.[43,44] Atopic dermatitis (eczema) patients have decreased levels of sebum-derived squalene and wax esters. Decreased sebum levels lead to an impaired skin barrier, diminished occlusive protection of the skin's surface, less substrate for lipases to generate FFAs, and attenuated antioxidant protection. Areas of the face with fewer SGs, such as the lips, are at an increased risk of dryness and skin cancer.

SG Count

SG count can reach as high as 400 to 900 glands per cm^2 on the face and less than 100 glands per cm^2 elsewhere on the body.[3] Several studies have used different techniques to evaluate SG count. Early studies that documented SG numbers used either of two techniques: the indirect or the direct. Benfenati and Brilliantini,[43] in their earliest study in 1939, and Powell and Beveridge in 1970,[44] used the indirect technique. The number of lipid-producing orifices per cm^2 of skin surface was measured using osmium tetroxide at room temperature to visualize the small areas of lipids on a collecting paper left over the skin surface for 7 minutes. Adding the osmium tetroxide produced tiny black spots that were counted under a dissecting microscope. The direct technique was used by Cunliffe et al. in 1974 using a surface microscope.[45] This involved staining the skin with Oil Red O (a lipophilic stain) and visualizing with a Leitz MZ surface microscope, which had a graticule attached to the eyepiece allowing the diameter of the pilosebaceous duct exit to be measured. A summary of the techniques and results is displayed in **Table 11-5**. As stated above, the number of SGs remains almost constant throughout life, whereas the size tends to increase with age.

Sebaceous Structure and Secretion

Synthesis and discharge of the lipid contents of sebocytes takes more than a week. The turnover of SGs is slower in older individuals than in young adults. The SG is composed of two types of cells: the lipid-producing cells (sebocytes) and the stratified squamous cells lining the ductal epithelium. Sebocytes pass through three stages to attain a full mature size, namely, the undifferentiated, differentiating, and mature stages. As the sebocytes pass through these stages, the sebaceous cells increase in size because of lipid accumulation and may undergo a 100- to 150-fold increase in volume.[46] The secretion mechanism of SGs is holocrine via rupture of individual sebocytes releasing the sebum,[47] which is discussed below. Sebum is the excretory product of the SGs. It is a mixture of nonpolar lipids synthesized by the SGs. Human sebum contains cholesterol,

TABLE 11-4	Sebaceous Gland Functions
Production of sebum[25]	
Integrity of skin barrier[34]	
Regulation of steroidogenesis[34,35]	
Expression of pro- and anti-inflammatory properties[34,39]	
Selective control on the action of cutaneous hormones[35]	
Regulation of neuropeptides[37]	
Transports antioxidants to skin surface: vitamin E and coenzmye Q_{10}[38]	
Protects keratinocytes against UVB irradiation[38]	
Innate antimicrobial activity[33]	

TABLE 11-5	Number of SGs per cm^2 of Skin in the Forehead of the Human Body		
Study and Year	Number of Subjects	Number of SGs Per cm^2	Technique Used for Sebaceous Count
Benfenati and Brilliantini[43]	4	560 ± 42	Indirect (osmium tetroxide)
Powell and Beveridge[44]	10	518 ± 91	Indirect (osmium tetroxide)
Cunliffe et al.[136]	120	334 ± 20	Direct (surface microscope)

cholesterol esters, fatty acids, diglycerides, and triglycerides in addition to two constituents that are unique to sebum and not produced anywhere else in the body: wax esters and squalene (see **Table 11-6** for the composition of human sebum as compared to other epidermal surface lipids).[48–51]

CIRCADIAN RHYTHM OF SEBUM SECRETION

Sebum production on the face has been revealed to follow a circadian rhythm. One study showed that sebum levels peaked at noon and were at a low at midnight, independent of skin temperature.[52] Other studies have also demonstrated a peak of sebum secretion at noon.[53,54] The rhythmicity of sebum has not been correlated to levels of free testosterone, DHEA, cortisol, or melatonin.[52,55]

EFFECTS OF HORMONES ON SEBOCYTES

Human sebocytes are a major site of hormone production in the skin (**Table 11-7**). Hormones have long been thought to play a role in lipogenesis because sebum secretion increases

TABLE 11-6	Composition of Human Sebum Compared to Epidermal Lipids	
Lipid	Sebum Weight (%)	Epidermal Surface Lipid Weight (%)
Triglycerides, diglycerides, and free fatty acids	57	65
Wax esters	26	–
Squalene	12	–
Cholesterol	2	20

TABLE 11-7	Effects on Sebum and Sebocytes of Various Hormones and Ligands	
Hormone/Ligand	Effects on Sebum	Effects on Sebocytes
2-arachidonoyl-glycerol	Increases lipid synthesis	Promotes differentiation
Acetylcholine	Increases lipid synthesis	
Arachidonic acid	Increases lipogenesis	Induces apoptosis, increases pro-inflammatory cytokines
Arachidonoylethanolamine	Increases lipid synthesis	Promotes differentiation
β-endorphin	Increases lipogenesis	
Cannabichromene (CBC)	Decreases lipid synthesis	

(Continued)

TABLE 11-7	Effects on Sebum and Sebocytes of Various Hormones and Ligands (Continued)	
Hormone/Ligand	Effects on Sebum	Effects on Sebocytes
Cannabidivarin (CBDV)	Decreases lipid synthesis	
Cannabigerol (CBG)	Increases lipid synthesis	
Cannabigerovarin (CBGV)	Increases lipid synthesis	
Cannabinol (CBD)	Decreases lipid synthesis	Decreases proliferation
Capsaicin	Decreases lipogenesis	Suppresses pro-inflammatory cytokines
Δ-9–tetra-hydrocannabivarin (THCV)	Decreases lipid synthesis	
Epidermal-derived growth factor	Inhibits differentiation	
Estrogen	Large doses decrease lipogenesis but physiologic doses do not	
GPR119	Suppresses OEA induction of lipogenesis	
Growth hormone	Increases lipogenesis	Differentiation
Insulin		Proliferation, differentiation
Insulin-like growth factor-1	Increases lipid synthesis	Proliferation, release of inflammatory cytokines
Leptin	Increases lipid synthesis	Induces pro-inflammatory response
Oleoylethanolamide (OEA)	Increases lipid synthesis	Promotes differentiation, induces apoptosis, induces pro-inflammatory response
PPAR agonists	Increase lipid synthesis	
Retinoids (larger dose)	Decrease lipid synthesis	Atrophy of SGs, inhibit proliferation and differentiation
Testosterone	Increases lipid synthesis	
TRPV agonists	Decrease lipid synthesis	Increase proliferation, TRPV3 induces pro-inflammatory response
Vitamin D (125-dihydroxyvitamin D₃ [125(OH)₂D₃])	Decreases lipid synthesis	Induces autophagy

when puberty begins and women with polycystic ovary syndrome exhibit acne. Acne breakouts tend to occur right before a woman's menstrual cycle and a recent study showed that menstruation is accompanied by dilatation of the pilosebaceous ducts reaching its maximum during ovulation and manifesting the maximum amount of sebum secretion.[13] Retinoids, hormones, and growth factors affect SG activity and differentiation. Although these processes are not completely understood, a brief discussion on what is known follows.

Peroxisome Proliferator-Activated Receptors

PPARs act as regulators of gene transcription for genes involved in lipid synthesis and induce sebocyte differentiation.[56–59] PPAR ligands, which stimulate lipid synthesis, include androgens, linoleic acid, retinoids, thiazolidinediones (glitazone drugs used for diabetes), and fibrates.[56,60]

Androgens

Testosterone is not thought to be directly related to sebum secretion because although men have much higher levels of testosterone than women do, their sebum secretion rates are only slightly higher.[61] Sebocytes express androgen receptors and contain multiple androgen-metabolizing enzymes. Androgens increase the proliferation of sebocytes, but this effect seems to depend upon the physical location of the SG (i.e., facial sebocytes are more affected than nonfacial sebocytes).[62] SGs are capable of producing testosterone and of converting testosterone to dihydroepiandrosterone sulfate (DHEAS), which may play a role in acne. DHEAS is converted to testosterone by several enzymes that are found in the SGs, including type 1 5-α-reductase. However, a type 1 5-α-reductase inhibitor was not found to be effective in the treatment of acne.[63] SGs can inactivate testosterone through conversion to androstenedione and 5-androstenedione. Androgens have been shown to increase the growth of SGs through actions on PPAR.

Estrogen

Estrogen receptors α and β are found on SGs. Large doses of estrogen decrease lipogenesis but physiologic doses do not. It seems that the effects of estrogen on SGs is not straightforward.[64] 17β-estradiol has been shown to induce metabolism of prostaglandin D2 to D12-prostaglandin J2, which is the most potent natural ligand for PPAR. Estrogen seems to regulate keratinocyte proliferation through the insulin-like growth factor-1 (IGF-1)/IGF-1 receptor pathway, so it may affect sebocytes through the same mechanism.[65] At this point the role of estrogen in sebum production remains unclear.

Insulin Growth Factor-1

IGF-1 expression is thought to play an important role in sebum production by stimulating SG lipogenesis.[66] IGF-1 increases expression of a transcription factor called sterol response element-binding protein-1 (SREBP-1). SREBP-1 regulates numerous genes involved in lipid biosynthesis and its expression stimulates lipogenesis in sebocytes.[67]

Other Hormones

Sebocytes also express receptors for corticotropin-releasing hormone, proopiomelanocortin (POMC), adrenocorticotropic hormone, α- and β-melanocyte-stimulating hormone, and β-endorphin. It is likely that SGs are affected by stress as many of these hormones are involved in the skin-stress axis.

Growth hormone affects sebocytes and increases sebum production. Increased growth hormone levels have been associated with very oily skin types.[68] Growth hormone accelerates the differentiation of sebocytes, but does not affect their proliferation. IGF-1 increases proliferation of sebocytes as well as the production of inflammatory cytokines and sebum.[69] Insulin stimulates both proliferation and differentiation of sebocytes. Epidermal-derived growth factor (EGF) receptors are found on sebocytes.[70] EGF acts differently on sebocytes *in vitro* versus *ex vivo* and effects on sebocytes have been shown to be species specific.[71] For these reasons, the exact effect of EGF on sebocytes is still not elucidated. Liver X receptors (LXR) play a critical role in cholesterol metabolism. They have been found in sebocytes and play a role in lipid metabolism.[72,73] **Table 11-7** lists a summary of what is known about various ligands and the sebocytes.

CANNABINOIDS AND SEBOCYTES

Sebocytes contain the CB_2 cannabinoid receptor, which mediates the lipogenic effect of endocannabinoids. Sebocytes produce the endocannabinoids arachidonoylethanolamine (anandamide or AEA) and 2-arachidonoylglycerol (2-AG). AEA and 2-AG increase lipid synthesis in sebocytes. Cannabidiol (CBD) decreases sebocyte proliferation and inhibits lipid synthesis.

Like CBD, cannabichromene (CBC), cannabidivarin (CBDV), and Δ-9-tetra-hydrocannabivarin (THCV) significantly reduce arachidonic acid-induced lipid synthesis whereas cannabigerol (CBG) and cannabigerovarin (CBGV) increase basal sebaceous lipid production.

The endocannabinoid-like substance oleoylethanolamide (OEA) is an endogenous activator of GPR119.[74] OEA increases lipid synthesis and induces apoptosis as well as a pro-inflammatory response from sebocytes. GPR119 is expressed in sebocytes and downregulates OEA-mediated lipogenesis. GPR119 is found to be downregulated in acne and therefore may play a role in the etiology of acne.

RETINOID RECEPTORS AND SEBOCYTES

SGs predominantly express RAR-γ and RXR-α. In trace amounts, retinoids promote the growth and differentiation of sebocytes; however, in larger amounts they induce SG atrophy and reduce lipid synthesis.[75] There are two groups of retinoid receptors RAR and RXR, which are discussed in Chapter 45, Retinoids.

RXRs stimulate sebum production. The retinoid X receptor not only stimulates lipid synthesis potently, but also promotes proliferation and differentiation of sebocytes via heterodimerization of RXR:PPAR leading to an increase in sebum production.[59]

All RAR agonists inhibit sebocyte growth and differentiation. At a high dose, the RAR-β,γ agonist adapalene completely obliterates cell growth and, consequently, sebocyte differentiation. Isotretinoin exerts robust suppressive effects on sebum production due to inhibition of sebocyte differentiation, and induction of sebocyte cell cycle arrest and apoptosis. These effects are partially mediated by autophagy.[76] Several studies have shown that isotretinoin increases the FOXO transcription factors that induce autophagy.[77]

AUTOPHAGY, LIPIDS, AND SEBOCYTES

Autophagy is a process that degrades cellular components and organelles. "Phagy" comes from the Greek word *phageîn* meaning to eat or devour. The three types of autophagy are discussed in Chapter 5, Intrinsic Aging. This process is thought to be extremely important in skin aging, especially autophagy of mitochondria and lysosomes. Autophagy that selectively degrades lipids is sometimes called lipophagy.[77]

Autophagy regulates lipid accumulation in sebocytes. The markers of autophagy are expressed in sebocytes in the differentiation phase but not during terminal differentiation. Autophagy markers have been demonstrated to be decreased in acne patients, suggesting that defective autophagy leads to increased lipids resulting in acne.[77] Autophagy in sebocytes declines with exposure to testosterone and IGF-1, both of which are known to contribute to the development of acne. Vitamin D (125-dihydroxyvitamin D_3 [$125(OH)_2D_3$]) induces autophagy and suppresses lipid production in sebocytes.[78] Acne patients have been shown to have lower levels of vitamin D. This may be due to decreased autophagy resulting from reduced vitamin D levels.

OTHER RECEPTORS AND SEBOCYTES

Transient receptor potential vallinoid (TRPV) receptors are found on sebocytes and differentiated sebocytes display a higher level of TRPV activity. TRPV1 and TRPV4 are heat receptors that modulate heat, pain, and itch. TRPV1 is the receptor that senses capsaicin, a component of chili peppers, and gives a sensation of heat. Activation of TRPV cation channels 1, 3, and 4 suppresses lipid synthesis in sebocytes, affects sebocyte proliferation, and mediates gene expression and cytokine production. Capsaicin, as expected, inhibits lipid synthesis in cell cultures of sebocytes.[79] TRPV1 is activated by several factors such as leukotrienes and CBD. TRPV1 and TRPV3 are activated by eugenol.

PPARs are lipid-activated nuclear receptors. They heterodimerize with retinoid X receptors, act as regulators of gene transcription for genes involved in lipid synthesis, and induce sebocyte differentiation.[56-59] PPAR-γ has a significant role in lipid metabolism and is expressed on differentiated sebocytes.

PPAR ligands that stimulate lipid synthesis include linoleic acid, thiazolidinediones (glitazone drugs used for diabetes), fibrates, and arachidonic acid (AA).[56] Activation of PPAR-γ by AA results in formation of neutral lipids and phospholipids. Keto metabolites of AA such as 5-KETE and 12-KETE act as endogenous ligands to activate PPAR-γ. PPAR's action on lipid synthesis may be decreased by TPRV activation.[79,80]

The SG is not innervated by the parasympathetic nervous system but has acetylcholine receptors.[81,82] Specifically, the nAchRa7 acetylcholine receptor has been found on sebocytes. Acetylcholine seems to play a role in skin hydration because patients with atopic dermatitis exhibit increased levels of acetylcholine.[83] Acetylcholine increases lipid synthesis via a MAPK/ERK pathway related to upregulation of PPAR-γ.[83] Decreased ERK signaling is associated with a reduction in PPAR-γ expression. Acetylcholine enhances ERK and PPAR expression leading to an increase in lipid synthesis. Botulinum toxin Type A is known to block acetylcholine activity. As expected, botulinum toxin reduces sebum production by interfering with acetylcholine activity.[81]

HOW TO DIAGNOSE OILY SKIN

Quantitative Evaluation of Sebum

As a determinant of the oiliness and greasiness of skin, evaluation of sebum has long been a target of interest. Sebum evaluation is performed on the skin surface; however, not all SSLs are sebum and, hence, understanding what SSLs are and taking them into consideration is crucial for an accurate estimation of sebum.

SSLs have a dual origin, resulting in a mixture of epidermal components and sebaceous components.[84] Epidermal lipids are secreted by the mature corneocytes and composed mainly of cholesterol, cholestryl esters, triglycerols, ceramides, and hydrocarbons (**Table 11-6**). The ratio of epidermal lipids to sebaceous lipids depends on the body region from which the sample is collected. In 1936, Emanuel reported regional variations of SSL concentrations in different regions of the body.[85] Body regions where the SSLs are predominantly sebum-derived are the forehead, scalp, the upper part of the trunk, and thorax. The epidermal lipid component only accounts for 3% to 6% in these areas, rendering such sites the most suitable for the evaluation of sebum parameters with minimal interference of epidermal lipids.[86-89]

Sebum quantities present on the skin surface may be as high as 100 to 500 $\mu g/cm^2$, compared with quantities as low as 25 to 40 $\mu g/cm^2$ of epidermal lipids.[85,87] Sebum can be measured many different ways as discussed in **Box 11-2** and shown in **Figs. 11-5** and **11-6**.

Diagnosis of Sebum Secretion Using a Questionnaire

Studies have shown that patients tend to underestimate their sebum secretion rates resulting in a self-diagnosis of dry skin or normal skin. In reality, they typically have sebum secretion rates of over 1.5 mg/10 cm^2 every 3 hours. Many people, including dermatologists, have been incorrect about their subjective perception of sebum secretion rates and surprised when objective measurements proved to them that they produced a normal or increased amount of sebum.[90] This self-misperception leads over 50% of people to choose the wrong cleansers and moisturizers for their skin type.[91,92]

BOX 11-2   Sebum Collection Techniques.

Several sebum collection techniques are available. Some of the primary methods employed during more than 50 years of research, which have contributed to the basic knowledge of sebum, are mentioned here.

Extraction: The earliest sebum collection technique. Based on the dissolution of SSLs in an applied solvent to the skin, followed by solvent evaporation and lipid residue analysis.[117,118]

Cigarette paper techniques: Ether-soaked cigarette papers applied in four sheets on the forehead and kept in place by a rubber band. This was followed by gravimetric measurement of sebum.[117,119]

Sebutape method: A more accurate and faster technique using a polymer film for lipid absorption. The polymer tape absorbs SSLs and becomes transparent to light afterwards. Sebutape can be analyzed in many ways, the easiest of which is the visual scoring of the tapes on a 1 to 5 scale (**Fig. 11-5**).[120]

Lipometre: A photometric instrument designed by a group from L'Oréal that utilized a diode light energy for evaluation of sebum lipids that proved fast; however, proper calibration of the device is required for optimal results.[121]

Sebumeter: A sebum-sensitive film attached to a probe is placed on the skin. The device gives the sebum quantification in $\mu g/cm^2$ and corresponds to the total amount of sebum collected on the film. The sampling period is as short as 30 seconds. The device can be interfaced with a computer for data management (**Fig. 11-6**).[122]

In comparing the Lipometre with the Sebumeter, the latter is more practical. The Lipometre must be washed between each application, whereas the Sebumeter procedure uses a new strip with each measurement. Moreover, the Sebumeter can be interfaced with a computer. The Sebumeter and Sebutape are both universally accepted as convenient instruments. Although these devices do not directly measure sebum, they are still useful as a research aid to extrapolate sebum levels.[123]

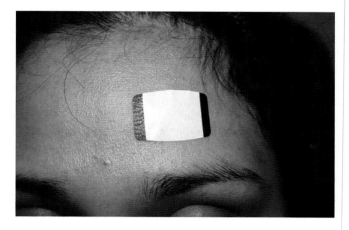

FIGURE 11-5. Sebutape easily measures skin surface lipids.

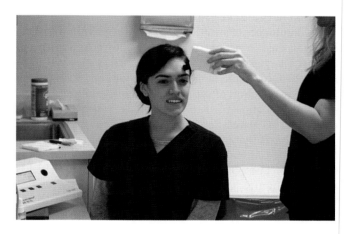

FIGURE 11-6. The Sebumeter is used to measure sebum on the skin.

A person's estimation of their skin type is subject to myriad biases and seasonal variations in sebum secretion can confuse the issue. When patients are asked the sole question, "Is your skin oily or dry?" the responses do not match objective measurements.[93] A scientifically validated questionnaire was developed by the author over a decade of research that involved testing questions against Sebutape and Sebumeter measurements to determine which questions would accurately reflect sebum secretion rates.[94] The BSTI Questionnaire was developed using these questions and has been shown to diagnose the skin type correctly in almost all cases except in patients who do not use any skincare products on their face (see Chapter 10).

In some cases, patients will be confused because they are habituated to using the imprecise terms "combination skin type" and "normal skin type," which are not skin type designations in the BSTS. In the BSTS, "normal skin types" are classified as oily as discussed below. Combination skin types have already been discussed. If patients are confused, explain that the BSTS is based on measurable sebum secretion rates and tewameter skin hydration measurements and the terminology is consistent with the science. Eventually they will learn the correct terminology.

FACTORS PREDISPOSING TO OILY SKIN

Stress and Sebum Production

In early 1972, stress was shown to be associated with an increase in the amount of FFAs on the skin.[95] Since then, much work has been accomplished to evaluate the role of stress in sebum production and acne. Corticotropin-releasing hormone (CRH), also known as a stress hormone, has been found in the SGs as has its receptor CRH-R.[96] CRH directly induces lipid synthesis and enhances the conversion of DHEAS to testosterone in sebocytes.[35,37] It is thought to play an important role in the link between stress and sebum production.[97] The SG also possesses receptors for substance P, which is a neuromediator released in response to stress.[98] *In vitro*, substance P stimulates sebaceous secretion.[99] It is postulated that substance P plays a role in acne as a response to stress.

Sebum and Genetics

Sebum production is also affected by genetic composition. In 1989, Walton et al. suggested in one study that acne development is *mediated* by genetic factors and only *modified* by environmental factors.[100] Their study of 20 pairs of homozygous twins versus 20 pairs of heterozygous twins demonstrated equal sebum excretion in the 20 identical pairs; however, the identical twins exhibited different acne severity revealing an environmental influence in acne development. Conversely, the acne severity and sebum excretion parameters in the 20 nonidentical pairs of twins varied significantly. This study suggested that sebum excretion is under genetic control, but that environmental factors influence acne development. In 2002, a study that examined 458 pairs of monozygotic twins and 1,099 pairs of dizygotic twins implied a strong genetic component in acne.[101] This study did not consider sebum secretion rates; however, many studies have demonstrated increased sebum secretion rates in acne patients.[102]

Predominance of an allele of the gene cytochrome P450 has been reported in patients with hyperseborrhea. Cytochrome P450 is a large supergene family of enzymes involved in the metabolism of a wide range of endogenous and foreign compounds. A mutation of cytochrome P450 could lead to accelerated degradation of natural retinoids, which could cause disordered SG maturation and secretion leading to oily skin.[103]

Notably, B lymphocyte-induced maturation protein 1 (Blimp1), a transcription factor, has been identified within the cells of SGs. One study revealed that Blimp1 acted by repressing c-myc gene expression in mice. Mice without Blimp1 c-myc expression demonstrated an increased number of sebaceous gland-containing cells that divided more frequently. Moreover, these SGs were enlarged, which in turn enhanced the numbers of sebum-producing sebocytes. The Blimp1-containing cells were shown to be the progenitors for the entire SG, and Blimp1 somehow controls this progenitor population, regulating how many cells are allowed into the gland. Blimp1 is thought to act as an inhibitor for SG formation and secretion through repressing the c-myc gene. This study strongly supports the genetic basis of sebum secretion rates.[104,105]

Diet and Sebum

Acne has been shown to worsen in individuals who consume a high-glycemic diet. It remains unclear why this is the case but there are clues. A high-glycemic diet can lead to mTORC1 overexpression and FOXO1 underexpression. Acne patients have been shown to have a similar imbalance in mTORC1 and FOXO1 signaling.[106–108] FOXO transcription increases induction of autophagy while mTORC1 decreases autophagy. This suggests that autophagy plays a role in sebum production and acne.[77]

OILY SKIN AND SKIN OF COLOR

Ethnic differences in sebum secretion have not been well studied. Most of the available reports on oily skin are based on the Caucasian human model; therefore, less is known about sebum secretion in darker skin types. In the few studies performed, one showed that sebum secretion and pore size may be higher in individuals with skin of color versus those with lighter skin.[26] However, a study by Grimes et al. compared instrumental measurements for sebum, pH, corneometry (skin moisture), or TEWL (barrier function) and found no difference between African Americans and Caucasians.[109]

A 2004 study at the University of Miami used the BSTS to look for ethnic differences in skin type.[110] This unpublished study included 399 subjects from four different ethnic groups: Caucasians, African Americans, Hispanics, and Asians. Categorization of skin type according to the BSTS was used and each of the study subjects was designated a skin type. The percentage of oily skin subjects among each ethnic group was in ascending manner: Caucasians (47.13%), Hispanics (55.88%), Asians (57.70%), and African Americans (61.9%). This study was the first to use the BSTS to compare ethnic differences and demonstrates some variability in skin types by ethnicity. Although it reports an increased incidence of oily skin among African Americans, it is important to realize that all subjects were being treated in a general dermatology clinic in Miami and therefore may not be representative of the general population.

Ethnic skin differences in skin lipids remain inconclusive given the discrepancies in study results. Further research is needed to identify the exact areas of differences in order to develop optimum regimens for targeting ethnic skin conditions.

CHANGES IN SEBUM PARAMETERS IN PATIENTS WITH ACNE

It is generally and scientifically accepted that the severity of acne correlates, and is directly proportional, to the sebum secretion level.[111] However, the correlation of sebum excretion rates and acne has been a subject of debate since the early 1960s when Fry and Ramsay measured sebum excretion in 17 acne patients and reported that there was no direct relation of the sebum excretion rate to acne severity.[112] Cunliffe and Shuster, using a superior collection technique in the late 1960s, demonstrated that sebum excretion is directly related to acne severity.[113] (See **Box 11-2** for a review of sebum collection techniques.) Many recent studies have indicated that sebum levels are indeed higher in the population with acne. Piérard et al. demonstrated a higher overall sebum excretion rate in acne subjects when studying it on the forehead using the Lipometre.[10] Piérard-Franchimont et al. noted a change in the rate of sebum excretion directly proportional to the severity of acne.[114] Harris et al. used disks of fine Dacron mesh embedded in fresh clay to report that inflammatory acne patients had a higher sustainable rate of sebum excretion.[115] In 2006, Kim et al. confirmed increased sebum secretion rates in subjects with acne using the Sebumeter in a study on 36 Asian patients.[116] However, it is important to realize that even though acne is associated with high sebum secretion rates, all patients with high sebum secretion rates do not develop acne. Patients with high sebum rates and no acne are classified as oily resistant types in the BSTS (see Chapter 9, Nutrition and the Skin).

Acne vulgaris is a disease of the pilosebaceous unit. Acne is a multifactorial condition with distinct pathologic factors including increased sebum production, ductal hypercornification, colonization of ducts by *Propionibacterium acnes*, and inflammation.[7] For a full review on acne vulgaris, refer to Chapter 16. PPARs α, β, and γ may play a role in acne and increased sebum production. These receptors have been identified in sebocytes, with the γ form deemed the most important. FFAs, linoleic acid, and androgens activate these receptors, which bind to RXR retinoid receptors (in the formation of heterodimers) inducing modifications of sebocyte proliferation and differentiation as well as the synthesis of FFAs. PPARs are therefore involved in the maturation of SGs and initiation of the inflammatory reaction in acne. The PPARs present in the SGs of hyperseborrheic patients are at a higher level, suggesting a disordered effect on the natural retinoids and leading to the development of acne.[26]

SKINCARE FOR OILY SKIN

Oily skin types start out with an advantage because dehydration is not an issue. The main goal in using a moisturizer for oily skin is to provide any needed hydration without causing comedones.

Normal oily types can use a light noncomedogenic moisturizer such as a serum containing hyaluronic acid that will help the other skincare products in the regimen penetrate the skin. Sebum can impede penetration of important ingredients, so the penetration boost provided by hyaluronic acid is a plus. Oily skin types with oiliness confined to the T-zone can use a light moisturizer on the sides of the face, skipping the sebaceous gland-laden T-zone.

Very oily skin types can eliminate the AM and PM moisturizer. It is often difficult to convince very oily skin types to wear a sunscreen; omitting a moisturizer may help increase sunscreen compliance. Layering a powder over sunscreen may help reduce the greasiness that occurs in oily skin patients with sunscreen use. Very oily skin types will benefit from a course of low-dose isotretinoin.

Changing skin types that vary from dry in the winter or dry climates to oily in the summer and warm climates need two completely different skincare routines. Treat for dry skin in cold, dry climates and for oily skin in the warm humid climates.

Topical Agents to Reduce Skin Oiliness

Although several products are touted for inhibiting sebum production, very few, if any, have been conclusively proven to work. Most oil-control products on the market contain talc and other oil-absorbing components that mask or absorb oil rather than function as sebum production inhibitors. Antiandrogens such as ketoconazole and spironolactone have shown some effects.[124,125] Progesterone has demonstrated a short-term effect (2–3 months) when applied topically in women. However, it has not reduced sebum excretion rates in

men.[126] Corticosteroids, erythromycin-zinc complex, elubiol (dichlorophenyl imidazoldioxolan), and an extract from saw palmetto, sesame seeds, and argan oil have all been used for this purpose.[127–130] Notably, topical retinoids have not been shown to decrease sebum secretion; however, oral retinoids have been found to confer such an effect.[131]

Oral Agents to Reduce Skin Oiliness

The most potent pharmacologic inhibitor of sebum secretion is the retinoid isotretinoin (13-*cis* retinoic acid). Reductions up to 90% in sebum excretion rates may be noted as early as 2 weeks after initiating treatment with isotretinoin. Its exact mechanism of action has not been fully described or understood yet, but histologically it shrinks the SG size and the sebocytes lose their characteristic interior accumulation of lipids.[7,132]

COSMETIC PROCEDURES TO TREAT OILY SKIN

In a 2006 study, chemical peels using 30% glycolic acid solution and Jessner's solution were not shown to decrease sebum secretion rates as measured by a Sebumeter.[133] Photodynamic therapy using blue light and 5-ALA (aminolevulinic acid) failed to demonstrate changes in sebum excretion rates, although improvement was observed in acne lesions, as reported in 2007.[134] Microdermabrasion has not been shown to decrease sebum excretion rates.

Botulinum Toxin Injections to Treat Oily Skin

In 2019, 20 patients were treated with intradermal BTX-A on one cheek and saline on the other in a split-face controlled study. Patients and three blinded investigators used a subjective numerical score: 0) dry skin, 1) mild oiliness, 2) moderate oiliness, or 3) severe oiliness. Pore size was scored as: 0) no visible pores, 1) visible pores, 2) enlarged pores, or 3) black heads embedded on facial pores. The total injected BTX-A dose was 10 units. Both sebum and pore size scores were significantly decreased ($P = .001$). When the saline-treated side sebum scores were compared to the side treated with BTX-A at 1 month, a significant difference was seen ($P = .008$). Pore size change was not statistically significant ($P = .05$).

In 2021, a study to determine the best dose of abobotulinum toxin A to reduce oiliness of the forehead was conducted comparing doses of 0, 15, 30, and 45 units. Subjects that received 30 or 45 units were scored by both investigators and subjects as less oily ($P < .05$), especially at months 2 and 3. Changes in Sebumeter measurements were statistically significant for the subjects who received 30 and 45 units ($P < 0.05$).[135] Subjects treated with 15 units did not have a significant difference in subject, investigator, or Sebumeter scores.

The mechanism by which BTX-A reduces sebum secretion can be explained by the effects of acetylcholine on sebum secretion as discussed above or decreased contraction of the arrector pili muscle, which is stimulated by acetylcholine (**Fig. 11-7**).

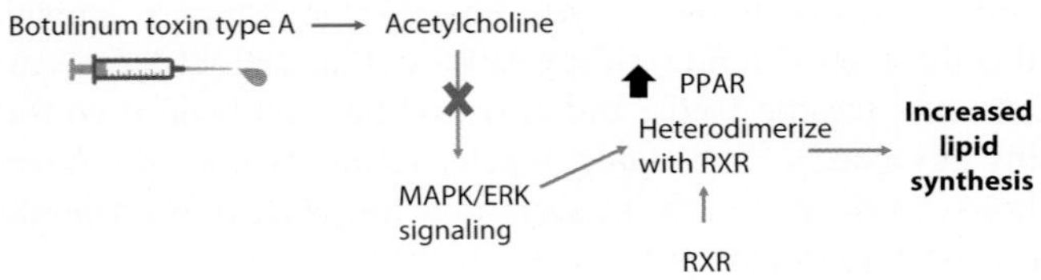

FIGURE 11-7. Botulinum toxin blocks the release of acetylcholine, which prevents MAPK/ERK signaling that results in decreased lipid synthesis.

CONCLUSION

A common condition that presents in varying degrees, oily skin can be divided into two subtypes, normal oily skin or very oily skin. The amount of sebum secretion determines the skin type. Oily skin ranges from the perfect healthy hydrated skin type to a mild cosmetic burden to a troublesome skin disease manifesting as acne. New understanding of sebocytes and how they are controlled by various receptors, hormones, cell signals, and other ligands will lead to novel ways to approach oily skin. For now, the best options, depending upon severity, are foaming and salicylic acid cleansers, noncomedogenic moisturizers, oral retinoids, and intradermal botulinum toxin.

References

1. Honari G. Skin structure and function. In: Honari G, Andersen R, Maibach HL, eds. *Sensitive Skin Syndrome*. Second Edition. CRC Press; 2017: 26–32.

2. Passi S, De Pità O, Puddu P, Littarru GP. Lipophilic antioxidants in human sebum and aging. *Free Radic Res*. 2002;36(4): 471–7.

3. Strauss J, Downing FJ, Ebling ME, Stewart ME. Sebaceous glands. In: Goldsmith LA, ed. *Physiology Biochemistry and Molecular Biology of the Skin*. New York, NY: Oxford University Press; 1991: 712–740.

4. Cunliffe WJ, Burton JL, Shuster S. The effect of local temperature variations on the sebum excretion rate. *Br J Dermatol*. 1970; 83(6):650–4.

5. Youn SW, Na JI, Choi SY, Huh CH, Park KC. Regional and seasonal variations in facial sebum secretions: a proposal for the definition of combination skin type. *Skin Res Technol*. 2005;11(3):189–95.

6. Nouveau-Richard S, Zhu W, Li YH, et al. Oily skin: specific features in Chinese women. *Skin Res Technol*. 2007;13(1):43–8.

7. Clarke SB, Nelson AM, George RE, Thiboutot DM. Pharmacologic modulation of sebaceous gland activity: mechanisms and clinical applications. *Dermatol Clin*. 2007;25(2):137–46.

8. Segot-Chicq E, Compan-Zaouati D, Wolkenstein P, et al. Development and validation of a questionnaire to evaluate how a cosmetic product for oily skin is able to improve well-being in women. *J Eur Acad Dermatol Venereol*. 2007;21(9):1181–6.

9. Thiboutot D. Regulation of human sebaceous glands. *J Invest Dermatol*. 2004;123(1):1–12.

10. Piérard GE, Piérard-Franchimont C, Lê T, Lapière C. Patterns of follicular sebum excretion rate during lifetime. *Arch Dermatol Res*. 1987;279(Suppl):S104–S107.

11. Daniel F. The seborrheic skin. *Rev Prat*. 1985;35(53):3215–24.

12. Lasek RJ, Chren MM. Acne vulgaris and the quality of life of adult dermatology patients. *Arch Dermatol*. 1998;134(4):454–8.

13. Roh M, Han M, Kim D, Chung K. Sebum output as a factor contributing to the size of facial pores. *Br J Dermatol*. 2006;155(5):890–4.

14. Pham DM, Boussouira B, Moyal D, Nguyen QL. Oxidization of squalene, a human skin lipid: a new and reliable marker of environmental pollution studies. *Int J Cosmet Sci*. 2015;37(4):357–65.

15. Lovászi M, Szegedi A, Zouboulis CC, Törőcsik D. Sebaceous-immunobiology is orchestrated by sebum lipids. *Dermatoendocrinol*. 2017;9(1):e1375636.

16. De Luca C, Valacchi G. Surface lipids as multifunctional mediators of skin responses to environmental stimuli. *Mediators Inflamm*. 2010;2010:321494.

17. Akaza N, Akamatsu H, Numata S, et al. Fatty acid compositions of triglycerides and free fatty acids in sebum depend on amount of triglycerides, and do not differ in presence or absence of acne vulgaris. *J Dermatol*. 2014;41(12):1069–76.

18. Katsuta Y, Iida T, Inomata S, Denda M. Unsaturated fatty acids induce calcium influx into keratinocytes and cause abnormal differentiation of epidermis. *J Invest Dermatol*. 2005;124(5):1008–13.

19. Yamamoto A, Serizawa S, Ito M, Sato Y. Effect of aging on sebaceous gland activity and on the fatty acid composition of wax esters. *J Invest Dermatol*. 1987;89(5):507–12.

20. Smith RN, Braue A, Varigos GA, Mann NJ. The effect of a low glycemic load diet on acne vulgaris and the fatty acid composition of skin surface triglycerides. *J Dermatol Sci*. 2008;50(1):41–52.

21. Ge L, Gordon JS, Hsuan C, Stenn K, Prouty SM. Identification of the delta-6 desaturase of human sebaceous glands: expression and enzyme activity. *J Invest Dermatol*. 2003;120(5):707–14.

22. Snodgrass RG, Huang S, Choi IW, Rutledge JC, Hwang DH. Inflammasome-mediated secretion of IL-1β in human monocytes through TLR2 activation; modulation by dietary fatty acids. *J Immunol*. 2013;191(8):4337–47.

23. Nakatsuji T, Kao MC, Zhang L, Zouboulis CC, Gallo RL, Huang CM. Sebum free fatty acids enhance the innate immune defense of human sebocytes by upregulating beta-defensin-2 expression. *J Invest Dermatol*. 2010;130(4):985–94.

24. Rawlings AV. Ethnic skin types: are there differences in skin structure and function? *Int J Cosmet Sci*. 2006;28(2):79–93.

25. Jacobsen E, Billings JK, Frantz RA, Kinney CK, Stewart ME, Downing DT. Age-related changes in sebaceous wax ester secretion rates in men and women. *J Invest Dermatol*. 1985;85(5):483–5.

26. Chiba K, Yoshizawa K, Makino I, Kawakami K, Onoue M. Comedogenicity of squalene monohydroperoxide in the skin after topical application. *J Toxicol Sci*. 2000;25(2):77–83.

27. Chiba K, Kawakami K, Sone T, Onoue M. Characteristics of skin wrinkling and dermal changes induced by repeated application of squalene monohydroperoxide to hairless mouse skin. *Skin Pharmacol Appl Skin Physiol*. 2003;16(4):242–51.

28. Chiba K, Sone T, Kawakami K, Onoue M. Skin roughness and wrinkle formation induced by repeated application of squalene-monohydroperoxide to the hairless mouse. *Exp Dermatol*. 1999; 8(6):471–9.

29. Ryu A, Arakane K, Koide C, Arai H, Nagano T. Squalene as a target molecule in skin hyperpigmentation caused by singlet oxygen. *Biol Pharm Bull*. 2009;32(9):1504–9.

30. De Luca C, Grandinetti M, Stancato A, Passi S. How antioxidants are sunscreen agents? in *Proceedings of the 7th Congress European Society for Photobiology*, Stresa, Italy, September 1997.

31. Thiele JJ, Weber SU, Packer L. Sebaceous gland secretion is a major physiologic route of vitamin E delivery to skin. *J Invest Dermatol*. 1999;113(6):1006–10.

32. Gebhart W, Metze D, Jurecka W. Identification of secretory immunoglobulin A in human sweat and sweat glands. *J Invest Dermatol*. 1989;92(4):648.

33. Zouboulis CC, Fimmel S, Ortmann J, et al. Sebaceous glands. In: Hoath SB, Maibach HI, eds. *Neonatal Skin:Structure and Function*. New York, NY: Marcel Dekker; 2003: 59–88.

34. Zouboulis CC. Human skin: an independent peripheral endocrine organ. *Horm Res*. 2000;54(5-6):230–42.

35. Fritsch M, Orfanos CE, Zouboulis CC. Sebocytes are the key regulators of androgen homeostasis in human skin. *J Invest Dermatol*. 2001;116(5):793–800.

36. Thiboutot D, Jabara S, McAllister JM, et al. Human skin is a steroidogenic tissue: steroidogenic enzymes and cofactors are expressed in epidermis, normal sebocytes, and an immortalized sebocyte cell line (SEB-1). *J Invest Dermatol*. 2003;120(6):905–14.

37. Zouboulis CC, Seltmann H, Hiroi N, et al. Corticotropin-releasing hormone: an autocrine hormone that promotes lipogenesis in human sebocytes. *Proc Natl Acad Sci U S A*. 2002;99(10):7148–53.

38. Zouboulis CC. Acne and sebaceous gland function. *Clin Dermatol*. 2004 Sep–Oct;22(5):360–6.

39. Zouboulis CC. Is acne vulgaris a genuine inflammatory disease? *Dermatology*. 2001;203(4):277–9.

40. Böhm M, Schiller M, Ständer S, et al. Evidence for expression of melanocortin-1 receptor in human sebocytes in vitro and in situ. *J Invest Dermatol*. 2002;118(3):533–9.

41. Passi S, Picardo M, Morrone A, De Luca C, Ippolito F. Skin surface lipids in HIV sero-positive and HIV sero-negative patients affected with seborrheic dermatitis. *J Dermatol Sci*. 1991;2(2):84–91.

42. Picardo M, Passi S, De Luca C, Morrone A, Bartoli F, Ippolito F. Skin surface lipids in patients affected with atopic dermatitis. In: Czernielewski JM, ed. *Immunological and Pharmacological Aspects of Atopic and Contact Eczema*. Vol. 4. Basel: Karger; 1991: 173–174.

43. Benfenati A, Brillanti F. Sulla distribuzione delle ghiandole sebacee nella cute del corpo umano. *Arch Ital Dermatol*. 1939;15:33–42.

44. Powell EW, Beveridge GW. Sebum excretion and sebum composition in adolescent men with and without acne vulgaris. *Br J Dermatol*. 1970;82(3):243–9.

45. Cunliffe WJ, Forster RA, Williams M. A surface microscope for clinical and laboratory use. *Br J Dermatol*. 1974;90(6):619–22.

46. Tosti A. A comparison of the histodynamics of sebaceous glands and epidermis in man: a microanatomic and morphometric study. *J Invest Dermatol*. 1974;62(3):147–52.

47. Jenkinson DM, Elder HY, Montgomery I, Moss VA. Comparative studies of the ultrastructure of the sebaceous gland. *Tissue Cell*. 1985;17(5):683–98.

48. Rajaratnam RA, Gylling H, Miettinen TA. Serum squalene in postmenopausal women without and with coronary artery disease. *Atherosclerosis*. 1999;146(1):61–4.

49. Pochi PE, Strauss JS, Downing DT. Age-related changes in sebaceous gland activity. *J Invest Dermatol*. 1979;73(1):108–11.

50. Stewart ME, Downing DT. Proportions of various straight and branched fatty acid chain types in the sebaceous wax esters of young children. *J Invest Dermatol*. 1985;84(6):501–3.

51. Stewart ME, Quinn MA, Downing DT. Variability in the fatty acid composition of wax esters from vernix caseosa and its possible relation to sebaceous gland activity. *J Invest Dermatol*. 1982;78(4):291–5.

52. Le Fur I, Reinberg A, Lopez S, Morizot F, Mechkouri M, Tschachler E. Analysis of circadian and ultradian rhythms of skin surface properties of face and forearm of healthy women. *J Invest Dermatol*. 2001;117(3):718–24.

53. Verschoore M, Poncet M, Krebs B, Ortonne JP. Circadian variations in the number of actively secreting sebaceous follicles and androgen circadian rhythms. *Chronobiol Int*. 1993;10(5):349–59.

54. Burton JL, Cunliffe WJ, Shuster S. Circadian rhythm in sebum excretion. *Br J Dermatol*. 1970;82(5):497–501.

55. Yosipovitch G, Xiong GL, Haus E, Sackett-Lundeen L, Ashkenazi I, Maibach HI. Time-dependent variations of the skin barrier function in humans: transepidermal water loss, stratum corneum hydration, skin surface pH, and skin temperature. *J Invest Dermatol*. 1998;110(1):20–3.

56. Trivedi NR, Cong Z, Nelson AM, et al. Peroxisome proliferator-activated receptors increase human sebum production. *J Invest Dermatol*. 2006;126(9):2002–9.

57. Wahli W, Braissant O, Desvergne B. Peroxisome proliferator activated receptors: transcriptional regulators of adipogenesis, lipid metabolism and more… *Chem Biol*. 1995;2(5):261–6.

58. Tontonoz P, Singer S, Forman BM, et al. Terminal differentiation of human liposarcoma cells induced by ligands for peroxisome proliferator-activated receptor gamma and the retinoid X receptor. *Proc Natl Acad Sci U S A*. 1997;94(1):237–41.

59. Rosenfield RL, Kentsis A, Deplewski D, Ciletti N. Rat preputial sebocyte differentiation involves peroxisome proliferator-activated receptors. *J Invest Dermatol*. 1999;112(2):226–32.

60. Makrantonaki E, Zouboulis CC. Testosterone metabolism to 5alpha-dihydrotestosterone and synthesis of sebaceous lipids is regulated by the peroxisome proliferator-activated receptor ligand linoleic acid in human sebocytes. *Br J Dermatol*. 2007;156(3):428–32.

61. Nelson AM, Thiboutot DM. Biology of sebaceous glands. In: Wolff K, Goldsmith LA, Katz SI, Gilchrest BA, Paller AS, Leffell DJ, eds. *Fitzpatrick's Dermatology in General Medicine*. 7th ed. New York, NY: McGraw-Hill; 2007: p. 689.

62. Szöllősi AG, Oláh A, Bíró T, Tóth BI. Recent advances in the endocrinology of the sebaceous gland. *Dermatoendocrinol*. 2018 Jan 23;9(1):e1361576.

63. Leyden J, Bergfeld W, Drake L, et al. A systemic type I 5 alpha-reductase inhibitor is ineffective in the treatment of acne vulgaris. *J Am Acad Dermatol*. 2004;50(3):443–7.

64. Smith KR, Thiboutot DM. Thematic review series: skin lipids. Sebaceous gland lipids: friend or foe? *J Lipid Res*. 2008;49(2):271–81.

65. Zouboulis CC, Boschnakow A. Chronological ageing and photoageing of the human sebaceous gland. *Clin Exp Dermatol*. 2001;26(7):600–7.

66. Smith TM, Cong Z, Gilliland KL, Clawson GA, Thiboutot DM. Insulin-like growth factor-1 induces lipid production in human SEB-1 sebocytes via sterol response element-binding protein-1. *J Invest Dermatol*. 2006;126(6):1226–32.

67. Smith TM, Gilliland K, Clawson GA, Thiboutot D. IGF-1 induces SREBP-1 expression and lipogenesis in SEB-1 sebocytes via activation of the phosphoinositide 3-kinase/Akt pathway. *J Invest Dermatol*. 2008;128(5):1286–93.

68. Deplewski D, Rosenfield RL. Growth hormone and insulin-like growth factors have different effects on sebaceous cell growth and differentiation. *Endocrinology*. 1999;140(9):4089–94.

69. Kim H, Moon SY, Sohn MY, Lee WJ. Insulin-Like Growth Factor-1 Increases the Expression of Inflammatory Biomarkers and Sebum Production in Cultured Sebocytes. *Ann Dermatol.* 2017;29(1):20–25.

70. Nanney LB, Magid M, Stoscheck CM, King LEJr. Comparison of epidermal growth factor binding and receptor distribution in normal human epidermis and epidermal appendages. *J Invest Dermatol.* 1984 Nov;83(5):385–93.

71. Zouboulis CC. Epidermal growth factor receptor and the sebaceous gland. *Exp Dermatol.* 2013;22(11):695–6.

72. Hong I, Lee MH, Na TY, Zouboulis CC, Lee MO. LXRalpha enhances lipid synthesis in SZ95 sebocytes. *J Invest Dermatol.* 2008;128(5):1266–72.

73. Schmuth M, Elias PM, Hanley K, et al. The effect of LXR activators on AP-1 proteins in keratinocytes. *J Invest Dermatol.* 2004;123(1):41–8.

74. Markovics A, Angyal Á, Tóth KF, et al. GPR119 Is a Potent Regulator of Human Sebocyte Biology. *J Invest Dermatol.* 2020;140(10):1909–1918.e8.

75. Kim MJ, Ciletti N, Michel S, Reichert U, Rosenfield RL. The role of specific retinoid receptors in sebocyte growth and differentiation in culture. *J Invest Dermatol.* 2000;114(2):349–53.

76. Tsukada M, Schröder M, Roos TC, et al. 13-cis retinoic acid exerts its specific activity on human sebocytes through selective intracellular isomerization to all-trans retinoic acid and binding to retinoid acid receptors. *J Invest Dermatol.* 2000;115(2):321–7.

77. Seo SH, Jung JY, Park K, Hossini AM, Zouboulis CC, Lee SE. Autophagy regulates lipid production and contributes to the sebosuppressive effect of retinoic acid in human SZ95 sebocytes. *J Dermatol Sci.* 2020;98(2):128–136.

78. Zouboulis CC, Seltmann H, Abdel-Naser MB, Hossini AM, Menon GK, Kubba R. Effects of Extracellular Calcium and 1,25 dihydroxyvitamin D3 on Sebaceous Gland Cells In vitro and In vivo. Acta Derm Venereol. 2017;97(3):313–320.

79. Tóth BI, Géczy T, Griger Z, et al. Transient receptor potential vanilloid-1 signaling as a regulator of human sebocyte biology. *J Invest Dermatol.* 2009;129(2):329–39.

80. Dozsa A, Dezso B, Toth BI, et al. PPARγ-mediated and arachidonic acid-dependent signaling is involved in differentiation and lipid production of human sebocytes. *J Invest Dermatol.* 2014;134(4):910–920.

81. Li ZJ, Park SB, Sohn KC, et al. Regulation of lipid production by acetylcholine signalling in human sebaceous glands. *J Dermatol Sci.* 2013;72(2):116–22.

82. Kurzen H, Berger H, Jäger C, et al. Phenotypical and molecular profiling of the extraneuronal cholinergic system of the skin. *J Invest Dermatol.* 2004;123(5):937–49.

83. Wessler I, Reinheimer T, Kilbinger H, et al. Increased acetylcholine levels in skin biopsies of patients with atopic dermatitis. *Life Sci.* 2003;72(18-19):2169–72.

84. Clarys P, Barel A. Quantitative evaluation of skin surface lipids. *Clin Dermatol.* 1995;13(4):307–21.

85. Saint-Léger D. Quantification of skin surface lipids and skin flora. In: Leveque JL, ed. *Cutaneous Investigation in Health and Disease: Non-invasive Methods and Instrumentations.* New York, NY: Basel, Marcel Dekker; 1989: 153–182.

86. Blume U, Ferracin J, Verschoore M, Czernielewski JM, Schaefer H. Physiology of the vellus hair follicle: hair growth and sebum excretion. *Br J Dermatol.* 1991;124(1):21–8.

87. Greene RS, Downing DT, Pochi PE, Strauss JS. Anatomical variation in the amount and composition of human skin surface lipid. *J Invest Dermatol.* 1970;54(3):240–7.

88. Vantrou M, Venencie PY, Chaumeil JC. Skin surface lipids in man: origins, synthesis and regulation. *Ann Dermatol Venereol.* 1987;114(9):1115–1129.

89. Verschoore M. Hormonal aspects of acne. *Ann Dermatol Venereol.* 1987;114(3):439–454.

90. Data on file by author. Based on author's clinical observations.

91. Data unpublished by author. Estimate is based on author's clinical experience and research.

92. Al-Niaimi F, Glagoleva E, Araviiskaia E. Pulsed dye laser followed by intradermal botulinum toxin type-A in the treatment of rosacea-associated erythema and flushing. *Dermatol Ther.* 2020;33(6):e13976.

93. Youn SW, Kim SJ, Hwang IA, Park KC. Evaluation of facial skin type by sebum secretion: discrepancies between subjective descriptions and sebum secretion. *Skin Res Technol.* 2002;8(3): 168–72.

94. Baumann LS, Penfield RD, Clarke JL, Duque DK. A validated questionnaire for quantifying skin oiliness. *J Cosmet Dermatol Sci App.* 2014;4:78–84.

95. Kraus SJ. Stress, acne and skin surface free fatty acids. *Psychosom Med.* 1970;32(5):503–8.

96. Kono M, Nagata H, Umemura S, Kawana S, Osamura RY. In situ expression of corticotropin-releasing hormone (CRH) and proopiomelanocortin (POMC) genes in human skin. *FASEB J.* 2001;15(12):2297–9.

97. Krause K, Schnitger A, Fimmel S, Glass E, Zouboulis CC. Corticotropin-releasing hormone skin signaling is receptor-mediated and is predominant in the sebaceous glands. *Horm Metab Res.* 2007;39(2):166–70.

98. Singh LK, Pang X, Alexacos N, Letourneau R, Theoharides TC. Acute immobilization stress triggers skin mast cell degranulation via corticotropin releasing hormone, neurotensin, and substance P: A link to neurogenic skin disorders. *Brain Behav Immun.* 1999;13(3):225–39.

99. Toyoda M, Morohashi M. Pathogenesis of acne. *Med Electron Microsc.* 2001;34(1):29–40.

100. Walton S, Wyatt EH, Cunliffe WJ. Genetic control of sebum excretion and acne—a twin study. *Br J Dermatol.* 1988;118(3):393–6.

101. Bataille V, Snieder H, MacGregor AJ, Sasieni P, Spector TD. The influence of genetics and environmental factors in the pathogenesis of acne: a twin study of acne in women. *J Invest Dermatol.* 2002;119(6):1317–22.

102. Stewart ME, Grahek MO, Cambier LS, Wertz PW, Downing DT. Dilutional effect of increased sebaceous gland activity on the proportion of linoleic acid in sebaceous wax esters and in epidermal acylceramides. *J Invest Dermatol.* 1986;87(6):733–6.

103. Paraskevaidis A, Drakoulis N, Roots I, Orfanos CE, Zouboulis CC. Polymorphisms in the human cytochrome P-450 1A1 gene (CYP1A1) as a factor for developing acne. *Dermatology.* 1998;196(1):171–5.

104. Horsley V, O'Carroll D, Tooze R, et al. Blimp1 defines a progenitor population that governs cellular input to the sebaceous gland. *Cell.* 2006;126(3):597–609.

105. Arnold I, Watt FM. c-Myc activation in transgenic mouse epidermis results in mobilization of stem cells and differentiation of their progeny. *Curr Biol.* 2001;11(8):558–68.

106. Agamia NF, Abdallah DM, Sorour O, Mourad B, Younan DN. Skin expression of mammalian target of rapamycin and forkhead box transcription factor O1, and serum insulin-like growth factor-1 in patients with acne vulgaris and their relationship with diet. *Br J Dermatol.* 2016;174(6):1299–307.

107. Melnik BC. Western diet-induced imbalances of FoxO1 and mTORC1 signalling promote the sebofollicular inflammasomopathy acne vulgaris. *Exp Dermatol.* 2016;25(2):103–4.

108. Melnik B. Dietary intervention in acne: Attenuation of increased mTORC1 signaling promoted by Western diet. *Dermatoendocrinol.* 2012;4(1):20–32.

109. Grimes P, Edison BL, Green BA, Wildnauer RH. Evaluation of inherent differences between African American and white skin surface properties using subjective and objective measures. *Cutis.* 2004;73(6):392–6.

110. Data on file with author.

111. Youn SW, Park ES, Lee DH, Huh CH, Park KC. Does facial sebum excretion really affect the development of acne? *Br J Dermatol.* 2005;153(5):919–24.

112. Fry L, Ramsay CA. Tetracycline in acne vulgaris. Clinical evaluation and the effect of sebum production. *Br J Dermatol.* 1966;78(12):653–60.

113. Cunliffe WJ, Shuster S. Pathogenesis of acne. *Lancet.* 1969;1(7597):685–7.

114. Piérard-Franchimont C, Piérard GE, Saint-Léger D, Lévêque JL, Kligman AM. Comparison of the kinetics of sebum secretion in young women with and without acne. *Dermatologica.* 1991;183(2):120–2.

115. Harris HH, Downing DT, Stewart ME, Strauss JS. Sustainable rates of sebum secretion in acne patients and matched normal control subjects. *J Am Acad Dermatol.* 1983;8(2):200–3.

116. Kim MK, Choi SY, Byun HJ, et al. Comparison of sebum secretion, skin type, pH in humans with and without acne. *Arch Dermatol Res.* 2006;298(3):113–9.

117. Piérard GE, Piérard-Franchimont C, Marks R, Paye M, Rogiers V. EEMCO guidance for the in vivo assessment of skin greasiness. The EEMCO Group. *Skin Pharmacol Appl Skin Physiol.* 2000;13(6):372–89.

118. Lavrijsen AP, Higounenc IM, Weerheim A, et al. Validation of an in vivo extraction method for human stratum corneum ceramides. *Arch Dermatol Res.* 1994;286(8):495–503.

119. Chivot M, Zeziola F, Saurat JH. The rate of sebum excretion in man. A study on the reproducibility and the accuracy of the gravimetric method. *Br J Dermatol.* 1981;105(6):701–5.

120. Serup J. Formation of oiliness and sebum output—comparison of a lipid-absorbant and occlusive-tape method with photometry. *Clin Exp Dermatol.* 1991;16(4):258–63.

121. Saint-Leger D, Berrebi C, Duboz C, Agache P. The lipometre: an easy tool for rapid quantitation of skin surface lipids (SSL) in man. *Arch Dermatol Res.* 1979;265(1):79–89.

122. Cunliffe WJ, Kearney JN, Simpson NB. A modified photometric technique for measuring sebum excretion rate. *J Invest Dermatol.* 1980;75(5):394–8.

123. Dikstein S, Zlotogorski A, Avriel E, Katz M, Harms M. Comparison of the Sebumeter® and the Lipometre®. *Bioeng Skin.* 1987;3(2):197–207.

124. Brown M, Evans TW, Poyner T, Tooley PJ. The role of ketoconazole 2% shampoo in the treatment and prophylactic management of dandruff. *J Dermatol Treat.* 1990;1(4):177–9.

125. Yamamoto A, Ito M. Topical spironolactone reduces sebum secretion rates in young adults. *J Dermatol.* 1996;23(4):243–6.

126. Simpson NB, Bowden PE, Forster RA, Cunliffe WJ. The effect of topically applied progesterone on sebum excretion rate. *Br J Dermatol.* 1979;100(6):687–92.

127. Lévêque JL, Piérard-Franchimont C, de Rigal J, Saint-Léger D, Piérard GE. Effect of topical corticosteroids on human sebum production assessed by two different methods. *Arch Dermatol Res.* 1991;283(6):372–6.

128. Piérard-Franchimont C, Goffin V, Visser JN, Jacoby H, Piérard GE. A double-blind controlled evaluation of the sebosuppressive activity of topical erythromycin-zinc complex. *Eur J Clin Pharmacol.* 1995;49(1-2):57–60.

129. Piérard GE, Ries G, Cauwenbergh G. New insight into the topical management of excessive sebum flow at the skin surface. *Dermatology.* 1998;196(1):126–9.

130. Dobrev H. Clinical and instrumental study of the efficacy of a new sebum control cream. *J Cosmet Dermatol.* 2007;6(2):113–8.

131. Cunliffe WJ, Macdonald-Hull S. Lack of effect of topical retinoic acid on sebum excretion rate in acne. *Lancet.* 1988;2(8609):503.

132. Nelson AM, Gilliland KL, Cong Z, Thiboutot DM. 13-cis Retinoic acid induces apoptosis and cell cycle arrest in human SEB-1 sebocytes. *J Invest Dermatol.* 2006;126(10):2178–89.

133. Lee SH, Huh CH, Park KC, Youn SW. Effects of repetitive superficial chemical peels on facial sebum secretion in acne patients. *J Eur Acad Dermatol Venereol.* 2006;20(8):964–8.

134. Akaraphanth R, Kanjanawanitchkul W, Gritiyarangsan P. Efficacy of ALA-PDT vs blue light in the treatment of acne. *Photodermatol Photoimmunol Photomed.* 2007;23(5):186–90.

135. Kesty K, Goldberg DJ. A Randomized, Double-Blinded Study Evaluating the Safety and Efficacy of AbobotulinumtoxinA Injections for Oily Skin of the Forehead: A Dose-Response Analysis. *Dermatol Surg.* 2021;47(1):56–60.

136. Cunliffe WJ, Perera WD, Thackray P, Williams M, Forster RA, Williams SM. Pilo-sebaceous duct physiology. III. Observations on the number and size of pilo-sebaceous ducts in acne vulgaris. *Br J Dermatol.* 1976;95(2):153–6.

CHAPTER 12

Dry Skin

Leslie S. Baumann, MD

SUMMARY POINTS

What's Important?

1. The water content of the SC should be greater than 10%.
2. The formation of fine wrinkles is associated with low water content in the skin.
3. Increasing water consumption will increase the water content of skin, especially in those who consume less than 2,500 mL/day of water.
4. The microbiome affects skin hydration and skin hydration affects the microbiome.
5. Relative humidity below 30% can lead to dry skin unless the patient has high levels of sebum production. The optimal relative humidity for skin hydration is 60%.
6. Increased humidity increases skin elasticity.
7. An elevated pH impairs barrier homeostasis and SC cohesion, decreasing skin protection from the environment.

What's New?

1. Cell phone-attached devices to measure skin hydration are inaccurate due to humidity and ambient air flow.
2. Use of moisturizers in newborns decreases the development of atopic dermatitis, food allergies, and asthma.

What's Coming?

1. The effects of cannabinoids on the skin barrier and skin hydration are unclear.

Dry skin, also known as xerosis, is due to genetics, environment, and lifestyle factors. It can be so mild that it is hardly noticed or so severe that it leads to skin breakdown, severe itching, and infection. Mild dry skin is a condition that affects many patients, especially women over 50. Fine wrinkles occur on the skin when water content is low,[1] resulting in billions of dollars a year spent worldwide on moisturizing skincare products. It is important, therefore, for dermatologists, medical providers, and cosmetic scientists to understand the underlying causes of dry skin and how current therapies treat this condition.

There are so many products on the market to treat skin dryness that one can become easily overwhelmed. The preponderance of them treat the symptoms rather than the underlying causes. This chapter will discuss what is known about the etiology of dry skin with an eye toward elucidating issues that must be understood in order to identify the most effective products or the ones best suited to particular skin types. Moisturizers are discussed in Chapter 43.

WHAT IS DRY SKIN?

Dry skin is characterized by the lack of water in the stratum corneum (SC). Water is the major plasticizer of the skin; when levels are low, skin becomes less resilient and cracks and fissures can occur.[2] For the skin to appear and feel normal, the water content of the SC must be greater than 10%.[3] The increase in transepidermal water loss (TEWL) that leads to dry skin results when a defect in the permeability barrier allows excessive water to be lost to the atmosphere (**Box 12-1**). This barrier perturbation is caused by several different factors such as anionic detergents, acetone and other solvents, water

Kligman discussed his observations on the efficiency of the epidermal water barrier as a structure to prevent TEWL in a text in 1964.[4] He described covering the orifice of an inverted vial of water with a sheet of SC. This sheet of SC tissue prevented water evaporation. TEWL is now used as a measure of the integrity of the SC and the skin barrier. TEWL is defined as water loss from evaporation from the skin's surface. It is not the same as active perspiration.

Skin hydration can be measured in four main ways. The first is to measure the amount of water evaporating off the skin's surface. The Tewameter® uses an open-chamber system with humidity and temperature sensors that calculate the water evaporation gradient at the skin's surface.[5] (Another instrument called the Evaporometer was similar but it is no longer on the market.) The TEWL measured value is expressed in $g/h/m^2$. The downside to Tewameter measurement is that the microenvironment effects, such as humidity and airflow, distort the measurements requiring controlled laboratory conditions for accuracy. This is why the Tewameter devices made for cell phones and portable devices are not very accurate.[6] For years, the Tewameter was the predominant device used but now there are other options. The Aquaflux™ uses a condenser chamber—rather than an open chamber—that prevents disturbance by ambient air movements.[7] The Vapometer™ uses a humidity sensor mounted in a measurement chamber that is closed by skin contact. The device, small and portable, is unaffected by ambient airflow. It is difficult to convert measurements across instruments so this should be considered when comparing research using different devices.[8]

The second way to measure skin hydration is to use devices that measure capacitance or conductance. These tools measure the changes in a dielectric constant in the skin that is altered by water content.[9] This is a measure of hydration of the SC rather than a measure of TEWL. The rate of water loss can be extrapolated using capacitance measurements. Both the Corneometer® and the MoistureMeter® measure capacitance. Newer devices such as the SkinChip®, developed by L'Oréal, and the MoistureMap use microprocessors to produce an image based on capacitance that is interpreted by computer software.

The third way is to measure skin conductance. A high water content increases electrical conductance. The Skicon® measures conductance.

The fourth way is to measure impedance. This evaluates the resistance of skin, which increases with dehydration. Skin composition can affect this measurement. Two devices that measure impedance are the Nova® Dermal Phase Meter and the Surface-Characterizing Impedance Monitor (SCIM).[10,11]

In order to increase the validity of skin hydration measurements, it is very important that all measurements are performed in climate-controlled conditions with minimal air currents. (This is most critical with open-chamber measurements.) Skin hydration is most accurately assessed using several methods including clinical correlation.

with high levels of calcium, hot water, and frequent bathing (Chapter 40, Cleansing Agents). Skin hydration is assessed using several types of measurements including TEWL and capacitance (**Box 12-2**).

When skin becomes too dry, the outer skin layers stiffen, the desquamation process is impeded, and dead layers of keratinocytes accrue on the skin's surface. This more uneven surface causes friction against rough fabrics. The friction puts mechanical stress on the stiff skin and cracks can develop. Scratching itchy dry skin can also increase cracks and fissures that become irritated and inflamed, rendering it more itchy. Bacteria from fingernails or the microbiome can lead to infection. Sebum can help protect the skin from dryness by providing an occlusive layer of lipids, which is why dry skin is worse in areas of the body with relatively few oil glands such as the arms, legs, and trunk.

Alterations in the epidermal lipid constituents of the skin can also cause xerosis. Some dermatologists believe that the incidence of dry skin has increased in recent years because people bathe and shower more frequently using hot water, foaming cleansers, fragranced bubble baths, and bath salts, which impair the skin's barrier by stripping away important lipids. Soap, detergents, and hard water can wash off the healthy and normal lipids that compose the barrier of the skin.

The preponderance of people who complain of having dry skin do not have an underlying genetic disorder but, rather, lack the ability to cope with environmental elements that adversely affect the water-binding capacity of the SC. **Table 12-1** lists agents in the environment that can cause dry skin. Generally, as people age their skin tends to become drier and produce less sebum. Dry skin occurs more during the fall and winter months because of low humidity and excessive bathing in hot water. Xerosis is often called "winter itch" because it is at its worst during that season.

CATEGORIZATION OF DRY SKIN TYPES

In the Baumann Skin Typing System, there are three subtypes of dry skin:

- Dry Skin
- Very Dry Skin
- Changing Skin Type

All these dry skin types have an impaired skin barrier. The difference between them is how well sebum compensates for the barrier deficiency. Dry skin types produce between 0.5 mg to 0.9 mg/10 cm² of sebum every 3 hours while those with very dry skin produce less than 0.5 mg/10 cm² of sebum every 3 hours. Another difference between a dry skin type and a very dry skin type is the status of the skin barrier. Dry skin types have a slightly impaired barrier with slightly increased TEWL, while very dry skin types have a significantly impaired barrier with a significantly increased TEWL (**Table 12-2**).

TABLE 12-1	Environmental Agents That Can Lead to Dry Skin
Air conditioning	
Air travel	
Chlorinated water	
Friction from clothing	
Hard water (high calcium content)	
Harsh detergents such as anionic detergents	
Hot water	
Low humidity	
Other chemicals	
Pollution	

TABLE 12-2	Bioengineering Measurements in Dry Skin		
	Dry Skin	Very Dry Skin	Changing Skin Type
Sebum production per 10 cm^2 of sebum every 3 hours	0.5–0.9 mg	< 0.5 mg	0.5–0.9 mg
Skin Barrier	Slightly impaired	Significantly impaired	Mildly impaired
TEWL	Increased	Very increased	Slightly increased

Changing Skin Type

Many patients self-report seasonal variability in self-perceived skin hydration. Changes in skin type from dry to oily due to seasonal variations in sebum secretion were demonstrated in a study that tracked sebum secretion in 46 patients over an entire year.[12] This changing skin type occurs when the skin barrier is mildly impaired but is producing enough sebum to form an occlusive coat on the skin's surface. The coat allows the skin to retain enough water in climates with a relative humidity of 40% or higher. When humidity levels drop below 30–40%, as seen in winter and dry environments, the sebum level is no longer sufficient to protect the skin and it becomes dry due to barrier impairment. Patients who have the changing skin type often state that they have "combination skin." In the Baumann Skin Typing System nomenclature, they are said to have dry skin in the winter and normal oily skin in the summer (see section below on Effects on Skin Barrier from Humidity and the Environment). Chapter 10 discusses the Baumann Skin Types in detail.

Diagnosing Dry Skin

Dry skin can be diagnosed clinically by the presence of rough dry skin with visible scales. **Box 12-2** lists the various bioengineering devices that can be used to measure skin hydration. There are advantages and disadvantages to each of these devices as each measures different skin qualities. For greatest

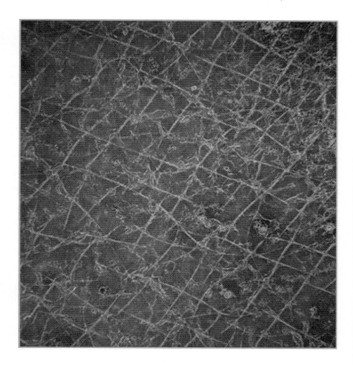

FIGURE 12-1. Increased skin markings seen in dry skin. This is called ashy skin when it occurs in darker skin types as shown.

accuracy, several of these measurements should be taken. It is difficult to ascribe a range of normal measurements to the devices because they can vary greatly by skin region, temperature and humidity of the room in which the measurements are taken, and other factors.[11] For this reason, questionnaires have been developed to simplify the process of diagnosing dry skin.

The Baumann Skin Type Indicator Questionnaire is used to identify dry skin types. The questions have been validated and shown to accurately identify dehydrated skin.[13,14] Dry skin types tend to answer questions a certain way as described in Chapter 10.

Clinical Signs of Dry Skin

The first clinical sign of skin dryness is dull skin with increased topographic skin markings.[15] In darker skin types, the surface of the skin can appear gray or ashy (**Fig. 12-1**). As xerosis worsens, the loss of water causes a reduction of cohesiveness between the corneocytes and abnormal retention of desmosomes. (A corneocyte is a keratinocyte in the SC layer.) The edges of the corneocytes curl up much like shingles on a roof in extremely arid conditions. The loosening of entire sheets of corneocytes results in scaling and flaking. The entire skin surface feels rough. Its appearance is dull because a rough surface is less able to refract light than a smooth surface. The skin may feel less pliable with stretching and bending; cracks and fissures can occur due to this reduced flexibility. Xerosis and an impaired epidermal barrier can also emerge due to genetic disorders or conditions with genetic predisposition, including ichthyosis and atopic dermatitis (AD). There are other diseases that manifest in dry skin that are beyond the scope of this chapter.

ETIOLOGY OF DRY SKIN

TEWL is the primary cause of skin dehydration. Evaporative losses can be as high as 0.5–1.0 mg/cm²/h, which can lead to a total loss of 500 mL of water from the skin per day. This is higher than the volume of water lost daily through sweat.[11] Dry skin is a result of decreased water content in the SC, which yields abnormal desquamation of corneocytes.[16] SC hydration is largely a property of corneocytes within the outer SC (stratum disjunctum), because corneocytes within the lower SC (stratum compactum) are relatively dehydrated and unable to absorb water when exposed to hypotonic stress.[17,18] Rawlings et al. demonstrated that desmosomes remain intact at higher levels of the SC and desmoglein I levels remain elevated in the superficial SC of individuals with dry skin as compared to controls.[19] This occurs because the enzymes necessary for desmosome digestion are impaired when the water level is insufficient, which leads to abnormal desquamation resulting in visible "clumps" of corneocytes that cause the skin to appear rough and dry (**Fig. 12-2A** and **B**).[20] These clumps of corneocytes manifest in the phenotype known as dry or scaled skin. In darker skin types, this perturbation of desquamation is associated with a grayish skin color and is labeled "ashy skin." Essentially, ashy skin is dry skin in a dark-skinned person.

The skin barrier resembles a brick-and-mortar type structure with the bricks representing the keratinocytes and the mortar mimicking the lipids that surround the keratinocytes in a protective coating. The lipids are arranged in lipid bilayers as illustrated in **Fig. 12-3**. The skin barrier exhibits several important functions such as preventing evaporation of water, which is known as TEWL. The barrier also helps keep out unwanted compounds such as allergens and irritants. Injured skin barriers render individuals more susceptible to contact and irritant dermatitis. Lastly, the barrier displays a defensive

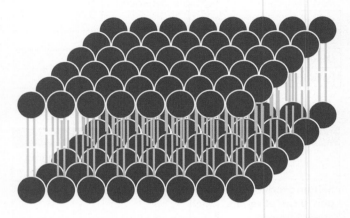

FIGURE 12-3. Lipid bilayers form when the blue hydrophilic heads line up. The yellow tails form a hydrophobic section in the center that prevents the movement of water across the bilayer membrane.

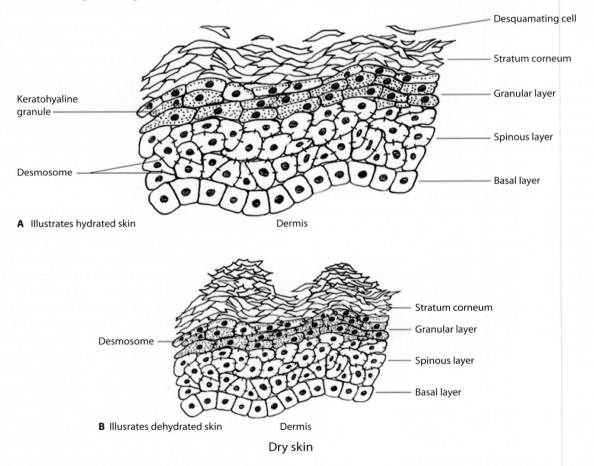

FIGURE 12-2A AND B. Dehydrated skin results in heaps of retained keratinocytes that make skin rough and decrease light reflection.

role or mechanism against infections and this SC defense depends on corneocyte function and the surrounding extracellular matrix (ECM).[21]

THE SKIN BARRIER

Cornified Cell Envelope

The cornified cell (CE) envelope that encases the corneocyte is a 10 nm insoluble layer composed of several highly crossed proteins. Loricrin, the main component of this envelope, and other proteins such as involucrin, small proline-rich proteins, desmoplakin, and periplakin are cross-linked by the calcium (Ca^{2+})-dependent transglutaminase-1 (TG-1) enzyme to form this structure.[22] Defects in CE envelope proteins or the TG-1 enzyme result in genetic disorders with impaired cornification, leading to the phenotype of severely dry skin. Lamellar ichthyosis and Vohwinkel's syndrome are examples of TG-1 and loricrin defects, where an impaired skin barrier is clearly present.

Extracellular Matrix and SC Lipids

The ECM surrounding the corneocyte is a lipid-rich component necessary for maintaining the epidermal barrier. Lamellar bodies that are secretory organelles located in the stratum granulosum play a key role in forming this lipid bilayer barrier by releasing their contents in the ECM of the stratum granulosum and SC. The lamellar bodies contain predominantly glucosylceramides, phospholipids, and cholesterol. The lipid mixture delivered by lamellar bodies is composed of 50% ceramides, approximately 15% fatty acids, and approximately 25% cholesterol.[23] These substances are converted by the enzymes β-glucocerebrosidase and phospholipases into ceramides and fatty acids once they are extruded. The 3D structure of the skin barrier is formed by a 1:1:1 ratio of ceramides, fatty acids, and cholesterol (**Fig. 12-4**). These extracellular lipids of the SC are responsible for the protective skin barrier function.[24] Alterations in any of these three components can cause a disruption in barrier function.

There are three rate-limiting enzymes involved in the synthesis of the primary lipids of epidermal skin (**Fig. 12-5A** and **B**). They are 3-hydroxy-3-methylglutarylcoenzyme A (HMG-CoA) reductase (the rate-limiting enzyme in cholesterol synthesis), acetyl Co-A carboxylase (ACC), and the fatty acid synthase involved in the synthesis of free fatty acids and palmitoyl transferase (SPT), which is the regulatory enzyme for the synthesis of ceramides.[25,26] As expected, when skin barrier disruption occurs, the activity of these enzymes is enhanced in

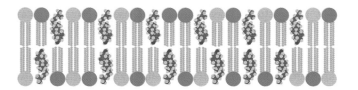

FIGURE 12-4. The lipid bilayer is made of fatty acids (green), cholesterol (purple), and ceramides (orange).

order to compensate for barrier dysfunction.[26] In addition, a group of transcription factors known as sterol regulatory element-binding proteins (SREBPs) regulate cholesterol and fatty acid production. When decreased epidermal sterols are noted, the SREBPs are activated via proteolytic processes, enter the cell nucleus, and stimulate genes leading to increased production of cholesterol and fatty acid synthesis enzymes.[21,27] There are three known types of SREBPs: SREBP-1a, SREBP-1c, and SREBP-2. In human keratinocytes, SREBP-2 has been shown to be the predominant one and is involved in regulating cholesterol and fatty acid synthesis.[28] Interestingly, the ceramide pathway is not affected by SREBPs.

An intact skin barrier consists of layers of bilayer membranes between keratinocytes (**Fig. 12-6**). When the proper 3D structure of lipids is in the same concentric multilamellar pattern as the natural skin barrier, anisotropy can be seen when viewed under a cross-polarized microscope.[29] Optical anisotropy is a pattern of light that resembles a Maltese cross (see Fig. 1–7 in Chapter 1, Basic Science of the Epidermis, for the Maltese cross image). The Maltese cross pattern of optical anisotropy demonstrates an intact skin barrier (**Fig. 12-7**).

Cholesterol

Basal cells are capable of absorbing cholesterol from the circulation; however, most cholesterol is synthesized from acetate in cells such as the keratinocytes. The synthesis of cholesterol is increased when the epidermal barrier is impaired.[30] Peroxisome proliferator-activated receptors (PPARs) and retinoid X receptors have been found to play a role in transporting cholesterol across keratinocyte cell membranes by increasing expression of ABCA1, a membrane transporter that regulates cholesterol efflux.[31]

Ceramides

Ceramides constitute 40% of the SC lipids in humans;[32] however, they are not found in significant amounts in lower levels of the epidermis such as the stratum granulosum or basal layer. This suggests that terminal differentiation is a key factor in ceramide production. Ceramides function as a water reservoir and play an important role in the development of multilayered lamellar structures that form the skin barrier.[33]

There are at least 12 classes of ceramides in the SC based on their fatty acid and sphingoid base structure.[34] In 1982, Ceramide 1 was the first ceramide identified. Subsequently, additional types of ceramides were found and named according to the polarity and composition of the molecule. The basic ceramide structure is a fatty acid covalently bound to a sphingoid base. Different classes are based on arrangements of sphingosine (S) versus phytosphingosine (P) versus 6-hydroxysphingosine (H) bases, to which an α-hydroxy (A) or nonhydroxy (N) fatty acid is attached, as well as the presence or absence of a distinct ω-esterified linoleic acid residue.[35] Ceramide 1 is unique because it is nonpolar and contains linoleic acid (a fatty acid). It is believed that the unique structure of Ceramide 1 gives it a special function in the SC. Many have proposed that this unique structure allows it to function as a molecular rivet to bind the multiple bilayers of the SC.[32] This

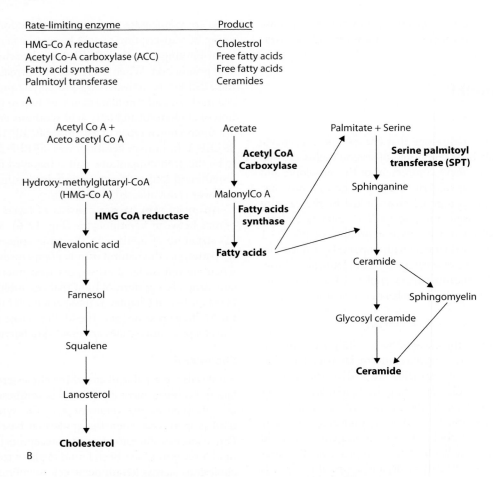

Rate-limiting enzyme	Product
HMG-Co A reductase	Cholestrol
Acetyl Co-A carboxylase (ACC)	Free fatty acids
Fatty acid synthase	Free fatty acids
Palmitoyl transferase	Ceramides

A

FIGURE 12-5A AND B. Enzymes that play a role in producing skin barrier lipids.

sort of interaction can account for the stacking of lipid bilayers that is observed. Ceramides 1, 4, and 7 play a vital role in epidermal integrity by serving as the main storage areas for linoleic acid, an essential fatty acid with key functions in the epidermal lipid barrier.[36] Although all epidermal ceramides are generated from a lamellar body-derived glucosylceramide precursor, sphingomyelin-derived ceramides (Ceramides 2 and 5) are also necessary for the integrity of the epidermal barrier.[37] Alkaline pH inhibits the activity of β-glucocerebrosidase and acid sphingomyelinase.[38] Therefore, alkaline soaps may contribute to poor barrier formation.

The regulatory enzyme for ceramide synthesis (SPT) is increased via exposure to UVB radiation and cytokines.[39] A study by L'Oréal researchers showed that total ceramide levels (especially Ceramide 2) are decreased in skin xerosis.[40] They did not see a difference in total lipid amount between xerotic patients and controls.

A study by Unilever demonstrated that exogenously applied sphingoid precursors (specifically tetraacetyl phytosphingosine or TAPS) increased ceramide levels in keratinocytes.[41] Another study by Unilever showed that TAPS combined with the fatty acids 1% linoleic acid and 1% juniperic acid further increased these ceramide levels.[42] In the second study,

barrier integrity was also assessed and shown to be improved in patients treated with TAPS, and even more improved in those treated with TAPS as well as linoleic and juniperic acids. These results suggest that topically applied lipid precursors are incorporated into ceramide biosynthetic pathways in the epidermis, increasing SC ceramide levels and thereby improving barrier integrity.

Pseudoceramides are now commonly used in skincare products because it is expensive and difficult to use naturally derived ceramides. Natural ceramides were originally extracted from animal products but that became unsafe when mad cow disease emerged, and other sources of ceramides were explored. Now natural ceramides are usually extracted from microorganisms. Most companies prefer the safety of pseudoceramides that are produced in the laboratory. Many studies have shown that pseudoceramides can replace natural ceramides to form the lipid bilayer in the SC.[34] The length of the chains can be customized to affect ceramide function, making pseudoceramides a popular skincare ingredient to treat dry skin and eczema. MLE-PC, also called myristoyl/palmitoyl oxostearamide/arachamide MEA, is an example of a pseudoceramide product shown to mimic natural ceramides.[29]

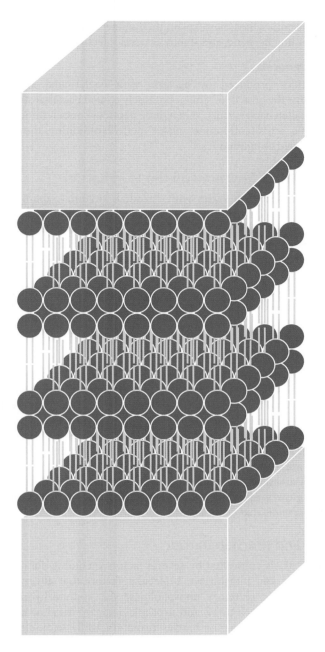

FIGURE 12-6. Lipids form a bilayer between keratinocytes and form the skin barrier.

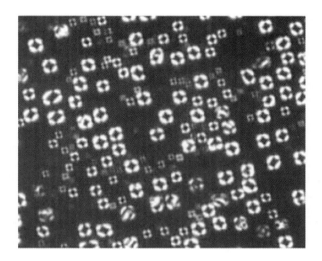

FIGURE 12-7. Anisotropy is seen with a cross-polarized microscope in the form of a Maltese cross when the multilamellar layers of the skin barrier are intact. (Courtesy of Dr. Jong-Kyung Youm.)

Fatty Acids

The skin contains free fatty acids and fatty acids bound in triglycerides, glycosylceramides, ceramides, and phospholipids. The free fatty acids in the SC are predominantly straight chained, with 24 to 24 carbon chain lengths being the most abundant.[30] Acetyl Co-A carboxylase (ACC) and fatty acid synthase are the rate-limiting enzymes in fatty acid synthesis. Barrier disruption increases the mRNA and activity levels of both these enzymes resulting in de novo fatty acid synthesis. (The increase in activity of these enzymes is likely caused by an increase in SREBPs.) Essential fatty acids such as linoleic acid can only be obtained through diet or topical application.

Changes in any of the three lipid components (ceramides, cholesterol, and fatty acids) or their regulatory enzymes result in impairment of the epidermal barrier. For example, lovastatin, an inhibitor of cholesterol synthesis (HMG-Co A reductase), slows barrier recovery,[43] and induces a defect in barrier function when applied topically.[44] Also, feeding mice with an essential fatty acid deficiency (EFAD) diet lacking in linoleic acid leads to barrier disruption, likely by lowering ceramide levels.[45] Therefore, it is clear that essential fatty acids and cholesterol play an integral role in dry skin conditions. It is currently believed that no single lipid alone mediates barrier function, and that normal levels of ceramides, cholesterol, and fatty acids, in the correct ratio, are necessary to achieve an intact barrier. Studies support this notion.[46] Man et al. showed that after altering the barrier with acetone, reapplication of ceramides, and fatty acids alone, or a combination of ceramides and fatty acids, further delayed barrier recovery. Only the application of a combination of all three components—ceramides, fatty acids, and cholesterol—resulted in normal barrier recovery.

Lipids on the skin's surface are degraded into fatty acids by bacterial enzymes. Some middle- to long-chain fatty acids have been shown to exert direct antibacterial activity against Gram-positive bacteria. In addition, the fatty acids lauric acid, palmitic acid, and oleic acid have been found to induce defensins in sebocytes.[47]

DEFECTS IN THE SKIN BARRIER

The skin barrier protects the skin in several ways. Although the term "skin barrier" usually applies to the lipid coating around the cells that prevents TEWL, it also pertains to other protective factors such as the microbiome, antimicrobial peptides, immune cells, and protective proteins. Defects in these barrier components not only allow loss of water but also permit entry of chemicals, allergens, and microorganisms that influence skin health. The skin barrier is affected by several factors including the microbiome, pH, humidity, calcium, chlorine and other elements in water, temperature, exposure to surfactants, pollution, light exposure, and friction. Inflammation, exposure to free radicals, and actions of cytokines can also modulate skin barrier function.

Aging and the Skin Barrier

Baseline barrier function has been found to be the same in aged skin as compared to young skin. However, the barrier is more easily disturbed and recovery is slower in older subjects.[48] This occurs due to a deficiency in lipid production. Acid sphingomyelinase activity was shown to be reduced in patients in the 8th decade of life as compared to younger subjects.[49] Serine palmitoyltransferase, 3-hydroxy-3-methylglutaryl-coenzyme A reductase, and acetyl coenzyme A carboxylase activity are also reduced.[50] Aged skin has about one-third less lipid weight percentage than younger skin.[48]

Antimicrobial Peptides and the Chemical Barrier of the Skin

Keratinocytes protect against infection by producing antimicrobial peptides (AMPs) that may be referred to as "the chemical barrier of the skin."[51] AMPs are part of the innate immune system of the skin. They are produced by keratinocytes, mast cells, neutrophils, and sebocytes. They are also produced by organisms on the skin, in which case they are called bacteriocins. AMPs exhibit a broad spectrum of antimicrobial activity against bacteria, viruses, and fungi. Levels of defensins and cathelicidins are low at steady state and upregulated during wounding or inflammation. Defensins, cathelicidins, and bacteriocins are three major groups of AMPs.

Defensins

Defensins are cysteine-rich cationic AMPs present in mammalians that are categorized into two subgroups: α-defensins and β-defensins. α-defensins are mostly found in neutrophils and paneth cells in the small intestines.[52–54] β-defensins, on the other hand, are present in the epidermis, and possess antimicrobial activity against Gram-positive and -negative bacteria, *Candida albicans,* and fungi.[55–60] Defensins are now used in anti-aging cosmeceutical products because they stimulate the stem cell LGR6+, leading to regeneration of the epidermal layer (see Chapter 37, Anti-Aging Ingredients).

Cathelicidins

Cathelicidins are another family of AMPs containing a C-terminal cationic segment with antimicrobial activity.[61] Cathelicidins can recruit inflammatory cells and stimulate the release of cytokines. Cathelicidin LL-37 has been shown to be especially important against viral skin infections: It can trigger inflammatory cell recruitment and cytokine release.[62] LL-37 has been demonstrated to increase in the keratinocytes of inflamed skin such as those with psoriasis and nickel allergy.[63,64] Patients with AD have been reported to have lower levels of LL-37 and human β-defensin 2 peptide in their epidermis, which may explain their vulnerability toward viral, including herpetic, and staphylococcal infections.[62,65]

Bacteriocins

Peptides produced by bacteria with bactericidal activity against the growth of similar or closely related bacterial strains are called bacteriocins. When these peptides contain thioether amino acids lanthionine and/or methyllanthionine, they are classified as lantibiotics.[47]

Circadian Rhythm and the Skin Barrier

Sebum secretion varies with circadian rhythm. Sebum can affect TEWL by forming an occlusive layer on the skin's surface. In 1971, Spruit showed that TEWL was higher on the forearm in the afternoon as compared to the morning.[66] The results changed depending upon the body area tested, which makes sense because sebum secretion levels also vary in different parts of the body. In 1998, Yosipovitch showed that TEWL is increased in the evening and at night as compared to the morning.[67]

Microbiome and the Skin Barrier

The microorganisms that live on the skin are affected by the amount of water in and on the skin. Water activity (a_w) varies from 0 (no free water) to 1.0 (all molecules of water are free). *Staphylococcus aureus* cannot grow once the a_w surpasses 0.83, which means that dry skin favors the growth of *S. aureus*. In contrast, *Pseudomonas fluorescens* prefer a wet environment and are unable to grow below an a_w of 0.97. Dry skin promotes the growth of potentially invasive Staphylococci and inhibits the growth of commensal organisms such as *Staphylococcus epidermidis* that cannot grow below an a_w of 0.87.[51]

pH and the Skin Barrier

Skin pH is controlled by several factors including choice of cleanser and moisturizer. Molecular factors that affect skin pH include secretory phospholipase A2, sodium/hydrogen exchanger-1 (NHE-1), and urocanic acid.[68,69] Alkaline soaps may contribute to poor barrier formation, while acidic cleansers such as hydroxy acid cleansers may help improve barrier lipid formation.

The skin's pH affects the skin barrier, cell adhesion, antimicrobial activity, and enzyme activity. An elevated pH impairs barrier homeostasis and SC cohesion, decreasing skin protection from the environment.[69] An elevated pH decreases conversion of phospholipids to free fatty acids and the actions of many different pH-dependent enzymes in the skin. Alkaline pH inhibits the activity of β-glucocerebrosidase and acid sphingomyelinase and decreases production of ceramides.[38]

Patients with AD tend to have an elevated pH, and studies have demonstrated that maintenance of an acidic pH reduces development of dermatitis.[70] Serine protease activity increases when pH rises. Kallikrein, thymic stromal lymphopoietin (TSLP), and PAR-2 also play a role.[71] Kallikrein is a regulator of protease cascades and is upregulated in AD. TSLP is secreted by keratinocytes when the skin barrier is perturbed and directly activates Langerhans cells triggering the differentiation of T cells into allergy-promoting Th2 cells. PAR-2 controls central inflammatory pathways. Increasing skin pH stimulates the expression of kallikrein, PAR-2, and TSLP leading to impairment of barrier function.

Light and the Skin Barrier

A single UVB exposure can result in an impaired barrier in aged skin.[48] Free amino acids derived from natural moisturizing factor (NMF), except proline, are increased after UV irradiation. *Trans*-urocanic acid, pyrrolidone carboxylic acid, lactate, and urea are decreased after UV irradiation. The amount of ceramide in the SC decreases after UV exposure, while cholesterol levels increase.[72]

Red and blue light can also affect the skin barrier. Tape-stripped skin in mice has been demonstrated to exhibit increased TEWL. When the murine skin was treated with blue light, the barrier repair was delayed. Blue light (430 nm–510 nm) was found to delay barrier recovery while red light accelerated barrier recovery.[73] The delayed barrier recovery is thought to be due to blue light's inhibitory effects on the release of lamellar granules.

Skin barrier disruption is associated with an increase in interleukin (IL)-1α, which stimulates the release of lamellar granules. When tape-stripped skin was treated with a 453 nm LED light, elevation of IL-1α was not seen.[74] Blue light's inhibition of IL-1α, thereby preventing release of lamellar granules, may be the mechanism by which blue light slows barrier recovery.

Stress and the Skin Barrier

Psychologic stress has long been known to be associated with skin conditions, such as AD, psoriasis, and seborrheic dermatitis (**Box 12-3**). Immune and neuroendocrine mechanisms likely play a role in these diseases, but studies have also shown

that barrier disruption occurs during stress, leading to the exacerbation of dry skin and other skin conditions. Studies have also demonstrated that glucocorticoids lead to disruption of the skin barrier.[75] Glucocorticoids inhibit lipid synthesis resulting in decreased production and secretion of lamellar bodies. "Stress hormones" are glucocorticoids produced in response to stress. It follows then that stress would lead to barrier disruption by increasing glucocorticoid levels. Choi et al. showed that psychologic stress led to a decrease of lipid synthesis as well as disruption of lamellar body formation, and was corrected by applications of exogenous physiologic lipids.[76]

How the Epidermis Responds to Epidermal Barrier Insult

Acute disruption of the epidermal barrier initiates a homeostatic repair response that results in the rapid recovery of permeability barrier function.[82] This repair mechanism is inhibited if the skin is covered with an occlusive dressing. Grubauer et al. showed that TEWL triggers lipid synthesis resulting in a repaired skin barrier. As TEWL decreases, lipid synthesis returns to normal levels.[83] Once initiated, this repair response begins within minutes with the rapid secretion of the contents of the lamellar bodies from the outer stratum granulosum cells. A marked decrease (50–80%) of pre-existing lamellar bodies is seen in the stratum granulosum cells initially but is soon followed by newly formed lamellar bodies. Accelerated lipid synthesis and lamellar body secretion continues until permeability barrier function returns toward normal.[84]

A calcium gradient seems to play a role in spurring lamellar body secretion. High levels of extracellular calcium are found in the upper epidermis surrounding the stratum granulosum cells.[85] Immediately after barrier disruption, the increased water movement through the compromised SC carries calcium outward toward the skin surface. This leads to a reduction in calcium concentration around the stratum granulosum cells, which precipitates lamellar body secretion.[86] It is postulated that skin calmodulin-related factor (SCARF) acts as a Ca^{2+} sensor, by binding target proteins and leading to barrier repair.[87] The important role of calcium flux is demonstrated when exogenous calcium is supplied to a disturbed barrier—lamellar body secretion does not occur, and permeability barrier repair is not initiated.[88] If the calcium surrounding the stratum granulosum cells is decreased experimentally by iontophoresis or sonophoresis, secretion of lamellar bodies is stimulated even if the barrier is undisturbed.[89]

Other factors likely play a role in lamellar body secretion as well. Keratinocytes can produce large amounts of cytokines and a store of IL-1α and IL-1β is kept available in the keratinocyte. In response to acute barrier disruption, IL-1α is released,[90] and an increase in the expression of tumor necrosis factor (TNF), IL-1, and IL-6 on messenger RNA and protein levels is seen.[91,92] Mice deficient in IL-1, IL-6, and TNF-α signaling exhibit a delay in permeability barrier repair after acute barrier disruption, indicating a role for these cytokines in regulating permeability barrier homeostasis.[93]

BOX 12-3   Atopic Dermatitis

Atopic dermatitis is a multifactorial disorder characterized by dry skin. Multiple studies have shown that an insufficiency of extracellular lipids in the SC is an important pathophysiologic factor in this condition.[77] There are several reasons for an impaired skin barrier. If there is a decrease in secretions of lamellar bodies, this leads to a decrease of fatty acids, cholesterol, or ceramides in the SC.[78] These important lipids can also be diminished by exposure to harsh surfactants, solvents, hard water, and other factors that strip these lipids from the epidermis. In some cases, use of improper skincare products can injure the skin barrier and lead to AD-like symptoms.

Mutations in the filaggrin gene have been described in patients with AD.[79,80] In fact, filaggrin mutation is the first strong genetic factor identified in AD. A defect in filaggrin leads to a decrease in NMF, a by-product of filaggrin that has hygroscopic properties.[81] NMF is present in keratinocytes in the top layers of the epidermis and helps cells hold onto intracellular water.

Each of these factors is thought to play an important role in barrier repair, and topical therapies using cytokines, growth factors, and calcium modulators are being studied.

OTHER COMPONENTS THAT PLAY A ROLE IN DRY SKIN

Natural Moisturizing Factor

SC hydration is highly regulated by NMF, a mixture of low-molecular-weight and water-soluble by-products of filaggrin found inside corneocytes (**Fig. 12-8**). Corneocytes are anucleated with no lipid content. They are composed of keratin filaments and filaggrin and encased by a cornified cell envelope. Filaggrin, also known as filament aggregating protein, plays a dynamic role in epidermal barrier function and hydration. In the lower levels of the skin, filaggrin has a structural role; however, higher up in the skin, it is broken down into amino acids that are hygroscopic and strongly bind water. Histidine, glutamine, and arginine are metabolites of filaggrin in the SC. Following deamination of the mentioned three amino acids to *trans*-urocanic acid, pyrrolidone carboxylic acid, and citrulline, respectively, an osmotically active compound that regulates skin hydration, known as NMF, is produced (**Fig. 12-9A** and **B**).[21,94]

Trans-urocanic acid, pyrrolidone carboxylic acid, and citrulline, all derived from filaggrin, generate an inward gradient of water into the SC. Other components of NMF are lactic acid and urea—also functioning as humectants—and inorganic ions such as sodium, potassium, calcium, and chloride, which contribute to epidermal hydration. The osmotically active and humectant properties of NMF allow the epidermis to retain

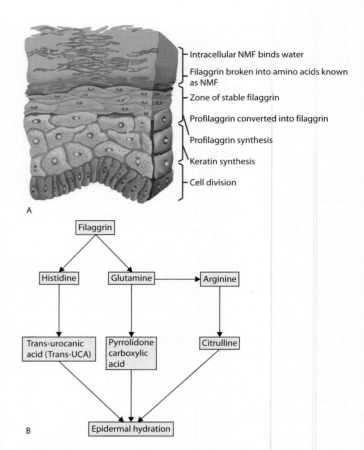

A

B

FIGURE 12-9A AND B. NMF forms from the breakdown of filaggrin. Filaggrin has multiple functions depending on where in the epidermis it is found. It has a structural role in lower layers and a hydration role in upper layers.

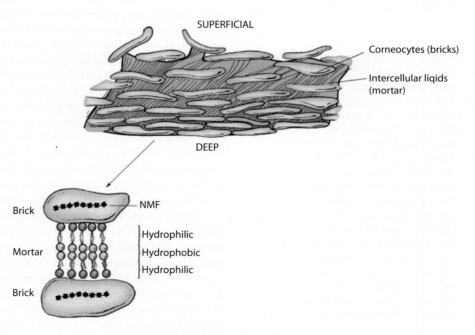

FIGURE 12-8. NMF is intracellular (inside keratinocytes).

hydration even in dry environments. Extraction of NMF components results in a decrease in the moisture accumulation rate (MAT) of the epidermis, emphasizing the importance of NMF in skin hydration.[95] Interestingly, NMF components undergo seasonal changes. While amino acid components of NMF have been shown to increase during winter, lactic acid, potassium, sodium, and chloride were significantly lower compared to their levels in summer.[96] Although there are numerous products on the market simulating NMF, formulating a product identical to it has been a challenge to researchers. This may be due to the natural adaptation of NMF to different environments, in every person.

AQUAPORINS AND THE EPIDERMIS

Water is well known to permeate through the lipid bilayers of epidermal skin. Until recently, simple diffusion was the only presumed mechanism for water conduction through the epidermis. Aquaporins (AQPs), which are a form of water channel, are integral membrane proteins that facilitate water transport in various organs such as skin, renal tubules, the eyes, the digestive tract, and even the brain. In 2003, Peter Agre and Roderick MacKinnon received the Nobel Prize in chemistry for discovering AQPs and for their structural studies of ion channels, respectively. There are 13 isoforms of AQPs found in mammals, classified as AQP 0 to 12. In the cell membrane they are arranged as homotetramers. Each subunit of the tetramer consists of six α helical domains and contains a distinct aqueous pore (**Fig. 12-10**). Functionally, they can be classified into two subtypes: AQPs 1, 2, 4, 5, and 8, which only transport water, and AQPs 3, 7, 9, and 10, which can conduct other substances such as glycerol or urea in addition to water.[97] AQP-3 is the predominant water channel found in human epidermis, and is permeable to both water and glycerin. Glycerin

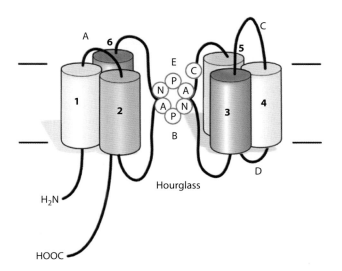

FIGURE 12-10. Aquaporin-1 structure. Each aquaporin-1 subunit contains six bilayer-spanning domains in an hourglass structure. (Reproduced with permission from Jung JS, Preston GM, Smith BL, Guggino WB, Agre P. Molecular structure of the water channel through aquaporin CHIP. The hourglass model. *J Biol Chem.* 1994;269(20):14648-14654.)

has been implicated as an endogenous humectant contributing to SC hydration.[98] Studies have shown that defects in AQP-3 in mouse models result in epidermal dryness, as well as decreased SC hydration and glycerol content of the epidermis, followed by decreased elasticity and impaired skin barrier recovery.[99,100] These studies emphasize the importance of glycerol in skin hydration. AQPs are thought to facilitate transport of water, glycerol, and solutes between keratinocytes.

Sebum

Sebum-derived lipids may also play a part in dry skin pathophysiology by preventing water loss through forming lipid films on the skin's surface that function as an emollient. However, low levels of sebaceous gland activity have not been consistently correlated with the occurrence of dry skin and the impact of sebum on dry skin conditions is poorly understood.[32] Choi et al. compared sebum production and SC hydration and found that even though males had sebum secretion levels 30% to 40% higher than women, the males did not show greater SC hydration on the sebaceous gland-enriched forehead sites than females. They also showed that prepubertal children whose sebaceous glands have not reached maximal function demonstrated normal levels of SC hydration. They did, however, find a correlation with glycerol levels and SC hydration that can help explain the role of the sebaceous glands in dry skin. The sebaceous glands utilize large amounts of triglycerides, leading to the production of glycerol. Supplying glycerol for skin hydration may be an important role for sebaceous glands.[98] This theory is supported by the fact that mice with hypoplastic sebaceous glands display poor SC hydration and low SC glycerol levels.[101] However, glycerol can originate from sources other than the sebaceous glands, which would explain the normal SC hydration in prepubertal children. Glycerol can be transported from the circulation into the basal cells via AQP-3 channels.[99] The importance of glycerol is highlighted by the fact that topical glycerol restores hydration to asebia mice while topical sebaceous lipids do not.[101]

WATER CONSUMPTION AND SKIN HYDRATION

Nutritional guidelines recommend that men drink at least 3.7 liters of water a day, and women 2.7. A study evaluated food diaries of 49 healthy females and grouped them into Group 1 (< 3200 mL/day of water consumption) and Group 2 (> 3200 mL/day).[102] Both groups were instructed to add 2000 mL water/day to their intake. Measurements of both groups were taken from multiple body sites. TEWL measurements made by a Tewameter showed no difference in TEWL between the groups, demonstrating that water supplementation did not change the skin barrier status. However, hydration measurements by the MoistureMeter SC showed an increase in hydration in both groups when water intake was increased. This difference was much more pronounced in the group with the baseline lower intake (Group 1), demonstrating that water intake has a direct effect on skin hydration but does not affect the skin barrier or TEWL.

CANNABINOIDS AND SKIN HYDRATION

Both CB-1 and CB-2 receptors are expressed in keratinocytes (see Chapter 1). Topical application of CB-1R agonists was shown to accelerate the recovery of an injured skin barrier.[103] It is unknown if this effect is due to some influence on the proliferation and differentiation of keratinocytes, or upon other aspects that control the skin barrier function. The endocannabinoid system (ECS) responds to xerosis by increasing lipid synthesis in the stratum granulosum.[103,104]

ANATOMICAL VARIATION IN WATER LOSS

Various body parts are known to regulate water loss differently. For example, the soles and palms regulate water loss poorly, while facial skin is relatively water impermeable. While the functions of the SC lipids are not fully understood, evidence supports the notion that lipids play a critical role in skin permeability. One study found no relationship between barrier function and the thickness or the number of cell layers in the SC.[105] However, an inverse relationship was discovered between lipid weight percent and permeability. Researchers gleaned that the lipid weight percent was higher in the face (less permeable) and lower in the plantar SC (more permeable). Another study was conducted to identify the components of this "lipid weight percent" and how they vary site to site.[106] Investigators compared characteristics from the abdomen, leg, face, and sole, and found that the areas with superior barrier properties contained a higher percent of neutral lipids and lower amount of sphingolipids. In other words, the neutral lipid to sphingolipid ratio was proportional to the known permeability of each site. Interestingly, the plantar surface, known to be the most permeable, contained the highest levels of sphingolipids.

EFFECTS ON SKIN BARRIER FROM HUMIDITY AND THE ENVIRONMENT

Exacerbations of AD, skin itching, hyperproliferation, and inflammation are seen in winter and in low-humidity environments.[107] (See **Box 12-4**.) The amount of water in the air

---

BOX 12-4	How the Skin Responds to Changes in the Environment

The skin can adjust to changes in humidity. This process takes several days, so skin may be dry and inflamed during the first few days of exposure to decreased humidity, but several mechanisms seem to allow skin to adjust to these environmental changes. Epidermal permeability function is increased in a low-humidity environment.[115]

Changes in hydration status signal several downstream responses, including epidermal DNA synthesis and catabolism of filaggrin into deiminated carboxylic acid metabolites.[116,117] NMF production is increased in low-humidity environments as well.[118,119]

---

affects the skin barrier and skin function. Relative humidity (RH) is the amount of water vapor in the air divided by how much water the air can hold. RH is expressed as a percent.[108] The optimal RH for lipids and protein organization is 60%.[109]

Human skin in 32% RH (considered low RH) is more susceptible to mechanical stress than skin in an RH of 96%.[108] Hydrated skin exhibits more elasticity than dehydrated skin.[1,110] Healthy subjects who are placed in a low RH for 6 hours show clinical signs of dry skin and have lower skin hydration.[111] One study of office workers compared skin symptoms at two different levels of humidity. The workers in an RH of 20–30% had more symptoms than those at 30–40% RH.[112]

The amount of water in the SC decreases with colder temperatures. This decline is even more pronounced in low humidity.[113] The skin becomes more permeable, less hydrated, and more fragile in winter.[114] In patients with high levels of sebum secretion that forms a protective occlusive surface on the skin, the TEWL level will remain the same and the skin will become hydrated. Thus, sebum secretion rates greatly affect the skin's ability to remain hydrated in low RH and cold temperatures. This is the basis for the changing skin type discussed above that patients incorrectly call "combination skin." The changing skin type is dry in cold climates and normal oily in warm climates (see Chapters 10, The Baumann Skin Typing System and 11, Oily Skin).

DRY SKIN AND INFLAMMATION

Dry skin is more likely to become inflamed than oily skin. One reason is that the barrier is not as effective at keeping out allergens, irritants, and microbes. Ceramides have been demonstrated to be disrupted in inflammation. Further, ceramide content has been shown to be reduced in patients with AD. This disruption is also seen in contact dermatitis.[120]

Disruption of skin barrier function induces the production of epidermal cytokines,[92] especially IL-1α.[121] IL-1α stimulates the release of lipid-filled lamellar granules needed for barrier repair. IL-1α has been shown to be pre-formed, stored, and released immediately when the barrier is disturbed.[91] Once IL-1α is expressed, it may also induce other cytokines or pro-inflammatory molecules such as IL-6, IL-8, granulocyte/macrophage colony-stimulating factor, and intercellular adhesion molecule-1. Ashida et al. showed that exposure to low humidity increased epidermal IL-1α synthesis and stimulated IL-1α release from the pre-formed pool in the epidermis after tape stripping.[107]

TREATMENT

The symptoms of dry skin can be treated by increasing the hydration state of the SC with occlusive or humectant ingredients and by smoothing the rough surface with an emollient. Moisturizers are products designed to increase hydration of the skin. They often contain lipids such as ceramides, fatty acids, and cholesterol. In addition, glycerin is a common ingredient. The most popular moisturizers are oil-in-water emulsions, such as creams and lotions, and water-in-oil emulsions such as hand creams. For more information on the range of topical dry skin treatment options, see Chapter 33, Choosing Skincare Products.

Supplements, Diet, and Dry Skin

Though lipids make up only approximately 10% of the total weight of the SC, their role in constructing a watertight barrier is crucial for survival. The epidermis is the main site of sterol and fatty acid synthesis and most lipids found in the epidermal barrier are produced in the epidermis itself and not dietarily derived. In fact, lipid synthesis occurs independently of serum sterol levels and the amount of dietary cholesterol.[83] Linoleic acid is a very important essential fatty acid that must be supplied through diet or topical application because it is not produced in the epidermis. It is a component of phospholipids, glucosylceramides, and Ceramides 1, 4, and 9.[122] In essential fatty acid deficiency, when linoleate is not present, it is replaced with oleate, which results in marked abnormalities in cutaneous permeability barrier function.[123,124] These observations indicate that essential fatty acids are required for the normal structure and permeability barrier function of the SC. An ω-3 fatty acid, α-linoleic acid is found in salmon and fish oils such as cod liver oil. Although no skin changes have been associated with a deficiency of ω-3 fatty acids, it is widely believed that they play an important role in regulating inflammation.

THE SKIN BARRIER, FOOD ALLERGY, AND THE ATOPIC MARCH

The atopic march is a progression from skin atopy to food allergies, allergies, and asthma. Children with an impaired skin barrier are more likely to develop peanut and other allergies. Studies show increased TEWL occurs in neonates 6–12 months before developing AD.[125] In a study of 227 healthy Asian babies, the proper use of moisturizers was associated with a decreased incidence of diaper dermatitis in the first month of life and fewer skin problems from birth to 3 months.[126] Many studies have demonstrated that moisturizing the skin in young babies will decrease the incidence of allergies and other atopic disorders.[127] Moisturizing newborns with barrier repair moisturizers should be considered the standard of care.

CONCLUSION

Dry skin is less elastic, ages faster, and is much more likely to become inflamed than normal skin. Dry skin is characterized by fine lines and an ashy, rough appearance. For this reason, dehydration is a barrier to skin health. Skin hydration can be improved by changing habits, such as using a different cleanser or type of water, increasing water consumption, using a humidifier to increase humidity to 40% or higher, and using a moisturizer.

References

1. Tsukahara K, Hotta M, Fujimura T, Haketa K, Kitahara T. Effect of room humidity on the formation of fine wrinkles in the facial skin of Japanese. *Skin Res Technol*. 2007;13(2):184–188.

2. Takahashi M, Kawasaki K, Tanaka M, et al. The mechanism of stratum corneum plasticization with water. *Bioeng Skin*. 1981; 67–72.

3. Draelos ZD. Therapeutic moisturizers. *Dermatol Clin*. 2000;18(4): 597–607.

4. Kligman A. The biology of the stratum corneum. In: Montagna W Jr., Lobitz W, eds. *The Epidermis*. New York, NY: Academic Press; 1964: 387–433.

5. Barel AO, Clarys P. Study of the stratum corneum barrier function by transepidermal water loss measurements: comparison between two commercial instruments: Evaporimeter and Tewameter. *Skin Pharmacol*. 1995;8(4):186–195.

6. Imhof RE, De Jesus ME, Xiao P, Ciortea LI, Berg EP. Closed-chamber transepidermal water loss measurement: microclimate, calibration and performance. *Int J Cosmet Sci*. 2009;31(2): 97–118.

7. BioX website: https://www.bioxsystems.com/products/aquaflux/. Accessed Jan 19, 2021.

8. Steiner M, Aikman-Green S, Prescott GJ, Dick FD. Side-by-side comparison of an open-chamber (TM 300) and a closed-chamber (Vapometer™) transepidermal water loss meter. *Skin Res Technol*. 2011;17(3):366–372.

9. Berardesca E; European Group for Efficacy Measurements on Cosmetics and Other Topical Products (EEMCO). EEMCO guidance for the assessment of stratum corneum hydration: electrical methods. *Skin Res Technol*. 1997;3(2):126–132.

10. Qassem M, Kyriacou P. Review of modern techniques for the assessment of skin hydration. *Cosmetics*. 2019;6(1):19.

11. Jansen van Rensburg S, Franken A, Du Plessis JL. Measurement of transepidermal water loss, stratum corneum hydration and skin surface pH in occupational settings: A review. *Skin Res Technol*. 2019;25(5):595–605.

12. Youn SW, Na JI, Choi SY, Huh CH, Park KC. Regional and seasonal variations in facial sebum secretions: a proposal for the definition of combination skin type. *Skin Res Technol*. 2005;11(3):189–195.

13. Baumann LS, Penfield RD, Clarke JL, Duque DK. A validated questionnaire for quantifying skin oiliness. *J Cosmet Dermatol Sci App*. 2014;4:78–84.

14. Baumann L. Validation of a questionnaire to diagnose the Baumann skin type in all ethnicities and in various geographic locations. *J Cosmet Dermatol Sci App*. 2016;6(1):34–40.

15. Chernosky ME. Clinical aspects of dry skin. *J Soc Cosmet Chem*. 1976;27:365–376.

16. Wildnauer RH, Bothwell JW, Douglass AB. Stratum corneum biomechanical properties. I. Influence of relative humidity on normal and extracted human stratum corneum. *J Invest Dermatol*. 1971;56(1):72–78.

17. Bouwstra JA, de Graaff A, Gooris GS, Nijsse J, Wiechers JW, van Aelst AC. Water distribution and related morphology in human stratum corneum at different hydration levels. *J Invest Dermatol*. 2003;120(5):750–758.

18. Richter T, Peuckert C, Sattler M, et al. Dead but highly dynamic—the stratum corneum is divided into three hydration zones. *Skin Pharmacol Physiol*. 2004;17(5):246–257.

19. Rawlings AV. Skin dryness-what is it? *J Invest Dermatol*. 1993; 100:510.

20. Orth D, Appa Y. Glycerine: a natural ingredient for rizing skin. In: Loden M, HMaibach H, eds. *Dry Skin and Moisturizers*. Boca Raton, FL, CRC Press; 2000: p. 214.

21. Elias PM. Stratum corneum defensive functions: an integrated view. *J Invest Dermatol.* 2005;125(2):183–200.

22. Kalinin A, Marekov LN, Steinert PM. Assembly of the epidermal cornified cell envelope. *J Cell Sci.* 2001;114(Pt 17):3069–3070.

23. Feingold KR, Elias PM. Role of lipids in the formation and maintenance of the cutaneous permeability barrier. *Biochim Biophys Acta.* 2014;1841(3):280–294.

24. Elias PM, Menon GK. Structural and lipid biochemical correlates of the epidermal permeability barrier. *Adv Lipid Res.* 1991;24:1–26.

25. Bigby M, Corona R, Szklo M. Evidence-based dermatology. In: Wolff K, Goldsmith LA, Katz SI, Gilchrest BA, Paller AS, Leffell DJ, eds. *Fitzpatrick's Dermatology in General Medicine.* 7th ed. New York, NY: McGraw-Hill; 2007: 13.

26. Holleran WM, Feingold KR, Man MQ, Gao WN, Lee JM, Elias PM. Regulation of epidermal sphingolipid synthesis by permeability barrier function. *J Lipid Res.* 1991;32(7):1151–1158.

27. Brown MS, Goldstein JL. Sterol regulatory element binding proteins (SREBPs): controllers of lipid synthesis and cellular uptake. *Nutr Rev.* 1998;56(2 Pt 2):S1–S3.

28. Harris IR, Farrell AM, Holleran WM, et al. Parallel regulation of sterol regulatory element binding protein-2 and the enzymes of cholesterol and fatty acid synthesis but not ceramide synthesis in cultured human keratinocytes and murine epidermis. *J Lipid Res.* 1998;39(2):412–422.

29. Park BD, Youm JK, Jeong SK, Choi EH, Ahn SK, Lee SH. The characterization of molecular organization of multilamellar emulsions containing pseudoceramide and type III synthetic ceramide. *J Invest Dermatol.* 2003;121(4):794–801.

30. Wertz PW. Biochemistry of human stratum corneum lipids. In: Elias PM, Feingold KR, eds. *Skin Barrier.* New York, NY: Taylor and Francis; 2006: 33–42.

31. Proksch E, Jensen J-M. Skin as an organ of protection. In: Wolff K, Goldsmith LA, Katz SI, Gilchrest BA, Paller AS, Leffell DJ, eds. *Fitzpatrick's Dermatology in General Medicine.* 7th ed. New York, NY: McGraw-Hill; 2007: 386–387.

32. Downing DT, Stewart ME, Wertz PW, Colton SW, Abraham W, Strauss JS. Skin lipids: an update. *J Invest Dermatol.* 1987; 88(3 Suppl):2s–6s.

33. Imokawa G, Kuno H, Kawai M. Stratum corneum lipids serve as a bound-water modulator. *J Invest Dermatol.* 1991;96(6):845–851.

34. Ishida K, Takahashi A, Bito K, Draelos Z, Imokawa G. Treatment with Synthetic Pseudoceramide Improves Atopic Skin, Switching the Ceramide Profile to a Healthy Skin Phenotype. *J Invest Dermatol.* 2020;140(9):1762–1770.e8.

35. de Jager MW, Gooris GS, Dolbnya IP, Bras W, Ponec M, Bouwstra JA. Novel lipid mixtures based on synthetic ceramides reproduce the unique stratum corneum lipid organization. *J Lipid Res.* 2004;45(5):923–932.

36. Elias PM, Brown BE, Ziboh VA. The permeability barrier in essential fatty acid deficiency: evidence for a direct role for linoleic acid in barrier function. *J Invest Dermatol.* 1980;74(4):230–233.

37. Uchida Y, Hara M, Nishio H, et al. Epidermal sphingomyelins are precursors for selected stratum corneum ceramides. *J Lipid Res.* 2000;41(12):2071–2082.

38. Hachem JP, Man MQ, Crumrine D, et al. Sustained serine proteases activity by prolonged increase in pH leads to degradation of lipid processing enzymes and profound alterations of barrier function and stratum corneum integrity. *J Invest Dermatol.* 2005;125(3):510–520.

39. Farrell AM, Uchida Y, Nagiec MM, et al. UVB irradiation up-regulates serine palmitoyltransferase in cultured human keratinocytes. *J Lipid Res.* 1998;39(10):2031–2038.

40. Nappé C, Delesalle G, Jansen A, Derigal J, Camus C. Decrease in ceramide-II in skin xerosis. *J Invest Dermatol.* 1993;100(4):530.

41. Carlomusto M, Pillai S, Rawlings AV. Human keratinocytes in vitro can utilize exogenously supplied sphingosine analogues for sphingolipid biosynthesis. *J Invest Dermatol.* 1996;4(106):871.

42. Davies A, Verdejo P, Feinberg C, Rawlings AV. Increased stratum corneum ceramide levels and improved barrier function following topical treatment with tetraacetylphytosphingosine. *J Invest Dermatol.* 1996;4(106):918.

43. Feingold KR, Man MQ, Menon GK, Cho SS, Brown BE, Elias PM. Cholesterol synthesis is required for cutaneous barrier function in mice. *J Clin Invest.* 1990;86(5):1738–1745.

44. Feingold KR, Man MQ, Proksch E, Menon GK, Brown BE, Elias PM. The lovastatin-treated rodent: a new model of barrier disruption and epidermal hyperplasia. *J Invest Dermatol.* 1991;96(2):201–209.

45. Prottey C. Essential fatty acids and the skin. *Br J Dermatol.* 1976;94(5):579–585.

46. Man MQ, Feingold KR, Elias PM. Exogenous lipids influence permeability barrier recovery in acetone-treated murine skin. *Arch Dermatol.* 1993;129(6):728–738.

47. Gallo RL, Nakatsuji T. Microbial symbiosis with the innate immune defense system of the skin. *J Invest Dermatol.* 2011; 131(10):1974–1980.

48. Choi EH. Aging of the skin barrier. *Clin Dermatol.* 2019;37(4): 336–345.

49. Yamamura T, Tezuka T. Change in sphingomyelinase activity in human epidermis during aging. *J Dermatol Sci.* 1990;1(2):79–83.

50. Ghadially R, Brown BE, Hanley K, Reed JT, Feingold KR, Elias PM. Decreased epidermal lipid synthesis accounts for altered barrier function in aged mice. *J Invest Dermatol.* 1996; 106(5):1064–1069.

51. Baldwin HE, Bhatia ND, Friedman A, Eng RM, Seite S. The Role of Cutaneous Microbiota Harmony in Maintaining a Functional Skin Barrier. *J Drugs Dermatol.* 2017;16(1):12–18.

52. Rice WG, Ganz T, Kinkade JM Jr, Selsted ME, Lehrer RI, Parmley RT. Defensin-rich dense granules of human neutrophils. *Blood.* 1987;70(3):757–765.

53. Harwig SSL, Park ASK, Lehrer RI. Characterization of defensin precursors in mature human neutrophils. *Blood.* 1992; 79(6):1532–1537.

54. Porter E, Liu L, Oren A, Anton PA, Ganz T. Localization of human intestinal defensin 5 in Paneth cell granules. *Infect Immun.* 1997;65(6):2389–2395.

55. Fulton C, Anderson GM, Zasloff M, Bull R, Quinn AG. Expression of natural peptide antibiotics in human skin. *Lancet.* 1997;350(9093):1750–1751.

56. Harder J, Bartels J, Christophers E, Schröder JM. A peptide antibiotic from human skin. *Nature.* 1997;387(6636):861.

57. Sahly H, Schubert S, Harder J, et al. Activity of human β-defensins 2 and 3 against ESBL-producing Klebsiella strains. *J Antimicrob Chemother.* 2006;57(3):562–565.

58. Meyer JE, Harder J, Görögh T, et al. Human beta-defensin-2 in oral cancer with opportunistic Candida infection. *Anticancer Res.* 2004;24(2B):1025–1030.

59. Harder J, Bartels J, Christophers E, Schroder JM. Isolation and characterization of human β-defensin-3, a novel human inducible peptide antibiotic. *J Biol Chem.* 2001;276(8):5707–5713.

60. Zanetti M, Gennaro R, Romeo D. Cathelicidins: a novel protein family with a common proregion and a variable C-terminal antimicrobial domain. *FEBS Lett.* 1995;374(1):1–5.

61. Niyonsaba F, Ushio H, Nakano N, et al. Antimicrobial peptides human β-defensins stimulate epidermal keratinocyte migration, proliferation and production of proinflammatory cytokines and chemokines. *J Invest Dermatol.* 2007;127(3):594–604.

62. Howell MD, Jones JF, Kisich KO, Streib JE, Gallo RL, Leung DY. Selective killing of vaccinia virus by LL-37: implications for eczema vaccinatum. *J Immunol.* 2004;172(3):1763–1767.

63. Frohm M, Agerberth B, Ahangari G, et al. The expression of the gene coding for the antibacterial peptide LL-37 is induced in human keratinocytes during inflammatory disorders. *J Biol Chem.* 1997;272(24):15258–15263.

64. Frohm Nilsson M, Sandstedt B, Sørensen O, Weber G, Borregaard N, Ståhle-Bäckdahl M. The human cationic antimicrobial protein (hCAP18), a peptide antibiotic, is widely expressed in human squamous epithelia and colocalizes with interleukin-6. *Infect Immun.* 1999;67(5):2561–2566.

65. Ong PY, Ohtake T, Brandt C, et al. Endogenous antimicrobial peptides and skin infections in atopic dermatitis. *N Engl J Med.* 2002;347(15):1151–1160.

66. Spruit D. The diurnal variation of water vapour loss from the skin in relation to temperature. *Br J Dermatol.* 1971;84(1):66–70.

67. Yosipovitch G, Xiong GL, Haus E, Sackett-Lundeen L, Ashkenazi I, Maibach HI. Time-dependent variations of the skin barrier function in humans: transepidermal water loss, stratum corneum hydration, skin surface pH, and skin temperature. *J Invest Dermatol.* 1998;110(1):20–23.

68. Jang H, Matsuda A, Jung K, et al. Skin pH Is the Master Switch of Kallikrein 5-Mediated Skin Barrier Destruction in a Murine Atopic Dermatitis Model. *J Invest Dermatol.* 2016;136(1):127–135.

69. Hachem JP, Crumrine D, Fluhr J, Brown BE, Feingold KR, Elias PM. pH directly regulates epidermal permeability barrier homeostasis, and stratum corneum integrity/cohesion. *J Invest Dermatol.* 2003;121(2):345–353.

70. Hatano Y, Man MQ, Uchida Y, et al. Maintenance of an acidic stratum corneum prevents emergence of murine atopic dermatitis. *J Invest Dermatol.* 2009;129(7):1824–1835.

71. Redhu D, Franke K, Kumari V, Francuzik W, Babina M, Worm M. Thymic stromal lymphopoietin production induced by skin irritation results from concomitant activation of protease-activated receptor 2 and interleukin 1 pathways. *Br J Dermatol.* 2020;182(1):119–129.

72. Yoon SH, Park JI, Lee JE, Myung CH, Hwang JS. In vivo Change of Keratin-Bound Molecules in the Human Stratum Corneum following Exposure to Ultraviolet Radiation. *Skin Pharmacol Physiol.* 2019;32(5):254–264.

73. Denda M, Fuziwara S. Visible radiation affects epidermal permeability barrier recovery: selective effects of red and blue light. *J Invest Dermatol.* 2008;128(5):1335–1336.

74. Falcone D, Uzunbajakava NE, van Abeelen F, et al. Effects of blue light on inflammation and skin barrier recovery following acute perturbation. Pilot study results in healthy human subjects. *Photodermatol Photoimmunol Photomed.* 2018;34(3):184–193.

75. Kao JS, Fluhr JW, Man MQ, et al. Short-term glucocorticoid treatment compromises both permeability barrier homeostasis and stratum corneum integrity: inhibition of epidermal lipid synthesis accounts for functional abnormalities. *J Invest Dermatol.* 2003;120(3):456–464.

76. Choi EH, Brown BE, Crumrine D, et al. Mechanisms by which psychologic stress alters cutaneous permeability barrier homeostasis and stratum corneum integrity. *J Invest Dermatol.* 2005;124(3):587–595.

77. Imokawa G, Abe A, Jin K, Higaki Y. Decreased level of ceramides in stratum corneum of atopic dermatitis: an etiologic factor in atopic dry skin? *J Invest Dermatol.* 1991;96(4):523–526.

78. Fartasch M, Bassukas ID, Diepgen TL. Disturbed extruding mechanism of lamellar bodies in dry non-eczematous skin of atopics. *Br J Dermatol.* 1992;127(3):221–227.

79. Weidinger S, Illig T, Baurecht H, et al. Loss-of-function variations within the filaggrin gene predispose for atopic dermatitis with allergic sensitizations. *J Allergy Clin Immunol.* 2006;118(1):214–219.

80. Irvine AD, McLean WH. Breaking the (un)sound barrier: filaggrin is a major gene for atopic dermatitis. *J Invest Dermatol.* 2006;126(6):1200–1202.

81. Chu DH. Development and structure of skin. In: Wolff K, Goldsmith LA, Katz SI, Gilchrest BA, Paller AS, Leffell DJ, eds. *Fitzpatrick's Dermatology in General Medicine.* 7th ed. New York, NY: McGraw-Hill; 2007: 61.

82. Proksch E, Holleran WM, Menon GK, Elias PM, Feingold KR. Barrier function regulates epidermal lipid and DNA synthesis. *Br J Dermatol.* 1993;128(5):473–482.

83. Grubauer G, Elias PM, Feingold KR. Transepidermal water loss: the signal for recovery of barrier structure and function. *J Lipid Res.* 1989;30(3):323–333.

84. Menon GK, Feingold KR, Mao-Qiang M, Schaude M, Elias PM. Structural basis for the barrier abnormality following inhibition of HMG CoA reductase in murine epidermis. *J Invest Dermatol.* 1992;98(2):209–219.

85. Menon GK, Elias PM. Ultrastructural localization of calcium in psoriatic and normal human epidermis. *Arch Dermatol.* 1991;127(1):57–63.

86. Lee SH, Elias PM, Proksch E, Menon GK, Mao-Quiang M, Feingold KR. Calcium and potassium are important regulators of barrier homeostasis in murine epidermis. *J Clin Invest.* 1992;89(2):530–538.

87. Hwang J, Kalinin A, Hwang M, et al. Role of Scarf and its binding target proteins in epidermal calcium homeostasis. *J Biol Chem.* 2007;282(25):18645–18653.

88. Menon GK, Elias PM, Feingold KR. Integrity of the permeability barrier is crucial for maintenance of the epidermal calcium gradient. *Br J Dermatol.* 1994;130(2):139–147.

89. Lee SH, Choi EH, Feingold KR, Jiang S, Ahn SK. Iontophoresis itself on hairless mouse skin induces the loss of the epidermal calcium gradient without skin barrier impairment. *J Invest Dermatol.* 1998;111(1):39–43.

90. Wood LC, Feingold KR, Sequeira-Martin SM, Elias PM, Grunfeld C. Barrier function coordinately regulates epidermal IL-1 and IL-1 receptor antagonist mRNA levels. *Exp Dermatol.* 1994;3(2):56–60.

91. Wood LC, Elias PM, Calhoun C, Tsai JC, Grunfeld C, Feingold KR. Barrier disruption stimulates interleukin-1 α expression

and release from a preformed pool in murine epidermis. *J Invest Dermatol.* 1996;106(3):397–403.

92. Wood LC, Jackson SM, Elias PM, Grunfeld C, Feingold KR. Cutaneous barrier perturbation stimulates cytokine production in the epidermis of mice. *J Clin Invest.* 1992;90(2):482–487.

93. Wang XP, Schunck M, Kallen KJ, et al. The interleukin-6 cytokine system regulates epidermal permeability barrier homeostasis. *J Invest Dermatol.* 2004;123(1):124–131.

94. Scott IR, Harding CR, Barrett JG. Histidine-rich protein of the keratohyalin granules. Source of the free amino acids, urocanic acid and pyrrolidone carboxylic acid in the stratum corneum. *Biochim Biophys Acta.* 1982;719(1):110–117.

95. Visscher MO, Tolia GT, Wickett RR, Hoath SB. Effect of soaking and natural moisturizing factor on stratum corneum water-handling properties. *J Cosmet Sci.* 2003;54(3):289–300.

96. Nakagawa N, Sakai S, Matsumoto M, et al. Relationship between NMF (lactate and potassium) content and the physical properties of the stratum corneum in healthy subjects. *J Invest Dermatol.* 2004;122(3):755–763.

97. Takata K, Matsuzaki T, Tajika Y. Aquaporins: water channel proteins of the cell membrane. *Prog Histochem Cytochem.* 2004;39(1):1–83.

98. Choi EH, Man MQ, Wang F, et al. Is endogenous glycerol a determinant of stratum corneum hydration in humans? *J Invest Dermatol.* 2005;125(2):288–293.

99. Hara M, Ma T, Verkman AS. Selectively reduced glycerol in skin of aquaporin-3-deficient mice may account for impaired skin hydration, elasticity, and barrier recovery. *J Biol Chem.* 2002;277(48):46616–46621.

100. Hara-Chikuma M, Verkman AS. Glycerol replacement corrects defective skin hydration, elasticity, and barrier function in aquaporin-3-deficient mice. *Proc Natl Acad Sci U S A.* 2003;100(12):7360–7365.

101. Fluhr JW, Mao-Qiang M, Brown BE, et al. Glycerol regulates stratum corneum hydration in sebaceous gland deficient (asebia) mice. *J Invest Dermatol.* 2003;120(5):728–737.

102. Palma L, Marques LT, Bujan J, Rodrigues LM. Dietary water affects human skin hydration and biomechanics. *Clin Cosmet Investig Dermatol.* 2015;8:413–421.

103. Proksch E, Soeberdt M, Neumann C, Kilic A, Abels C. Modulators of the endocannabinoid system influence skin barrier repair, epidermal proliferation, differentiation and inflammation in a mouse model. *Exp Dermatol.* 2019;28(9):1058–1065.

104. Yuan C, Wang XM, Guichard A, et al. N-palmitoylethanolamine and N-acetylethanolamine are effective in asteatotic eczema: results of a randomized, double-blind, controlled study in 60 patients. *Clin Interv Aging.* 2014;9:1163–1169.

105. Elias PM, Cooper ER, Korc A, Brown BE. Percutaneous transport in relation to stratum corneum structure and lipid composition. *J Invest Dermatol.* 1981;76(4):297–301.

106. Lampe MA, Burlingame AL, Whitney J, et al. Human stratum corneum lipids: characterization and regional variations. *J Lipid Res.* 1983;24(2):120–130.

107. Ashida Y, Ogo M, Denda M. Epidermal interleukin-1 α generation is amplified at low humidity: implications for the pathogenesis of inflammatory dermatoses. *Br J Dermatol.* 2001;144(2):238–243.

108. Engebretsen KA, Johansen JD, Kezic S, Linneberg A, Thyssen JP. The effect of environmental humidity and temperature on skin barrier function and dermatitis. *J Eur Acad Dermatol Venereol.* 2016;30(2):223–249.

109. Vyumvuhore R, Tfayli A, Duplan H, Delalleau A, Manfait M, Baillet-Guffroy A. Effects of atmospheric relative humidity on Stratum Corneum structure at the molecular level: ex vivo Raman spectroscopy analysis. *Analyst.* 2013;138(14):4103–4111.

110. Kim E, Han J, Park H, et al. The effects of regional climate and aging on seasonal variations in Chinese Women's skin characteristics. *J Cosmet Dermatol Sci App.* 2017;7(2):164–172.

111. Egawa M, Oguri M, Kuwahara T, Takahashi M. Effect of exposure of human skin to a dry environment. *Skin Res Technol.* 2002;8(4):212–218.

112. Reinikainen LM, Jaakkola JJ, Seppänen O. The effect of air humidification on symptoms and perception of indoor air quality in office workers: a six-period cross-over trial. *Arch Environ Health.* 1992;47(1):8–15.

113. Spencer TS, Linamen CE, Akers WA, Jones HE. Temperature dependence of water content of stratum corneum. *Br J Dermatol.* 1975;93(2):159–164.

114. Andersen F, Andersen K, Kligman A. Xerotic skin of the elderly: a summer versus winter comparison based on biophysical measurements. *Exog Dermatol.* 2003;2(4):190–194.

115. Denda M, Sato J, Masuda Y, et al. Exposure to a dry environment enhances epidermal permeability barrier function. *J Invest Dermatol.* 1998;111(5):858–863.

116. Denda M, Sato J, Tsuchiya T, Elias PM, Feingold KR. Low humidity stimulates epidermal DNA synthesis and amplifies the hyperproliferative response to barrier disruption: implication for seasonal exacerbations of inflammatory dermatoses. *J Invest Dermatol.* 1998;111(5):873–878.

117. Sato J, Denda M, Chang S, Elias PM, Feingold KR. Abrupt decreases in environmental humidity induce abnormalities in permeability barrier homeostasis. *J Invest Dermatol.* 2002;119(4):900–904.

118. Katagiri C, Sato J, Nomura J, Denda M. Changes in environmental humidity affect the water-holding property of the stratum corneum and its free amino acid content, and the expression of filaggrin in the epidermis of hairless mice. *J Dermatol Sci.* 2003;31(1):29–35.

119. Scott IR, Harding CR. Filaggrin breakdown to water binding compounds during development of the rat stratum corneum is controlled by the water activity of the environment. *Dev Biol.* 1986;115(1):84–92.

120. Kim D, Lee NR, Park SY, et al. As in Atopic Dermatitis, Nonlesional Skin in Allergic Contact Dermatitis Displays Abnormalities in Barrier Function and Ceramide Content. *J Invest Dermatol.* 2017;137(3):748–750.

121. Barker JN, Mitra RS, Griffiths CE, Dixit VM, Nickoloff BJ. Keratinocytes as initiators of inflammation. *Lancet.* 1991;337(8735):211–214.

122. Uchida Y, Hamanaka S. Stratum corneum ceramides: function, origins, and therapeutic implications. In: Elias PM, Feingold KR, eds. *Skin Barrier.* New York, NY: Taylor and Francis; 2006: 43.

123. Elias PM, Brown BE. The mammalian cutaneous permeability barrier: defective barrier function is essential fatty acid deficiency correlates with abnormal intercellular lipid deposition. *Lab Invest.* 1978;39(6):574–583.

124. Hansen HS, Jensen B. Essential function of linoleic acid esterified in acylglucosylceramide and acylceramide in maintaining the

epidermal water permeability barrier. Evidence from feeding studies with oleate, linoleate, arachidonate, columbinate and alpha-linolenate. *Biochim Biophys Acta.* 1985;834(3):357–363.

125. Kelleher M, Dunn-Galvin A, Hourihane JO, et al. Skin barrier dysfunction measured by transepidermal water loss at 2 days and 2 months predates and predicts atopic dermatitis at 1 year. *J Allergy Clin Immunol.* 2015;135(4):930–935.e1.

126. Yonezawa K, Haruna M, Matsuzaki M, Shiraishi M, Kojima R. Effects of moisturizing skincare on skin barrier function and the prevention of skin problems in 3-month-old infants: A randomized controlled trial. *J Dermatol.* 2018;45(1):24–30.

127. Lowe AJ, Leung DYM, Tang MLK, Su JC, Allen KJ. The skin as a target for prevention of the atopic march. *Ann Allergy Asthma Immunol.* 2018;120(2):145–151.

Sensitive Skin

Leslie S. Baumann, MD

SUMMARY POINTS

What's Important?

1. People mean different things when they say they have sensitive skin, so a standardized classification system should be adopted.
2. There are four subtypes of sensitive skin in the Baumann Skin Typing System: acne, rosacea, stinging, and allergic.

What's New?

1. Inflammation plays such a large role in aging that the term "inflammaging" is now used.
2. Seventy-two percent of patients who have seen a medical doctor for skincare recommendations were diagnosed with sensitive skin.

What's Coming?

1. Studies looking at neuroimmunology and the effects of skin inflammation are being conducted and will provide insights into the causes and treatments of inflammation.

Sensitive skin, which can be very distressing to those who have it, is a condition characterized by hypersensitivity to stimuli that often results in inflammation. When patients develop a reaction to a product, they may blame the doctor, aesthetician, or skincare brand, so it is important for the physician-patient relationship to identify underlying susceptibility to inflammation before prescribing any skincare routine for sensitive skin. A strong majority (78%) of consumers who have sensitive skin state that they have avoided a particular product or brand because of past skin reactions.[1] Those with frequent skin reactions often learn to limit their use of skin products to the few that do not cause inflammation in order to avoid the annoyance of acne, redness, and itching that can interfere with everyday activities. Those with frequent skin reactions report a decrease in quality of life and frustration is a common complaint. In a French study of more than 2000 individuals, it was found using the SF-12 questionnaire that those with sensitive skin reported a poorer quality of life compared to those without sensitive skin.[2]

PREVALENCE OF SENSITIVE SKIN

Epidemiologic surveys show a high prevalence of sensitive skin. In a phone survey of 800 ethnically diverse women in the US, 52% described having sensitive skin.[1] In a UK mail survey of 2058 people, 51.5% of the women and 38.2% of the men reported having sensitive skin.[3] Sensitive skin is most commonly reported on the face. However, one study showed that 85% of the 400 subjects evaluated described sensitive skin on the face, while 70% reported sensitive skin in other areas: hands (58%), scalp (36%), feet (34%), neck (27%), torso (23%), and back (21%).[4]

The Baumann Skin Type Indicator Questionnaire was used to skin type patients seen in medical practices and found that of the 102,216 patients who took the questionnaire, 72% had at least one type of sensitive skin.[5] These were patients seen in a medical practice, usually a dermatology practice, so the survey was skewed towards those with a skin complaint, leaving this high number of sensitive skin reports unsurprising.

INFLAMMATION

Sensitive skin types are characterized by inflammation. The exception is Type 3, the stinging type, which may occur without any visible changes. Inflammation is detrimental because it can cause barriers to skin health such as dehydration or pigmentation and lead to aging. Aging is discussed in Chapters 5 (Intrinsic Aging) and 6 (Extrinsic Aging). Inflammation is such a known cause of aging that the term "inflammaging" is now used to describe a state of chronic inflammation with increased levels of inflammatory cytokines like IL-6, IL-8 and TNF-α.[6] Inflammation can engender cutaneous aging via multiple mechanisms that are beyond the scope of this chapter (**Table 13-1**).[6]

CLASSIFICATION OF SENSITIVE SKIN

Sensitive skin has been difficult to characterize because there is confusion about its definition. It has been classified in several ways, and sensitive skin is often self-diagnosed. It may not be accompanied by visible skin changes and testing can show inconsistent results. It is important to standardize the language used to describe the condition so that there is agreement on how to classify sensitive skin.

Yokota et al. classified sensitive skin into three different types based on their physiologic parameters.[7] Type 1 was defined as the low-barrier function group. Type 2 was labeled as the inflammation group with normal barrier function and inflammatory changes. Type 3 was termed the "pseudohealthy group" in terms of normal barrier function and no inflammatory changes. In all of the Yokota sensitive skin types, a higher content of nerve growth factor was observed in the stratum corneum (SC). In both types 2 and 3, sensitivity to electrical stimuli was high.

These data suggest that the hypersensitive reaction seen in these types is closely related to nerve fibers innervating the epidermis.

Pons-Guiraud divided sensitive skin into three subgroups.[8] "Very sensitive skin" was described as reactive to a wide variety of both endogenous and exogenous factors. This type was associated with both acute and chronic symptoms and a robust psychologic component. The second type was called "environmentally sensitive" and described as clear, dry, thin skin with a tendency to blush or flush in reaction to environmental factors. The final group was "cosmetically sensitive skin," which was transiently reactive to specific and definable cosmetic products.

Muizzuddin and others from the Estée Lauder Companies defined three sensitive skin subgroups as well.[9] The first subgroup was called "delicate skin," distinguished by easily disrupted barrier function not accompanied by a rapid or intense inflammatory response. The second subgroup was "reactive skin," characterized by a strong inflammatory response without a significant increase in transepidermal water loss. The third group was known as "stingers" (a term coined by Kligman in 1977), which was described as a heightened neurosensory perception to minor cutaneous stimulation.

THE BAUMANN SKIN TYPING SYSTEM CLASSIFICATION OF SENSITIVE SKIN

The Baumann Skin Typing System is determined by historical data gathered in a questionnaire form.[10] It divides sensitive skin into four types based on diagnosis (**Table 13-2**). Type 1 sensitive skin is prone to developing papules and pustules and is known as the acne type or S1 type. Type 2 sensitive skin is characterized by facial redness triggered by heat, spicy

TABLE 13-1	[i,ii]This Very Abbreviated Chart Shows Which Signs of Aging Are Affected by Inflammation. Column 1 lists signs of aging. Column 2 is the role of inflammation in causing column 1. And column 3 is what happens once column 1 and 2 occur. TLR = toll-like receptor. (See chapter 5 and the References for details.)		
Evidence of Aging	**Role of inflammation**	**Results in**	
Senescence of keratinocytes	Decreased ECM production, Increased IL-1α and altered secretome	Repercussions are unclear	
Senescence of fibroblasts	Increase in proinflammatory cytokines such as prostaglandin E$_2$ (PGE)[iii]	Detrimental effect on nearby cells	
Senescence of fibroblasts	P38-MAPK	Dysregulation of immunity	
Dysfunctional T cells with loss of CD8+ cells	Proinflammatory T helper (Th)17 phenotype	Increase TNF-α production	
Defective B cells	Not yet known	Secrete IL-6	
Fragments of ECM: Matrikines	Chemoattractant for immune cells	TLR activation	
Damaged mitochondria	Free radicals	Decreased ATP	
Damaged lysosomes	Free radicals	Increase in cellular junk	
Defective regulation of compliment pathway	Dysregulation of homeostasis	Build up of apoptotic cells	
Antimicrobial peptides	Overexpression of immune pathways	Shortened life span	

[i]O'Malley, J. T., Clark, R. A., & Widlund, H. R. (2019). Skin Inflammation in Human Health and Disease: 2018 International Conference. *Journal of Investigative Dermatology*, 139(5), 991–994.
[ii]Pilkington, S. M., Bulfone-Paus, S., Griffiths, C. E., & Watson, R. E. (2020). Inflammaging and the Skin. *Journal of Investigative Dermatology*.
[iii]Yang, H. H., Kim, C., Jung, B., Kim, K. S., & Kim, J. R. (2011). Involvement of IGF binding protein 5 in prostaglandin E 2-induced cellular senescence in human fibroblasts. *Biogerontology*, 12(3), 239–252.

TABLE 13-2	Baumann Sensitive Skin Classification
Type 1 Acne Type: Papules and Pustules	
Type 2 Rosacea Type: Redness, Flushing	
Type 3 Stinging Type: Burning, Stinging or Itching	
Type 4 Allergic/Irritant Type: Susceptible to contact and irritant dermatitis	

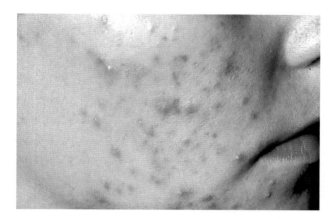

FIGURE 13-1. Inflammatory pustules seen in acne.

food, emotion, or vasodilation of any cause and is known as the flushing rosacea type or S2 type. Type 3 sensitive skin, or the S3 type, is characterized by burning, itching, or stinging of any cause. Type 4 sensitive skin is the phenotype susceptible to developing contact dermatitis and irritant dermatitis (see Chapters 11–19). An individual may suffer from combinations of the sensitive skin subtypes. For example, a person may burn and sting and develop acne from certain skincare products. In this case, they would be designated as an S1S3 sensitive skin type.

S1 Type: Acne

Baumann S1 sensitive skin is characterized by acne breakouts manifesting as papules and pustules (**Fig. 13-1**). When this occurs from exposure to makeup the term "acne cosmetica" is used.[11] Ingredients in skincare and hair care products such as coconut oil and isopropyl myristate may contribute to acne. Blushes, lipstick, and other color cosmetics that contain D & C (Drug & Cosmetic) red dyes, which are coal tar derivatives, are comedogenic (**Table 13-3**). Sunscreen ingredients have been known to cause acneiform eruptions as well.[12] For a detailed explanation of acne and its causes and treatment, see Chapter 16, Acne.

S2 Type: Rosacea

Baumann S2 sensitive skin is manifested by flushing and facial redness (**Fig. 13-2**). Not all individuals who fall into this category have true rosacea; however, they all suffer from facial flushing that may be a predictor of future rosacea. Patients with the S2 sensitive skin type should be treated with anti-inflammatory skincare products to reduce inflammation (see Chapters 17, Rosacea, and 38, Anti-Inflammatory Ingredients).

TABLE 13-3	Topical Ingredients in Skincare and Hair Care Products That May Cause Acne[12–14]
Acetylated Lanolin Alcohol	
Algin	
Almond Oil	
Anhydrous Lanolin	
Arachidic Acid	
Ascorbyl Palmitate	
Azulene	
Beeswax	
Benzaldehyde	
Benzoic Acid	
Beta Carotene	
BHA	
Bubussa Oil	
Butyl Stearate	
Butylated Hydroxyanisole (BHA)	
Cajeput Oil	
Calendula	
Camphor	
Capric Acid	
Carbomer 940	
Carnuba Wax	
Carotene	
Carrageenan	
Castor Oil	
Ceteareth- 20	
Cetearyl Alcohol	
Cetyl acetate	
Cetyl Alcohol	
Chaulomoogra Oil	
Cocoa Butter	
Coconut Butter	
Coconut Oil	
Colloidal Sulfur	
Corn Oil	
Cotton Seed Oil	
D & C Red # 17	
D & C Red # 19	
D & C Red # 21	
D & C Red # 27	
D & C Red # 3	
D & C Red # 30	
D & C Red # 36	
D & C Red # 4	

(continued)

TABLE 13-3	Topical Ingredients in Skincare and Hair Care Products That May Cause Acne[12–14](Continued)
D & C Red # 40	
Decyl Oleate	
Dioctyl Succinate	
Disodium Monooleamido	
Emulsifying Wax NF	
Ethoxylated Lanolin	
Ethylhexyl Palmitate	
Evening Primrose Oil	
Glyceryl-3-Diisostearate	
Hexadecyl Alcohol	
Hydrogenated Castor Oil	
Hydrogenated Vegetable Oil	
Hydroxypropylcellulose	
Isocetyl alcohol	
Isodecyl Oleate	
Isodecyl Oleate	
Isopropyl Isosterate	
Isopropyl lanolate	
Isopropyl linoleate	
Isopropyl Myristate	
Isopropyl Palmitate	
Isostearyl Isostearate	
Isostearyl Neopentanoate	
Laneth 10	
Lanolin acid	
Lanolin Alcohol	
Lanolin Oil	
Lanolin Wax	
Laureth 23	
Laureth 4	
Menthyl Anthranilate	
Mink Oil	
Myristic Acid	
Myristyl Lactate	
Octyl Palmitate	
Octyl Stearate	
Oleth-10	
Oleth-3	
Oleyl Alcohol	
Palmitic Acid	
Peach Kernal Oil	
Peanut Oil	

TABLE 13-3	Topical Ingredients in Skincare and Hair Care Products That May Cause Acne[12–14](Continued)
PEG 100 Distearate	
PEG 150 Distearate	
PEG 16 Lanolin	
PEG 200 Dilaurate	
PEG 2-Sulfosuccinate	
PEG 8 Stearate	
Pentarythrital Tetra Isostearate	
PG Caprylate/Caprate	
PG Dicaprylate/Caprate	
PG Dipelargonate	
PG Monostearate	
Polyethylene Glycol (PEG 400)	
Polyethylene Glycol 300	
Polyglyceryl-3-Diisostearate	
Potassium Chloride	
PPG 2 Myristyl Propionate	
PPG-5 ceteth-10 phosphate	
Propylene Glycol Monostearate	
Red Algae	
Sandelwood Seed Oil	
Sesame Oil	
Shark Liver Oil	
Solulan 1	
Solulan 16	
Sorbitan Oleate	
Soybean Oil	
Steareth 10	
Steareth 10	
Steareth 2	
Steareth 2	
Steareth 20	
Steareth 20	
Stearyl Heptanoate	
Stearyl Heptanoate	
Sulfated Castor Oil	
Sulfated Jojoba Oil	
Syearyl Heptanoate	
Synthetic Dyes, (Especially, D&C Red #S 3, 4, 6, 7, 9, 17, 40)	
Triethanolamine	
Vitamin A Palmitate	
Wheat Germ Glyceride/Oil	
Xylene	

(continued)

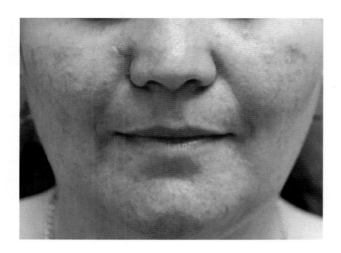

FIGURE 13-2. Facial redness in the rosacea type patient.

S3 Type: Burning and Stinging

Baumann S3 sensitive skin is characterized by burning and stinging upon application of skincare products or exposure to environmental factors such as wind, cold, or heat. In some cases, the skin stings when washed with water or touched. These subjective signs are usually not accompanied by facial flushing unless the individual also suffers from Baumann S2 sensitive skin with a tendency to flush (see Chapter 17). Fifty percent of patients with sensitive skin manifest their uncomfortable symptoms without accompanying visible signs of inflammation.[13]

Stinging may be due to a new skincare product such as a retinoid or benzoyl peroxide that causes an irritant dermatitis as seen in the Baumann S4 subtype. This will easily resolve by stopping the product use, reducing the amount applied, decreasing the frequency of application, changing the cleanser to a creamy nonfoaming formulation, or adding a barrier repair moisturizer. Patients that are stingers should avoid any low-pH skincare products such as hydroxy acids and ascorbic acid (see Chapter 18, Burning and Stinging Skin).

S4 Type: Contact Dermatitis and Irritant Dermatitis

Baumann S4 sensitive skin is exhibited by individuals who have a history of frequent scaling, redness, or reaction to allergens and irritants. Atopic dermatitis sufferers fall into this category. These patients are more susceptible to react to substances that are not commonly considered irritants, likely caused by an impaired skin barrier. These substances include many cosmetics ingredients such as dimethyl sulfoxide, benzoyl peroxide preparations, salicylic acid, propylene glycol, amyldimethylaminobenzoic acid, and 2-ethoxyethyl methoxycinnamate. The current theory is that molecules bind receptors in the skin or enter into the skin, leading to vasodilatation, itching, scaling, and other symptoms. Several studies have supported the idea that an impaired barrier predisposes an individual to develop this type of sensitive skin; therefore, dry skin types are more likely to develop this type of sensitive skin than oily skin types who are protected by sebum. One elegant study used

methyl nicotinate (MN), a water-soluble compound widely deployed to investigate transcutaneous penetration. Topical application of MN in humans induces vasodilatation because of the action of the drug on smooth muscle cells.[14] This study demonstrated that lactic acid stingers and those that showed susceptibility to SLS patch-testing irritation were more likely to develop vasodilatation when MN was applied, revealing increased transcutaneous absorption in those labeled as sensitive skin types or "reactors."

OTHER ISSUES THAT SENSITIVE SKIN TYPES ASK ABOUT

Seborrheic Dermatitis

Seborrheic dermatitis is redness and scaling in areas with hair follicles such as the face, scalp, eyebrows, and chest (**Fig. 13-3A and 13-3B**). This is known by patients as "dandruff." Half of the adult population has suffered from "seb derm." *Malassezia* yeasts play a role in causing this inflammatory disorder. Treatments are geared towards reducing *Malassezia* yeasts and reducing inflammation.[15] This condition is very closely associated with stress, so stress reduction is encouraged.

Razor Rash

Many men develop a rash after shaving referred to as a "razor rash" or "razor burn." Sensitivity of the skin after shaving can have many sources. A thorough history is needed to elucidate the cause and best treatment. Ingrown hairs can be treated with salicylic acid cleansers and retinoids, but it is more important to teach the patient the proper way to shave. The angle at which the hair is cut plays a role in this disorder because a hair with a sharp edge is more likely to penetrate into the skin and cause ingrown hairs. Acne can occur due to ingredients in shaving cream or the use of a dirty razor blade. Seborrheic dermatitis arises when the beard is allowed to grow out. Contact or irritant dermatitis can emerge as a reaction to the ingredients in shaving cream or aftershave products. There are also patients with rosacea that flush red after shaving. In summary, razor rash can be caused by many different underlying skin disorders.

Gluten Sensitivity

Dermatitis herpetiformis (DH) is a skin disorder caused by ingesting gluten. Eating gluten will cause pruritus but applying topical products with gluten has not been shown to cause a problem unless ingested orally.

As fears of gluten sensitivity have emerged, patients often ask if gluten is in various skincare products. This is really not an issue because gluten must be ingested into the GI tract to cause a problem in gluten-sensitive individuals. Skincare should not cause a reaction with gluten-sensitive patients unless they use the product on their lips, which often leads to ingestion via lip licking. However, many gluten-sensitive patients are still concerned. Gluten is found in wheat (*Triticum vulgare*), barley (*Hordeum vulgare*), rye (*Secale cereal*), and oats (*Avena sativa*) but these can be labeled differently on a cosmetic product. **Table 13-4** lists ingredients that may have gluten. It is very likely

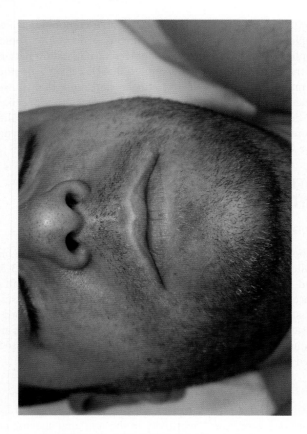

FIGURE 13-3A. Seborrheic dermatitis c on the face. (Courtesy of Nilfredo Orozco.)

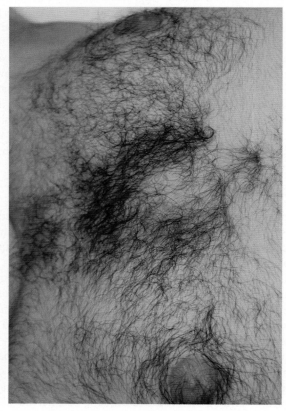

FIGURE 13-3B. Seborrheic dermatitis c on the chest . (Courtesy of Nilfredo Orozco.)

TABLE 13-4	Ingredients With the Words Wheat, Malt, Barley or Rye Have Gluten. These Skincare ingredients also have gluten	
Gluten Ingredient Name List		
Avena Sativa (Oat)		
Cyclodextrin		
Dextrin		
Dextrin Palmitate		
Extract/Glycine Soja Seed Ferment Extract		
Extract/Xanthium Strumarium Fruit		
Fagopytum (Buckwheat) Leaf Extract		
Fermented grain extract		
Hydrolyzed Vegetable Protein		
Hydroxypropyltrimonium Corn/Wheat/Soy Amino Acids		
Hydroxypropyltrimonium Hydrolyzed Wheat Protein/ Siloxysilicate		
Lactobacillus/Oat/Rye/Wheat Seed Extract Ferment		
Lactobacillus/Rye Flour Ferment		
Lactobacillus/Rye Flour Ferment Filtrate		
Laurdimonium Hydroxypropyl Hydrolyzed Wheat Amino Acids		
Malt Extract		
Maltodextrin		
Oat Amino Acids		
Oat Beta-Glucan		
OAT FLOURSODIUM LAUROYL		
Phytosphingosine Extract		
Polygonum G		
Potassium Cocoyl Hydrolyzed Oat Protein		
Rye Extract		
Rye Flour		
Saccharomyces/Barley Seed Ferment Filtrate		
Samino Peptide Complex		
Secale Cereale (Rye) Phytoplacenta Placenta Culture Extract Filtrate		
Sodium C8-16 Isoalkylsuccinyl		
Sodium Wheat Germanphoacetate		
Stearyl Dimonium Hydroxypropyl		
Steardmnonium Hydroxypropyl Hydrolyzed Wheat Protein		
Tocopherol Acetate		
Triticale		
Triticum Aestivum (Wheat) Flour		
Triticum Boeoticum		
Triticum Carthlicum		
Triticum lipids		
Triticum Monococcum		
Triticum Turgidum Durum (Wheat) Seed Extract		
Triticum Vulgare		

Gluten-sensitive individuals do not need to avoid gluten in skincare for two reasons:

1. Gluten must be ingested into the GI tract to cause symptoms.
2. Most gluten is removed from skincare products during processing.

However, those with gluten sensitivity are very distressed by the symptoms and often prefer to avoid skincare with gluten (see Table 13-4). The Food Allergen Labeling and Consumer Protection Act of 2004 does not apply to skincare products; therefore, these products are not required to notify consumers if they contain gluten, nuts, or other allergens.

Skincare ingredients with gluten are derived from wheat, barley, and rye. Reading ingredient labels can be difficult because one ingredient can have multiple names. The INCI name is the official International Nomenclature Cosmetic Ingredient description used to standardize ingredient labeling. However, knowing the name alone is not sufficient. How an ingredient is produced can affect whether it contains gluten. Vitamin E, also called tocopherol, is an example. Tocopherol is a fat-soluble vitamin that can contain gluten depending on its source. Most vitamin E is derived from wheat germ oil, in which case it would contain gluten. The tocopherol used in cosmeceuticals is refined, removing most, if not all, of the gluten. The quality of the tocopherol depends on the source and how it is refined. Cheaper products will be more likely to have gluten due to lower quality in the refining process. Regardless of where the tocopherol is derived from, it is labeled as tocopherol or Vitamin E on the product and it is impossible to know the source unless the manufacturer reveals it. The best recommendation for gluten-sensitive individuals is to avoid Vitamin E-containing products on the lips unless the manufacturer reveals the Vitamin E source.

that even if these ingredients contain gluten, the elements that lead to gluten allergy are usually removed during product manufacturing. In a study published in the *Journal of the Academy of Nutrition and Dietetics*, researchers evaluated skincare products that contained at least one ingredient derived from wheat, barley, rye, or oats. They reported that none of the skincare products contained measurable levels of gluten.[16]

SEASONALITY AND SENSITIVE SKIN

"Sensitive skin" of the burning, stinging, and itching type was found to be more frequent during the summer than the winter in one study.[2] Some rosacea patients report worsening symptoms when seasons change. Normal oily skin types (see Chapter 11, Oily Skin) may become dry skin types in cold, dry months. When the skin barrier is impaired, sensitive skin types 2, 3, and 4 are more likely. Therefore, skin dehydration may be in part responsible for the seasonality seen with sensitive skin.

GENDER AND SENSITIVE SKIN

Women have been found to be more likely than men to have sensitive skin. This may reflect the fact that women have a much higher exposure, in terms of frequency and variety, to personal care products than do men.[2] The thickness of the epidermis was observed to be greater in males than in females, which may mean that men have a stronger barrier to entry of irritants and allergens.[17] Hormonal differences may produce increased inflammatory sensitivity in females.[18]

ETHNICITY AND SENSITIVE SKIN

Research suggests that black skin is less reactive than white skin. Asians report sensitive skin more often than do Caucasians. However, no studies comparing ethnicity and sensitive skin are conclusive.[19,20] A French study based on questionnaires showed that a fair skin type was more commonly associated with sensitive or very sensitive skin.[2] An American study, by Jourdain et al., used telephone surveys of approximately 200 each of African Americans, Asians, European Americans, and Hispanics and did not find any differences in the prevalence of sensitive skin among ethnic groups.[1] In a German–Japanese investigation, Japanese women reported subjective feelings of skin irritation more frequently than German women. This study demonstrated that Japanese women report skin stinging of greater severity than do Caucasian women.[21]

A normal SC, as measured in Caucasians, has been reported to consist of around 15 cell layers.[22,23] The SC appears to be equally thick in black and white skin.[24,25] However, black skin types have been shown to have a higher lipid content in the SC, more SC cell layers, and required more tape strips to remove the SC as compared to light skin types.[26,27] This was purported to be the reason that several studies have reported decreased erythema in black skin after topical application of known irritants.[28–30] Large-scale global studies looking at ethnic differences in the incidence of the various types of sensitive skin have not been performed. At this time, the precise role of ethnicity in skin sensitivity remains to be elucidated.

TESTING FOR SENSITIVE SKIN

Baumann S1 Type Skin

For years, the rabbit ear model was used to test cosmetic ingredients for their potential to cause comedones.[31,32] Based on the rabbit ear model, it appeared that many ingredients used in cosmetics evoked a comedogenic response in animals. As animal testing fell into disfavor, new methods of comedogenicity testing were developed. Subsequently, Mills and Kligman published a study exploring the effects of these chemicals in human beings and found that the results were dissimilar to those observed in the rabbit ear model.[33] Human models of comedogenicity are currently used.[34]

Baumann S2 Type Skin

Vasoreactive tests examine vasodilatation of the skin to ascertain susceptibility to flushing. The most popular test uses methyl nicotinate, a potent vasodilator. MN is applied to the upper third of the ventral forearm in concentrations varying between 1.4% and 13.7% for a period of 15 seconds.

The vasodilatory effect is assessed by observing the induced erythema and measuring it with various devices such as a spectrometer or laser Doppler velocimeter (LDV). Another test used to measure the propensity for facial flushing is the red wine provocation test; however, this test is not very specific. Susceptible patients report a sense of warmth beginning around the head or neck area and moving upward on the face 10 to 15 minutes after ingestion of 6 ounces of red wine. Within 30 minutes, flushing becomes clinically evident.[35] The disadvantage of this test, though, is that it lacks specificity for S2 sensitive skin types; it may be positive when other conditions, such as alcohol dehydrogenase syndrome, are present.

Baumann S3 Type Skin

The sensory reactivity test focuses on the neurosensory component of the sensitive skin response. The most popular has been the sting test,[36] in which lactic acid or other agents including capsaicin, ethanol, menthol,[37] sorbic acid, and benzoic acid[38] are applied to the skin (see Chapters 17 and 38).

Baumann S4 Type Skin

To test for this type of skin, an irritant reactivity test is performed. This is also called a "patch test." In this test, an irritant or allergen is applied to the skin for a certain amount of time, usually 48 to 72 hours, and objective measures of irritation such as erythema and scaling are gauged. Primary irritants such as SLS or suspected allergens may be applied (see Chapter 18).

SUMMARY

Sensitive skin is a very common complaint globally. It has several presentations that have led to different classification systems. The Baumann Skin Typing System divides those with sensitive skin into four subtypes, which are discussed at length in other chapters. Using this system can help provide insights into the causes of these various subgroups of sensitive skin, including the potential roles of gender and ethnicity pertaining to subtype, and should help lead to advances in the treatment of these subtypes.

References

1. Jourdain R, de Lacharrière O, Bastien P, et al. Ethnic variations in self-perceived sensitive skin: epidemiological survey. *Contact Dermatitis*. 2002;46:162.

2. Misery L, Myon E, Martin N, et al. Sensitive skin: psychological effects and seasonal changes. *J Eur Acad Dermatol Venereol*. 2007;21:620.

3. Willis CM, Shaw S, De Lacharrière O, et al. Sensitive skin: an epidemiological study. *Br J Dermatol*. 2001;145:258.

4. Saint-Martory C, Roguedas-Contios AM, Sibaud V, et al. Sensitive skin is not limited to the face. *Br J Dermatol*. 2008;158:130.

5. Data on file Skin Type Solutions Inc. Data collected on 1/15/2021.

6. Pilkington SM, Bulfone-Paus S, Griffiths CEM, Watson REB. Inflammaging and the Skin. *J Invest Dermatol*. 2020;S0022-202X (20)32294–6.

7. Yokota T, Matsumoto M, Sakamaki T, et al. Classification of sensitive skin and development of a treatment system appropriate for each group. *IFSCC Mag*. 2003;6:303.

8. Pons-Guiraud A. Sensitive skin: a complex and multifactorial syndrome. *J Cosmet Dermatol*. 2004;3:145.

9. Muizzuddin N, Marenus KD, Maes DH. Factors defining sensitive skin and its treatment. *Am J Contact Dermat*. 1998;9:170.

10. Baumann L. Cosmetics and skin care in dermatology. In: Wolff K, Goldsmith LA, Katz SI, Gilchrest BA, Paller AS, Leffell DJ, eds. *Fitzpatrick's Dermatology in General Medicine*. 7th ed. New York, NY: McGraw-Hill; 2007:2357–2364.

11. Kligman AM, Mills OH. Acne cosmetica. *Arch Dermatol*. 1972;106:893.

12. Foley P, Nixon R, Marks R, et al. The frequency of reactions to sunscreens: results of a longitudinal population-based study on the regular use of sunscreens in Australia. *Br J Dermatol*. 1993; 128:512.

13. Simion FA, Rau AH. Sensitive skin. *Cosmet Toilet*. 1994;109:43.

14. Berardesca E, Cespa M, Farinelli N, et al. In vivo transcutaneous penetration of nicotinates and sensitive skin. *Contact Dermatitis*. 1991;25:35.

15. Borda LJ, Wikramanayake TC. Seborrheic Dermatitis and Dandruff: A Comprehensive Review. *J Clin Investig Dermatol*. 2015;3(2).doi:10.13188/2373-1044.1000019.

16. Thompson T, Grace T. Gluten in cosmetics: is there a reason for concern? *J Acad Nutr Diet*. 2012;112(9):1316–1323.

17. Sandby MJ, Poulsen T, Wulf HC. Epidermal thickness at different body sites: relationship to age, gender, pigmentation, blood content, skin type and smoking habits. *Acta Derm Venereol*. 2003;83:410.

18. Farage MA. Vulvar susceptibility to contact irritants and allergens: a review. *Arch Gynecol Obstet*. 2005;272:167.

19. Modjtahedi SP, Maibach HI. Ethnicity as a possible endogenous factor in irritant contact dermatitis: comparing the irritant response among Caucasians, blacks and Asians. *Contact Dermatitis*. 2002;47:272.

20. Berardesca E, Maibach H. Ethnic skin: overview of structure and function. *J Am Acad Dermatol*. 2003;48:S139.

21. Aramaki J, Kawana S, Effendy I, et al. Differences of skin irritation between Japanese and European women. *Br J Dermatol*. 2002;146:1052.

22. Christophers E, Kligman AM. Visualization of the cell layers of the stratum corneum. *J Invest Dermatol*. 1964;42:407.

23. Blair C. Morphology and thickness of the human stratum corneum. *Br J Dermatol*. 1968;80:430.

24. Freeman RG, Cockerell EG, Armstrong J, et al. Sunlight as a factor influencing the thickness of epidermis. *J Invest Dermatol*. 1962;39:295.

25. Thomson ML. Relative efficiency of pigment and horny layer thickness in protecting the skin of Europeans and Africans against solar ultraviolet radiation. *J Physiol*. 1955;127:236.

26. Weigand DA, Haygood C, Gaylor JR. Cell layers and density of Negro and Caucasian stratum corneum. *J Invest Dermatol*. 1974;62:563.

27. Reinertson RP, Wheatley VR. Studies on the chemical composition of human epidermal lipids. *J Invest Dermatol*. 1959;32:49.

28. Weigand DA, Gaylor JR. Irritant reaction in Negro and Caucasian skin. *South Med J*. 1974;67:548.

29. Marshall EK, Lynch V, Smith HV. Variation in susceptibility of the skin to dichlorethylsulphide. *J Pharmacol Exp Ther.* 1919;12:291.

30. Weigand DA, Mershon GE. The cutaneous irritant reaction to agent O-chlorobenzylidene malonitrile (CS). Quantitation and racial influence in human subjects. *Edgewood Arsenal Technical Report 4332.* February, 1970.

31. Kligman AM, Kwong T. An improved rabbit ear model for assessing comedogenic substances. *Br J Dermatol.* 1979;100:699.

32. Morris WE, Kwan SC. Use of the rabbit ear model in evaluating the comedogenic potential of cosmetic ingredients. *J Soc Cosmet Chem.* 1983;34:215.

33. Mills OH, Kligman AM. Human model for assessing comedogenic substances. *Arch Dermatol.* 1982;118:903.

34. Draelos ZD, DiNardo JC. A re-evaluation of the comedogenicity concept. *J Am Acad Dermatol.* 2006;54:507.

35. Mills OH, Berger RS. Defining the susceptibility of acne prone and sensitive skin populations to extrinsic factors. *Dermatol Clin.* 1991;9:93.

36. Frosch P, Kligman AM. Method for appraising the sting capacity of topically applied substances. *J Soc Cosmet Chem.* 1977; 28:197.

37. Marriott M, Holmes J, Peters L, et al. The complex problem of sensitive skin. *Contact Dermatitis.* 2005;53:93.

38. Seidenari S, Francomano M, Mantovani L. Baseline biophysical parameters in subjects with sensitive skin. *Contact Dermatitis.* 1998;38:311.

39. O'Malley JT, Clark RA, Widlund HR. Skin Inflammation in Human Health and Disease: 2018 International Conference. *J Invest Dermatol.* 2019;139(5):991–994.

40. Yang HH, Kim C, Jung B, Kim KS, Kim JR. Involvement of IGF binding protein 5 in prostaglandin E(2)-induced cellular senescence in human fibroblasts. *Biogerontology.* 2011;12(3): 239–252.

41. Nguyen SH, Dang TP, Maibach HI. Comedogenicity in rabbit: some cosmetic ingredients/vehicles. *Cutan Ocul Toxicol.* 2007;26(4):287–292.

CHAPTER 14

Uneven Skin Tone

Leslie S. Baumann, MD

SUMMARY POINTS

What's Important?
1. Skin can become pigmented from UV, blue, or infrared light.
2. Patient education and compliance are critical for treatment success.
3. Treating pigmentation is a multifaceted approach.

What's New?
1. Oral tranexamic acid is used to treat pigmentation disorders.
2. Iron oxides in tinted sunscreens block blue light.

What's Coming?
1. There are recent questions about the safety of the sunless tanner DHA that need to be explored.
2. Topical SIK2 inhibitors are being developed to increase skin pigmentation.
3. Hydroquinone was banned in cosmetic products in 2020 leading to the pursuit of new options.

Several factors play a role in the perception of age, health, and attractiveness. Patients often focus on fine lines or skin radiance and are less cognizant of evenness of skin tone. However, many studies have shown that evenness of skin tone plays an important role in perceived skin health, age, and beauty. This chapter will discuss what colors contribute to skin tone, the importance of an even skin tone, and designing the best skincare routine to even skin tone.

REDHEADS AND FRECKLES

Redheads have polymorphic changes in the MCIR gene that affect the ability of the melanocortin receptor to stimulate production of eumelanin. This MCIR polymorphism results in red hair, freckles, nevi, and an increased risk of melanoma. Redheads who avoid the sun have fewer nevi than those with more sun exposure. However, the number of freckles seems to be entirely determined by genetics as shown in a twin study.[1] For this reason, many redheads consider freckles as part of their identity and want to keep them. Freckles do not cause a perception of poor health as other pigmented lesions do.

The studies described below did not evaluate the presence of freckles; rather, they considered solar lentigos, melasma, and post-inflammatory hyperpigmentation that lead to an uneven skin tone.

VITILIGO

Vitiligo is an autoimmune skin condition in which antibodies destroy melanocytes leading to depigmented patches of white skin. This frequently affects the face and can affect self-esteem. Recognizing and treating vitiligo early improves the prognosis. Discussion of the diagnosis and treatment of vitiligo is beyond the scope of this book but it is mentioned here because those with vitiligo need excellent sun protection and options to camouflage the white patches with cosmetics.[2] In extensive vitiligo, some patients choose to depigment the remaining pigmented areas with agents discussed in Chapter 41 (Depigmenting Ingredients) but this can lead to health risks. Fortunately, the recent popularity of models with vitiligo has led to a decreased stigma and increased acceptance of this skin disorder.

THE IMPORTANCE OF AN EVEN SKIN TONE

An even skin tone is perceived as healthier than an uneven skin tone. A 2011 study looked at two different facial images of 61-year-old British women. In one image, the skin surface topography of fine lines was removed ("smoothed"), while the other image had "smoothing" of the uneven color distribution.[3] A panel of 160 German men assessed the photos and were asked to choose which images looked younger and which images looked healthier. The images with less visible fine lines were judged to be younger. The images with even color distribution were perceived to be healthier. This study buttresses the results seen in a similar 2007 study that also suggested an association between evenness of skin color and perception of health.[4] In this study, smoothing the fine lines in images resulted in a decrease in perception of age by 10 years, while smoothing the unevenness of color yielded a decrease in perceived age by 5 years. When both fine lines and unevenness of color were smoothed, the perception of age dropped 15 years. Similar results were seen in a 2008 study demonstrating that men's eyes lingered longer on photos of female faces that had an even skin tone.[5]

Studies in various cultures have shown that uneven skin tone causes a decrease in self-esteem and quality of life.[6-9] Patients are usually very motivated to treat these dyschromia, but treatments can take 4–6 months or longer and compliance can wane without follow-up visits and consistent encouragement.

PIGMENTED AND NONPIGMENTED BAUMANN SKIN TYPES

The Baumann Skin Typing System (BSTS) divides skin into 16 Baumann Skin Types® (BSTs) based on skincare needs (see Chapter 10, The Baumann Skin Typing System). Eight of the BSTs are pigmented skin types (P), while the remaining eight are nonpigmented (N) skin types. An easy way to understand the distinction of these skin types is:

P Skin Types = include pigment-reducing ingredients in the skincare regimen (**Fig. 14-1A**).
N Skin Types = do not include skin-lightening ingredients in the skincare regimen (**Fig. 14-1B**).

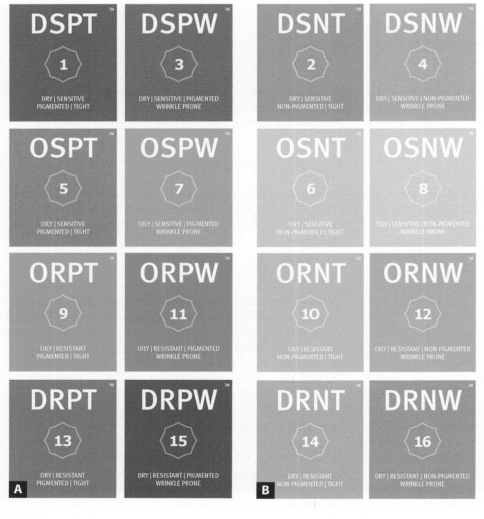

FIGURE 14-1. Pigmented and nonpigmented Baumann Skin Types. There are 16 Baumann Skin Types®. Eight of these have uneven skin tone.
A. Pigmented skin types with uneven skin tone.
B. Individuals who are nonpigmented skin types have an even skin tone or do not want to lighten any hyperpigmented areas. Note that the colors of the nonpigmented skin types are a lighter hue than the pigmented skin types and have an even number in the Baumann Skin Typing System to denote an even skin tone.

The definition of pigmented skin type in the BSTS differs from the Fitzpatrick Skin Typing System, which is based on the skin's pigmentation and erythematous response to UV light as discussed in Chapter 10. Although darker skin types are more likely to develop dyschromia such as melasma or post-inflammatory pigment alteration (PIPA), the "pigmented skin type" in the BSTS does not refer to overall skin color; rather, it describes the presence of unevenness of skin color due to the presence of hyperpigmented macules or patches and the patient's desire to lighten these hyperpigmented lesions. The distinction of "patient's desire to treat" is important because some patients have freckles that give them an uneven skin tone but unless they want to remove the freckles, they do not need skin-lightening ingredients in their skincare regimen. A redhead who has freckles and does not want to remove them is considered an N skin type, while another patient with solar lentigos who wants to remove them would be considered a P skin type. The P designation is based on:

1. The presence of pigmented lesions that are darker than most of the skin tone.
2. The desire to remove these pigmented lesions.

The designation of a P skin type does not correlate with ethnicity or sun reactivity and only provides limited predictive ability about the risk for hyperpigmentation after cosmetic procedures. Pigmented BSTs benefit from the use of tinted sunscreens, skin-lightening ingredients, and camouflage cosmetics. How to treat uneven skin tone will be discussed later in this chapter.

PERCEPTION AND MEASUREMENT OF SKIN COLOR

Lighting affects the perception of color, which makes it difficult to purchase color cosmetics online. Colors look different depending upon whether they are viewed on the computer or phone or in person. The characteristics of the light that color is viewed in also influences the perception of color. This explains why makeup foundation looks like a different color when applied in a store under florescent lights and then the color changes outside in natural light. Color perception also changes depending on the colors that surround it. Consequently, it is difficult for patients to match tinted sunscreens and cover foundations to their skin color.

Reflection of light also affects skin tone. Smooth surfaces reflect more light and appear brighter than rough surfaces. Therefore, smooth hydrated skin looks radiant, while patients with dry rough skin complain of dull skin. Darker skin types manifest an ashy skin tone when dry due to the way light reflects off the retained corneocytes on the skin's surface.

SKIN COLOR

There are several nomenclature systems used to classify color (**Box 14-1**). Conversion tools can be found online to convert one color system to another. The CIELAB color system is the one most commonly used in skincare research and the

---

BOX 14-1 Color Classification Systems

RYB System

This is used by artists working with color cosmetics and paints. The system is based on the amounts of red, yellow, and blue, which make up skin tone. When fully saturated versions of R, Y, and B are mixed, pure white results. When all three colors are completely removed, black results. RYB is also used in digital applications such as computers, games, and television. RYB colors require illumination for vibrancy.

CMY or CMYK System

This uses combinations of tiny dots of cyan, magenta, yellow, and black. These dots overlap each other to form colors. When a CMYK printed piece is viewed with a magnifying glass, different dots of color are seen rather than a uniform color as seen in Pantone colors. This system is used most often in printing.

The RGB System

This is deployed in systems that use light such as photography, television, and digital graphic interfaces.

Hex (Hexadecimal color) Code

The hex code is also used for digital interfaces. It is basically R, G, B simplified by providing one number overall rather than one number each corresponding to an R, G, and B tone.

Pantone®

Pantone colors are patented standardized ink colors produced by the Pantone company. It is the first standardized comprehensive system used to match colors in the graphics and design community. Pantone has color swatches with assigned codes that help ensure colors are standardized.

Commission Internationale de l'Eclairage (CIE)

CIE is an international authority on light and color. The CIELAB expresses color in three values. Lightness (L*) measures the gray scale with values from 0 (white) to 100 (black). This is what artists call "tone." Red/green intensity (a*) is measured as the red values being positive and the green values being negative. The yellow/blue intensity (b*) has positive values for yellow and negative values for blue.

---

cosmetic industry. In the CIELAB system, melanin correlates with the score labeled L*; lighter skin types have a higher L* value, while darker skin types have a lower L* value. Erythema correlates with a positive a* value and is due partly to the amount of hemoglobin and its saturation in the dermis.[10]

Skin tone, also referred to as the "complexion," is the surface color of the skin. It is derived from combinations of melanin pigment, hemoglobin (oxyhemoglobin and deoxyhemoglobin), bilirubin, and carotene. Most human skin tone results from the visual impact of the two kinds of melanin scattered in the keratinocytes and melanocytes of the skin: eumelanin and pheomelanin. Eumelanin is derived from tyrosine and is brown/black while pheomelanin is derived from tyrosine and cysteine and is yellow/red. The production of melanin vacillates between eumelanin and pheomelanin based on MCIR activity, the presence of glutathione, and the availability of cysteine.

The top layer of the epidermis, a normal stratum corneum (SC), does not play much of a role in skin color. An unhealthy SC does affect perception of skin tone. In healthy skin of light-skinned individuals, the SC does not have melanin in the corneocytes so the SC is clear and translucent like plastic wrap. The SC of dark-skinned individuals is slightly yellow due to the presence of "melanin" dust in the corneocytes. See Chapter 15, Skin of Color, for a more complete description.

The major chromophore (in the visible range of light) in the *epidermis* is melanin and its metabolites and precursors. Melanin granules both absorb and scatter light. The skin tone of healthy human skin depends upon the melanin concentration in the epidermis. The dominant chromophore in the *dermis* is hemoglobin (either oxyhemoglobin or deoxyhemoglobin), which is usually contained in capillaries (except in the case of trauma or bruising). This explains why areas of the skin with more capillaries look pink or reddish as compared to other areas of the skin. The perceived erythema of inflammation is a result of the number of capillaries involved, their diameter, and blood flow rate.

Tanning

The amount of melanin in the skin is increased upon UV exposure. When UV light causes DNA damage in keratinocytes, proteolytic cleavage of the pro-opiomelanocortin gene is triggered. This leads to production of α-melanocyte-stimulating hormone, which binds the melanocortin receptor-1 subsequently activating cAMP. Increased cAMP activates protein kinase A, which then phosphorylates cAMP-responsive-element-binding protein resulting in stimulation of the microphthalmia-associated transcription factor gene, ultimately leading to an increase in melanin production (**Fig. 14-2**).

The skin color change produced by UVA is different from that provoked by UVB (**Table 14-1**).[11] Melanin pigments produced by UVA light appear gray while those caused by UVB light appear brown. This is thought to be due to the level of the epidermis and dermis that the light hits: UVA penetrates deeper than UVB.

After UVA exposure, immediate pigment darkening (IPD) occurs in the skin. The result, a gray/black color, is believed to be caused by oxidation of melanin and the colorless melanogenic precursors (such as polymers of DHICA or 6H5MICA) found in melanosomes.[11] The pigment produced by oxidized polymers of DHICA and 6H5MICA does not provide the same level of photoprotection that melanin does and this should *not* be considered a protective tan. IPD is followed by persistent pigment darkening (PPD), which is a separate stage and results in pigmentation that is brown and lasts for several weeks corresponding with the epidermal turnover time of around 40 days. Note that tanning beds use UVA and the "tan" achieved from tanning beds does not deliver the same protection as a tan from UVB. This is one of the many reasons that tanning beds are so harmful—they give a false sense of security.

UVB exposure engenders a different color response than UVA. UVB first results in erythema. Brown tanning occurs a day or two later and is caused by an increase in tyrosinase activity, increased melanin production, and melanosome transfer.[12]

SKIN OPTICS

Light affects how color is perceived. Also, various wavelengths of light act differently upon contact with the skin. When light strikes the skin, some is absorbed, some is reflected, and some is scattered. This phenomenon is elegantly described in a 1995 paper by Kollias, who was a leader in the field of skin optics.[13]

TABLE 14-1	Difference in Skin Tone Changes Caused by UVA and UVB	
	UVA	**UVB**
	Immediate color change	Delayed color change
	No erythema	Erythema
	Immediate gray color	No immediate pigment
	Delayed brown color	Delayed brown color
	Oxidation of melanogenic precursors	Increased tyrosinase
		Increased melanosome transfer

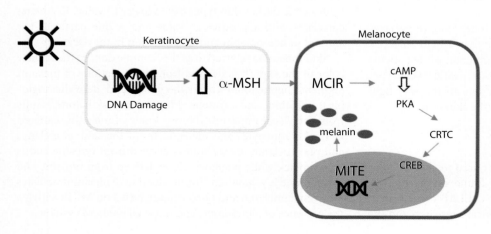

FIGURE 14-2. The cAMP-MITF eumelanin pathway.
MSH = Melanocyte-stimulating hormone, MCIR = Melanocortin receptor-1, PKA = protein kinase A, CRTC = CREB-regulated transcription co-activator, CREB = cAMP-responsive-element-binding protein (CREB), MITF = microphthalmia-associated transcription factor gene.
Proteolytic cleavage of the pro-opiomelanocortin gene produces α-MSH, which binds the MCIR subsequently activating cAMP. Increased cAMP activates PKA, which then phosphorylates CREB resulting in stimulation of the MITF gene, yielding melanin production.

The SC and epidermis of normal skin do not produce enough scattering to render a significant effect on the skin's appearance. Most of the perceived skin color comes from light reflected from the dermis. However, abnormal epidermis with dryness, inflammation, or unusual pigment distribution will influence how light absorbs, reflects, and scatters. Kollias and Bager explained that scales on the skin from xerosis and psoriasis contain numerous surfaces and edges resulting in multiple reflections of light at various angles off the skin. This accounts for why a very scaly skin surface as seen in psoriasis appears white, while a smooth SC appears clear.

The dermis incorporates several components that contribute to skin optics. Dermal collagen is the main scatterer of visible light in the skin. This is one reason that younger skin with larger amounts of collagen has a healthier looking skin tone than photoaged skin.

PHEOMELANIN AND EUMELANIN

There are two distinct forms of melanin in human skin (**Table 14-2**). Eumelanin is considered photoprotective, while pheomelanin is considered phototoxic because it is a pro-oxidant (causes free radicals), especially when exposed to UVA.[14,15] Human skin, regardless of Fitzpatrick Skin Type, has a consistent ratio of 74% eumelanin to 26% pheomelanin.[16]

Pheomelanin is derived from the oxidative polymerization of 5-S- and 2-S-cysteinyldopa and consists of benzothiazine and benzothiazole derivatives.[17] Benzothiazine is the portion of pheomelanin that renders it a pro-oxidant that promotes free radicals. Pheomelanin formation depends on sulfur, which is found in L-cysteine, and the presence of L-cysteine. A major storage pool of cysteine is the natural antioxidant glutathione. Glutathione is used intravenously as a skin-lightening ingredient, as discussed in Chapter 41, because pheomelanin is lighter than eumelanin. Increasing the amount of glutathione

favors production of pheomelanin over eumelanin. Increased production of pheomelanin can deplete glutathione stores, decreasing the skin's natural antioxidant defenses and contributing to the pro-oxidant capabilities of pheomelanin. Pheomelanin plays a role in carcinogenesis, especially in the presence of UVA radiation, due to the production of free radicals that damage DNA and deplete glutathione, NAD(P)H, and other cellular antioxidants that protect DNA from damage.[14]

Eumelanin is a polymer of 5,6-dihydroxyindole (DHI) and DHICA and exhibits robust antioxidant activity. Eumelanin protects skin from sun exposure.[18] Melanosomes, which contain more eumelanin than pheomelanin, localize to areas around the cell nucleus where they form a protective cap to shield cellular DNA from UV radiation and resulting mutations. Eumelanin is the primary determinant of skin color and directly correlates with total melanin content.[18] It is the decreased amount of eumelanin seen in redheads (they have a mutation of the MCIR gene) that increases their risk of melanoma.

SKINCARE FOR PIGMENTED SKIN TYPES

Skin types with uneven skin tone due to areas of hyperpigmentation will benefit from tyrosinase inhibitors, antioxidants, anti-inflammatories, retinoids, protease-activated receptor 2 (PAR-2) blockers, exfoliation, and sun protection. These ingredients are discussed at length in Chapter 41, while skin disorders that cause skin pigmentation are discussed in Chapter 20, Pigmentation Disorders.

Treating pigmented skin types is frustrating because it requires patient compliance and patience. Results are typically not seen for 8–16 weeks because it takes around 40 days to renew all the epidermal keratinocytes. Managing patient expectations, giving written instructions, and scheduling monthly follow-ups can improve compliance. Taking baseline photographs and telling patients that at each visit photos will be taken, assessed, and compared to baseline helps motivate them to use the products properly (**Fig. 14-3A** and **Box 14-2**).

Pigmented skin types as defined in the BSTS will benefit from a skincare routine to lighten skin and even skin tone. The approach to treating pigmented skin types is multifaceted and involves two or more phases.

Phase 1 Skincare for "P" Baumann Skin Types

The first approach to treating any skin type is to evaluate if there is underlying dryness, inflammation, or lifestyle habits that can be contributing to the dyspigmentation. Skin dryness can lead to inflammation, and an impaired skin barrier can contribute to increased side effects from skin-lightening ingredients and retinoids. Skin dryness should be treated with cleansers and moisturizers that protect and repair the skin barrier. At the same time, if inflammation manifested as skin sensitivity is present, it should be addressed before beginning a pigmentation treatment regimen. Inflammation contributes to both skin pigmentation and skin aging. If inflammation is not addressed prior to beginning skincare products for pigmentation, it is likely that the pigmentation will worsen. Phase 1

TABLE 14-2	Differences between Eumelanin and Pheomelanin[36]
EUMELANIN	**PHEOMELANIN**
Photoprotective	Phototoxic, generating free radicals
Made of polymers of DHI and DHICA	Made of benzothiazine
74% of melanin in human skin	25% of melanin in human skin
Brown or black	Reddish-yellow
Production stimulated by α-MSH	Requires sulfur in form of L-cysteine
Formation regulated by MCR1	Formation favored by glutathione
Has antioxidant capacity	Reduces glutathione stores
	Reduces antioxidants
	Depletes NAD(P)H
	Plays a role in carcinogenesis

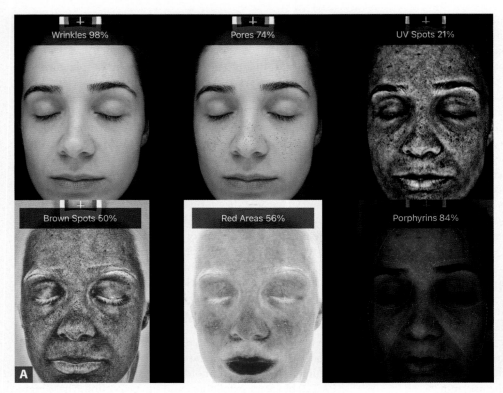

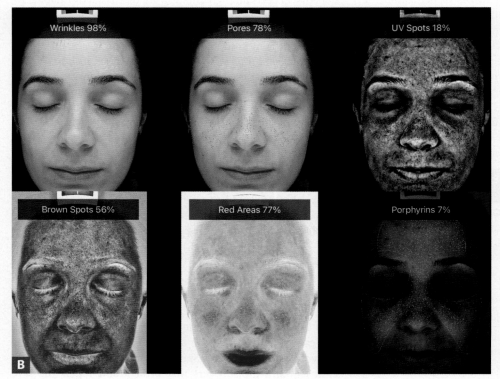

FIGURE 14-3. Progression of pigmentation treatment regimen Images.
A. This baseline image shows skin prior to beginning a pigmentation treatment regimen. The numbers represent how "good" the image is compared with others of the same skin color, age, and gender. In other words, a high % number is better. In Figure A, the UV spot % shows that the patient has an excess of pigment in the upper layer of the epidermis and they score in the 21st percentile. The goal is to raise this number to 70% or higher. The brown spot %, which illustrates pigment deeper in the epidermis, is 50%. The goal is to raise this number to 70% or higher while maintaining a red area score of 50% or higher. **B.** This one-month image shows the expected effect of a patient using their regimen as prescribed. After 1 month of a pigmentation treatment regimen, as described in Fig. 14-5, the UV % number actually worsens from 21% to 18% because melanin has moved from deeper layers of the epidermis to the surface. How fast this occurs depends on how often the patient uses a low-pH cleanser and the TCC product. There is evidence that the patient is being compliant with the regimen because the brown spot % rose from 50% to 56% showing that the pigment is rising to the surface, without an increase in new pigment production. The red area % rose to 77% (decreased erythema) because the patient is on the proper cleansers and a soothing barrier repair moisturizer to minimize retinoid side effects and is only using the low-pH cleanser once daily and the TCC every other night on top of a moisturizer. (continued)

skincare should target dryness and inflammation and be used for 2–4 weeks before beginning phase 2. If a patient is an oily, resistant skin type, then phase 1 is not necessary because there is no underlying dryness or inflammation.

Phase 2 Skincare for "P" Baumann Skin Types

Ingredients that target pigmentation, such as retinoids and tyrosinase inhibitors, can be irritating to the skin and lead to inflammation. Completing phase 1 first

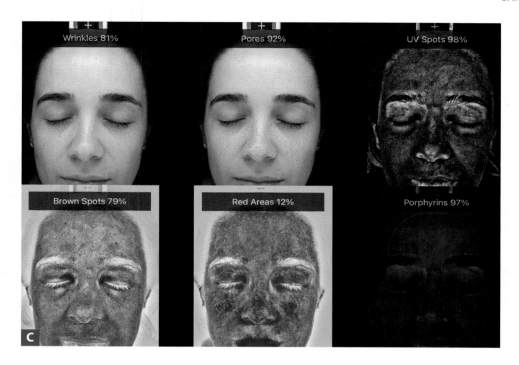

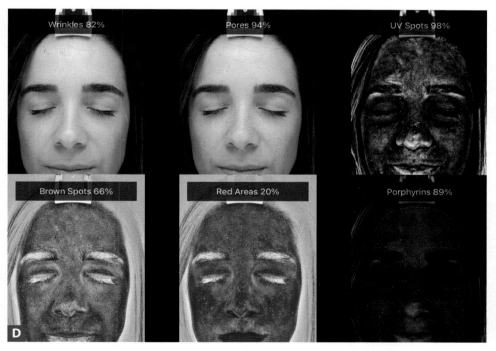

FIGURE 14-3. (continued) **C.** This four-month image shows a huge improvement in pigmentation both superficial and deep with an increase in erythema. The patient has been on a low-pH cleanser twice daily and the TCC in Step 4 with a moisturizer in Step 5 since the Month 3 visit. The mild inflammation can lead to an increase in pigmentation when the tyrosinase inhibitors are stopped as part of the pigmentation maintenance regimen. **D.** This five-month image shows a continued improvement of the UV spot number and as seen by the naked eye. However, this patient was not treated with oral tranexamic acid and has been on the pigmentation maintenance regimen for 4 weeks without tyrosinase inhibitors. The brown spots % shows that melanin production has increased, and pigment can be seen in the lower layers of the epidermis. (Valeria M. Abello.)

should allow dry and sensitive skin types to better tolerate products to treat their skin pigmentation. Once phase 1 has been completed, as ascertained by the medical provider, phase 2 can be started. Phase 2 is also known as the pigmentation treatment regimen. The pigmentation treatment regimen is used for 3 months or until the unwanted pigmentation is cleared. It will then be followed by a pigmentation maintenance regimen (which can be referred to as phase 3). There are two scenarios to consider

at the completion of the first Pigmentation Treatment Regimen:

1. The pigment has disappeared, and the skin is even toned: the patient should be treated with a pigmentation maintenance skincare regimen.
2. The pigmentation is still present: the patient will use the maintenance skincare regimen for 4 weeks and then return to the Pigmentation Treatment Regimen.

BOX 14-2	Complexion Analysis Measurements

The Canfield Visia CF can be used effectively to track the progress of pigmentation change and encourage patients even when they cannot yet see a difference with the naked eye. The Canfield Visia complexion analysis software provides several measurements. The UV spots and brown spots measurements in addition to the inflammation measurements are the most helpful when tracking skin pigmentation changes.

UV Spots Measurement

Epidermal melanin just below the skin's surface absorbs UV light, resulting in a measurement of melanin. This measurement is used to gauge the amount of melanin in the upper levels of the epidermis. It is important to explain to patients at the baseline visit that this number will get worse (due to an increase in superficial melanin) before it gets better as melanin rises from the lower layers and becomes visible here.

Brown Spots Measurement

The brown spot measurement shows melanin on the skin's surface and in deeper layers of the epidermis. This number will improve first before the UV spot number does because it shows melanin levels deeper in the skin.

Red Areas Measurement

This measurement can be used to track side effects from retinoids, hydroxy acids, and other agents used to even skin tone. The goal is to mitigate inflammation to prevent triggering the production of new melanin. See **Fig. 14-4** for an example of how to use the camera system to track progress.

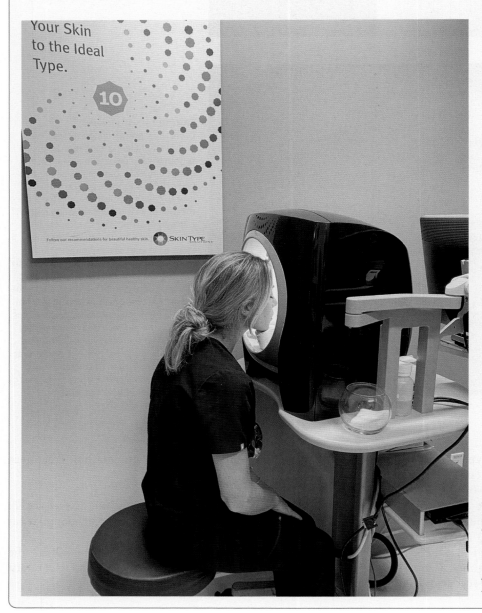

FIGURE 14-4. The Canfield Visia Camera system is a useful instrument for tracking progress of skincare routines designed to even skin tone. Photos help the medical provider assess compliance and efficacy. Photos also serve to motivate patients to use recommended products because they look forward to seeing the result and getting their "scores" that the camera provides.

Phase 3 Skincare for "P" Baumann Skin Types: The Pigmentation Maintenance Regimen

Baseline Visit

Once the patient's skin is hydrated and less inflamed, the pigmentation treatment regimen can be started. **Fig. 14-5** shows a sample regimen format for treating melasma.

Step 1: Cleanser

Two different cleansers should be prescribed, an AM cleaner and a PM cleanser. In patients with sensitive skin, or retinoid-naïve patients, a soothing cleanser with anti-inflammatory ingredients can be chosen for the AM, or they can use the same cleanser as in the PM.

The PM cleanser should have the ability to remove sunscreen and makeup but confer minimal exfoliation effects. Further, the PM cleanser should be a foaming cleanser for oily skin types or a creamy nonfoaming cleanser for dry skin types. Consider the PM cleanser as the "rescue cleanser." If the skin gets irritated, the patient will use the PM cleanser in both the morning and evening until the skin calms down.

In resistant skin types or for patients already acclimated to a retinoid, the AM cleanser should help exfoliate the skin to accelerate the keratinization cycle, so results are visible sooner. This AM cleanser can be a low-pH cleanser or a mechanical exfoliating scrub (Chapter 40, Cleansing Agents). Oily skin patients do well with a salicylic acid cleanser, while dry skin patients should use an alpha hydroxy acid cleanser with humectant properties such as glycolic acid.

Step 2: Eye Product

After the cleanser, in both the AM and PM, a protective barrier repair eye cream should be used to protect the delicate eye area from the other products. This is especially important at night when retinoids can be rubbed onto the pillowcase and transfer onto eyelid skin.

Step 3: Treatment Product

After the eye cream, the pigmentation treatment formulation should be applied. This product should contain tyrosinase inhibitors, PAR-2 blocking agents, and antioxidants that are not included in PM Step 5. It is preferred that Step 3 not contain retinoids because retinoids will be introduced in Step 5 in the PM.

Step 4: Moisturizer

Depending on the BST, moisturizers in the pigmentation treatment regimen may contain anti-inflammatory or anti-aging ingredients but should not contain retinoids or hydroxy acids because the moisturizer will be used to soothe skin in the case of retinoid dermatitis or irritation from the depigmenting ingredients.

Oily skin patients can use a hyaluronic acid or other light humectant-containing moisturizer that does not have barrier repair ingredients. Very oily skin types can omit a moisturizer.

In dry skin patients, it is important to choose a barrier repair moisturizer with unsaturated fatty acids that help decrease melanin synthesis and tyrosinase activity.[19,20] Free fatty acids cause regulatory effects on melanogenesis (Chapter 43, Moisturizers). Linoleic acid, an ω-6 fatty acid found in argan oil and other oils, has been shown to inhibit tyrosinase activity in melanocytes and decrease UVB-induced pigmentation.[20,21] Using barrier repair moisturizers containing grape seed oil, borage seed oil, and argan oil, which are all are good sources of linoleic acid, may help increase efficacy of skin-lightening products.

The moisturizer is applied after the Step 3 products to help increase penetration of the Step 3 products into the skin.

Step 5: Sunscreen in AM and Retinoid in PM

The last step in the AM is a tinted sunscreen. This should contain iron oxide pigments that help block blue light and prevent activation of melanocytes. Step 5 in the PM should be a triple combination cream (TCC) as discussed in Chapter 41. TCCs contain a corticosteroid, a tyrosinase inhibitor, and a retinoid. The combination of these three ingredients has been established as the most successful topical treatment for melasma and other causes of hyperpigmentation. In retinoid-naïve patients, the TCC product should be applied after the moisturizer. Have the patient use the TCC every third night for 2 weeks and then every other night for 2 weeks so they can acclimate to the retinoid without developing inflammation.

Month 1 Visit

At this visit there is usually minimal change in pigmentation to the naked eye and patients may be experiencing some retinoid side effects, such as erythema or scaling. This visit serves as a "cheerleading visit" because patients are often discouraged. The Canfield photos should be compared to baseline. This will help assess compliance, side effects, and efficacy. In many cases the photos will show an improvement in the brown spot %, which will help motivate the patient to continue as instructed. **Fig. 14-3B** demonstrates typical findings at this visit. When compared with Fig. 14-3A taken at baseline, an increase in melanin is seen at the skin's surface in the UV spots image. The pigment is more easily visualized when it is at the skin's surface, which is why patients may see an increase in pigmentation with the naked eye at this visit that is discouraging. Showing the patient that the deeper layer is improved, as seen in the brown spots image, can help encourage them to be compliant and stay on course.

Step 1: Cleanser

If the patient is experiencing redness or peeling or an increase in inflammation is seen in the photos, the low-pH cleanser can be temporarily stopped. In this case, the PM cleanser should be used twice daily. Another option is to change the low-pH cleanser in the AM to a soothing cleanser with anti-inflammatory ingredients.

If the patient is using the retinoid every other night and not experiencing any retinoid dermatitis, keep the cleanser the same as the baseline regimen.

If the patient is tolerating the retinoid every night, then add the low-pH cleanser in the PM so they are using it twice daily.

Step 2: Eye Product, Step 3: Treatment Product, and Step 5: Sunscreen

These steps are unchanged from baseline.

Step 4: Moisturizer

In most cases this step will be unchanged. However, some normal oily skin types that produce a normal rather than excess amount of sebum (see Chapter 11, Oily Skin) will require a barrier repair moisturizer until their skin acclimates

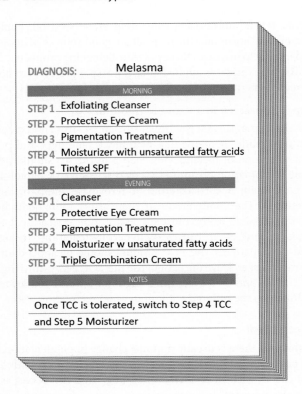

DIAGNOSIS:	Melasma

MORNING

STEP 1 Exfoliating Cleanser
STEP 2 Protective Eye Cream
STEP 3 Pigmentation Treatment
STEP 4 Moisturizer with unsaturated fatty acids
STEP 5 Tinted SPF

EVENING

STEP 1 Cleanser
STEP 2 Protective Eye Cream
STEP 3 Pigmentation Treatment
STEP 4 Moisturizer w unsaturated fatty acids
STEP 5 Triple Combination Cream

NOTES

Once TCC is tolerated, switch to Step 4 TCC
and Step 5 Moisturizer

FIGURE 14-5. Sample pigmentation treatment regimen for melasma.

to the retinoid. If retinoid dermatitis is seen, ensure that a barrier repair moisturizer is used. This will be their "rescue moisturizer." Choose a barrier repair moisturizer with anti-inflammatory ingredients to soothe the skin if the patient has redness or peeling or if the "red areas" % on the Canfield camera is below 50%.

Step 5: Retinoid

If no redness or peeling is visible and the patient does not report any skin stinging, the retinoid in the PM should be increased to every night and applied over the moisturizer. The "red areas" image from the Canfield camera can be used to assess whether the patient has underlying erythema, but the clinical presentation is more important to consider when deciding on whether to increase the frequency of retinoid application. If no inflammation is seen, continue the same dose of retinoid in a TCC product and increase application to nightly.

If the patient was already tolerating the retinoid/TCC every night, then switch the regimen so the TCC is applied in Step 4 and the moisturizer is applied in Step 5. This will allow more retinoid to penetrate into the skin, thereby increasing the delivered dose.

Month 2 Visit

Assess the skin for redness and scaling as discussed above. At this visit, the patient may be seeing an improvement in skin pigmentation if they have been able to use the TCC every night. If the patient has been tolerating the TCC every night, then switch the regimen so the TCC is applied in Step 4 and the moisturizer is applied in Step 5. If the patient has been tolerating the TCC every night in Step 4 with the moisturizer

applied in Step 5, then increase the low-pH cleanser to twice daily.

If the patient is not tolerating the TCC every night, discontinue the low-pH cleanser and ensure that the moisturizer is a soothing formulation with anti-inflammatory ingredients.

Normal oily skin types who were placed on a barrier repair moisturizer may feel that it is too heavy if they are tolerating the retinoid well every night. If so, change to a light moisturizer with hyaluronic acid. This will help increase penetration of the retinoid. Make this change only if they are tolerating the retinoid every night.

The photos at this visit should begin to show some improvement in the UV spots % in addition to the brown spots % if the patient is compliant with the regimen.

Month 3 Visit

Follow the recommendations of the Month 2 visit until the patient is using a low-pH cleanser twice a day and a TCC in Step 4 every night. Most patients will see a difference in skin pigmentation with the naked eye by this visit; however, it can take 16 weeks to see improvement so do not be discouraged.

If the pigmentation is not improving or the patient is getting discouraged, consider oral tranexamic acid, as discussed in Chapter 41.

In the Canfield photos, it is normal to see some erythema (increase in the red areas %) if the patient is using a low-pH cleanser twice daily, a skin lightener in Step 3 twice daily, and a TCC in Steps 3 or 5. If this is the case, confirm that the patient is using a moisturizer with anti-inflammatory ingredients.

Month 4 Visit

The first pigmentation treatment regimen phase has been completed. Many patients see improvement at this visit both with the naked eye and with the Canfield camera (**Fig. 14-3C**). There are two scenarios to consider at the completion of the first pigmentation treatment regimen phase:

1. The pigment has disappeared, and the skin is even toned: the patient should be treated with a pigmentation maintenance skincare regimen unless pigment returns.
2. The pigmentation is still present: the patient will use the maintenance skincare regimen for 4 weeks and then return to the pigmentation treatment regimen.

The pigmentation treatment regimen should be followed for a total of 3 months and stopped at the Month 4 visit. Although there are no studies that prove patients develop tachyphylaxis from tyrosinase inhibitors, it is a common practice to take a one-month holiday from tyrosinase inhibitors that have a chemical structure similar to hydroquinone (HQ) such as kojic acid and arbutin. There is a widespread belief that halting HQ and other similar tyrosinase inhibitors for 4 weeks will improve their effectiveness when restarted. During this four-week period, the patient should use the pigmentation maintenance regimen. Oral tranexamic acid can be used during this period to help prevent recurrence of pigmentation.

The Pigmentation Maintenance Regimen: 4 Weeks

Whether the patient has remaining pigment or is clear, the pigmentation maintenance regimen should start at the beginning of Month 4. At this point, the patient should be adjusted to the retinoid, so a low-pH (exfoliating) cleanser can be used twice daily. The same eye cream can be used as in the pigmentation treatment regimen. The same moisturizer can also be used. It is Step 3 AM and PM and Step 5 PM that are different in the pigmentation maintenance regimen (**Fig. 14-6**).

In the pigmentation maintenance regimen, tyrosinase inhibitors that share a similar chemical structure to HQ should be avoided. PAR-2 blocking agents such as niacinamide or myristyl nicotinate should be used to block melanosome transfer during this period so that even if melanin is produced, it does not transfer to keratinocytes. Use antioxidants such as flavonoids that chelate copper to decrease tyrosinase activity (see Chapter 39, Antioxidants). Ascorbic acid can be used because it can prevent pigmentation from UV exposure.[22,23] Polypodium leucotomos oral supplements may help prevent recurrence.[24,25] Other oral supplements used to prevent recurrence include melatonin and pycnogenol.[26,27] Oral tranexamic acid can be used during the pigmentation maintenance regimen to prevent recurrence or to continue clearing in the absence of tyrosinase inhibitors. Retinoids should be continued so that when the TCC is restarted, there is no need to adjust to the retinoid.

It is common to see a recurrence of pigmentation during the pigmentation maintenance regimen (**Fig. 14-3D**). Patients should be instructed to adhere to strict heat, sun, and light avoidance. The Canfield camera can detect the increase of pigment formation in the brown spots % prior to changes seen with the naked eye.

If the pigmentation is still present at the end of 1 month, the cycle should be repeated as follows: Pigmentation Treatment Regimen – 4 months → Pigmentation Maintenance Regimen – 1 month → Pigmentation Treatment Regimen – 4 months → Pigmentation Maintenance Regimen – 1 month. It may take three or four cycles in severe cases. In some cases, especially when heat and light cannot be avoided and/or the patient is on estrogen, the pigmentation never completely clears. However, when patients have been educated or are compliant, good results are usually achieved.

COLOR COSMETICS AND COLOR THEORY

One of the most significant obstacles to patient satisfaction with cosmetic procedures is the prevention and treatment of bruising (Chapter 36, Pre- and Post-Procedure Skincare). Covering bruising with a makeup concealer is somewhat complicated because bruises change color over time from red → red-violet → green → yellow → yellow brown. Different concealer shades are needed to cover each of these colors. **Box 14-3** discusses color theory as it pertains to skin (**Fig. 14-7**). Birthmarks and scars that remain one color are easier to conceal than bruises.

Box 14-3	Color Theory as It Pertains to Skin

Complementary colors are on opposite sides of each other on the color wheel. Complementary colors cancel each other out to form gray. Most makeup artists recommend using a complementary color over a discolored skin area and then covering the resulting gray with a foundation that matches the skin tone. A red-violet bruise should be covered with yellow-green concealer. This should yield a gray tone that can then be covered with foundation. The color of bruises changes from red to red-violet, then green, and followed by yellow in a progression over 3–10 days. Each day the color concealer should be adjusted to the color that is complementary to the skin color.

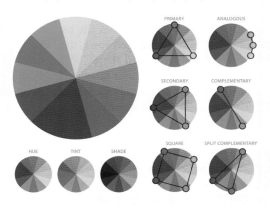

FIGURE 14-7. The color wheel (Macrovector/Shutterstock).

Pigmentation Maintenance Regimen

DIAGNOSIS: _____

MORNING
STEP 1 Exfoliating Cleanser
STEP 2 Protective Eye Cream
STEP 3 Ascorbic acid or PAR-2 blocker
STEP 4 Moisturizer with unsaturated fatty acids
STEP 5 Tinted SPF

EVENING
STEP 1 Cleanser
STEP 2 Protective Eye Cream
STEP 3 Ascorbic acid or PAR-2 blocker
STEP 4 Moisturizer w unsaturated fatty acids
STEP 5 Retinoid

NOTES

If retinoid is tolerated, switch Step 4 to
Retinoid and Step 5 to Moisturizer

FIGURE 14-6. Sample pigmentation maintenance regimen.

COSMETIC PROCEDURES TO EVEN SKIN TONE

Uneven skin tone benefits from treatments that remove dark spots. These should be chosen based on the underlying cause of the altered pigmentation (Chapter 20). Options include lasers, intense pulsed light (IPL), and chemical peels. In the author's experience in sunny Miami, melasma patients do best with skincare alone because they often experience rebound effects from lasers and IPL 3 to 6 months after treatment.

AGENTS TO AUGMENT SKIN PIGMENTATION

In some cases, patients may have vitiligo, idiopathic guttate hypomelanosis, light scars, stretch marks, or other light areas that they want to conceal. Tinted sunscreens and foundations can be used. Henna and vegetable dyes have been used to color light areas of the skin. The most commonly used ingredient to increase skin pigmentation is dihydroxyacetone (DHA), but other solutions may soon be available. Tanning beds are often used to pigment the skin, but they cause lasting damage to skin health.

Iron Oxide Pigments

Iron oxide (FeO) pigments are found in makeup foundations, cosmetic powders, and some tinted sunscreens. The darker the sunscreen tint or makeup color, the more iron oxide is in the formulation. Tinted sunscreens with iron oxides help block visible as well as UV light and should be included in skincare routines designed to lighten facial pigmentation and prevent skin aging.[28]

Dihydroxyacetone

DHA is the component used in sunless tanners to darken skin color by causing a color change of corneocytes in the SC. DHA is a three-carbon sugar that undergoes glycation with the amino acids in corneocytes. This results in an orange/brown skin appearance seen under the microscope as clumps of pigment distributed irregularly in the keratin layer. The Maillard reaction (glycation) responsible for the pigment change also causes the distinctive odor of self-tanner.

The skin color that results from the use of sunless tanner is an unnatural tone of orange/brown that emerges from an increase in yellow pigment in the SC.[29] The color change is usually noticeable about 1 hour after application. The addition of antioxidants, specifically caffeic acid phenethyl ester (CAPE), yields a less yellow, more natural-looking skin tone.[30] DHA is most stable at a pH from 4 to 6 and should not be combined with oxygen- or nitrogen-containing compounds, collagen, urea derivatives, amino acids, peptides, or proteins due to stability issues.[31]

The color change of skin seen with sunless tanners is independent of the melanin pathway and the DHA pigmentation does not provide cell nucleus protection the way that melanin

does. Although a few reports have shown that some DHA products have an SPF of around 3,[32] data are inconsistent as the SPF depends on concentration of DHA, amount used, and number of applications. Sunless tanners should not be considered as sun protectant. The minimal sun protection seen with a 20% DHA cream is temporary and was shown to have an SPF of 3 on Day 1, SPF 2 on Day 5, and SPF 1.7 on Day 7.[33] Although DHA-containing products are in widespread use, there are emerging questions about their long-term safety.[34]

Salt-Inducible Kinase Inhibitors

When UV-induced DNA damage occurs in keratinocytes, p53-mediated transcription of the pro-opiomelanocortin gene results in production of melanocyte-stimulating hormone (MSH). A series of steps lead to activation of the MITF gene leading to melanin synthesis (**Fig. 14-8A**). The activation of MITF is inhibited by salt-inducible kinase 2 (SIK2).[35] (See **Fig. 14-8B**.)

SIK2 inhibitors are being studied to increase skin pigmentation as a skin-protective mechanism against skin cancer. When SIK2 inhibitors are applied to human skin explants, skin becomes darker. This occurs because of the increase in MITF expression as well as an increase in melanosome transfer from melanocytes to keratinocytes.[35]

Enhancing skin pigmentation by increasing eumelanin content imparts several advantages. An increase in melanin content around the cell nucleus provides protection against

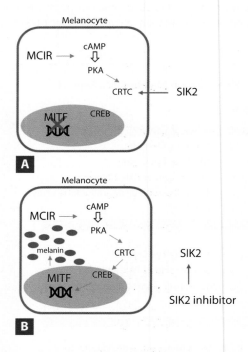

FIGURE 14-8. Steps leading to MITF-activated melanin synthesis and its inhibition by salt-inducible kinase 2 (SIK2).
A. The activation of MITF is inhibited by salt-inducible kinase 2 (SIK2) leading to a decrease in MITF activation and a reduction in melanin production.[35] **B.** SIK2 inhibition leads to MITF expression resulting in an increase in melanin formation and an increase in transport of melanosomes to keratinocytes. This causes an increase in skin pigmentation.

mutations and skin cancers. Generalized use of a product that increases eumelanin content in the skin should greatly reduce the incidence of skin cancers annually. This protection results from both increased protective eumelanin content in the skin, and reduced intentional skin tanning by tanning beds and natural UV light. Applying an SIK2 inhibitor to depigmented skin as seen in albinism and vitiligo would greatly increase sun protection in addition to evening skin tone. Other purported benefits include reducing melanoma risk in redheads, preventing skin aging, and concealing rosacea. These agents are under investigation and were not available at the time this chapter was completed.

Tanning Beds

It is more harmful to the skin to go to a tanning bed than it is to sunbathe on the beach. Tanning beds use UVA to darken the skin. As discussed above, IPD occurs in the skin subsequent to UVA exposure. This gray/black color is caused by oxidation of melanin and the melanogenic precursors and does not provide photoprotection like melanin does. UVA rays penetrate deeper into the dermis than UVB rays do, causing much more damage. UVA rays do not cause the erythema that UVB does, so the skin's early warning system that the skin has had too much sun exposure does not come into play. Sunscreens that block only UVB rays can lead to an accidental increase of UVA exposure by blocking the erythema response to sunlight, enticing sunbathers into a false sense of security resulting in extended time of exposure to UVA. A broad-spectrum sunscreen, sun-protective clothing, and avoidance of tanning beds is the best way to protect skin from UVA. UVA exposure sets the stage for skin cancers, unwanted skin pigmentation such as solar lentigos, and skin aging.

CONCLUSION

Even skin tone is desirable and associated with healthy skin. Skin tone results from complex interactions between light, eumelanin, pheomelanin, hemoglobin, and carotenoids. Smoothness of the SC and collagen content in the dermis also affect perception of skin color. Skin tone depends upon regulation of melanin production and melanosome transfer, as well as the passage of time for the epidermis to repopulate with new keratinocytes.

Patient education is particularly critical on the subject of even skin tone: it cannot be accomplished without vigilant compliance. Exposure to UV light, blue light from cell phones and computer screens, infrared light (heat), estrogen, and stress all influence skin pigmentation. Compliance with daily sunscreen, sun protection, and avoidance of sun and heat is required to even skin tone.

References

1. Bataille V, Snieder H, MacGregor AJ, Sasieni P, Spector TD. Genetics of risk factors for melanoma: an adult twin study of nevi and freckles. *J Natl Cancer Inst.* 2000;92(6):457–63.

2. Rodrigues M, Ezzedine K, Hamzavi I, Pandya AG, Harris JE; Vitiligo Working Group. Current and emerging treatments for vitiligo. *J Am Acad Dermatol.* 2017;77(1):17–29.

3. Samson N, Fink B, Matts P. Interaction of skin color distribution and skin surface topography cues in the perception of female facial age and health. *J Cosmet Dermatol.* 2011;10(1):78–84.

4. Fink B, Matts PJ. The effects of skin colour distribution and topography cues on the perception of female facial age and health. *J Eur Acad Dermatol Venereol.* 2008;22(4):493–8.

5. Fink B, Matts PJ, Klingenberg H, Kuntze S, Weege B, Grammer K. Visual attention to variation in female facial skin color distribution. *J Cosmet Dermatol.* 2008;7(2):155–61.

6. Pawaskar MD, Parikh P, Markowski T, McMichael AJ, Feldman SR, Balkrishnan R. Melasma and its impact on health-related quality of life in Hispanic women. *J Dermatolog Treat.* 2007;18(1):5–9.

7. Freitag FM, Cestari TF, Leopoldo LR, Paludo P, Boza JC. Effect of melasma on quality of life in a sample of women living in southern Brazil. *J Eur Acad Dermatol Venereol.* 2008;22(6):655–62.

8. Yalamanchili R, Shastry V, Betkerur J. Clinico-epidemiological Study and Quality of Life Assessment in Melasma. *Indian J Dermatol.* 2015;60(5):519.

9. Jiang J, Akinseye O, Tovar-Garza A, Pandya AG. The effect of melasma on self-esteem: A pilot study. *Int J Womens Dermatol.* 2017;4(1):38–42.

10. Ly BCK, Dyer EB, Feig JL, Chien AL, Del Bino S. Research Techniques Made Simple: Cutaneous Colorimetry: A Reliable Technique for Objective Skin Color Measurement. *J Invest Dermatol.* 2020;140(1):3–12.e1.

11. Maeda K, Hatao M. Involvement of photooxidation of melanogenic precursors in prolonged pigmentation induced by ultraviolet A. *J Invest Dermatol.* 2004;122(2):503–9.

12. Rosen CF, Seki Y, Farinelli W, et al. A comparison of the melanocyte response to narrow band UVA and UVB exposure in vivo. *J Invest Dermatol.* 1987;88(6):774–9.

13. Kollias N, Baqer AH. Absorption mechanisms of human melanin in the visible, 400–720 nm. *J Invest Dermatol.* 1987;89(4):384–8.

14. Tanaka H, Yamashita Y, Umezawa K, Hirobe T, Ito S, Wakamatsu K. The Pro-Oxidant Activity of Pheomelanin is Significantly Enhanced by UVA Irradiation: Benzothiazole Moieties Are More Reactive than Benzothiazine Moieties. *Int J Mol Sci.* 2018;19(10):2889.

15. Maresca V, Flori E, Briganti S, et al. UVA-induced modification of catalase charge properties in the epidermis is correlated with the skin phototype. *J Invest Dermatol.* 2006;126(1):182–90.

16. Del Bino S, Ito S, Sok J, et al. Chemical analysis of constitutive pigmentation of human epidermis reveals constant eumelanin to pheomelanin ratio. *Pigment Cell Melanoma Res.* 2015;28(6):707–17.

17. Ito S, Wakamatsu K, Sarna T. Photodegradation of Eumelanin and Pheomelanin and Its Pathophysiological Implications. *Photochem Photobiol.* 2018;94(3):409–420.

18. Swope VB, Abdel-Malek ZA. MC1R: Front and Center in the Bright Side of Dark Eumelanin and DNA Repair. *Int J Mol Sci.* 2018;19(9):2667.

19. Ando H, Watabe H, Valencia JC, et al. Fatty acids regulate pigmentation via proteasomal degradation of tyrosinase: a new aspect of ubiquitin-proteasome function. *J Biol Chem.* 2004;279(15):15427–33.

20. Ando H, Ryu A, Hashimoto A, Oka M, Ichihashi M. Linoleic acid and alpha-linolenic acid lightens ultraviolet-induced hyperpigmentation of the skin. *Arch Dermatol Res.* 1998;290(7):375–81.

21. Sarkar R, Bansal A, Ailawadi P. Future therapies in melasma: What lies ahead? *Indian J Dermatol Venereol Leprol.* 2020;86(1): 8–17.

22. De Dormael R, Bastien P, Sextius P, et al. Vitamin C Prevents Ultraviolet-induced Pigmentation in Healthy Volunteers: Bayesian Meta-analysis Results from 31 Randomized Controlled versus Vehicle Clinical Studies. *J Clin Aesthet Dermatol.* 2019;12(2): E53–E59.

23. Oresajo C, Stephens T, Hino PD, et al. Protective effects of a topical antioxidant mixture containing vitamin C, ferulic acid, and phloretin against ultraviolet-induced photodamage in human skin. *J Cosmet Dermatol.* 2008;7(4):290–7.

24. Middelkamp-Hup MA, Pathak MA, Parrado C, et al. Oral Polypodium leucotomos extract decreases ultraviolet-induced damage of human skin. *J Am Acad Dermatol.* 2004;51(6):910–8.

25. Goh CL, Chuah SY, Tien S, Thng G, Vitale MA, Delgado-Rubin A. Double-blind, Placebo-controlled Trial to Evaluate the Effectiveness of Polypodium Leucotomos Extract in the Treatment of Melasma in Asian Skin: A Pilot Study. *J Clin Aesthet Dermatol.* 2018;11(3):14–19.

26. Zhou LL, Baibergenova A. Melasma: systematic review of the systemic treatments. *Int J Dermatol.* 2017;56(9):902–908.

27. Ni Z, Mu Y, Gulati O. Treatment of melasma with Pycnogenol. *Phytother Res.* 2002;16(6):567–71.

28. Lyons AB, Trullas C, Kohli I, Hamzavi IH, Lim HW. Photoprotection beyond ultraviolet radiation: A review of tinted sunscreens. *J Am Acad Dermatol.* 2020:S0190–9622(20) 30694-0.

29. Amano K, Xiao K, Wuerger S, Meyer G. A colorimetric comparison of sunless with natural skin tan. *PloS One.* 2020;15(12): e0233816.

30. Muizzuddin N, Marenus KD, Maes DH. Tonality of suntan vs sunless tanning with dihydroxyacetone. *Skin Res Technol.* 2000; 6(4):199–204.

31. Levy SB. Dihydroxyacetone-containing sunless or self-tanning lotions. *J Am Acad Dermatol.* 1992;27(6 Pt 1):989–93.

32. Faurschou A, Janjua NR, Wulf HC. Sun protection effect of dihydroxyacetone. *Arch Dermatol.* 2004;140(7):886–7.

33. Faurschou A, Wulf HC. Durability of the sun protection factor provided by dihydroxyacetone. *Photodermatol Photoimmunol Photomed.* 2004;20(5):239–42.

34. Perer J, Jandova J, Fimbres J, et al. The sunless tanning agent dihydroxyacetone induces stress response gene expression and signaling in cultured human keratinocytes and reconstructed epidermis. *Redox Biol.* 2020;36:101594.

35. Mujahid N, Liang Y, Murakami R, et al. A UV-Independent Topical Small-Molecule Approach for Melanin Production in Human Skin. *Cell Rep.* 2017;19(11):2177–2184.

36. Nasti TH, Timares L. MC1R, eumelanin and pheomelanin: their role in determining the susceptibility to skin cancer. *Photochem Photobiol.* 2015;91(1):188–200.

SECTION 3

Specific Skin Problems

CHAPTER 15

Skin of Color

Kiyanna Williams, MD
Daniel Gutierrez, MD
Heather Woolery-Lloyd, MD

SUMMARY POINTS

What's Important?

1. There is little variation in number of melanocytes between light- and dark-skinned individuals. Skin color is determined by the type of melanin produced and the size and distribution of melanosomes within melanocytes and keratinocytes.
2. There are several scales and typing systems used to classify patients by skin color. The most commonly used system is the Fitzpatrick skin typing system; however, it does not fully delineate darker-skinned individuals and other systems may be deemed more appropriate for use with skin of color patients.
3. Stratum corneum thickness appears to be the same across skin types; however, darker skin may be more compact and cohesive. Mast cell granule size has been shown to be larger and ceramides have been shown to be in lower concentration in darker skin.
4. Data regarding racial differences in lipid content, transepidermal water loss, barrier function, spontaneous corneocyte desquamation, water content and skin irritancy are inconclusive and often contradictory.
5. Darker pigmented skin provides photoprotective effects including delayed photoaging; however, it also confers greater risk of dyschromia including procedure-related dyschromia.

What's New?

1. As the US population continues to grow more ethnically and racially diverse there is an increased interest in skin of color. The practicing dermatologist will need to develop increased awareness of the similarities and differences in skin structure and function in different racial/ethnic groups to better diagnose and treat a diverse patient population.

What's Coming?

1. Interpretation and application of existing data is limited by small sample size, varying methodologies, varying definitions of racial/ethnic groups, and lack of standardization of study protocols. These limitations demonstrate the need for newer studies.
2. New, large, comprehensive, and standardized studies with clear methodologies and classifications of patients by skin types are currently taking place. These studies will be most useful to address the current limitations seen in this research area.

Skin of color (SOC) describes individuals with increased epidermal pigment and darker skin. This subset of patients has unique cosmetic concerns and often require special consideration for cosmetic procedures. SOC often collectively refers to those of African, Native American, Asian, and Hispanic descents.

BIOLOGY OF SKIN COLOR

There is little variation in the number of epidermal melanocytes between light- and dark-skinned individuals. There are approximately 2000 epidermal melanocytes/mm^2 on the head and forearm and 1000 epidermal melanocytes/mm^2 on the rest of the body. These differences are present at birth.[1] Thus, total number of melanocytes is relatively equivalent among all people.

Melanin is classified into two types: eumelanin and pheomelanin. Eumelanin is darker and exerts a greater photoprotective effect than pheomelanin which is lighter. Eumelanin is characteristically found in darker individuals where it serves as a photoprotectant and free radical scavenger. Pheomelanin is predominantly found in lighter-skinned individuals where it is a less effective UV filter and serves as an endogenous photosensitizer.

Although increased epidermal pigmentation results in a darker skin phenotype, there are more distinct ultrastructural characteristics that correlate with skin color. Specifically, the density and distribution of melanosomes translocated into keratinocytes correlate with skin color. In white skin, melanosomes are small and aggregated in complexes. In black skin, there are larger melanosomes, which are singly distributed within keratinocytes.[2]

Interestingly, the distribution of melanosomes in darker skin varies with the location on the body. In lighter skin, keratinocytes of both the thigh and volar skin exhibit complexed melanosomes. However, keratinocytes from the thighs of dark-skinned patients display singly dispersed melanosomes, while keratinocytes from the lighter volar skin of these patients have complexed melanosomes.[3] Thus, the melanosomes in the minimally pigmented volar skin of dark-skinned individuals closely resemble the melanosomes of lighter-skinned individuals. This finding further supports the theory that skin color correlates with the distribution of melanosomes. From such studies, one can conclude that melanosome distribution correlates with the color of skin; however, skin color is also determined by other factors.

Researchers have examined the contribution of melanin, oxyhemoglobin, and deoxyhemoglobin on pigmentation observed clinically after ultraviolet B (UVB) exposure. Investigators found that the clinical evaluation of skin complexion was affected both by epidermal melanin concentration and deoxyhemoglobin residing in the superficial venous plexus. Additionally, altering the concentration of deoxyhemoglobin in the skin with pressure or with topical therapies also significantly altered what is visually perceived as skin pigmentation.[4,5]

CATEGORIZING SKIN OF COLOR

There continues to be an increasing interest in categorizing skin type based on its response to an inciting agent whether it

be injury, UV light, laser, or cosmetic procedures. Skin typing has several practical considerations in the field of dermatology and cosmetic dermatology; however, the classification systems used vary widely.

Fitzpatrick Skin Typing System

Skin phototyping refers to classification of skin based on its response to UV light. In 1975, Fitzpatrick proposed a phototyping scale most commonly used today. Skin of color is most frequently defined as Fitzpatrick skin phototypes (SPT) IV through VI. These skin types, by definition, tan easily or profusely and burn minimally, rarely, or never. The Fitzpatrick SPT system was originally developed to assess a patient's response to UV exposure for the purpose of treating skin conditions with phototherapy.[6] Using this system, patients are assigned a skin type based on the self-reported ability to tan or burn. The SPT defines a minimum erythema dose (MED) for each skin type, which is then used to guide dosing of UV phototherapy for various skin diseases. This skin typing system has since evolved into a way to describe a patient's skin color. Dermatologists often assign a patient's SPT based on their clinical assessment of skin color and not necessarily after obtaining a patient's history of sun tanning or burning (**Table 15-1**).

The Fitzpatrick SPT system originally categorized only white skin and included skin types I to IV. All skin of color (brown or dark brown skin) was identified as SPT V skin. SPT VI skin was later added to further classify skin of color.[7] Although this system is widely accepted and used frequently in dermatology, it does not fully address certain issues related to darker skin types.

There are two key issues that arise when using the Fitzpatrick SPT system. First, some authors have challenged the ability to predict a patient's MED based on the reported ability to tan and burn. In one study involving white patients, there was a poor correlation between SPT (as determined by self-reported tanning history) and MED. This study found a better correlation between MED and skin complexion characteristics such as eye and hair color, freckling tendency, and number of nevi.[8] Other studies in Asian and Arab patients have also demonstrated a poor correlation between skin phototype (based on tanning history) and MED.[9–12] These authors have suggested that the SPT system, which was originally developed for white skin, is not applicable in patients of other ethnicities.

The second issue with the SPT system involves the correlation of visually assessed skin color with MED. As mentioned above, most dermatologists often assign a patient's SPT based on their clinical assessment of skin color, and rarely obtain a

TABLE 15-1	**Fitzpatrick Skin Phototype Scale**				
TYPE I	**TYPE II**	**TYPE III**	**TYPE IV**	**TYPE V**	**TYPE VI**
Very fair, pale white	Fair, white	Medium, olive	Olive, moderate brown	Brown, dark brown	Very dark brown
Always burns, never tans	Usually burns, tans with difficulty	Sometimes burns, gradually tans	Rarely burns, tans with ease	Very rarely burns, tans very easily	Never burns, tans very easily, deeply pigmented

patient's skin tanning history. Some authors have proposed that SPT (as determined by observed skin color) does not correlate with the MED in ethnic skin. They suggest that in skin of color, the constitutive pigment does not correlate with MED, as is suggested by the current conventional application of SPT.[4]

For example, most patients of African descent are conventionally labeled as Fitzpatrick skin type V (brown) or VI (dark brown). However, upon questioning, some of these patients report frequently burning. This subset of patients would therefore be classified as having a skin type of III or IV, if they were truly categorized based on a self-reported tanning history. One study compared skin pigmentation as measured by diffuse reflectance spectroscopy (DRS) of MEDs.[4] This study confirmed that epidermal pigmentation was not an accurate predictor of skin sensitivity to UVB radiation.

Such research highlights the limitation of the SPT, which was originally designed to evaluate lighter skin types. Although the Fitzpatrick SPT continues to be widely used, other systems have been proposed to more clearly define skin of color.

Japanese Skin Type Scale

A Japanese skin type (JST) scale has been used to classify Japanese patients based on personal history of sun-reactivity.[13] This scale, which ranges from JST-I to JST-III, has been correlated with MEDs and minimal melanogenic dose (MMD) in Japanese patients. The MED and the MMD have been shown to increase with increasing JST. The MMD was shown to be greater than corresponding MED for all JST types.[14] These data are in contrast to data in Caucasian skin, revealing that the MED was the same as MMD in SPT II and MMD was less than MED in SPT III and IV.[15] The authors proposed that UVB may elicit more erythema than pigmentation in Japanese patients.

Taylor Hyperpigmentation Scale

The Taylor Hyperpigmentation Scale is a validated scale to describe skin of color and to monitor treatment of hyperpigmentation.[16] It consists of 15 plastic cards representing different hues in skin phototypes IV through VI. Each card also has 10 bands of progressively darker gradations of skin hue. Clinicians can use this system to assess and define skin color in a given patient. The Taylor Hyperpigmentation Scale also provides a simple, convenient tool to measure improvement after treatment of hyperpigmentation (**Fig. 15-1**).

Lancer Ethnicity Scale

The Lancer Ethnicity Scale (LES) was specifically developed to assess risk and outcome in the cosmetic laser patient.[17] After completing a detailed history of the patient's ethnicity, an LES skin type ranging from 1 to 5 is assigned to each grandparent. The LES skin type is based on the geographic origin of the grandparent, ranging from type 5 (African) to type 1 (Nordic). The number is totaled for all four grandparents and then divided by four to determine the LES skin type of the patient. The author suggests that the lower the LES skin type, the lower the risk of scarring and uneven pigment alteration after laser and surgical procedures. The LES is a novel approach to

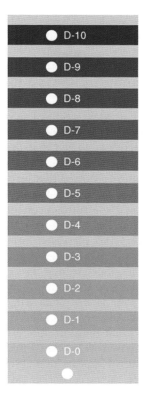

FIGURE 15-1. An example of one of the cards used to measure color in the Taylor Hyperpigmentation Scale.

treating the cosmetic patient. It places a greater emphasis on ethnicity and country of origin than the patient's skin color. This concept is insightful but more studies are needed to validate this novel skin typing system.

Baumann Skin Typing System

Baumann's Skin Typing System addresses a very important cosmetic concern in skin of color, namely, the propensity to develop hyperpigmentation.[18] It does not define ethnicity or skin color. Rather, this questionnaire aids in predicting which patients are most likely to develop hyperpigmentation after a given procedure. It also addresses the fact that there are some patients with Fitzpatrick skin types IV to VI who do not have a strong tendency to hyperpigment despite their constitutive pigment. Thus, certain procedures may propose less of a risk in this special group. At the same time, there are some patients with Fitzpatrick skin type III with a strong propensity to develop hyperpigmentation. By determining each individual patient's hyperpigmentation tendencies, this survey provides an excellent tool to the cosmetic dermatologist. It can offer further insight into treatment options for a given patient that transcends the visual assessment of skin complexion (see Chapter 14, Uneven Skin Tone).

DEFINING STRUCTURE AND FUNCTION IN SKIN OF COLOR

Comparative studies of skin structure and function in skin of color are limited. It is important to note that most studies on this subject involve small numbers of patients. Much of the data are contradictory and can be difficult to interpret. In the following section, these findings will be summarized.

Stratum Corneum: Thickness and Compaction

The stratum corneum (SC) has been extensively studied in black and white skin. Most studies confirm that SC thickness does not differ between black and white individuals.[19–23] However, studies have suggested that the SC of black skin is more compact than white skin.[22,24] Using repeated tape stripping, investigators reported that black skin required an average of 16.6 strips to remove the SC compared to 10.3 strips in white skin.[22] The authors concluded that although SC thickness was equal in both groups, the SC in black skin had more cell layers and increased intracellular adhesion. Subsequent studies confirmed these findings.[25] The investigators in one of these later studies also examined recovery time after barrier damage and found that darker skin recovered more quickly after barrier damage from tape stripping.[24] This study included African American, Asian, and Hispanic subjects and found that the skin differences in SC cell layers and barrier function were related to skin color and not related to race. Thus, it appears that although SC thickness is the same between the races, darker skin is more compact and more cohesive.

Stratum Corneum: Lipid Content, Ceramides, and Barrier Function

Lipids in the SC play an important role in the barrier function of the skin with optimal lipid composition being essential for ideal barrier function. The major lipids of the epidermis are ceramides, cholesterol, and free fatty acids. Studies have shown that there is greater lipid content in black SC when compared to white SC.[26,27] Once the lipids are removed from the SC, the weight of delipidized SC is equal in black and white patients.[22]

Controversial findings have been reported regarding the SC lipid levels of varying ethnic groups. Although greater overall lipid content has been reported in black SC, subsequent studies have showed that ceramide levels were lowest in black skin. Sugino et al. found ceramide levels existed in decreasing order in Hispanic and Asian, white, and black skins. Ceramide levels were inversely correlated with transepidermal water loss (TEWL). Additionally, ceramide levels directly correlated with the water content of the SC.[28] This was again demonstrated by Hellemans et al. who quantified ceramide levels using hydrolysis and found the lowest level of lipid in the SC in black skin.[29] Another study found African Americans to have significantly few ceramides compared to Caucasian and Asian American subjects.[25]

Data is limited in Asian patients. Scalp lipids in British and Thai subjects were compared, with investigators finding no difference in scalp lipids between the two groups.[30] More recently, SC lipid profiles in Asian, black, and white subjects have been evaluated by high-performance thin layer chromatography. The highest ceramide/cholesterol ratio was seen in the Asian group while the lowest was seen in Africans. However, no significant differences were found in the ceramide subgroups.[31]

Based on the various studies discussed, the data regarding racial differences in lipid content are unclear; however, ceramides appear to be consistently lower in Black subjects.

Stratum Corneum: TEWL and Barrier Function

TEWL is one measure of SC barrier function. Five studies of TEWL in black skin indicate that TEWL is greater in black skin than white skin.[28,32–35] There are also nine studies that contradict these findings. Seven reported no difference in baseline TEWL between the black and white subjects,[36–42] and two reported decreased TEWL in black patients.[25,43] The variations in these results may be influenced by the location of the skin examined.[44]

Data on TEWL of Asian skin are inconclusive. Studies have reported that TEWL in Asian skin is greater than, equal to, and less than TEWL in Caucasian skin.[25,28,34,45] One study comparing Chinese, Malay, and Indian subjects demonstrated no differences in TEWL (as measured by skin vapor water loss) among the three groups.[46] There has been no difference demonstrated in TEWL between Hispanic and white skin.[33,37]

From the studies involving black subjects, 5 out 14 studies concluded that TEWL was increased in black skin either at baseline or after irritation. The significance of these data while inconclusive could be far reaching. If skin color truly does impact barrier function, these data would imply that acquired dyschromias may alter skin barrier properties.[44] It also has implications regarding the ability of people with different skin colors to tolerate environmental insults and to absorb topical agents.

Stratum Corneum: Corneocyte Surface Area and Spontaneous Desquamation

Corneocytes are the nonnucleated cells that comprise the SC. Corneocyte surface area has been demonstrated to influence skin permeabilty.[48] A study examining corneocyte surface area in black, white, and Asian subjects demonstrated no differences in corneocyte surface area among the groups.[49]

In the same study, spontaneous desquamation was measured in black, white, and Asian subjects. The investigators found that spontaneous corneocyte desquamation was equal in white and Asian patients; however, spontaneous corneocyte desquamation was greatest in black patients.[49] The increased desquamation seen in this study may explain the dry "ashy" skin often seen clinically in black patients (**Fig. 15-2**). However, subsequent studies have not confirmed these data. Two studies reported a greater desquamation index in white subjects.[43] One study demonstrated the greatest desquamation activity in Caucasians, intermediate activity in Asians, and the least activity in African Americans.[25] Another study reported no difference in the desquamation index between black and white patients.[50] The data on the differences in spontaneous corneocyte desquamation between these populations remain unclear.

Stratum Corneum: Water Content

Water content in the skin can be measured by capacitance, conductance, impedance, and resistance. There are few studies

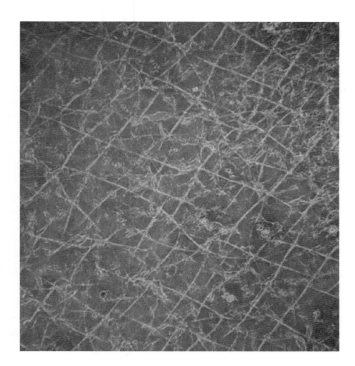

FIGURE 15-2. Dry skin presents as "ashy skin" in dark-skinned patients.

in the literature using these methods to compare water content in the skin of black, white, Hispanic, and Asian subjects.

Seven studies examined black and white skin. Four studies showed no significant differences.[33,40,41,50] In one of these studies, skin hydration correlated with clinical scaliness. One study showed increased water content in black skin while another suggested decreased water content in black skin.[43,51] Another study showed no statistical difference in skin hydration between Africans and Caucasians except for the palms that demonstrated a greater level of SC hydration in Caucasians.[42]

One study examined Hispanic and white subjects and found no difference in water content at baseline.[47] Later work contradicts these data. This subsequent study showed racial variability in SC water content among white, black, and Hispanic patients.[37] The water content values also varied by anatomic site. In the only study that included Asian patients, Asian skin was found to have higher water content than white, black, and Hispanic subjects.[29]

Based on a summation of the research, there does not appear to be a clear trend in the difference in water content among various ethnic groups. Indeed, the data on this subject are contradictory and inconclusive.

Percutaneous Absorption

Percutaneous absorption has been studied in black and white patients. Three studies estimated absorption via urinary excretion of a topically applied substance. Two studies saw no difference between black and white patients, while the other showed decreased urinary excretion in black patients.[52–54] All of these studies had a limited sample size. One additional study examined

absorption in white and black cadaveric skin.[55] The authors reported decreased absorption in the black cadaveric skin.

Based on a summation of the studies, it is difficult to confirm any differences in percutaneous absorption in skin of color. The studies measuring urinary excretion are limited by other possible variables such as incomplete urine collections, renal function, and metabolism differences. In addition, the study of cadaveric skin may not reflect in vivo absorption. Thus, the data regarding percutaneous absorption in skin of color are inconclusive.

Cutaneous Blood Vessel Reactivity

Cutaneous blood vessel reactivity can be measured via Laser Doppler Velocimetry (LDV) or photoplethysmography (PPG). LDV is a noninvasive method to measure the flow of red blood cells in vasculature. PPG measures the pulsative changes in dermal vasculature and is synchronized with pulse rate.[44] These methods have been used to measure skin irritancy to topical products, absorption of topicals, and efficacy of topical medications. Nine studies compared blood vessel reactivity among ethnic groups via LDV. One of these studies also examined blood vessel reactivity via PPG. In all studies, a topical agent was applied (i.e., vasodilator, vasoconstrictor, or irritant) and then reactivity to the given agent was measured.

In the six studies that included black subjects, two showed no difference,[33,56] three showed decreased blood vessel reactivity in black subjects,[34,57,58] and one showed increased blood vessel reactivity in black subjects when compared to white subjects.[59]

Two studies compared Hispanic and white subjects and found no difference in LDV response to a topical irritant or nicotinate.[47,60]

Three studies included Asian patients. Two studies demonstrated increased blood vessel reactivity in Asian patients,[34,59] and one showed no difference in blood vessel reactivity when compared with white patients.[45]

Much of the data on blood vessel reactivity in skin of color are difficult to interpret because in each study different topical agents were used. However, in five of the nine studies, the authors concluded that there was no significant difference between the subjects studied. Further research is needed to clarify the data on cutaneous blood vessel reactivity in skin of color.

Skin Irritancy

The impact of ethnicity on skin irritancy is controversial. Original studies used visual perception of erythema as a primary endpoint.[61–63] This method of assessing cutaneous irritancy has obvious limitations in darker skin types. The earlier studies suggested that black subjects were less sensitive to irritants than white subjects.[33,47] As described in previous sections, much of this research revealed inconsistent and contradictory data. Subsequent authors have reviewed and reexamined the research on skin irritancy in an effort to determine if definitive conclusions can be made regarding skin irritancy in skin of color.[44,64,65] Most authors agree, from the current data, there does not appear to be a clear increase or decrease in skin irritancy in skin of color.

Stinging, a manifestation of sensory irritation, has also been studied in different skin types. Early reports suggested that stinging was most frequent in fair-skinned persons of Celtic ancestry.[66] A subsequent study showed no skin type propensity for stinging. The authors reported that increased stinging was most related to a history of sensitivity to soaps, cosmetics, and drugs (see Chapter 18, Burning and Stinging Skin).[67]

Most epidemiologic studies of allergic contact dermatitis demonstrate equal incidence among ethnicities.[68–71] Thus, based on current objective data, there does not appear to be any clear difference in skin irritancy in skin of color when compared to white skin (see Chapter 19, Contact Dermatitis).

pH, Elastic Recovery/Extensibility, Mast Cell Granules, Epidermal Innervation

Three studies have examined pH in skin of color.[34,39,40] One demonstrated decreased pH in black skin after three tape strips but not at baseline, or after 9, 12, or 15 tape strips.[34] Another showed decreased pH in black skin when compared to white skin on the cheeks but not the legs.[43] A recent study revealed no difference in pH between black and white subjects.[40] The data from these three studies are insufficient to draw any definitive conclusions on pH in skin of color.

Elastic recovery and extensibility have also been studied in black and white skin.[37,43] The current data are inconsistent and conflicting. Based on the data, no conclusion can be made regarding skin biomechanics in different races.

Mast cell size and characteristics have been studied in black skin. In one study, no histologic differences in the number and size of mast cells were identified.[23] However, electron microscopy of mast cells in black skin demonstrated larger granules, more parallel-linear striations, and less curved lamellae. Tryptase was localized to the parallel-linear striations in black skin and localized to the curved lamellae in white skin. In this small study, significant structural differences were demonstrated in mast cells of black subjects.[72]

Pruritus, atopic dermatitis, and macular amyloid are frequently described in many Asian populations. Epidermal innervation has been studied in Asian and Caucasian patients to investigate differences in skin innervation. No differences in innervation as measured by confocal microscopy were found between European Caucasian, Japanese American, and Chinese American subjects.[73]

Melanin and Melanosome Distribution

As described previously, it is well established that differences in pigmentation are caused by the size and distribution of melanosomes within the keratinocytes.[2] Darker-skinned subjects have large, singly dispersed melanosomes while lighter-skinned subjects have small grouped melanosomes within keratinocytes. Subsequent research confirmed and expanded on the role of melanosomes in skin color. These studies demonstrated that melanosome grouping correlates with the degree of pigmentation in white, black, and Asian subjects.[74,75] Darker-skinned black subjects had large, singly dispersed melanosomes while lighter-skinned black subjects had both large, singly distributed melanosomes and small grouped melanosomes. Similarly, dark-skinned white subjects had singly dispersed melanosomes on sun-exposed skin, while light-skinned white subjects with minimal sun exposure had grouped melanosomes. Melanosome grouping was also correlated with sun exposure. Asian forearm skin primarily had singly distributed melanosomes while unexposed abdominal skin had grouped melanosomes.[74,75]

Further research has determined that the ability of a melanosome to form aggregates is determined by its size. Research suggests that melanosomes greater than 0.35 μm cannot form groups.[74,75]

Basal cell layer melanosomes and total melanin content also correlate with the degree of pigmentation. Darkly pigmented skin has increased melanin as measured by cell culture.[76] Darkly pigmented skin also has increased density of basal cell layer melanosomes.[74] Fewer basal layer melanosomes were observed in fair-skinned Asian patients when compared to darker-skinned individuals.[77] Additional studies have shown that, in black skin, melanosomes are not only increased in the basal layer but also distributed throughout all layers of the epidermis.[23,78] This is in contrast to white skin where melanosomes are primarily limited to the basal layer.

The protease-activated receptor-2 (PAR-2) expressed on keratinocyte plays a role in melanosome uptake via phagocytosis. Trypsin activates PAR-2 in vivo. Investigators have demonstrated that PAR-2 and trypsin have greater expression in darkly pigmented skin when compared to lighter skin. In addition, PAR-2-induced phagocytosis is more efficient in darker skin types. These data suggest that PAR-2 expression may play a role in darker skin phenotypes (see Chapter 14).[79]

Epidermis: Overall Architecture

It is well established that SC thickness does not differ among ethnicities.[19–23] Overall skin thickness as measured by calipers also does not differ between white and black subjects.[80] Differences in the architecture of the epidermis between racial groups involve melanin and melanosome distribution as described above. Other differences in epidermal architecture are related to UV damage. These changes are described below.

PHOTOAGING IN SKIN OF COLOR

UV Reactivity and Photoprotection

The photoprotection conferred by melanin greatly influences the UV-induced differences seen in darkly pigmented skin when compared to lighter pigmented skin. Epidermal architecture in black and white subjects supports this notion. One study demonstrated an intact, compact stratum lucidum in sun-exposed black skin, in contrast to a swollen, cellular stratum lucidum in sun-exposed white skin. Black skin rarely exhibited atrophy, while white skin had numerous focal areas of atrophy, necrosis, vacuoles, and dyskeratosis.[23]

Melanin clearly offers protection from UV radiation. It acts as a neutral density filter to equally reduce penetration of various wavelengths of light.[81] In a study using skin samples from blacks and whites, investigators found that five times as much UV light reached the upper dermis of white skin when compared to black skin. The authors determined that the main site of UV filtration in white patients was the SC, compared to the malpighian layer in black patients. The average protection offered by melanin in black skin was calculated to be equivalent to a sun protective factor (SPF) of 13.4 compared to 3.4 for white skin. They concluded that the photoprotection observed in black skin was due to both increased melanin content and the unique distribution of melanosomes in dark skin.[81]

Another study examined biopsies in black and white skin before and after solar-simulating radiation (SSR). After SSR, white skin displayed epidermal and dermal DNA damage, an influx of neutrophils, active proteolytic enzymes, and diffuse keratinocyte activation. Black skin only demonstrated DNA damage in the suprabasal dermis. This study of acute changes after SSR confirms the significance of UV protection imparted by melanin.[82]

Racial differences in MED have been described. Darkly pigmented black skin has been determined to have an MED up to 33 times greater than that of individuals with white skin.[75] In Japanese subjects, MED has also been correlated with skin color. In this study, the investigators found that the greater the epidermal melanin content, the less severe the reaction to the sun.[83] It is important to note, however, that darker skin is not always predictive of MED. As mentioned previously, in darker skin, pigmentation does not consistently correlate with MED.[4] Other factors may influence the ability to tan or burn in skin of color.

The process of skin tanning in different racial ethnic groups has been studied. The most significant change noted after one MED exposure was an upward shift in the distribution of melanin to the middle layers of the epidermis. This change was most dramatic in darker skin. Such data provide the basis for a better understanding of tanning in the darker skin types.[84]

One study examined skin in Korean subjects and the cumulative response to sun exposure. Investigators compared constitutive and facultative (acquired) pigmentation in different age groups. Facultative pigment of sun-exposed skin in Caucasians appears to reflect cumulative lifetime UV exposure. In this study, constitutive pigment was highest during the first decade of life, decreased during the second decade, and was maintained during the third decade of life in Korean subjects. In contrast to Caucasians, facultative pigmentation did not increase with age.[87]

Recently, the role of visible light in causing skin pigmentation has more clearly been evaluated. When compared with those of lighter skin phenotypes, visible light irradiation in darker skin individuals elicits more immediate and sustained skin hyperpigmentation.[85] Combination UVA1 and visible light, however, will synergistically cause greater pigment intensity compared to visible light alone in darker

skin types.[86] In light of such findings, it is prudent to discuss appropriate photoprotection. Organic (chemical) sunscreens work by absorbing light and are not effective against visible light. Inorganic (physical blocking metal oxides) provide the broadest spectrum of protection as photons are reflected and scattered. The reflection and scattering of visible light, however, can result in an aesthetically displeasing white hue on those with darker basal skin pigmentation. Micronized metal oxides alleviate this cosmetic concern, but provide less protection against visible light.[88] Iron oxides, however, can be added to sunscreens which provide a red-tinted color and not only increase cosmesis, but also provide increased visible light protection.[89]

Histologic Findings

Despite the photoprotection conferred by darker skin, chronologic aging has been observed in black skin. In one study, older black subjects demonstrated flattening of the dermal-epidermal junction when compared to younger subjects.[78] Elastic fiber degeneration and an increase in the superficial vascular plexus were also noted in the aged group. The skin of older black subjects was also characterized by a decrease in the number of melanocytes.[78]

A study in older Thai patients with a history of high sun exposure also showed epidermal atrophy, cell atypia, poor polarity, and disorderly differentiation.[90] In a study of Japanese patients, the relationship between skin phototype and facial wrinkling was examined. As expected, higher scores were recorded for deep wrinkles in individuals with Fitzpatrick SPT I. Interestingly, the same tendency was not demonstrated for fine wrinkle scores.[91]

Clinical Findings

The clinical signs of aging in skin of color have been described. In a study of French Caucasian and Chinese subjects, wrinkle onset was delayed by approximately 10 years in Chinese women. Hyperpigmentation was a much more important sign of aging in Chinese women.[92]

In a study of Japanese and Caucasian patients, young Japanese patients had significantly lower wrinkle scores. The sagging score was also significantly lower in Japanese subjects older than 40 years when compared with Caucasian subjects. Lower face aging was more common in Caucasian subjects.[93]

In African Americans, the clinical signs of aging are less pronounced and tend to be delayed at least a decade when compared to Caucasian skin. Many patients complain of dark circles and hollowing beneath the eyes, while others experience lower eyelid bags. Lower-eyelid signs of aging usually start with midface aging during the 30s. In midface aging, the malar fat pad descends from its location overlying the infraorbital rim and accumulates along the nasolabial fold. This can lead to a hollowed appearance beneath the eyes and an apparent deepening of the nasolabial fold.[94] It is important to note that these changes occur with intrinsic aging and are less related to photodamage. Photoaging in darker skin is manifested primarily by skin dyspigmentation, which is one of the most common cosmetic complaints in skin of color. While increased melanin is advantageous in delaying photoaging in those with darker skin, labile melanocytes also confer a greater risk of pigment alteration which can ultimately contribute to photoaging.

The presence of seborrheic keratoses and dermatosis papulosa nigra is another common clinical sign of aging in such patients.

Based on these studies, photoaging, although delayed, does occur in skin of color. Despite the significant protection offered by melanin in darker skin types, these data suggest that photoprotection should still be emphasized in patients with skin of color.

ADDITIONAL CONSIDERATIONS REGARDING STRUCTURE AND FUNCTION IN SKIN OF COLOR

Dermis: Overall Architecture

In a comparison of black and white facial skin, dermal differences are evident. Some of these changes are related to UV damage and include decreased elastosis in black skin.[23]

Other differences appear to be primary variations in the fibroblasts, macrophages, and giant cells. In one study, black skin was reported to contain more fiber fragments composed of collagen fibrils and glycoproteins. Fibroblasts were more numerous and larger in size. They were frequently binucleated and multinucleated. Additionally, there were more binucleated and multinucleated macrophages and giant cells.[23]

The changes described in fibroblasts are especially significant in skin of color because of the increased risk of keloids and scarring in these patients. Other differences in dermal structures reported between the races are described below.[23]

Eccrine glands

Research on ethnic differences in eccrine sweat glands are contradictory. Of the four studies measuring sweat production in black and white subjects, two reported decreased sweating in black subjects and two reported no difference.[95–99]

Four other studies have measured resistance to indirectly assess eccrine gland activity. They have shown increased resistance in darker-skinned patients, which suggests increased eccrine gland activity.[55,99–101]

Based on these studies, no conclusion can be made on eccrine gland activity between different ethnic groups.

APOCRINE glands

Research on ethnic differences in apocrine glands are limited. Two small nonblinded studies suggest that apocrine glands are larger in black subjects.[102,103] One larger histologic analysis reported that apocrine glands are more numerous in black skin.[99] Based on these data, apocrine glands may be increased in black individuals.

Apocrine-eccrine glands

Apocrine-eccrine sweat glands have features of both eccrine and apocrine glands. One study of facial skin reported more numerous apocrine-eccrine glands in black skin when compared to white skin.[23]

Sebaceous glands

Studies of sebaceous glands and sebaceous gland activity reveal contradictory findings. One study reported increased sebaceous gland size in black patients.[104] Another study reported increased sebum production in black patients.[105] Three studies indicated no difference in sebaceous gland activity between black and white subjects.[40,106,107] Research in Japanese subjects, however, found a correlation between skin surface lipids and increased pigmentation (see Chapter 10, The Baumann Skin Typing System).[83]

Hair

Hair composition and structure has been studied between the races. There is no difference in keratin between black and white subjects.[108] One study has shown some differences in amino acid composition; however, a follow-up study demonstrated no difference.[109,110]

Vellus hair follicular density has been studied in African American, Asian, and Caucasian subjects. It has been proposed that vellus hair follicles are a potential reservoir for topically applied substances. In one study, vellus follicular hair density was lower in African Americans and Asians when compared to white subjects. The authors suggested that this difference may impact skin absorption in different ethnic groups.[111] Another study showed vellus hair density to be the greatest in Asians followed by African Americans and whites.[41]

Differences in terminal hair structure between the races have been well studied and are described below.

African hair

In subjects of African descent, four distinct hair types are recognized: straight, wavy, helical, and spiral. The spiral hair type is the most common subtype.[112] African hair has a flattened elliptical shape in cross-section with a ribbon-like appearance.[113] The hair is typically coiled tightly, and most naturally shed hairs have a frayed tip. Spontaneous knotting is often seen. Longitudinal splitting, fissures, and breaking of the hair shaft are also observed.[114]

Other studies of black hair have revealed that black subjects had fewer elastic fibrils anchoring the hair to the dermis.[23] This has implications in several forms of alopecia frequently seen in black patients, particularly traction alopecia. Additionally, there is decreased hair density in African American subjects when compared to white subjects.[115]

White hair

White hair is typically straight or slightly curved. The hair is elliptical in cross-section. It has the smallest cross-sectional area among ethnic groups and naturally shed hairs usually have the original or cut tip.[109] Spontaneous knotting is rarely observed.[114] Moisture content is known to be higher in whites compared to Africans or Asians.[116]

Asian hair

Asian hair is typically straight. The hair is round in cross-section. It has the largest cross-sectional area and naturally shed hairs usually have original or cut tips.[113] No spontaneous knotting is observed.[9114] Asian hair has a faster rate of growth when compared to African and white hair.[117]

SUMMARY

Understanding the unique characteristics of skin of color is extremely important in dermatology. The most well-defined and distinct differences in skin of color pertain to melanin in the skin. Increased melanin in skin of color offers a relative delay in photoaging.

The disadvantage of melanin, however, has great impact in those with darker skin types as this constitutive pigment increases the risk of dyspigmentation from many cosmetic procedures.

Apparent differences in fibroblasts in skin of color also greatly impact the practice of dermatology. These differences likely place those with skin of color at increased risk of hypertrophic scars and keloids after surgical and laser procedures.

More than half of the world's population has skin of color. Despite this fact, our understanding of skin structure and function is limited in these patients. Research to date has been quite compelling; however, most research on skin of color is preliminary. Further research and larger population studies are necessary to definitively describe the similarities and differences in skin structure and function among the various ethnic groups.

References

1. Jimbow K, Quevedo W, Prota G, Fitzpatrick T. Biology of melanocytes. In: Freedberg I, Eisen A, Wolff K, et al. eds. *Fitzpatrick's Dermatology in General Medicine*. 5th ed. New York, NY: McGraw Hill; 1999:192–200.

2. Gupta V, Sharma VK. SKin typing: Fitzpatrick graiding and others. *Clin Dermatol*. Sep–Oct 2019;37(5):430–436.; Szabó G, Gerald AB, Pathak MA, Fitzpatrick TB. Racial Differences in the Fate of Melanosomes in Human Epidermis. *Nature*. 1969;222:1081–1082.

3. Milburn PB, Sian CS, Silvers DN. The color of the skin of the palms and soles as a possible clue to the pathogenesis of acral-lentiginous melanoma. *Am J Dermatopathol*. 1982;4:429–434.

4. Smith G, Kollias N, Wallo W. Estimating the ability of melanin to proect skin of color from UV exposure. Paper presented at: Program and abstracts of the 64th Annual Meeting of the American Academy of Dermatology; March 3–7, 2006; San Francisco, CA.

5. Stamatas GN, Kollias N. Blood stasis contributions to the perception of skin pigmentation. *J Biomed Opt*. 2004;9:315.

6. Fitzpatrick TB. Soleil et Peau. *J Med Esthet*. 1975;2:33–34.

7. Fitzpatrick TB. The Validity and Practicality of Sun-Reactive Skin Types I Through VI. *Arch Dermatol*. 1988;124:869.

8. Rampen F, Fleuren B, de Boo T, Lemmens W. Unreliability of self-reported burning tendency and tanning ability. *Arch Dermatol*. 1988;124(6):885–888.

9. Youn J, Oh J, Kim B, et al. Relationship between skin phototype and MED in Korean, brown skin. *Photodermatol Photoimmunol Photomed*. 1997;13(5-6):208–211.

10. Park SB, Suh DH, Youn JI. Reliability of self-assessment in determining skin phototype for Korean brown skin. *Photodermatol Photoimmunol Photomed*. 1998;14(5-6):160–163.

11. Stanford D, Georgouras K, Sullivan E, Greenoak G. Skin phototyping in Asian Australians. *Australas J Dermatol*. 1996;37 (Suppl 1):S36–S38.

12. Venkataram MN, Haitham AA. Correlating skin phototype and minimum erythema dose in Arab skin. *Int J Dermatol*. 2003;42(3):191–192.

13. Satoh Y, Kawada A. Action spectrum for melanin pigmentation to ultraviolet light, and Japanese skin typing. In: Fitzpatrick TB WM, Tada K, ed. *Brown Melanoderma: Biology and Disease of Epidermal Pigmentation*. Tokyo, Japan: University of Tokyo Press; 1986:87–95.

14. Kawada A. UVB-induced erythema, delayed tanning, and UVA-induced immediate tanning in Japanese skin. *Photodermatol*. 1986;3(6):327–333.

15. Pathak MA, Fanselow DL. Photobiology of melanin pigmentation: dose/response of skin to sunlight and its contents. *J Am Acad Dermatol*. 1983;9(5):724–733.

16. Taylor SC, Arsonnaud S, Czernielewski J. The Taylor Hyperpigmentation Scale: a new visual assessment tool for the evaluation of skin color and pigmentation. *Cutis*. 2005;76(4):270–274.

17. Wolbarsht M, Urbach F. The Lancer Ethnicity Scale. *Lasers Surg Med*. 1999;25(2):105–106.

18. Baumann L. *The Skin Type Solution*. New York, NY: Bantam Dell; 2006.

19. Thomson ML. Relative efficiency of pigment and horny layer thickness in protecting the skin of Europeans and Africans against solar ultraviolet radiation. *J Physiol*. 1955;127(2):236–246.

20. Freeman RG, Cockerell EG, Armstrong J, Knox JM. Sunlight as a factor influencing the thickness of epidermis. *J Invest Dermatol*. 1962;39:295–298.

21. Mitchell R. The skin of the Australian Aborigine; a light and electronmicroscopical study. *Australas J Dermatol*. 1968;9(4):314–328.

22. Weigand DA, Haygood C, Gaylor JR. Cell layers and density of Negro and Caucasian stratum corneum. *J Invest Dermatol*. 1974;62(6):563–568.

23. Montagna W, Carlisle K. The architecture of black and white facial skin. *J Am Acad Dermatol*. 1991;24(6 Pt 1):929–937.

24. Reed J, Ghadially R, Elias P. Effect of race, gender, and skin type of epidermal permeability barrier function [abstract]. *J Invest Dermatol*. 1994(102):537.

25. Muizzuddin N, Hellemans L, Van Overloop L, Corstjens H, Declercq L, Maes D. Structural and functional differences in barrier properties of African American, Caucasian and East Asian skin. *J Dermatolog Science*. 2010;59(2):123–128.

26. Reinertson RP, Wheatley VR. Studies on the chemical composition of human epidermal lipids. *J Invest Dermatol*. 1959;32(1):49–59.

27. La Ruche G, Cesarini JP. [Histology and physiology of black skin]. *Ann Dermatol Venereol*. 1992;119(8):567–574.

28. Sugino K, Imokawa G, Maibach H. Ethnic difference of stratum corneum lipid in relation to stratum corneum function [abstract]. *J Invest Dermatol.* 1993(100):597.

29. Hellemans L, et al. Characterization of stratum corneum properties in human subjects from a different ethnic background. *J Invest Dermatol.* 2005;124(S4):A62.

30. Harding CR, Moore AE, Rogers JS, Meldrum H, Scott AE, McGlone FP. Dandruff: a condition characterized by decreased levels of intercellular lipids in scalp stratum corneum and impaired barrier function. *Arch Dermatol Res.* 2002;294(5):221–230.

31. Jungersted JM, Høgh JK, Hellgren LI, Jemec GB, Agner T. Ethnicity and stratum corneum ceramides. *Br J Dermatol.* 2010;163(6):1169–1173.

32. Wilson D, Berardesca E, Maibach HI. In vitro transepidermal water loss: differences between black and white human skin. *Br J Dermatol.* 1988;119(5):647–652.

33. Berardesca E, Maibach HI. Racial differences in sodium lauryl sulphate induced cutaneous irritation: black and white. *Contact Dermatitis.* 1988;18(2):65–70.

34. Kompaore F, Marty JP, Dupont C. In vivo evaluation of the stratum corneum barrier function in blacks, Caucasians and Asians with two noninvasive methods. *Skin Pharmacol.* 1993;6(3):200–207.

35. Berardesca E, Pirot F, Singh M, Maibach H. Differences in stratum corneum pH gradient when comparing white Caucasian and black African-American skin. *Br J Dermatol.* 1998;139(5):855–857.

36. Reed JT, Ghadially R, Elias PM. Skin type, but neither race nor gender, influence epidermal permeability barrier function. *Arch Dermatol.* 1995;131(10):1134–1138.

37. Berardesca E, de Rigal J, Leveque JL, Maibach HI. In vivo biophysical characterization of skin physiological differences in races. *Dermatologica.* 1991;182(2):89–93.

38. De Luca R, Balestrieri A, Dinle Y. [Measurement of cutaneous evaporation. 6. Cutaneous water loss in the people of Somalia]. *Boll Soc Ital Biol Sper.* 1983;59(10):1499–1501.

39. Pinnagoda J, Tupker RA, Agner T, Serup J. Guidelines for transepidermal water loss (TEWL) measurement. A report from the Standardization Group of the European Society of Contact Dermatitis. *Contact Dermatitis.* 1990;22(3):164–178.

40. Grimes P, Edison BL, Green BA, Wildnauer RH. Evaluation of inherent differences between African American and white skin surface properties using subjective and objective measures. *Cutis.* 2004;73(6):392–396.

41. Luther N, Darvin ME, Sterry W, Lademann J, Patzelt A. Ethnic Differences in Skin Physiology, Hair Follicle Morphology and Follicular Penetration. *Skin Pharmacol Physiol.* 2012;25:182–191

42. Young MM, Franken A, du Plessis JL. Transepidermal water loss, stratum corneum hydration, and skin surface pH of female African and Caucasian nursing students. *Skin Res Technol.* 2019;25:88–95

43. Warrier A, Kligman A, Harper RA, Bowman J, Wickett RR. A comparison of black and white skin using noninvasive methods. *J Cosmet Sci.* 1996;47:229–240.

44. Wesley NO, Maibach HI. Racial (ethnic) differences in skin properties: the objective data. *Am J Clin Dermatol.* 2003;4(12):843–860.

45. Aramaki J, Kawana S, Effendy I, Happle R, Löffler H. Differences of skin irritation between Japanese and European women. *Br J Dermatol.* 2002;146(6):1052–1056.

46. Goh CL, Chia SE. Skin irritability to sodium lauryl sulphate—as measured by skin water vapour loss—by sex and race. *Clin Exp Dermatol.* 1988;13(1):16–19.

47. Berardesca E, Maibach HI. Sodium-lauryl-sulphate-induced cutaneous irritation. Comparison of white and Hispanic subjects. *Contact Dermatitis.* 1988;19(2):136–140.

48. Rougier A, Lotte C, Corcuff P, Maibach H. Relationship between skin permeability and corneocyte size according to anatomic site, age, and sex in man. *J Soc Cosmet Chem.* 1988;39:15–26.

49. Corcuff P, Lotte C, Rougier A, Maibach HI. Racial differences in corneocytes. A comparison between black, white and oriental skin. *Acta Derm Venereol.* 1991;71(2):146–148.

50. Manuskiatti W, Schwindt DA, Maibach HI. Influence of age, anatomic site and race on skin roughness and scaliness. *Dermatology.* 1998;196(4):401–407.

51. Johnson LC, Corah NL. Racial Differences in Skin Resistance. *Science.* 1963;139(3556):766–767.

52. Wickrema Sinha AJ, Shaw SR, Weber DJ. Percutaneous absorption and excretion of tritium-labeled diflorasone diacetate, a new topical corticosteroid in the rat, monkey and man. *J Invest Dermatol.* 1978;71(6):372–377.

53. Wedig J, Maibach H. Percutaneous penetration of dipyrithione in man: effect of skin color (race). *J Am Acad Dermatol.* 1981;5(4):433–438.

54. Lotte C, Wester RC, Rougier A, Maibach HI. Racial differences in the in vivo percutaneous absorption of some organic compounds: a comparison between black, Caucasian and Asian subjects. *Arch Dermatol Res.* 1993;284(8):456–459.

55. Stoughton R. Bioassay methods for measuring percutaneous absorption. In: Montagna W SR, van Scott EJ, eds. *Pharmacology of the Skn.* New York, NY: Appleton-Century-Crofts; 1969:542–544.

56. Guy RH, Tur E, Bjerke S, Maibach HI. Are there age and racial differences to methyl nicotinate-induced vasodilatation in human skin? *J Am Acad Dermatol.* 1985;12(6):1001–1006.

57. Berardesca E, Maibach H. Cutaneous reactive hyperaemia: racial differences induced by corticoid application. *Br J Dermatol.* 1989;120(6):787–794.

58. Berardesca E, Maibach HI. Racial differences in pharmacodynamic response to nicotinates in vivo in human skin: black and white. *Acta Derm Venereol.* 1990;70(1):63–66.

59. Gean CJ, Tur E, Maibach HI, Guy RH. Cutaneous responses to topical methyl nicotinate in black, oriental, and caucasian subjects. *Arch Dermatol Res.* 1989;281(2):95–98.

60. Berardesca E, Maibach HI. Effect of race on percutaneous penetration of nicotinates in human skin: A comparison of whites and Hispano-Americans. *Bioeng Skin.* 1988;4(1):31–38.

61. Marshall E, Lynch V, Smith HW. On dichlorethylsulphide (mustard gas) II. Variations in susceptibility of the skin to dichlorethylsulphide. *J Pharmacol Exp Ther.* 1918;12(5):291.

62. Weigand DA, Mershon GE. The cutaneous irritant reaction to agent O-chlorobenzylidene malonitrile (CS). Quantitation and racial influence in human subjects. *Edgewood Arsenal Technical Report 4332*, February 1970.

63. Weigand DA, Gaylor JR. Irritant reaction in Negro and Caucasian skin. *South Med J.* 1974;67(5):548–551.

64. Taylor SC. Skin of color: biology, structure, function, and implications for dermatologic disease. *J Am Acad Dermatol.* 2002;46(2 Suppl Understanding):S41–S62.

65. Frosch P, Kligman A. A method for appraising the stinging capacity of topically applied substances. *J Soc Cosmet Chem.* 1977;28:197–209.

66. Grove GL, Soschin DM, Kligman AM. Adverse subjective reactions to topical agents. In: Drill VA, Lazar P, eds. *Cutaneous Toxicology.* New York, NY: Raven Press; 1984:200–210.

67. Berardesca E, Maibach H. Ethnic skin: Overview of structure and function. *J Am Acad Dermatol.* 2003;48(6, Supplement):S139–S142.

68. Kligman AM, Epstein W. Updating the maximization test for identifying contact allergens. *Contact Dermatitis.* 1975; 1(4):231–239.

69. Fisher AA. Contact dermatitis in black patients. *Cutis.* 1977;20(3):303, 308–309, 316 passim.

70. Deleo VA, Taylor SC, Belsito DV, et al. The effect of race and ethnicity on patch test results. *J Am Acad Dermatol.* 2002;46(2 Suppl Understanding):S107–S112.

71. Epidemiology of Contact Dermatitis in North America: 1972. *Arch Dermatol.* 1973;108(4):537–540.

72. Sueki H, Whitaker-Menezes D, Kligman AM. Structural diversity of mast cell granules in black and white skin. *Br J Dermatol.* 2001;144(1):85–93.

73. Reilly DM, Ferdinando D, Johnston C, Shaw C, Buchanan KD, Green MR. The epidermal nerve fibre network: characterization of nerve fibres in human skin by confocal microscopy and assessment of racial variations. *Br J Dermatol.* 1997;137(2):163–170.

74. Toda K, Pathak MA, Parrish JA, Fitzpatrick TB, Quevedo WCJr. Alteration of racial differences in melanosome distribution in human epidermis after exposure to ultraviolet light. *Nat New Biol.* 1972;236(66):143–145.

75. Olson RL, Gaylor J, Everett MA. Skin color, melanin, and erythema. *Arch Dermatol.* 1973;108(4):541–544.

76. Smit NP, Kolb RM, Lentjes EG, et al. Variations in melanin formation by cultured melanocytes from different skin types. *Arch Dermatol Res.* 1998;290(6):342–349.

77. Goldschmidt H, Raymond JZ. Quantitative analysis of skin color from melanin content of superficial skin cells. *J Forensic Sci.* 1972;17(1):124–131.

78. Herzberg AJ, Dinehart SM. Chronologic aging in black skin. *Am J Dermatopathol.* 1989;11(4):319–328.

79. Babiarz-Magee L, Chen N, Seiberg M, Lin CB. The expression and activation of protease-activated receptor-2 correlate with skin color. *Pigment Cell Res.* 2004;17(3):241–251.

80. Whitmore SE, Sago NJ. Caliper-measured skin thickness is similar in white and black women. *J Am Acad Dermatol.* 2000;42(1 Pt 1):76–79.

81. Kaidbey KH, Agin PP, Sayre RM, Kligman AM. Photoprotection by melanin—a comparison of black and Caucasian skin. *J Am Acad Dermatol.* 1979;1(3):249–260.

82. Rijken F, Bruijnzeel PL, van Weelden H, Kiekens RC. Responses of black and white skin to solar-simulating radiation: differences in DNA photodamage, infiltrating neutrophils, proteolytic enzymes induced, keratinocyte activation, and IL-10 expression. *J Invest Dermatol.* 2004;122(6):1448–1455.

83. Abe T, Arai S, Mimura K, Hayakawa R. Studies of physiological factors affecting skin susceptibility to ultraviolet light irradiation and irritants. *J Dermatol.* 1983;10(6):531–537.

84. Tadokoro T, Yamaguchi Y, Batzer J, et al. Mechanisms of skin tanning in different racial/ethnic groups in response to ultraviolet radiation. *J Invest Dermatol.* 2005;124(6):1326–1332.

85. Mahmoud BH, Ruvolo E, Hexsel CL, et al. Impact of long-wavelength UVA and visible light on melanocompetent skin. *J Invest Dermatol.* 2010;130(8):2092–2097.

86. Kohli I, Chaowattanapanit S, Mohammad TF, et al. Synergistic effects of long-wavelength ultraviolet A1 and visible light on pigmentation and erythema. *Br J Dermatol.* 2018;178(5):1173–1180.

87. Roh K, Kim D, Ha S, Ro Y, Kim J, Lee H. Pigmentation in Koreans: study of the differences from caucasians in age, gender and seasonal variations. *Br J Dermatol.* 2001;144(1):94–99.

88. Narla S, Kohli I, Hamzavi IH, Lim HW. Visible light in photodermatology. *Photochemical & photobiological sciences: Official journal of the European Photochemistry Association and the European Society for Photobiology.* 2020;19(1):99–104.

89. Lyons AB, Trullas C, Kohli I, Hamzavi IH, Lim HW. Photoprotection beyond ultraviolet radiation: A review of tinted sunscreens. *J Am Acad Dermatol.* 2021 May;84(5):1393–1397. doi:10.1016/j.jaad.2020.04.079. Epub 2020 Apr 23. PMID: 32335182.

90. Kotrajaras R, Kligman AM. The effect of topical tretinoin on photodamaged facial skin: the Thai experience. *Br J Dermatol.* 1993;129(3):302–309.

91. Nagashima H, Hanada K, Hashimoto I. Correlation of skin phototype with facial wrinkle formation. *Photodermatol Photoimmunol Photomed.* 1999;15(1):2–6.

92. Nouveau-Richard S, Yang Z, Mac-Mary S, et al. Skin ageing: a comparison between Chinese and European populations. A pilot study. *J Dermatol Sci.* 2005;40(3):187–193.

93. Tsukahara K, Fujimura T, Yoshida Y, et al. Comparison of age-related changes in wrinkling and sagging of the skin in Caucasian females and in Japanese females. *J Cosmet Sci.* 2004;55(4):351–371.

94. Harris MO. The aging face in patients of color: minimally invasive surgical facial rejuvenation-a targeted approach. *Dermatol Ther.* 2004;17(2):206–211.

95. Robinson S, Dill DB, Wilson JW, Nielsen M. Adaptations of White Men and Negroes to Prolonged Work in Humid Heat. *Am J Trop Med.* 1941;s1-21(2):261–287.

96. McCance RA, Purohit G. Ethnic differences in the response of the sweat glands to pilocarpine. *Nature.* 1969;221(5178):378–379.

97. Herrmann F, Prose PH, Sulzberger MB. Studies on sweating. V. Studies of quantity and distribution of thermogenic sweat delivery to the skin. *J Invest Dermatol.* 1952;18(1):71–86.

98. Rebel G, Kirk D. Patterns of eccrine sweating in the human axilla. In: Montagna W, Ellis R, Silver A, eds. *Advances in Biology of Skin.* Vol 3. New York, NY: Pergamon Press; 1962:108–126.

99. Homma H. On Apocrine Sweatglands in White and Negro Men and Women. *Bull Johns Hopkins Hosp.* 1926;38(5):365–371.

100. Janes CL, Worland J, Stern JA. Skin potential and vasomotor responsiveness of black and white children. *Psychophysiology.* 1976;13(6):523–527.

101. Juniper KJr., Dykman RA. Skin resistance, sweat-gland counts, salivary flow, and gastric secretion: age, race, and sex differences, and intercorrelations. *Psychophysiology*. 1967;4(2):216–222.

102. Schiefferdecker P. Dsaael be (vollkomin. Mitt.). *Zoologica*. 1922;27:1.

103. Hurley HJ, Shelley WB. The physiology and pharmacology of the apocrine sweat gland. The Human Apocrine Sweat Gland in Health and Disease. Springfield, IL: Charles Thompson; 1960:64.

104. Champion RH, Gillman T, Rood AS, et al. *An Introduction to the Biology of the Skin*. Philadelphia, PA: FA Davis; 1970:418.

105. Kligman AM, Shelley WB. An investigation of the biology of the human sebaceous gland. *J Invest Dermatol*. 1958;30(3):99–125.

106. Pochi PE, Strauss JS. Sebaceous gland activity in black skin. *Dermatol Clin*. 1988;6(3):349–351.

107. Abedeen SK, Gonzalez M, Judodihardjo H, et al. Racial variation in sebum excretion rate. Program and abstracts of the 58th Annual Meeting of the American Academy of Dermatology; March 10–15, 2000; San Francisco, CA. Abstract 559.

108. Hrdy D, Baden HP. Biochemical variation of hair keratins in man and non-human primates. *Am J Phys Anthropol*. 1973;39(1):19–24.

109. Menkart J, Mao I. Caucasian Hair, Negro Hair, and Wool: Similarities and Differences. *J Soc Cosmetic Chemists*. 1966;17:769–787

110. Gold RJ, Scriver CG. The amino acid composition of hair from different racial origins. *Clin Chim Acta*. 1971;33(2):465–466.

111. Mangelsdorf S, Otberg N, Maibach HI, Sinkgraven R, Sterry W, Lademann J. Ethnic variation in vellus hair follicle size and distribution. *Skin Pharmacol Physiol*. 2006;19(3):159–167.

112. Halder RM. Hair and scalp disorders in blacks. *Cutis*. 1983;32(4):378–380.

113. Vernall DG. A study of the size and shape of cross sections of hair from four races of men. *Am J Phys Anthropol*. 1961;19(4):345–350.

114. Khumalo NP, Doe PT, Dawber RP, Ferguson DJ. What is normal black African hair? A light and scanning electron-microscopic study. *J Am Acad Dermatol*. 2000;43(5 Pt 1):814–820.

115. Sperling LC. Hair density in African Americans. *Arch Dermatol*. 1999;135(6):656–658.

116. Martí M, Barba C, Manich AM, Rubio L, Alonso C, Coderch L. The influence of hair lipids in ethnic hair properties. *Int J Cosmet Sci*. 2016;38(1):77–84.

117. Leerunyakul K, Suchonwanit P. Asian Hair: A Review of Structures, Properties, and Distinctive Disorders. *Clin Cosmet Investig. Dermatology*. 2020;13:309–318.

CHAPTER 16

Acne (Type 1 Sensitive Skin)

Rachel Sally, BA
Evan A. Rieder, MD

SUMMARY POINTS

What's Important?

1. Acne is the most common condition of the skin worldwide and a common complaint among aesthetic patients of a broad age range due to its highly visible nature on the skin.
2. The etiology of acne is complex and multifactorial, involving an interplay between *Cutibacterium acnes* (formerly known as *Propionibacterium acnes*), inflammation, sebaceous gland hypersecretion, and changes in follicular keratinization.
3. Though there is not one panacea for acne treatment, staple medications include oral and topical retinoids, comedolytics like salicylic acid, topical and oral antibiotics, and benzoyl peroxide.

What's New?

1. There has been increasing evidence of widespread antibiotic resistance among *C. acnes*, though combination therapy with benzoyl peroxide is an effective way to prevent resistance. The newest FDA-approved narrow-spectrum tetracycline, sarecycline, has promising efficacy with fewer systemic side effects and less potential for inducing resistance.
2. The oral anti-androgen agent spironolactone continues to be incorporated into regimens for female patients. However, the novel topical anti-androgen clascoterone has been shown to have minimal systemic absorption and is thus safe for all patients.
3. A recent uptrend of acne mechanica and acne cosmetica is likely to continue with increased mask-wearing due to airborne pathogens like SARS-CoV-2 and the rapid trend cycle of skincare products in a burgeoning marketplace that has many start-up companies with less established research and development.

What's Coming?

1. Future treatment routines may include light and laser therapy, which use photosensitive adjuncts to target *C. acnes* or the sebaceous gland and reduce inflammation and sebum production with minimal systemic effects. Gold microparticle-mediated photothermal therapy is a newly FDA-cleared modality to decrease sebum production that uses gold microspheres as the adjunct.
2. There is increasing interest and understanding of the role of diet in acne and how lifestyle modification, including plant-based diets, could play a role in treating and preventing acne.

Any discussion of the practice of cosmetic dermatology must include a discussion of acne. Although acne is not typically considered to be a "cosmetic" problem, its highly visible nature makes it a very common complaint among aesthetic patients who are by definition concerned about their appearance. Acne often has a profound psychosocial impact on patients. Patients with acne may experience tremendous impairment in self-image and a decrease in quality of life equivalent to disorders such as asthma, epilepsy, and diabetes.[1,2] Acne can be especially troublesome to adults who perceive themselves as too old to have this condition most often associated with adolescence.

Acne vulgaris is a common, multifactorial process involving the pilosebaceous unit. More than 50 million people[3] and

75 to 95% of all teens[4] are affected by some form of acne each year in the United States alone. Acne is estimated to affect 9.4% of the global population, making it the eighth most prevalent disease worldwide.[5] The majority of patients outside this age range are adult women who typically exhibit a hormonal component to their acne. Approximately 12 to 22% of women will have acne until the age of 44, whereas only 3% of men will have acne until the same age.[6–8] In many cases, adults are more surprised and upset by acne onset than are teenagers. In all cases, though, early and individually tailored treatment is necessary to achieve a satisfactory cosmetic appearance for the patient. This chapter will include a brief survey of the salient aspects of acne pathophysiology as well as suggestions for treatment and prevention. The psychosocial aspects of acne, or the significant psychological distress that this condition provokes, are beyond the scope of this chapter. It is worth noting, however, that many patients seeking treatment only for acne report substantial anxiety associated with this disease. Regardless of acne severity, acne is also one of the chief concerns of patients with body dysmorphic disorder.[9]

PATHOPHYSIOLOGY OF ACNE

Comedogenesis and acnegenesis are actually discrete processes, but they are usually associated with one another, with the latter often succeeding the former. Inflammation of the follicular epithelium, which loosens hyperkeratotic material within the follicle creating pustules and papules, characterizes acnegenesis (**Fig. 16-1**). Comedogenesis is best described as a noninflammatory follicular reaction manifested by a dense compact hyperkeratosis of the follicle, and usually precedes acnegenesis. Because the etiology of such lesions varies from person to person and also within individuals, it is difficult to categorically identify or isolate a basic cause of acne; however,

four principal factors have been identified. The primary causal factors in acne work interdependently and are mediated by such important influences as heredity and hormonal activity.

Sebaceous Gland Hyperactivity

Sebum is continuously synthesized by the sebaceous glands and secreted to the skin surface through the hair follicle pores. The excretion of lipids by the sebaceous glands is controlled hormonally. Sebaceous glands are located all over the body but are largest and most numerous in the face, back, chest, and shoulders. These glands become more active during puberty because of the increase in androgens, particularly testosterone, which spurs sebum production. This imbalance between sebum production and the secretion capacity leads to a blockage of sebum in the hair follicle followed by inflammation.

Hormones continue to affect sebaceous gland activity into adulthood. In males, lipid secretion is regulated by the action of testosterone. In females, the immediate increase in luteinizing hormone following ovulation incites acceleration in sebaceous gland activity. The higher sebum secretion then stimulates or exacerbates acne breakouts, usually 2 to 7 days prior to menstruation. Women experiencing excessive androgen states, such as those seen in polycystic ovarian disease, frequently suffer from acne as well.

The notion that sebum plays a key role in acnegenesis is buttressed by several facts including its comedogenicity, data showing that it causes inflammation when injected into the skin, and the reportedly higher level of sebum production in people with severe acne.[10] Researchers have also reported that acne lesions are associated with sebaceous glands that produce abnormally high amounts of sebum.[11,12] Furthermore, drugs that cause sebaceous gland shrinkage and reduced sebum production, such as anti-androgens, estrogens, and oral retinoids, are integral treatment modalities in the successful control of acne.

There is a growing body of evidence that the composition of sebum associated with acne is distinct from that of healthy skin and that the degree of difference correlates to acne severity.[13] For example, linoleic acid has been consistently demonstrated to be diminished in concentration in acne.[14] Downing et al. theorized that the lower concentration of linoleic acid, which correlated with the high sebum secretion rates of acne patients, leads to a localized deficiency of essential fatty acid of the follicular epithelium.[15] This deficiency then contributes to diminished epithelial barrier function and follicular hyperkeratosis, which aggravates acne.

Diet has increasingly been implicated in acnegenesis through sebum production, partially underscored by the fact that sebum contains linoleic acid, which is an essential fatty acid that must be obtained from the diet. A typical "Western" diet, comprised of dairy—particularly skim milk—and high glycemic index foods, is thought to play a role in the pathogenesis of acne by increasing insulin and insulin-like growth factor 1 (IGF-1) signaling, thus inducing sebaceous lipogenesis and sebocyte and keratinocyte proliferation.[16,17]

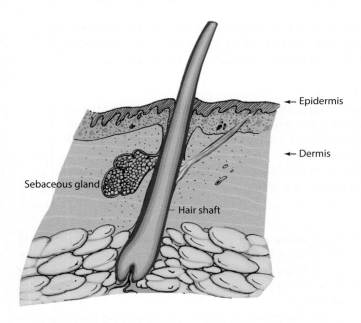

← Epidermis

← Dermis

Sebaceous gland

Hair shaft

FIGURE 16-1. The hair follicle or "pore" is the site where acne occurs.

Changes in Follicular Keratinization

In the lower portion of the follicular infundibulum, the normal process of keratinization occurs in the same way that it occurs on the skin's surface. This maturing of keratinocytes and subsequent exfoliation into the follicle marks the beginning of the formation of comedones. In acne patients, these keratinocytes tend to stick together because of the effects of positive and negative charges, the actions of transglutaminase, and the stickiness of sebum. Hyperproliferative keratins are expressed at elevated levels in acne lesions.[18] Filaggrin (filament aggregating protein) expression and IL-1α have also been implicated in abnormal keratinization.[19-21] However, the precise pathogenesis of follicular hyperkeratinization remains uncertain. Clumped keratinocytes block the pore/follicle, creating a blackhead if the pore is open ("open comedone") or a whitehead if it is closed ("closed comedone") (**Fig. 16-2**). The clogged pore is a great nutritional source for bacteria, so *Cutibacterium acnes* (*C. acnes*, formerly known as *Propionibacterium acnes*) gravitate to the blocked pores. The immune system recognizes the presence of bacteria and mounts an immune response resulting in redness, pus, as well as inflammation, and the typical "pimple" results (**Fig. 16-3**).

The Influence of Bacteria

C. acnes is a commensal bacterium long implicated in acnegenesis, though it is commonly found in the normal skin microbiome.[22] There is no quantitative difference in *C. acnes* between people with acne and those without. However, recent phylogenetic typing of *C. acnes* has revealed discrete strain profiles highly associated with acne.[22,23]

It is known that sebum accumulation because of excess lipid secretion and hyperkeratosis at the infundibulum leads to an increase in *C. acnes* around the hair follicles. *C. acnes* macrocolonies or biofilms are more frequently observed in skin biopsies of patients with acne.[24] Similar biofilms have been observed in other cutaneous diseases. What precise role

C. acnes biofilms play in the pathogenesis of acne is a developing area of interest.

Inflammation

C. acnes stimulates the release of pro-inflammatory cytokines from follicular keratinocytes, sebocytes, and monocytic cells in a Toll-like receptor 2 (TLR2) dependent manner.[25] This leads to activation of the local immune response and subsequently, inflammation. Additionally, *C. acnes* triggers inflammasome activation, leading to significant IL-1β (a key inflammatory mediator) release and thus further upregulating the host inflammatory response. A third mechanism by which *C. acnes* elicits inflammation is through upregulation of matrix metalloproteinases (MMPs), possibly in a TLR dependent manner, which increases inflammation and contributes to tissue injury and scar formation.[26]

In vitro work on monocytes has shown that all-*trans*-retinoic acid led to down-regulation of TLR2 and modulation of MMP induction, yielding more details regarding the retinoid mechanism of action (see Chapter 4, The Skin Microbiome).[26,27]

DIFFERENTIAL DIAGNOSIS

There are several acne variants and disorders with similar presentations. A brief survey of these conditions appears near the conclusion of this chapter. In addition, many other dermatologic conditions can be confused with acne (**Box 16-1**). These are unrelated conditions but can be mimics.

The Basic Lesion

The fundamental acne lesion is the microcomedo, or microcomedone, an enlarged hair follicle full of sebum and *C. acnes*. Although there is a long list of materials that can cause comedones, the mechanism of spontaneous comedone formation remains unclear. The comedo that remains beneath the skin is colloquially referred to as a "whitehead"; a comedo that opens to the surface of the skin is labeled a "blackhead" because it appears black on the epidermis due to an oxidation reaction. The diverse array of other acne lesions includes papules (small, inflamed lesions presenting as pink, tender, nonpustular bumps); pustules (small, inflamed, tender, pustular lesions, usually red at the base); nodules (relatively large, spherical, painful lesions located deeper in the dermis); and cysts (even deeper, inflamed, pustular, painful lesions that can cause scarring) (**Figs. 16-4** and **16-5**).

TREATMENT

There are several therapeutic regimens for acne, most of which focus on prevention of future eruptions rather than treatment of present lesions. This is the reason that the majority of treatments take 6+ weeks to work. *Only topical retinoids, salicylic acid, benzoyl peroxide, and steroids treat lesions already visible on the skin.* Steroids, although occasionally used, are not advised because they can actually worsen or bring about new acne lesions. Five basic principles govern the successful treatment of acne.

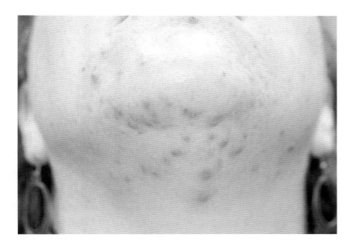

FIGURE 16-2. Open comedones and inflammatory papules on the neck.

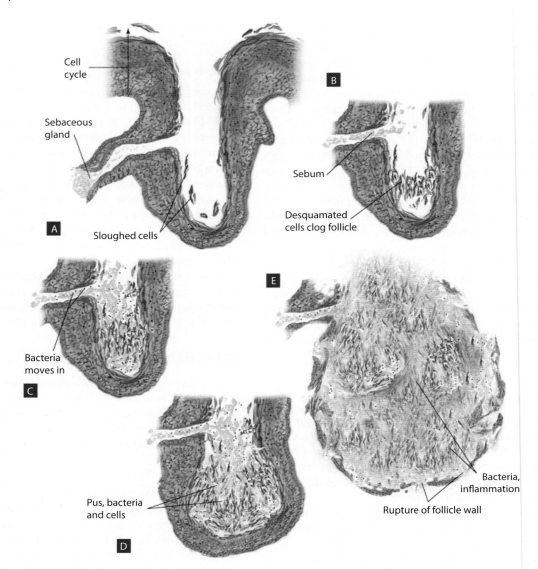

FIGURE 16-3. A close-up of the hair follicle and sebaceous gland demonstrating the different stages of acne. **A.** Desquamation of keratinocytes occurs in the same way that it does on the skin's surface. However, instead of sloughing into the environment, the keratinocytes slough into the hair follicle. This is a continuous and normal process that represents the culmination of the cell cycle. **B.** The first stage of acne is also known as comedogenesis. The sloughed cells stick together inside the hair follicle, resulting in a clogged pore or comedone. This is caused by several factors including increased amounts of sebum, inflammation of the sides of the hair follicle preventing the release of the desquamated keratinocytes, and increased cohesion of keratinocytes. **C.** The keratinocyte plug and sebum is an excellent food source for bacteria. The bacteria invade the comedone and release inflammatory factors that lead to the next stage of acne. **D.** Inflammation continues with increased redness and pus. This is clinically detectable as a papule or pustule. **E.** Continued inflammation may lead to so much inflammation that the hair follicle ruptures and the bacteria and debris are released into the dermis. When severe, this can lead to scarring.

BOX 16-1	Conditions That Can Be Confused with Acne

Adenoma sebaceum
Keratosis pilaris
Perioral dermatitis
Pityrosporum folliculitis
Rosacea
Seborrheic dermatitis
Steroid abuse/use dermatitis
Tinea barbae

The Five Steps

Normalizing Keratinization/Exfoliation

The first step in controlling acne is to normalize the desquamation of keratinocytes (**Box 16-2**). Retinoids exhibit strong inhibitory effects on keratinocyte proliferation and differentiation, which is what gives them strong comedolytic activity.[28] Ultrastructural studies examining tretinoin use have demonstrated the loosening of follicular impactions and loss of cohesiveness within microcomedones.[29] Retinoids are also anti-inflammatory, exerting effects on numerous inflammatory pathways, including suppression of TLR2 expression.[12] Topical retinoids are effective against existing comedonal and inflammatory acne lesions and are

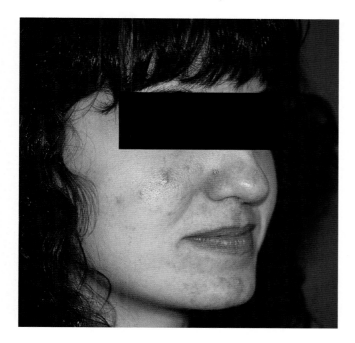

FIGURE 16-4. Multiple papules and pustules in an acne patient.

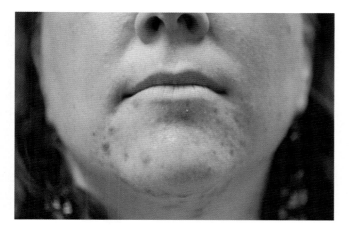

FIGURE 16-5. Acne on the chin. Patients with this presentation should be asked if they are plucking or waxing hairs on the chin because this distribution mimics folliculitis.

preventative for future lesions. Currently, available topical retinoids include tretinoin, tazarotene, adapalene, and trifarotene. Each active is available in several concentrations and formulations. Additionally, adapalene 0.1% gel is available over the counter. Topical retinoids should be considered a first-line therapy for acne because they enhance the efficacy of other topical and oral regimens in combination.[30]

Patients with cystic, scarring, or severely dyspigmenting acne, as well as those who are unresponsive to all other regimens, can be treated with oral retinoids such as isotretinoin (**Fig. 16-6**). Oral retinoids are the only class of drugs that normalize keratinization as well as reduce sebaceous gland function. It has been shown that a marked decrease in sebum production—up to 90%—occurs within 6 weeks after the initiation of therapy.[31] All oral retinoids have teratogenic effects and patients should be cautioned to avoid pregnancy while taking these medications.

Eliminating or reducing C. Acnes *bacteria*

Antibiotics or benzoyl peroxide attack the bacterial population, thereby decreasing the level of inflammation induced by *C. acnes* (**Box 16-3**). The two antibiotics that are most commonly used in the treatment of acne are topical erythromycin and clindamycin. In addition to being antibacterial, these agents exhibit anti-inflammatory activity as they lower the

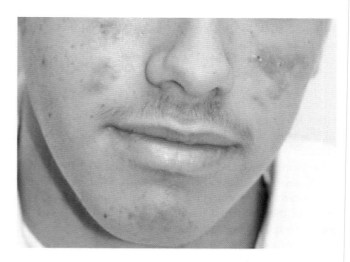

FIGURE 16-6. Cystic acne on cheeks.

BOX 16-2	Products That Block Step 1 (Retinoids)

Tretinoin (Altreno®, Avita™, Renova™, Retin-A™, Retin-A Micro™, Atralin™)
Adapalene (Differin™)
Tazarotene (Arazlo™, Tazorac™)
Triferotene (Aklief®)
Retinol, retinyl linoleate, retinyl palmitate
Oral retinoids: isotretinoin (Accutane™, Claravis, Sotret, Amnesteen)

BOX 16-3	Products That Affect Step 2

Topical antibiotics: clindamycin, erythromycin solution
Combination products with benzoyl peroxide and either clindamycin or erythromycin
Benzoyl peroxide
Azelaic acid (Azelex™, Finacea™)
Sodium sulfacetamide
Sulfur
Oral antibiotics (doxycycline, minocycline, sarecycline)
Light Therapy

percentage of inflammatory free fatty acids produced by bacterial digestion of surface lipids.[32]

The escalating incidence of antibiotic resistance is an important consideration when treating the bacterial aspect of acne. Recent research suggests that as many as 60% of acne patients exhibit antibiotic-resistant strains of *C. acnes*.[33] Clindamycin is preferred over erythromycin as *C. acnes* resistance to the latter has decreased its clinical efficacy. Cunliffe et al. found monotherapy with topical clindamycin resulted in profound increases in resistant strains as early as 2 months; however, in combination with 5% benzoyl peroxide, no increase in resistance occurred in that time period.[34]

Benzoyl peroxide kills bacteria by generating reactive oxygen species in the sebaceous follicle; it also demonstrates mild comedolytic properties.[35] Benzoyl peroxide has synergistic anti-inflammatory and clinical effects when combined with topical retinoids.[36] However, it is important to note that tretinoin (but not microsphere formulation tretinoin, adapalene, tazarotene, or trifarotene) is oxidized and inactivated by benzoyl peroxide and thus the two should not be applied together.[37,38]

Although standard dosing regimens of oral antibiotics—commonly doxycycline or minocycline—remain a mainstay of treatment, newer lower-dose antibiotic formulations are submicrobial and may be a prudent approach to combating bacterial resistance. With such low-dose antibiotics, drugs work as anti-inflammatory agents rather than antimicrobials. Sarecycline is a novel tetracycline with a narrow spectrum of activity targeted at *C. acnes* with little to no activity against Gram-negative bacteria, thus reducing the potential development of resistant strains and disruption of normal gut microflora.[39] Though sarecycline has not yet been compared head–to-head with doxycycline or minocycline, early clinical trials demonstrate that it is well tolerated, with a lower rate of common adverse events of tetracyclines such as vestibular effects, phototoxicity, and gastrointestinal effects.[40]

Sodium sulfacetamide and sulfur are present in a variety of combination products. Though their mechanisms of action are not certain, sodium sulfacetamide is an antibacterial agent, while the mechanism of action of sulfur is also thought to be both antibacterial and keratolytic.

A promising addition to acne regimens is light and laser therapy. Endogenous or exogeneous (applied) photosensitive adjuncts are excited by light, creating reactive oxidative species that either target *C. acnes* or the sebaceous gland, thus reducing inflammation and sebum production.[41] There is evidence that heat-killed *C. acnes* can still cause inflammation, so laser and light therapy should be combined with anti-inflammatories.[42]

Removing the material that clogs the pores

Comedolytics, such as salicylic acid (BHA) and AHAs, are used to loosen the keratinocytes and "unclog" the pores (**Box 16-4**). BHA may be more effective in reducing the number of comedones than are AHAs (see "AHAs versus BHA"). Comedone extractions and acne surgery can also be performed.

AHAs versus BHA

There is a significant chemical distinction between salicylic acid and the alpha hydroxy acids. The AHAs are water soluble, while salicylic acid is lipid soluble. Consequently, the distinct hydroxy acid families enter and function in different areas of the skin; salicylic acid usually effects change only in the upper epidermis while AHAs are believed to penetrate the dermis.[49,50] This difference might account for the longer duration of stinging reported by patients using AHAs as compared to those using BHA.

Because BHA is lipophilic, it is suited, unlike AHAs, to penetrate the sebaceous material in the follicles and thus able to induce exfoliation within the infundibula.[51] The comedolytic properties of BHA have been well-documented, though the extent to which its lipophilicity confers increased comedolytic and anti-acne effects in comparison to AHAs remains unclear.[52] Salicylic acid is marketed to patients in a variety of formulations including gels, lotions, masks, and cleansers.

Due to its anti-inflammatory activity, salicylic acid is also widely used in acne peels. A recent study showed salicylic acid suppresses the sebocyte inflammatory response induced by *C. acnes* in addition to increasing sebocyte apoptosis (and therefore decreasing hyperseborrhea).[53]

Anecdotally, salicylic acid has been reported to work better than AHAs in the treatment of rosacea because the anti-inflammatory properties of BHA induce less erythema. As of the date of this publication, however, there have been no double-blind studies to address this purported benefit.

BOX 16-4   Products That Affect Step 3

Retinoids
Salicylic acid (BHA)
Alpha hydroxy acids (primarily glycolic and lactic)
Azelaic acid

BOX 16-5   Products That Affect Step 4

Salicylic acid (OTC acne wash, lotion, gel, mask)
Topical retinoids
In-office BHA peels
Oral NSAIDs

Attacking the inflammatory response

The use of anti-inflammatory products, such as salicylic acid and topical retinoids, is an effective approach to the most physically troublesome symptom of acne (**Box 16-5**). Steroid injections and topical corticosteroids, especially potent topical corticosteroids, pose important risks such as steroid atrophy and steroid acne. However, in severe cystic, scarring acne, oral corticosteroids and intralesional steroids may be warranted and necessary to rapidly decrease inflammation and prevent scarring. Finally, in-office BHA peels are effective in reducing the inflammation seen in acne (**Table 16-1**).

TABLE 16-1	Anti-Inflammatory Agents
Aloe vera	
Chamomile	
Coenzyme q10	
Cucumber extract	
Feverfew	
Green tea	
Licorice extract	
Mushrooms	
Niacinamide	
Pycnogenol	
Silymarin	

BOX 16-6 Products That Affect Step 5

Oral contraceptives
Spironolactone
Clascoterone
Gold microparticle phototherapy
Retinoids (see Step 1)

Decreasing the level of sebum

The use of oral and topical retinoids decreases sebaceous gland activity. Hormonal stabilization using oral contraceptives, is also an effective way for females to reduce sebaceous secretions (**Box 16-6**). Although there are currently only four oral contraceptive pills approved by the FDA in the United States for the treatment of acne (Ortho Tri-Cyclen, Estrostep, Beyaz, and Yaz), other such pills can be used. Yaz is a combination product of ethinyl estradiol and drospirenone. The drospirenone in this product is an anti-androgen and has about the same anti-androgen effect as 25 mg of spironolactone. Yaz and Yasmin, another oral contraceptive, are similar in that both contain drospirenone, but differ in the amount of estrogen, with Yaz having lower estrogen content.

Other non-contraceptive medications can also modulate sebum. Spironolactone is an aldosterone receptor antagonist that acts as an anti-androgen by competing with testosterone and dihydrotestosterone at androgen receptors in the skin, and by reducing testosterone production. Though the medical literature evidence base for the use of spironolactone is somewhat sparse, it is widely accepted as a safe and effective modality for the treatment of adult female acne. Note that this medication is a known teratogen that is only appropriate for use in women who do not wish to conceive during treatment. Clascoterone is a novel topical androgen receptor inhibitor with minimal systemic activity that has been shown to reduce inflammatory and noninflammatory acne lesions in both male and female patients.[41,43]

Finally, gold microparticle-mediated photothermal therapy is a newly FDA-cleared modality to decrease sebum production. Light absorbing gold microparticles are selectively taken up by sebaceous glands and *C. acnes*, followed by irradiation which damages the sebaceous glands and reduces bacteria.[44]

MOISTURIZATION AND ACNE

In 1980, Swinyer reported on the differences between treating acne patients in a climate with relatively normal humidity in comparison to treatment in a dry climate. He identified skin dryness as an important factor in exacerbating the pathogenetic cycle of acne, thus hampering its treatment.[45] In a subsequent four-cell study that tested Swinyer's hypothesis, Jackson et al. conducted a 3-month evaluation of the influence of cleansing regimens on the effectiveness of acne therapy using 10% benzoyl peroxide lotion, isolating the type of cleanser as the only variable. An emollient facial wash clearly outperformed pure soap and a benzoyl peroxide wash in decreasing open comedones, papules, and in overall global assessment.[46] (Soap and placebo comprised one cell of the study; in each of the others, the variable—soap, an emollient, or benzoyl peroxide wash—was matched with 10% benzoyl peroxide lotion.)

Washing the skin with a noncomedogenic agent appears to act against acne and serves as a suitable alternative to cleansing with relatively abrasive products while satisfying the acne patient's typical desire to wash one's face. In hydrating while cleansing, use of an emollient facial cleanser will accelerate the pace of acne resolution and contribute to overall response regardless of the patient's treatment regimen.[46]

ACNE PREVENTION REGIMEN

Regimens should contain products that affect each of the five steps of acne formation described above. One such program utilizing topicals only is the following:

AM

1. Washing with a 2.5% benzoyl peroxide cleanser.
2. Applying a topical antibiotic solution or azelaic acid.
3. Applying a sunscreen SPF 45 with moisturizing cream (unless the skin is very oily, in which case the patient should try a lotion or gel).

PM

1. Washing with a mild salicylic acid cleanser if comedone volume is high. If skin is irritated or dry, washing with a mild hydrating cleanser is recommended.
2. Applying a topical retinoid.
3. Applying the same moisturizing agent used in the morning.

The physician might consider adding in-office salicylic acid peels, oral antibiotics and retinoids, and oral contraceptives (or other sebum decreasing agents) in recalcitrant cases. Some make-up foundations contain salicylic acid as an additive to aid in the prevention or amelioration of acne.

COMMON ACNE VARIANTS

Acne Cosmetica

Developing acne as a result of cosmetics use is not as common today as it was just a couple of decades ago. Manufacturers test their products for comedogenicity now before putting them on the market. If a person chooses non-greasy, non-occlusive products, the cosmetic choice is unlikely to be a source of acne. With increased competition in the skin-care marketplace, particularly from start-up companies without sufficient budgets for appropriate research and development, acne cosmetica is beginning to occur with greater frequency. See Chapter 43, Moisturizers for more information.

Acne Mechanica

In 2019, a novel coronavirus (SARS-CoV-2), which causes an acute severe respiratory illness, rapidly spread throughout the globe. Necessitating the regular use of masks to prevent the airborne transmission of infection, the COVID-19 pandemic resulted in a surge in the phenomenon of acne mechanica, or "maskne." Typically limited to the distribution of worn items (e.g., bra straps, casts, sports helmets) causing pilosebaceous unit irritation and subsequent comedone formation, acne mechanica developed as a sequela of frequent face mask wearing. The primary treatment for acne mechanica is the removal of occlusive masks. Additional treatment involves the stepwise use of topical and oral acne medications as described above.

Acne Detergicans

The obsessive use of soaps by patients may lead to acne. Many facial cleansers and shampoos contain unsaturated fatty acids that have been shown to be comedogenic.[47] Other components such as bacteriostatic agents and botanical ingredients may irritate the hair follicle and cause acne as well. Therefore, it is important to educate patients that washing does not necessarily improve acne because the detergents used are only capable of removing surface oil and do not affect the sebum in the follicles, where the disease originates. (Of course, one exception to this would be cleansers containing salicylic acid, which has been shown to penetrate into the comedones and improve them.) Acne detergicans is uncommon but should be considered in patients that wash their face or skin more than four times daily.[48]

Rosacea

This is an acneiform condition typically presenting in adults between 25 and 60 years of age that is characterized by facial redness, flushing, papules and pustules, and the formation of prominent blood vessels in the face. These patients usually worsen with AHAs and retinoids but do well with antibiotics, BHA, and laser or light treatment of telangiectasias. The exact cause is unknown, but rosacea is a condition distinct from acne, although a patient may have both conditions at the same time (see Chapter 17, Rosacea).

SUMMARY

Acne is the most common condition of the skin and directly affects the pilosebaceous unit, comprising the hair follicle, the lining cells, and nearby sebaceous gland. Acne is a function of a complex interplay of hereditary, hormonal, and occasional exogenous factors. A change in the inner lining of the hair follicle—with cells turning over too quickly and clumping together—results in an inhibition of the usual passage of sebum and a blockage at the follicular opening. This sets the stage for the involvement of *C. acnes* and subsequent inflammation.

Just as the etiology is complex and multifactorial, the approach to treatment is variable and typically requires several steps tailored to the individual patient. There is not, to date, one isolated cause or a panacea—a medication that works for all patients. Early intervention and preventative treatment are largely effective in resolving all but the most recalcitrant cases of this common, cosmetically altering, and distressing condition.

References

1. Mallon E, Newton JN, Klassen A, Stewart-Brown SL, Ryan TJ, Finlay AY. The quality of life in acne: a comparison with general medical conditions using generic questionnaires. *Br J Dermatol*. 1999;140(4):672–676. doi:10.1046/j.1365-2133.1999.02768.x

2. Thomas DR. Psychosocial effects of acne. *J Cutan Med Surg*. 2004;8(Suppl 4):3–5. doi:10.1007/s10227-004-0752-x

3. Bickers DR, Lim HW, Margolis D, et al. The burden of skin diseases: 2004. *J Am Acad Dermatol*. 2006;55(3):490–500. doi:10.1016/j.jaad.2006.05.048

4. Cordain L, Lindeberg S, Hurtado M, Hill K, Eaton SB, Brand-Miller J. Acne vulgaris: a disease of Western civilization. *Arch Dermatol*. 2002;138(12):1584–1590. doi:10.1001/archderm.138.12.1584

5. Tan JKL, Bhate K. A global perspective on the epidemiology of acne. *Br J Dermatol*. 2015;172(Suppl 1):3–12. doi:10.1111/bjd.13462

6. Goulden V, Stables GI, Cunliffe WJ. Prevalence of facial acne in adults. *J Am Acad Dermatol*. 1999;41(4):577–580.

7. Perkins AC, Maglione J, Hillebrand GG, Miyamoto K, Kimball AB. Acne vulgaris in women: prevalence across the life span. *J Womens Health*. 2012;21(2):223–230. doi:10.1089/jwh.2010.2722

8. Poli F, Dreno B, Verschoore M. An epidemiological study of acne in female adults: results of a survey conducted in France. *J Eur Acad Dermatol Venereol: JEADV*. 2001;15(6):541–545. doi:10.1046/j.1468-3083.2001.00357.x

9. Marron SE, Miranda-Sivelo A, Tomas-Aragones L, et al. Body dysmorphic disorder in patients with acne: a multicentre study. *J Eur Acad Dermatol Venereol: JEADV*. 2020;34(2):370–376. doi:10.1111/jdv.15954

10. Harris HH, Downing DT, Stewart ME, Strauss JS. Sustainable rates of sebum secretion in acne patients and matched normal control subjects. *J Am Acad Dermatol*. 1983;8(2):200–203. doi:10.1016/s0190-9622(83)70023-x

11. Clayton RW, Göbel K, Niessen CM, Paus R, Steensel MAM, Lim X. Homeostasis of the sebaceous gland and mechanisms

of acne pathogenesis. *Br J Dermatol.* 2019;181(4):677–690. doi:10.1111/bjd.17981

12. Gollnick H. Current Concepts of the Pathogenesis of Acne: Implications for Drug Treatment. *Drugs.* 2003;63(15):1579–1596. doi:10.2165/00003495-200363150-00005

13. Camera E, Ludovici M, Tortorella S, et al. Use of lipidomics to investigate sebum dysfunction in juvenile acne. *J Lipid Res.* 2016;57(6):1051–1058. doi:10.1194/jlr.M067942

14. Ottaviani M, Camera E, Picardo M. Lipid mediators in acne. *Mediators Inflamm.* 2010;2010. doi:10.1155/2010/858176

15. Downing DT, Stewart ME, Wertz PW, Strauss JS. Essential fatty acids and acne. *J Am Acad Dermatol.* 1986;14(2 Pt 1):221–225. doi:10.1016/s0190-9622(86)70025-x

16. Melnik BC, Schmitz G. Role of insulin, insulin-like growth factor-1, hyperglycaemic food and milk consumption in the pathogenesis of acne vulgaris. *Exp Dermatol.* 2009;18(10):833–841. doi:10.1111/j.1600-0625.2009.00924.x

17. Çerman AA, Aktaş E, Altunay İK, Arıcı JE, Tulunay A, Ozturk FY. Dietary glycemic factors, insulin resistance, and adiponectin levels in acne vulgaris. *J Am Acad Dermatol.* 2016;75(1):155–162. doi:10.1016/j.jaad.2016.02.1220

18. Hughes BR, Morris C, Cunliffe WJ, Leigh IM. Keratin expression in pilosebaceous epithelia in truncal skin of acne patients. *Br J Dermatol.* 1996;134(2):247–256. doi:10.1111/j.1365-2133.1996.tb07609.x

19. Kurokawa I, Mayer-da-Silva A, Gollnick H, Orfanos CE. Monoclonal antibody labeling for cytokeratins and filaggrin in the human pilosebaceous unit of normal, seborrhoeic and acne skin. *J Invest Dermatol.* 1988;91(6):566–571. doi:10.1111/1523-1747.ep12477026

20. Guy R, Ridden C, Kealey T. The improved organ maintenance of the human sebaceous gland: modeling in vitro the effects of epidermal growth factor, androgens, estrogens, 13-cis retinoic acid, and phenol red. *J Invest Dermatol.* 1996;106(3):454–460. doi:10.1111/1523-1747.ep12343608

21. Kurokawa I, Nakase K. Recent advances in understanding and managing acne. *F1000Research.* 2020;9:792. doi:10.12688/f1000research.25588.1

22. Fitz-Gibbon S, Tomida S, Chiu B-H, et al. Propionibacterium acnes Strain Populations in the Human Skin Microbiome Associated with Acne. *J Invest Dermatol.* 2013;133(9):2152–2160. doi:10.1038/jid.2013.21

23. Platsidaki E, Dessinioti C. Recent advances in understanding Propionibacterium acnes (Cutibacterium acnes) in acne. *F1000Research.* 2018;7. doi:10.12688/f1000research.15659.1

24. Jahns AC, Lundskog B, Ganceviciene R, et al. An increased incidence of Propionibacterium acnes biofilms in acne vulgaris: a case-control study: Increased incidence of P. acnes biofilms in acne vulgaris. *Br J Dermatol.* 2012;167(1):50–58. doi:10.1111/j.1365-2133.2012.10897.x

25. Kim J, Ochoa M-T, Krutzik SR, et al. Activation of Toll-Like Receptor 2 in Acne Triggers Inflammatory Cytokine Responses. *J Immunol.* 2002;169(3):1535–1541. doi:10.4049/jimmunol.169.3.1535

26. Ray Jalian H, Liu PT, Kanchanapoomi M, Phan JN, Legaspi AJ, Kim J. All-Trans Retinoic Acid Shifts Propionibacterium acnes-Induced Matrix Degradation Expression Profile toward Matrix Preservation in Human Monocytes. *J Invest Dermatol.* 2008;128(12):2777–2782. doi:10.1038/jid.2008.155

27. Liu PT, Krutzik SR, Kim J, Modlin RL. Cutting edge: all-trans retinoic acid down-regulates TLR2 expression and function. *J Immunol Baltim Md 1950.* 2005;174(5):2467–2470. doi:10.4049/jimmunol.174.5.2467

28. Czernielewski J, Michel S, Bouclier M, Baker M, Hensby JC. Adapalene biochemistry and the evolution of a new topical retinoid for treatment of acne. *J Eur Acad Dermatol Venereol: JEADV.* 2001;15(Suppl 3):5–12. doi:10.1046/j.0926-9959.2001.00006.x

29. Lavker RM, Leyden JJ, Thorne EG. An ultrastructural study of the effects of topical tretinoin on microcomedones. *Clin Ther.* 1992;14(6):773–780.

30. Gollnick H, Cunliffe W, Berson D, et al. Management of Acne. *J Am Acad Dermatol.* 2003;49(1):S1–S37. doi:10.1067/mjd.2003.618

31. Layton A. The use of isotretinoin in acne. *Dermatoendocrinol.* 2009;1(3):162–169. doi:10.4161/derm.1.3.9364

32. Strauss JS, Stranieri AM. Acne treatment with topical erythromycin and zinc: effect of Propionibacterium acnes and free fatty acid composition. *J Am Acad Dermatol.* 1984;11(1):86–89. doi:10.1016/s0190-9622(84)70139-3

33. Simonart T, Dramaix M. Treatment of acne with topical antibiotics: lessons from clinical studies. *Br J Dermatol.* 2005;153(2):395–403. doi:10.1111/j.1365-2133.2005.06614.x

34. Cunliffe WJ, Holland KT, Bojar R, Levy SF. A randomized, double-blind comparison of a clindamycin phosphate/benzoyl peroxide gel formulation and a matching clindamycin gel with respect to microbiologic activity and clinical efficacy in the topical treatment of acne vulgaris. *Clin Ther.* 2002;24(7):1117–1133. doi:10.1016/S0149-2918(02)80023-6

35. Fulton JE, Farzad-Bakshandeh A, Bradley S. Studies on the Mechanism of Action of Topical Benzoyl Peroxide and vitamin A Acid in Acne Vulgaris. *J Cutan Pathol.* 1974;1(5):191–200. doi:10.1111/j.1600-0560.1974.tb00628.x

36. Leyden J, Stein-Gold L, Weiss J. Why Topical Retinoids Are Mainstay of Therapy for Acne. *Dermatol Ther.* 2017;7(3):293–304. doi:10.1007/s13555-017-0185-2

37. Marson JW, Baldwin HE. An Overview of Acne Therapy, Part 1. *Dermatol Clin.* 2019;37(2):183–193. doi:10.1016/j.det.2018.12.001

38. Trifarotene (Aklief)—A New Topical Retinoid for Acne. *JAMA.* 2020;323(13):1310. doi:10.1001/jama.2019.22507

39. Moore A, Green LJ, Bruce S, et al. Once-Daily Oral Sarecycline 1.5 mg/kg/day Is Effective for Moderate to Severe Acne Vulgaris: Results from Two Identically Designed, Phase 3, Randomized, Double-Blind Clinical Trials. *J Drugs Dermatol.* 2018;17(9):987–996.

40. Moore AY, Del Rosso J, Johnson JL, Grada A. Sarecycline: A Review of Preclinical and Clinical Evidence. *Clin Cosmet Investig Dermatol.* 2020;13:553–560. doi:10.2147/CCID.S190473

41. Barbieri JS. A New Class of Topical Acne Treatment Addressing the Hormonal Pathogenesis of Acne. *JAMA Dermatol.* 2020;156(6):619. doi:10.1001/jamadermatol.2020.0464

42. Lyte P, Sur R, Nigam A, Southall MD. Heat-killed *Propionibacterium acnes* is capable of inducing inflammatory responses in skin. *Exp Dermatol.* 2009;18(12):1070–1072. doi:10.1111/j.1600-0625.2009.00891.x

43. Hebert A, Thiboutot D, Stein Gold L, et al. Efficacy and Safety of Topical Clascoterone Cream, 1%, for Treatment in Patients With Facial Acne: Two Phase 3 Randomized Clinical Trials. *JAMA Dermatol.* 2020;156(6):621. doi:10.1001/jamadermatol.2020.0465

44. Paithankar DY, Sakamoto FH, Farinelli WA, et al. Acne Treatment Based on Selective Photothermolysis of Sebaceous Follicles with Topically Delivered Light-Absorbing Gold Microparticles. *J Invest Dermatol.* 2015;135(7):1727–1734. doi:10.1038/jid.2015.89

45. Swinyer LJ. Topical Agents Alone in Acne: A Blind Assessment Study. *JAMA.* 1980;243(16):1640. doi:10.1001/jama.1980.03300420024019

46. Draelos Z, Jackson E. The Effects of Cleansing in an Acne Treatment Regimen. *Cosmet Dermatol-CEDAR KNOLLS-.* 1999;12(1):9–10.

47. Kligman AM, Wheatley VR, Mills OH. Comedogenicity of human sebum. *Arch Dermatol.* 1970;102(3):267–275.

48. Mills OH. Acne Detergicans. *Arch Dermatol.* 1975;111(1):65. doi:10.1001/archderm.1975.01630130067007

49. Arif T. Salicylic acid as a peeling agent: a comprehensive review. *Clin Cosmet Investig Dermatol.* 2015;8:455–461. doi:10.2147/CCID.S84765

50. Ditre CM, Griffin TD, Murphy GF, et al. Effects of alpha-hydroxy acids on photoaged skin: a pilot clinical, histologic, and ultra-structural study. *J Am Acad Dermatol.* 1996;34(2 Pt 1):187–195. doi:10.1016/s0190-9622(96)80110-1

51. Rendon MI, Berson DS, Cohen JL, Roberts WE, Starker I, Wang B. Evidence and considerations in the application of chemical peels in skin disorders and aesthetic resurfacing. *J Clin Aesthetic Dermatol.* 2010;3(7):32–43.

52. Kessler E, Flanagan K, Chia C, Rogers C, Anna Glaser D. Comparison of α- and β-hydroxy acid chemical peels in the treatment of mild to moderately severe facial acne vulgaris: comparison of α- and β-hydroxy acid chemical peels. *Dermatol Surg.* 2007;34(1):45–51. doi:10.1111/j.1524-4725.2007.34007.x

53. Lu J, Cong T, Wen X, et al. Salicylic acid treats acne vulgaris by suppressing AMPK/SREBP 1 pathway in sebocytes. *Exp Dermatol.* 2019;28(7):786–794. doi:10.1111/exd.13934

CHAPTER 17

Rosacea

Joshua Zeichner, MD
Krystal Mitchell, MD, MBA

SUMMARY POINTS

What's New

1. The potential role of probiotics in rosacea given the innate/adaptive immunity dysregulation and the contribution of commensal and pathogenic bacteria.
2. Transient receptor potential channels, vanilloid (TRPV) and ankyrin (TRPA), may contribute to the role of flushing and burning in rosacea.
3. Zonulin, a human protein that regulates intestinal permeability, is significantly higher in patients with rosacea.
4. Topical minocycline foam (Zilxi) has recently received FDA approval for the treatment of rosacea.

What's important

1. Treatment of rosacea focuses on patient education, skincare, and pharmacologic/procedural interventions.
2. Distinguishing rosacea from other conditions and initiation of early treatment when a patient reports flushing and burning.
3. Treatment of rosacea involves addressing both background facial redness and inflammatory lesions.

What We Don't Know

1. The pathogenesis of rosacea has yet to be fully elucidated and it is unclear whether the four rosacea subtypes are truly variants of the same condition.
2. The mechanism by which TLR2 is activated by *Demodex* mites.
3. The potential virulence factors of *S. epidermidis* in patients with rosacea.

What's Coming

1. The use of cromolyn, a mast cell stabilizer, in patients with rosacea.
2. The use of protease serine inhibitors to prevent the formation of the abnormal cathelicidin (LL-37) in patients with rosacea.

INTRODUCTION

Rosacea is a well-recognized, chronic, cutaneous condition presenting as central facial erythema, telangiectasia, papules, and pustules. A Swedish study demonstrated a prevalence of approximately 10% in the general population.[1] In the United States, it is believed that there are 13 million people affected by rosacea. It is usually diagnosed between the ages of 30 and 50 years, and although both genders are affected, it is more common in women. However, more men experience phymatous changes than women. Rosacea is also more prevalent in fair-skinned than dark-skinned individuals. Sun damage, a propensity to facial flushing, and genetic predisposition are risk factors for developing rosacea.

ETIOLOGY

While the precise cause of rosacea remains unknown, genetic factors, immune system overactivity, environmental and internal triggers, and abnormal vascular response all play a role.

No single causative gene has been identified through genomic studies in rosacea patients.[2] However, three human leukocyte antigens (HLA-DRB1*03:01, HLA-DQB1*02:01, and HLA-DQA1*05:01) have been identified in rosacea as well as Type 1 diabetes, multiple sclerosis, rheumatoid arthritis, and celiac disease. This raises the question of a possible association with autoimmune diseases.[3]

Environmental factors including ultraviolet light, heat, alcohol, hot beverages, and spicy food are all known triggers for rosacea flares.[2] They are thought to induce abnormal vascular responses and flushing, along with the production of pro-inflammatory cytokines. UV radiation is known to cause exaggerated expression of MMPs, collagen denaturation, production of fibroblast growth factor 2 and vascular endothelial growth factor 2, and reactive oxygen species (ROS).[2]

Overactivity of the innate immune system has been shown to be directly involved in the development of rosacea. In 2007, Gallo and colleagues observed that individuals with rosacea express abnormally high cathelicidin levels. Cathelicidins are antimicrobial peptides important in mounting an immune response to various bacterial, viral, and fungal pathogens.[4] Cathelicidins are enzymatically processed by the stratum corneum tryptic enzyme (SCTE), also called kallikrein 5 (KLK5), a serine protease. In rosacea, overactivity of KLK5 leads to the production of high levels of the biologically active cathelicidin, known as LL-37. This leads to inflammation, erythema, and cutaneous vascular dilatation. Cathelicidin production is strongly induced by vitamin D, helping to explain why UV light may serve as a trigger for rosacea. Increased activity of toll-like receptor 2 (TLR2) has also been implicated as a driving factor in rosacea. TLR2 is thought to be activated by *Demodex* mites with subsequent increases in KLK5 levels.[2]

Skin flora including *Demodex folliculorum* mites, *Staphylococcus epidermidis* organisms, and *Bacillus oleronius* have all been shown to be stimulating factors in rosacea.[5–7] Expression of matrix metalloproteinase-9 (MMP-9) is increased in the fibroblasts of rosacea patients with *Demodex folliculorum*.[8] It is thought that unchecked activity of MMP-9 propagates the inflammatory response and degradation of collagen. Afonso et al. demonstrated that MMP-9 is also increased in patients with ocular rosacea.[9] Furthermore, the *Demodex* mites have been shown to harbor bacteria known as *Bacillus olenorium,* thought to be a driver of inflammation in rosacea.[2] Strains of *S. epidermidis* are also thought to secrete virulence factors causing immune dysregulation, although these virulence factors do not cause the same type of immune dysregulation in patients without rosacea. Finally, elevated mast cell levels are observed in rosacea patients and are thought to secrete MMP-9 and trigger inflammatory cytokines.

Rosacea is associated with neurovascular dysregulation. Facial skin in rosacea shows increased superficial cutaneous vasculature, higher blood flow rates, and exaggerated vascular responses.[10–13] Prostaglandins, histamine, serotonin, and substance P have all been shown to cause abnormal vasodilation in rosacea patients leading to flushing.[13–15] Vascular endothelial growth factor (VEGF), a cytokine involved in angiogenesis and vasodilation, may play a role as well.[16–18] Neurovascular

---

BOX 17-1

The kinin-kallikrein system or "kinin system" is a poorly delineated system of blood proteins that plays a role in inflammation, blood pressure control, coagulation, and pain. Its important mediators, bradykinin and kallidin, are vasodilators.

---

communication is thought to be mediated in part by transient receptor potential channels, vanilloid (TRPV) and ankyrin (TRPA) types, found on neuronal tissue.[2] These receptors are stimulated by factors such as environmental heat and spicy foods, and contribute to the flushing and burning sensations rosacea patients experience. Protease-activated receptor 2 (PAR2), a receptor found in inflammatory cells and epithelial tissue, is thought to be involved in communication between sensory nerves and the immune system.[2,17]

While controversial, rosacea has been linked to alterations in digestive tract bacteria. It has been suggested that alterations of intestinal microflora increase gut permeability leading to systemic inflammation.[5] The plasma kallikrein-kinin pathway has been implicated, with the production of bradykinin, a well-known vasodilator, leading to sensitization of cutaneous nerves and blood vessels (Box 17-1).[6] Zonulin, a protein produced in the gut in response to gluten, is involved in regulating small intestinal permeability and has been found to be elevated in rosacea patients.[19] Small intestinal bacterial overgrowth (SIBO) may also be involved, as clearance of SIBO has been associated with improvement of rosacea symptoms.[20,21] *Helicobacter pylori* infection of the stomach has been implicated in the development of rosacea, but there is data supporting both sides of the argument.[22–24] Finally, there is data implicating inflammatory gastrointestinal diseases such as Celiac disease, Crohn's disease, ulcerative colitis, and irritable bowel as causative factors.[25]

CLINICAL MANIFESTATION

Diagnostic Criteria

Rosacea has traditionally been categorized into four different subtypes. However, in 2016, the Global ROSacea COnsensus (ROSCO) panel of 17 international dermatologists re-evaluated the diagnostic criteria and classification of rosacea. According to the panel, persistent erythema of the midface with periodic exaggeration is sufficient for a diagnosis of rosacea.[26] Telangiectasias, papules, and pustules are often seen in rosacea patients, but they are not enough on their own to make the diagnosis[26] Phymatous changes, however, are also considered to be independently diagnostic of rosacea (**Table 17-1**).[26] The panel concluded that patients should be diagnosed and treated based on their individual symptoms rather than placing them into a particular subtype.[26]

TRADITIONAL ROSACEA SUBTYPES

The characteristics of the four rosacea subtypes are listed in **Table 17-2**. The condition may progress from the milder

TABLE 17-1	Guidelines for the Diagnosis of Rosacea	
One or More of the Following Sufficient for Diagnosis	**Additional Symptoms and Signs**
Flushing (transient erythema)	Burning/stinging
Persistent erythema	Facial edema
Telangiectasia	Facial dryness
Papules/pustules	Plaques
	Ocular symptoms
	Peripheral involvement (+/− facial roscea)
	Phymatous changes

Adapted from Wilkin J, Dahl M, Detmar M, et al.; National Rosacea Society Expert Committee. Standard grading system for rosacea: report of the National Rosacea Society Expert Committee on the classification and staging of rosacea. *J Am Acad Dermatol.* 2004;50(6):907-912.

TABLE 17-2	Clinical Subtypes and Variants of Rosacea
Erythemotelangiectatic subtype
Facial flushing
Erythema/edema of central face
Telangiectasias on face
Papulopustular subtype
Persistent erythema of central face
Episodic papules and pustules on face
Phymatous subtype
Thickened skin of nose
Nodularities of nose
Irregular skin surface of nose
Ocular subtype
Burning and stinging of eyes
Foreign body sensation
Photosensitivity
Conjunctivitis/blepharitis/inflamed meibomian glands
Granulomatous variant
Yellow, brown, or red papules and nodules on face
Possible scarring

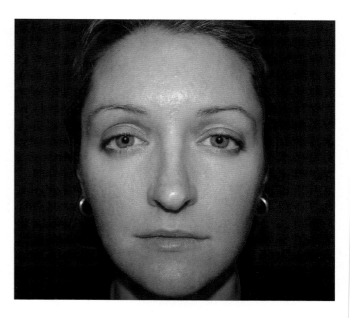

FIGURE 17-1. Facial flushing is a characteristic of rosacea and its presence alone is enough to diagnose the disorder. Patients with this form of rosacea often do not realize that they have rosacea and do not seek treatment.

the mentioned signs and symptoms. Many patients describe worsening of their symptoms with aggravating factors such as hot beverages, spicy food, sunlight, and heat. These patients have sensitive and irritable skin types. Therefore, complaints of burning and stinging with topical skin regimens are common[27] Many patients in this subtype do not realize that they have rosacea and therefore may not be using the proper skincare to minimize progression. Consequently, it is important for dermatologists to screen patients and ask them about facial flushing symptoms. Telangiectasias are common but are not required for diagnosis.

Subtype 2: Papulopustular Rosacea (Fig. 17-2)

Papulopustular rosacea, also called "classic rosacea," presents with papules, pustules, and erythema on the central face. Patients describe the erythema as persistent with episodic breakouts of papules and pustules. This type may be misdiagnosed as acne. Age of onset (older than 30 years), absence of comedones, development after precipitating factors such as spicy food, and the presence of telangiectasias may help the practitioner to distinguish the papulopustular form of rosacea from acne. Severe cases can lead to chronic facial edema.

Subtype 3: Phymatous Rosacea (Fig. 17-3)

Phymatous changes are well recognized by thickened and uneven skin on the nose with an irregular surface and nodularities. This is commonly known as the "W.C. Fields' nose." Although it most commonly affects the nasal area, it also occurs in the malar area and chin. This type is seen more commonly in men and typically develops after patients have been affected for many years. Treatment modalities include isotretinoin, laser resurfacing, and surgical intervention.

subtypes such as flushing, to papulopustular and phymatous rosacea. Patients may have more than one subtype. It is important to diagnose and treat rosacea early to try to avoid the progression of the disorder. The four traditional subtypes of rosacea are discussed below.

Subtype 1: Erythematelangiectatic Rosacea (Fig. 17-1)

This subtype is characterized by erythema of the central face typically sparing the periocular skin, in addition to telangiectasias and flushing. The patient may only present with one of

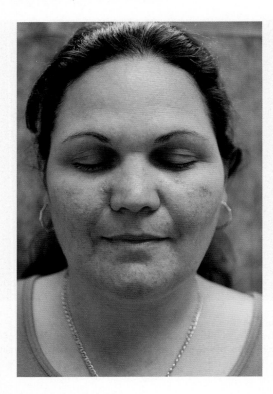

FIGURE 17-2. Papulopustular rosacea.

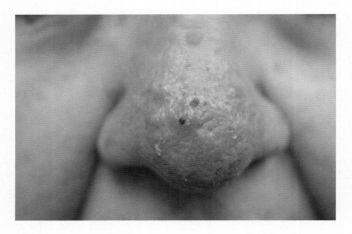

FIGURE 17-3. Phymatous rosacea. Thickened, irregular skin on the nose. This individual exhibits the papulopustular form of rosacea as well.

Subtype 4: Ocular Rosacea (Fig. 17-4)

The ocular manifestations of rosacea are usually nonspecific. Most patients with ocular rosacea complain of burning, stinging, itching, a gritty sensation, and watering of their eyes. Ocular rosacea is often undiagnosed since symptoms are misdiagnosed as seasonal allergies. Ocular rosacea should be considered if a patient complains of or exhibits one of the following: interpalpebral conjunctival hyperemia, burning or stinging of the eyes, photosensitivity, telangiectasias of the lid margin or conjunctiva, foreign body sensation, and periocular

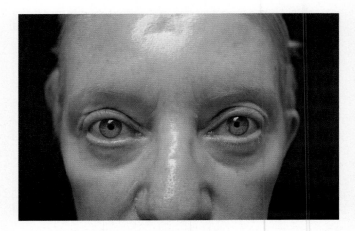

FIGURE 17-4. Ocular rosacea is characterized by bilateral erythema of the conjunctiva and/or eyelids.

erythema.[2] Patients may also present with clinical pictures of conjunctivitis, blepharitis, inflamed meibomian glands (or tarsal glands), chalazion, or irregularity of the eyelid margins.[2,28,29] Notably, the symptoms of ocular rosacea may precede the cutaneous signs, although most patients have some cutaneous manifestation of this condition. Interestingly, children who have styes are more likely to develop rosacea as adults. In rare cases, scarring and surface irregularities may lead to decreased visual acuity.[2]

VARIANTS OF ROSACEA

The National Rosacea Society Expert Committee has only recognized one variant for rosacea, which is the granulomatous form.[30] It is worth noting that pyoderma faciale (also called rosacea fulminans), steroid-induced rosacea, and perioral dermatitis are now considered to be different entities and are no longer classified as subtypes of rosacea.

Granulomatous Rosacea

The granulomatous variant of rosacea is characterized by plaques of red to yellow-brown firm papules and nodules usually on the periorificial and malar areas of the face.[30] The papules and nodules appear to be less inflamed than in the papulopustular subtype. The presence of other subtypes is not necessary for the diagnosis of this variant.

Differential Diagnosis

Facial erythema and flushing are seen in many dermatologic and systemic disorders. Clinical history and physical examination are very important aspects of patient evaluation, including historical questions about facial flushing. Laboratory tests may be needed to rule out systemic diseases, such as collagen vascular disorders, if these are suspected. In older patients, it is important to distinguish rosacea from a photoaging associated with telangiectasias. This entity is characterized by less transient and non-transient erythema, more lateral distribution of erythema, telangiectasia, lack of flushing and burning, and features of photoaging, including atrophy, facial wrinkling,

TABLE 17-3	Differential Diagnosis of Rosacea
Benign cutaneous flushing	
Allergic contact dermatitis	
Lupus erythematosus	
Dermatomyositis	
Mixed connective tissue disease	
Carcinoid syndrome	
Pheochromocytoma	
Medullary carcinoma of the thyroid	
Pancreatic cell tumor (VIPoma)	
Mastocytosis	
Photosensitivity from medications	
Climacterium/postmenopausal	

TABLE 17-4	Rosacea Aggravating Factors
Food	
Hot temperature beverages	
Spicy food	
Chocolate	
Dairy products	
Vanilla	
Soy sauce	
Environmental factors	
Heat	
UV light	
Cold	
Humidity	
Chemicals	
Alcoholic beverages	
Medications	
Physical exertions	
Stress	
Chronic cough	
Heavy exercise	

TABLE 17-5	Rosacea Treatment Modalities
Topical treatments	
Antibiotics	
Metronidazole	
Clindamycin	
Erythromycin	
Anti-inflammatories	
Azelaic acid	
Feverfew	
Green tea	
Licochalcone	
Licorice extract	
Immunomodulators	
Pimecrolimus	
Tacrolimus	
Sulfur products	
Sulfur	
Sodium sulfacetamide	
Oral antibiotics	
Tetracyclines (Tetracycline, doxycycline, minocycline)	
Macrolides (Erythromycin, azithromycin, clarithromycin)	
Metronidazole	
Ampicillin	
Trimethoprim/sulfamethoxazole	
Other oral treatments	
Isotretinoin	
Aspirin	
Beta-blockers	
Selective serotonin reuptake inhibitors (SSRIs)	
Clonidine	
Hormones (oral contraceptives)	
Laser and light treatments	
Intense, pulsed-light therapy	
Vascular lasers (Pulsed dye laser, Dornier 940 nm, KTP laser)	
Carbon dioxide resurfacing laser	
Other treatments (for phymatous subtype)	
Hot loop electrocoagulation	
Dermabrasion	

dyspigmentation, poikiloderma, and history of premalignant or malignant neoplasms.[31] **Table 17-3** lists the differential diagnosis of rosacea.[32]

TREATMENT

Treatment of rosacea involves proper skincare, prescription medications, and avoidance of triggers, see Table 17-4. Gentle cleansers and moisturizers are important to maintain skin barrier function. Given the triggering effects of UV light, sunscreen and sun avoidance are very important. Since rosacea patients typically have sensitive skin, selecting the right sunscreen may be challenging. Physical blockers (e.g., zinc oxide and titanium dioxide) may be better tolerated than chemical filters by rosacea patients. Also, green-tinted cosmetics can be used to conceal facial erythema.[33]

When selecting a prescription regimen, the two main treatment components to consider are inflammatory papules and erythema. For papules and pustules, several topical and oral antibiotics may be used based on the severity of symptoms. Commonly prescribed topical agents include metronidazole, azelaic acid, and ivermectin cream.[34] Recently, topical minocycline 1.5% foam (Zilxi) was FDA-approved for the treatment of rosacea.[35] Oral therapies include extended-release sub-antimicrobial dose doxycycline (10 mg extended/30 mg immediate) and off-label use of microbial dose doxycycline or minocycline. Oral ivermectin use has also been reported in some patients, especially in those with severe inflammatory papules. In severe or recalcitrant cases, isotretinoin may be effective. Emerging therapies include serine protease inhibitors that prevent the formation of abnormal cathelicidin (LL-37) and topical cromolyn, a mast cell stabilizer.[34]

Although antibiotic therapy controls the inflammatory component of rosacea and may prevent its exacerbation, antibiotics do not improve the persistent erythema nor telangiectatic lesions on the face. Persistent erythema of rosacea can be addressed with topical alpha-adrenergic receptors (e.g., oxymetazoline and brimonidine), and systemic beta-blockers in refractory cases.[34] In recent years, light and laser treatments have been widely and successfully used to target telangiectatic lesions. In a study of 60 patients affected with rosacea who were treated with intense pulsed light (IPL), there was a mean clearance of almost 78% of the telangiectasias. In this study, the mean number of treatments was about four, and the wavelength, pulse duration, and energy were adjusted according to patients' skin color.[36,37] Pulsed dye laser (PDL) is another alternative. It is reasonable to consider a treatment plan combining both IPL and PDL. **Table 17-5** summarizes different treatment modalities for rosacea.[38,39]

CONCLUSION

The complex etiology and wide spectrum of clinical manifestations of rosacea render it a challenging condition for both dermatologists and patients. There is no single and universal approach to treating patients affected by this condition. However, diagnosing rosacea early in the flushing stage and treating it with anti-inflammatory modalities may prevent its progression. Treatment regimens should be individualized and tailored to address patients' concerns.

References

1. Berg M, Liden S. An epidemiological study of rosacea. *Acta Dermatol Venereol*. 1989;69:419.

2. Two AM, Wu W, Gallo RL, Hata TR. Rosacea: part I. Introduction, categorization, histology, pathogenesis, and risk factors. *J Am Acad Dermatol*. 2015 May;72(5):749–758.

3. Chang ALS, Raber I, Xu J, et al. Assessment of the genetic basis of rosacea by genome-wide association study. *J Invest Dermatol*. 2015;135(6):1548–1555.

4. Schwab VD, Sulk M, Seeliger S, Nowak P, Aubert J, et al. Neurovascular and neuroimmune aspects in the pathophysiology of rosacea. *J Investig Dermatol Symp Proc*. 2011 Dec;15(1):53–62.

5. Sharma JN, Zeitlin IJ, Mackenzie JF, et al. Plasma kinin-precursor levels in clinical intestinal inflammation. *Fundam Clin Pharmacol*. 1988;2:399.

6. Kendall SN. Remission of rosacea induced by reduction of gut transit time. *Clin Exp Dermatol*. 2004;29:297.

7. Nam JH, Yun Y, Kim HN, et al. Rosacea and its association with enteral microbiota in Korean females. *Exp Dermatol*. 2018;27(1):37–42.

8. Egeberg A, Weinstock LB, Thyssen EP, et al. Rosacea and gastrointestinal disorders: a population-based cohort study. *Br J Dermatol*. 2017;176(1):100–106.

9. Crawford GH, Pelle MT, James WD. Rosacea: I. Etiology, pathogenesis, and subtype classification. *J Am Acad Dermatol*. 2004;51:327.

10. Bonamigo RR, Bakos L, Edelweiss M, et al. Could matrix metalloproteinase-9 be a link between Demodex folliculorum and rosacea? *J Eur Acad Dermatol Venereol*. 2005;19:646.

11. Afonso AA, Sobrin L, Monroy DC, et al. Tear fluid gelatinase B activity correlates with IL-1alpha concentration and fluorescein clearance in ocular rosacea. *Invest Ophthalmol Vis Sci*. 1999;40:2506.

12. Ryan TJ. The blood vessels of the skin. *J Invest Dermatol*. 1976;67:110.

13. Tur E, Tur M, Maibach HI, et al. Basal perfusion of the cutaneous microcirculation: measurements as a function of anatomic position. *J Invest Dermatol*. 1983;81:442.

14. Wilkin JK. Flushing reactions: consequences and mechanisms. *Ann Intern Med*. 1981;95:468.

15. Wilkin JK. Why is flushing limited to a mostly facial cutaneous distribution? *J Am Acad Dermatol*. 1988;19:309.

16. Pelwig G, Jansen T. Rosacea. In: Freedberg IM, Eisen AZ, Wolff K, Austen K, Goldsmith L, et al. eds. *Fitzpatrick's Dermatology in General Medicine*. New York: McGraw-Hill; 1999: 785.

17. Bates DO, Harper SJ. Regulation of vascular permeability by vascular endothelial growth factors. *Vascul Pharmacol*. 2003;39:225.

18. Smith JR, Lanier VB, Braziel RM, et al. Expression of vascular endothelial growth factor and its receptors in rosacea. *Br J Ophthalmol*. 2007;91:226.

19. Rufli T, Büchner SA. T-cell subsets in acne rosacea lesions and the possible role of Demodex folliculorum. *Dermatologica*. 1984;169:1.

20. Powell FC. Rosacea and the pilosebaceous follicle. *Cutis*. 2004;74:9.

21. Yukel M, Ulfer G. Measurement of the serum zonulin levels in patients with acne rosacea. 2020.

22. Rebora A, Drago F, Picciotto A. Helicobacter pylori in patients with rosacea. *Am J Gastroenterol*. 1994;89:1603.

23. Utaş S, Ozbakir O, Turasan A, et al. Helicobacter pylori eradication treatment reduces the severity of rosacea. *J Am Acad Dermatol*. 1999;40:433.

24. Gedik GK, Karaduman A, Sivri B, et al. Has Helicobacter pylori eradication therapy any effect on severity of rosacea symptoms? *J Eur Acad Dermatol Venereol*. 2005;19:398.

25. Porubsky CF, Glass AB, Comeau V, Buckley C, et al. Probiotics - Current Knowledge and Future Prospects: The Role of Probiotics in Acne and Rosacea. London, IntechOpen, 2018 p. 93.

26. Yamasaki K, Di Nardo A, Bardan A, et al. Increased serine protease activity and cathelicidin promotes skin inflammation in rosacea. *Nat Med*. 2007;13:975.

27. Ong PY, Ohtake T, Brandt C, et al. Endogenous antimicrobial peptides and skin infections in atopic dermatitis. *N Engl J Med*. 2002;347:1151.

28. Tan J, Almeida L, Bewley A, et al. Updating the diagnosis, classification and assessment of rosacea: recommendations from the global ROSacea COnsensus (ROSCO) panel. *Br J Dermatol.* 2017 Feb;176(2):431–438.

29. Lonne-Rahm SB, Fischer T, Berg M. Stinging and rosacea. *Acta Derm Venereol.* 1999;79:460.

30. Quarterman MJ, Johnson DW, Abele DC, et al. Ocular rosacea. Signs, symptoms, and tear studies before and after treatment with doxycycline. *Arch Dermatol.* 1997;133:49.

31. Ghanem VC, Mehra N, Wong S, et al. The prevalence of ocular signs in acne rosacea: comparing patients from ophthalmology and dermatology clinics. *Cornea.* 2003;22:230.

32. Wilkin J, Dahl M, Detmar M, et al. National Rosacea Society Expert Committee. Standard grading system for rosacea: report of the National Rosacea Society Expert Committee on the classification and staging of rosacea. *J Am Acad Dermatol.* 2004;50:907.

33. Helfrich YR, Maier LE, Cui Y, Fisher GJ, Chubb H, et al. Clinical, Histologic, and Molecular Analysis of Differences Between Erythematotelangiectatic Rosacea and Telangiectatic Photoaging. *JAMA Dermatol.* 2015 Aug;151(8):825–836.

34. Izikson L, English JC III, Zirwas MJ. The flushing patient: differential diagnosis, workup, and treatment. *J Am Acad Dermatol.* 2006;55:193.

35. Draelos ZD. Cosmeceuticals for rosacea. *Clin Dermatol.* 2017 Mar-Apr;35(2):213–217.

36. Two AM, Wu W, Gallo RL, Hata TR. Rosacea: part II. Topical and systemic therapies in the treatment of rosacea. *J Am Acad Dermatol.* 2015 May;72(5):761–770.

37. Schroeter CA, Haaf-von Below S, Neumann HA. Effective treatment of rosacea using intense pulsed light systems. *Dermatol Surg.* 2005;31:1285.

38. United States Food and Drug Administration. Zilxi (Minocycline Hydrochloride). https://www.accessdata.fda.gov/drugsatfda_docs/label/2020/213690s000lbl.pdf. Silver Spring, MD, 2020.

39. Pelle MT, Crawford GH, James WD. Rosacea: II. therapy. *J Am Acad Dermatol.* 2004;51:499.

CHAPTER 18

Burning and Stinging Skin (Type 3 Sensitive Skin)

Leslie S. Baumann, MD

SUMMARY POINTS

What's Important?

1. "Stingers" are a subset of people who feel stinging, burning, or other painful sensations upon exposure to certain chemical (e.g., skincare ingredients) and/or physical factors.
2. In the Baumann Skin Typing System, stingers are classified as having Baumann S3 sensitive skin. Identifying this skin type using the Baumann Skin Type Indicator (BSTI) is important to prevent patient discomfort and noncompliance.

What's New?

1. Mechanisms of burning and stinging work through an increased nervous system response, mediated by sensory nerve fibers connected to specialized receptors in the superficial skin layer.
2. Though causes of stinging vary by individual, common ingredients include those with a low pH (e.g., lactic, glycolic, salicylic, and sorbic acids, among others), alcohol, and capsaicin.

What's Coming?

1. Future research exploring associations between stinging, burning, and itch, as well as the pathophysiology of diseases such as rosacea, are needed to improve treatment options for this subtype of sensitive skin.
2. Large-scale studies of stinging in non-white populations are needed to better understand the relationship between stinging and ethnicity.

A subset of people feel stinging and burning when exposed to certain skincare products. These people have traditionally been called "stingers" since Kligman coined the term in 1977. This skin type has also been called reactive skin, hyperreactive skin, intolerant skin, or irritable skin. In the Baumann Skin Typing System, stingers are designated as having Baumann S3 sensitive skin (see Chapter 10, The Baumann Skin Typing System); the "3" denotes burners and stingers rather than other types of sensitive skin that develop such as acne (S1), rosacea (S2), or contact dermatitis (S4). One patient can demonstrate one to four different types of sensitive skin. For example, many rosacea (S2) patients are also burners and stingers (S3). Although this skin type is referred to as stingers in the context of applying chemical factors such as skincare ingredients, this skin type also includes those who feel the onset of a prickling, tingling sensation, or slight pain because of physical factors such as ultraviolet radiation, heat, cold, and wind. Psychologic stress or hormonal factors such as menstruation may play a role as well. It is important to know a patient's susceptibility to S3 sensitive skin because this may lead to noncompliance with certain medications and vehicles that cause discomfort to the patient. Finacea is an example of a rosacea medication that causes stinging in a small proportion of users. Retin-A Micro contains benzyl alcohol (a derivative of benzoic acid) that can cause stinging in certain people. This chapter will discuss what is known about the mechanisms of burning and stinging, what ingredients are most likely to cause it, and how to identify a potential "stinger."

EPIDEMIOLOGY

Type 3 sensitive skin is common worldwide. In a British study, 57% of women and 31.4% of men reported that they had experienced an adverse reaction to a personal skincare product at some stage in their lives, with 23% of women and 13.8% of men having had a problem in the last 12 months.[1] Another study demonstrated that women showed a greater tendency toward being more sensitive to the subjective effects elicited by lactic acid than males.[2]

MECHANISMS OF BURNING AND STINGING

Stinging is a problem reported to occur primarily on the face, particularly on the nasolabial folds and cheeks. The extreme sensitivity of this region is thought to be caused by a more permeable horny layer, a high density of sweat glands and hair follicles, and an elaborate network of sensory nerves.[3] There is specificity of the stinging response that is not understood. In other words, an individual may be a lactic acid stinger, but not experience such a reaction to other ingredients such as benzoic acid and azelaic acid. One study showed that there was no correlation between patients who stung from lactic acid and those who stung from azelaic acid.[4] This suggests that there is some sort of specificity involved that has not yet been deciphered.

The Role of the Sensory Nervous System

It is likely that the sensory system in the epidermis is involved in this process, rather than the dermal sensory system. In the epidermis, sensory nerves are linked to keratinocytes, melanocytes, Langerhans cells, and Merkel cells (**Box 18-1**). Sensory nerves are categorized into two groups: the epidermal and the dermal sensory organs. It is the Merkel cells in the epidermis that are thought to play a role in sensory perception; however, the exact role of Merkel cells and their possible involvement in mechanosensation is unclear.[5] Merkel cells consist of neurosecretory granules that contain neurotransmitter-type substances such as met-enkephalin, vasoactive intestinal peptide, neuron-specific enolase, and synaptophysin.[6] The Merkel cell-nerve complex has been referred to by other names including touch domes, hederiform endings, Iggo's capsule, Pinkus corpuscles, and Haarsheibe. Merkel cell-nerve complexes have been found to be associated with hair follicles and eccrine sweat ducts. Little is known about the effects of chemical agents upon the excitability of sensory units such as Merkel cells.

It is believed that those with a predilection toward stinging have an increased nerve response. Capsaicin, the irritant ingredient found in red pepper and used commercially as "pepper spray," causes pain and burning on skin contact on all subjects. Its mechanisms of action have been studied in the pursuit of a better understanding of chemogenic pain. Although it is not known if these same pathways play a role in the skin burning that patients feel when they apply skincare products, it is possible that these follow a similar mechanism; therefore, the actions of capsaicin will be explored here. The C polymodal nociceptor is stimulated by capsaicin and other chemicals. The effects of capsaicin are dependent on

---

BOX 18-1	Sensory Nerves in the Skin

The superficial skin layer includes sensory nerve fibers connected to specialized receptors such as Merkel cells.

Three types of fibers are generally recognized in the sensory subclass of fibers:

- Beta fibers, which are the largest fibers and myelinated, mediate the touch, vibration, and pressure sensations (conduction velocity of $2–30$ m s^{-1}).
- Delta fibers, smaller and myelinated, mediate the cold and pain sensations (conduction velocity of > 30 m s^{-1}).
- C fibers, the slowest, smaller and nonmyelinated, mediate the warm and itching sensations (conduction velocity of < 2 m s^{-1}). C fibers mediate most of the autonomic peripheral functions.

---

concentration. Topical application of 1% capsaicin on intact skin typically produces sensitization to heat.[7] Findings of differential capsaicin effects on heat perception and mechanical stimuli perception have led to the belief in the existence of two categories of functionally different nociceptors in human skin.[8] Much more research needs to be conducted in this area; however, it is plausible that the heat-sensitive nociceptors play a role in this stinging and burning skin type.

Transient Receptor Proteins

Transient receptor protein (TRP) receptors in keratinocytes have the ability to sense a variety of environmental factors. TRP receptors may play a role in the skin stinging seen in sensitive skin. Transient receptor potential vallinoid 1 (TRPV1) and TRPV4 are heat receptors and integral in pain and itch. TRPV1 is the receptor that senses capsaicin, a component of chili peppers, and provides a sensation of heat. TRPV1 is also activated by a low pH.[9] TRPV1 may be one of the mechanisms by which stingers sting from the application of lactic acid.

VASODILATATION AND ITCHING

Type 3 sensitive skin patients complain of abnormal sensations and may or may not exhibit vasodilatation. C nonmyelinated fibers likely play a role because they are known to mediate warm sensations. Although the stinging and burning that characterize this skin type are not always associated with inflammation, inflammation may occur as well. Neurogenic inflammation may result from neuromediators such as substance P, calcitonin gene-related peptide (CGRP), and vasoactive intestinal peptide, leading to vasodilatation and mast cell degranulation.[10] Nonspecific inflammation may also be associated with the release of IL-1, IL-8, PgE2, PgF2, and TNF.[11] Sorbic acid, a known cause of skin stinging, has been found to release prostaglandin D2 (PGD2) from a cellular source in the skin resulting in cutaneous vasodilatation.[12]

Itching

Itching seems to be a different process than burning or stinging; however, there may be some overlap. A detailed explanation of itching is beyond the scope of this chapter, but a good recent review was reported by Chen.[13] An itch response can be experimentally induced by topical or intradermal injections of various substances such as proteolytic enzymes, mast cell degranulators, and vasoactive agents. Grove compared the cumulative lactic acid sting scores with the histamine itch scores in 32 young subjects; all the subjects who were stingers were also moderate to intense itchers, whereas 50% of the moderate itchers experienced no stinging.[14] Recent studies suggest that a new class of C fibers with an exceptionally lower conduction velocity and insensitivity to mechanical stimuli likely can be considered as afferent units that mediate the itchy sensation.[15]

The Skin Barrier and Stinging

The skin barrier plays an important role in both keeping water from evaporating from the skin as well as keeping out allergens and irritants (see Chapter 19, Contact Dermatitis to Cosmetic Ingredients). It has been postulated that an impaired skin barrier allows excessive penetration of applied ingredients, which may lead to stinging. A recent study evaluated 298 women with 5% lactic acid solution and measured transepidermal water loss, skin hydration, sebum content, and pH.[16] A positive correlation between stinging and increased transepidermal water loss was found, suggesting that skin barrier perturbation played a role in the development of stinging. No correlation was observed between stinging responses and other parameters such as skin hydration, sebum content, or pH. However, not all studies show stingers to have impaired barriers. One study examining the relationship between stingers (Baumann S3 type) and those who develop an irritant reaction to a 0.3% sodium dodecyl sulfate patch test (Baumann S4 type) found that stingers were no more likely to develop an irritant response than nonstingers.[3]

Rosacea and Skin Stinging

Patients with rosacea (Baumann S2 type) have a tendency to flush. This flushing is often accompanied by a warm sensation. Many rosacea patients also complain of intolerance to skincare products. One study examined this relationship. Thirty-two patients with rosacea and 32 controls were given the lactic acid stinging test. Twenty-four patients and six controls reacted positively as stingers ($P < 0.001$). This study suggests that patients with rosacea may be more likely to be stingers.[17]

ETHNICITY AND STINGING

Although there is a clinical consensus that blacks are less reactive and Asians are more reactive than whites, the data supporting this hypothesis rarely reach statistical significance.[18] Frosch reported that most common stingers were light-complexioned persons of Celtic ancestry who sunburned easily and tanned poorly.[19] Grove et al. found that stinging was not related to ethnicity, but was associated mainly with a person's history of sensitivity to soaps, cosmetics, and drugs.[20] Aramaki et al. found significant subjective sensory differences between Japanese and German women even though they had significant differences in reactions to sodium lauryl sulfate testing.[21] They concluded that Japanese women might be more likely to report stronger stinging sensations, reflecting a different cultural behavior. Large-scale studies of ethnic differences in this skin type have not been performed.

INGREDIENTS THAT CAUSE STINGING

A list of common stinging ingredients is found in **Table 18-1**. However, new ingredients are being developed every day, so it is impossible to have a complete list. Patients with a proclivity to experience stinging should be advised to make a list of the ingredients found in products that evoke the stinging response. The dermatologist can help the patient identify the responsible ingredient(s) to be avoided in the future. As a general rule, products with a low pH such as any acids (e.g., glycolic, salicylic, lactic) will cause stinging. Vitamin C is formulated with a low pH to enhance absorption, so some forms may cause stinging. In addition, alcohols that are often found in toners and astringents can cause stinging.

HOW TO IDENTIFY A POTENTIAL STINGER

The Baumann Skin Type Indicator (BSTI) contains a series of questions that are designed to identify those with the Baumann S3 skin type (see Chapter 10). This questionnaire can be accessed online by registering at www.SkinIQ.com. Using the online version of the questionnaire will allow data to be collected in order to examine issues such as the roles of gender, ethnicity, and climate in skin stinging. It is imperative to collect large amounts of worldwide data to identify the factors relevant in this condition.

Objective measures in the research and clinical settings may be used to identify stingers. However, it is important to note that not all stingers react to all known stinging agents. Clinical tests can give insight into this distressing condition, though. The lactic acid stinging test was first described by Kligman in 1977.[19] This method is now used with various stinging agents besides lactic

TABLE 18-1	Ingredients Known to Cause Stinging in Some People
Alcohol	
Avobenzone (Parsol)	
Azelaic acid	
Benzoic acid	
Capsaicin	
Eucalyptus oil	
Fragrance	
Glycolic acid	
Lactic acid	
Menthol	
Peppermint	
Salicylic acid	
Sorbic acid	
Vitamin C	
Witch hazel	

acid. The agent of choice is applied to the cheek using a cotton swab. The stingers experience a moderate to severe sensation within a few minutes. These subjects are then asked to describe the intensity of the sensation using a point scale.[22] It is important to note that substances cannot be simultaneously tested on both cheeks. Strong stinging on one side may enhance the perception of stinging on the opposite cheek. In a laboratory setting, stingers are easy to identify. The problem is that not all people sting in response to the same substance. For example, a lactic acid stinger may sting to lactic acid but not to benzoic acid. For this reason, it is very difficult to predict outside the laboratory setting which ingredients will make a patient sting. The BSTI can help identify susceptible subpopulations who are more likely to develop a stinging response based on historical data.

HOW TO PREVENT STINGING

At this point, identification and avoidance of agents that cause stinging is the most prudent approach. Patients should be instructed to keep a list of ingredients that cause stinging and avoid agents that contain such components. This includes shampoos, conditioners, and shaving products as well as skincare products. It is likely that improving the skin barrier will decrease the incidence of the stinging response. Anti-inflammatory products such as antioxidants, aloe vera, and chamomile can help decrease inflammation that may coincide with the stinging response. It is important to remember that stinging not accompanied by inflammation is not necessarily detrimental to the skin. In fact, chemical peel agents, glycolic acid, and lactic acid agents cause stinging in many because of their low pH. However, these agents have been shown to be very useful in increasing skin hydration and improving the appearance of photodamaged skin.

SUMMARY

Baumann S3 sensitive skin is a poorly understood skin type. Those who exhibit such a skin type find that they are intolerant to some skincare products. This likely affects their brand and product choices. Although stinging skin is usually not accompanied by inflammation, it can be very uncomfortable for the patient and can lead to noncompliance with skincare regimens for other conditions. More research is needed into the mechanisms and associations of this intellectually intriguing skin type so that treatment options can be improved and/or expanded for the patients who suffer symptoms because of this subtype of sensitive skin.

References

1. Willis CM, Shaw S, De Lacharrière O, et al. Sensitive skin: an epidemiological study. *Br J Dermatol.* 2001;145:258.

2. Marriott M, Whittle E, Basketter DA. Facial variations in sensory responses. *Contact Dermatitis.* 2003;49:227.

3. Basketter DA, Griffiths HA. A study of the relationship between susceptibility to skin stinging and skin irritation. *Contact Dermatitis.* 1993;29:185.

4. Draelos ZD. Noxious sensory perceptions in patients with mild to moderate rosacea treated with azelaic acid 15% gel. *Cutis.* 2004;74:257.

5. Hitchcock IS, Genever PG, Cahusac PM. Essential components for a glutamatergic synapse between Merkel cell and nerve terminal in rats. *Neurosci Lett.* 2004;362:196.

6. Chu DH. Development and structure of skin. In: Wolff K, Goldsmith LA, Katz SI, Gilchrest BA, Paller AS, Leffell DJ, eds. *Fitzpatrick's Dermatology in General Medicine.* 7th ed. New York, NY: McGraw-Hill; 2007:62.

7. LaMotte RH, Lundberg LE, Torebjörk HE. Pain, hyperalgesia and activity in nociceptive C units in humans after intradermal injection of capsaicin. *J Physiol.* 1992;448:749.

8. Schmelz M, Schmid R, Handwerker HO, et al. Encoding of burning pain from capsaicin-treated human skin in two categories of unmyelinated nerve fibres. *Brain.* 2000;123:560.

9. Denda M, Tsutsumi M. Roles of transient receptor potential proteins (TRPs) in epidermal keratinocytes. In: *Transient Receptor Potential Channels.* Dordrecht: Springer; 2011:847–860.

10. Misery L, Myon E, Martin N, et al. Sensitive skin: psychological effects and seasonal changes. *J Eur Acad Dermatol Venereol.* 2007;21:620.

11. Reilly DM, Parslew R, Sharpe GR, et al. Inflammatory mediators in normal, sensitive and diseased skin types. *Acta Derm Venereol.* 2000;80:171.

12. Morrow JD, Minton TA, Awad JA. Release of markedly increased quantities of prostaglandin D2 from the skin in vivo in humans following the application of sorbic acid. *Arch Dermatol.* 1994;130:1408.

13. Chen XJ, Sun YG. Central circuit mechanisms of itch. *Nat Commun.* 2020;11(1):3052.

14. Grove GL. Age-associated changes in integumental reactivity. In: Léveque JL, Agache PG, eds. *Aging Skin: Properties and Functional Changes.* New York, NY: Marcel Dekker; 1993:189–192.

15. Schmelz M, Schmidt R, Bickel A, et al. Specific C-receptors for itch in human skin. *J Neurosci.* 1997;17:8003.

16. An S, Lee E, Kim S, et al. Comparison and correlation between stinging responses to lactic acid and bioengineering parameters. *Contact Dermatitis.* 2007;57:158.

17. Lonne-Rahm SB, Fischer T, Berg M. Stinging and rosacea. *Acta Derm Venereol.* 1999;79:460.

18. Modjtahedi SP, Maibach HI. Ethnicity as a possible endogenous factor in irritant contact dermatitis: comparing the irritant response among Caucasians, blacks and Asians. *Contact Dermatitis.* 2002;47:272.

19. Frosch PJ, Kligman AM. A method for appraising the stinging capacity of topically applied substances. *J Soc Cosmet Chem.* 1981;28:197.

20. Grove GL, Soschin DM, Kligman AM. Adverse subjective reactions to topical agents. In: Drill VA, Lazar P, eds. *Cutaneous Toxicology.* New York, NY: Raven Press; 1984:200–210.

21. Aramaki J, Kawana S, Effendy I, et al. Differences of skin irritation between Japanese and European women. *Br J Dermatol.* 2002;146:1052.

22. Christensen M, Kligman AM. An improved procedure for conducting lactic acid stinging tests on facial skin. *J Soc Cosmet Chem.* 1996;47:1.

CHAPTER 19

Contact Dermatitis (Type 4 Sensitive Skin)

Alina Goldenberg, MD, MAS
Sharon E. Jacob, MD

SUMMARY POINTS

What's Important

1. Contact dermatitis, including irritant and allergic variants, affects up to 20% of the population at some point in their life. Personal hygiene and cosmetic products are the culprits behind the majority of the non-occupational cases of contact dermatitis involving the face, neck and hands.
2. Allergic Contact Dermatitis (ACD) can develop to a chemical ingredient in a product that has been in routine use for years. The cutaneous response of ACD, with erythema, scale and pruritus, can extend beyond the area of direct contact with the allergen.
3. Fragrances and preservatives are common agents causing ACD. Package labeling of "fragrance free" may mislead the consumer, if the manufacturer includes the fragrance-based ingredient for a non-fragrance function, eg: as a preservative.
4. Essential oils are the building blocks of fragrances. Natural is not synonymous with safe.

What's New

1. Methylisothiozolinone (MI) overtook formaldehyde-releasing preservatives and fragrances as the leading prevalent sensitizing allergen. Moreover, MI was found to be the most clinically relevant allergen, with the highest ever recorded relevance value.
2. Dillarstone effect describes the development of new contact dermatitis epidemics following 2–3 years after introduction of an allergenic compound to the market.
3. Although cautioned by the media, parabens are consistently found to be weak sensitizers and play a very minor role in ACD. Moreover, epidemiologic data has failed to show a direct connection between parabens and hormonal effects or the development of breast cancer.

What's Coming

1. The COVID-19 pandemic dampened, but saw a rise in index cases of ACD associated with personal protective equipment (masks, gloves and hand sanitizers) both in the health care industry and the public realm.
2. Open dialogue between consumers and industry members on social media has sparked a movement toward more "clean," ethically transparent, allergen-free cosmetics which may be the focus of the next decade.

OVERVIEW OF CONTACT DERMATITIS

Contact dermatitis (CD) comprises a group of cutaneous reactions that are triggered by the epidermis coming into contact with an allergen or an irritant. There are three main clinical forms of CD: (1) irritant contact dermatitis (ICD); (2) contact urticaria (CU); and (3) allergic contact dermatitis (ACD). CD is highly prevalent and is estimated to affect approximately 15–20% of the general population[1] and cost over $1.5 billion in medical expenditure in the United States alone.[2] CD clinically presents with debilitating rashes, sleep-depriving itch, and incessant irritability. Such presentations often lead to significant morbidity and inability to participate in activities of daily life, thus directly affecting patients' quality of life.[3,4] CD due to suspected personal hygiene products (PHP) and cosmetic products is an extremely common cause for patients to seek medical care, and thus, must be a condition that cosmetic dermatologists are knowledgeable in diagnosing and treating.

Irritant Contact Dermatitis

The most common type of CD, totaling approximately 80% of all CD cases,[5] is ICD. ICD represents a nonspecific, non-immunologic inflammatory response to an irritant or a chemical that is directly toxic to the skin. Wet work—immersing in detergents, water, or frequent hand washing during a pandemic[6]—predisposes an individual to these irritant-type reactions (see Chapter 11) because it weakens the skin barrier. ICD can also occur due to exposure to physiologically natural substances such as saliva (lip-licking), and urine or feces (as in diaper dermatitis). With prolonged contact, the natural acids and alkalis within the fluids directly break down the skin barrier and incite cutaneous inflammation. Physical irritation with friction and occlusion may also induce ICD. Cosmetic products were found to be the most common cause of ICD among 1066 patients.[7] An example of an inducible ICD is epidermal keratinocyte damage following a cosmetic peel (**Fig. 19-1**).

The severity of ICD is dependent on various factors including the duration, frequency and concentration of the irritant chemical on the exposed skin. Additionally, environmental factors such as humidity and temperature can mediate the severity.[8] Clinically, ICD may present with non-specific redness, burning, or stinging. Itching is not as common with ICD as it is with ACD and may be used as a diagnostic clue.[8]

Contact Urticaria

At the other end of the spectrum is CU, which accounts for approximately 0.5% of CD. This type of reaction may be immunologic or nonimmunologic. Immunologic CU is IgE-mediated and represents an immediate-type hypersensitivity response.[9] Clinically, CU manifests with classic wheals and flares (hives); in extreme cases the clinical symptoms may progress to severe respiratory compromise, anaphylaxis, and, in very rare cases, death. Immunologic CU is primarily seen in occupational settings, with a primary example being latex hypersensitivity in healthcare workers. Nonimmunologic CU is more common and much less severe. It is induced by a direct induction of vasoactive substances including prostaglandins, histamines, leukotrienes, and substance P.[10] Clinically, it presents within an hour of application of the product with tingling, stinging, and rarely hives. Cosmetic products which include fragrances and preservatives may be common culprits,[11] as well as glycolic acid peels.[12] As CU is among the less common forms of CD, further discussion is outside of the scope of this chapter, those interested may find supplementary information in the aforementioned references.

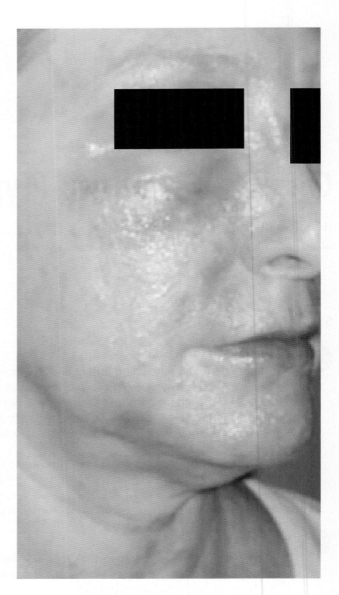

FIGURE 19-1. Glycolic acid is an irritant that can result in keratinolysis. In this figure, pink tender plaques occurred on the cheeks 1 day after a 30% glycolic acid peel.

Allergic Contact Dermatitis

ACD is the primary etiology behind CD related to PHP and cosmetics. The pathophysiology of ACD is remarkably different from the other types of CD. The key difference is that ACD is an immunologic reaction which implies cutaneous memory and the ability to be re-triggered. ACD is a consequence of lymphocyte activation via a T cell-mediated Type IV delayed-type hypersensitivity reaction. Cutaneous exposure to an allergen, which molecularly is just a protein antigen, elicits a clonal proliferation of T lymphocytes capable of recognizing and responding to the same antigen upon future exposure. These processes are deemed sensitization and elicitation, respectively.

Sensitization occurs through repeated exposure to an allergen, by which that exposure reaches beyond a certain physiologic threshold. This is vital to understand clinically as it is a common misconception that a product used for years without a reaction would not be the culprit. Sensitivity to the product can develop over many years. Certain allergens are stronger sensitizers than others and thus, are associated with more deleterious effects on consumers.[13] With each subsequent exposure to some antigen, the immune system is boosted and the ability of the immune system to remember that antigen for future interactions becomes more likely. As an example, albeit in a different pathophysiologic response, for the hepatitis B vaccine, three shots are required for establishing long-lasting and effective "immunity," or memory to this agent. Conversely, a tetanus vaccine may be "boosted" every 10 years to guarantee memory. Likewise, the more potent the allergen, the less boost-dose may be required in an exposure to trigger ACD, such as poison ivy and MI. In most cases of ACD, however, the boosts or exposures are mini-*doses* that, when taken sequentially over a given period of time, result in the individual being *sensitized* to that chemical.

DEVELOPMENT OF ALLERGIC CONTACT DERMATITIS

The chemicals likely to elicit an ACD are generally small lipophilic compounds to which an individual is routinely exposed. These chemicals usually have a molecular weight less than 500 Da, allowing them to penetrate the skin or mucous membranes and activate an immunologic cascade.[14,15] Subsequent to entry into the skin, these chemicals are taken up by antigen-presenting dendritic immunologic cells and further processed for presentation to naïve T lymphocytes. This process of chemical capture and presentation is known as the induction phase of sensitization.

Repeat exposures to allergenic chemicals stimulate clonal expansion of memory T cells, each inheriting the capability to mount an immune response. With each re-exposure, or challenge, the elicitation phase of sensitization is enhanced until the process becomes clinically apparent. This involves a complex interplay between immune cells (i.e. antigen-presenting cells, lymphocytes, and keratinocytes) and their respective cytokine repertoire. It is important to note that overcoming the energy of activation to trigger the initial sensitization process may take days to years, but once established subsequent re-exposure of the sensitized individual to the allergenic chemical will characteristically lead to the development of a rechallenge reaction within 48 to 120 hours.[15] This is important clinically, as patients may have used a product for years before becoming sensitized to an ingredient and may not be able to temporally associate an exposure with a delayed dermatitis presentation.

THE CLINICAL EXPRESSION OF ALLERGIC CONTACT DERMATITIS

Typically ACD occurs in the distribution of the contact with the instigating allergen, but unlike ICD (which is classically confined to the exposure site), ACD can extend beyond.

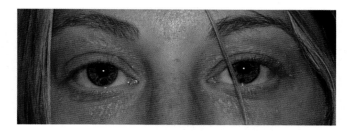

FIGURE 19-2. Contact dermatitis to fragrance presenting on eyelids.

Classic localizations for PHP and cosmetic contact allergy are the face, neck, hands, and axillae relating to the chemical agents used in the products for these areas, e.g., fragrances, preservatives, emulsifiers, and solvents (**Fig. 19-2**).[16] In addition, flavorants such as peppermint, cinnamon, and chamomile can cause ACD, most associated with reactions around the mouth, aka perioral dermatitis. In some cases, "consort" or "connubial" contact dermatitis occurs when the contact dermatitis is caused by contact with products used by partners, coworkers or co-sleeping companions (as in toddler-parent).

Differences in the moisture and frictional exposure of the skin, the potency of the allergen, and the duration of the contact may lead to variability in the expression of the dermatitis.[17] Furthermore, ACD has been classified into three main categories: subacute, acute, and chronic subtypes to notate the extent and/or duration of the presentation and the associated findings.[15] In subacute presentations, clinically the skin exhibits macular erythema and scaling. The acute presentation typically displays pruritic erythematous, edematous, and papulovesicular changes in the skin. When the dermatitis is chronic, however, the clinical presentation involves lichenification and fissuring and may not be distinguishable from other chronic dermatoses, such as atopic dermatitis.[18]

ACD reactions tend to follow the cutaneous distribution of where epidermal contact with the allergen occurred, as this is the site of heightened immunity. That said, it is also important to note that auto-eczematization can occur at distant sites and "recall reactions" can occur at sites of previous sensitization that are remotely activated when contact with the chemical is initiated at a new and potentially distant site. The confounding factors of delay and recall pose a unique challenge in the diagnosis of ACD.

As a case point example, a patient with known paraphenylenediamine (PPD) hair dye allergy developed severe face and scalp erythema, pain, itching and scaling a day after hyaluronic acid (HA) filler injection. She suspected that she had a reaction to the HA. Notably, the erythema followed the areas where HA was injected, including the nasolabial folds, lateral temples, chin and cheeks; however, there was also erythema along the frontal and vertex scalp, hairline, and posterior neck—areas where no cosmetic procedures occurred. On review of the case, the patient's target skin sites had been "prepared" with 70% ethyl alcohol and compounded tetracaine-benzocaine topical anesthetic applied for 1 hour prior to the procedure. The vital clinical pearl herein is that ester-based topical anesthetics and PPD are both para-aminobenzoic acid derivatives. Due to the recall-reaction phenomenon, although she was only exposed to the anesthetic on the face, other areas of her skin previously sensitized to PPD also reacted. Additionally, her dermatitis onset was quick, only after 1 day, due to the high memory recall power of her prior sensitization to a strong allergen.

DIAGNOSIS OF ALLERGIC CONTACT DERMATITIS

In order to elucidate the cause of ACD in most patients, a thorough history is crucial (as retrospectively this will be important in the determining the clinical relevance of source allergens). Having the patients bring in their routinely used skincare products, when known, is also often helpful. The epicutaneous patch test is the *gold standard* testing tool in the diagnosis of ACD.[19] Appropriate use of patch testing paired with education of the patient has been shown to improve patient's quality of life, and thus is recommended in patients with suspected ACD. It is also recommended in recalcitrant or worsening chronic dermatitis that has been present for 2 or more months, has failed to improve following standard treatment protocols, or requires systemic immunosuppressant medications.[20,21,23] Patch testing is often performed by dermatologists and allergists trained in the selection and application of allergens, as well as evaluation and analysis of the results.

Patch testing may be performed with a limited 35 allergen pre-made commercial test—Thin-layer Rapid Use Epicutaneous Test (T.R.U.E. Test™ by SmartPractice, Phoenix, AZ), or via unlimited customized panels of standardized reagents, aka comprehensive testing. Comprehensive testing allows for tailoring the selection of the allergens to include various fragrances, cosmetics, vehicles, and preservatives to test on the patient based on their personal exposure history and clinical distribution of the dermatitis. Additionally, clinicians may test the patient's own PHP and cosmetic products via repeat open application testing and closed or open chamber testing to provide a personalized definitive approach.

In comprehensive testing, suspect chemical substances are, per standard procedure, hand-loaded into chambers and placed in contact with the clinically unaffected epidermis of the back and/or inner arm for 48 hours (**Figs. 19-3 and 19-4**). These patches are then removed, marked, and evaluated after the initial 48-hour application period. The patch sites are assessed at both 48 hours and at a delayed reading between 72 and 120 hours post application. Compared to ICD reactions which peak within 24 h (and improve by 72–96 h), contact hypersensitivity reactions typically evolve over the testing period and worsen by the delayed reading. In addition, ICD reactions tend to clinically appear as patches of erythema, rather than induration and eczematization.[19] Reactions are graded per the International Contact Dermatitis Research Group (ICDRG) protocol from 0 to 3+ and irritant.[22]

The sodium lauryl sulfate (SLS) test has been historically used as a positive control for irritancy reactions, in conjunction with the epicutaneous allergen patch test, especially in the sensitive skin patient, as it may help the reader to differentiate

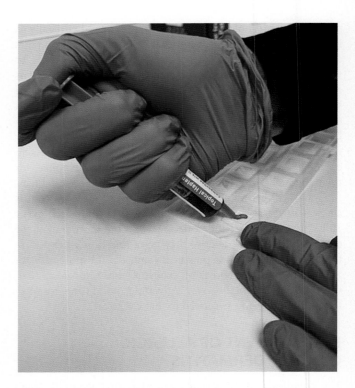

FIGURE 19-3. Comprehensive chamber preparation — standard tray and some cosmetic vehicles

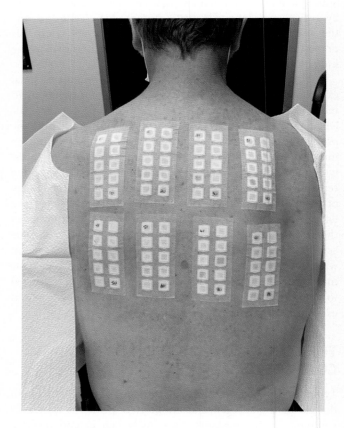

FIGURE 19-4. Application of the patch to the patient.

between allergic and irritant reactions.[23] A reaction in the SLS application patch during patch testing indicates that macular erythema in the patch test sample on that patient more likely reflects an irritant etiology. Conversely, if the SLS test fails to demonstrate a reaction upon patch testing, it is more likely that macular erythematous reactions may be allergic in nature. While the SLS testing may be useful, it is important to note that clinical correlation of the presentation and exposure history are crucial for the correct diagnosis of allergic versus irritant contact dermatitis.

TREATMENT

The first step in the treatment of any contact dermatitis is to identify the offending agent, whether an allergen or a caustic irritating chemical. Once identification has been made, the subsequent step is **avoidance** of the culprit agent and, in the case of ACD, cross-reacting substances. Alternative product substitution is imperative for the well-being of the patient. Furthermore, measures should be taken to ensure barrier integrity (e.g., decreased hand washing with soaps and increased emollient use) for both allergic- and irritant-based dermatiditis. The use of emollients to help heal the skin is important, especially with regard to reactions that are irritant in nature (see Chapter 31).

In the interim, while the avoidance regimen is being instituted and the immune system is being given a chance to "forget" (reduce the memory) the sensitization, symptomatic treatment may be needed. Topical corticosteroids and/or topical immunomodulators and at times, in severe acute or chronic extensive involvement, the use of systemic agents such as prednisone, cyclosporine, mycophenolate, methotrexate, or ultraviolet light treatments may be indicated.[24] Recently, dupilumab, a monoclonal antibody that binds to the interleukin-4 receptor and inhibits the IL-4 and IL-13 pathways, has been reported to improve clinical ACD to weak allergens eliciting Th2 axis reactions and may emerge as a future first-line treatment.[25,26]

COSMETIC IMPLICATIONS OF CONTACT DERMATITIS

As defined by the US Food and Drug Administration (FDA), a cosmetic product is "an article intended to be rubbed, poured, sprinkled, sprayed on, introduced to the skin, or otherwise applied to the human body for cleansing, beautifying, promoting attractiveness, or altering the appearance (excluding soap)".[27] Under the Federal Food Drug and Cosmetic Act, cosmetic products and ingredients, with the exception of color additives, do not require FDA approval before they go on the market. Thus, legally, the potential risk of CD from cosmetic ingredients is not a determinant of their inclusion.

However, clinically, cosmetic products may pose potential for morbidity due to the sensitizing properties of their ingredients. Cosmetic products including eye and facial makeup, moisturizers, and hair products have been continuously reported as the most common sources of ACD.[28,29] In a review of over 30 000 ACD patients in seven pooled studies, 9.8% of positive reactions were due to cosmetic allergens.[30]

Almost any ingredient in topical products, *sin* water and purified petrolatum, has the potential to cause an allergy or a skin reaction in some person, at some point. The majority of the culprits are the added preservatives, vehicles, and fragrances.[11] Products with expiration dates have preservatives to fend off microbial activity and decomposition. Cosmetic clinicians and manufacturers must possess the knowledge of which chemicals pose the highest risk for CD and instruct, guide and develop products which confer the highest safety measures to protect consumers.

In the following sections we will provide the core information on the top allergens within the cosmetic industry with the goals of educating clinicians and manufacturers, improving the quality of cosmetic products, and protecting our patients and our families from potentially debilitating skin reactions of CD.

TOP SENSITIZERS IN COSMETIC PRODUCTS

A full discussion of the wide range of sensitizing chemicals found in cosmetic-based products is beyond the scope of this chapter, however a list of the most common allergens is found in **Table 19-1**. Three categories deserve special attention, however, with regard to cosmetic-based contact allergies, most notably fragrances, preservatives and vehicle ingredients.

Fragrances (Table 19-2)

Since the first report of allergy to fragrance-based chemicals in 1957, fragrances have continued to remain on the top 10 allergen list for contact sensitization.[31,32] In fact, fragrances are the third most common allergen family identified to cause ACD, and notably the most frequent cause of contact allergy to cosmetics.[7] Specifically, cosmetics account for 30% to 45% of these allergic contact reactions, while perfumes and deodorants/antiperspirants account for 4% to 18% and 5% to 17% of cases, respectively.[16] It has been estimated that an "average" woman will use approximately 12 personal care products each day, with over 160 ingredients, and an "average" man will use six products with 85 ingredients.[33] Thus, most likely due to these exposure habits, fragrance allergy tends to occur more frequently in women, with a female to male ratio of 3.5:1.[34,35] Data from the North American Contact Dermatitis Group (NACDG) obtained from 10 983 positive allergic reactions between 2015–2016 showed the most recent estimates of prevalence of fragrance allergy to be 11.3%.[7] If one was to extrapolate this prevalence rate to the current US population, it would equate to over 37 million affected individuals.

Fragrances are well known to be significant allergens. There is a wide range of potential exposure to them from PHP and cosmetic preparations (e.g., perfumes and colognes, to skin and hair products, deodorants, laundry products, and cleansing products) as their presence is almost ubiquitous within the developed and developing worlds.[16,34] This is why fragrance allergy is emerging as a significant problem among pediatric patients as well.[36] Detection of fragrance allergy may be quite

		POSITIVE REACTIONS (%)	POTENTIAL COSMETIC IMPLICATIONS
ORDER	**SUBSTANCE**		
1	Nickel sulfate (2.5%)	17.5	Metal: eyelash curlers, razors, tweezers, mineral makeup
2/5	Methylisothizolinone/Methylchloroisothiozolinone+Methylisothizolinone	13.4/7.3	Makeup, shampoos, soaps, wipes
3	Fragrance mix (8%) (α-amyl cinnamic aldehyde, cinnamic alcohol, cinnamic aldehyde, eugenol, geraniol, hydroxycitronellal, isoeugenol, oak moss absolute)	11.3	Fragrance & Flavorant
4/9	Formaldehyde (2% aqs)/(1%aqs)	8.4/6.4	Preservative—cleansers, cosmetics
6	Balsam of Peru (25%)	7	Fragrance & Flavorant—perfume, cosmetics, lotions, makeup removers
7	Neomycin (20%)	11.6	Antibiotic
8	Bacitracin (20%)	7.9	Antibiotic—Obagi Nuderm step 7
10	4-Phenylenediamine	6.4	Hair dyes, temporary tattoos

TABLE 19-1 Cosmetically Implicated Top Allergens 2015–2016

Adapted from DeKoven JG, Warshaw EM, Zug KA, et al. North American Contact Dermatitis Group Patch Test Results: 2015–2016. *Dermatitis: contact, atopic, occupational, drug.* 2018;29(6):297–309.

complex. More than 5000 fragrance materials and chemicals are available for use, many of which have several known different names.[37,38] Ascertaining which fragrances are actually used in a given cosmetic product is sometimes almost impossible. Many of the specific fragrance ingredients are protected by the Fair Packaging and Labeling Act as they are considered trade secrets.[39] If the ingredients are listed, they are often non-specific such as simply "fragrance" without any further specification. An average of 30 to 50 (and upward of 200) chemicals may be used to create a perfume's fragrance composition![40]

Increasing rates of sensitization prompted calls for fragrance identification measures to be established. In 1977, Larsen proposed a mixture of eight ingredients (isoeugenol, eugenol, cinnamic aldehyde, cinnamic alcohol [also called cassia oil], geraniol [base substance of the essential oils: geranium, rose, jasmine, lavender, and citronella], oak moss absolute [tree lichen], hydroxycitronellal [synthetic], and a-amyl cinnamic aldehyde [synthetic]) as a screening tool for fragrance contact allergy.[15,41] This component mix, aka Fragrance Mix 1, is currently used in both the commercially available FDA-approved T.R.U.E. Test™ (SmartPractice, Phoenix, AZ) screening panel and in comprehensive testing to screen for fragrance allergy. Notably, Fragrance Mix I in conjunction with balsam of Peru were thought to detect approximately 90% of fragrance allergies.[42] However, it has become common to patch test to an array of supplemental fragrance allergens suggesting that the original combination of Fragrance Mix I and balsam of Peru is not sufficient alone. Studies show that a combination of Fragrance Mix 1, balsam of Peru and two additional allergen combinations (Fragrance Mix II and cinnamic aldehyde) only identified 73.2% of the patients with fragrance-induced eyelid dermatitis.[43] **Table 19-2** provides a compilation of estimated sensitization rates from several fragrance sources. Of note,

patients may be allergic to more than one fragrance, and several cross-react.

It is also important to note that the top four sensitizers of the eight ingredients in Fragrance Mix 1 are also natural cross-sensitizers/components of balsam of Peru or *Myroxylon pereirae.*[15] Balsam of Peru is a dark brown, complex viscid fluid harvested from the mature *Myroxylon balsamum* tree primarily found in El Salvador. The balsam contains the volatile oil cinnamein, a combination of cinnamic acid, benzoyl cinnamate, benzoyl benzoate, benzoic acid, vanillin, and nerodilol, all of which have wide utility in the pharmaceutical, cosmetic, and flavoring industries.[44] In 2005, cinnamic alcohol was found to naturally occur in both tomatoes and balsam of Peru, providing proof to support the common claim that tomatoes were a trigger in patients with a known allergy to balsam of Peru.[45]

Because it confers mild bactericidal and capillary-bed stimulant effects, balsam of Peru is widely used in topical medicines for wounds, burns, hemorrhoids, and diaper salves. Furthermore, balsam of Peru components, such as benzyl alcohol, are used widely in cosmetics (i.e., BOTOX™-reconstituted) for their mild anesthetic and preservative properties (no fragrance indications). Although there are no reported cases of delayed-type allergic reactions to Botox during neurologic or dermatologic procedures,[46] this risk would be one to consider discussing in a patient with significant fragrance allergies. Likewise it could be included in any consent form prior to the cosmetic procedure.[47]

Medical providers should be cognizant of the use of these covert fragrance chemicals. The FDA Code of Federal Regulations, Title 21, Volume 7, Section 700.3 (d), states that the term "fragrance" applies to any natural or synthetic substance or substances used solely to impart an odor to a cosmetic

TABLE 19-2	Fragrance-Based Allergens	
ALLERGEN MIX	ALLERGEN	ESTIMATED SENSITIZATION %
Balsam of Peru[a,d]		7
Fragrance Mix 1[b,d]		11.3
Fragrance Mix 2[c,d]		5.3
	Cinnamic alcohol[a,b]	0.6
	Eugenol[a,b]	1
	Cinnamic aldehyde[a,b]	1
	Isoeugenol[a,b]	1.1
	Geraniol[b]	2.8[3]
	Lyral[c]	2.7[57]–0.4[56]
	Ylang-ylang[d]	1.3
	Hydroxycitronellal[b]	1.3
	Oak moss absolute[b]	2
	Benzyl Alcohol[a,d]	0.3
	Narcissus	1.3[55]
	Jasmine	1.2[55]–0.4[56]
	Citral[c]	0.6
	Sandalwood	0.9[55]
	Farnesol[c]	0.9
	Citronellol[c]	0.5
	Tea tree[d]	1.2
	a-Hexyl-cinnamic aldehyde[c,d]	0.1
	Coumarin[c]	0.4
	α-amyl cinnamic aldehyde[b]	0.1

[a]Indicates component/cross-sensitization with balsam of Peru.
[b]Indicates component of Fragrance Mix 1.
[c]Indicates component of Fragrance Mix 2.
[d]Current inclusion on 2007 NACDG screening panel.
DeKoven JG, Warshaw EM, Zug KA, et al. North American Contact Dermatitis Group Patch Test Results: 2015–2016. *Dermatitis: contact, atopic, occupational, drug.* 2018;29(6):297–309.]
Frosch PJ, Johansen JD, Menne T, et al. Further important sensitizers in patients sensitive to fragrances. *Contact Dermatitis.* 2002;47(5):279
Schnuch, A., Uter, W., Geier, J., Lessmann, H. and Frosch, P.J. (2007), Sensitization to 26 fragrances to be labelled according to current European regulation. *Contact Dermatitis.* 57: 1–10. doi:10.1111/j.1600-0536.2007.01088.x

product.[48] By this definition, a product can be labeled as "fragrance-free" if fragrance-based ingredients are added to serve a purpose other than affecting the odor of a product, such as for preservation.[49]

Consumers and providers alike should be aware that packaging monikers of "fragrance-free" and "unscented" are often not evidence based. In general, "fragrance-free" refers to the absence of aroma-enhancing chemicals, whereas unscented means 'the absence of detectable aroma' and could mean that

a fragrance-masking chemical has been added. However, neither label confirms that fragrances will be truly excluded from the ingredient list, as they can be included still as preservatives. "Hypoallergenic" labels are additional unregulated marketing tools with minimal to no substantiation which confuse consumers as the products commonly include highly allergenic ingredients.[50]

As a clinical example, a patient exquisitely sensitized to balsam of Peru may turn to easily recognizable "fragrance-free" products as alternatives due to their front package labeling. Unbeknownst to the patient, these products could contain, for example, the fragrance benzyl alcohol, which cross-reacts with balsam of Peru, and which has a secondary preservative function allowing it to be used in products with "fragrance-free" labeling. In this example, the patient using a benzyl alcohol-containing "fragrance-free" product could end up with severe widespread dermatitis in areas where they applied the "fragrance-free" product, as well as recall-type dermatitis in the distributions of prior fragrance sensitivity responses. Thus, knowledge of the clinical capacity for ACD among various fragrances and their cross-reactors is vital for cosmetic patient counseling and education.

Lastly, essential oils must be mentioned as their use among patients has skyrocketed due to the erroneous belief of their "natural" composition. It must be emphasized that there is nothing "essential" in essential oils and the connotation of their purity and safety is a major social misconception.[51] Essential oils are composed of processed hydrophobic volatile compounds from raw plant material with various stabilizing additives and solvents, including methanol, which is a toxic pesticide.[52] Over 80 essential oils have been reported to induce ACD, while certain essential oils when ingested can be potentially lethal.[51] Tea tree oil, specifically, makes up the majority of the reported ACD reactions to essential oils.[53] Thus, as medical providers we must continue to educate and protect our patients from misinformation and potentially harmful cosmetic products.

Preservatives (Tables 19-3 and 19-4)
FORMALDEHYDE AND FORMALDEHYDE-RELEASING PRESERVATIVES

Formaldehyde and formaldehyde-releasing preservatives are in the top five of the most common sources of cosmetic-associated contact dermatitis.[54] Of 5597 patients patch tested between 2015–2016, the reported sensitization rate to formaldehyde was 8.4%.[7] Formaldehyde itself is rarely used in modern cosmetics due to its infamous publicity in relation to its potential carcinogenic events.[55] However, as it is a powerful preservative, manufacturing companies have switched to the use of other ingredients in which formaldehyde is a byproduct after degradation—termed, formaldehyde-releasing preservative (FRPs).[56] Examples of FRPs are listed in **Table 19-4**. It is important to note, however, that the FRPs are the most sensitizing of the preservative class. Cases of contact dermatitis to formaldehyde/FRPs commonly present as eyelid dermatitis,

TABLE 19-3	Preservatives Found in Cosmetic Products with Estimated Sensitization Rates (%)
Thimerosal (merthiolate)	10.2
Quaternium 15 (Dowicil®) (FRP)	3.6
Bronopol (Bronopol®) (FRP)	1.3
DiadUrea (Germall 11®) (FRP)	1.2
Imidurea (Germall 115) (FRP)	1.1
DMDM Hydantoin (Glydant®) (FRP)	0.8
Methyldibromo glutaronitrile and phenoxyethanol (Euxyl K 400)	3.5
Methylisothiazolinone/ Methylchloroisothiazolinone and Methylisothiazolinone (Euxyl K100)	13.4/7.3
Benzyl alcohol	=
Parabens	0.6
Iodopropynyl butyl carbamate	3.9

DeKoven JG, Warshaw EM, Zug KA, et al. North American Contact Dermatitis Group Patch Test Results: 2015–2016. *Dermatitis: contact, atopic, occupational, drug.* 2018;29(6):297–309.]

TABLE 19-4	Preservatives That Can Cause Contact Dermatitis
Benzoic acid	
Benzyl alcohol	
Euxyl K 400 (Methyldibromo glutaronitrile and phenoxyethanol)	
Formaldehyde	
Formaldehyde-releasing-preservatives	
(FRPs):	
Quaternium 15	
Imidazolidinyl urea (Germall)	
Diazolidinyl urea (Germall II)	
Bromonitropropane diol (Bronopol)	
DMDM hydantoin	
Methylchloroisothiazolinone and Methylisothiozolinone (MCI/MI)	
P-tert-Butylphenol formaldehyde resin	
Parabens	
Propylene glycol	
Sodium benzoate	
Toluenesulphonamide Formaldehyde	
Resin (tosylamide)	

which is often associated with the use of nail hardeners/lacquers/cosmetics that contain formaldehydes. Several mascaras, blushes, eye shadows, foundations, and shampoos also contain the FRPs that can contribute to the development of eyelid and facial dermatitis in the areas of sensitization. Other important potential sources of exposure to formaldehyde-based chemicals and FRPs include permanent press clothing, cleaning agents, baby wipes, disinfectants, cigarette smoke, and the sweetener aspartame.[57] Moreover, with the widespread use of personal protective equipment including surgical and N-95 masks during the COVID-19 pandemic, the incidence of ACD secondary to head and face coverings and gowns containing formaldehyde rose.[58,59]

METHYLCHLOROISOTHIAZOLINONE AND METHYLISOTHIAZOLINONE (EUXYL K100)

In 1977, methylchloroisothiazolinone (MCI, 5-chloro-2-methyl-4-isothiazolin-3-one) and methylisothiazolinone (MI, 2-methyl-4-isothiazolin-3-one) were first registered in the United States as Kathon CG and Euxyl K100 ((Dow Chemical, Midland, MI).[60] These two chemical preservatives were combined in a ratio of 3:1 (MCI:MI) and were extensively added to bubble bath preparations, cosmetics, and soaps.[61,62] Because of their chemical nature of having polarity (being lipophilic at one end and lipophobic at the other), MCI and MI are compatible with a large number of surfactants and emulsifiers. Furthermore, the isothiazolinones are biocidal, as they interact and oxidize accessible cellular thiols on microbials.[63] This versatility, and its ability to replace formaldehyde-releasing preservatives, solidified its uses in millions of personal care products.

With the widespread use of the MCI/MI mixture, an epidemic of ACD began to emerge in the 1980s with sensitization rates of 5%.[64] The Cosmetic Ingredient Review panel made recommendations to lower the maximum level of MCI/MI to 15 ppm (from 300 ppm) in rinse-off products and 7.5 ppm in leave-on products.[15] In addition, MI, which was thought to be a less potent sensitizer than MCI, was approved as a sole preservative. However, MI is a less effective biocide than MCI, and thus, higher concentrations were used to achieve efficacy.[65,66] Not surprisingly in hindsight, repeat reports of rising MI sensitization rates began to be reported soon after.[65,67,68] MI was named the 2013 Contact Allergen of the Year by the American Contact Dermatitis Society and its rates of sensitization have continued to increase every year since.[60]

The latest North American Contact Dermatitis Group (NACDG) report of over 10 000 patch test results showed a sensitization rate of 13.4%, second only to nickel.[7] Moreover, MI ranked first in the NACDG SPIN calculations, which reflect the current clinical relevance of an allergen, with a highest ever recorded value, over 50% higher than the second highest allergen.[7]

Thus, cosmetic providers and manufacturers must be aware of the heightened potential of sensitization and high risk of ACD from MCI and MI preservatives. Of note, there may be a potential for MCI or MI to cross-react with metronidazole, as the chemicals have similar molecular structures.[69] Thus, the provider may need to be aware of this when prescribing formulations for rosacea, such as Noritate™ (Bausch Health US, LLC, Bridgewater, NJ USA) and Metrogel™ (GALDERMA HOLDING S.A.) in an MCI- or MI-allergic patient.

BENZOPHENONES

Benzophenones are chemical absorbers of ultraviolet (UV) light. Their increased use in cosmetics and sunscreens led to them being named the ACDS 2014 Allergen of the Year.[70] They were initially designed to be used in paints and plastics to protect them from UV degradation, but in the 1950s they were Introduced as sunscreens. In addition to cosmetic products, benzophenones may be found in moisturizers, and hair and nail products.

Benzophenone-3 is also known as oxybenzone and is the most common UV filter to cause ACD.[71] However, benzophenones have been documented to cause various other adverse reactions including photocontact dermatitis, CU, and anaphylaxis.[70,72] Additionally, studies evaluating the safety of benzophenones have reported systemic absorption of oxybenzone within breast milk, amniotic fluid, urine and blood.[73–75] Thus, clinicians should be aware of the potential cutaneous systemic adverse effects of benzophenones.

PARABENS

The **para**-hydroxy**ben**zoic acids (parabens) are a family of five alkyl esters that differ in para-position chemical composition substitutions on the benzene ring (methyl paraben, ethyl paraben, propyl paraben, butyl paraben, and benzyl paraben). These chemical substitutions impart on each paraben ester a different solubility and antimicrobial activity spectrum. Frequently, manufacturers take advantage of this and use the parabens in conjunction with each other to enhance antimicrobial efficacy.[33] Moreover, parabens are odorless, tasteless, pH neutral and do not discolor or harden over time, making them ideal preservatives in topical, industrial, and dietary products.[76] In fact, parabens are ubiquitous in our products and our environment.[76,77] It is estimated that an average American is exposed to about 76 mg/day of paraben, with cosmetics accounting for two thirds of this exposure.[78]

The FDA considers parabens to be generally regarded as safe, and are used in cosmetics at a concentration of up to 0.4% and in mixtures of parabens of up to 0.8%.[79,80]

The utilization of parabens in cosmetic products has been extensively studied. Of 4000 German products, 39% contained at least one paraben,[81] and 99% of leave-on products and 77% of rinse-off products tested in a European study were found to have at least one paraben.[82] The ACDS evaluated over 5400 cosmetic products and found a range of 66–87% prevalence of parabens in cosmetics, 30% of shampoos, 77–82% of lip products, 30% of sunscreens, and 23% of skin wipes.[83] However, despite their remarkable prevalence, paraben sensitization and ACD rates have remained low, underlined by its naming as the 2019 "Non-Allergen of the Year" by the ACDS.[76]

The overall estimated sensitization and allergy rate among numerous paraben ACD reviews is 1%.[76] Fransway et al. reviewed literature from the NACDG from 1992 to 2016 and calculated the mean positivity rate of parabens in over 55 000 patients to be 1.1%, equivalent to only 618 patients.[76]

Cosmetic products specifically have been reviewed for paraben sensitization extensively, and the overall data suggests that parabens are weak sensitizers and very rarely cause ACD despite their frequent use.[84] Fransway et al. calculated that in a total of 14 studies evaluating cosmetics, involving 21 132 patients, only 508 patients or 2.3% were found to be allergic to parabens.[76]

The parabens, when absorbed through the skin, are partially metabolized by carboxyl esterases in the skin, liver, and kidney.[85] It has been demonstrated that a portion of parabens may be retained in human body tissues without hydrolysis by tissue esterases, which has raised concern over the potential for adverse side effects.[86] Special regard has been given to the estrogen-like effects, which were first described by Routledge et al. in 1998 and have been further substantiated by several studies.[87–89]

Since estrogen is a major etiologic factor in the development of human breast tissue and breast cancers, Darbre et al. proposed that parabens and other chemicals that are used in underarm cosmetics may have contributed to what was then, in 2003, the increasing incidence of breast cancer.[90] In an uncontrolled study of 20 patients with breast tumors, parabens were found in 90% of the breast tumor samples; however, it has been suggested that there may have been "contamination" of the glassware that the samples were processed in from the detergents used by the technicians.[87,91]

The close proximity of the axilla and the breast has further fueled queries as to the possibility of an association of parabens with breast cancer.[92] This led the Cosmetic Ingredient Review board to reevaluate the safety of parabens in 2005, 2016, and 2019.[93] The panel determined that the original conclusion on the safety of parabens in cosmetics withstood, and that there was "no significant association of parabens exposure with diseases or other adverse health conditions." They also determined that "cosmetic product use is a major source of parabens exposure." However, the vast quantity of biomonitoring data indicates that "systemic exposure to these ingredients is very low to have much less estrogenic activity than the body's naturally-occurring estrogen."[93] An extensive review of the literature was undertaken by Fransway et al. in 2018 to summarize parabens' overall safety despite their extreme frequency in our environment.[76] Overall, multiple peer-reviewed extensive epidemiologic studies conclude that there is no direct link between underarm products and breast cancer, and parabens have 100,000-fold less estrogen effects than naturally occurring hormones.[93–96] Moreover, spurious reports of assumed paraben risk has led the cosmetic industry to specifically exclude parabens with eye-catching "paraben-free" labeling. This does not incur true product safety as instead of the tried and tested low-sensitizing parabens, manufacturers have turned to other preservatives such as isothizolinones, which are extremely strong sensitizers, driving new ACD epidemics.[97]

Thus, cosmetic practitioners should be aware of the controversial nature of parabens, media misinformation, and the scientific data behind parabens in order to provide the highest level of guidance and education to their patients.

Vehicles and surfactants
PROPYLENE GLYCOL

Propylene glycol is an emollient and emulsifier (solvent) used for its odorless quality, and stability in various settings including water oils and acetone. It is used in various cosmetic products, but most noteworthy is its extensive use in prescription and over-the-counter topical medicines due to its ability to enhance product penetration.[94] Of 746 analyzed topical corticosteroids in 2020, 56.6% contained propylene glycol.[98] ACD to propylene glycol has been reported since the 1950s.[99] Estimates of current sensitization are estimated to be as high as 3.5%.[100] Propylene glycol was deemed the 2018 Allergen of the Year by the ACDS due to its increased use.[101] As various "anti-itch" and soothing medicines are often prescribed in concordance with various cosmetic treatments (such as topical steroids post chemical peels), cosmetic clinicians should be aware of the role propylene glycol may play in sensitization and both irritant and allergic CD.

GLUCOSIDES

Alkyl gluocosides are surfactants (SURFace ACTive AgeNTS), which, as a category, are molecules which permit oil and water to mix, allow for foaming (lathering) of water by reducing the surface tension between air and water, and are most often used for cleaning.[102] The most common glucosides used are decyl and lauryl glucoside; they are frequently found in shampoos, disinfectants, lotions, creams, sunscreens and cosmetics. The Cosmetic Ingredient Review Expert Panel has deemed glucosides safe for use.[103] The rates of ACD have been around 2% over the last decade.[7] As glucosides are considered weak sensitizers, their use in cosmetic products has increased. This has led to their designation as the 2017 Allergen of the Year by the ACDS to prompt awareness of their risk to certain populations, specifically patients with eczema.[104] Studies show that 86% of the patients sensitized to decyl- or lauryl-glucoside have a history of atopy.[104] Thus, as glucosides continue to be used in various products, especially those deemed for "sensitive skin," we may see an emergence of new sensitizations, especially among individuals with an impaired skin barrier, such as those with eczema.

OTHER ALLERGENS IN SKIN, HAIR, AND NAIL CARE PRODUCTS (Table 19-5)

Skin reactions have been described (see **Table 19-6**) with hair care products as well as hair processing and coloring chemicals. Natural botanicals (see **Table 19-7**), which are major fragrance additives, have also been reported to cause skin allergy. Toluene sulfonamide formaldehyde (see **Table 19-8**) resin in nail polish is such a common cause of contact dermatitis that companies such as Sally Hansen™ (Coty Inc, New York, NY) and Revlon™ (The Estée Lauder Companies Inc, New York, NY) have developed "formaldehyde- and toluene-free" nail polish. In fact, in some countries such as Switzerland, "formaldehyde resins" are banned in nail care products. Nevertheless, contact dermatitis from nail products often affects other areas, most commonly the eyelids and the face. Acrylic nails, gel nails nail wraps and shellac

TABLE 19-5	Other Sensitizers Found in Skin Products
2,6-Ditert-butyl-4-cresol (BHT)	
2-tert-Butyl-4-methoxyphenol (BHA)	
4-Chloro-3-cresol (PCMC)	
Benzyl alcohol	
Benzyl salicylate	
Cetyl alcohol	
Chloracetamide	
Chlorhexidine digluconate	
Isopropyl myristate	
Lanolin alcohol	
Propyl gallate	
Sorbic acid	
Sorbitan monooleate (Span 80)	
Sorbitan sesquioleate	
Stearyl alcohol	
tert-Butylhydroquinone	
Triclosan (Irgasan DP 300)	
Triethanolamine	
Benzoyl peroxide	
Cocamide DEA	
Cocamidopropyl Betaine	
Di-alpha-tocopherol acetate (vitamin E)	
Methyl methacrylate	
Potassium dichromate	

polish have become more common in the last decade. They contain many different types of acrylates which, before they harden, can drive ACD. Although preformed plastic nails do not cause ACD, the adhesive they come with to apply to the nail plate often contains cyanoacrylate which can be an allergen.[105,106]

A LOOK TO THE FUTURE

ACD to PHP and cosmetics is common. The face, neck, and hands are the most likely affected cutaneous surfaces. The list of potential allergenic chemicals is extensive, but fragrances and preservatives continue to be the most common culprits. Patch testing is the gold standard diagnostic method to diagnose ACD, and subsequent allergen avoidance is the principal treatment. As older, or controversial preservatives are phased out of cosmetics and replaced with newer chemicals, longitudinal monitoring for new sensitization epidemics is vital to protect our patients.

Consumers (through perception, advocacy and litigation) also play a vital role in manufacturing changes. Through direct consumer feedback on the open digital platform of social media, consumers' voices have begun to rise seeking greater safety and transparency of their cosmetic ingredients and environmentally responsible manufacturing practices. It is the role of clinical and academic clinicians to continue to educate

TABLE 19-6	Botanicals That Can Cause Allergy in Skin and Hair Care Products
Aloe vera	
Angelica	
Arnica	
Balsam of Peru (*Myroxylon pereirae*)	
Beeswax	
Bladderwrack	
Catnip	
Chamomile	
Colophony (rosin)	
Compositae Mix	
Coriander	
Cucumber	
Dog rose hips	
Echinacea	
Ginkgo	
Goldenseal	
Gotu kola (*Centella asiatica*)	
Green tea	
Hops	
Kelp	
Lavender	
Licorice	
Marigold	
Propolis (bee's glue)	
Rosemary	
Sage	
Sesquiterpene lactone	
St. John's wort	
Tea tree oil	
Witch hazel	
Ylang-ylang oil	

TABLE 19-7	Products in Hair Coloring and Processing and Nail Products That Can Cause Skin Sensitization	
Hair	2,5 Diaminotoluene sulfate	
	2-Nitro-P-phenylenediamine	
	3-Aminophenol	
	4-Aminophenol	
	Ammonium persulfate	
	Ammonium thioglycolate	
	Glyceryl thioglycolate	
	Hydrogen peroxide	
	Hydroquinone	
	Paraphenylenediamine (PPD)[+]	
	Resorcinol	
Nails	Ethyl acrylate 0.1% pet	
	Ethyl cyanoacrylate 10% pet	
	2-Hydroxy-4-methoxybenzo-phenone-5-sulfonic acid	
	Hydroxymethyl methacrylate 2% pet	
	Methyl methacrylate 2% pet	
	Tosylamide formaldehyde resin 10% pet	

TABLE 19-8	Sunscreen Ingredients That Can Cause Sensitization
2-Ethylhexyl-4-dimethylaminobenzoate (Eusolex 6007) (Padimate O) (Octyl Dimethyl paba)	
2-Ethylhexyl-4-methoxycinnamate (Parsol MCX)	
2-Hydroxy-4-methoxy-4-methylbenzophenone (Mexenone)	
2-Hydroxy-4-methoxy-benzophenon-5-sulfonic acid (Suliso-benzone)	
2-Hydroxy-4-methoxybenzophenone (Eusolex 4360)	
3-(4-Methylbenzyliden)camphor (Eusolex 6300)	
4-Aminobenzoic acid (PABA)	
4-tert-Butyl-4′-methoxydibenzoylmethane (Parsol 1789) (Avobenzone)	
Benzophenone-3 (oxybenzone)	
Homomenthylsalicylate (Homosalate)	
Isoamyl-p-methoxycinnamate	
Octyl salicylate (Octisalate)	
Phenylbenzimidazol-5-sulfonic acid (Eusolex 232)	

patients and industry manufacturers on the potential risks of various ingredients in developing ACD, and the potential safety of their alternatives.

The COVID-19 pandemic of 2019–2022, has left a mark on the cosmetic industry. Social distancing and quarantine restrictions discouraged people from seeking not only cosmetic treatments, but also medical care—often delaying vital evaluation of serious medical conditions, including ACD. Consumers were more inclined to perform self "at-home" cosmetic peels, masks and other treatments, often using unregulated, imported and unlabeled cosmetics which pose high risks of CD.[106] Moreover, government mandates of wearing a mask in public settings created a new physical facial irritant which increased humidity and skin barrier breakdown in the perioral area, and led to increased cases of ICD and ACD.

As the cosmetic industry reels back over the next few years, it remains to be seen if the focus will re-adjust to a more scientifically driven basis for ingredient selection, with, in addition to evaluation of systemic toxicity, an inclusion of CD risk consideration.

References

1. Peiser M, Tralau T, Heidler J. et al. Allergic contact dermatitis: epidemiology, molecular mechanisms, in vitro methods and regulatory aspects. *Cell Mol Life Sci.* 212:763–781.

2. Lim HW, Collins SAB, Resneck JSJr., et al. The burden of skin disease in the United States. *J Am Acad Dermatol.* 2017;76(5):958–972.e952.

3. Ramirez F, Chren M-M, Botto N. A review of the impact of patch testing on quality of life in allergic contact dermatitis. *J Am Acad Dermatol.* 2017;76(5):1000–1004.

4. Bickers DR, Lim HW, Margolis D, et al. The burden of skin diseases: 2004 a joint project of the American Academy of Dermatology Association and the Society for Investigative Dermatology. *J Am Acad Dermatol.* 2006;55(3):490–500.

5. Jakasa I, Thyssen JP, Kezic S. The role of skin barrier in occupational contact dermatitis. *Exp Dermatol.* 2018;27(8):909–914.

6. Rundle CW, Presley CL, Militello M, et al. Hand hygiene during COVID-19: Recommendations from the American Contact Dermatitis Society. *J Am Acad Dermatol.* 2020.

7. DeKoven JG, Warshaw EM, Zug KA, et al. North American Contact Dermatitis Group Patch Test Results: 2015–2016. *Dermatitis: contact, atopic, occupational, drug.* 2018;29(6):297–309.

8. Rietschel RL. Clues to an accurate diagnosis of contact dermatitis. *Dermatol Ther.* 2004;17(3):224–230.

9. Kligman AM. The spectrum of contact urticaria. Wheals, erythema, and pruritus. *Dermatolo Clin.* 1990;8(1):57–60.

10. Lahti A. Non-immunologic contact urticaria. *Acta dermatovenereologica. Supplementum.* 1980;Suppl 91:1–49.

11. Emmons WW, Marks JG.Jr. Immediate and delayed reactions to cosmetic ingredients. *Contact Dermatitis.* 1985;13(4):258–265.

12. Vishal B, Rao SS, Pavithra S, Shenoy MM. Contact urticaria to glycolic acid peel. *J Cutan Aesthet Surg.* 2012;5(1):58–59.

13. Basketter DA, Gerberick GF, Kimber I. Measurement of allergenic potency using the local lymph node assay. *Trends Pharmacol Sci.* 2001;22(6):264–265.

14. Jacob SE, Amado A, Cohen DE. Dermatologic surgical implications of allergic contact dermatitis. *Dermatol Surg.* 2005;31(9):1116–1123.

15. Rietschel RFJ. Fisher's Contact Dermatitis. 6th ed. Hamilton, ON: BC Decker Inc.

16. de Groot AC, Frosch PJ. Adverse reactions to fragrances. A clinical review. *Contact Dermatitis.* 1997;36(2):57–86.

17. Camarasa JG, Lluch M, Serra-Baldrich E, Zamorano M, Malet A, García-Calderón PA. Allergic contact dermatitis from 3-(aminomethyl)-pyridyl salicylate. *Contact Dermatitis.* 1989;20(5):347–351.

18. Jacob SE, Goldenberg A, Nedorost S, Thyssen JP, Fonacier L, Spiewak R. Flexural eczema versus atopic dermatitis. *Dermatitis: contact, atopic, occupational, drug.* 2015;26(3):109–115.

19. Goldenberg A, Ehrlich A, Machler BC, Jacob SE. Patch Test Clinic Start-up: From Basics to Pearls. *Dermatitis: contact, atopic, occupational, drug.* 2020;31(5):287–296.

20. Admani S, Jacob SE. Allergic contact dermatitis in children: review of the past decade. *Curr Allergy Asthma Rep.* 2014;14(4):421.

21. Jacob SE, Burk CJ, Connelly EA. Patch testing: another steroid-sparing agent to consider in children. *Pediatr Dermatol.* 2008;25(1):81–87.

22. Wilkinson DS, Fregert S, Magnusson B, et al. Terminology of contact dermatitis. *Acta Derm Venereol.* 1970;50(4):287–292.

23. Uter W, Geier J, Becker D, Brasch J, Löffler H. The MOAHLFA index of irritant sodium lauryl sulfate reactions: first results of a multicentre study on routine sodium lauryl sulfate patch testing. *Contact Dermatitis.* 2004;51(5-6):259–262.

24. Sheehan MP. Therapeutics in Allergic Contact Dermatitis, when Avoidance Fails. *Curr Treat Options Allergy.* 2014;1(4):337–347.

25. Jacob SE, Sung CT, Machler BC. Dupilumab for Systemic Allergy Syndrome With Dermatitis. *Dermatitis: contact, atopic, occupational, drug.* 2019;30(2):164–167.

26. Raffi J, Suresh R, Botto N, Murase JE. The impact of dupilumab on patch testing and the prevalence of co-morbid ACD in recalcitrant atopic dermatitis: a retrospective chart review. *J Am Acad Dermatol.* 2019.

27. Available at https://www.fda.gov/cosmetics/cosmetics-laws-regulations/it-cosmetic-drug-or-both-or-it-soap. Accessed October 22, 2020.

28. Salverda JGW, Bragt PJC, de Wit-Bos L, et al. Results of a cosmetovigilance survey in The Netherlands. *Contact Dermatitis.* 2013;68(3):139–148.

29. Berne B, Tammela M, Färm G, Inerot A, Lindberg M. Can the reporting of adverse skin reactions to cosmetics be improved? A prospective clinical study using a structured protocol. *Contact Dermatitis.* 2008;58(4):223–227.

30. Biebl KA, Warshaw EM. Allergic contact dermatitis to cosmetics. *Dermatol Clin.* 2006;24(2):215–232, vii.

31. Warshaw EM, Belsito DV, Taylor JS, et al. North American Contact Dermatitis Group patch test results: 2009 to 2010. *Dermatitis: contact, atopic, occupational, drug.* 2013;24(2):50–59.

32. Thyssen JP, Menné T, Linneberg A, Johansen JD. Contact sensitization to fragrances in the general population: a Koch's approach may reveal the burden of disease. *Br J Dermatol.* 2009;160(4):729–735.

33. Hamilton T, de Gannes GC. Allergic contact dermatitis to preservatives and fragrances in cosmetics. *Skin Therapy Lett.* 2011;16(4):1–4.

34. Johansen JD. Fragrance contact allergy: a clinical review. *Am J Clin Dermatol.* 2003;4(11):789–798.

35. Scheinman PL. Allergic contact dermatitis to fragrance: a review. *Am J Contact Dermat: official journal of the American Contact Dermatitis Society.* 1996;7(2):65–76.

36. Goldenberg A, Mousdicas N, Silverberg N, et al. Pediatric Contact Dermatitis Registry Inaugural Case Data. *Dermatitis: contact, atopic, occupational, drug.* 2016;27(5):293–302.

37. de Groot AC. *Patch testing: test concentrations and vehicles for 4350 chemicals.* Acdegroot Publ.; 2008.

38. Winter R. *A Consumer's Dictionary of Household, Yard and Office Chemicals: Complete Information About Harmful and Desirable Chemicals Found in Everyday Home Products, Yard Poisons, and Office Polluters.* iUniverse; 2007.

39. Scheman A, Jacob S, Zirwas M, et al. Contact Allergy: alternatives for the 2007 North American contact dermatitis group (NACDG) Standard Screening Tray. *Disease-a-month: DM.* 2008;54(1-2):7–156.

40. Kumar M, Devi A, Sharma M, Kaur P, Mandal UK. Review on perfume and present status of its associated allergens. *Journal of Cosmetic Dermatology.* 2021;20:391–399.

41. Larsen WG. Perfume Dermatitis: A Study of 20 Patients. *Arch Dermatol.* 1977;113(5):623–626.

42. Larsen W, Nakayama H, Lindberg M, et al. Fragrance contact dermatitis: a worldwide multicenter investigation (Part I). *Am J Contact Dermat: official journal of the American Contact Dermatitis Society.* 1996;7(2):77–83.

43. Wenk KS, Ehrlich A. Fragrance series testing in eyelid dermatitis. *Dermatitis: contact, atopic, occupational, drug.* 2012;23(1):22–26.

44. Hjorth N. Eczematous allergy to balsams, allied perfumes and flavouring agents, with special reference to balsam of Peru. *Acta dermato-venereologica. Supplementum.* 1961;41(Suppl 46):1–216.

45. Srivastava D, Cohen DE. Identification of the constituents of balsam of peru in tomatoes. *Dermatitis: contact, atopic, occupational, drug.* 2009;20(2):99–105.

46. Wang C, Sun T, Li H, Li Z, Wang X. Hypersensitivity Caused by Cosmetic Injection: Systematic Review and Case Report. *Aesthetic Plast Surg.* 2020.

47. Amado A, Jacob SE. Benzyl Alcohol Preserved Saline Used to Dilute Injectables Poses a Risk of Contact Dermatitis in Fragrance-Sensitive Patients. *Dermatol Surg.* 2007;33(11).

48. Available at https://www.accessdata.fda.gov/scripts/cdrh/cfdocs/cfcfr/CFRSearch.cfm?CFRPart=700%20&showFR=1 Accessed October 22, 2020.

49. Scheinman PL. The foul side of fragrance-free products: what every clinician should know about managing patients with fragrance allergy. *J Am Acad Dermatol.* 1999;41(6):1020–1024.

50. Xu S, Kwa M, Lohman ME, Evers-Meltzer R, Silverberg JI. Consumer Preferences, Product Characteristics, and Potentially Allergenic Ingredients in Best-selling Moisturizers. *JAMA Dermatol.* 2017;153(11):1099–1105.

51. de Groot AC, Schmidt E. Essential Oils, Part IV: Contact Allergy. *Dermatitis: contact, atopic, occupational, drug.* 2016;27(4).

52. Reeder MJ. Allergic Contact Dermatitis to Fragrances. *Dermatol Clin.* 2020;38(3):371–377.

53. de Groot AC, Schmidt E. Tea tree oil: contact allergy and chemical composition. *Contact Dermatitis.* 2016;75(3):129–143.

54. Adams RM, Maibach HI. A five-year study of cosmetic reactions. *J Am Acad Dermatol.* 1985;13(6):1062–1069.

55. Squire RA, Cameron LL. An analysis of potential carcinogenic risk from formaldehyde. *Regul Toxicol Pharmacol.* 1984;4(2):107–129.

56. de Groot A, Flyvholm M-A. Formaldehyde and Formaldehyde-Releasers. In: John SM, Johansen JD, Rustemeyer T, Elsner P, Maibach HI, eds. *Kanerva's Occupational Dermatology.* Cham: Springer International Publishing; 2018:1–32.

57. Hill AM, Belsito DV. Systemic contact dermatitis of the eyelids caused by formaldehyde derived from aspartame? *Contact Dermatitis.* 2003;49(5):258–259.

58. Lan J, Song Z, Miao X, et al. Skin damage among health care workers managing coronavirus disease-2019. *J Am Acad Dermatol.* 2020;82(5):1215–1216.

59. Donovan J, Skotnicki-Grant S. Allergic contact dermatitis from formaldehyde textile resins in surgical uniforms and nonwoven textile masks. *Dermatitis: contact, atopic, occupational, drug.* 2007;18(1):40–44.

60. Castanedo-Tardana MP, Zug KA. Methylisothiazolinone. *Dermatitis: contact, atopic, occupational, drug.* 2013;24(1):2–6.

61. Mowad CM. Methylchloro-isothiazolinone revisited. *American journal of contact dermatitis : official journal of the American Contact Dermatitis Society.* 2000;11(2):115–118.

62. Isaksson M, Gruvberger B, Bruze M. Occupational contact allergy and dermatitis from methylisothiazolinone after contact with wallcovering glue and after a chemical burn from a biocide. *Dermatitis: contact, atopic, occupational, drug.* 2004;15(4):201–205.

63. Collier PJ, Ramsey A, Waigh RD, Douglas KT, Austin P, Gilbert P. Chemical reactivity of some isothiazolone biocides. *J Appl Bacteriol.* 1990;69(4):578–584.

64. Wilkinson JD, Shaw S, Andersen KE, et al. Monitoring levels of preservative sensitivity in Europe. *Contact Dermatitis.* 2002;46(4):207–210.

65. Geier J, Lessmann H, Schnuch A, Uter W. Recent increase in allergic reactions to methylchloroisothiazolinone/methylisothiazolinone: is methylisothiazolinone the culprit? *Contact Dermatitis.* 2012;67(6):334–341.

66. Yim E, Baquerizo Nole KL, Tosti A. Contact dermatitis caused by preservatives. *Dermatitis: contact, atopic, occupational, drug.* 2014;25(5):215–231.

67. Lundov MD, Krongaard T, Menné TL, Johansen JD. Methylisothiazolinone contact allergy: a review. *Br J Dermatol.* 2011;165(6):1178–1182.

68. Urwin R, Wilkinson M. Methylchloroisothiazolinone and methylisothiazolinone contact allergy: a new 'epidemic'. *Contact Dermatitis.* 2013;68(4):253–255.

69. Wolf R, Orion E, Matz H. Co-existing sensitivity to metronidazole and isothiazolinone. *Clin Exp Dermatol.* 2003;28(5):506–507.

70. Heurung AR, Raju SI, Warshaw EM. Benzophenones. *Dermatitis: contact, atopic, occupational, drug.* 2014;25(1):3–10.

71. Scheman A, Jacob S, Katta R, et al. Part 4 of a 4-part series Miscellaneous Products: Trends and Alternatives in Deodorants, Antiperspirants, Sunblocks, Shaving Products, Powders, and Wipes: Data from the American Contact Alternatives Group. *J Clin Aesthet Dermatol.* 2011;4(10):35–39.

72. Yesudian PD, King CM. Severe contact urticaria and anaphylaxis from benzophenone-3(2-hydroxy 4-methoxy benzophenone). *Contact Dermatitis.* 2002;46(1):55–56.

73. Schlumpf M, Kypke K, Wittassek M, et al. Exposure patterns of UV filters, fragrances, parabens, phthalates, organochlor pesticides, PBDEs, and PCBs in human milk: correlation of UV filters with use of cosmetics. *Chemosphere.* 2010;81(10):1171–1183.

74. Gonzalez H, Farbrot A, Larkö O, Wennberg AM. Percutaneous absorption of the sunscreen benzophenone-3 after repeated whole-body applications, with and without ultraviolet irradiation. *Br J Dermatol.* 2006;154(2):337–340.

75. Food U, Administration D. Sunscreen drug products for over-the-counter human use: proposed rule. *Fed Regist.* 2019;84(38):6204–6275.

76. Fransway AF, Fransway PJ, Belsito DV, et al. Parabens: Contact (Non)Allergen of the Year. *Dermatitis: contact, atopic, occupational, drug.* 2018.

77. Ramírez N, Marcé RM, Borrull F. Determination of parabens in house dust by pressurised hot water extraction followed by stir bar sorptive extraction and thermal desorption-gas chromatography-mass spectrometry. *J Chromatogr A.* 2011;1218(37):6226–6231.

78. Soni MG, Burdock GA, Taylor SL, Greenberg NA. Safety assessment of propyl paraben: a review of the published literature. *Food and chemical toxicology: an international journal published for the British Industrial Biological Research Association.* 2001;39(6):513–532.

79. FDA (Food and Drug Administration), 2013. GRAS substances (SCOGS) database. 2013. Available at: https://www.fda.gov/food/ingredientspackaginglabeling/gras/scogs/default.htm. Accessed October 29, 2020.

80. Safety Assessment of Parabens as Used in Cosmetics. Available at: https://www.cir-safety.org/sites/default/files/parabens.pdf. Accessed October 29, 2020.

81. Uter W, Yazar K, Kratz EM, Mildau G, Lidén C. Coupled exposure to ingredients of cosmetic products: II. Preservatives. *Contact Dermatitis.* 2014;70(4):219–226.

82. Rastogi SC, Schouten A, de Kruijf N, Weijland JW. Contents of methyl-, ethyl-, propyl-, butyl- and benzylparaben in cosmetic products. *Contact Dermatitis.* 1995;32(1):28–30.

83. Scheman A, Jacob S, Katta R, et al. Part 1 of a 4-part series Facial Cosmetics: Trends and Alternatives: Data from the American Contact Alternatives Group. *J Clin Aesthet Dermatol.* 2011;4(6):25–30.

84. Alani JI, Davis MD, Yiannias JA. Allergy to cosmetics: a literature review. *Dermatitis: contact, atopic, occupational, drug.* 2013;24(6):283–290.

85. Lee CH, Kim HJ. A study on the absorption mechanism of drugs through biomembranes. *Arch Pharm Res.* 1994;17(3):182–189.

86. Oishi S. Lack of spermatotoxic effects of methyl and ethyl esters of p-hydroxybenzoic acid in rats. *Food and chemical toxicology : an international journal published for the British Industrial Biological Research Association.* 2004;42(11):1845–1849.

87. Routledge EJ, Parker J, Odum J, Ashby J, Sumpter JP. Some alkyl hydroxy benzoate preservatives (parabens) are estrogenic. *Toxicol Appl Pharmacol.* 1998;153(1):12–19.

88. Blair RM, Fang H, Branham WS, et al. The estrogen receptor relative binding affinities of 188 natural and xenochemicals: structural diversity of ligands. *Toxicological sciences: an official journal of the Society of Toxicology.* 2000;54(1):138–153.

89. Darbre PD, Byford JR, Shaw LE, et al. Oestrogenic activity of benzylparaben. *J Appl Toxicol: JAT.* 2003;23(1):43–51.

90. Darbre PD. Underarm cosmetics and breast cancer. *J Appl Toxicol: JAT.* 2003;23(2):89–95.

91. Darbre PD, Aljarrah A, Miller WR, Coldham NG, Sauer MJ, Pope GS. Concentrations of parabens in human breast tumours. *J Appl Toxicol: JAT.* 2004;24(1):5–13.

92. Darbre PD. Environmental oestrogens, cosmetics and breast cancer. *Best Pract Res Clin Endocrinol Metab.* 2006;20(1):121–143.

93. Final amended report on the safety assessment of Methylparaben, Ethylparaben, Propylparaben, Isopropylparaben, Butylparaben, Isobutylparaben, and Benzylparaben as used in cosmetic products. *International journal of toxicology.* 2008;27(Suppl 4):1–82.

94. Fowler JF, Zirwas MJ. *Fisher's contact dermatitis.* BookBaby; 2019.

95. Mirick DK, Davis S, Thomas DB. Antiperspirant use and the risk of breast cancer. *J Natl Cancer Inst.* 2002;94(20):1578–1580.

96. Golden R, Gandy J, Vollmer G. A review of the endocrine activity of parabens and implications for potential risks to human health. *Crit Rev Toxicol.* 2005;35(5):435–458.

97. Castelain F, Castelain M. Parabens: a real hazard or a scare story? *Eur J Dermatol: EJD.* 2012;22(6):723–727.

98. Tran JM, Reeder MJ. When the treatment is the culprit: Prevalence of allergens in prescription topical steroids and immunomodulators. *J Am Acad Dermatol.* 2020;83(1):228–230.

99. Warshaw TG, Herrmann F. Studies of skin reaction to propylene glycol. *J Invest Dermatol.* 1952;19(6):423–430.

100. Warshaw EM, Botto NC, Maibach HI, et al. Positive patch-test reactions to propylene glycol: a retrospective cross-sectional analysis from the North American Contact Dermatitis Group, 1996 to 2006. *Dermatitis: contact, atopic, occupational, drug.* 2009;20(1):14–20.

101. Jacob SE, Scheman A, McGowan MA. Propylene Glycol. *Dermatitis: contact, atopic, occupational, drug.* 2018;29(1):3–5.

102. Alfalah M, Loranger C, Sasseville D. Alkyl Glucosides. *Dermatitis: contact, atopic, occupational, drug.* 2017;28(1):3–4.

103. Fiume M, Bergfeld WF, Belsito DV, et al. Final report on the safety assessment of sodium cetearyl sulfate and related alkyl sulfates as used in cosmetics. *Int J Toxicol.* 2010;29(3 Suppl):115s–132s.

104. Sasseville D. Alkyl Glucosides: 2017 "Allergen of the Year". *Dermatitis: contact, atopic, occupational, drug.* 2017;28(4):296.

105. Zirwas MJ. Contact Dermatitis to Cosmetics. *Clin Rev Allergy Immunol.* 2019;56(1):119–128.

106. Galadari H, Gupta A, Kroumpouzos G, et al. COVID 19 and its impact on cosmetic dermatology. *Dermatol Ther.* 2020:e13822–e13822.

CHAPTER 20

Skin Pigmentation Disorders

Daniel Gutierrez, MD

SUMMARY POINTS

What's Important

1. Disorders of pigmentation are commonly seen, can cause significant distress, and often require a multi-modal approach in order to provide satisfactory outcomes.
2. Dyspigmentation is often multifactorial and can stem from a combination of both environmental (photo-induced) and intrinsic (constitutional skin pigmentation) factors.
3. The melanin biosynthesis pathway is complex and improved knowledge regarding these mechanisms may yield additional targets for therapy in the future.

What's New

1. The effect of light outside of the ultraviolet spectrum is becoming better elucidated. Visible light is able to illicit dyspigmentation in darker-skin individuals. Therefore, it is crucial to protect against the visible light spectrum when counseling patients on management of their pigmentary disorders.
2. For treatment of melasma, new skin-lightening options are becoming available and being integrated into clinical practice. These include methimazole, flutamide, cysteamine, and tranexamic acid.

What's Coming

1. Newer protocols for treatment of dyschromia are continually being developed as technology advances. Picosecond lasers represent one of the newer advances in treatment of melasma. Best practices for integration of these devices in clinical practice are currently underway.
2. Larger studies in diverse populations comparing medical and procedural interventions are occurring to determine the optimal combination of interventions for treatment of various dyschromia.

SKIN PIGMENTATION AND PIGMENTATION DISORDERS

Disorders of pigmentation can cause significant stress to patients, so available treatment options should be well-understood. Ultraviolet as well as visible light-induced changes to the skin may contribute to cutaneous pigmentation. In this chapter, the mechanisms involved in pigment formation will be detailed and the pigmentary conditions most likely to be seen by a cosmetic dermatologist will be discussed. There is a wide array of rarer dyschromia (lichen planus pigmentosus, erythema dyschromicum perstans) that is beyond the scope of this chapter. Cosmetic dermatologists are often faced with patients presenting with melasma, lentigines, postinflammatory hyperpigmentation, and periorbital hyperpigmentation. These conditions will be addressed in addition to some common treatment options. Depigmenting agents will be discussed in greater detail in Chapter 41 while energy-based devices will be discussed in greater detail in Chapter 26.

SKIN COLOR

Although many factors contribute to skin color, including carotenoids or hemoglobin,[1] the amount, quality, and distribution of melanin present in the epidermis are principally responsible for human skin color. The number of melanocytes in human skin is equal in all races. However, melanocyte activity and interaction with the keratinocytes account for skin color.[2] In darker-pigmented individuals, melanocytes produce more melanin; the melanosomes are larger and more heavily concentrated, and they undergo degradation at a slower rate as compared to lighter-skinned individuals.[3] Skin color is related to a combination of intrinsic and extrinsic factors. Experts refer to *Constitutive skin color* (CSC) as the genetically influenced color, whereas *facultative skin color* (FSC) will denote pigmentation influenced by environmental factors, most often referring to sunlight.[4] Key concepts related to skin of color will be explored further in Chapter 15.

MELANIN BIOSYNTHESIS AND MELANOSOME TRANSFER

Melanin is produced in the melanosome, a cytoplasmic organelle in melanocytes. Melanin production within melanosomes begins with hydroxylation of tyrosine to 3,4-dihydroxyphenylalanine (DOPA) using the copper-dependent enzyme tyrosinase. Tyrosine then oxidizes DOPA to dopaquinone. After processing of intermediate products, melanin is eventually formed (**Fig. 20-1**).[5] Two types of melanin are produced through this pathway: eumelanin and pheomelanin. The relative amounts of these two types determine hair color and skin tone. Individuals with darker skin tones have mostly eumelanin and a lesser amount of pheomelanin, while the opposite is true in people with a lighter skin color.

Tyrosinase is the rate-limiting step for melanin production and is stimulated by factors including ultraviolet (UV) radiation through production of DNA fragments such as thymidine dinucleotides,[6] melanocyte-stimulating hormone (MSH), and growth factors such as bFGF and endothelin. Activation of protein kinase C[7] and the cyclic adenosine monophosphate (cAMP) ± protein kinase A pathway[6] plays a role in increasing melanin production as do prostaglandins D2, E2, and F2, tumor necrosis factor (TNF)-α, interleukins 1 α, IL1 β, and IL6.[8] Vitamin D may also play a role in stimulating melanogenesis.[9]

Melanosomes in human skin undergo four stages of development inside the melanocyte. The first two stages lack pigment. In stage I, premelanosomes are characterized by their spherical structure and amorphous matrix. Intraluminal formation begins during this stage and is completed by stage II. During stage II, the melanosome becomes more oval shaped. In stage III, melanin production begins due to tyrosinase activity and continues to stage IV at which point the organelle contains such a high concentration of melanin that internal structures are obscured due to the pigment. Fully formed melanosomes are then transferred into melanocyte dendrites along microtubules using myosin V filaments[10] as well as a dynein and kinesin motor.[11] Each melanocyte is in contact with roughly 36 keratinocytes which constitutes the "epidermal melanin unit"[1,12] (**Fig. 20-2**). The process by which melanin is incorporated into keratinocytes is poorly understood but four potential transfer mechanisms have been proposed: (i) keratinocyte phagocytosis of the melanosome-filled tip of the melanocytes (cytophagocytosis model), (ii) melanosome movement through a cellular membrane connection between keratinocytes and melanocytes (membrane fusion model), (iii) melanocyte shedding of membrane-enclosed vesicles with highly concentrated amounts of melanosomes (shedding-phagocytosis model), and (iv) melanocyte release of the melanosome's melanin core by exocytosis with subsequent phagocytosis by keratinocytes (exocytosis-endocytosis model).[13]

New discoveries are continually made to better understand cellular mechanisms for melanin transfer. Sieberg et al. found that the protease-activated receptor 2 (PAR-2), expressed on keratinocytes, is important in regulating the ingestion of melanosomes by keratinocytes in culture.[14] PAR-2 is a G-protein-coupled receptor that is activated by a serine protease cleavage,[15] and is able to enhance the capacity of keratinocytes to ingest melanosomes. The PAR-2 can be up- or downregulated but is upregulated by UV radiation.[16] It is thought to be important in hyperpigmentation disorders because it has been found that serine protease inhibitors that interfere with PAR-2 activation induce depigmentation by reducing melanosome transfer and distribution.[17] Soybeans, which contain the serine protease inhibitors soybean trypsin inhibitor (STI) and Bowman-Birk protease inhibitor (BBI), have been shown to inhibit melanosome transfer, resulting in an improvement of facial pigmentation.[18] In addition, activation of PAR-2 with trypsin and other synthetic peptides has been shown to result in visible skin darkening.[17]

Other systems play a role in melanosome transfer as well. For example, the soluble portion of the N-terminal of β-amyloid precursor protein (APP), called sAPP, is an epidermal growth factor that has been shown to increase the release of melanin as well as enhance the movements of the melanocyte dendritic tips.[19] Keratinocyte growth factor (KGF/FGF7) also promotes melanosome transfer by stimulating the phagocytic process.[20]

MELANOCYTE-STIMULATING HORMONE AND PIGMENTATION

MSH is derived from the proopiomelanocortin (POMC) gene. Among the three forms of MSH (α, β, and γ), α-MSH is the most active form in humans and will bind to the melanocortin 1 receptor (MC1R) on melanocytes. The binding of MSH to MC1R leads to activation of adenylate cyclase which increases cAMP levels, activates tyrosinase, and leads to production of eumelanin (**Fig. 20-3**). When MC1R is mutated or improperly functioning, production of pheomelanin is increased. Mutations in MC1R, causing increased levels of pheomelanin are seen in individuals with red hair[21]. This pathway is intriguing for several reasons. MSH is implicated in the tanning

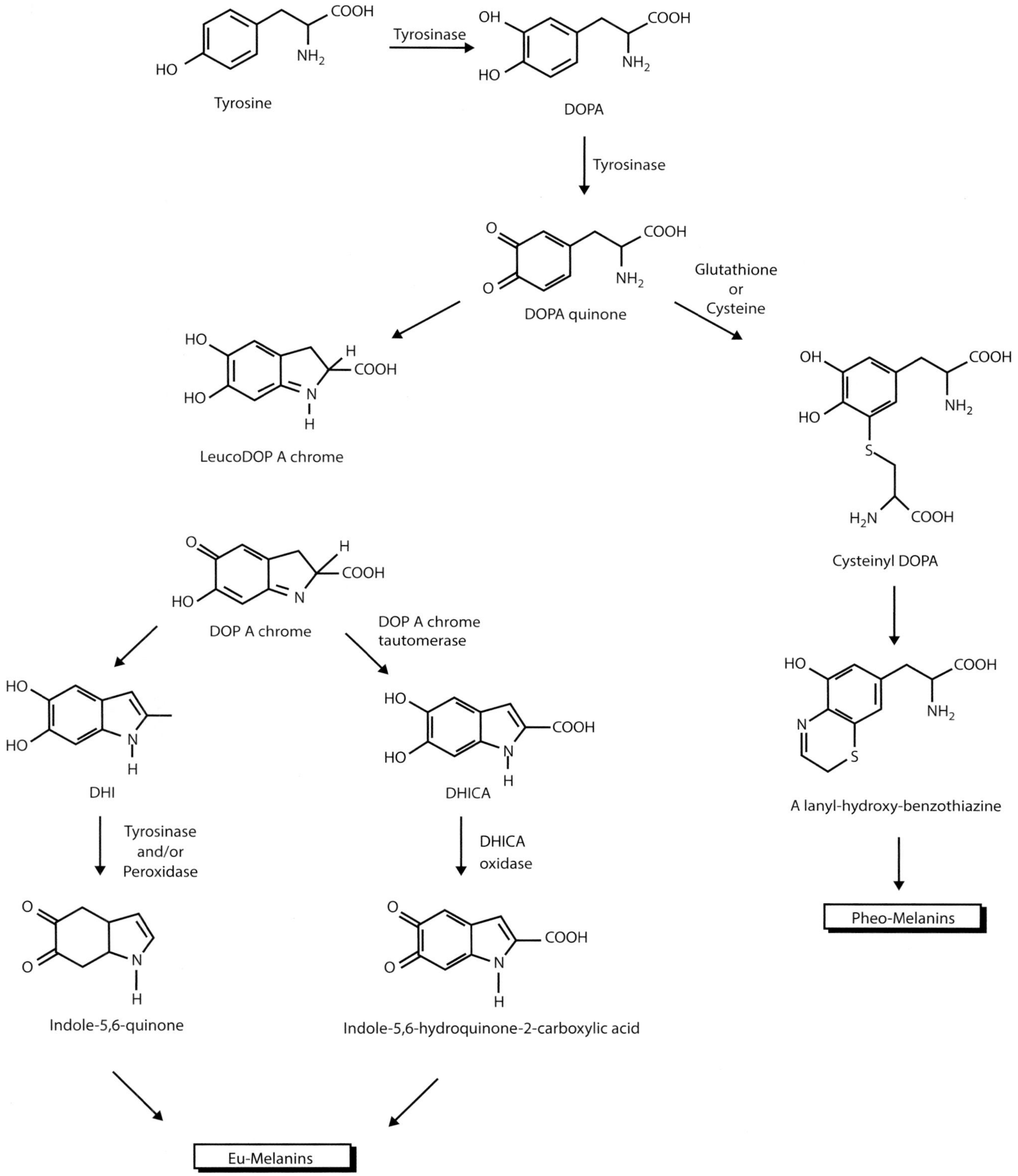

FIGURE 20-1. The melanin biosynthesis pathway. Many depigmenting agents work by inhibiting tyrosinase.

mechanism. Those with red hair have defects in MC1R and are poor tanners.[22] In addition, MSH production is regulated by the adrenocorticotropic hormone (ACTH) which stimulates POMC transcription. Hyperpigmentation can be seen in endocrinopathies causing ACTH levels. Physiologic stress can also activate the hypothalamic-pituitary-adrenal access of the sympathetic nervous system which may contribute to pigmentation. In a murine study, increased hyperpigmentation was seen in stressed mice exposed to UVB which was then inhibited when treated with corticostatin, an ACTH inhibitor.[23]

THE EFFECT OF LIGHT ON PIGMENTATION

Solar energy plays a significant impact on skin. Infrared radiation (IR), visible light (VL), and UVR (ultraviolet radiation) all have effects on the skin. IR exists from 700 to 2500 nm, VL ranges from 400 to 700 nm, and UVR encompasses wavelengths from 100 to 400 nm. UVR is divided into UVC (100–290 nm), UVB (290–320 nm), and UVA (320–400 nm). UVA can be further subdivided into UVA1 (340 to 400 nm) and UVA2 (320 to 340 nm). UVC is filtered by the earth's atmosphere and is not implicated in perpetuating common cutaneous conditions. When exposed skin is subjected to UV light, melanogenesis occurs as a means to limit UV-induced photodamage. With UVA exposure, an *immediate pigmentary*

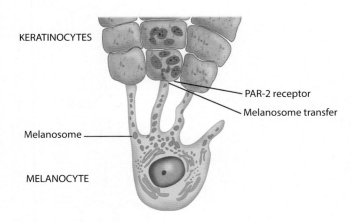

FIGURE 20-2. Epidermal—melanin unit. One melanocyte can interact with many keratinocytes.

darkening is seen which is caused by the photo-oxidation of the existing melanin. This results in a new-onset, effervescent gray discoloration, which appears within a few minutes of UVA exposure and rapidly disappears after 6 to 8 hours. Both UVB and UVA are involved in the process of *delayed tanning* which is seen 2 to 3 days after UV exposure and lasts for approximately 10 to 14 days. With delayed tanning, melanin synthesis and melanosome transfer is enhanced[24] and protects against further UV damage by absorbing reactive oxygen species before cellular damage occurs.

The presence of DNA damage or DNA repair intermediates themselves can stimulate melanogenesis in the absence of UV radiation.[25] In fact, small, single-stranded DNA fragments such as thymidine dinucleotides (pTpT) are able to stimulate tanning through activation of p53, a well-known tumor suppressor gene.[6,26] Once DNA damage occurs, p53 induces cell-cycle arrest and facilitates DNA repair or triggers apoptosis if DNA damage is irreparable. Some propose a link between skin darkening and p53 expression that may account for the positive sensations, reported by those who frequently tan.[27] When p53 is stimulated by UVR, POMC gene transcription is activated which increases production of both MSH and β-endorphin, an endogenous opioid neuropeptide. This may lend credence to the theory that some individuals develop a rewarding response to tanning[28] (**Fig. 20-4**).

Recent studies have shown differences between skin phenotypes and the response to light. Furthermore, the role of wavelengths of light outside the UV spectrum have become better elucidated. Both long-wavelength UVA1 and VL are able to elicit hyperpigmentation in those with darker skin pigmentation; this effect, however, is not seen in more lightly

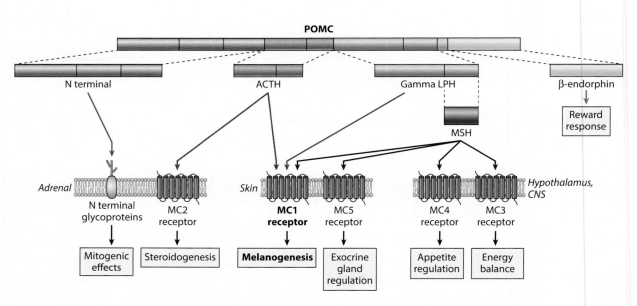

FIGURE 20-3. The POMC gene is found in keratinocytes, adrenal tissue, the hypothalamus, and CNS. When POMC is activated, it transcribes four main sequences: the N terminus, adrenocorticotrophin (ACTH), gamma lipotrophin (gamma LPH), and β-endorphins. These sequences subsequently lead to activation of the melanocortin receptors as shown. Activation of the MC1R receptor leads to melanogenesis.

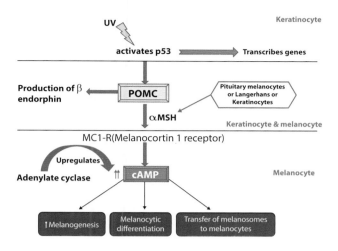

FIGURE 20-4. UV radiation activates p53, which stimulates the POMC gene to transcribe alpha melanocyte-stimulating hormone. αMSH binds the MC1-R receptor located on the melanocytes, which triggers adenylate cyclase to produce cAMP. cAMP then stimulates tyrosinase to produce melanin. Interestingly, when POMC transcription is stimulated, β-endorphin production also increases, leading to a potential rewarding response.

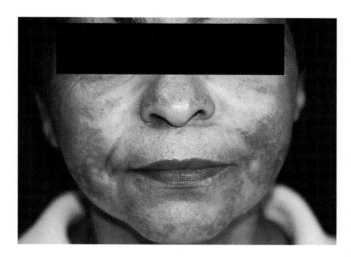

FIGURE 20-5. Patient with diffuse melasma. The patient has not improved despite multiple therapies including depigmenting agents, chemical peels, and good sun protection.

pigmented individuals.[29] Infrared light, which causes fleeting erythema lasting less than an hour, does not seem to contribute to long-lasting skin pigmentation.[30] Knowledge of these biological effects of the different wavelengths of light will provide more tailored guidance on photoprotection with photo-aggravated skin conditions.

MELASMA

Melasma is a common pigmentary disorder that is routinely seen in the dermatology clinics (**Fig. 20-5**). Although melasma more commonly occurs in women with darker skin types, it may also be seen in men. Melasma typically presents as irregularly shaped, but often distinctly defined, light- to dark-brown patches on the forehead, cheeks, nose, upper lip, chin, and neck. There are four patterns of clinical distribution: centrofacial, malar, mandibular, and extrafacial. The centrofacial pattern involving the forehead, upper lip, nose, and chin is most common.[31] While it is most commonly seen in photo-exposed sites, extrafacial melasma has been reported in relatively photo-protected sites including the areola and external genitalia.[32,33]

Melasma can be grouped into two general categories based on location of pigment in the skin: epidermal or dermal disease. Epidermal melasma appears as brown to black patches. Dermal melasma may appear more blue-gray. Epidermal melasma is more amenable to treatment as the melanin is at a higher level and therefore can be more easily reached by topical products. Because dermal melasma is much more difficult to treat, it is helpful to determine the extent of the dermal component in order to provide proper expectations and predict a likely treatment response. A Wood's light can be used to determine the extent of the dermal component[34] (**Fig. 20-6**). In epidermal melasma, the epidermal component will appear darker under Wood's light examination while the dermal component

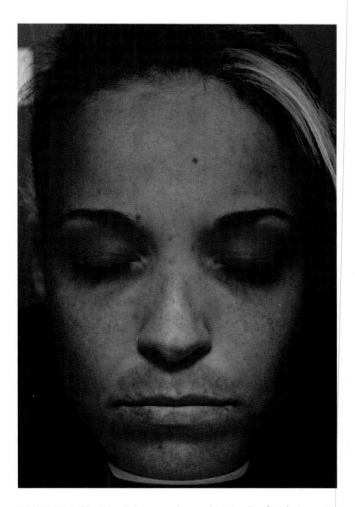

FIGURE 20-6. The Wood's lamp can be used to visualize facial pigment.

is less notable. Some, however, feel that Wood's lamp examination may not able to accurately predict clinical response, particularly if mixed epidermal/dermal melasma is suspected.[35]

The etiology of melasma is multifactorial. UV and VL exposure, hormonal influences, and genetic factors are thought to contribute to overall pathogenesis.[36] Although there have been a few familial cases reported, the evidence that melasma can be inherited is sparse.[37] Sun exposure is well known to exacerbate melasma and seems to be necessary for its development.[5,34] In fact, melasma has been reported to be less noticeable in the winter months when the average sun exposure is typically lower.[5] UVR- and VL-induced pigmentation is thought to be perpetuated by secretion of stem cell factor (SCF), the ligand for c-kit located on the melanocytes, by dermal fibroblasts and keratinocytes which is supported as there is known to be increased levels of SCF and c-kit of lesional skin of patients with melasma.[38]

It is currently unknown as to how hormonal influences directly play into overall melasma pathophysiology. The hormone, 17 β-estradiol, which is known to affect other cells of neural crest origin, has been shown to significantly increase the activity of tyrosinase when added to melanocyte cultures.[39] Many have also noted the development of melasma on younger women taking oral contraceptives.[32,33] Melasma is also common among pregnant women or those with prior pregnancy; together these two conditions comprise a significant proportion of cases. Menopausal and premenstrual presentations occasionally occur as well. Although melasma may diminish in the months following a patient's pregnancy or after the patient discontinues oral contraceptives, the condition often persists.[33,37] Given hormonal influences, melasma can occur with some ovarian disorders. Some have also proposed that certain exogenous agents may worsen the disease. For example, antiepilepsy medications such as hydantoin and phenytoin have been implicated in contributing to melasma in both women and men.[33,37]

Histopathology

In epidermal melasma, the basal and suprabasal layers have higher melanin levels.[5,32] The melanocytes appear larger with more noticeable dendritic processes; however, the total number of melanocytes is equal to unaffected skin.[40] In dermal melasma, melanin-laden macrophages emerge in a perivascular arrangement in the superficial and middle level of the dermis. In the mixed form elements from the epidermal and dermal subtypes are seen together.

Electron microscopy of skin from patients with melasma shows increased melanosomes and dendritic processes in the hyperpigmented area of the skin.[40]

Treatment

Melasma is very difficult to treat and often requires a multimodal approach to treatment in order to achieve satisfactory results. Topical treatments include skin-lightening agents like hydroquinone and kojic acid, retinoids, glucocorticoids, hydroxy acids. Procedural treatments may also be used with good cosmetic outcomes. Regardless of therapies employed, serial photography with a regular camera and a UV camera should be used to document treatment response.[41]

Topical therapies remain a cornerstone of therapy. Often, multiple medications can be compounded together in order to inhibit different aspects of the melanin biosynthesis and transfer pathways. Together, these work synergistically to improve hyperpigmentation. One of the earliest and most well-known combination treatments, the "Kligman formula" consisted of a mixture of 0.1% tretinoin, 4% hydroquinone, 0.1% dexamethasone, and hydrophilic ointment which was popular for treatment since its creation in 1975.[42] This formula, however, is currently not commercially available and must be compounded by a pharmacy. In light of this, a prescription combination formulation containing hydroquinone 4%, tretinoin 0.05%, and fluocinolone 0.01% has been approved by the FDA, is commercially available, and remains popular for melasma treatment.

Hydroquinone has long been a staple of treatment for pigmentary disorders and works through inhibiting tyrosinase. It is available without prescription in the United States as a 2% formulation. Caution should be used when using concentrations of 4% or higher for long periods. High concentrations can cause irritant contact dermatitis with resultant postinflammatory changes that may be more noticeable than a patient's melasma. Further, extended periods of use may predispose an individual to developing exogenous ochronosis. It is therefore recommended that hydroquinone-containing products be used in a cyclical fashion with periods of break. An example of such a regimen involves daily use for 3 months with a 1-month period using non-hydroquinone products before resuming hydroquinone use.

Topical tretinoin improves epidermal hyperpigmentation by decreasing tyrosinase activity, slowing melanin production, and enhancing epidermal desquamation.[43] Although tretinoin 0.1% has been studied as monotherapy for melasma treatment,[44,45] the time to improvement can be lengthy and may require 10 months. Therefore, most physicians utilize a combination of topical products. A tretinoin peel is another acceptable option in patients with melasma. In a study of 10 Asian women with melasma, a 1% tretinoin peel was as effective and better tolerated compared to a 70% glycolic acid peel in patients.[46]

Kojic acid also improves the efficacy of combination topical agents according to other recent studies. In a split face trial comparing 10% glycolic acid and 2% hydroquinone with or without 2% kojic acid over a 12-week period, the side treated with the combination containing kojic acid showed more improvement.[47]

Topical glucocorticoids are known to induce hypopigmentation with continued use and are helpful for treatment of hyperpigmentation. It has been proposed that they decrease both production and secretion of melanin in the melanocytes.[42] Given additional adverse effects including skin atrophy, lower potency topical glucocorticoids are recommended for regular use on the face unless they are combined with retinoids; studies have demonstrated that retinoids help prevent the atrophy caused by topical glucocorticoids.[48]

Other promising therapeutics have been investigated recently including: topical methimazole 5% daily,[49] topical flutamide 1% daily,[50] topical cysteamine 5% daily,[51] and topical tranexamic acid 2–5% twice daily.[52] Oral tranexamic acid, a medication used for the treatment of menorrhagia, has been trialed at doses ranging from 500 mg to 750 mg daily with impressive results in those with recalcitrant disease. Thrombosis remains a significant side effect when utilizing this medication. Prior to use, patients should be screened for either a personal or family history of thromboembolic disease, disorders predisposing a patient to develop thromboembolic disease including hypercoagulable states, including those induced by smoking or using hormonal contraceptives renal insufficiency, or conditions; side effects range from mild gastrointestinal discomfort to myalgias, headaches, and dysmenorrhea.[52] Patient should be closely monitored while on the medication and reevaluated after 3 months of use.

Hydroxy acids promote keratinocyte turnover in melasma. They are also beneficial in enhancing the effectiveness of other topical agents as they facilitate penetration, therefore promoting efficacy.[53] Glycolic acid peels alone or in combination with Jessner's peels can be used in combination with topical agents to hasten the resolution of melasma (see Chapter 24). Jessner's solution and 70% glycolic acid (combined with tretinoin and hydroquinone between peels) work equally well in the treatment of melasma.[35]

Lasers and light-based devices are commonly used in dermatology for treatment of a myriad conditions. Their use for treatment of melasma has been documented and results are promising. However, energy-delivering treatments should be used as adjuncts alongside appropriate topical therapies. Patients should be counseled on expectations from procedural therapies, risk of rebound of disease, and that durable response from therapy may be variable.

Intense pulsed light (IPL), a noncoherent broadband light source ranging from 500 to 1200 nm, is another available option for melasma treatment with minimal downtime and low number of adverse effects in properly trained physicians. In a study of 31 Asian women with dermal and mixed melasma, monthly IPL treatment was compared with topical 4% hydroquinone use; 35% of patients in the IPL group had greater than 50% improvement compared to 14% in the hydroquinone group.[54] The initial cutoff filter was 570 nm, and 590 to 615 filters were used for the remaining treatments to target deeper components. As expected, epidermal components of melasma treated with IPL responded better than dermal melasma.[55] Although IPL is considered a safe treatment, postinflammatory changes remains a possibility.

The Q-switched 755 nm laser has also been successfully used to treat melasma.[56] In addition, this laser has been used in conjunction with the UltraPulse CO_2 laser.[57,58] In one study, the combination of the Q-switched 755 nm laser and UltraPulse CO_2 was associated with more side effects than the Q-switched 755 nm laser alone, though the combination treatment was more effective.[58]

Fractional photothermolysis is an option for lightening hyperpigmented areas of the face. In one study 10 patients with refractory melasma and Fitzpatrick skin types III to V received four to six treatments with a 1535 and 1550 nm Fraxel laser at 1- to 2-week intervals; 60% showed 75% to 100% clearance of their melasma based on the physician evaluation[59] (see Chapter 26).

Picosecond lasers (755 nm and 1064 nm) have been trialed for the treatment of melasma in a total of seven studies to date with a cumulative total of 140 patients.[60] This technology is promising as adverse effects are low, though presently, it is not recommended as monotherapy.[60]

Post-treatment care and prevention of worsening of disease should be discussed with patients. Proper photoprotection is paramount as UVA, UVB, and VL can all worsen melasma.[61] Inorganic (physical) sunscreens are recommended as they reflect a wider spectrum of light (UV and VL) in comparison to organic (chemical) sunscreens which absorb light and are not protective against VL. In patients with dyspigmentation, use of inorganic sunscreens may be cosmetically displeasing as it may impart a white hue over applied areas. Micronized formulations, while improving the cosmesis and minimizing this white hue, are not as protective against VL. Iron oxide, which is added to sunscreens to provide a better color match, enhances photoprotective effects by providing additional VL blocking properties.[62] Patients should be counseled on the repeated reapplication of sunscreens, use of photoprotective clothing, sun avoidance, and adherence to topical therapies to ensure effective responses.

Although there have been many new advances in the therapies utilized for melasma, many of these studies have smaller sample sizes and varying methodologies. Larger comparative studies regarding these medications and treatment devices in diverse populations are needed to determine the most optimal combination of interventions.

SOLAR LENTIGINES

Up to 90% of elderly patients have solar lentigines.[63] Solar lentigines present as brown macules and patches most commonly on the face and dorsal hands (**Fig. 20-7**). They develop as a result of cumulative sun exposure and the presence of a large number can constitute a significant risk factor for melanoma and nonmelanoma skin cancer.[64,65] A patient with high numbers of solar lentigines should be routinely be followed with skin examinations for screening of cutaneous malignancies.

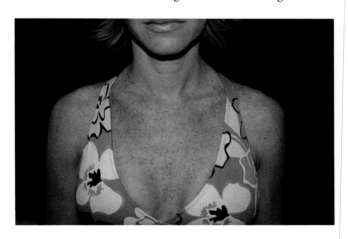

FIGURE 20-7. Clinical photo of solar lentigines.

Histopathology

Solar lentigines exhibit elongated rete ridges that contain pigmented basaloid cells intermingled with melanocytes (**Fig. 20-8**). They are characterized by an increased melanin retention by keratinocytes with lack of change in the number of melanocytes. The melanin content of the epidermis in facial solar lentigines has been demonstrated to be 2.2 times higher than that in photodamaged skin.[66]

Treatment

Treatment for solar lentigines is based primarily on which therapy is most convenient for a patient. Some may choose a more conservative treatment with less recovery time while others may wish for swift and aggressive removal. For patients who want faster and more visible results, chemical peels, lasers, intense pulsed light dermabrasion, and cryotherapy can all be used.

Chemical peeling agents such as TCA (trichloroacetic acid), glycolic acid, and combination peels have been used for many years for treatment of solar lentigines.[67-69] Although effective, the pain and burning sensation when treating large surface areas may be a limiting factor. Several studies have compared the efficacy of these various treatments. In a study comparing liquid nitrogen to 35% TCA in the treatment of solar lentigines of hands in 25 patients, cryotherapy was found to be superior with 71% of subjects showing 50% or more improvement compared to 47% improvement with TCA peel.[70] In this study, although most patients believed that TCA peel had the fastest healing time, liquid nitrogen was rated more efficacious. When treating a patient with cryotherapy, only a single freeze thaw is recommended, since an aggressive treatment may lead to scarring and dyspigmentation.[71]

Dermabrasion is also an effective destructive therapy for treatment of lentigines.[72] When compared to cryotherapy, the risks of hypopigmentation are less—more than 50% of the patients treated with cryotherapy continued to display hypopigmentation in the treated areas 6 months after

treatment compared with 11% of the patients treated with dermabrasion.

Lasers targeting epidermal pigment are particularly successful for treatment of lentigines. These include the Q-switched and long pulse 755 nm,[73] Q-switched 532 nm, 1550/1927 nm Fraxel Dual,[75] and IPL[76] which have all been used in the treatment of solar lentigines with success. Newer picosecond lasers[74] (532 nm, 755 nm) have shown excellent results in the treatment of lentigines with minimal adverse effects.[60] Specifics regarding laser treatments will be discussed more thoroughly in Chapter 26. Although lasers are very effective for these lesions, patients should be warned that treated areas will be erythematous and can crust for approximately 7 to 10 days depending on the type of laser used. The most common side effect of laser treatment is postinflammatory pigment alteration.

Topical agents are good alternatives for patients who do not wish to undergo procedurally based interventions. Topical retinoids (tretinoin, tazarotene, adapalene, and potentially trifarotene) are effective options and can be used alone or in combination with other skin-lightening. Retinoids have the ability to increase the penetration of skin-lightening agents and chemical peels in addition to decreasing melanin production. Tretinoin 0.01% in combination with 4-hydroxyanisole (Mequinol) has been shown to be effective in the treatment of solar lentigines.[77,78] Ortonne et al. reported the effect of 4-hydroxyanisole 2%/tretinoin 0.01% solution, and sunscreen in 406 patients with solar lentigines for up to 24 weeks; 325 patients (88%) had an almost complete fading of their facial lesions and 298 (81%) experienced the same in targeted forearm lesions.[79] In another study, Kang et al. treated 90 patients exhibiting solar lentigines and actinic keratoses with adapalene gel (0.1% or 0.3%) and compared the results to its vehicle; 1 month following the treatment, patients treated with adapalene gel showed significant improvement of photodamage.[80] In addition, the use of tazarotene 0.1% cream once daily in 562 patients with facial photoaging for 24 weeks showed improvement of the lentigines and mottled hyperpigmentation by at least 1 point using a 7-point scale when compared to its vehicle.[81] This treatment was followed by an additional 28 weeks of tazarotene 0.1% cream treatment and continuing improvement was observed without plateau effect.[82] Accordingly, it is important to inform patients that it may take months for topical retinoids to show results.

"TANNING-BED" LENTIGINES

The development of unusual melanocytic lesions after exposure to UVA tanning beds has been reported. These lesions commonly appear on the chest and upper back, and look similar to the lentigines that occur after psoralen photochemotherapy.[83] The histologic examination of these lentigines has revealed melanocytic hyperplasia and cytologic atypia.[84] Patients with these lesions may be at an increased risk of skin cancer. These patients should be cautioned about the hazards of tanning bed use and should have annual skin examinations.

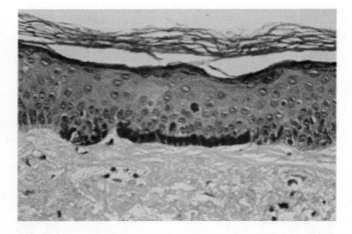

FIGURE 20-8. Hematoxylin and eosin (H&E) stain of a solar lentigo. (*Photo courtesy of George Ioannides, MD.*)

POSTINFLAMMATORY HYPERPIGMENTATION

Postinflammatory hyperpigmentation (PIH or postinflammatory pigment alteration, PIPA) occurs as direct result of skin inflammation—it is a consequence of increased melanin synthesis and pigmentary incontinence as a result of cutaneous injury. It presents as brown macules and patches located in areas of prior inflammation or cutaneous injury. It can be diffused or localized depending on the extent of the prior inflammatory response. Although postinflammatory hyperpigmentation appears most frequently among patients with darker skin types, it can afflict those of any skin phototype.[85–87] Those of Asian ancestry tend to be susceptible to PIH even when their skin tone is light. Unfortunately, this phenomenon tends to recur in susceptible individuals.[88] It is one of the most common conditions responsible for spurring patients to visit a dermatologist, especially in patients of color.[89]

A patient's pigmentation risk can be assessed based on historical information by utilizing the Baumann Skin Typing System discussed in Chapter 10.

Histopathology

PIH is characterized by numerous melanophages in the superficial dermis. An infiltrate of lymphohistiocytes may be seen around superficial blood vessels and in dermal papillae with active inflammation.[90]

Treatment

This condition is difficult to treat because it occurs in individuals susceptible to hyperpigmentation following inflammation. The primary cause of these postinflammatory changes should be addressed. The inflammation, if induced by cosmetic procedures aimed toward improving dyspigmentation, can potentially turn into PIH. Therefore, risks and benefits of further procedural therapies for treatment should be weighed and discussed with the patient. Evidence of active inflammation should be swiftly treated with topical anti-inflammatory medications. While topical products such as hydroquinone and retinoids are potentially useful to treat PIH, they may cause irritant contact dermatitis. Because of this, it is recommended that lower concentrations of retinoids and hydroquinone be used at onset. Strict photoprotection and sun avoidance should be stressed. Patient should be counseled on expectations. Clearance of postinflammatory changes requires many months.

PERIORBITAL HYPERPIGMENTATION

Periorbital hyperpigmentation is a common cosmetic concern. The cause of this is poorly understood but may be contributed by one or several factors including constitutional skin pigmentation, dermal melanocytosis, postinflammatory pigmentary alteration, edema, increased vascularity, and shadowing from skin laxity and tear trough deformity due to photoaging.[91] It was demonstrated that the lower and lateral parts of the internal canthus have high blood mass and low velocity and therefore contribute to dark circles around eyes.[92]

Medications can also have significant effect in inducing pigmentary changes. Prostaglandin analogs such as latanoprost and bimatoprost, used for the treatment of glaucoma, are a common cause of periorbital hyperpigmentation.[93–95] Bimatoprost-induced hyperpigmentation is noted 3 to 6 months after initiation of treatment and may resolve within 3 to 12 months following discontinuation of the medication.[95] Eyelid biopsies of patients with hyperpigmentation following bimatoprost treatment revealed increased melanosomes and melanin production,[96] which can be explained by the effects of prostaglandins in the melanin synthesis pathway.

Topical lightening agents are useful and can be combined with non-invasive approaches to treat each different factor contributing to pigmentation. Q-switched and Picosecond 532, 755, and 1064 nm lasers have all been found effective in reducing the pigmentary and vascular components in periorbital hyperpigmentation.[60,91] Autologous fat transplantation can aid in providing volume when volume loss is thought to be contributory.[91] Recently, platelet-rich plasma delivered in by dermal injection can help correct tear trough deformity and rhytides.[97] Blepharoplasty can also be trialed if non-invasive treatment fails.

CAMOUFLAGE COSMETICS

In recalcitrant pigmentary disorders, camouflaging agents can be recommended to provide a more natural appearance during the treatment process. These opaque products are formulated to match the normal skin color of a patient and prevent the underlying dyspigmented skin from being visualized. Some companies have developed advanced techniques using spectrophotometers to measure skin color which is then used to create a pigment-rich foundation exactly matching the desired skin color. If such an approach is not possible, camouflaging using complementary colors to hide the unwanted color is suggested. Green can be used to cover red discoloration, while purple is used to cover yellow discoloration. Yellow and white camouflage products are the most effective in treating melasma and brown pigmentation disorders. Patients should then apply their normal facial foundation over the color camouflage in order to achieve the most natural look.

SUMMARY

All skin types are susceptible to disorders of pigmentation. Dyspigmentation can be particularly prominent in people with dark skin tones. Therapy is difficult as it mandates adherence to topical medications, strict photoprotection, and often requires adjunctive procedural interventions.

References

1. Jimbow K, Quevedo WC Jr., Fitzpatrick TB, Szabo G. Some aspects of melanin biology: 1950–1975. *J Invest Dermatol.* 1976; 67(1):72–89.
2. Bolognia JL, Pawelek JM. Biology of hypopigmentation. *J Am Acad Dermatol.* 1988;19(2 Pt 1):217–255.
3. Szabó G, Gerald AB, Pathak MA, Fitzpatrick TB. Racial differences in the fate of melanosomes in human epidermis. *Nature.* 1969;222(5198):1081–1082.

4. Quevedo WC, Fitzpatrick TB, Pathak MA, Jimbow K. Role of light in human skin color variation. *Am J Phys Anthropol.* 1975; 43(3):393–408.

5. Mosher D, Fitzpatrick T, Ortonne J, Hori Y. Hypomelanoses and Hypermelanoses. In: IM F, AZ E, K W, eds. *Fitzpatrick's Dermatology in General Medicine.* 5th ed. New York, NY: McGraw-Hill; 1999:996.

6. Khlgatian MK, Hadshiew IM, Asawananda P, et al. Tyrosinase gene expression is regulated by p53. *J Invest Dermatol.* 2002; 118(1):126–132.

7. Park HY, Russakovsky V, Ohno S, Gilchrest BA. The beta iso-form of protein kinase C stimulates human melanogenesis by activating tyrosinase in pigment cells. *J Biol Chem.* 1993;268(16): 11742–11749.

8. Lee JH, Park JG, Lim SH, et al. Localized intradermal microinjec-tion of tranexamic acid for treatment of melasma in Asian patients: a preliminary clinical trial. *Dermatol Surg.* 2006;32(5):626–631.

9. Tomita Y, Torinuki W, Tagami H. Stimulation of human mela-nocytes by vitamin D3 possibly mediates skin pigmentation after sun exposure. *J Invest Dermatol.* 1988;90(6):882–884.

10. Wei Q, Wu X, Hammer JA 3rd. The predominant defect in dilute melanocytes is in melanosome distribution and not cell shape, supporting a role for myosin V in melanosome transport. *J Muscle Res Cell Motil.* 1997;18(5):517–527.

11. Ogawa K, Hosoya H, Yokota E, et al. Melanoma dynein: evidence that dynein is a general "motor" for microtubule-associated cell motilities. *Eur J Cell Biol.* 1987;43(1):3–9.

12. Nordlund JJ. The melanocyte and the epidermal melanin unit: an expanded concept. *Dermatol Clin.* 2007;25(3):271–281, vii.

13. Van Den Bossche K, Naeyaert JM, Lambert J. The quest for the mechanism of melanin transfer. *Traffic.* 2006;7(7):769–778.

14. Seiberg M, Paine C, Sharlow E, et al. Inhibition of melano-some transfer results in skin lightening. *J Invest Dermatol.* 2000;115(2):162–167.

15. Nystedt S, Emilsson K, Larsson AK, Strömbeck B, Sundelin J. Molecular cloning and functional expression of the gene encod-ing the human proteinase-activated receptor 2. *Eur J Biochem.* 1995;232(1):84–89.

16. Seiberg M. Keratinocyte-melanocyte interactions during mela-nosome transfer. *Pigment Cell Res.* 2001;14(4):236–242.

17. Seiberg M, Paine C, Sharlow E, et al. The protease-activated receptor 2 regulates pigmentation via keratinocyte-melanocyte interactions. *Exp Cell Res.* 2000;254(1):25–32.

18. Wallo W, Nebus J, Leyden JJ. Efficacy of a soy moisturizer in photoaging: a double-blind, vehicle-controlled, 12-week study. *J Drugs Dermatol.* 2007;6(9):917–922.

19. Quast T, Wehner S, Kirfel G, Jaeger K, De Luca M, Herzog V. sAPP as a regulator of dendrite motility and melanin release in epidermal melanocytes and melanoma cells. *FASEB J.* 2003;17(12):1739–1741.

20. Cardinali G, Bolasco G, Aspite N, et al. Melanosome transfer promoted by keratinocyte growth factor in light and dark skin-derived keratinocytes. *J Invest Dermatol.* 2008;128(3):558–567.

21. Valverde P, Healy E, Jackson I, Rees JL, Thody AJ. Variants of the melanocyte-stimulating hormone receptor gene are asso-ciated with red hair and fair skin in humans. *Nat Genet.* 1995; 11(3):328–330.

22. Rees JL. The genetics of sun sensitivity in humans. *Am J Hum Genet.* 2004;75(5):739–751.

23. Inoue K, Hosoi J, Ideta R, Ohta N, Ifuku O, Tsuchiya T. Stress aug-mented ultraviolet-irradiation-induced pigmentation. *J Invest Dermatol.* 2003;121(1):165–171.

24. Hermanns JF, Petit L, Martalo O, Piérard-Franchimont C, Cauwenbergh G, Piérard GE. Unraveling the patterns of sub-clinical pheomelanin-enriched facial hyperpigmentation: effect of depigmenting agents. *Dermatology.* 2000;201(2):118–122.

25. Goukassian DA, Eller MS, Yaar M, Gilchrest BA. Thymidine dinu-cleotide mimics the effect of solar simulated irradiation on p53 and p53-regulated proteins. *J Invest Dermatol.* 1999;112(1):25–31.

26. Gilchrest BA, Eller MS. DNA photodamage stimulates melano-genesis and other photoprotective responses. *J Investig Dermatol Symp Proc.* 1999;4(1):35–40.

27. Cui R, Widlund HR, Feige E, et al. Central role of p53 in the suntan response and pathologic hyperpigmentation. *Cell.* 2007;128(5):853–864.

28. Barsh G, Attardi LD. A healthy tan? *N Engl J Med.* 2007; 356(21):2208–2210.

29. Mahmoud BH, Ruvolo E, Hexsel CL, et al. Impact of long-wave-length UVA and visible light on melanocompetent skin. *J Invest Dermatol.* 2010;130(8):2092–2097.

30. Sklar LR, Almutawa F, Lim HW, Hamzavi I. Effects of ultraviolet radiation, visible light, and infrared radiation on erythema and pig-mentation: a review. *Photochem Photobiol Sci.* 2013;12(1):54–64.

31. Mandry Pagán R, Sánchez JL. Mandibular melasma. *P R Health Sci J.* 2000;19(3):231–234.

32. Kelleher MB, Christopherson WA, Macpherson TA. Disseminated granulomatous disease (BCGosis) following chemoimmu-notherapy for ovarian carcinoma. *Gynecol Oncol.* 1988;31(2): 321–326.

33. Tan SY, Buzney E, Mostaghimi A. Trends in phototherapy utili-zation among Medicare beneficiaries in the United States, 2000 to 2015. *J Am Acad Dermatol.* 2018.

34. Sanchez NP, Pathak MA, Sato S, Fitzpatrick TB, Sanchez JL, Mihm MC Jr. Melasma: a clinical, light microscopic, ultrastruc-tural, and immunofluorescence study. *J Am Acad Dermatol.* 1981;4(6):698–710.

35. Lawrence N, Cox SE, Brody HJ. Treatment of melasma with Jessner's solution versus glycolic acid: a comparison of clinical efficacy and evaluation of the predictive ability of Wood's light examination. *J Am Acad Dermatol.* 1997;36(4):589–593.

36. Ogbechie-Godec OA, Elbuluk N. Melasma: an Up-to-Date Comprehensive Review. *Dermatol Ther.* 2017;7(3):305–318.

37. Goyal K, Nguyen MO, Reynolds RV, et al. Perceptions of U.S. dermatology residency program directors regarding the ade-quacy of phototherapy training during residency. *Photodermatol Photoimmunol Photomed.* 2017;33(6):321–325.

38. Kang HY, Hwang JS, Lee JY, et al. The dermal stem cell factor and c-kit are overexpressed in melasma. *Br J Dermatol.* 2006;154(6): 1094–1099.

39. McLeod SD, Ranson M, Mason RS. Effects of estrogens on human melanocytes in vitro. *J Steroid Biochem Mol Biol.* 1994;49(1):9–14.

40. Grimes PE, Yamada N, Bhawan J. Light microscopic, immuno-histochemical, and ultrastructural alterations in patients with melasma. *Am J Dermatopathol.* 2005;27(2):96–101.

41. Fulton JE Jr. Utilizing the ultraviolet (UV detect) camera to enhance the appearance of photodamage and other skin condi-tions. *Dermatol Surg.* 1997;23(3):163–169.

42. Kligman AM, Willis I. A new formula for depigmenting human skin. *Arch Dermatol.* 1975;111(1):40–48.

43. Orlow SJ, Chakraborty AK, Pawelek JM. Retinoic acid is a potent inhibitor of inducible pigmentation in murine and hamster melanoma cell lines. *J Invest Dermatol.* 1990;94(4):461–464.

44. Griffiths CE, Finkel LJ, Ditre CM, Hamilton TA, Ellis CN, Voorhees JJ. Topical tretinoin (retinoic acid) improves melasma. A vehicle-controlled, clinical trial. *Br J Dermatol.* 1993;129(4): 415–421.

45. Kimbrough-Green CK, Griffiths CE, Finkel LJ, et al. Topical retinoic acid (tretinoin) for melasma in black patients. A vehicle-controlled clinical trial. *Arch Dermatol.* 1994;130(6):727–733.

46. Khunger N, Sarkar R, Jain RK. Tretinoin peels versus glycolic acid peels in the treatment of Melasma in dark-skinned patients. *Dermatol Surg.* 2004;30(5):756–760; discussion 760.

47. Lim JT. Treatment of melasma using kojic acid in a gel containing hydroquinone and glycolic acid. *Dermatol Surg.* 1999;25(4): 282–284.

48. McMichael AJ, Griffiths CE, Talwar HS, et al. Concurrent application of tretinoin (retinoic acid) partially protects against corticosteroid-induced epidermal atrophy. *Br J Dermatol.* 1996;135(1): 60–64.

49. Gheisari M, Dadkhahfar S, Olamaei E, Moghimi HR, Niknejad N, Najar Nobari N. The efficacy and safety of topical 5% methimazole vs 4% hydroquinone in the treatment of melasma: A randomized controlled trial. *J Cosmet Dermatol.* 2020;19(1):167–172.

50. Adalatkhah H, Sadeghi-Bazargani H. The first clinical experience on efficacy of topical flutamide on melasma compared with topical hydroquinone: a randomized clinical trial. *Drug Des Devel Ther.* 2015;9:4219–4225.

51. Mansouri P, Farshi S, Hashemi Z, Kasraee B. Evaluation of the efficacy of cysteamine 5% cream in the treatment of epidermal melasma: a randomized double-blind placebo-controlled trial. *Br J Dermatol.* 2015;173(1):209–217.

52. Zhang L, Tan W-Q, Fang Q-Q, et al. Tranexamic Acid for Adults with Melasma: A Systematic Review and Meta-Analysis. *BioMed Research International.* 2018;2018:1683414–1683414.

53. Lim JT, Tham SN. Glycolic acid peels in the treatment of melasma among Asian women. *Dermatol Surg.* 1997;23(3):177–179.

54. Wang CC, Hui CY, Sue YM, Wong WR, Hong HS. Intense pulsed light for the treatment of refractory melasma in Asian persons. *Dermatol Surg.* 2004;30(9):1196–1200.

55. Moreno Arias GA, Ferrando J. Intense pulsed light for melanocytic lesions. *Dermatol Surg.* 2001;27(4):397–400.

56. Rusciani A, Motta A, Rusciani L, Alfano C. Q-switched alexandrite laser-assisted treatment of melasma: 2-year follow-up monitoring. *J Drugs Dermatol.* 2005;4(6):770–774.

57. Nouri K, Bowes L, Chartier T, Romagosa R, Spencer J. Combination treatment of melasma with pulsed CO2 laser followed by Q-switched alexandrite laser: a pilot study. *Dermatol Surg.* 1999;25(6):494–497.

58. Angsuwarangsee S, Polnikorn N. Combined ultrapulse CO2 laser and Q-switched alexandrite laser compared with Q-switched alexandrite laser alone for refractory melasma: split-face design. *Dermatol Surg.* 2003;29(1):59–64.

59. Rokhsar CK, Fitzpatrick RE. The treatment of melasma with fractional photothermolysis: a pilot study. *Dermatol Surg.* 2005;31(12): 1645–1650.

60. Wu DC, Goldman MP, Wat H, Chan HHL. A Systematic Review of Picosecond Laser in Dermatology: Evidence and Recommendations. *Lasers Surg Med.* 2021;53(1):9–49.

61. Alcantara GP, Esposito ACC, Olivatti TOF, Yoshida MM, Miot HA. Evaluation of ex vivo melanogenic response to UVB, UVA, and visible light in facial melasma and unaffected adjacent skin. *Anais brasileiros de dermatologia.* 2020;95(6):684–690.

62. Boukari F, Jourdan E, Fontas E, et al. Prevention of melasma relapses with sunscreen combining protection against UV and short wavelengths of visible light: a prospective randomized comparative trial. *J Am Acad Dermatol.* 2015;72(1):189–190.e181.

63. Hodgson C. Senile lentigo. *Arch Dermatol.* 1963;87:197–207.

64. Bliss JM, Ford D, Swerdlow AJ, et al. Risk of cutaneous melanoma associated with pigmentation characteristics and freckling: systematic overview of 10 case-control studies. The International Melanoma Analysis Group (IMAGE). *Int J Cancer.* 1995;62(4):367–376.

65. Naldi L, DiLandro A, D'Avanzo B, Parazzini F. Host-related and environmental risk factors for cutaneous basal cell carcinoma: evidence from an Italian case-control study. *J Am Acad Dermatol.* 2000;42(3):446–452.

66. Andersen WK, Labadie RR, Bhawan J. Histopathology of solar lentigines of the face: a quantitative study. *J Am Acad Dermatol.* 1997;36(3 Pt 1):444–447.

67. Humphreys TR, Werth V, Dzubow L, Kligman A. Treatment of photodamaged skin with trichloroacetic acid and topical tretinoin. *J Am Acad Dermatol.* 1996;34(4):638–644.

68. Collins PS. Trichloroacetic acid peels revisited. *J Dermatol Surg Oncol.* 1989;15(9):933–940.

69. Newman N, Newman A, Moy LS, Babapour R, Harris AG, Moy RL. Clinical improvement of photoaged skin with 50% glycolic acid. A double-blind vehicle-controlled study. *Dermatol Surg.* 1996;22(5):455–460.

70. Lugo-Janer A, Lugo-Somolinos A, Sanchez JL. Comparison of trichloroacetic acid solution and cryosurgery in the treatment of solar lentigines. *Int J Dermatol.* 2003;42(10):829–831.

71. Ortonne JP, Pandya AG, Lui H, Hexsel D. Treatment of solar lentigines. *J Am Acad Dermatol.* 2006;54(5 Suppl 2):S262–S271.

72. Hexsel DM, Mazzuco R, Bohn J, Borges J, Gobbato DO. Clinical comparative study between cryotherapy and local dermabrasion for the treatment of solar lentigo on the back of the hands. *Dermatol Surg.* 2000;26(5):457–462.

73. Ho SG, Yeung CK, Chan NP, Shek SY, Chan HH. A comparison of Q-switched and long-pulsed alexandrite laser for the treatment of freckles and lentigines in oriental patients. *Lasers Surg Med.* 2011;43(2):108–113.

74. Chan HH, Fung WK, Ying SY, Kono T. An in vivo trial comparing the use of different types of 532 nm Nd:YAG lasers in the treatment of facial lentigines in Oriental patients. *Dermatol Surg.* 2000;26(8):743–749.

75. Narurkar VA, Alster TS, Bernstein EF, Lin TJ, Loncaric A. Safety and Efficacy of a 1550nm/1927nm Dual Wavelength Laser for the Treatment of Photodamaged Skin. *J Drugs Dermatol.* 2018;17(1):41–46.

76. Wang CC, Sue YM, Yang CH, Chen CK. A comparison of Q-switched alexandrite laser and intense pulsed light for the treatment of freckles and lentigines in Asian persons: a randomized, physician-blinded, split-face comparative trial. *J Am Acad Dermatol.* 2006;54(5):804–810.

77. Fleischer AB Jr., Schwartzel EH, Colby SI, Altman DJ. The combination of 2% 4-hydroxyanisole (Mequinol) and 0.01% tretinoin is effective in improving the appearance of solar lentigines and related hyperpigmented lesions in two double-blind multicenter clinical studies. *J Am Acad Dermatol.* 2000;42(3):459–467.

78. Colby SI, Schwartzel EH, Huber FJ, et al. A promising new treatment for solar lentigines. *J Drugs Dermatol.* 2003;2(2):147–152.

79. Ortonne JP, Camacho F, Wainwright N, Bergfelt L, Westerhof W, Roseeuw D. Safety and efficacy of combined use of 4-hydroxy-anisole (mequinol) 2%/tretinoin 0.01% solution and sunscreen in solar lentigines. *Cutis.* 2004;74(4):261–264.

80. Kang S, Goldfarb MT, Weiss JS, et al. Assessment of adapalene gel for the treatment of actinic keratoses and lentigines: a randomized trial. *J Am Acad Dermatol.* 2003;49(1):83–90.

81. Phillips TJ, Gottlieb AB, Leyden JJ, et al. Efficacy of 0.1% tazarotene cream for the treatment of photodamage: a 12-month multicenter, randomized trial. *Arch Dermatol.* 2002;138(11): 1486–1493.

82. Phillips TJ. Tazarotene 0.1% cream for the treatment of photodamage. *Skin Therapy Lett.* 2004;9(4):1–2.

83. Salisbury JR, Williams H, du Vivier AW. Tanning-bed lentigines: ultrastructural and histopathologic features. *J Am Acad Dermatol.* 1989;21(4 Pt 1):689–693.

84. Roth DE, Hodge SJ, Callen JP. Possible ultraviolet A-induced lentigines: a side effect of chronic tanning salon usage. *J Am Acad Dermatol.* 1989;20(5 Pt 2):950–954.

85. Burns RL, Prevost-Blank PL, Lawry MA, Lawry TB, Faria DT, Fivenson DP. Glycolic acid peels for postinflammatory hyperpigmentation in black patients. A comparative study. *Dermatol Surg.* 1997;23(3):171–174; discussion 175.

86. Grimes PE, Stockton T. Pigmentary disorders in blacks. *Dermatol Clin.* 1988;6(2):271–281.

87. Ruiz-Maldonado R, Orozco-Covarrubias ML. Postinflammatory hypopigmentation and hyperpigmentation. *Semin Cutan Med Surg.* 1997;16(1):36–43.

88. Fairley JA. Tretinoin (retinoic acid) revisited. *N Engl J Med.* 1993;328(20):1486–1487.

89. Gaulding JV, Gutierrez D, Bhatia BK, et al. Epidemiology of Skin Diseases in a Diverse Patient Population. *J Drugs Dermatol.* 2018;17(10):1032–1036.

90. Wong SN, Khoo LS. Chronic actinic dermatitis as the presenting feature of HIV infection in three Chinese males. *Clin Exp Dermatol.* 2003;28(3):265–268.

91. Roh MR, Chung KY. Infraorbital dark circles: definition, causes, and treatment options. *Dermatol Surg.* 2009;35(8):1163–1171.

92. Tojo N, Yoshimura N, Yoshizawa M, et al. Vitiligo and chronic photosensitivity in human immunodeficiency virus infection. *Jpn J Med.* 1991;30(3):255–259.

93. Kook MS, Lee K. Increased eyelid pigmentation associated with use of latanoprost. *Am J Ophthalmol.* 2000;129(6):804–806.

94. Wand M. Latanoprost and hyperpigmentation of eyelashes. *Arch Ophthalmol.* 1997;115(9):1206–1208.

95. Doshi M, Edward DP, Osmanovic S. Clinical course of bimatoprost-induced periocular skin changes in Caucasians. *Ophthalmology.* 2006;113(11):1961–1967.

96. Kapur R, Osmanovic S, Toyran S, Edward DP. Bimatoprost-induced periocular skin hyperpigmentation: histopathological study. *Arch Ophthalmol.* 2005;123(11):1541–1546.

97. Mehryan P, Zartab H, Rajabi A, Pazhoohi N, Firooz A. Assessment of efficacy of platelet-rich plasma (PRP) on infraorbital dark circles and crow's feet wrinkles. *J Cosmet Dermatol.* 2014;13(1): 72–78.

CHAPTER 21

Wrinkled Skin

Mary D. Sun, MSCR, MA
Edmund M. Weisberg, MS, MBE
Leslie S. Baumann, MD

SUMMARY POINTS

What's Important?

1. Facial wrinkles are a common, yet frequently distressing, consequence of physiological aging processes.
2. Wrinkles are most commonly treated with injections of botulinum neurotoxin type A, which are commercially available in multiple preparations. These treatments are now the most frequently performed cosmetic procedures in the United States.

What's New?

1. Soft tissue fillers, also delivered via facial injection, have become increasingly popular for midface augmentation and the treatment of facial wrinkles.
2. New evidence supports the potential efficacy of topical products containing antioxidants, peptides, and various growth factors in treating skin aging.

What's Coming?

1. Additional research is needed to determine the effects of multiple treatment cycles, frequency of significant adverse events, and duration of the effects of botulinum neurotoxin injections.
2. Future treatment mechanisms may result from an improved understanding of the mechanisms underlying age-related changes to neuroendocrine pathways, thyroid function regulation, and lipid metabolism.

The desire to maintain or restore a youthful appearance has become a significant concern for many people in today's world. Evidently, "wrinkles" are considered one of the major obstacles in this arena. Studies of differently aged men and women across multiple ethnicities have found that facial wrinkles (as a measure of skin texture) were a major factor in the assessment of perceived age and tiredness, providing some context for one of the most popular cosmetic dermatology procedures.[1,2] Injections of botulinum neurotoxin type A, more commonly known as Botox Cosmetic™ injections, are the most frequently performed cosmetic procedure in the United States.[3] A 2021 systematic review of 65 randomized controlled trials involving 14,919 participants found that botulinum toxin type A reduced wrinkles within 4 weeks of treatment but probably increased the risk of ptosis; evidence was absent on the effects of multiple cycles of botulinum toxin type A use, the frequency of adverse events, the duration of effects, and comparisons with other treatments.[4] Aesthetic concerns also remain regarding the use of Botox for the neck, where it has not been found to be particularly effective.[5]

Cutaneous wrinkles, defined as furrows or ridges on the skin surface, appear to be multifactorial in etiology and a consequence of intrinsic and extrinsic aging (discussed in Chapters 5, Intrinsic Aging, and 6, Extrinsic Aging). While genetic predisposition is an important factor in developing wrinkles, engaging in particular lifestyle behaviors such as excessive sun exposure and smoking are also known causes of cutaneous aging (see Chapter 6). This chapter will concentrate on wrinkles not caused by sun exposure, but rather by intrinsic aging. Treatment approaches focus more on the condition itself, but also address behavioral elements pertaining to extrinsic aging.

AGING

Aging is a process that occurs in all organs but is most visible in the skin. The skin may very well reflect or act as an outward sign of processes occurring in the internal organs. Notably, wrinkles are one aspect of a validated photonumeric assessment scale used to evaluate the quality of female facial skin (the other five aspects are skin elasticity, age, pigmentation, erythema, and overall skin quality).[6] Further, the amount of facial wrinkling, the formation of which is associated with solar (actinic) elastosis,[7] has been shown to correlate with the extent of lung disease in COPD.[8] Diminished skin elasticity has also been linked to pulmonary emphysema, biomarkers of inflammation, and matrix metalloproteinase (MMP) activity in smokers.[9] In addition to COPD, wrinkle scores are correlated with lung function/airflow obstruction, with facial wrinkle scores related to oxidative stress.[10,11]

The naturally occurring functional decline of organs with age can be exacerbated by environmental factors, but there is certainly a genetic component that influences the aging process. In fact, data compiled in just the last few years suggest that genes are implicated in premature aging beyond their known involvement in premature aging syndromes such as Werner's syndrome (**Table 21-1**).[12-14] Human collagen alpha-2 type I (encoded by the COL1A2 gene) stimulates collagen synthesis, wound healing, and elastin production in normal human dermal fibroblasts.[15] Some soluble factors, such as IL-6, IL-8, and monocyte chemotactic protein-3 are induced by solar radiation *in vitro* and may be involved in facial subcutaneous fat loss that manifests as skin atrophy and wrinkle formation.[16,17] Ribosomal protein S3-derived repair domain peptides regulate ultraviolet (UV)-induced MMP-1 and could help prevent UV-induced wrinkle formation.[18] MicroRNAs (specifically the miR-34 family) are upregulated by UVB irradiation and degrade collagen in the extracellular matrix (ECM) due to the activation of MMPs, thus potentiating wrinkle formation.[19] Menopause, UV exposure, and low water intake may interact with genetic variants related to collagen metabolism to influence skin wrinkle risk in middle-aged women.[20] Mammalian cells can undergo only a certain number of cell divisions before replicative senescence occurs and they are no longer able to divide.[21] This may be nature's way of preventing these cells from becoming cancerous; however, this process plays a role in aging as well.

Pathology and Etiology

The histopathology of wrinkles is a combination of interesting findings. Epidermal thinning is an outstanding microscopic feature, where the atrophy is more prominent in the deepest area of the wrinkle (Fig. 6–8). Other changes include flattening of the dermal-epidermal junction, atrophy of the subcutaneous adipose tissue of the hypodermis, as well as the loss of collagen, glycosaminoglycans, and elastin tissue.

Collagen Loss

Abnormal and reduced collagen is a major finding in the pathology of wrinkles, both in sun-exposed and non-sun-exposed skin.[22] Collagen modification in wrinkled skin can be characterized in terms of the multifaceted signaling pathways and molecules playing important regulatory roles in the skin aging process. It is well known that collagen synthesis is decreased in aging skin. In addition, with higher MMP levels collagen degradation appears to increase with aging. This is because MMPs can degrade almost all ECM constituents that maintain the structural integrity of skin components, including collagen, fibronectin, elastin, and proteoglycan.[23] UV radiation also activates MMPs and induces their expression in skin, thus linking sun exposure/oxidative damage and skin photoaging.[24] Further, cyclic adenosine monophosphate (cAMP) regulates MMP expression by affecting the MAPK/AP-1 pathway, leading to collagen degradation.[25] Another explanation for abnormal dermal collagen in cutaneous aging is collagen glycation.[26] As discussed in Chapter 2, Basic Science of the Dermis, glycation of collagen is a nonenzymatic process that involves the addition of a reducing sugar molecule to ECM collagen and proteins. Following an oxidative reaction, the end products of glycated collagen and proteins, known as advanced glycation end products (AGEs), are formed. The AGEs are then deposited on the collagen and elastin tissue, rendering them stiffer and less susceptible to contracture and remodeling.[27] In addition, glycated collagen modifies the actin cytoskeleton of fibroblasts and inhibits their contracture effect on the collagen.[28] Glycated elastin fibers abnormally aggregate and interact with lysozymes in the skin of sun-exposed skin, indicating that glycation is involved in photoaging.[29] AGEs can interact with certain receptors to induce intracellular signaling that leads to enhanced oxidative stress and elaboration of key pro-inflammatory cytokines. The resulting free radicals and cytokines lead to a breakdown of collagen.[30]

Decorin, a small leucine-rich proteoglycan (SLRP) found in the ECM protein, is involved in "decorating" the collagen (see Chapter 2). It is shaped in a "horseshoe" pattern and holds collagen fibers in the proper arrangement.[31] Interestingly, a fragment of decorin known as "decorunt" has been shown to be higher in adult versus fetal skin.[32] Since decorunt has a lower affinity for collagen fibers, the breakdown of decorin to decorunt may play a role in the disorganization of the dermal collagen network seen in aged skin.

Both versican and decorin show age-related differences in human skin, with versican in the size and sulfation pattern of its glycosaminoglycans and decorin in the size of its glycosaminoglycans. Catabolic fragments of versican are detected in skin of all ages but are lower in adult skin compared with fetal skin. In contrast, catabolic fragments of decorin are present in adult skin but nearly absent from fetal skin. This suggests that

TABLE 21-1.	Premature Aging Syndromes[a]
Syndrome	Defect
Werner's syndrome[12]	DNA helicase
Cockayne syndrome[13]	DNA helicase
Progeria[14]	Lamin A

[a]These premature aging syndromes suggest that DNA repair capacity is very important to mitigate aging.

there are age-related differences in the catabolism of proteo-glycans in human skin that play a role in age-related changes.[33]

Elastin Degradation

Wrinkled skin is known to exhibit decreased resilience because of abnormal elastic tissue. In the setting of UV exposure, the quantity of elastase, the enzyme responsible for degrading elastin, increases and leads to "elastosis," a hallmark of photoaged skin. However, studies have demonstrated that nonexposed aged skin also displays less elastin tissue.[34,35] The aging of elastin fibers is a convoluted process involving enzymatic degradation, oxidative damage, glycation, calcification, and mechanical fatigue.[36]

Telomere Shortening

Telomeres are the terminal portions of mammalian chromosomes that are composed of hundreds of short sequences of repeating TTAGGG base pairs. They cap the ends of chromosomes preventing fusion.[37] During cell division, when the chromosomes divide, the enzyme DNA polymerase cannot replicate the final base pairs of the chromosome. Therefore, these terminal sequences are continuously lost on replication, resulting in shortening of the chromosome. When telomeres get "too short," apoptosis of the cells is triggered. For this reason, telomeres are thought to play a role in aging. Telomerase is a reverse transcriptase enzyme found in stem cells that can replicate the terminal base pairs, but this enzyme is not found in most cells. Many ongoing studies are looking at the role of telomerase in aging and cancer.

UV exposure may contribute to telomere shortening. Telomeres normally exist in a loop configuration, with the loop held in place by the final 150 to 200 bases on the 3' strand that form a single-stranded overhang (**Figs. 21-1A and B**). It is believed that when the loop is disrupted and the overhang becomes exposed, p53 (a tumor suppressor protein) and other DNA damage response proteins are induced,[38] resulting in apoptosis or senescence. Telomeres are also strong signals of autocrine and paracrine DNA damage that occur during skin aging.[39] UV light leads to the bonding together of thymine dimers, which may lead to disruption of the telomere loop (**Fig. 21-2**). This is one way to explain the overlap seen in intrinsic and extrinsic aging. It is also worth noting that a genome-wide association study (GWAS) for self-reported facial aging with 417,772 participants drawn from the UK Biobank found an association between genetically predicted telomere length and facial skin aging.[40]

The Immune System

Aging is associated with an increase in pro-inflammatory cytokines (see Chapter 8, Immunology of Skin Aging). These cytokines result in inflammation, which plays a role in degrading collagen and elastin as well as other vital skin components. The role of cytokines in aging has not been completely elucidated, but this will likely be an area of extreme interest in upcoming research. The functioning of antigen-presenting cells, T cells, and B cells declines with age. T cells are particularly susceptible to age-related changes, which can be accelerated due to thymic degeneration, metabolic abnormalities, telomere shortening, and epigenetic changes associated with aging. In addition to reducing immune function, T cell loss can induce inflammation (referred to as immunosenescence) that disrupts biological homeostasis and leads to the progression of pathologies such as cardiovascular disease.[41] These changes are thought to contribute to the higher risk of infections and cancer observed in older patients.[42]

The Endocrine System

The endocrine system may contribute to aging. Cutaneous neuroendocrine pathways that regulate the production of

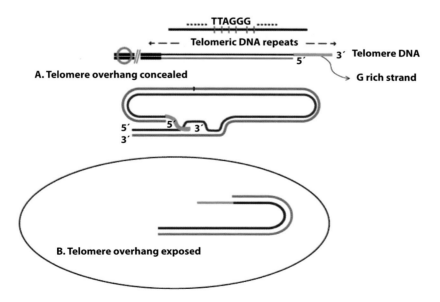

FIGURE 21-1. A. Telomeres in normal loop configuration. The 3-prime end is held in place by the last 150 to 200 base pairs on the 3-prime strand. **B.** Once damaged, the loop structure opens and the 3-prime end is exposed. (Adapted from p. 965 *Fitzpatrick's, 7th edition.*)

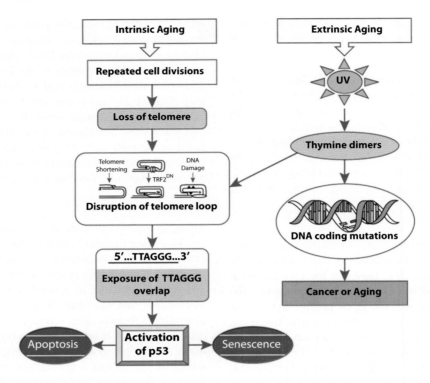

FIGURE 21-2. Extrinsic aging and intrinsic aging can both result in the same outcome—cellular apoptosis or senescence. This diagram shows the proposed mechanisms in which these two processes overlap to lead to aging. Repeated cell division, thymine dimers, and other causes of telomere damage cause disruption of the telomere loop. This leads to exposure of the TTAGGG overlap and activation of p53. (*Yaar M, Gilchrest BA. Photoageing: mechanism, prevention and therapy. Br J Derm. 2007;157(5):874–87.*)

neuropeptides, neurohormones, and neurotransmitters can decay with age/pathological malfunctions.[43] Hormones, especially estrogens and androgens, are significant factors in the aging of skin (see Chapter 5). The loss of estrogens with age generally leads to a decline in cutaneous health, whereas hormone therapy helps to restore it.[44] Additionally, epigenetic mechanisms that directly regulate skin homeostasis and regeneration also mark cell senescence and are believed to play important roles in aging processes.[45] Further, recent findings are beginning to elucidate the ways in which insulin, vitamin D, and thyroid hormone levels influence skin aging.

Insulin

Animal models suggest that age-related changes may interact antagonistically with insulin/IGF-1-like signaling necessary for the maintenance of lipid stores.[46]

Vitamin D

Two 2021 studies suggest that the demand for vitamin D (calcitriol) increases with age, as the depleted stores of vitamin D in older adults have been shown to be less able to exert protective anti-aging effects, which has been correlated with inflammatory markers in overweight older adults.[47,48]

Thyroid Hormone

Thyroid hormones are central to muscle function and energy metabolism. A 2021 study by Di Iorio et al. found that nonagenarians with higher FT3/FT4 ratios had lower levels of muscle aging.[49]

PREVENTION AND TREATMENT

Identifying skin types predisposed to wrinkling is the first step in patient management. The Baumann Skin Typing System (Chapter 10) is a useful classification approach, aiding physicians and patients to understand and manage their skin needs to prevent and treat wrinkles. Other classification systems also help physicians quantify the amount of wrinkling. After assessing the degree of wrinkling, patient education is the next essential step. Patients must understand that prevention of additional wrinkling is the mainstay of managing wrinkled skin. Effects of certain behaviors such as excessive sun exposure and smoking should be discussed, and treatment plans with expected and realistic results should be explained in detail with patients.

It is well known that sunscreen and sun avoidance are key elements in preventing extrinsic photoaging. Although UVA is more often implicated in cutaneous aging, coverage for both UVA and UVB is recommended when selecting a sunscreen. A routine skin regimen containing retinoid application is also valuable in both the prevention and treatment of aging skin. Topical retinoids have been shown to both increase collagen synthesis[50] and decrease the MMPs involved in collagen and elastin degradation.[51] Since oxidative stress resulting from UV irradiation and free radicals are implicated in skin aging, antioxidants have an important role in the prevention and treatment of wrinkles (see Chapter 39, Antioxidants). Of the numerous antioxidants, vitamin C (ascorbic acid) deserves special attention. Vitamin C is well recognized for its role in the collagen synthesis pathway via the prolyl hydroxylase enzyme. Studies have revealed a reduction of wrinkles following topical application of ascorbic acid,[52–54] correlating with increased collagen on histology of the treated areas.[53] Recently, studies of topical serums consisting of vitamins C and E combined with green tea polyphenols have found them able to ameliorate the visual condition of photoaged facial skin.[55–57]

Other antioxidants such as retinol, peptides, growth factors, and coenzyme Q_{10} (ubiquinone), as we as polyphenols such as green tea are also believed to be of value in the prevention and treatment of aging.[58–60] A double-blind, placebo-controlled study by Heinrich et al. in 2011 found that supplementation with green tea polyphenols significantly reduced UV-induced erythema in facial skin, and also improved elasticity, roughness, density, as well as water homeostasis, and increased blood flow to the skin.[61]

In recent years, photorejuvenation has become a popular approach to wrinkle reduction. Procedures with intense pulsed light (IPL) and light emitting diodes (LEDs) have also shown promising results in the treatment of wrinkled skin and photoaging (see Chapter 26, Lasers and Light Devices).[62–65] Further, the use of soft tissue fillers, particularly those containing hyaluronic acid, has become an increasingly popular way to correct facial wrinkles, especially of the midface.[66,67] Polymethylmethacrylate (PMMA), poly-L-lactic acid (PLLA), calcium hydroxyapatite (CaHA), and autologous fat are among the non-hyaluronic acid fillers used.

CONCLUSION

Much remains to be learned regarding the science or biomechanics of aging. However, the field is rapidly progressing with increased knowledge about the roles of genetics, stem cells, telomeres, the immune system, and hormones. Advances in these theoretical realms and in the laboratory will likely lead to novel therapies in the future. Specific preventive measures and treatment modalities are well recognized and discussed at length in various chapters of this book, including the roles of diet and cigarette smoking. Sunscreen and topical retinoids are the basic treatment options, proven to be valuable in treating wrinkled skin. Retinoids improve skin texture in intrinsically aged skin as well as photodamaged skin. Patient education and compliance, which are crucial in this matter, may be achieved by providing thorough information, including illustrations of the benefits of treatments and behavioral changes and the disadvantages of noncompliance.

References

1. Flament F, Abric A, Prunel A, et al. The respective weights of facial signs on the perception of age and a tired-look among differently aged Korean men. *Skin Res Technol.* 2021;27(5):909–917.

2. Flament F, Abric A, Adam AS. Evaluating the respective weights of some facial signs on perceived ages in differently aged women of five ethnic origins. *J Cosmet Dermatol.* 2021;20(3):842—853.

3. Galadari H, Galadari I, Smit R, et al. Use of AbobotulinumtoxinA for Cosmetic Treatments in the Neck, and Middle and Lower Areas of the Face: A Systematic Review. *Toxins* (Basel). 2021;13(2):169.

4. Camargo CP, Xia J, Costa CS, et al. Botulinum toxin type A for facial wrinkles. *Cochrane Database Syst Rev.* 2021;7(7):CD011301.

5. Qiu H, Zhao R, Cao L, et al. The Aesthetic Concerns of Botulinum Toxin Type A in the Treatment of Neck Wrinkles: A Systematic Review. *Aesthet Surg J.* 2021;41(6):NP592–NP601.

6. Eiben-Nielson C, Kerscher M. Development and validation of a global photonumeric scale for evaluating skin quality of aged female facial skin. *J Cosmet Dermatol.* 2021 Mar 10. Online ahead of print.

7. Tsukahara K, Tamatsu Y, Sugawara Y, et al. Morphological study of the relationship between solar elastosis and the development of wrinkles on the forehead and lateral canthus. *Arch Dermatol.* 2012;148(8):913–917.

8. Patel BD, Loo WJ, Tasker AD, et al. Smoking related COPD and facial wrinkling: is there a common susceptibility? *Thorax.* 2006;61(7):568–571.

9. O'Brien ME, Chandra D, Wilson RC, et al. Loss of skin elasticity is associated with pulmonary emphysema, biomarkers of inflammation, and matrix metalloproteinase activity in smokers. *Respir Res.* 2019;20(1):128.

10. Vierkötter A, Schikowski T, Sugiri D, et al. MMP-1 and -3 promoter variants are indicative of a common susceptibility for skin and lung aging: results from a cohort of elderly women (SALIA). *J Invest Dermatol.* 2015;135(5):1268–1274.

11. Tsuchida K, Kobayashi M. Oxidative stress in human facial skin observed by ultraweak photon emission imaging and its correlation with biophysical properties of skin. *Sci Rep.* 2020;10(1):9626.

12. Yu CE, Oshima J, Fu YH, et al. Positional cloning of the Werner's syndrome gene. *Science.* 1996;272(5259):258–262.

13. Troelstra C, van Gool A, de Wit J, et al. ERCC6, a member of a subfamily of putative helicases, is involved in Cockayne's syndrome and preferential repair of active genes. *Cell.* 1992;71(6):939–953.

14. De Sandre-Giovannoli A, Bernard R, Cau P, et al. Lamin A truncation in Hutchinson-Gilford progeria. *Science.* 2003;300(5628):2055.

15. Hwang SJ, Ha GH, Seo WY, et al. Human collagen alpha-2 type I stimulates collagen synthesis, wound healing, and elastin production in normal human dermal fibroblasts (HDFs). *BMB Rep.* 2020;53(10):539–544.

16. Li WH, Pappas A, Zhang L, et al. IL-11, IL-1α, IL-6, and TNF-α are induced by solar radiation in vitro and may be involved in facial subcutaneous fat loss in vivo. *J Dermatol Sci.* 2013;71(1):58–66.

17. Geng R, Kang SG, Huang K, et al. Boosting the Photoaged Skin: The Potential Role of Dietary Components. *Nutrients.* 2021;13(5):1691.

18. Yang HW, Jung Y, Kim HD, et al. Ribosomal protein S3-derived repair domain peptides regulate UV-induced matrix metalloproteinase-1. *Biochem Biophys Res Commun.* 2020;530(1):149–154.

19. Gerasymchuk M, Cherkasova V, Kovalchuk O, et al. The Role of microRNAs in Organismal and Skin Aging. *Int J Mol Sci.* 2020;21(15):5281.

20. Park S, Kang S, Lee WJ. Menopause, Ultraviolet Exposure, and Low Water Intake Potentially Interact with the Genetic Variants Related to Collagen Metabolism Involved in Skin Wrinkle Risk in Middle-Aged Women. *Int J Environ Res Public Health.* 2021;18(4):2044.

21. Campisi J. Replicative senescence: an old lives's tale? *Cell.* 1996;84(4);497–500.

22. Varani J, Fisher GJ, Kang S, et al. Molecular mechanisms of intrinsic skin aging and retinoid-induced repair and reversal. *J Investig Dermatol Symp Proc.* 1998;3(1):57–60.

23. Quan T, Qin Z, Xia W, et al. Matrix-degrading metalloproteinases in photoaging. *J Investig Dermatol Symp Proc.* 2009;14(1):20–24.

24. Lu J, Guo JH, Tu XL, et al. Tiron Inhibits UVB-Induced AP-1 Binding Sites Transcriptional Activation on MMP-1 and MMP-3 Promoters by MAPK Signaling Pathway in Human Dermal Fibroblasts. *PLoS One.* 2016;11(8):e0159998.

25. Kang W, Choi D, Park T. Decanal Protects against UVB-Induced Photoaging in Human Dermal Fibroblasts via the cAMP Pathway. *Nutrients.* 2020;12(5):1214.

26. Dyer DG, Dunn JA, Thorpe SR, et al. Accumulation of Maillard reaction products in skin collagen in diabetes and aging. *J Clin Invest.* 1993;91(6):2463–2469.

27. Iwamura M, Yamamoto Y, Kitayama Y, et al. Epidermal expression of receptor for advanced glycation end products (RAGE) is related to inflammation and apoptosis in human skin. *Exp Dermatol.* 2016;25(3):235–237.

28. Howard EW, Benton R, Ahern-Moore J, et al. Cellular contraction of collagen lattices is inhibited by nonenzymatic glycation. *Exp Cell Res.* 1996;228(1):132–137.

29. Zhang S, Duan E. Fighting against Skin Aging: The Way from Bench to Bedside. *Cell Transplant.* 2018;27(5):729–738.

30. Goh SY, Cooper ME. Clinical review: The role of advanced glycation end products in progression and complications of diabetes. *J Clin Endocrinol Metab.* 2008;93(4):1143–1152.

31. Scott JE. Proteodermatan and proteokeratan sulfate (decorin, lumican/fibromodulin) proteins are horseshoe shaped. Implications for their interactions with collagen. *Biochemistry.* 1996;35(27):8795–8799.

32. Carrino DA, Onnerfjord P, Sandy JD, et al. Age-related changes in the proteoglycans of human skin. Specific cleavage of decorin to yield a major catabolic fragment in adult skin. *J Biol Chem.* 2003;278(19):17566–17572.

33. Carrino DA, Calabro A, Darr AB, et al. Age-related differences in human skin proteoglycans. *Glycobiology.* 2011;21(2):257–268.

34. El-Domyati M, Attia S, Saleh F, et al. Intrinsic aging vs. photoaging: a comparative histopathological, immunohistochemical, and ultrastructural study of skin. *Exp Dermatol.* 2002;11(5):398–405.

35. Seite S, Zucchi H, Septier D, et al. Elastin changes during chronological and photo-ageing: the important role of lysozyme. *J Eur Acad Dermatol Venereol.* 2006;20(8):980–987.

36. Heinz A. Elastic fibers during aging and disease. *Ageing Res Rev.* 2021;66:101255.

37. Blackburn EH. Switching and signaling at the telomere. *Cell.* 2001;106(6):661–673.

38. Eller MS, Puri N, Hadshiew IM, et al. Induction of apoptosis by telomere 3′ overhang-specific DNA. *Exp Cell Res.* 2002;276(2):185–193.

39. Victorelli S, Passos JF. Telomeres: beacons of autocrine and paracrine DNA damage during skin aging. *Cell Cycle.* 2020;19(5):532–540.

40. Zhan Y, Hägg S. Association between genetically predicted telomere length and facial skin aging in the UK Biobank: a Mendelian randomization study. *Geroscience.* 2021;43(3):1519–1525.

41. Shirakawa K, Sano M. T Cell Immunosenescence in Aging, Obesity, and Cardiovascular Disease. *Cells.* 2021;10(9):2435.

42. Yaar M, Gilchrest BA. Aging of skin. In: Wolff K, Goldsmith LA, Katz SI, Gilchrest BA, Paller AS, Leffell DJ, eds. *Fitzpatrick's Dermatology in General Medicine.* 7th ed. New York, NY: McGraw-Hill; 2007: 963.

43. Bocheva G, Slominski RM, Slominski AT. Neuroendocrine Aspects of Skin Aging. *Int J Mol Sci.* 2019;20(11):2798.

44. Lephart ED. A review of the role of estrogen in dermal aging and facial attractiveness in women. *J Cosmet Dermatol.* 2018;17(3):282–288.

45. Orioli D, Dellambra E. Epigenetic Regulation of Skin Cells in Natural Aging and Premature Aging Diseases. *Cells.* 2018;7(12):268.

46. Clark JF, Ciccarelli EJ, Kayastha P, et al. BMP pathway regulation of insulin signaling components promotes lipid storage in Caenorhabditis elegans. *PLoS Genet.* 2021;17(10):e1009836.

47. Li W, Che X, Chen X, et al. Study of calcitriol anti-aging effects on human natural killer cells in vitro. *Bioengineered.* 2021 Dec;12(1):6844–6854.

48. Dewansingh P, Reckman GAR, Mijlius CF, et al. Protein, Calcium, vitamin D Intake and 25(OH)D Status in Normal Weight, Overweight, and Obese Older Adults: A Systematic Review and Meta-Analysis. *Front Nutr.* 2021;8:718658.

49. Di Iorio A, Paganelli R, Abate M, et al. Thyroid hormone signaling is associated with physical performance, muscle mass, and strength in a cohort of oldest-old: results from the Mugello study. *Geroscience.* 2021;43(2):1053–1064.

50. Woodley DT, Zelickson AS, Briggaman RA, et al. Treatment of photoaged skin with topical tretinoin increases epidermal-dermal anchoring fibrils. A preliminary report. *JAMA.* 1990;263(22):3057–3059.

51. Fisher GJ, Datta SC, Talwar HS, et al. Molecular basis of sun-induced premature skin ageing and retinoid antagonism. *Nature.* 1996;379(6563):335–339.

52. Humbert PG, Haftek M, Creidi P, et al. Topical ascorbic acid on photoaged skin. Clinical, topographical and ultrastructural evaluation: double-blind study vs. placebo. *Exp Dermatol.* 2003;12(3):237–244.

53. Fitzpatrick RE, Rostan EF. Double-blind, half-face study comparing topical vitamin C and vehicle for rejuvenation of photodamage. *Dermatol Surg.* 2002;28(3):231–236.

54. Traikovich SS. Use of topical ascorbic acid and its effects on photodamaged skin topography. *Arch Otolaryngol Head Neck Surg.* 1999;125(10):1091–1098.

55. Jagdeo J, Kurtti A, Hernandez S, et al. Novel vitamin C and E and Green Tea Polyphenols Combination Serum Improves Photoaged Facial Skin. *J Drugs Dermatol.* 2021;20(9):996–1003.

56. Serra M, Bohnert K, Narda M, et al. Brightening and Improvement of Facial Skin Quality in Healthy Female Subjects With Moderate Hyperpigmentation or Dark Spots and Moderate Facial Aging. *J Drugs Dermatol.* 2018;17(12):1310–1315.

57. Enescu CD, Bedford LM, Potts G, et al. A review of topical vitamin C derivatives and their efficacy. *J Cosmet Dermatol.* 2021 Sep 24. Epub ahead of print.

58. Farris P, Draelos ZD, Felipe de Oliveira Stehling L. Novel Facial Treatment Regimen Improves Aging Skin Appearance. *J Drugs Dermatol.* 2021;20(3):274–278.

59. Miller-Kobisher B, Suárez-Vega DV, Velazco de Maldonado GJ. Epidermal Growth Factor in Aesthetics and Regenerative Medicine: Systematic Review. *J Cutan Aesthet Surg.* 2021;14 (2):137–146.

60. Kafi R, Kwak HS, Schumacher WE, et al. Improvement of naturally aged skin with vitamin A (retinol). *Arch Dermatol.* 2007;143(5):606–612.

61. Heinrich U, Moore CE, De Spirt S, et al. Green tea polyphenols provide photoprotection, increase microcirculation, and modulate skin properties of women. *J Nutr.* 2011;141(6):1202–1208.

62. Sadick NS, Weiss R, Kilmer S, et al. Photorejuvenation with intense pulsed light: results of a multi-center study. *J Drugs Dermatol.* 2004;3(1):41–49.

63. Brazil J, Owens P. Long-term clinical results of IPL photorejuvenation. *J Cosmet Laser Ther.* 2003;5(3-4):168–174.

64. Trelles MA, Allones I, Velez M. Non-ablative facial skin photorejuvenation with an intense pulsed light system and adjunctive epidermal care. *Lasers Med Sci.* 2003;18(2):104–111.

65. Trelles MA. Phototherapy in anti-aging and its photobiologic basics: a new approach to skin rejuvenation. *J Cosmet Dermatol.* 2006;5(1):87–91.

66. Trinh LN, Gupta A. Non-Hyaluronic Acid Fillers for Midface Augmentation: A Systematic Review. *Facial Plast Surg.* 2021;37(4):536–542.

67. Trinh LN, Gupta A. Hyaluronic Acid Fillers for Midface Augmentation: A Systematic Review. *Facial Plast Surg.* 2021;37 (5):576–584.

SECTION 4

Cosmetic Procedures

CHAPTER 22

Non-Surgical Body Contouring

Leslie S. Baumann, MD
Paula Purpera, MSHS, PA-C

SUMMARY POINTS

What's Important?
1. Patient selection is critical.
2. All modalities work best in someone who is exercising and dieting and is only about 10–15 pounds overweight.
3. Results are not immediate.

What's New?
1. Heat, cold, and ultrasound devices are used to remove body fat.
2. Injectable deoxycholic acid can be used to diminish body fat.

What's Coming?
1. Studies are evaluating if removing body fat has any effect on the fat-burning hormone adiponectin or insulin sensitivity.
2. Doctors are beginning to combine injectable deoxycholic acid with body contouring devices to enhance results.

INTRODUCTION

The popularity of non-invasive body contouring has risen in recent years. Increasing numbers of patients are seeking a non-invasive way to sculpt their bodies because of the greater risk of complications, prolonged downtime, as well as the cost of liposuction and surgical body contouring.[1] According to the American Society of Plastic Surgeons, a total of 427,965 non-surgical body contouring procedures were performed in 2017 compared to 388,742 in 2016.[2] The American Society of Aesthetic Plastic Surgery reported a 217% increase in non-invasive body contouring procedures from 2012 to 2017.[3]

There are numerous modalities for non-invasive body contouring, including several injectable and device-oriented options. The choice of technique depends on various factors: anatomical location of the treatment area, cost, number of treatments needed, and amount of skin laxity in the treatment area. The most commonly treated areas are the abdomen, lumbar rolls, hip rolls/flanks, inner thighs, submental area, and bra fat area.[4]

Proper selection of patients is imperative. Patients who are poor candidates for any type of body contouring are those with excessive skin laxity, and those with unrealistic expectations. While these treatments are effective, combining them with lifestyle changes such as exercise and improved diet will greatly improve the results.[5,6] Some physicians suggest using supplements to speed the liver's breakdown of fat, but this approach has not been conclusively proven to be effective.[7]

Regardless of the modality used, it is crucial to accurately and precisely measure the changes throughout the treatment process using standardized and reproducible methods. Standardized pre-procedure photos with consistent positioning and lighting are essential. Using a tape measure, while effective, can be affected by positioning, posture, lighting, weight changes, as well as respiration. Repeated measurements, taking measurements at the same time of the day, or using an apparatus that standardizes tension may be necessary. Ultrasound has also been used as a method for quantifying changes in fat reduction. It is widely accessible and can visualize the fat layer. Designation of landmarks is critical for reproducibility and may be user dependent. It is also unclear how much of a change in fat layer thickness can induce a detectable change in the ultrasound. In addition, magnetic resonance imaging has been used to measure reduction in fat but is very costly and not readily accessible. Measurements in this case should be limited to extremities. Subjective measures such as blinded observer ratings or patient-reported outcomes also have value; while all are not formally validated, those validated are generally considered reliable.[8]

Practitioners should monitor patients' baseline and post-treatment weights. Most physicians require their patients to maintain weight or keep BMI within a narrow range during the treatment period in order to control for weight fluctuations.[9,10]

METABOLIC BENEFITS OF BODY CONTOURING TREATMENTS

Obesity is associated with diabetes, heart disease, and other health issues. The risk declines with weight loss. Although liposuction has not been shown to improve risk factors for heart disease,[11] large volume liposuction has been demonstrated to increase adiponectin levels.[12] Adiponectin is a hormone produced by fat cells. It is a desirable hormone because it has been shown to reduce inflammation and atherogenesis, as well as enhance the response of cells to insulin. High levels of adiponectin are associated with a lower risk of heart disease while lower levels are associated with obesity and cellulite.[13] Adiponectin levels have not been studied in patients who have received body contouring modalities besides large volume liposuction.

INJECTABLES

Deoxycholic Acid

Studies have shown that excess submental fat can have a detrimental effect on a person's feelings of attractiveness and emotional well-being.[14] Until recently, patients with excess submental fact who desired a contoured jawline had to rely on either surgical procedures or targeted liposuction.[15] There were no non-invasive treatment options for the submental area.

Injectable deoxycholic acid (DCA), marketed as Kybella (Kythera Biopharmaceuticals, Westlake Village, CA, acquired by Allergan, Inc.), was approved in 2015 for adults with moderate-to-severe submental fullness.[16] DCA is a naturally occurring bile acid that emulsifies fat for absorption in the intestine. It acts by irreversibly disrupting the adipocyte membrane causing adipocytolysis.[17]

Kybella is injected in the pre-platysmal fat in the submental area using an area-adjusted dose of 2 mg/cm². Each 0.2 mL injection is spaced 1 cm apart, for up to a maximum of 50 injections, using a grid (**Fig. 22-1**). Up to six treatment sessions approximately 4 weeks apart may be administered. Some practitioners space them further apart using swelling as a guide for when to perform the next round of injections. The total number of treatments needed depends on the amount of fat present in the submental area (**Fig. 22-2**). Proper injection

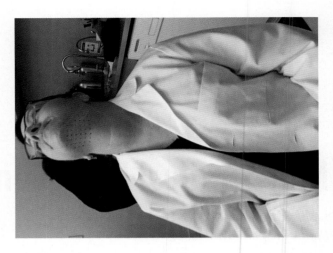

FIGURE 22-1. The Kybella kit comes with a pre-made grid that can be placed on the patient's submental area as shown.

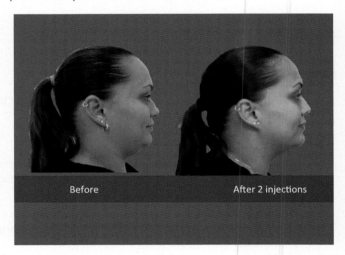

Before   After 2 injections

FIGURE 22-2. This amount of chin fat required two injections of 3 cc of Kybella spaced 4 weeks apart.

technique and knowledge of anatomy are necessary to avoid injecting in vulnerable structures such as the marginal mandibular nerve, the platysma, or lymph nodes.[18] The swelling associated with Kybella injections can be significant and depends on the amount of fat present and amount of Kybella used. The first treatment episode is usually accompanied by more swelling than subsequent episodes, possibly because there is less fat present. Arnica pads or oral arnica can be used to diminish swelling and discomfort. Patients should be warned about swelling when the submental area is treated because it is a difficult area to conceal and swelling may last 10–14 days. In most cases, swelling resolves in 5–7 days (**Fig. 22-3**). In the author's experience, it takes at least two treatments before results are seen. The results for the patient in **Fig. 22-3** are unusual because they occurred after one treatment.

Phase I trials of Kybella revealed no effect on systemic lipid profiles or inflammatory markers such as C-reactive protein or IL-6.[19] Common adverse effects include discomfort, swelling that may last up to 14 days, and bruising/ecchymosis.[20] Associated complications entail possible marginal mandibular

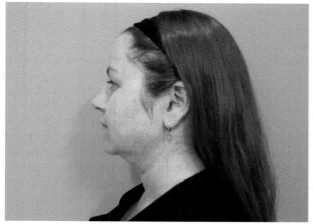

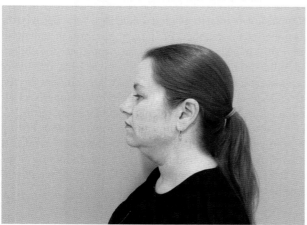

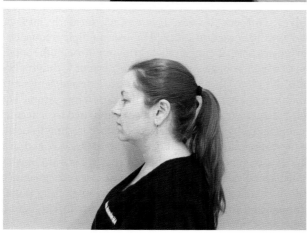

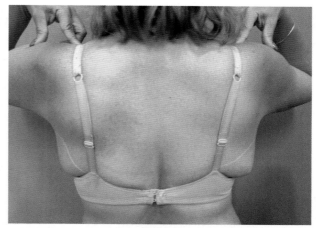

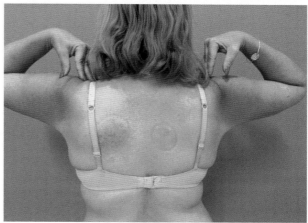

FIGURE 22-4A and B. A. before Kybella to bra fat area. **B.** After three treatments of 5 cc each side (10 cc total per treatment visit). The round bruises are due to an unrelated cupping procedure.

FIGURE 22-3A, B, and C. A. Before Kybella to submental area. **B.** Swelling 1 day after injections. This swelling is mild and occurred after 2 cc of Kybella. **C.** Day 25 after one Kybella injection.

nerve (MMN) injury, dysphagia, injection-site alopecia, and skin ulceration. MMN injury, which presents in an asymmetric smile, has occurred in 4.3% of patients and resolved after a median duration of 42 days. Dysphagia often associated with injection volumes or post-injection swelling has emerged in 1.9% of patients and resolved after a median duration of 3 days. Injection site alopecia has been reported in 0.4% of patients with a median duration of 151 days. Skin ulceration,

likely due to inappropriate injection technique, has been seen in 0.2% of patients and resolved within 23 days.[21]

Patients treated with Kybella who presented with mild-to-moderate skin laxity were shown to have significant skin tightening after treatment.[18] The resulting skin tightening is initiated by an acute inflammatory response from adipocytolysis. This inflammatory process is cleared by M1 macrophages that reduce the synthesis of pro-inflammatory cytokines and induce the production of anti-inflammatory cytokines as well as M2 macrophages. M2 macrophages yield growth factors that engender granulation tissue, leading to the deposition of actin microfilaments and a collagen matrix with the subsequent contraction of tissue.[22]

Because of the success and efficacy of DCA injections for submental fullness, it is reasonable to extrapolate the usefulness of Kybella for other areas of the body with localized adiposity.[23] DCA injections have been used with success with localized adiposity in the "bra-line" (upper arm and the anterior and posterior axillary area in females) (**Fig. 22-4**, A and B).[24,25] Other areas where DCA could be used are the medial and lateral knee fat, and for subcutaneous abdominal fat.[23] Injections in the cheeks, chin, jaw fat pads, jowls, lipoma, and male breasts for pseudogynecomastia have also been reported.[20,26]

Collagenase *Clostridium histolyticum*

Cellulite is a major concern for many patients, especially in post-pubertal women. The appearance of cellulite is believed to arise from fat deposition mediated by hormones, reduced venous return due to the compression of capillary vessels by fat lobules, and deposition of proteins around clumped fat lobules.[28] From a histological standpoint, cellulite presents as irregular herniations of subdermal fat into the reticular and papillary dermis with the presence of thinner, radially oriented fibrous septae in the deep subcutis.[29]

Collagenase *Clostridium histolyticum*, or CCH (Endo Pharmaceuticals, Malvern, PA), is an enzyme that can cleave the triple-helical region of collagen.[30] Pending FDA approval, this injectable collagenase is being investigated to treat cellulite in women by lysing the dermal septa, the underlying cause of skin dimpling in women.[31]

RADIOFREQUENCY

Velashape

Velashape (Syneron-Candela, Wayland, MA) is the first US Food and Drug Administration class II medical device to receive approval for cellulite reduction and for circumferential reduction of the abdomen, flanks, buttocks, thighs, and upper arm regions.[32,33] This system incorporates four treatment modalities including pulsed vacuum, mechanical massage, bipolar radiofrequency (RF) technology, and infrared (IR) light. The pulsed vacuum combined with the action of the massage rollers causes vasodilation and increased blood flow, oxygen, and lymphatic drainage to the treatment area. Application of the IR and RF boosts the existing oxygen, which facilitates an increase in localized fat metabolism.[32] This combination technology induces deep heating of the connective tissue, including the fibrous septae, promoting an increase in collagen deposition, cellular metabolism, and localized reduction in skin laxity and volume.[34] Treatment regimens are usually once weekly for 6 weeks.[35]

This modality is not recommended for patients who are pregnant or nursing, have a history of keloids, cancer in the treatment area, known photosensitivity disorders, or have used isotretinoin within 6 months of treatment. It is safe for all phototypes as RF and IR energies are neither scattered nor absorbed by epidermal melanin.[33] Associated complications have included transient erythema/edema, bruising/ecchymosis, and superficial crusting/burning.[32,33]

Vanquish

Approved by the FDA in 2015, Vanquish (BTL Industries, Framingham, MA) is a non-contact RF device in which the applicator is placed approximately 1 cm above the skin.[36] This selective-field RF instrument uses electromagnetically-induced rapid oscillations of electrical dipoles to heat fatty tissue with subsequent adipocyte tissue destruction. A patented Energy Flow Control (EFC) System selectively delivers the energy to the adipose tissue layer while minimizing the risk of overheating the skin, muscles, and other internal structures.[37] A multipolar broad field applicator shapes the electromagnetic field to optimize penetration and maximize the treatment area. The treatment protocol is four 45-minute, once weekly sessions for 4 weeks.[38]

The Vanquish system is equipped with two types of applicators: the EX applicator, to treat the abdomen and flanks, and the AB applicator, to treat thighs and saddlebags. Vanquish is particularly preferred for treatment of a large surface area in patients with a high BMI in a single application, as it can cover the abdomen and flanks simultaneously with a spot size as large as 2,100 cm². The most frequently reported side effects are transient erythema and tenderness, occasional skin blistering due to superficial sweat accumulation, small area panniculitis, and localized burns.[39]

Fat reduction has been clinically proven to be long lasting, if not permanent. A small study in Germany demonstrated that patients maintained circumferential waist reduction 4 years after treatment.[40] This therapy is not ideal for a patient with a lower BMI due to a thinner subcutaneous fat layer.[41]

BodyFX

BodyFX (InMode Invasix, Irvine, CA), formerly known as TiteFX, utilizes suction-coupled bipolar multiple frequency RF that creates permanent fat cell destruction through the application of a high-voltage pulsed electrical current with ultra-short pulse duration. The handpiece has an external temperature monitor that continuously reads the skin temperature. These high-voltage, ultra-short RF pulses are designed to deliver irreversible fat cell membrane electroporation, leading to delayed apoptosis and adipocyte cell death. The "pores" created in the adipocyte membrane lead to the egress of lipids from the intracellular space, causing significant volume loss and signaling cell death.[42] Histological examination after treatment has revealed shrunken and withered adipocytes with partially ruptured cell membranes, but no evidence of necrosis.[43]

In addition to circumferential reduction, this device has also been shown to decrease cellulite due to the RF-related dermal thickening of the reticular dermis. This provides more resistance to re-herniation of adipose tissue into the subdermal fat as well as relaxation of the vertical fibrous septae leading to a smoother-appearing contour.[44] The prescribed treatment regimen is once a week for 6 weeks. Associated adverse effects are erythema, strong sensation of heat, transient and mild bruising, and slight discomfort.[35]

General contraindications include pregnancy and nursing, pacemakers, epilepsy, thyroid dysfunction, diabetes, cardiac arrhythmias, heart disease, uncontrolled hypertension, history of cancer, liver or kidney disease, use of immunosuppressive medications, use of isotretinoin within the previous 6 months, abnormal wound healing, diuretic use, and anticoagulant use.[43]

CRYOLIPOLYSIS

Coolsculpting

It has been shown that adipose tissue is preferentially sensitive to cold injury. A rare clinical phenomenon called popsicle panniculitis is characterized by cold-induced fat necrosis in the cheeks of infants after prolonged exposure to frozen treats.[45] This mechanism of cold injury is the basis of cryolipolysis.

Coolsculpting (Zeltiq Aesthetics, Pleasanton, CA, acquired by Allergan, Inc.) employs selective cryolipolysis with no adverse effects to the epidermis, dermis, or underlying muscle tissue.[46] Controlled, selective extraction of heat from the adipocytes along with vacuum suction impedes blood flow and results in fat cell destruction by inducing crystallization of the target tissue.[4] This gradual apoptosis is characterized by lipid-ice crystallization, inflammatory panniculitis, phagocytosis, then gradual clearance. Additional fat cell injury is provoked by the subsequent rewarming of adipose tissue after treatment due to ischemic reperfusion injury.[47] Importantly, this controlled cooling of subcutaneous fat has been demonstrated as safe in studies of peripheral nerve function, serum lipids, and liver function tests.[48–50]

The Coolsculpting device has an applicator that allows tissue to be vacuumed in between two cooling panels for 30–60 minutes.[39] Because of the different areas that can be treated with cryolipolysis, the applicator has been fashioned to create a contoured surface to maximize tissue contact with the cooling surface. There are specially designed applicators based on the size, shape, and accessibility of the treatment area.[51]

The most common complication of the procedure is decreased sensation of the treated area lasting greater than 4 weeks. Another notable complication is paradoxical adipose hyperplasia (PAH) with visible contour irregularities.[52] PAH is a phenomenon observed after cryolipolysis in which gradual, non-tender growth of tissue the size and shape of the treatment area occurs at the treatment site. It is hypothesized that this arises as a result of reactive fibrosis to the damaged adipocytes. To date, 33 confirmed cases of PAH have been reported to the device manufacturer as part of post-marketing surveillance data. No single common characteristic has been identified in affected individuals, but the incidence seems to be higher in men.[53] Other associated adverse reactions include pain, erythema, swelling, sensitivity, and purpura in the treated area.[54]

Contraindications include known history of cryoglobulinemia, cold urticaria, cold agglutinin disease, paroxysmal cold hemoglobinuria, and Raynaud's disease.[26] Cryolipolysis should be avoided in areas with severe varicose veins, dermatitis, or other cutaneous lesions.[55] This procedure is not for obese patients with significant skin laxity.[56]

Studies have shown enhanced clinical outcomes with post-treatment manual massage. This synergistic effect is probably due to an additional mechanism of damage immediately following treatment, likely from tissue reperfusion

injury.[57,58] Multiple treatments in the same location can yield additional fat reduction but efficacy appears to diminish with subsequent treatments.[4] Results are long lasting, if not permanent. Case reports show durability of clinical effects from 2 to 5 years after treatment.[59]

ULTRASOUND

Liposonix

High-intensity focused ultrasound (HIFU) has been used in numerous therapeutic applications. In HIFU, the ultrasound beam is precisely focused to deliver acoustic energy to a target area in a non-invasive manner. The intention is to heat a large volume of tissue without affecting the tissue in the ultrasound propagation pathway. HIFU can increase the temperature of a target area above 55°C, which results in coagulative necrosis and immediate cell death.[60] The two underlying mechanisms of adipocyte destruction are the disruption of the cell membrane due to the mechanical effects of ultrasonic energy, and the coagulative necrosis that results from the increased temperature.[61]

Liposonix (Solta Medical, Pleasanton, CA) has been approved by the FDA for circumferential waist reduction using HIFU. This device has a hemispherically shaped transducer with a ceramic element that generates HIFU energy with a fixed frequency of 2 MHz. The amount of energy delivered is controlled by adjusting the peak power and duration of emitted energy, with water acting as a coupling agent between the skin and the transducer. Accurate delivery of ultrasonic energy is ensured by a programmable pattern generator that scans the transducer head over the treatment area at a mechanically adjusted, predetermined depth while preventing excessive overlap.[62]

This device provides the advantage of a single treatment session comprising two passes, which can result in a mean circumference reduction of 4.6 cm from baseline after 3 months.[63] Significant waist reduction has been reported as early as 4 weeks after a single treatment.[64]

The most common adverse events associated with the treatment are procedural pain, postprocedural pain, swelling, and ecchymosis. There have been no reports of skin dimpling, indurations, scars, burns, or increased skin laxity. Contraindications include pregnancy and lactation, coagulation disorders as well as the use of anticoagulants, diabetes, and cardiovascular disease.[65]

UltraShape

The UltraShape (Syneron-Candela, Wayland, MA) system uses focused ultrasound technology that emits acoustic sound waves in the 200±30 KHz frequency range that converge into a confined focal point at a depth of 1.5 cm below the skin surface, targeting subcutaneous fat. This focused, pulsed ultrasound enables selective mechanical fat cell destruction by creating rapid changes in pressure, which leads to bubbles in the interstitial fluid that implode and rupture the adipocyte cell membrane.[66,67] This cavitation effect appears to be restricted to adipocytes, with other surrounding tissues and cells showing normal features.[68,69] See **Table 22-1** for a review of the mechanisms of action, approved

TABLE 22-1

Modality	Mechanism of Action	Approved Areas	Caution*	Adverse Effects	Downtime
Injectables					
Deoxycholic Acid	Cytolytic drug that destroys the cell membrane, causing adipolysis	Submental area	Infection at the injection site; Use with caution in patients being treated with anticoagulants; Possible marginal mandibular nerve injury	Edema, erythema, itching, numbness, induration, bruising	2–3 weeks of swelling
CCH	CCH is a proteinase that can hydrolyze the triple-helical region of collagen and has the potential to lyse the dermal septa	Thighs and buttocks (not FDA approved yet)	Data not currently available	Bruising	Data not currently available
Radiofrequency					
Velashape	Bipolar RF uses the impedance of tissue to generate heating of the target tissue with the addition of pulsed vacuum, mechanical massage and infrared light[84]	Thighs, hips, abdomen	History of photosensitivity[33]	Erythema	None
Vanquish	Contactless selective RF	Abdomen, flanks, thighs, saddlebags	None	Erythema, tenderness, skin irritation, abdominal discomfort, hyperesthesia Uncommon: blistering, small area panniculitis, localized burns	None
BodyFX/TiteFX	Use of two different RF frequencies with coupled suction provides bulk heating causing electroporation of adipocyte cell membranes	Abdomen, flanks, anterior and posterior thighs[44]	None	Erythema, edema, discomfort especially near bony prominences, petechiae[42]	None
Cryolipolysis					
Coolsculpting	Cold temperature triggers apoptosis of adipocytes	Abdomen, inner thighs, flanks, brassiere rolls, medial knees, peritrochanteric areas (saddlebags), arms, ankles[4,39]	Contraindicated in patients with PCH, cryoglobulinemia, and Raynaud's disease	Paradoxical adipose hyperplasia	
Ultrasound					
Liposonix	HIFU heating adipocytes from 56°C to 70°C leading to thermal necrosis	Abdomen and flanks; buttocks, inner and outer thighs, lower chest[61]		Severe treatment discomfort; bruising, erythema, edema, hard lumps[35]	
UltraShape	Nonthermal pulsed ultrasound cavitation	Abdomen, flanks, thighs[70]			None

(Continued)

TABLE 22-1   *(Continued)*

Modality	Mechanism of Action	Approved Areas	Caution*	Adverse Effects	Downtime
Laser Therapy					
Zerona	Using 635 nm diode laser to create transient pores in the adipocyte cell membrane, leading to efflux of lipids from adipocytes; LLLT stimulates the production of cytosolic lipase	Hips, waist, thighs		Well tolerated; No adverse events reported in studies	None
Sculpsure	Using 1060 nm diode laser to elevate temperature of fat tissue from 42°C to 47°C resulting in adipocyte injury (Hyperthermic laser lipolysis)	Abdomen, flanks		Treatment discomfort, edema, erythema, blistering, bruising, subcutaneous nodules	
HIFEM Therapy					
EMSculpt	Production of supra-maximal contractions of abdominal muscles, inducing muscular hypertrophy and lipolysis	Abdomen		None to mild discomfort	None

*All of the treatment modalities are contraindicated in pregnant and lactating females, users of Accutane within the previous 6 months, individuals with infection/malignancy in the treatment area, those with any condition that delays wound healing (diabetes mellitus, uncontrolled hypertension, immunosuppression, and the use of anticoagulants).

CCH: Collagenase *Clostridium histolyticum*; HIFEM: High-intensity focused electromagnetic; PCH: Paroxysmal cold hemoglobinuria; HIFU: High-intensity focused ultrasound; LLLT: Low-level laser therapy.

areas, cautions, adverse effects, and downtime of the modalities discussed in this chapter.

In contrast to the Liposonix, this device utilizes a nonthermal pulsed wave, rendering it more comfortable without the need for anesthesia or analgesia. After fat cell disruption by mechanical ultrasound waves, the contents of the adipocytes leak into the interstitial space and are transported through the lymphatic system to the liver where the triglycerides are metabolized into glycerol and free fatty acids. To date, there have been no abnormal changes in serum lipids in treated patients.[70]

The treatment protocol is three sessions 2 weeks apart.[9] A medical grade, transducer-compatible oil is used to ensure optimal acoustic contact between the transducer and the patient's skin during treatments. A generous layer of the acoustic contact oil must be maintained over the area to ensure efficient energy delivery as well as to prevent discomfort.[71] The treatment is generally well tolerated with most patients reporting minimal to no discomfort during the procedure (**Figs. 22-5** A and B, **22-6** A and B). The most common complication is transient erythema. Other associated complications include a mild tingling sensation, purpura, and blistering. No hyperpigmentation or hypopigmentation, nodules, or contour irregularities have been reported. Contraindications include pregnancy, cardiac pacemakers, abdominal wall hernias, diabetes, and coagulation disorders or the use of anticoagulants.[72]

One drawback with this device is the decreased efficacy of the treatment in Asian patients. Objective measurements by ultrasound as well as circumferential and caliper measurements have failed to show significant improvement, leading to poor overall satisfaction among patients. This is likely due to the smaller body size and frame of Asian patients compared to Caucasians.[73]

LASER THERAPY

Zero LipoLaser

Laser devices have been used in medicine for decades. More recently, low-level laser devices have been deployed for therapeutic purposes, particularly to relieve pain, inflammation, and swelling in degenerative diseases and orthopedic injuries.[74] Exposure of subcutaneous fat to low-level laser therapy (LLLT) has been shown to cause an increase in reactive oxygen species (ROS), initiating a process called lipid peroxidation. The generated ROS react with the lipids found on the cellular membrane of adipocytes and temporarily damage them by creating pores in the cell membrane, allowing the release of intracellular lipids. It is also proposed that LLLT activates cyclic adenosine monophosphate, triggering a secondary cascade that stimulates the release of cytoplasmic lipase, breaking

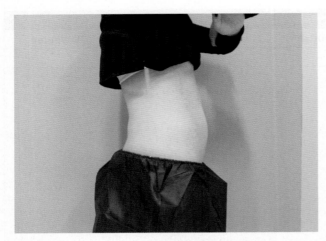

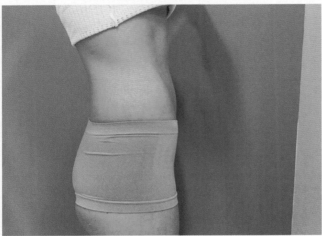

FIGURE 22-5A and B. **A.** Before Ultrashape to abdomen. **B.** One month after the third treatment spaced 2 weeks apart. (Photos courtesy of Ali Dispazio.)

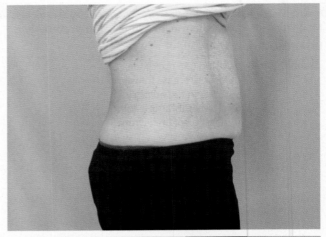

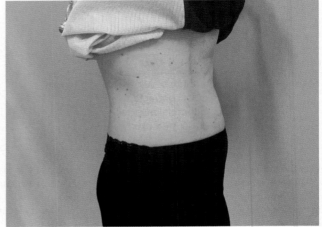

FIGURE 22-6A and B. **A.** Before Ultrashape to abdomen. **B.** One month after the third treatment spaced 2 weeks apart. (Photos courtesy of Ali Dispazio.)

down intracellular triglycerides into fatty acids and glycerol, causing shrinkage in the adipocytes.[10,75]

The Zerona LipoLaser (Erchonia Medical, Inc., Melbourne, FL) is a device with four to six rotating diode laser heads, each emitting 17 mW of 635 nm laser light. The device uses internal mechanics, which collect the light emitted from each laser diode, and processes it through a lens system that redirects the beam with a line refractor. The refracted light is bent into a random circular pattern independent of other individual diodes. Each diode emits a line of light approximately 9 mm long and 3 mm wide with an energy of approximately 0.0002 joules per cm^2/minute/treated area at a distance of 3 inches (7.62 cm) and approximately 0.0001 joules per cm^2/minute/treated area at a distance of 4 inches (10.16 cm).[76]

The device was approved by the FDA in 2010 for fat circumferential reduction of the hips, waist, and thighs but has also been shown to be effective in decreasing upper arm circumference.[7,77] Most treatment protocols call for three weekly sessions for 2 to 4 weeks.[7,78]

Complications associated with LLLT are generally less common than with all other non-invasive body contouring modalities, with several studies reporting no adverse events.[79]

Contraindications include pregnancy/nursing, renal failure, liver failure, and uncontrolled diabetes.[80]

Interestingly, LLLT has also been demonstrated to decrease both cholesterol and leptin blood levels. This is likely due to the modulation of transcription factors that contribute to the reduction of cholesterol levels as well as inhibition of cholesterogenesis.[80,81] See **Table 22-2** for a review of advantages, and disadvantages, and treatment details of the modalities described in this chapter.

Sculpsure

Approved by the FDA in 2017 for non-invasive fat removal in the abdomen and flanks, Sculpsure (Cynosure, Westford, MA) also uses laser energy to reduce subcutaneous fat. This device activates a 1,060 nm diode laser that directly heats subcutaneous fat at around 42–47°C.[82] At this temperature the cell membranes of the adipocytes lose their structural integrity, leading to subsequent cell death. While hyperthermic laser lipolysis is responsible for the fat reduction, the selected wavelength enables the energy to penetrate to the appropriate depth to adequately target the adipocytes while achieving very

TABLE 22-2

Modality	Advantages	Drawbacks	Number of Treatments/ Interval between Treatments	Treatment Time
Injectables				
Deoxycholic Acid	Able to treat areas that are difficult to treat with the device handpieces; Subsequent skin retraction	Prolonged swelling	Up to six treatments, at least 4 weeks apart	No data
CCH Collagenase	First in class to treat fibrous septae	No data	No data	No data
Radiofrequency				
Velashape	Clinically shown to also improve cellulite as well as circumference reduction		Six treatments one to two times per week;[32] Once weekly for 4–5 weeks[33]	Varies until thermal endpoint is reached, around 25–45 mins[32,33]
Vanquish	Ideal for large areas in patients with higher BMI (≥ 25);[39] "Hands-free" once positioned; Skin can be additionally cooled by circulating air[84]	Not recommended for patients with lower BMI[41]	4	45 mins
TiteFX/BodyFX	No down time		Six treatments once a week[44]	45 mins
Cryolipolysis				
Coolsculpting	Significant reduction after one treatment;[35] Several different treatment applicators of various size/shape; "Hands-free" once positioned; Long-lasting 2- and 5-year data[59]	Can be uncomfortable; Efficacy appears to be attenuated with subsequent treatments[4]	1–3[39]	30–60 mins
Ultrasound				
Liposonix	Significant reduction after one treatment;[35] Concurrent circumference reduction as well as skin tightening	Painful	Single treatment	60–90 mins
UltraShape		Not very effective in Asian patients; Fixed size of treatment applicator	Three treatments 2 weeks apart	30–120 mins
Laser Therapy				
Zerona	Been shown to reduce cholesterol and leptin levels;[85] Maximal results seen immediately;[35] Comfortable treatment	Lost volume may rebound if patient does not adhere to lifestyle changes		

(Continued)

TABLE 22-2 (Continued)

Modality	Advantages	Drawbacks	Number of Treatments/ Interval between Treatments	Treatment Time
Sculpsure	Safe for darker-skinned patients; Can adjust number of treatment heads based on size and shape of target area; "Hands-free" once positioned		Two treatments 4–6 weeks apart	25 mins
HIFEM				
EMSculpt	Improves diastasis recti; Patients with low BMI can be treated with good results		Four treatments spaced 2–3 days apart	30 mins

CCH: Collagenase *Clostridium histolyticum*; HIFEM: High-intensity focused electromagnetic; HIFU: High-intensity focused ultrasound.

low absorption within the dermis, rendering it safe for all skin types.[83]

This laser device has four applicator heads that users arrange in a customized manner. Each applicator has a water-cooled sapphire window that comes in direct contact with the skin, keeping the skin cool at 15°C throughout the treatment. The most common adverse event reported has been treatment discomfort. Other complications include erythema, transient edema, blistering, bruising, and subcutaneous nodules. Optimal treatment time ranges between 20–25 minutes. Treatment times longer than 30 minutes have been associated with developing palpable nodules.[86] The therapeutic protocol is usually one to three sessions spaced at least 4 weeks apart.[39,83]

Ideal patients for this procedure are non-obese (a BMI less than 30) with discrete areas of adiposity that are resistant to diet and exercise.[83]

HIGH INTENSITY FOCUSED ELECTROMAGNETIC THERAPY

EMSculpt

Surgical body contouring and the non-invasive body contouring devices primarily focus on fat reduction. None of the procedures specifically target the underlying musculature, which is highly responsible for the toned and chiseled abdominal contour typically considered aesthetically pleasing. Other than physical exercise, electromagnetic stimulation has been used for muscle training and muscle strengthening.[87]

EMSculpt (BTL Industries, Framingham, MA) is a new device that utilizes high intensity focused electromagnetic (HIFEM) technology using frequencies that induce tonic muscle contractions. The device delivers pulses that produce supramaximal contractions not ordinarily achieved voluntarily. This triggers a stress response in the tissue. The energy supplying the contractions is thought to be taken from the

fat cells through lipolysis. The waist circumference reduction is attributed to both fat reduction via lipolysis as well as strengthening and tightening of the abdominal wall.[88] Research on high-intensity muscle training has shown that lipolysis occurs in the fat tissue adjacent to the contracting muscle.[89] Histological studies reveal that adipocyte apoptosis occurs after subcutaneous fat treatment with HIFEM.[84]

Treatments with this device reduce waist circumference, increase muscle mass, and have been demonstrated to improve diastasis recti by diminishing abdominal separation.[90] It has been used in the abdomen as well as for non-invasive buttock lifting and toning. The therapeutic protocol usually consists of four treatment sessions spaced 2 to 3 days apart.[91]

One advantage of this modality is that it can be used in patients with lower BMI who may not be candidates for other body contouring procedures. This treatment is contraindicated in pregnant and breastfeeding mothers, patients with any medical condition contraindicating the application of an electromagnetic field, and those with heart disorders.[88]

References

1. Talasila S, Evers-Meltzer R, Xu S. Social media ratings of minimally invasive fat reduction procedures: benchmarking against traditional liposuction. *Dermatol Surg*. 2018;44(7):971–975.
2. American Society of Plastic Surgeons. (2018). 2017 Complete Plastic Surgery Statistics Report. Retrieved from https://www.plasticsurgery.org/documents/News/Statistics/2017/plastic-surgery-statistics-full-report-2017.pdf
3. American Society for Aesthetic Plastic Surgery. (2018). 2017 Cosmetic Surgery National Data Bank Statistics. Retrieved from https://www.surgery.org/sites/default/files/ASAPS-Stats2017.pdf
4. Ingargiola MJ, Motakef S, Chung MT, Vasconez HC, Sasaki GH. Cryolipolysis for fat reduction and body contouring: safety and efficacy of current treatment paradigms. *Plast Reconstr Surg*. 2015;135(6):1581–1590.
5. Sarwer DB, Polonsky HM. Body image and body contouring procedures. *Aesthet Surg J*. 2016;36(9):1039–1047.

6. Pinto H, Arredondo E, Ricart-Jane D. Evaluation of adipocytic changes after a simil-lipocryolysis stimulus. *Cryo Letters.* 2013;34(1):100–105.

7. McRae E, Boris J. Independent evaluation of low-level laser therapy at 635 nm for non-invasive body contouring of the waist, hips, and thighs. *Lasers Surg Med.* 2013;45(1):1–7.

8. Auh SL, Iyengar S, Weil A, et al. Quantification of noninvasive fat reduction: A systematic review. *Lasers Surg Med.* 2018;50(2)96–110.

9. Ascher B. Safety and efficacy of UltraShape Contour I treatments to improve the appearance of body contours: multiple treatments in shorter intervals. *Aesthet Surg J.* 2010;30(2):217–224.

10. Caruso-Davis MK, Guillot TS, Podichetty VK, et al. Efficacy of low-level laser therapy for body contouring and spot fat reduction. *Obes Surg.* 2011;21(6):722–729.

11. Klein S, Fontana L, Young VL, et al. Absence of an effect of liposuction on insulin action and risk factors for coronary heart disease. *N Engl J Med.* 2004;350(25):2549–2557.

12. Giugliano G, Nicoletti G, Grella E, et al. Effect of liposuction on insulin resistance and vascular inflammatory markers in obese women. *Br J Plast Surg.* 2004;57(3):190–194.

13. Emanuele E, Minoretti P, Altabas K, Gaeta E, Altabas V. Adiponectin expression in subcutaneous adipose tissue is reduced in women with cellulite. *Int J Dermatol.* 2011;50(4):412–416.

14. Baumann L, Shridharani SM, Humphrey S, Gallagher CJ. Personal (self) perceptions of submental fat among adults in the United States. *Dermatol Surg.* 2019;45(1):124–130.

15. Ascher B, Hoffmann K, Walker P, Lippert S, Wollina U, Havlickova B. Efficacy, patient-reported outcomes and safety profile of ATX-101 (deoxycholic acid), an injectable drug for the reduction of unwanted submental fat: results from a phase III, randomized, placebo-controlled study. *J Eur Acad Dermatol Venereol.* 2014;28(12):1707–1715.

16. Rzany B, Griffiths T, Walker P, Lippert S, McDiarmid J, Havlickova B. Reduction of unwanted submental fat with ATX-101 (deoxycholic acid), an adipocytolytic injectable treatment: results from a phase III, randomized, placebo-controlled study. *Br J Dermatol.* 2014;170(2):445–453.

17. Shridharani SM. Early experience in 100 consecutive patients with injection adipocytolysis for neck contouring with ATX-101 (deoxycholic acid). *Dermatol Surg.* 2017;43(7):950–958.

18. Shamban AT. Noninvasive submental fat compartment treatment. *Plast Reconstr Surg Glob Open.* 2016 Dec 14;4(12 Suppl Anatomy and Safety in Cosmetic Medicine: Cosmetic Bootcamp):e1155.

19. Kamalpour S, Leblanc KJr. Injection adipolysis: Mechanisms, agents, and future directions. *J Clin Aesthet Dermatol.* 2016;9(12):44–50.

20. Talathi A, Talathi P. Fat busters: Lipolysis for face and neck. *J Cutan Aesthet Surg.* 2018;11(2):67–72.

21. Dayan SH, Schlessinger J, Beer K, et al. Efficacy and safety of ATX-101 by treatment session: Pooled analysis of data from the Phase 3 REFINE trials. *Aesthet Surg J.* 2018;38(9):998–1010.

22. Pereira JX, Cavalcante Y, Wanzeler de Oliveira R. The role of inflammation in adipocytolytic nonsurgical esthetic procedures for body contouring. *Clin Cosmet Investig Dermatol.* 2017;10:57–66.

23. Sykes JM, Allak A, Klink B. Future applications of deoxycholic acid in body contouring. *J Drugs Dermatol.* 2017;16(1):43–46.

24. Jegasothy SM. Deoxycholic acid injections for bra-line lipolysis. *Dermatol Surg.* 2018;44(5):757–760.

25. Verma KD, Somenek MT. Deoxycholic acid injection as an effective treatment for reduction of posterior upper torso brassiere strap adiposity. *Plast Reconstr Surg.* 2018;141(1):200e–202e.

26. Carruthers JD, Humphrey S, Rivers JK. Cryolipolysis for reduction of arm fat: Safety and efficacy of a prototype CoolCup applicator with flat contour. *Dermatol Surg.* 2017;43(7):940–949.

27. Jones DH, Kenkel JM, Fagien S, et al. Proper technique for administration of ATX-101 (deoxycholic acid injection): Insights from an injection practicum and roundtable discussion. *Dermatol Surg.* 2016 Nov;42(Suppl 1):S275–S281.

28. Draelos ZD. The disease of cellulite. *J Cosmet Dermatol.* 2005;4(4):221–222.

29. Rosenbaum M, Prieto V, Hellmer J, et al. An exploratory investigation of the morphology and biochemistry of cellulite. *Plast Reconstr Surg.* 1998;101(7):1934–1939.

30. Azmi W, Chauhan S, Gautam M. An overview on therapeutic potential and various applications of microbial collagenases. *J Microb Biotechnol Res.* 2017;7(6):17–29.

31. Endo Pharmaceuticals. Injection technique of Collagenase Clostridium Histolyticum (CCH) for the treatment of EFP (cellulite). 2018. Retrieved from: https://clinicaltrials.gov/ct2/show/NCT03632993. Accessed 9/8/2019.

32. Adatto MA, Adatto-Neilson RM, Morren G. Reduction in adipose tissue volume using a new high-power radiofrequency technology combined with infrared light and mechanical manipulation for body contouring. *Lasers Med Sci.* 2014;29(5):1627–1631.

33. Brightman L, Weiss E, Chapas AM, et al. Improvement in arm and post-partum abdominal and flank subcutaneous fat deposits and skin laxity using a bipolar radiofrequency, infrared, vacuum and mechanical massage device. *Lasers Surg Med.* 2009;41(10):791–798.

34. Sadick N. Tissue tightening technologies: fact or fiction. *Aesthet Surg J.* 2008;28(2):180–188.

35. Kennedy J, Verne S, Griffith R, Falto-Aizpurua L, Nouri K. Non-invasive subcutaneous fat reduction: a review. *J Eur Acad Dermatol Venereol.* 2015;29(9):1679–1688.

36. Nassab R. The evidence behind noninvasive body contouring devices. *Aesthet Surg J.* 2015;35(3):279–293.

37. Weiss R, Weiss M, Beasley K, Vrba J, Bernardy J. Operator independent focused high frequency ISM band for fat reduction: porcine model. *Lasers Surg Med.* 2013;45(4):235–239.

38. Downie J, Kaspar M. Contactless abdominal fat reduction with selective RF™ evaluated by magnetic resonance imaging (MRI): case study. *J Drugs Dermatol.* 2016;15(4):491–495.

39. Chilukuri S, Mueller G. "Hands-free" noninvasive body contouring devices: Review of effectiveness and patient satisfaction. *J Drugs Dermatol.* 2016;15(11):1402–1406.

40. Fritz K, Salavastru C. Long-term follow-up on patients treated for abdominal fat using a selective contactless radiofrequency device. *J Cosmet Dermatol.* 2017;16(4):471–475.

41. Fajkošová K, Machovcová A, Onder M, Fritz K. Selective radiofrequency therapy as a non-invasive approach for contactless body contouring and circumferential reduction. *J Drugs Dermatol.* 2014;13(3):291–296.

42. Duncan DI, Kim TH, Temaat R. A prospective study analyzing the application of radiofrequency energy and high-voltage, ultrashort pulse duration electrical fields on the quantitative reduction of adipose tissue. *J Cosmet Laser Ther.* 2016;18(5):257–267.

43. Boisnic S, Divaris M, Nelson AA, Gharavi NM, Lask GP. A clinical and biological evaluation of a novel, noninvasive radiofrequency device for the long-term reduction of adipose tissue. *Lasers Surg Med.* 2014;46(2):94–103.

44. Mulholland RS, Kreindel M. Non-surgical body contouring: introduction of a new non-invasive device for long-term localized fat reduction and cellulite improvement using controlled, suction coupled, radiofrequency heating and high voltage ultra-short electrical pulses. *J Clin Exp Dermatol Res.* 2012;3(4):157–165.

45. Epstein EHJr, Oren ME. Popsicle panniculitis. *N Engl J Med.* 1970;282(17):966–967.

46. Manstein D, Laubach H, Watanabe K, Farinelli W, Zurakowski D, Anderson RR. Selective cryolysis: a novel method of noninvasive fat removal. *Lasers Surg Med.* 2008;40(9):595–604.

47. Sasaki GH, Abelev N, Tevez-Ortiz A. Noninvasive selective cryolipolysis and reperfusion recovery for localized natural fat reduction and contouring. *Aesthet Surg J.* 2014;34(3):420–431.

48. Klein KB, Zelickson B, Riopelle JG, et al. Non-invasive cryolipolysis for subcutaneous fat reduction does not affect serum lipid levels or liver function tests. *Lasers Surg Med.* 2009;41(10):785–790.

49. Stevens WG, Bachelor EP. Cryolipolysis conformable-surface applicator for nonsurgical fat reduction in lateral thighs. *Aesthet Surg J.* 2015;35(1):66–71.

50. Meyer PF, da Silva RM, Oliveira G, et al. Effects of cryolipolysis on abdominal adiposity. *Case Rep Dermatol Med.* 2016;216:60522194.

51. Allergan, Inc. Coolsculpting User Manual.

52. Derrick CD, Shridharani SM, Broyles JM. The safety and efficacy of cryolipolysis: a systematic review of available literature. *Aesthet Surg J.* 2015;35(7):830–836.

53. Jalian HR, Avram MM, Garibyan L, Mihm MC, Anderson RR. Paradoxical adipose hyperplasia after cryolipolysis. *JAMA Dermatol.* 2014;150(3):317–319.

54. Wanitphakdeedecha R, Sathaworawong A, Manuskiatti W. The efficacy of cryolipolysis treatment on arms and inner thighs. *Lasers Med Sci.* 2015;30(8):2165–2169.

55. Pinto H. Local fat treatments: classification proposal. *Adipocyte.* 2015;5(1):22–26.

56. Alizadeh Z, Halabchi F, Mazaheri R, Abolhasani M, Tabesh M. Review of the mechanisms and effects of noninvasive body contouring devices on cellulite and subcutaneous fat. *Int J Endocrinol Metab.* 2016;14(4):e36727.

57. Kilmer SL, Burns AJ, Zelickson BD. Safety and efficacy of cryolipolysis for non-invasive reduction of submental fat. *Lasers Surg Med.* 2016;48(1):3–13.

58. Krueger N, Mai SV, Luebberding S, Sadick NS. Cryolipolysis for noninvasive body contouring: clinical efficacy and patient satisfaction. *Clin Cosmet Investig Dermatol.* 2014;7:201–205.

59. Bernstein EF. Longitudinal evaluation of cryolipolysis efficacy: two case studies. *J Cosmet Dermatol.* 2013;12(2):149–152.

60. Izadifar Z, Babyn P, Chapman D. Mechanical and biological effects of ultrasound: A review of present knowledge. *Ultrasound Med Biol.* 2017;43(6):1085–1104.

61. Fatemi A. High-intensity focused ultrasound effectively reduces adipose tissue. *Semin Cutan Med Surg.* 2009;28(4):257–262.

62. Gadsden E, Aguilar MT, Smoller BR, Jewell ML. Evaluation of a novel high-intensity focused ultrasound device for ablating subcutaneous adipose tissue for noninvasive body contouring: safety studies in human volunteers. *Aesthet Surg J.* 2011;31(4):401–410.

63. Fatemi A, Kane MA. High-intensity focused ultrasound effectively reduces waist circumference by ablating adipose tissue from the abdomen and flanks: a retrospective case series. *Aesthetic Plast Surg.* 2010;34(5):577–582.

64. Robinson DM, Kaminer MS, Baumann L, et al. High-intensity focused ultrasound for the reduction of subcutaneous adipose tissue using multiple treatment techniques. *Dermatol Surg.* 2014;40(6):641–651.

65. Jewell ML, Weiss RA, Baxter RA, et al. Safety and tolerability of high-intensity focused ultrasonography for noninvasive body sculpting: 24-week data from a randomized, sham-controlled study. *Aesthet Surg J.* 2012;32(7):868–876.

66. Gold MH, Khatri KA, Hails K, Weiss RA, Fournier N. Reduction in thigh circumference and improvement in the appearance of cellulite with dual-wavelength, low-level laser energy and massage. *J Cosmet Laser Ther.* 2011;13(1):13–20.

67. Weinstein Velez M, Ibrahim O, Petrell K, Dover JS. Nonthermal pulsed ultrasound treatment for the reduction in abdominal fat: a pilot study. *J Clin Aesthet Dermatol.* 2018;11(9):32–36.

68. Bani D, Quattrini Li A, Freschi G, Russo GL. Histological and ultrastructural effects of ultrasound-induced cavitation on human skin adipose tissue. *Plast Reconstr Surg Glob Open.* 2013 Oct 7;1(6):e41.

69. Brown SA, Greenbaum L, Shtukmaster S, Zadok Y, Ben-Ezra S, Kushkuley L. Characterization of nonthermal focused ultrasound for noninvasive selective fat cell disruption (lysis): technical and preclinical assessment. *Plast Reconstr Surg.* 2009;124(1):92–101.

70. Coleman KM, Coleman WP, Benchetrit A. Non-invasive, external ultrasonic lipolysis. *Semin Cutan Med Surg.* 2009;28(4):263–267.

71. Moreno-Moraga J, Valero-Altés T, Riquelme AM, Isarria-Marcosy MI, de la Torre JR. Body contouring by non-invasive transdermal focused ultrasound. *Lasers Surg Med.* 2007;39(4):315–323.

72. Teitelbaum SA, Burns JL, Kubota J, et al. Noninvasive body contouring by focused ultrasound: safety and efficacy of the Contour I device in a multicenter, controlled, clinical study. *Plast Reconstr Surg.* 2007;120(3):779–789; discussion 790.

73. Shek S, Yu C, Yeung CK, Kono T, Chan HH. The use of focused ultrasound for non-invasive body contouring in Asians. *Lasers Surg Med.* 2009;41(10):751–759.

74. Jang H, Lee H. Meta-analysis of pain relief effects by laser irradiation on joint areas. *Photomed Laser Surg.* 2012;30(8):405–417.

75. Avci P, Nyame TT, Gupta GK, Sadasivam M, Hamblin MR. Low-level laser therapy for fat layer reduction: A comprehensive review. *Lasers Surg Med.* 2013;45(6):349–357.

76. Thornfeldt CR, Thaxton PM, Hornfeldt CS. A six-week low-level laser therapy protocol is effective for reducing waist, hip, thigh, and upper abdomen circumference. *J Clin Aesthet Dermatol.* 2016;9(6):31–35.

77. Nestor MS, Zarraga MB, Park H. Effect of 635nm low-level laser therapy on upper arm circumference reduction: A double-blind,

randomized, sham-controlled trial. *J Clin Aesthet Dermatol.* 2012;5(2):42–48.

78. Gold MH, Coleman WP, Coleman W, Weiss R. A randomized, controlled multicenter study evaluating focused ultrasound treatment for fat reduction in the flanks. *J Cosmet Laser Ther.* 2019;21(1):44–48.

79. Rzepecki AK, Farberg AS, Hashim PW, Goldenberg G. Update on noninvasive body contouring techniques. *Cutis.* 2018;101(4);285–288.

80. Jackson RF, Stern FA, Neira R, Ortiz-Neira CL, Maloney J. Application of low-level laser therapy for noninvasive body contouring. *Lasers Surg Med.* 2012;44(3):211–217.

81. Jackson RF, Roche GC, Wisler K. Reduction in cholesterol and triglyceride serum levels following low-level laser irradiation: a noncontrolled, nonrandomized pilot study. *Am J Cosmet Surg.* 2010;27(4):177–184.

82. Decorato JW, Chen B, Sierra R. Subcutaneous adipose tissue response to a non-invasive hyperthermic treatment using a 1,060 nm laser. *Lasers Surg Med.* 2017;49(5):480–489.

83. Schilling L, Saedi N, Weiss R. 1060 nm diode hyperthermic laser lipolysis: The latest in non-invasive body contouring. *J Drugs Dermatol.* 2017;16(1):48–52.

84. Weiss RA, Bernardy J. Induction of fat apoptosis by a non-thermal device: Mechanism of action of non-invasive high-intensity electromagnetic technology in a porcine model. *Lasers Surg Med.* 2019;51(1):47–53.

85. Nestor MS, Newburger J, Zarraga MB. Body contouring using 635-nm low level laser therapy. *Semin Cutan Med Surg.* 2013;32(1):35–40.

86. Katz B, Doherty S. Safety and efficacy of a noninvasive 1,060-nm diode laser for fat reduction of the flanks. *Dermatol Surg.* 2018;44(3):388–396.

87. Abulhasan J, Rumble Y, Morgan E, Slatter W, Grey M. Peripheral electrical and magnetic stimulation to augment resistance training. *J Funct Morphol Kinesiol.* 2016;1(3):328–342.

88. Jacob CI, Paskova K. Safety and efficacy of a novel high-intensity focused electromagnetic technology device for noninvasive abdominal body shaping. *J Cosmet Dermatol.* 2018;17(5): 783–787.

89. Stallknecht B, Dela F, Helge JW. Are blood flow and lipolysis in subcutaneous adipose tissue influenced by contractions in adjacent muscles in humans? *Am J Physiol Endocrinol Metab.* 2007;29(2):E394–E399.

90. Kinney BM, Lozanova P. High intensity focused electromagnetic therapy evaluated by magnetic resonance imaging: Safety and efficacy study of a dual tissue effect based non-invasive abdominal body shaping. *Lasers Surg Med.* 2019;51(1):40–46.

91. Jacob C, Kinney B, Busso M, et al. High intensity focused electro-magnetic technology (HIFEM) for non-invasive buttock lifting and toning of gluteal muscles: a multi-center efficacy and safety study. *J Drugs Dermatol.* 2018;17(11):1229–1232.

CHAPTER 23

Botulinum Toxins

Paula Purpera, MSHS, PA-C
Leslie S. Baumann, MD

SUMMARY POINTS

What's Important?

1. All BTX-A work the same way and are basically interchangeable.

What's New?

1. A new BTX-A with a stabilizing peptide called RTP004 from Revance has joined the market.
2. BTX-A tends to "prejuvenate" the skin and prevent aging when used consistently.

What's Coming?

1. More research is necessary to determine how to titrate diffusion and how much diffusion is preferred for cosmetic indications.
2. More studies are needed to determine the safety of intradermal BTX-A to treat fine lines.
3. Preliminary data suggest BTX-A has an anti-aging effect separate from its ability to immobilize muscles. More data are needed to understand the "prejuvenation" abilities of BTX-A.
4. Shorter acting toxins are coming.
5. Studies evaluating the use of BTX-A to treat rosacea and acne as well as to reduce oil secretion are on the horizon.

Botulinum toxin (BTX), an exotoxin produced by the bacteria *Clostridium botulinum,* occurs in nature. BTX induces a bilaterally symmetric descending neuroparalytic condition called botulism. The word "botulinum" is derived from the Latin word for sausage, *botulus*. Botulism was so named during the Napoleonic era in the early 1800s when it was noted to be triggered by the ingestion of spoiled sausages. Later, German physician Justinus Kerner described food-borne botulism and its clinical symptoms during the period between 1817 and 1822. In 1946, Schantz reported isolating BTX type A in its crystalline form, and nearly a quarter of a century later, Alan Scott became the first to harness the effects of BTX for medicinal use in monkey strabismus.[1]

The use of *C. botulinum* A exotoxin, commonly known as botulinum toxin type A (BTX-A), has emerged over the last 20 years as one of the most popular methods of combating cutaneous signs of aging, particularly the dynamic wrinkles of the face. The therapeutic application of this potent neurotoxin has carved a comfortable niche in the cosmetic realm of dermatology practice for practical reasons: Results appear within several days of administration, the procedure itself is short in duration and relatively uncomplicated, and side effects are minimal.

Although medicinal use of BTX by physicians is widespread, professional opinions vary as to the best ways to administer the treatment. For instance, the ideal dilution of the toxin, the number of units to inject, and the longevity of prepared and refrigerated BTX remain debated issues (**Box 23-1**). The methods described in this chapter are those used most frequently by the authors. The novice injector should try the various methods espoused by experienced specialists to determine which yields the best results in his/her own practice.

MECHANISM OF ACTION

Acetylcholine (Ach) is the neurotransmitter associated with induction of muscle movement. BTX achieves chemical denervation of striated muscles by cleaving one or more of

TABLE 23-1	Binding Sites of Various Toxin Serotypes
Toxin Serotype	Binding Site
BTX-A	SNAP-25
BTX-B	Synaptobrevin
BTX-C1	SNAP-25 and syntaxin
BTX-D	Synaptobrevin
BTX-E	SNAP-25
BTX-F	Synaptobrevin
BTX-G	Synaptobrevin

> **BOX 23-2** Composition of Botulinum Toxin
>
> BTX is composed of three domains: the binding domain, the translocation domain, and the enzymatic domain. The binding domain is responsible for attaching to the presynaptic nerve terminal. (These receptors are specific to each BTX serotype and the serotypes do not bind to each other's acceptors.) Binding of the toxin initiates endocytosis and internalization of the molecule. Once inside the endosome, the acidic environment is believed to create a change in the conformation of the translocation domain of the toxin that allows the light chain to cross the membrane of the endosome and enter the cytosol.[3] Once released into the cytosol, the enzymatic domain residing in the light chain cleaves a protein in the SNARE complex that inactivates this complex, preventing the fusion of Ach vesicles and blocking the release of Ach into the synaptic cleft. The specific cleaved SNARE complex protein depends on the BTX serotype. BTX-A cleaves the SNAP-25 molecule at the peptide bond between glutamine 197 and arginine 198 and BTX-B cleaves synaptobrevin between the amino acid residues glutamine 76 and phenylalanine 77.[4] Interestingly, tetanus toxin also cleaves synaptobrevin, but uses a different enzyme.

the proteins required for the release of Ach. The target protein depends on the serotype of toxin used (**Table 23-1**). The result is temporary flaccid paralysis of the injected muscles, which persists approximately 3 to 5 months. As new neuromuscular junctions form, muscle function returns. There are seven BTX serotypes (A–G). Serotype A is the most potent and was the first to be made available in the United States U.S. for medical use. Botox Cosmetic™ (Allergan Inc., Irvine, CA), Dysport® (Ipsen Products, Maidenhead, Berkshire, UK), Xeomin® (Merz Pharmaceuticals, Frankfurt, Germany), Jeuveau (Evolus, Newport Beach, CA), and a new BTX-A coming from Revance Therapeutics, Inc. (Newark, CA) were formed from serotype A, which functions by cleaving the SNAP-25 protein, a component of the SNARE (soluble N-ethylmaleamide-sensitive factor attachment protein receptor) complex (**Box 23-2**). The presence of an intact SNARE complex, composed of synaptobrevin, SNAP-25, and syntaxin, is necessary for vesicles containing Ach to fuse with the cell membrane and to release Ach into the neuromuscular junction (**Fig. 23-1**). BTX-B, available in the U.S. as Myobloc™ (known as Neurobloc in Europe), cleaves synaptobrevin, thus preventing the release of Ach.

CLINICAL INDICATIONS

In the 1970s, Dr. Alan Scott became the first scientist to use BTX to treat strabismus in monkeys. Within 7 years, he had performed the first human trials.[2] Subsequently, ophthalmologists began using BTX to treat strabismus, nystagmus, and blepharospasm.[5,6] In 1990, the first paper reporting the use of BTX for cosmetic purposes was published.[7] Since that time, the use of BTX has become increasingly widespread and is currently the most popular nonsurgical cosmetic procedure, with 1.8 million injections performed in 2018.[8]

The cosmetic indications for BTX currently include the prevention and treatment of dynamic wrinkles (wrinkles "in motion") and amelioration of excessive sweating (hyperhidrosis). BTX is also used to correct platysmal banding in the neck, which leads to a condition commonly known as "turkey neck." In addition, some practitioners have obtained satisfactory results in treating the signs of aging in the lower face.[9,10] New indications are frequently reported.

BOTULINUM TOXIN TYPE A

Botox Cosmetic (OnabotulinumtoxinA)

Initially introduced as Botox™ (Allergan, Inc., Irvine, California), this product was first used for cosmetic purposes in 1981. Botox Cosmetic, still usually referred to as "Botox," was approved by the U.S. Food and Drug Administration (FDA) in 2002 for treatment of (glabellar) frown lines. Botox is formed from fermented cultures of *C. botulinum*. The cultures are subjected to autolysis, releasing a 900 kD toxic complex. Prior to placement in storage vials, the compound is diluted with human serum albumin. The manufacturers then freeze-dry and seal the toxin. One vial of Botox contains 100 U of BTX-A.

> **BOX 23-1** Units of Botulinum Toxin
>
> One unit (U) of BTX is the dose that would be lethal to 50% (LD_{50}) of the specific mouse species tested. For a 70-kg person, the LD_{50} of Botox is 2500 to 3000 U. However, manufacturers use different mouse models, so a unit of one brand is not equivalent to a unit of another brand. Because of these variations, it is important to know which type of BTX was used when evaluating dosing information in the literature. For cosmetic indications, injection of approximately 20 to 75 U doses of Botox is typical. Practitioners have used doses as high as 1000 Botox units to treat cerebral palsy and other neurologic conditions.

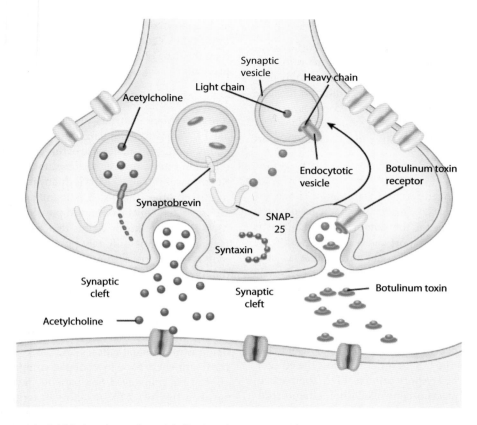

FIGURE 23-1. Botulinum toxins inhibit the release of acetylcholine into the neuromuscular junction.

Dilution and Storage

Physicians do not agree on the optimal dilution ratio for the toxin or on how long the toxin retains its potency after dilution. However, Klein published a survey of expert Botox users and found that most of them use a dilution of 2.5 cc per 100-U vial.[11] This dilution was used in the Allergan glabellar FDA trials as well. Reports in the literature support the use of 1 cc to 10 cc dilutions.[11] See **Table 23-2** for dilution guidelines or download a mobile app called "Dilution Calc!" from the app store that calculates how to dilute any of the toxins to get the correct dose.

The 100-U bottle of Botox is diluted with 0.9% saline. Preservative-free saline was recommended initially until studies showed that pain perception diminished when preservative-containing saline was used.[12] When diluting the bottle, care must be taken to gently inject the saline into the bottle to prevent foaming and bubbles, which may denature the toxin and decrease its potency. Many physicians remove the rubber stopper before adding the saline, which prevents the rapid addition of saline to the bottle because of the vacuum of the bottle and helps avoid leaving a few expensive drops of BTX-A in the vial. Novice practitioners should be advised to never insert the needle of the syringe that is to be used for injection into the rubber stopper. This would render it dull and increase the pain on injection. In addition, it is important not to shake the bottle or "flick" the syringe to eliminate air bubbles as agitation of the toxin may lead to loss of potency.

TABLE 23-2	Dilution Table for Botox
Volume of Diluent Added (cc)	Number of Units Per 0.1 cc
1.0	10
2.0	5
2.5	4
3.0	3.3

The amount of saline used to dilute Botox, Xeomin, and Jeuveau determines the number of units in each 0.1 cc. Another option is to use the DilutionCalc! app found on the app store.

Once the BTX-A has been diluted with saline, it begins to lose potency, but the point at which the potency losses become clinically significant is unknown. Many authors suggest that BTX-A should be used within 48 hours; however, some state that Botox may remain in the refrigerator up to 4 weeks.[13] If one plans to keep Botox for an extended period of time, preservative-containing saline should be used, and the reconstituted Botox should be kept in a refrigerator. In the authors' experience, the best Botox is "fresh" Botox and should be used within 24 hours of dilution. Botox should not be refrozen once prepared as this also causes a definite loss of potency, due to the formation of ice crystals.

Dysport (AbobotulinumtoxinA)

Dyspor® (Ipsen, Ltd., Paris, France) is sold in bottles containing 500 U of BTX-A. Similar to Botox, this neurotoxin is produced from *C. botulinum*. One unit of Botox is equivalent to 2.5 to 4 U of Dysport.[14,15] The units and dilution must be adjusted accordingly. Dysport is manufactured as freeze-dried 300-U and 500-U vials and preserved as a powder.[16] One bottle of Botox contains 5 ng of protein while a vial of Dysport contains 4.35 ng.[17]

Dilution and Storage

The shelf life of the packaged Dysport vial is approximately 1 year, if refrigerated at 2°–8°C.[16] The vial should be used within 24 hours of reconstitution, for the same reasons that this is recommended with Botox. Dysport can be diluted with 0.9% preservative-free or preservative-containing saline as suggested in **Table 23-3**. Using a dilution with 2.5 mL provides 20 U of Dysport per 0.1 mL. Reconstituted Dysport should not be frozen. In the authors' clinical practice, Dysport is diluted with 3.0 mL of diluent so the volume injected is the same for all neurotoxins regardless of the brand selected.

Separate studies on glabellar lines were carried out at major cosmetic centers across the U.S. in order to assess the efficacy, tolerability, and safety of Dysport prior to FDA approval. In two parallel groups of placebo-controlled double-blind studies including 300 and 158 patients, respectively, subjects were randomized to either Dysport (50 U) or placebo. The study durations were 150 and 180 days, respectively. Based on visual response scales assessed by investigators and patients, both studies concluded that at 30 days post-injection, Dysport significantly reached study-designed improvement endpoints in 90% of patients and reduced the severity of glabellar lines significantly better than placebo ($P < 0.001$). The median time of onset was either 2 or 3 days for both studies. The median duration of effect was 85 days, with significant efficacy through Day 120.[18]

A larger multicenter open-label study was carried out in 21 centers across the U.S. and enrolled 1,200 patients over a 13-month duration. Dysport (50 U) was used for glabellar lines to assess effectiveness and duration. Results suggested an onset of action within 3 days and a median duration of 88 days for effect. In all series, Dysport was deemed safe with negligible adverse effects.[19] Dysport performs similarly to Botox and is injected in the same sites and manner as Botox. It is important to remember that the dose of Dysport is different than the dose of Botox; otherwise, these are virtually identical products.

Xeomin (IncobotulinumtoxinA)

Xeomin® (Merz Pharmaceuticals, Frankfurt, Germany) is also a BTX-A product containing only the 150 kDa neurotoxin component. The smaller size of this compound may increase its diffusion rates; however, this has not been clearly established. Xeomin was introduced in Germany in 2005 and was approved in 2010 by the USFDA. It is manufactured as 50 Units, 100 Units, or 200 Units lyophilized powder in a single-dose vial.[20] Merz Pharmaceuticals claims that the product is highly purified and contains only 600 pg of bacterial proteins,[21] which may result in lower immune response. In addition, Xeomin differs from Botox and Dysport in one of its constituent elements. While Botox and Dysport contain sodium chloride and lactose, respectively, Xeomin contains saccharose. The clinical conversion rate of Botox to Xeomin is reported as 1:1.[22] Several major studies conducted and reported by Jost et al. demonstrated equal efficacy and safety profiles of Xeomin in the treatment of focal dystonias as compared to Botox. The five clinical trials involved 862 patients and found no difference between the two BTX-A toxins in terms of onset of action, duration, or waning of effect.[23] Further research is needed to evaluate efficacy in cosmetic dermatology and antigenic response of this product.

Dilution and Storage

Xeomin can remain stable when stored unreconstituted at room temperature for up to 48 months.[24] Reconstituted Xeomin should be administered within 24 hours after dilution. During this time period, unused reconstituted Xeomin may be stored in the original container in a refrigerator at 2°–8°C (36°–46°F) for up to 24 hours until time of use.[20] A 2015 study showed that efficacy was maintained for 1 week after reconstitution when stored at 25°C (77°F).[25] Xeomin is diluted in the same manner as Botox with 2.5 mL of diluent.

A multicenter, randomized, Phase III study investigated the efficacy and safety of incobotulinumtoxinA to treat the glabellar lines of 276 patients. The patients were randomized 2:1 to receive a single injection of 20 U of incobotulinumtoxinA or placebo, respectively. The results showed incobotulinumtoxinA to be significantly superior to placebo in the treatment of glabellar frown lines at Day 30 ($P < .001$), with investigators and patients assessing glabellar frown lines as significantly more improved after incobotulinumtoxinA injection than with placebo ($P < .001$).[26] Another multicenter study with 271 subjects with moderate to severe glabellar frown lines showed similar results over 120 days.[27]

The lack of complexing proteins may convey an advantage from a clinical standpoint. The complexing proteins have been shown to elicit an immune response.[28] Antibody-induced treatment failure is a well-known phenomenon in the therapeutic setting, with reported ranges from 4%–9.5% of patients treated.[29,30] The development of neutralizing antibodies in

TABLE 23-3	Dysport Dilution Table[a]	
Diluent:		
0.9% Saline	**300-U Vial**	**125-U Vial**
1.0 mL	30 U	12.5 U
2.0 mL	15 U	6.25 U
2.5 mL	12 U	5 U
3.0 mL	10 U	4.1 U

[a]Units per 0.1 mL.
Another option is to use the DilutionCalc! app found on the app store.

humans following aesthetic use of BoNT-A products is rare. There have been several reports of treatment failure with abobotulinumtoxinA and onabotulinumtoxinA.[31,32]

Jeuveau (PrabotulinumtoxinA)

Jeuveau® (Evolus, Inc., Newport Beach, CA) received FDA approval on February 1, 2019, for the treatment of moderate to severe glabellar lines. PrabotulinumtoxinA is a 900-kDa BTX-A preparation that was originally developed by Daewoong Pharmaceutical Co., Ltd. of Seoul, South Korea and licensed to Evolus for clinical development and distribution in the U.S., Europe, and Canada.[33] Jeuveau is being marketed as the only BTX-A product with an exclusively aesthetic indication, as the only FDA-approved indication is for the treatment of glabellar frown lines.[34]

Dilution and Storage

Jeuveau comes in 100-U vials and is reconstituted with 2.5 mL of 0.9% sterile saline with a resulting dose of 4 U per 0.1 mL. Jeuveau should be administered within 24 hours after reconstitution. During this time period, unused reconstituted Jeuveau should be stored in a refrigerator between 2°–8°C (36°–46°F).[34]

A multicenter, double-blind, controlled, single-dose Phase III study with 540 patients with moderate to severe glabellar lines at maximum frown was conducted for 150 days. This study compared the efficacy and safety of prabotulinumtoxinA compared to onabotulinumtoxinA and placebo for the treatment of glabellar frown lines. Results showed no statistically significant difference between the two BTX-A products in terms of efficacy and safety.[33] Additionally, two multicenter, randomized, double-blind, placebo-controlled, single-dose Phase III studies (EV-001 and EV-002) were conducted to investigate the safety and efficacy of prabotulinumtoxinA for the treatment of glabellar frown lines in 330 adult subjects. The studies revealed a 66.3% response rate and 69.1% response rate in EV-001 and EV-002, respectively, as compared to placebo ($P < 0.001$).[35]

DAXI (Daxibotulinumtoxin A)

DAXI (Revance Therapeutics Inc., Newark, CA) is a novel BTX-A product consisting of a purified 150 kDa molecule devoid of accessory proteins and formulated with a proprietary stabilizing peptide called RTP004 in a lyophilized powder. The peptide is constructed on a backbone of consecutive lysines, which carry a positive charge, resulting in the peptide binding strongly to the BTX-A molecule through electrostatic bonds.[36] In preclinical studies, daxibotulinumtoxinA has been shown to exhibit less diffusion than onabotulinumtoxinA, suggesting that it could confer a greater duration of effect after injection. Preclinical studies indicate that the duration to full recovery of muscle force generation for the DAXI group and the Botox group were 31.6 and 15.8 weeks, respectively. These data demonstrate that the limited diffusion may permit safe administration of higher and more efficacious doses.[37] DaxibotulinumtoxinA is currently pending FDA approval for treatment of glabellar lines, cervical dystonia, upper limb spasticity, and plantar fasciitis.[38]

Dilution and Storage

DaxibotulinumtoxinA is stable at room temperature and is produced without albumin or any other animal or human blood products. It is supplied in vials containing 160 U of lyophilized product. It is diluted to a 100 U/mL solution using 1.6 mL of sterile non-preserved 0.9% sodium chloride solution.[29]

Pooled results from two Phase III pivotal studies with 609 adults to evaluate the safety and efficacy of daxibotulinumtoxinA to treat moderate to severe glabellar lines showed a responder rate of 72.6% at 16 weeks and 32.3% at 24 weeks in the DAXI group respectively versus 4.4% and 2.0% in the placebo group respectively. Of the DAXI subjects, 98% had improvement of glabellar lines at maximum frown at 4 weeks versus 3.1% of placebo subjects. Furthermore, the median time to return to baseline glabellar line status was 27.1 weeks with DAXI. Treatment-related adverse events were reported in <20% of subjects and were predominantly mild. There were no new or unexpected safety findings observed and no subjects developed neutralizing antibodies to DAXI.[39]

BOTULINUM TOXIN TYPE B

Myobloc

Myobloc™ (Solstice Neurosciences, South San Francisco, CA) received FDA approval for use in the U.S. in December 2000. Myobloc is composed of BTX-B, which acts by cleaving the protein synaptobrevin preventing Ach release in the synaptic cleft. The drug is available in a ready-to-use formula that does not require reconstitution, but it should be kept refrigerated. Myobloc is stable for up to 21 months in refrigerator storage. This product is available in three-vial configurations of 2500, 5000, and 10,000 U, with a composition of 5000 U BTX-B/mL. Once the bottle has been opened, Myobloc begins to lose its potency. A physician who performs few Myobloc injections per week can opt to use a smaller size bottle to avoid wasting the residual toxin, thus ensuring that the toxin is as potent as possible.

The FDA has approved Myobloc for the treatment of cervical dystonia; however, its use in cosmetics has not yet been approved. Phase III clinical trials of the drug for the treatment of cervical dystonia reported a 12- to 16-week duration of effect. In a study by Baumann et al., 20 patients were treated for crow's feet with Myobloc and the maximum efficacy was determined to be at Day 30, with the effect beginning to dissipate at a mean of 67.5 days.[40]

Approximately 50 U of Myobloc are equivalent to 1 U of Botox. Although Myobloc is shipped in a reconstituted form, preservative-free saline may be added to change the number of units in 0.1 cc. When diluting a bottle of Myobloc, it is important to recognize that the bottles are overfilled and actually contain slightly more Myobloc than the label states in order to compensate for the volume that may be lost in the needle tip and on the edges of the bottle.

BOTULINUM TOXIN TYPE E

Botulinum toxin serotype E (BTX-E) is the predominant serotype causing botulism associated with native Arctic foods.[41] As opposed to BTX-A, which cleaves SNAP-25 between residues 197 and 198, BTX-E cleaves SNAP-25 between residues 180 and 181.[42] The therapeutic effects of BTX-A last from 3 to 12 months, whereas the effects of BTX-E last less than 4 weeks in trials. Confocal microscopy has determined that the BTX-E long chain stays in the cytoplasm of neurons and is more accessible to degradation. The BTX-E-cleaved SNAP-25 protein is cleared and replaced by intact SNAP-25 relatively quickly.[43] The long chain of BTX-A and BTX-A-cleaved SNAP-25 is retained at the plasma membrane. This accounts for the persistence of BTX-A-cleaved SNAP-25 in presynaptic endings.[44]

DIFFUSION CHARACTERISTICS OF BOTULINUM TOXINS

With the emergence of multiple brands of BTX, differences in preparations and effects need to be assessed for optimal patient benefit with minimal complications. Although the various BTX preparations impart very similar results, there are a few differences to take into account. Diffusion rates may result in different "fields of effects" or surface area affected by the toxin.

The diffusion potential of botulinum neurotoxins and their migration depends on several factors such as the size and structure of the molecule,[45] the subtype of the toxin,[46,47] the volume of saline in injections,[48] the protein load as well as the formulation's excipient content,[49] and finally on the muscle and site of injection.[19] The field of effects or diffusion of BTX-A and BTX-B have been characterized and targeted in a few studies concerned with their extent of diffusion and potential complications.

Myobloc appears to have a greater field of effect than Botox. One study compared the radius of diffusion of Myobloc to Botox in eight patients with moderate to severe forehead wrinkles. Patients were injected with 5 U of Botox on one side of their frontalis muscle and with 500 U of Myobloc to the other side (1:100 Botox: Myobloc conversion rate). The field of effect of Myobloc was assessed using a digital micrometer on traced scanned images and demonstrated a higher diffusion.[50] In another comparative study of Botox and Myobloc, Matarasso showed that treating crow's feet with Myobloc produces more sensation of tightness and freezing in comparison to Botox and he speculated that the observation is caused by increased Myobloc diffusion.[51] An increased field of effect may be advantageous in that it would allow fewer injection points to produce the same effect. This is particularly beneficial when treating hyperhidrosis of the palms, where the pain of injection is significant. In fact, in the primary author's experience,

Myobloc is the most efficacious toxin in the treatment of hyperhidrosis because of the greater amount of diffusion.[52]

Dysport may also have a greater field of effect than Botox. In a 2007 study, the diffusions of Botox and Dysport were compared in 20 patients with forehead hyperhidrosis.[53] Patients were randomly injected with 3 U of Botox or Dysport (conversion rate of 1:2.5, 1:3, and 1:4 correlating to 7.5, 9, or 12 U, respectively) in four areas of the forehead. The injection volume was consistent in all treatments. The anhidrotic area was assessed by using the starch-iodine test. Subjects who received Dysport had a significantly higher mean area of anhidrosis on their forehead as compared to patients treated with Botox. Another study compared 12 healthy volunteers who were randomly assigned to receive three 0.1-mL intradermal injections in their forehead: 4 U Botox on one side, 12 U Dysport (conversion rate of 1:3) on the contralateral side, and saline in the center. The anhidrotic area was assessed by using the starch-iodine test. A higher mean area of anhidrosis was observed in 11 of the 12 subjects who received Dysport and the authors concluded that Dysport has a higher migration potential than Botox.[54] A higher migration potential would likely result in fewer injections required in a treated area. (See **Box 23-3** for a brief discussion related to the number of injections and the business aspects of these treatments.) This would be beneficial in areas such as crow's feet, where bruising from the needle is common. More studies need to be performed to determine if an increased field of effect provides an advantage. Xeomin is the smallest of the BTX-A preparations because it is composed of the neurotoxin component alone and not the surrounding complexing proteins.[21] For this reason, it may diffuse more than the other BTX-A preparations. More research is necessary to determine how much diffusion is preferred for cosmetic indications.

BOTULINUM TOXIN FOR BEGINNERS: CLINICAL USES

In this section the focus is on BTX injections for beginners. This will cover commonly used indications and what is currently FDA approved (with the exception of nasalis). Becoming

---

BOX 23-3 The Business Side of Botulinum Toxin

The amount of BTX needed per site depends on the musculature of the individual patient. Therefore, many practitioners choose to charge by the number of units and not by the area treated. When using a consistent dilution technique, one can charge by the number of units used. The price per unit varies geographically. The patient should understand that additional injections (and charges) may occur at the next visit because individual musculature varies. In other words, if you charge by the number of units, you will likely need to charge for touch-ups as well. Charging by the number of units used simplifies keeping track of inventory and when to re-order.

proficient at these techniques for at least a year before moving to the advanced techniques that will be discussed in the next section is recommended.

Dynamic Wrinkles

BTX can be injected into specific muscles to induce temporary paralysis resulting in an inability to move and wrinkle the skin overlying the treated muscle. BTX is only beneficial for dynamic wrinkles (wrinkles in motion). It is not as effective for static wrinkles (wrinkles at rest), although prolonged use of BTX may help prevent wrinkles in motion from becoming wrinkles at rest. BTX can be combined with dermal fillers (Chapter 25), microneedling (Chapter 27), lasers and lights (Chapter 26), and retinoids (Chapter 45) to optimize patient satisfaction. The upper part of the face contains distinct muscle groups that can be selectively paralyzed by a knowledgeable injector. In the lower part of the face, the muscle groups are less discrete and thus more difficult to inject accurately (**Fig. 23-2**). The paralytic effects of BTX appear approximately 3 to 7 days after injection. However, the effects may take up to 2 weeks. In the authors' experience, the effects are the strongest at Days 14–15 and tend to relax slightly after Day 15. For this reason, it is suggested to evaluate new patients between Days 14–17 if possible.

To use Botox, dilute the 100-U vial with 2.5 cc of preservative-free saline. This yields 4 U per 0.1 cc. To use Dysport, dilute the 500-U vial with 2.5 mL of 0.9% preservative-free saline. This provides 20 U per 0.1 mL. To use Myobloc, dilute a 2500-U vial with 1.2 cc of saline. This yields 200 U per 0.1 cc. Inject with a 1-cc syringe and a 30-gauge needle. You may also use a 3.0 cc dilution for Dysport, yielding 30 U per 0.1 cc.

BTX toxin binding to cholinergic receptor sites is complete by 64 minutes post-injection.[55] Historically, clinicians advise their patients to perform post-injection facial exercises for 4 hours after the procedure. Some studies suggest that post-injection exercises are helpful in achieving an earlier onset of clinical effect of BTX injections but do not affect the longevity of correction.[56]

Glabellar Region

To treat the glabellar region, inject 0.1 cc (4 U of Botox, Xeomin, or Jeuveau; or 200 U Myobloc; or 10 U of Dysport) into each corrugator muscle along with 0.1 cc into the procerus muscle (**Figs. 23-3 to 23-5**). The glabellar indication is also the FDA-approved cosmetic indication for Dysport. Rzany et al. studied the effect of Dysport in a double-blinded, placebo-controlled study of 221 subjects with glabellar lines. Participants were injected with 30 U, 50 U, or placebo in the glabellar area and followed for 16 weeks. After 4 weeks, there was little statistical difference between the treatment groups. The response rate among those who received 30 U and 50 U compared to placebo was 86.1% versus 18.9% and 86.3% versus 7.9%, respectively.[57]

The injection sites for female and male patients are shown in **Fig. Fig. 23-6, A and B**. In men or patients with stronger musculature, two sites superior to the corrugator muscle may need to be injected. The authors have found that doses of 20 U in the glabella work for most men while retaining a natural look; one study showed that 40 to 60 U in the glabellar area was more effective in males.[58] The injector should avoid hitting the periosteum with the needle tip as this can induce post-injection headache. After injecting the procerus muscle,

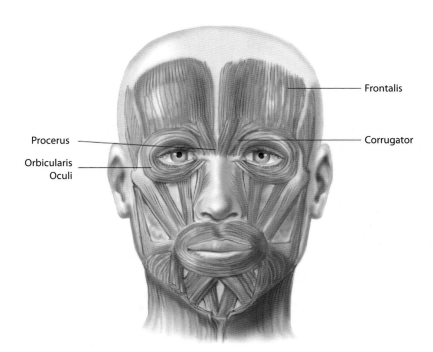

FIGURE 23-2. The muscles of the face. Each can be deliberately relaxed with an injection of botulinum toxin. Note that the muscles of the upper face are more distinct and separate from each other than the muscles in the lower face.

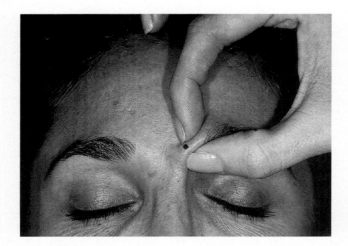

FIGURE 23-3. Corrugator injection site.

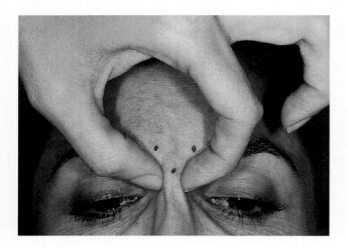

FIGURE 23-4. Procerus injection site.

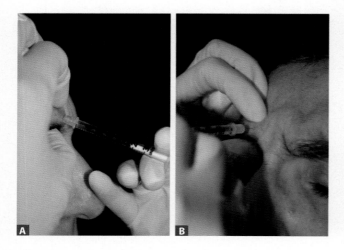

FIGURE 23-5. Angle of injection of the corrugator muscle. **A.** Use one hand to isolate the corrugator muscle. **B.** Rest the finger of the other hand on the nose as shown in **A** to stabilize the hand.

massage the area laterally across the bridge of the nose to ensure that the toxin enters the depressor supercilii portion of the corrugator muscle (**Fig. 23-7**), which will subtly lift the patient's medial brow, resulting in a more youthful appearance. Proper treatment of the glabellar area or "brow furrow" prevents the patient from frowning, leading to a more relaxed, less angry look (**Figs. 23-8 and 23-9, A and B**). In addition, relaxation of these muscles for long periods of time may prevent or reduce wrinkle formation in the brow area.

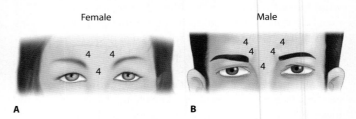

FIGURE 23-6. Each 4 represents 0.1 cc of medication that contains 4 units of Botox, Xeomin, or Jeuveau. **A.** Younger women aged 18 to 25 usually need only the three depicted injection sites. **B.** Women with increased musculature and men often need two extra injection sites as depicted, because they have increased muscle mass.

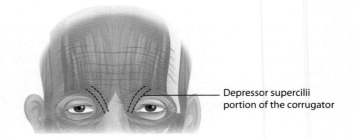

FIGURE 23-7. The depressor supercilii is a branch of the corrugator muscle responsible for depressing the medial eyebrow. Massaging the toxin into this area usually causes elevation of the medial brow.

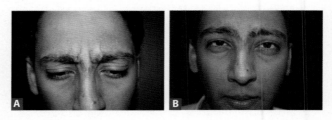

FIGURE 23-8. Male patient. **A.** before and **B.** after 20 units to the glabella. Note that he is recruiting facial muscles in the center of the brow in order to frown.

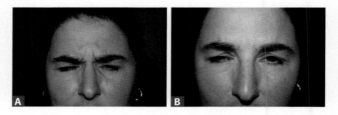

FIGURE 23-9. Female patient. **A.** before and **B.** after 12 units to the glabella. Note that she is recruiting facial muscles in the center of the brow in order to frown.

Forehead Region

In 2017, the FDA approved the use of BTX to treat horizontal forehead lines created by hyperdynamic frontalis muscles. A multicenter, randomized, controlled trial established the safety and efficacy for treating crow's feet alone or in combination with glabellar lines.[59] To treat wrinkles of the forehead, inject 0.1 cc (4 U Botox, Xeomin, or Jeuveau; 10 U Dysport; or 200 U Myobloc) across the forehead as demonstrated in **Figs. 23-10 and 23-11**. Injection of the forehead is an art as well as a science as it can dramatically affect eyebrow shape. Therefore, prior to injecting the forehead, the physician should consider whether s/he wants to enhance the arch of the eyebrow or to create a more horizontal eyebrow shape. Generally, women prefer a more arched brow because it imparts a more feminine look, while men prefer a more horizontal brow (**Table 23-4**). The forehead should be injected about every two square centimeters where movement of the muscles is seen on eyebrow elevation. It is important not to inject all patients in the same way. Forehead injections should be tailored or customized to the patient's forehead size and shape. In addition, one must consider the placement of the eyebrow over the superior orbital rim. Low brows will become even lower after injections of BTX to the forehead; therefore, forehead injections should be avoided in some patients. Alternatively, injections can be performed in the higher regions of the forehead in patients with low brows.

Use the recommendations in this chapter as rough guidelines and vary injection technique to suit the needs of each individual patient's anatomy. The major pitfalls with forehead injections are the following: (1) unwanted eyebrow shape (**Fig. 23-12**), (2) brow ptosis, (3) missed areas (**Figs. 23-13 and 23-14**), and (4) drooping eyelids. It is important not to over-inject the forehead area as this may lead to brow ptosis. Additionally, one must take care to avoid the area 1 cm above the eyebrows to reduce the chances of brow ptosis (**Fig. 23-15**). The physician should warn the patient with low forehead wrinkles within this 1-cm area that these wrinkles cannot be treated with BTX and will remain after treatment as demonstrated in **Figs. 23-16 and 23-17**. Care must be taken to avoid forehead injections in individuals with low-set brows and/or excessive eyelid skin. In older patients and patients with excess eyelid skin, overtreatment of the forehead area may result in drooping eyelids. Hooding of the upper eyelids by the descending eyebrow tissue results in a neural reflex that increases the activity of the frontalis muscle in an effort to keep the vision clear of the descending tissue that would otherwise obstruct vision or interfere with eyelid function.[60] In this population, the upward pulling of the frontalis muscle is needed to raise the baggy upper eye skin. These patients are better treated

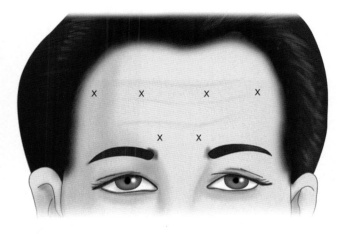

FIGURE 23-10. The pattern of injection to encourage arched brows. This pattern is used to promote a more feminine brow shape. Each x denotes 4 units of Botox, Xeomin, or Jeuveau.

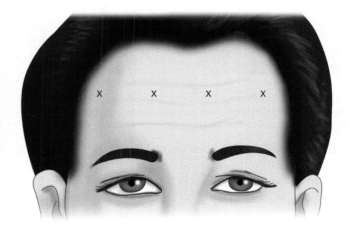

FIGURE 23-11. The pattern of injection to encourage horizontal brows. This pattern is used to cause a more masculine brow shape. Each x denotes 4 units of Botox, Xeomin, or Jeuveau.

TABLE 23-4	Feminine and Masculine Characteristics of Brow Shape	
Feminine Brows	**Masculine Brows**	
Arched	Horizontal	
Longer lid to brow distance	Lower lid to brow distance	
Thinner brow	Thicker brow	

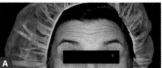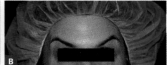

FIGURE 23-12. Before (**A**) and after (**B**) injection of Botox in the V-shaped pattern taught by many BTX experts. However, in this patient, significant use of the lateral forehead muscles is seen in **A.** Using the V-shaped injection technique in a patient with this forehead muscle function results in an unpopular "Diablo eyebrow" as seen in **B.** This can be avoided or corrected by injecting 4 units of Botox, Xeomin, or Jeuveau 2 cm above the lateral brow in the area of muscle movement.

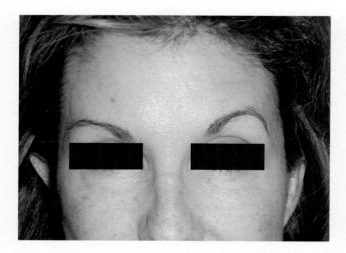

FIGURE 23-13. This patient was treated with Botox in the forehead by a beginning BTX injector. On her right side the lateral forehead was treated. On the left side it was not. It is crucial to inject the forehead equally on both sides to prevent asymmetry.

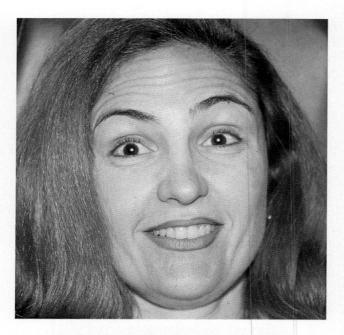

FIGURE 23-16. Forehead with eyebrows elevated prior to injection of botulinum toxin.

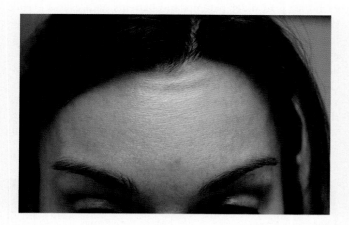

FIGURE 23-14. The physician who injected this female missed the area just below the hairline. In men, this can often occur laterally in areas of hair loss, so men may need to be injected in the upper lateral regions just below the receding hairline.

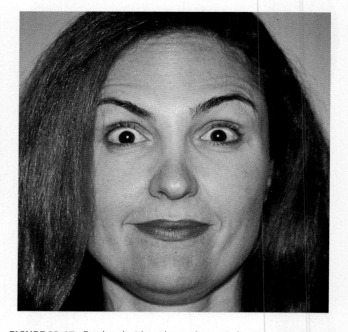

FIGURE 23-17. Forehead with eyebrow elevated after injection of botulinum toxin. Note that lower forehead wrinkles are still present. However, they are not apparent when eyebrows are not elevated.

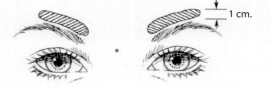

FIGURE 23-15. The 1-cm area above the medial portion of the eyebrow is a "danger zone" and, to avoid ptosis, should not be injected.

with blepharoplasty first, then with BTX. The ideal patient for BTX treatment in the forehead is a young patient (20s–40s) with no excess upper eyelid skin (**Figs. 23-18 and 23-19**).

Crow's Feet

In 2013, the FDA approved the use of BTX to treat the lateral canthal lines, also known as "crow's feet." A multicenter, randomized, controlled trial established the safety and efficacy for treating crow's feet alone or in combination with glabellar

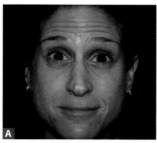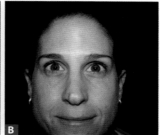

FIGURE 23-18. Before (**A**) and after (**B**) Botox injections.

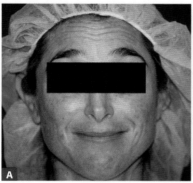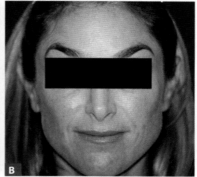

FIGURE 23-19. Before (**A**) and after (**B**) Botox injections to the forehead, glabella, and crow's feet.

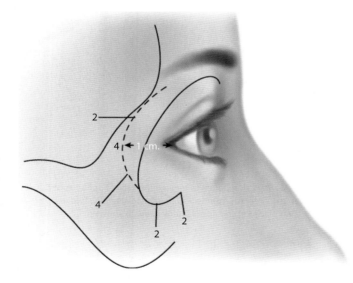

FIGURE 23-20. Injection points in the crow's feet area. The injection technique depends on the field of effect of the substances used. If Dysport is used, fewer injection sites (two) may be required because of an increased field of effect. Botox, Xeomin, or Jeuveau should be injected as shown in this diagram. The exact placement of injection is determined by the patient's facial anatomy, but this is a rough guide of placement.

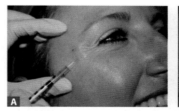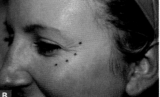

FIGURE 23-21. To inject Botox into crow's feet, have patients gently smile **A**. Inject at sites of maximal muscle contraction, which will be about 1.0 to 1.5 cm lateral to the corner of the eye **B**.

and **23-21**. If wrinkles progress medially, one can inject 0.05 cc approximately 1 cm apart along the orbital rim to the mid-pupillary line. When using Dysport, fewer injection sites may be required because of increased diffusion. Injecting medial to the midpupillary line does not correct medial wrinkles and can lead to an ectropion; therefore, this area should be avoided. Most patients do not notice these wrinkles prior to BTX injections and sometimes mistakenly believe that BTX "caused" these previously unobserved wrinkles. When used properly, BTX can temporarily erase lateral crow's feet lines (**Fig. 23-22**).

Nasalis ("Bunny Lines")
Expanded use is permissible for licensed physicians and aesthetic providers and is referred to as "off-label" use. The upper nasalis muscle across the bony dorsum of the nose causes

lines.[61] To treat crow's feet with Botox, inject 0.1 cc 1 cm lateral to the lateral canthus. Then inject 0.05 cc 1 cm above the first injection and 0.1 cc 1 cm below as shown in **Figs. 23-20**

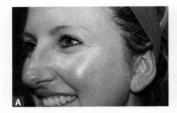 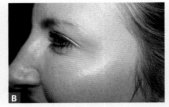

FIGURE 23-22. Before (**A**) and after (**B**) Botox injections.

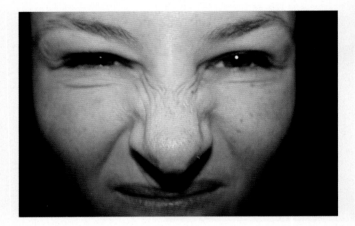

FIGURE 23-23. Wrinkling of the nasalis muscle or "bunny lines" leads to medial wrinkling under the eyes.

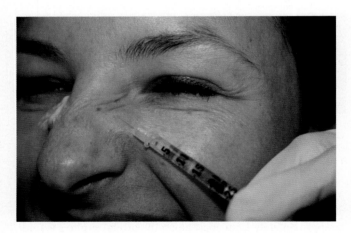

FIGURE 23-24. Injection site to treat bunny lines.

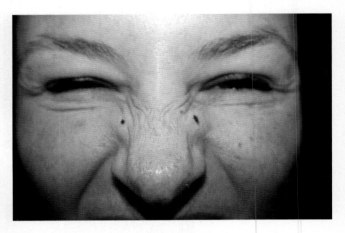

FIGURE 23-25. Injection sites to treat nasal bunny lines.

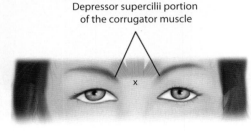

Depressor supercilii portion
of the corrugator muscle

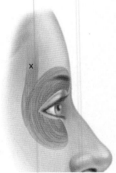

FIGURE 23-26. Injection points to elevate the brow. Four units of Botox are placed in the procerus muscle and massaged laterally. Two units of Botox are then placed in the upper lateral brow as shown.

fanning wrinkles at the radix of the nose and can lead to medial wrinkling around the eyes.[62] Two to four units of Botox can be injected into the nasalis muscle as shown to reduce or eliminate these lines. Many physicians inject into the wrinkles rather than into the nasalis muscle resulting in an incomplete correction. The correct injection points are in the belly of the muscle, inferior to the angular vein as shown in **Figs. 23-23 to 23-26**. If the injection is too low, the levator labii superioris will be relaxed, which leads to unwanted upper lip ptosis.

ADVANCED USE OF BOTULINUM TOXINS

Brow Lift and the Microdroplet Technique

BTX has been used to elevate eyebrow position by treating between the eyebrows as well as the lateral eyebrow with relatively few injection sites,[63] and with relatively large quantities of BTX (1.5–2.5 U BTX-A).[64] This technique is limited by the possibility of inducing the undesired side effect of upper eyelid ptosis caused by the unwanted diffusion of BTX into the levator palpebrae superioris muscle, which is responsible for eyelid elevation.[65]

The position and appearance of the eyebrows is determined at rest and dynamically by the opposing action of several groups of muscles that act on the eyebrow. The frontalis muscle primarily performs eyebrow elevation. Brow elevation is opposed by the septal and orbital portions of the orbicularis oculi muscle, including the depressor supercilii component of the orbicularis oculi muscle, and the procerus muscle.[66] The medial position of the eyebrow is also influenced by the activity of the corrugator supercilii muscle. Additionally, the shape of the brows is affected by the activities of the eyebrow elevators and the eyebrow depressor muscles where they interdigitate along the eyebrow to create facial expression.[67] With age there is a gradual fall in the position of the eyebrows, which is known as brow ptosis, resulting in smaller appearing eyes that is not aesthetically desirable.

BTX can also be used to elevate the brows, resulting in a more youthful appearance. This has been referred to in the literature as a chemical brow lift. The technique of lifting the brow includes injection of the glabellar area as described above. After injecting the procerus muscle with 0.1 cc of Botox the nasal bridge should be massaged to ensure that the toxin enters the depressor supercilii portion of the corrugator muscle as shown in **Fig. 23-8**. This can be used to try and correct an asymmetry of the medial brow. Injecting 0.05 cc of Botox into the lateral brow depressor muscles as shown in **Fig. 23-26** can raise the lateral aspect of the eyebrow.[68] Ahn et al. showed that treatment of the lateral depressors of the brow results in an average brow elevation of 4.83 mm when measured from the lateral canthus.[69] Injections of Botox into the glabellar area and lateral brow have also been shown to yield brow elevations of 1 to 3 mm when measured from the eyebrow to the midpupillary point.[68] However, it is the authors' experience that the lateral brow lift with Botox provides inconsistent results and leads to lateral brow lowering in some patients. (The procerus injection consistently raises the brows.)

A novel technique introduced by Steinsapir is intended to temporarily elevate the eyebrows without provoking any undesirable side effects. This "microdroplet technique" uses small quantities of BTX dissolved in microdroplets of injectable saline carrier to treat the septal and orbital orbicularis muscles on each side of the patient's face. He treats the frontalis at and below the brow by injecting very small volumes of fluid in multiple locations.[70] These microdroplets have volumes of 10 to 50 μL of injectable saline containing as little as 0.001 to 1 U Botox. Treatment is based on 100 U Botox and 3 mL of injectable saline, which equals approximately 0.33 U of Botox per 10 μL. A typical treatment involves a total of approximately 100 microdroplets placed in double or triple rows just above, in, and below the brow, stopping around the level of the lowest brow cilia. The microdroplet injections are placed superficially approximately 1 mm into the skin to trap the Botox at the interface between the orbicularis oculi and the skin. For crow's feet, the needle is inserted before the midline of the lateral palpebral raphe. The glabellar area is also treated. The combination of these treatments produces a uniform brow-lift effect.[14]

Dr. Woffles Wu expanded the use of Microbotox for a variety of applications. Injection of Microbotox into the dermis of the skin is used to reduce sweat and sebaceous gland activity, leaving a smooth, lustrous texture to the skin along with the reduction of superficial facial muscle activity. This leads to a marked reduction of surface wrinkling.[71] This technique is used in the upper face as well as in the platysma. In this technique, between 20–28 U (0.5–0.7 mL of a 100-U BTX vial diluted with 2.5 mL saline) is drawn into a 1-mL syringe. To produce a total of 1.0 mL of solution, 0.5–0.3 mL of 0.5% lidocaine is added. To treat the entire forehead, 20 U of BTX are sufficient. In the lower face and neck, 1 mL of solution containing 28 U is used per side (total of 56 U) to reduce superficial platysma activity and achieve better cervicomental and jawline contours.[72]

Treating Nasal Tip Ptosis

BTX has been used for lifting the nasal tip. More than one technique exists but there is no consensus on an optimal method. The main muscles that influence the nasal tip are the nasalis, the depressor septi nasi, the levator labii superioris, and the alaeque nasi muscle. Atamoros in 2003 described the injection of 4 U of Botox into each of the alar portions of the nasalis and 4 U into the depressor septi.[73] Dayan and Kempiners later described the injection of 5 U of Botox into each depressor septi nasi and 3 U into each levator labii superioris.[74] Ghavami et al. demonstrated similar results as Dayan and Kempiners with only 1 to 2 U injected to each of the depressor septi nasi and further stressed that proper studies excluding confounding variables, such as concomitant rhinoplasty or chemodenervation of synergistic muscles, are required before Botox injection alone can be recommended as a treatment for dynamic nasal tip ptosis.[75] The primary author uses 2 to 3 U injected at the base of the columella.[76] This procedure is most effective for those with a short- or normal-sized upper lip. Those with a long length between the top of the columella and the top of the lip, that is, long upper lip, do not receive good results from this procedure (**Fig. 23-27**). Those with a long upper lip will benefit from a dermal filler to raise the nasal tip (Chapter 25, Dermal Fillers).

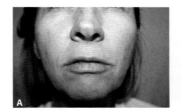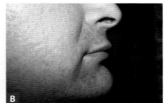

FIGURE 23-27. A. Patient with a long upper lip. **B.** Patient with a short upper lip. This patient is a better candidate for Botox injection to raise the nasal tip.

Cosmetic Use of Botulinum Toxin Type A in the Lower Face

Cosmetic treatments with BTX-A have focused mainly on the upper face, particularly the glabellar, forehead, and periocular areas. With the steep rise in the number of cosmetic BTX injections delivered each year and its clinical effectiveness, various off-label interventions using BTX-A for the lower face have emerged.[77] However, this area has an increased incidence of side effects and should only be treated by experienced BTX users.

As such, BTX-A is now more widely used in lower face and neck rejuvenation, in treating the chin and corners of the mouth, as well as in recontouring of the jawline. Yet another area where BTX-A has shown promise cosmetically is in the treatment of facial and chest wall flushing. The response of the lower facial muscles to BTX-A is greater than upper facial muscles. Moreover, it has been established that the lower facial muscles will have a longer-lasting response to BTX-A than upper facial musculature. The dose for the lower muscles therefore needs to be adjusted to the muscle size and patient's gender to be approximately half or one-third the dose injected in the upper facial muscles.

Upper Gum Show

The levator labii superioris alaeque nasi muscle retracts the upper lip. In some individuals, this muscle is overactive and pulls the lip back excessively, allowing visualization of the upper gums and upper incisors. Injecting 1 to 2 U into the levator labii superioris alaeque nasi muscle on each side of the bony nasal prominence will slightly drop the lip, preventing the upper gum show. This procedure works better in young patients because it causes vertical elongation of the lip. This can be used in combination with dermal fillers in the vermilion border to prevent the elongated lip (**Fig. 23-28**).

Melomental Folds

The melomental folds are also called marionette lines. They extend from the downturned corner of the mouth to the lateral chin. The depressor anguli oris pulls down the corner of the mouth in opposition to the zygomaticus major and minor contributing to these folds. Marionette lines are often corrected by dermal fillers (the primary author's preferred approach); however, some physicians prefer to combine dermal fillers with BTX injections. BTX can be injected into the depressor anguli oris to weaken it, allowing the zygomaticus to elevate the corners of the mouth and return them to a horizontal position.[10] For reducing the melomental folds, a dose of 2 to 4 U should be injected at the depressor anguli oris immediately above the angle of the mandible and 1 cm lateral to the lateral oral commissure.[78] Care must be taken not to use too high of a dose as this can lead to drooping of the lateral lower lip, flaccid cheeks, an incompetent mouth, or an asymmetric smile.

Perioral Lines

Several factors are implicated in the formation of perioral lines. Smoking, photoaging, loss of subcutaneous tissue in the lower face, and the purse string-like action of the orbicularis oris muscles are the most important causes. BTX-A injection is usually reserved for deep perioral lines exacerbated with muscular pursing of the lips. The dosage depends on the depth of lines but generally 1 U of BTX-A injected into each site with a total of 2 U per half of the upper lips is sufficient. The middle upper lip should be avoided in patients wanting to retain their cupid bow. It is critical to measure the placement on the upper lips first so that the sides are treated in exactly the same spot to preserve symmetry (**Fig. 23-29**). The best results occur when BTX is combined with laser resurfacing or lip fillers to enhance the vermilion border and smooth the surface of the skin.

Mentalis for Chin Puckering

Relaxing the hyperkinetic muscle fibers of the chin and the mentalis muscle with BTX-A can reduce and eliminate chin puckering (**Fig. 23-30**). A single dose of 4 to 6 U of BTX-A placed in the exact center of the point of the chin is effective.[76] An overdose in this area can result in the inability to approximate the lower lips tightly against the teeth, ultimately leading to involuntary dribbling from the lip when drinking or drooling from the corners of the mouth[79] (**Fig. 23-30**).

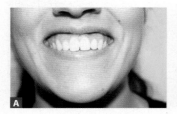
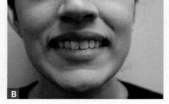

FIGURE 23-28. Upper gum shown (**A**) prior to Botox injections and (**B**) after Botox injections.

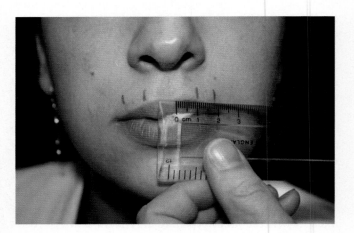

FIGURE 23-29. Placement of Botox, Xeomin, or Jeuveau on the upper lip to treat smoker's lines (now commonly called "bar code lines" as fewer people smoke). Only 1 unit should be used in each injection site for a total of 4 units for the entire upper lip.

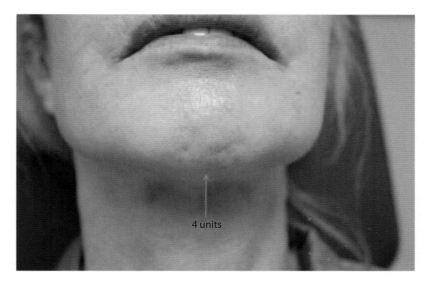

FIGURE 23-30. Chin puckering or Peau d'orange can be treated with BTX.

Masseter Hypertrophy/Bruxism

Benign masseter hypertrophy is an uncommon clinical condition characterized by unilateral or bilateral enlargement of the masseter muscle near the angle of the mandible. Masseter hypertrophy is associated with bruxism, temporomandibular disorders, and malocclusion.[80] It is also associated with muscular disfigurement and facial asymmetry. Traditional treatment is surgical resection of the masseter muscle.[81] Treatment of masseter hypertrophy using BTX was first reported in 1994.[82] It is a non-invasive alternative to treat this condition (**Fig. 23-31, A and B**).

Injections consist of 24 U to 30 U of BTX per side injected at five to six points into the prominent portions of the mandibular angle.[83,84] A study by Ahn et al. in 2004 had patients initially receive 25 U injected in the inferior masseter, and an additional 25 U per side was injected as needed at 1-week intervals. Maximum reduction was seen in 1–2 months.[85]

Neck and Chest

Brandt and Bellman were the first to report using BTX to treat aging of the neck.[86] Platysmal bands and neck vertical lines represent an accurate gauge of chronological age specifically for those people with exaggerated outdoor sun exposure. Separation of the platysma anteriorly occurs with aging, resulting in banding or "turkey neck." Vertical platysmal bands may be successfully treated with BTX-A. The extended or marked platysmal bands are grasped between the thumb and index fingers and the needle is vertically inserted into the muscle band. The dose is usually 2 to 4 U spaced 4 cm apart with an overall cumulative dose of 8 to 12 U per band and a total maximum in the neck of 25 to 30 U. Because of the nature of the muscle and the site of injection, complications such as dysphagia and dysphonia can be encountered if the toxin is placed

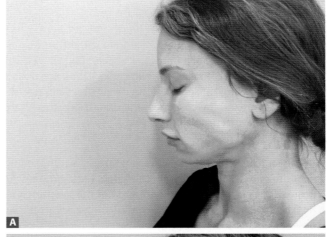
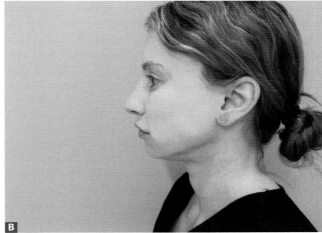

FIGURE 23-31. A and **B**, Masseter muscles seen while biting down before and after 12 units of Botox per side. (Courtesy of Tiffany faust.)

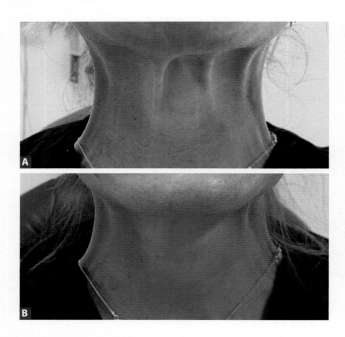

FIGURE 23-32. **A** and **B**, Platysmal bands before and after 12 units to each band totaling 24 units of Botox to the neck. (Courtesy of Ilanit Samuels, PA-C, MCMS.)

too deeply or in high volumes.[87] Patients should be warned about the possibility of such untoward effects (**Fig. 23-32**). The authors have noticed that when platysmal bands are treated there is less "jowling" observed along the jawline lateral to the marionette lines and the corners of the mouth slightly elevate, both of which are desirable outcomes.

Nefertiti Lift

The platysma muscle pulls downward with age, leading to jowl formation and frequent rhytides. Jawline redefinition with neurotoxin has not been widely reported in the literature and there is a range of opinions on the exact dosing and techniques to best define this area. A technique described in 2007 by Levy was named the "Nefertiti Lift" (after the perfect jawline of the ancient queen).[88] This technique releases the downward tension of the depressor effect of the aging platysma and releases the skin to the elevator muscles for lifting action. The "mini-lift" technique requires an injection of 2 to 3 U of BTX-A along and under each mandible and to the upper part of the posterior platysmal band for a total of 15 to 20 U per side.[88]

Chest

The upper area of the chest is a site of predilection for photodamage. Textural, pigmented, and photodamage changes are frequently seen in the V-shaped area of the chest. Static and dynamic wrinkles are caused by both photodamage and muscular sagging of the upper chest. Anatomically, the platysma is known to originate at the second rib; however, it can still present as far down as the fourth rib after which it traverses the pectoralis major and inserts in the mandible.[89] To date there is no consensus or indication for upper chest injection of BTX-A; however, there are various ways to inject BTX

in the upper chest. The techniques used are the curved, the "V," and the triangular approaches, during which BTX is injected over a curved, V-shaped, or triangular area with "5 to 10" sites identified within, each targeted with 2 to 8 U of BTX.[73] The recommended depths for these injections are superficially in the deep dermis or in the dermal-subcutaneous junction around 4 mm deep.[79,90] For complete reduction of skin wrinkling in the décolleté area, widespread diffusion of the injected BTX is necessary to achieve total coverage. This can be achieved with high volumes of hyperdilute concentrations of BTX.[79]

BOTULINUM TOXIN FOR PERSISTENT FACIAL FLUSHING AND ROSACEA

Facial flushing is not an uncommon problem in fair-skinned individuals of Celtic and northern European descent. A vasomotor phenomenon that results in increased erythema, persistent facial flushing can be accompanied by facial telangiectasias and gustatory sweating. Facial flushing is categorized as either autonomic neural-mediated (wet) or direct vasodilator-mediated (dry). The method by which BTX-A works to affect vasodilation is unknown, and the results regarding its efficacy for this indication are inconclusive. One theory is that BTX might work through reduction of local subclinical inflammation, which contributes to persistent erythema. Moreover, the anti-inflammatory role of BTX-A in blocking substance P, vanilloid receptor 1 (TRPV-1), and calcitonin gene-related peptide (CGRP) is important in decreasing the subclinical inflammation that might present as erythema.[91] Only Yuraitis et al. have described an improvement related to facial flushing in limited case reports.[92] Alexandroff et al. as well as Kranendonk et al. failed to show an effective response to BTX-A for facial flushing in three published cases.[93,94]

Chemical denervation by blocking Ach release from the neuromuscular junction has been seen to directly inhibit vasodilation and subsequent facial flushing.[95,96] The typical dose is a hyperdilute solution of BTX (concentration of 1.4–2 U/0.1 mL) injected over bilateral cheeks 0.5–1 cm apart.[96,97] Mast cells are also upregulated in patients with rosacea and recent studies have demonstrated that both BTX-A and BTX-B inhibit degranulation of mast cells.[98] Further studies are required to better assess the safety and efficacy of this procedure, but numerous case reports show promise.

BOTULINUM TOXINS AND ACNE VULGARIS

Acne, which most commonly occurs during adolescence, is influenced by several factors (Chapter 16, Acne). The pathology centers on the pilosebaceous follicle (comprising the sebaceous gland), the follicle (pore), and vellus hair. Factors that promote the formation of comedones (whiteheads or blackheads) include the following: (1) increased sebum production, (2) inflammation of the dermis and follicles by inflammatory mediators, (3) hyperkeratinization and obstruction of the upper region of the follicle, and (4) colonization of the follicle by the bacterium *Propionibacterium acnes.* Adolescence is marked by an increase in levels of circulating androgens, particularly dehydroepiandrosterone sulfate (DHEAS). Elevated androgen levels are thought to cause sebaceous glands to enlarge and increase sebum production. While most acne patients have normal hormone levels, increased sebum production plays an important role in acne. A correlation exists between the rate of sebum production and the severity of acne. In addition, acne patients typically produce sebum deficient in linoleic acid, which is a potential cause of abnormal keratinization and follicular obstruction. Increased sebum levels can also irritate keratinocytes, causing the release of interleukin-1, which in turn can cause follicular hyperkeratinization. The final common pathway in each of these acne-causing routes, which are not mutually exclusive, is follicular obstruction.[99]

BTX may inhibit the cascade of events leading to acne. This is likely achieved through parasympathetic effects, inhibiting sweat gland activity, and sebaceous gland secretion as well as stimulating keratinocyte locomotion. Associated anti-inflammatory and antiandrogenic effects may also contribute. It has been hypothesized that BTX-A toxin inhibits the formation of acne through at least three different pathways. First, BTX inhibits sebum production by sebaceous glands through cholinergic inhibition and sebocyte differentiation. Cholinergic secretions normally attributed to increased sebum production are inhibited by BTX resulting in a lowered sebum potential across the ducts and skin.[100] Moreover, decreased sebocyte promoter differentiation and lower sebum levels may clinically improve acne by decreasing the growth of *P. acnes.* Thus, the ability to lower sebum production decreases *P. acnes* growth and acne development. Additionally, BTX inhibits sweat production by sweat glands. Decreased perspiration may clinically improve acne by reducing the growth of *P. acnes.*[101] Furthermore, follicular occlusion by keratinocytes is the final common pathway in each of the various routes leading to acne. Keratinocyte migration is inhibited by the high-dose stimulation of nicotinic Ach receptors. By inhibiting the release of Ach, BTX may indirectly increase the migration of keratinocytes, thus reducing follicular occlusion.[102] The androgen surge during puberty is a known instigator of acne, and studies have shown that androgens increase the number of Ach receptors. Interestingly, androgen receptors are found on pilosebaceous duct keratinocytes, which are important in follicular occlusion. It is postulated that during puberty androgens increase the number of Ach receptors on the pilosebaceous keratinocytes, leading to further inhibition of keratinocyte locomotion through increased Ach stimulation. By inhibiting the release of Ach, BTX decreases the number of Ach receptors on the pilosebaceous keratinocytes, thereby increasing keratinocyte locomotion through decreased Ach stimulation.[103]

Further, surprising results from research alluded to above have shown that holocrine gland secretions are controlled by various neuropeptides, with substance P playing a significant role.[104] BTX-A blocks substance P, TRPV-1, and CGRP, which are important mediators in inflammation, and therefore helps decrease the inflammatory aspect of acne development.

BTX-A has been used to improve facial pore size and sebum production. There are three different techniques used to achieve this. The first one is the traditional intramuscular injection, utilizing about 10–45 U distributed over the forehead area.[105,106] An intradermal injection technique using a hyperdiluted concentration (5 cc of bacteriostatic saline per 100 U of BTX) has also been shown to be effective.[107] Lastly, intradermal delivery of a hyperconcentrated BTX-A solution using an electrical needling device at 3–3.5 mm has yielded improvements on sebum production, pore size, skin elasticity, and reduced laxity.[108]

BTX-A AND COSMETIC SURGERY

BTX-A can be used before or after the surgical manipulation to either enhance or sustain benefits. If injected in the pre-operative period, the toxin may allow improved tissue manipulation and reduced incisional tension leading to improved healing. Prior to endoscopic brow lift or a face lift using endoscopy, BTX-A injections help in raising the position of the brow and can reduce the number of surgical manipulations necessary. Finally, when used after surgery, BTX-A weakens the musculature, prolonging the anticipated effect.[109]

The authors recommend BTX-A injections prior to surgery. Tension exerted perpendicular to the wound during the healing phase can result in ongoing microtrauma, exacerbating inflammation, which leads to overproduction of collagen as well as glycosaminoglycans, and delayed healing.[110] Immobilization of facial wounds with BTX-A ameliorates wound healing and improves the eventual appearance of the surgical scar.[111]

COMBINATION THERAPIES: BTX-A AND OTHER REJUVENATION MODALITIES

In the authors' cosmetic dermatology practice, BTX-A injections are usually combined with other rejuvenation modalities such as dermal filler injections, skin tightening, skin resurfacing, peels, and more. Studies show that a combination of BTX-A injections with dermal fillers may achieve a greater durability of effect.[110]

It is recommended that BTX-A injections be performed 2 weeks before any resurfacing treatment such as microneedling or CO_2 laser. Pretreatment of hyperdynamic facial wrinkles with BTX-A prior to skin-resurfacing treatment prevents recurrence of wrinkling during re-epithelialization, resulting in a more optimal aesthetic result.[112] A similar protocol is used 2 weeks prior to skin-tightening treatments such as microfocused ultrasound and radiofrequency tightening. Expert consensus recommends the use of neuromodulators first, followed by soft-tissue fillers on the same visit. Then on a second visit, at least 3 days later, if possible, a skin-tightening procedure can be performed. Spacing these treatments 1 to 2 weeks apart to allow for the resolution of swelling, bruising, and other complications is ideal.[113] However, due to practical purposes (e.g., time constraints, patient schedules, patient is not local and had planned to return home), BTX-A injections may need to be performed the same day as other modalities. Skin tightening and laser modalities should be performed before any injectables on the same visit. It is recommended that BTX-A injections be performed first, then dermal filler injections because swelling of the fillers can interfere with BTX-A placement.

OTHER CLINICAL APPLICATIONS

Hyperhidrosis

Hyperhidrosis is a troublesome problem leading to awkward social situations for those affected. Unfortunately, topical and oral medications, iontophoresis, and surgery have not proven efficacious for most patients. The eccrine glands are innervated by sympathetic nerves that use Ach as the neurotransmitter. Therefore, BTX is effective in temporarily reducing or abolishing sweat production. Botox is the only BTX that is approved by the FDA for axillary hyperhidrosis.

Botox for hyperhidrosis is diluted with 5.0 cc of preservative-free saline, yielding 2 U per 0.1 cc. Dysport can also be diluted with 5.0 cc of preservative-free saline, providing 10 U per 0.1 cc. To use Myobloc, dilute a 5000-U vial with 2.1 cc of saline. This yields 200 U per 0.1 cc. Using a 1-cc tuberculin syringe with a 30-gauge needle, subcutaneously inject 0.05 cc with an approximate depth of 3 mm with care to avoid intramuscular injections. The palm or sole, including the webs of the hands and feet, should be injected every square centimeter. When treating the axilla, ask patients which areas bother them to determine how far beyond the hair-bearing area to inject. A starch-iodine test may be performed prior to injections to ascertain which areas need to be injected. The iodine solution is applied to the affected area and then covered with starch. The areas that produce sweat will turn black, indicating where to inject (**Fig. 23-33, A–E**). Although this test is messy, it is a useful technique for evaluating the efficacy of the injections and for determining which areas to inject. The primary author injects the tips of the fingers and toes as well to avoid compensatory sweating in these areas (**Figs. 23-34 and 23-35**). It is usually necessary to inject 100 U Botox, Xeomin, or Jeuveau, 300 U Dysport, or 5000 U Myobloc per palm or sole and 50 U Botox or 2500 U Myobloc per axilla. The effects last approximately 4 months although there are reports in the literature of longer-lasting results.[114] Lowe et al. studied 322 patients with axillary hyperhidrosis in a multicenter, double-blind trial for 52 weeks.[115] Subjects received 50 or 75 U of Botox and were compared to a control group of placebo injection. Seventy-five percent of the patients who received Botox noticed a reduction of hyperhidrosis, while only 25% of the placebo group noticed a difference. The median duration of effect was also significantly higher in patients who received Botox when compared to the placebo group. There was no statistically significant difference between the two groups receiving toxin. Following the first treatment, the median duration of effect was 205 days for the patients receiving 50 U and 197 days in patients injected with 75 U of Botox.

Baumann et al. studied Myobloc in the treatment of 20 patients with axillary hyperhidrosis in a double-blind, randomized, placebo-controlled trial. Subjects received either Myobloc (2500 U, or 0.5 mL, per axilla) or 0.5 mL vehicle (100 mmol NaCl, 10 mmol succinate, and 0.5 mg/mL human albumin) into the bilateral axillae. The onset and duration of action were determined to be 5 to 7 days and 2.2 to 8.1 months (mean of 5 months), respectively.[116] In another study conducted by Baumann et al., Myobloc was used to treat 20 patients with palmar hyperhidrosis. Participants were injected with either Myobloc (5000 U per palm) or a 1.0 mL vehicle (100 mM NaCl, 10 mM succinate, and 0.5 mg/mL human albumin) into bilateral palms. The duration of action of Myobloc in these patients ranged from 2.3 to 4.9 months, with a mean of 3.8 months.[40]

Inguinal Hyperhidrosis

Inguinal hyperhidrosis (IH) is a focal and primary form of hyperhidrosis in which the individual has intense sweating in the inguinal region. Appearing in adolescence, usually not later than the age of 25, the condition continues into adulthood. IH is characterized by chronic, intense sweating in the inguinal region, a situation that is potentially embarrassing for the patient. IH symmetrically affects the groin region, including the suprapubic area, the shallow depression that lies immediately below the fold of the groin (corresponding to the femoral triangle), the medial surfaces of the upper inner thighs, and the genital area. It may also include the lower part of the gluteus maximus, gluteal fold, and natal cleft.[117] No study to date has described the ideal doses of BTX for the treatment of IH. The threshold doses of BTX-A for the treatment of hyperhidrosis depend on the severity of the condition.[118] Two or three units of BTX-A per cm^2 can be used to treat the hyperhidrotic area in the inguinal region. The only side effects reported in the sparse literature are those related to the injections, such as rare small hematomas and temporary edema.[119]

Other Neuroglandular Disorders

The effects of BTX-A at the neuroglandular junction have not been explored as extensively as those occurring at the neuromuscular junction. Clinical studies examining the effect of intracutaneous BTX for focal hyperhidrosis have found complete abolition of sweating in the injected area within 3 to 7 days. No adverse effects were reported, and in a 5-month follow-up there were no clinical recurrences of the hyperhidrosis.[120] Gustatory sweating is another area of neuroglandular dysfunction in which BTX-A has proven effective. Gustatory sweating (or Frey's syndrome) is a disabling disorder in which the cheek skin sweats profusely during eating. The syndrome may occur after parotidectomy and is likely due to the misdirection of regenerating parasympathetic fibers that innervate the sweat glands of the face. Intracutaneous BTX-A has been reported to significantly decrease or prevent sweating for more than 6 months, with no clinical evidence of facial weakness in any patients.[121] BTX-A injected into the submandibular glands has been reported to significantly decrease salivation resulting from stimulation of the lingual nerves. The decreased salivation was temporary and did not appear to be directly toxic to the acinar

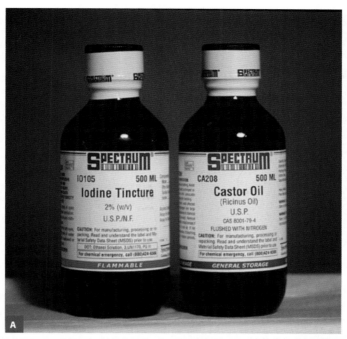

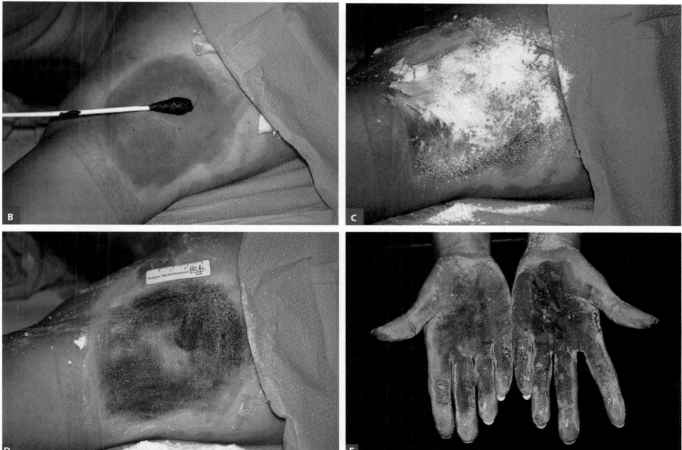

FIGURE 23-33. **A.** The starch-iodine test solution is made by combining nine parts of iodine with one part of castor oil. **B.** The iodine solution is then applied to the affected area using a swab. **C.** Potato starch is sprinkled over the iodine solution. **D.** Sweat turns the starch black, delineating the affected areas. **E.** This test is useful to determine which areas to inject. In this patient, the fingertips can be avoided because the iodine-starch test indicates that there is no sweating on the fingertips.

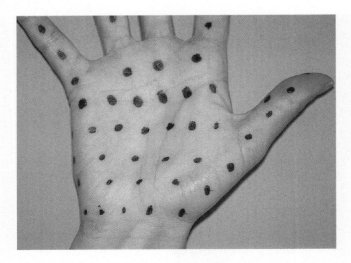

FIGURE 23-34. Injection sites on hands are approximately 1.5 cm apart.

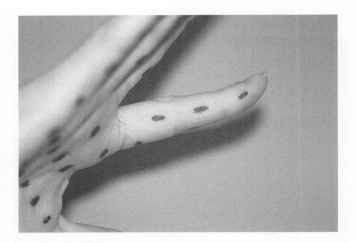

FIGURE 23-35. Injection sites on fingers.

cells of the gland.[122] Canine studies have also shown that vasomotor rhinorrhea, a parasympathetically controlled phenomenon, responds favorably to topical BTX-A. While the duration of action of BTX-A at the neuromuscular junction appears to be approximately 3 months, a longer-lasting effect may occur at the glandular level. BTX-A has produced anhydrosis for more than 12 months in patients with gustatory sweating. The reason for the difference in duration of action is uncertain; hypotheses include a higher rate of resynthesis of SNAP-25 (the protein cleaved by BTX) in neuromuscular synapses, and a higher area of axonal sprouting and consecutive reinnervation of muscle fibers as compared to that in glandular tissue.[123,124]

PAIN CONTROL

With the expanding use of botulinum toxins in cosmetic practice, pain alleviation remains an important aspect of the injection. Pain sensation depends on several factors, most importantly the concentration of the neuropeptides (substance P) at the site of injection, the tissue density (higher tissue density implies more pain), and the density of the nociceptor distribution at the site of injection. Other factors include the volume injected, the bore of the needle used, the layer of skin within which the toxin is injected, the rate of fluid injection, and, of course, the physician's level of experience.[125]

Differences in pain perception among patients treated with the commercially available toxin preparations have not been studied extensively; however, results from the only comparative study of three available preparations of the toxin showed that the pain induced by Neurobloc/Myobloc (BTX-B) was found to be significantly higher than that induced by Botox and Dysport (BTX-A), between which no significant difference was found. The study concluded that the different chemical properties and pharmaceutical adjuvants in toxins A and B likely affect pain sensation and speculated that the pH difference of Neurobloc/Myobloc (pH 5.6) and Botox/Dysport (pH 6.8) influences pain perception.

Pain sensation during toxin injections is usually fleeting, and simple measures can improve patient comfort.[126] For facial wrinkles, anesthesia is not necessary unless the patient prefers it. The 30-gauge needles used to inject the medication are the same size as acupuncture needles and cause minimal pain in a calm patient. Allowing the BTX to reach room temperature may decrease the level of pain otherwise felt by the patient. When the physician approaches the patient in a soothing and reassuring manner, not allowing the patient to see the needles prior to and during the injections, the patient's anxiety is significantly reduced as is the perception of pain.

Topical anesthetic creams containing lidocaine can be applied prior to injection to mitigate the sensation of pain. BTX should not be mixed with local anesthetics because they can alter the pH of the preparation and deplete its potency. Ice packs can be applied prior to injections, which may decrease the pain and encourage vasoconstriction, resulting in less bruising.

For hyperhidrosis, pain control is a necessity, especially for the palms and soles. Although some physicians perform nerve blocks, the primary author uses the following method: at least 1 hour prior to treating for hyperhidrosis, the topical anesthetic is applied to the area to be treated. Next, these areas are occluded with plastic bags or gloves when treating hands and feet or with tape when treating axillae. Numerous tools have been deployed to attenuate the pain associated with the use of BTX for palmar hyperhidrosis, including topical anesthetics, intravenous regional anesthesia, nerve blocks, ice, Frigiderm spray,[127] and others. The use of nitrous oxide ("laughing gas") requires office training and can induce an anxiolytic rather than an analgesic effect.[127] Ongoing trials to assess the effects of different anesthetics for an optimal injection with minimal pain are needed to establish the full potential of the various approaches to reducing the pain of BTX injections.

POTENTIAL BENEFIT OF BOTULINUM TOXIN TYPE A FOR HEADACHE TREATMENT

Migraine headaches occur in approximately 18% of women and 6% of men, resulting in a significant disability and decreased quality of life.[128] A subset of patients who have undergone BTX therapy for cosmetic indications have also reported improvement in migraine and chronic headache symptoms. Studies of the effects of BTX on headaches are controversial. While a few investigations failed to reveal a positive effect of Botox in the prevention of migraine or chronic headaches,[129–131] BTX may have a role in diminishing the severity of headaches experienced by some patients.[131] Some studies specifically designed to target headaches and chronic migraines have demonstrated efficacy of botulinum toxins in patients with chronic migraines and suggested further trials to reach an ideal optimal consensus on the safety and efficacy of this toxin in migraine/headache therapy.[132] In October 2010, Botox was approved by the FDA for prophylaxis of headaches in adults with chronic migraines.[133]

BOTOX AND GENDER

Interest among men seeking cosmetic procedures is increasing every year. Men had nearly 1.1 million cosmetic procedures performed in 2007, accounting for 9% of the total cosmetic procedures carried out in the U.S. As of 2019, the number of cosmetic procedures for men has increased 17% from 2006.[8] The BTX injection technique in men and women is similar; however, it is important to appreciate that higher doses are often required by men in comparison to women.[134] One study compared the muscle mass differences among 468 men and women aged 18 to 88 years and demonstrated a significantly higher amount of skeletal muscle in men than women in the muscles of the face, potentially because of the hypertrophic effect of testosterone.[135] Moreover, Monks et al. found androgen receptors to be abundant in the vicinity of the neuromuscular junction.[136] They speculated that androgens may even increase the number of junctions. The primary author's recommendation is to use a total of 20 U of BTX for glabellar injection in men as a starting dose. Five injection sites of 4 U each is the preferred method to preserve a more natural look. Significant care must be taken when injecting brows in men to avoid cosmetically undesired effects such as feminization of the brow or arching. With temporalis and masseter injections, men likely need an additional 25%–100% as compared to women. Furthermore, men need higher doses for orbicularis oculi paralysis owing to its broader circumference.

ETHNIC DIFFERENCES IN RESPONSES TO BOTULINUM TOXIN

There is a dearth of information available regarding the possible ethnic differences in the clinical effects of BTX or for dosing considerations. To date there is a lack of consensus on dosing considerations for different skin types and there exists a discrepancy regarding whether certain skin types require higher or lower doses for an optimal response.[137] Several variables must be taken into consideration, such as skin thickness, skin musculature, and circumference of bony prominences. Skin thickness and texture contribute to dosing decisions. Although the injections are generally muscular, the thickness of the dermis might influence the delivery technique. For instance, some studies have suggested that the skin of Asians tends to be thicker than that of Caucasians with more collagen fibers, which might demand a higher dose of injection.[138] However, other studies in Asians have found that lower doses may be needed than in Caucasians.[139] Arimura et al. evaluated the differences in the muscle-relaxing effect of BTX-B using electrophysiologic measurements in 48 Asian and Caucasian volunteers. They concluded that the muscle-relaxing effects of BTX-B were similar in both Asian and Caucasian study populations.[140] Racial differences in BTX responses remain unclear. More studies are required to determine any potential variations in the response of different skin types to botulinum toxins. The primary author has not noted any consistent differences among the various ethnicities treated in her practice.

The Asian Aesthetic Patient and Botulinum Toxin

Most studies and publications discuss aesthetic recommendations for Western populations. Asian patients differ not only in facial appearance, rate of facial aging, and structural anatomy but, more importantly, their concept of facial beauty and youth.

Facial shape is essential to a beautiful face, with the oval-shaped face considered universally attractive and youthful in all races.[141] The female Asian ideal is characterized by an oval-shaped face, V-shaped jawline, a smooth, convex forehead, large eyes, a petite nose with a raised bridge, and full but not prominent lips. In the past, these have been perceived as an attempt to westernize Asian features, but this is now understood to optimize the appearance of the aesthetic patient regardless of ethnicity.[138]

Compared with the Caucasian face, the Asian face is characterized by greater intercanthal width, the presence of epicanthal folds, increased bizygomatic and bigonial width, retruded forehead and orbital rims, lower nasal bridge, retruded piriform margin, and a hypoplastic mandible. Slower rate and onset of aging compared to Caucasians is not only attributed to anatomic differences such as denser fat and fibrous connective tissues between the superficial muscular aponeurotic system and the deep fascia, but also to sociocultural factors such as diets rich in antioxidants, skincare practices, and muscle use during articulation and facial expressivity.[142]

In 2015, a group of aesthetic providers (dermatologists and plastic surgeons) in Asia established a consensus on the aesthetic applications of BTX-A in Asians. In general, a lower dose of BTX-A in the upper face is recommended because of the weaker frontalis, orbicularis oculi, and glabellar muscles in the Asian population. In the midface and lower face, widespread use of Microbotox to reduce sweat and sebaceous gland activity is common in Asia, as is the long-established use of BTX-A to narrow the masseters.[72,143] It has also been used to reduce the size and activity of the parotid gland, to further accentuate this V-shaped ideal. BTX-A injections in this area seldom result in xerostomia, as studies show that the majority of salivary production originates in the submandibular gland.[144] Notably, the use of BTX-A for body-shaping in Asia is becoming more popular, with calf-shaping the most common indication. Most Asian patients tend to have shorter legs relative to their torsos and a thinner calf renders a more elegant appearance. BTX-A injections have also been used to slim down other body parts such as the deltoids.[143]

RESISTANCE TO BOTULINUM TOXIN

Development of Antibodies

Botulinum neurotoxins may be immunogenic, and antibodies may inactivate the molecule. The BTX molecule is composed of a light chain and a heavy chain. The toxin is embedded in a protein complex that protects the toxin's binding site until the desired pH is reached and the toxin is released. Antibodies to this critical binding site on the heavy chain of the BTX molecule will prevent binding of the toxin to its receptor, thereby crippling the actions of the toxin. Neutralizing antibodies have been reported in patients treated with high doses of BTX for neurologic disorders such as cerebral palsy. It is important to understand that there are many types of antibodies that can interact with BTX; however, the only antibodies that can affect the efficacy of the toxin are neutralizing antibodies. Antibodies may develop to BTX that are inconsequential to the patient, yet the antibodies capable of neutralizing the toxin are a concern as they have the potential to decrease the efficacy of the toxin. By definition, antibodies that neutralize BTX-A would not neutralize BTX-B and vice versa. Patients who develop antibodies to BTX-A can still enjoy the benefits of BTX-B. For this reason, it is recommended that practitioners have several different BTX serotypes available.

The incidence of antibody-mediated resistance to BTX, as determined by the mouse lethality assay, is reported between 3% and 9.5% and is accepted generally to be approximately 5%. The only apparent symptom of the development of antibodies is lack of response to further injections. The use of other serotypes (B or F) may benefit those who have developed antibody resistance. There are two types of therapy resistance to BTX, primary and secondary. A patient who does not respond to the first injection of BTX-A is referred to as a "primary nonresponder," but reasons for nonresponse can include inappropriate site of injection, poor technique, and/or insufficient dose.[145,146]

Immunogenicity should be suspected in a patient who no longer responds to BTX-A ("secondary nonresponder") following a successful course of earlier injections. Antibody formation could be targeted against the neurotoxin component of BTX or against its nontoxic protein component. The recommended approach is to inject 20 U BTX into the hypothenar or forehead muscles. If the patient responds to BTX, then transient weakness will develop in the muscle 1 to 2 weeks after

TABLE 23-5	Factors of Proteins That Increase Immunogenicity
Foreign instead of endogenous	
Large rather than small size	
Denatured rather than native	
Presence of adjuvants	
Aggregated rather than unaggregated	
Quantity present	
Frequency encountered	

injection. An alternative is to take blood for an antibody assay that is rarely used. In secondary nonresponders, the problem can be further overcome by using a different BTX serotype, BTX-B for example, if resistance develops to BTX-A.

Risk factors for the development of antibodies include higher doses, shorter intervals between injections, booster doses, and young age. Recommendations to help prevent development of antibodies include the following: (1) use of the smallest possible dose to achieve relief, (2) an interval between injections of at least 1 month (the preferred interval is 3 months), and (3) "touch-up injection" avoidance.

Several researchers have postulated that the risk of antibody formation is due in part to the quantity of protein or the "protein load" of the toxin, the type of protein present in the toxin, and to other factors listed in **Table 23-5**. Manufacturers of BTX have attempted to minimize each of these factors to create a less immunogenic product. For example, the original Botox that was used until December 1997 contained a higher level of protein than the Botox currently in use; therefore, it should lead to a lower incidence of antibody formation. As previously discussed, Merz Pharmaceuticals, the manufacturer of the new BTX product Xeomin, claims that its product contains a negligible level of bacterial proteins (0.6 ng) with lower immune response. In spite of the concerns regarding immunogenicity, there are no known or published reports of antibody production in patients treated with doses of any of the available BTX products for cosmetic indications, which may be explained by the lower doses used in comparison with neurologic and cervical dystonia indications where reports of resistance are centered.[147]

SIDE EFFECTS

Complications from the use of BTX injections occur infrequently and are transient and reversible. Bruising at the injection site(s) is one of the most common adverse events and the incidence can be reduced by avoiding aspirin, NSAIDs, green tea, vitamin E, and other anticoagulants for 10 days prior to treatment. Anecdotal reports reveal that application of ice packs to the area prior to injection alleviates the pain of the procedure and lowers the incidence of bruising. Some studies have shown an association with flu-like symptoms (Botox and Myobloc) and dry mouth (Myobloc) after injection of these products in larger doses used for neurologic indications.

The most serious side effects of BTX treatment in the upper face are asymmetry, ptosis, and, very rarely, diplopia or ectropion.[148] Proper injection technique and placement of the toxin will drastically reduce the incidence of these temporary side effects. In fact, many experts anecdotally state that physicians just learning to perform BTX injections in the upper face have approximately a 4% incidence of inducing ptosis, which, with practice, falls to 0.5%.

Adverse effects from injection into the platysma can include bruising, drooling, downturning of the corner of the mouth, weakness in the neck muscles, and dysphagia. Lip ptosis or mouth asymmetry may result from injections in this area.

Treatment of the palms and soles for hyperhidrosis can induce temporary muscle weakness. One should exercise caution when treating patients that require a strong grip (e.g., tennis players) and manual dexterity (e.g., piano players) and these patients should be aware of the risks of treating the palms. One other cautionary note: the use of Botox has been reported, in one patient, to have unmasked underlying myasthenia gravis;[149] therefore, its use is contraindicated in patients with myasthenia gravis, systemic lupus, and other autoimmune disorders associated with a pre-existing neuromuscular condition. Dysport is the only brand of BTX that contains lactose. Its use has been blamed for a fixed drug eruption in one patient.[150] Care should be taken to label all syringes containing BTX to avoid inadvertent administration of the toxin.

Postmarketing reports indicate that the effects of BTX products may spread from the area of injection. These may include asthenia, generalized muscle weakness, diplopia, ptosis, dysphagia, dysphonia, dysarthria, urinary incontinence, and breathing difficulties. These symptoms have been reported hours to weeks after injection. Swallowing and breathing difficulties can be life threatening and there have been reports of death.[133]

CONCLUSION

The injection of the *C. botulinum* A exotoxin is a safe, fast, and nontraumatic approach to correcting wrinkles, raising eyebrows, and improving hyperhidrosis. A significant number of physicians worldwide perform this procedure for cosmetic purposes. There are myriad new forms and brands of BTX entering the market. Some of these are longer lasting or shorter lasting than those currently on the market. Scientists are working on substances to reverse the effects of botulinum toxins. It is certain that we will see much more research examining these interesting agents in the near future.

References

1. Savardekar P. Botulinum toxin. *Indian J Dermatol Venereol Leprol*. 2008;74(1):77–79.
2. Scott A. Clostridial toxins as therapeutic agents. In: Simpson LL, ed. *Botulinum Neurotoxin and Tetanus Toxin*. New York, NY: Academic Press; 1989: 399–412.
3. Finkelstein A. Channels formed in phospholipid bilayer membranes by diphtheria, tetanus, botulinum and anthrax toxin. *J Physiol (Paris)*. 1990;84(2):188–190.
4. Setler P. The biochemistry of botulinum toxin type B. *Neurology*. 2000;55(12 Suppl 5):S22–S28.
5. Blitzer A, Binder WJ, Aviv JE, Keen MS, Brin MF. The management of hyperfunctional facial lines with botulinum toxin. A collaborative study of 210 injection sites in 162 patients. *Arch Otolaryngol Head Neck Surg*. 1997;123(4):389–392.
6. Carruthers JD, Carruthers JA. Treatment of glabellar frown lines with C. botulinum-A exotoxin. *J Dermatol Surg Oncol*. 1992;18(1):17–21.
7. Carruthers A, Carruthers J. History of the cosmetic use of Botulinum A exotoxin. *Dermatol Surg*. 1998;24(11):1168–1170.
8. The American Society for Aesthetic Plastic Surgery. Cosmetic surgery national data bank statistics 2019. https://www.surgery.org/sites/default/files/ASAPS-Stats2018.pdf. Accessed March 9, 2021.
9. Ocampo J. Indicaciones cosméticas de la toxina botulínica. *Piel*. 1997;12:434–441.
10. Carruthers A, Carruthers J. Clinical indications and injection technique for the cosmetic use of botulinum A exotoxin. *Dermatol Surg*. 1998;24(11):1189–1194.
11. Klein AW. Dilution and storage of botulinum toxin. *Dermatol Surg*. 1998;24(11):1179–1180.
12. Sarifakioglu N, Sarifakioglu E. Evaluating effects of preservative-containing saline solution on pain perception during botulinum toxin type-a injections at different locations: a prospective, single-blinded, randomized controlled trial. *Aesthetic Plast Surg*. 2005;29(2):113–115.
13. Hui JI, Lee WW. Efficacy of fresh versus refrigerated botulinum toxin in the treatment of lateral periorbital rhytids. *Ophthal Plast Reconstr Surg*. 2007;23(6):433–438.
14. Sampaio C, Ferreira JJ, Simões F, et al. DYSBOT: a single-blind, randomized parallel study to determine whether any differences can be detected in the efficacy and tolerability of two formulations of botulinum toxin type A--Dysport and Botox--assuming a ratio of 4:1. *Mov Disord*. 1997;12(6):1013–1018.
15. Odergren T, Hjaltason H, Kaakkola S, et al. A double blind, randomised, parallel group study to investigate the dose equivalence of Dysport and Botox in the treatment of cervical dystonia. *J Neurol Neurosurg Psychiatry*. 1998;64(1):6–12.
16. Ipsen Biopharmaceuticals, Inc. Dysport (AbobotulinumtoxinA) [package insert]. U.S. Food and Drug Administration website https://www.accessdata.fda.gov/drugsatfda_docs/label/2016/125274s107lbl.pdf. Revised December 2016. Accessed March 9, 2021.
17. Pickett A, O'Keeffe R, Panjwani N. The protein load of therapeutic botulinum toxins. *Eur J Neurol*. 2007;14(4):e11.
18. Brandt F, Swanson N, Baumann L. A phase III randomized double-blind, placebo-controlled study to assess the efficacy and safety of Dysport in the treatment of glabellar lines. Poster presented at Winter Clinical Dermatology Conference-Hawaii®, March 14–18, 2008, The Ritz Carlton, Kapalua, Maui, Hawaii.
19. Data on file, Medicis Corporation.
20. Merz Pharmaceuticals. Xeomin (IncobotulinumtoxinA) [package insert]. U.S. Food and Drug Administration website. https://www.accessdata.fda.gov/drugsatfda_docs/label/2018/125360s073lbl.pdf. Revised July 2018. Accessed August 8, 2019.
21. Wohlfarth K, Müller C, Sassin I, Comes G, Grafe S. Neurophysiological double-blind trial of a botulinum neurotoxin

type a free of complexing proteins. *Clin Neuropharmacol.* 2007;30(2):86–94.

22. Dressler D. Pharmacological aspects of therapeutic botulinum toxin preparations. *Nervenarzt.* 2006;77(8):912–921.

23. Jost WH, Blümel J, Grafe S. Botulinum neurotoxin type A free of complexing proteins (XEOMIN) in focal dystonia. *Drugs.* 2007;67(5):669–683.

24. Grein S, Mander GJ, Fink K. Stability of botulinum neurotoxin type A, devoid of complexing proteins. *Botulinum J.* 2011;2(1):49–58.

25. Soares DJ, Dejoseph LM, Zuliani GF, Liebertz DJ, Patel VS. Impact of postreconstitution room temperature storage on the efficacy of incobotulinumtoxinA treatment of dynamic lateral canthus lines. *Dermatol Surg.* 2015;41(6):712–717.

26. Carruthers A, Carruthers J, Coleman WP3rd, et al. Multicenter, randomized, phase III study of a single dose of incobotulinumtoxinA, free from complexing proteins, in the treatment of glabellar frown lines. *Dermatol Surg.* 2013;39(4):551–558.

27. Hanke CW, Narins RS, Brandt F, et al. A randomized, placebo-controlled, double-blind phase III trial investigating the efficacy and safety of incobotulinumtoxinA in the treatment of glabellar frown lines using a stringent composite endpoint. *Dermatol Surg.* 2013;39(6):891–899.

28. Lee JC, Yokota K, Arimitsu H, et al. Production of anti-neurotoxin antibody is enhanced by two subcomponents, HA1 and HA3b, of Clostridium botulinum type B 16S toxin-haemagglutinin. *Microbiology (Reading).* 2005;151(Pt 11):3739–3747.

29. Jankovic J, Vuong KD, Ahsan J. Comparison of efficacy and immunogenicity of original versus current botulinum toxin in cervical dystonia. *Neurology.* 2003;60(7):1186–1188.

30. Greene P, Fahn S, Diamond B. Development of resistance to botulinum toxin type A in patients with torticollis. *Mov Disord.* 1994;9(2):213–217.

31. Dressler D, Wohlfahrt K, Meyer-Rogge E, Wiest L, Bigalke H. Antibody-induced failure of botulinum toxin a therapy in cosmetic indications. *Dermatol Surg.* 2010;36(Suppl 4):2182–2187.

32. Stengel G, Bee EK. Antibody-induced secondary treatment failure in a patient treated with botulinum toxin type A for glabellar frown lines. *Clin Interv Aging.* 2011;6:281–284.

33. Rzany BJ, Ascher B, Avelar RL, et al. A Multicenter, Randomized, Double-Blind, Placebo-Controlled, Single-Dose, Phase III, Non-Inferiority Study Comparing PrabotulinumtoxinA and OnabotulinumtoxinA for the Treatment of Moderate to Severe Glabellar Lines in Adult Patients. *Aesthet Surg J.* 2020;40(4):413–429.

34. Evolus, Inc. Jeuveau (PrabotulinumtoxinA) [package insert]. U.S. Food and Drug Administration website. https://www. accessdata.fda.gov/drugsatfda_docs/label/2019/761085s000lbl. pdf. Revised April 2019. Accessed March 9, 2021.

35. Beer KR, Shamban AT, Avelar RL, Gross JE, Jonker A. Efficacy and Safety of PrabotulinumtoxinA for the Treatment of Glabellar Lines in Adult Subjects: Results From 2 Identical Phase III Studies. *Dermatol Surg.* 2019;45(11):1381–1393.

36. Glogau RG, Waugh JM. Preclinical transcutaneous flux experiments using a macromolecule transport system (MTS) peptide for delivery of botulinum toxin type A. Poster presented at the 66th annual meeting of the American Academy of Dermatology, San Antonio, TX, 2008.

37. Stone HF, Zhu Z, Thach TQ, Ruegg CL. Characterization of diffusion and duration of action of a new botulinum toxin type A formulation. *Toxicon.* 2011;58(2):159–167.

38. Revance Therapeutics. Our Latest. Available at: https://www. revance.com/news/?category=our-latest. Updated December 22, 2020. Accessed March 9, 2021.

39. Kaufman-Janette JA, Solish N, Liu Y, Rubio RG, Gallagher CJ. Pooled results from 2 phase 3 pivotal studies of daxibotulinumtoxinA for the treatment of glabellar lines. *Toxicon.* 2018;156:S59.

40. Baumann L, Slezinger A, Vujevich J, et al. A double-blinded, randomized, placebo-controlled pilot study of the safety and efficacy of Myobloc (botulinum toxin type B)-purified neurotoxin complex for the treatment of crow's feet: a double-blinded, placebo-controlled trial. *Dermatol Surg.* 2003;29(5):508–515.

41. Horowitz BZ. Type E botulism. *Clin Toxicol (Phila).* 2010;48(9):880–895.

42. Baldwin MR, Tepp WH, Pier CL, et al. Characterization of the antibody response to the receptor binding domain of botulinum neurotoxin serotypes A and E. *Infect Immun.* 2005;73(10):6998–7005.

43. Fernández-Salas E, Steward LE, Ho H, et al. Plasma membrane localization signals in the light chain of botulinum neurotoxin. *Proc Natl Acad Sci U S A.* 2004;101(9):3208–3213.

44. Bajohrs M, Rickman C, Binz T, Davletov B. A molecular basis underlying differences in the toxicity of botulinum serotypes A and E. *EMBO Rep.* 2004;5(11):1090–1095.

45. Aoki KR, Ranoux D, Wissel J. Using translational medicine to understand clinical differences between botulinum toxin formulations. *Eur J Neurol.* 2006;13(Suppl 4):10–19.

46. Dolly JO, Black J, Williams RS, Melling J. Acceptors for botulinum neurotoxin reside on motor nerve terminals and mediate its internalization. *Nature.* 1984;307(5950):457–460.

47. Black JD, Dolly JO. Interaction of 125I-labeled botulinum neurotoxins with nerve terminals. I. Ultrastructural autoradiographic localization and quantitation of distinct membrane acceptors for types A and B on motor nerves. *J Cell Biol.* 1986;103(2):521–534.

48. Gracies JM, Weisz DJ, Yang BY, Flanagan S, Simpson DM. Impact of botulinum toxin A (BTX-A) dilution and end plate targeting technique in upper limb spasticity. *Ann Neurol.* 2002;52(3):S87.

49. Wohlfarth K, Göschel H, Frevert J, Dengler R, Bigalke H. Botulinum A toxins: units versus units. *Naunyn Schmiedebergs Arch Pharmacol.* 1997;355(3):335–340.

50. de Almeida AT, De Boulle K. Diffusion characteristics of botulinum neurotoxin products and their clinical significance in cosmetic applications. *J Cosmet Laser Ther.* 2007;9(Suppl 1):17–22.

51. Matarasso SL. Comparison of botulinum toxin types A and B: a bilateral and double-blind randomized evaluation in the treatment of canthal rhytides. *Dermatol Surg.* 2003;29(1):7–13.

52. Baumann L, Slezinger A, Halem M, et al. Double-blind, randomized, placebo-controlled pilot study of the safety and efficacy of Myobloc (botulinum toxin type B) for the treatment of palmar hyperhidrosis. *Dermatol Surg.* 2005;31(3):263–270.

53. Trinidade de Almeida AR, Marques E, de Almeida J, Cunha T, Boraso R. Pilot study comparing the diffusion of two formulations of botulinum toxin type A in patients with forehead hyperhidrosis. *Dermatol Surg.* 2007;33(1 Spec No.):S37–S43.

54. Cliff SH, Judodihardjo H, Eltringham E. Different formulations of botulinum toxin type A have different migration characteristics: a double-blind, randomized study. *J Cosmet Dermatol.* 2008;7(1):50–54.

55. Alam M, Geisler A, Warycha M, et al. Effect of postinjection facial exercise on time of onset of botulinum toxin for glabella and forehead wrinkles: A randomized, controlled, crossover clinical trial. *J Am Acad Dermatol.* 2019;80(4):1144–1147.

56. Hsu TS, Dover JS, Kaminer MS, Arndt KA, Tan MH. Why make patients exercise facial muscles for 4 hours after botulinum toxin treatment? *Arch Dermatol.* 2003;139(7):948.

57. Rzany B, Ascher B, Fratila A, Monheit GD, Talarico S, Sterry W. Efficacy and safety of 3- and 5-injection patterns (30 and 50 U) of botulinum toxin A (Dysport) for the treatment of wrinkles in the glabella and the central forehead region. *Arch Dermatol.* 2006;142(3):320–326.

58. Carruthers A, Carruthers J. Prospective, double-blind, randomized, parallel-group, dose-ranging study of botulinum toxin type A in men with glabellar rhytids. *Dermatol Surg.* 2005;31(10):1297–1303.

59. Fagien S, Cohen JL, Coleman W, et al. Forehead line treatment with onabotulinumtoxinA in subjects with forehead and glabellar facial rhytids: a phase 3 study. *Dermatol Surg.* 2017;43 (Suppl 3):S274–S284.

60. Teske SA, Kersten RC, Devoto MH, Kulwin DR. Hering's law and eyebrow position. *Ophthalmic Plast Reconstr Surg.* 1998;14(2):105–106.

61. Moers-Carpi M, Carruthers J, Fagien S, et al. Efficacy and safety of onabotulinumtoxinA for treating crow's feet lines alone or in combination with glabellar lines: a multicenter, randomized, controlled trial. *Dermatol Surg.* 2015;41(1):102–112.

62. Carruthers J, Carruthers A. The adjunctive usage of botulinum toxin. *Dermatol Surg.* 1998;24(11):1244–1247.

63. Package insert. Neuronox®. Medy-Tox Inc. South Korea, 2006.

64. Huang W, Rogachefsky AS, Foster JA. Browlift with botulinum toxin. *Dermatol Surg.* 2000;26(1):55–60.

65. de Almeida AR, Cernea SS. Regarding browlift with botulinum toxin. *Dermatol Surg.* 2001;27(9):848.

66. Knize DM. Limited-incision forehead lift for eyebrow elevation to enhance upper blepharoplasty. *Plast Reconstr Surg.* 1996;97(7):1334–1342.

67. Karacalar A, Korkmaz A, Kale A, Kopuz C. Compensatory brow asymmetry: anatomic study and clinical experience. *Aesthetic Plast Surg.* 2005;29(2):119–123.

68. Huilgol SC, Carruthers A, Carruthers JD. Raising eyebrows with botulinum toxin. *Dermatol Surg.* 1999;25(5):373–375; discussion 376.

69. Ahn MS, Catten M, Maas CS. Temporal brow lift using botulinum toxin A. *Plast Reconstr Surg.* 2000;105(3):1129–1135; discussion 1136–9.

70. Evans J. Microdroplets provide less aggressive brow lift. *Skin and Allergy News.* 2007;3:42.

71. Wu WTL. Microbotox of the Lower Face and Neck: Evolution of a Personal Technique and Its Clinical Effects. *Plast Reconstr Surg.* 2015;136(5 Suppl):92S–100S.

72. Wu WT, Liew S, Chan HH, et al. Consensus on Current Injectable Treatment Strategies in the Asian Face. *Aesthetic Plast Surg.* 2016;40(2):202–214.

73. Atamoros FP. Botulinum toxin in the lower one third of the face. *Clin Dermatol.* 2003;21(6):505–512.

74. Dayan SH, Kempiners JJ. Treatment of the lower third of the nose and dynamic nasal tip ptosis with Botox. *Plast Reconstr Surg.* 2005;115(6):1784–1785.

75. Ghavami A, Janis JE, Guyuron B. Regarding the treatment of dynamic nasal tip ptosis with botulinum toxin A. *Plast Reconstr Surg.* 2006;118(1):263–264.

76. Carruthers J, Carruthers A. Aesthetic botulinum A toxin in the mid and lower face and neck. *Dermatol Surg.* 2003;29(5):468–476.

77. Wise JB, Greco T. Injectable treatments for the aging face. *Facial Plast Surg.* 2006;22(2):140–146.

78. Foster JA, Wulc AE, Hoick DE. Cosmetic indications for botulinum A toxin. *Semin Ophthalmol.* 1998;13(3):142–148.

79. Benedetto AV. Cosmetic uses of botulinum toxin A in the lower face, neck and upper chest. In: Benedetto AV, ed. *Botulinum Toxin in Clinical Dermatology.* Boca Raton, FL: Taylor & Francis Group; 2005: 3–12.

80. Al-Ahmad HT, Al-Qudah MA. The treatment of masseter hypertrophy with botulinum toxin type A. *Saudi Med J.* 2006;27(3):397–400.

81. Castro WH, Gomez RS, Da Silva Oliveira J, Moura MD, Gomez RS. Botulinum toxin type A in the management of masseter muscle hypertrophy. *J Oral Maxillofac Surg.* 2005;63(1):20–24.

82. Smyth AG. Botulinum toxin treatment of bilateral masseteric hypertrophy. *Br J Oral Maxillofac Surg.* 1994;32(1):29–33.

83. Park MY, Ahn KY, Jung DS. Botulinum toxin type A treatment for contouring of the lower face. *Dermatol Surg.* 2003;29(5):477–483; discussion 483.

84. Chang CS, Kang GC. Achieving ideal lower face aesthetic contours: Combination of tridimensional fat grafting to the chin with masseter botulinum toxin injection. *Aesthet Surg J.* 2016;36(10):1093–1100.

85. Ahn J, Horn C, Blitzer A. Botulinum toxin for masseter reduction in Asian patients. *Arch Facial Plast Surg.* 2004;6(3):188–191.

86. Brandt FS, Bellman B. Cosmetic use of botulinum A exotoxin for the aging neck. *Dermatol Surg.* 1998;24(11):1232–1234.

87. Lowe NJ. Botulinum toxin: combination treatments for the face and neck. In: Lowe NJ, ed. *Textbook of Facial Rejuvenation.* London, England: Martin Dunitz/Taylor and Francis; 2002: 158–170.

88. Levy PM. The 'Nefertiti Lift': a new technique for specific re-contouring of the jawline. *J Cosm Laser Ther.* 2007;9(4):249–252.

89. Becker-Wegerich PM, Rauch L, Ruzicka T. Botulinum toxin A: successful décolleté rejuvenation. *Dermatol Surg.* 2002;28(2):168–171.

90. Ascher B, Talarico S, Cassuto D, et al. International consensus recommendations on the aesthetic usage of botulinum toxin type A (Speywood Unit)--Part II: Wrinkles on the middle and lower face, neck and chest. *J Eur Acad Dermatol Venereol.* 2010;24(11):1285–1295.

91. Bansal C, Omlin KJ, Hayes CM, Rohrer TE. Novel cutaneous uses for botulinum toxin type A. *J Cosmet Dermatol.* 2006;5(3):268–272.

92. Yuraitis M, Jacob CI. Botulinum toxin for the treatment of facial flushing. *Dermatol Surg.* 2004;30(1):102–104.

93. Alexandroff AB, Sinclair SA, Langtry JA. Successful use of botulinum toxin A for the treatment of neck and anterior chest wall flushing. *Dermatol Surg.* 2006;32(12):1536.

94. Kranendonk SK, Ferris LK, Obagi S. Re: Botulinum toxin for the treatment of facial flushing. *Dermatol Surg.* 2005;31(4):491.

95. Kim MJ, Kim JH, Cheon HI, et al. Assessment of skin physiology change and safety after intradermal injections with botulinum toxin: A randomized, double-blind, placebo-controlled, split-face pilot study in rosacea patients with facial erythema. *Dermatol Surg.* 2019;45(9):1155–1162.

96. Park KY, Hyun MY, Jeong SY, Kim BJ, Kim MN, Hong CK. Botulinum toxin for the treatment of refractory erythema and flushing of rosacea. *Dermatology.* 2015;230(4):299–301.

97. Dayan SH, Pritzker RN, Arkins JP. A new treatment regimen for rosacea: onabotulinumtoxin A. *J Drugs Dermatol.* 2012;11(12):e76–e79.

98. Choi JE, Werbel T, Wang Z, Wu CC, Yaksh TL, Di Nardo A. Botulinum toxin blocks mast cells and prevents rosacea like inflammation. *J Dermatol Sci.* 2019;93(1):58–64.

99. Simonart T, Dramaix M, De Maertelaer V. Efficacy of tetracyclines in the treatment of acne vulgaris: a review. *Br J Dermatol.* 2008;158(2):208–216.

100. Yosipovitch G, Reis J, Tur E, Sprecher E, Yarnitsky D, Boner G. Sweat secretion, stratum corneum hydration, small nerve function and pruritus in patients with advanced chronic renal failure. *Br J Dermatol.* 1995;133(4):561–564.

101. Kurzen H, Schallreuter KU. Novel aspects in cutaneous biology of acetylcholine synthesis and acetylcholine receptors. *Exp Dermatol.* 2004;13(Suppl 4):27–30.

102. Chernyavsky AI, Arredondo J, Wess J, Karlsson E, Grando SA. Novel signaling pathways mediating reciprocal control of keratinocyte migration and wound epithelialzation through M_3 and M_4 muscarinic receptors. *J Cell Biol.* 2004;166(2):261–272.

103. Shapiro E, Miller AR, Lepor H. Down regulation of the muscarinic cholinergic receptor of the rat prostate following castration. *J Urol.* 1985;134(1):179–182.

104. Toyoda M, Morohashi M. Pathogenesis of acne. *Med Electron Microsc.* 2001;34(1):29–40.

105. Rose AE, Goldberg DJ. Safety and efficacy of intradermal injection of botulinum toxin for the treatment of oily skin. *Dermatol Surg.* 2013;39(3 Pt 1):443–448.

106. Min P, Xi W, Grassetti L, et al. Sebum production alteration after botulinum toxin type a injections for the treatment of forehead rhytides: A prospective randomized double-blind dose-comparative clinical investigation. *Aesthet Surg J.* 2015;35(5):600–610.

107. Shah AR. Use of intradermal botulinum toxin to reduce sebum production and facial pore size. *J Drugs Dermatol.* 2008;7(9):847–850.

108. Calvani F, Santini S, Bartoletti E, Alhadeff A. Personal technique of microinfiltration with botulin toxin: The SINB technique (Superficial Injection Needling Botulinum). *Plast Surg (Oakv).* 2019;27(2):156–161.

109. Carruthers A, Carruthers J. Botulinum toxin type A in facial aesthetics—an update. *US Dermatol Rev.* 2006:69–73.

110. Schlessinger J, Gilbert E, Cohen JL, Kaufman J. New uses of abobotulinumtoxinA in aesthetics. *Aesthet Surg J.* 2017;37(suppl_1):S45–S58.

111. Gassner HG, Brissett AE, Otley CC, et al. Botulinum toxin to improve facial wound healing: A prospective, blinded, placebo-controlled study. *Mayo Clin Proc.* 2006;81(8):1023–1028.

112. Zimbler MS, Holds JB, Kokoska MS, et al. Effect of botulinum toxin pretreatment on laser resurfacing results: a prospective, randomized, blinded trial. *Arch Facial Plast Surg.* 2001;3(3):165–169.

113. Carruthers J, Burgess C, Day D, et al. Consensus recommendations for combined aesthetic interventions in the face using botulinum toxin, fillers, and energy-based devices. *Dermatol Surg.* 2016;42(5):586–597.

114. Heckmann M, Ceballos-Baumann AO, Plewig G; Hyperhidrosis Study Group. Botulinum toxin A for axillary hyperhidrosis (excessive sweating). *N Engl J Med.* 2001;344(7):488–493.

115. Lowe NJ, Glaser DA, Eadie N, Daggett S, Kowalski JW, Lai PY; North American Botox in Primary Axillary Hyperhidrosis Clinical Study Group. Botulinum toxin type A in the treatment of primary axillary hyperhidrosis: a 52-week multicenter double-blind, randomized, placebo-controlled study of efficacy and safety. *J Am Acad Dermatol.* 2007;56(4):604–611.

116. Baumann LS, Halem ML. Botulinum toxin-B and the management of hyperhidrosis. *Clin Dermatol.* 2004;22(1):60–65.

117. Barankin B, Wasel N. Treatment of inguinal hyperhidrosis with botulinum toxin type A. *Int J Dermatol.* 2006;45(8):985–986.

118. Goldman A. Treatment of axillary and palmar hyperhidrosis with botulinum toxin. *Aesthetic Plast Surg.* 2000;24(4):280–282.

119. Moraru E, Voller B, Auff E, Schnider P. Dose thresholds and local anhidrotic effect of botulinum A toxin injections (Dysport). *Br J Dermatol.* 2001;145(2):368.

120. Kinkelin I, Hund M, Naumann M, Hamm H. Effective treatment of frontal hyperhidrosis with botulinum toxin A. *Br J Dermatol.* 2000;143(4):824–827.

121. Pomprasit M, Chintrakarn C. Treatment of Frey's syndrome with botulinum toxin. *J Med Assoc Thai.* 2007;90(11):2397–2402.

122. Suskind DL, Tilton A. Clinical study of botulinum-A toxin in the treatment of sialorrhea in children with cerebral palsy. *Laryngoscope.* 2002;112(1):73–81.

123. Marchese Ragona R, Blotta P, Pastore A, Tugnoli V, Eleopra R, De Grandis D. Management of parotid sialocele with botulinum toxin. *Laryngoscope.* 1999;109(8):1344–1346.

124. Laskawi R, Drobik C, Schönebeck C. Up-to-date report of botulinum toxin type A treatment in patients with gustatory sweating (Frey's syndrome). *Laryngoscope.* 1998;108(3):381–384.

125. Kranz G, Sycha T, Voller B, Gleiss A, Schnider P, Auff E. Pain sensation during intradermal injections of three different botulinum toxin preparations in different doses and dilutions. *Dermatol Surg.* 2006;32(7):886–890.

126. Carruthers A, Carruthers J, Said S. Dose-ranging study of botulinum toxin type A in the treatment of glabellar rhytids in females. *Dermatol Surg.* 2005;31(4):414–422; discussion 422.

127. Baumann L, Frankel S, Welsh E, Halem M. Cryoanalgesia with dichlorotetrafluoroethane lessens the pain of botulinum toxin injections for the treatment of palmar hyperhidrosis. *Dermatol Surg.* 2003;29(10):1057–1059; discussion 1060.

128. Lipton RB, Bigal ME. Migraine: epidemiology, impact, and risk factors for progression. *Headache.* 2005;45(Suppl 1):S3–S13.

129. Aurora SK, Gawel M, Brandes JL, Pokta S, Vandenburgh AM; BOTOX North American Episodic Migraine Study Group. Botulinum toxin type a prophylactic treatment of episodic migraine: a randomized, double-blind, placebo-controlled exploratory study. *Headache.* 2007;47(4):486–499.

130. Silberstein SD, Stark SR, Lucas SM, Christie SN, Degryse RE, Turkel CC; BoNTA-039 Study Group. Botulinum toxin type A for the prophylactic treatment of chronic daily headache: a randomized, double-blind, placebo-controlled trial. *Mayo Clin Proc.* 2005;80(9):1126–1137.

131. Vo AH, Satori R, Jabbari B, et al. Botulinum toxin type-a in the prevention of migraine: a double-blind controlled trial. *Aviat Space Environ Med.* 2007;78(5 Suppl):B113–B118.

132. Freitag FG, Diamond S, Diamond M, Urban G. Botulinum toxin type A in the treatment of chronic migraine without medication overuse. *Headache.* 2008;48(2):201–209.

133. Allergan. Botox (onabotulinumtoxinA) [package insert]. U.S. Food and Drug Administration website https://www.accessdata.fda.gov/drugsatfda_docs/label/2011/103000s5236lbl.pdf. Revised October 2010. Accessed March 11, 2021.

134. Flynn TC. Botox in men. *Dermatol Ther.* 2007;20(6):407–413.

135. Flynn TC. Update on botulinum toxin. *Semin Cutan Med Surg.* 2006;25(3):115–121.

136. Monks DA, O'Bryant EL, Jordan CL. Androgen receptor immunoreactivity in skeletal muscle: enrichment at the neuromuscular junction. *J Comp Neurol.* 2004;473(1):59–72.

137. Carruthers J, Fagien S, Matarasso SL; Botox Consensus Group. Consensus recommendations on the use of botulinum toxin type a in facial aesthetics. *Plast Reconstr Surg.* 2004;114(6 Suppl):1S–22S.

138. Ahn KY, Park MY, Park DH, Han DG. Botulinum toxin A for the treatment of facial hyperkinetic wrinkle lines in Koreans. *Plast Reconstr Surg.* 2000;105(2):778–784.

139. Kim J. Cosmetic treatments for ethnic skin. Paper presented at: 65th Annual summer meeting of American Academy of Dermatology, focus session 872; February 2007; Washington, DC.

140. Arimura K, Arimura Y, Takata Y, Nakamura T, Kaji R. Comparative electrophysiological study of response to botulinum toxin type B in Japanese and Caucasians. *Mov Disord.* 2008;23(2):240–245.

141. Swift A, Remington K. BeautiPHIcation™: a global approach to facial beauty. *Clin Plast Surg.* 2011;38(3):347–377, v.

142. Liew S, Wu WT, Chan HH, et al. Consensus on changing trends, attitudes, and concepts of Asian beauty. *Aesthetic Plast Surg.* 2016;40(2):193–201.

143. Sundaram H, Huang PH, Hsu NJ, et al.; Pan-Asian Aesthetics Toxin Consensus Group. Aesthetic applications of botulinum toxin A in Asians: An international, multidisciplinary, pan-Asian consensus. *Plast Reconstr Surg Glob Open.* 2016;4(12):e872.

144. Elluru RG, Kumar M. Physiology of the salivary glands. In: Flint PW, Haughey BH, Lund LJ. *Cummings Otolaryngology: Head & Neck Surgery.* 6th ed. Philadelphia, PA: Elsevier Saunders; 2015.

145. Lee SK. Antibody-induced failure of botulinum toxin type A therapy in a patient with masseteric hypertrophy. *Dermatol Surg.* 2007;33:S105–S110.

146. Pellett S, Tepp WH, Clancy CM, Borodic GE, Johnson EA. A neuronal cell-based botulinum neurotoxin assay for highly sensitive and specific detection of neutralizing serum antibodies. *FEBS Lett.* 2007;581(25):4803–4808.

147. Dressler D. Clinical presentation and management of antibody-induced failure of botulinum toxin therapy. *Mov Disord.* 2004;19(Suppl 8):S92–S100.

148. Guyuron B, Huddleston SW. Aesthetic indications for botulinum toxin injection. *Plast Reconstr Surg.* 1994;93(5):913–918.

149. Borodic G. Myasthenic crisis after botulinum toxin. *Lancet.* 1998;352(9143):1832.

150. Cox NH, Duffey P, Royle J. Fixed drug eruption caused by lactose in an injected botulinum toxin preparation. *J Am Acad Dermatol.* 1999;40(2 Pt 1):263–264.

CHAPTER 24

Chemical Peels

Jennifer M. Rullan, MD

SUMMARY POINTS

What's Important?

1. Superficial peels induce epidermal injury and are indicated for mild acne, melasma, pores, texture, and mild photodamage.
2. Superficial peels include the water-soluble alpha-hydroxy acids (AHA) (which include lactic acid, mandelic acid, glycolic acid (GA) and pyruvic acid (PA)), the lipid-soluble acids, beta-hydroxy acid (which includes salicylic acid), retinoic acid, Jessner's solution (JS), and trichloroacetic acid (TCA) 10% to 35%.
3. GA and PA require neutralization by removal with water or 10% sodium bicarbonate.
4. Medium depth peels penetrate into or through the papillary dermis when a level II frost (confluent white frost with background erythema) or a level III frost (confluent white frost without background erythema).
5. The classic combination medium depth peels for the face and scalp include solid CO_2 plus TCA 35%, JS plus TCA 35%, and GA 70% plus TCA 35%.
6. Baker-Gordon's formula (2.1% croton oil) was the standard phenol-croton oil peel from 1962 to 2000, but since 2000 Hetter's formulas (less than or equal to 1.6% croton oil) have been the standard.
7. Segmental phenol/croton oil peels limited to one or two cosmetic units, over 10–15 minutes per unit, do not require cardiac monitoring.

What's New?

1. Medium and deep chemical peels: updated safety and patient selection information, histology, techniques, healing stages and endpoints.
2. Chemical peels for acne scars.

What's Coming?

1. More publications on deep chemical peels (segmental and full face) showing safety protocols, procedures, and technique.

INTRODUCTION

Chemical peels are safe and inexpensive methods of resurfacing the skin. Peels have been utilized since ancient Egyptian times but the science behind chemical peeling has evolved significantly over the last 30 years. Recent scientific studies investigating the histologic and long-term effects of peels support their effective controlled wounding for medical and aesthetic improvement.[1] Chemical peeling is an art, and successful outcomes depend on tailoring the peel to the patient's skin needs,

with the correct technique, patient education, and safety standards. When the appropriate peel is selected and the desired end point is achieved, the risks of complications are minimized. Supervised hands-on training is of utmost importance and provides the highest quality of education.

Chemical peels are categorized based on the depth of the procedure: superficial, medium or deep (**Table 24-1**).[2] Superficial peels induce necrosis of all or parts of the epidermis, from the stratum granulosum to the basal cell layer (**Figs. 24-1**) and can be used in all skin types. These peels can

TABLE 24-1

Peel Depth	Wounding Spectrum (depth)	Peeling Time
Superficial	Stratum granulosum to papillary dermis (< 0.45 mm)	0–7 days
Medium	Through the papillary dermis to the upper reticular dermis (0.45–0.60 mm)	7–10 days
Deep	To the mid reticular dermis (0.60–0.80 mm)	10–14 days

treat melasma, acne, acne scars, thin seborrheic keratoses, and post-inflammatory hyperpigmentation, with subtle improvement in texture and pores.[2] Medium-depth peels, safest in skin types I–III, create necrosis of the epidermis and the papillary dermis. These peels can be used to treat actinic keratoses, fine lines, laxity, melasma, seborrheic keratoses, solar lentigines, acne scars, and skin texture. Deep peels, safest in skin types I–II, can dramatically improve deep facial rhytids, acne scarring, and photoaging. The depth of injury for deep peels is the mid-reticular dermis.[3,4]

Patient Selection

The success of a peel depends on careful selection of patients and individualization of treatment. The first step is careful examination of skin type and complexion. When one pinches the skin (where the cheekbone is most prominent), the thickness of the pinched skin is considered thin if less than 1 cm, normal if 1 cm, or thick if greater than 1 cm. Thinner skinned patients have higher risks of both lasers and peels due to a decrease in adnexal structures. Thin skin requires less coats to produce frosting.[5] Oily skin, on the other hand, can be a barrier to peeling solution absorption and will require more prepeel treatment. Medium to deep peels should be avoided in patients with darker skin types (unless one is an expert peeler), residual xerosis from isotretinoin, and radiation. Patients with a recent insult to the stratum corneum, such as beginning a regimen with tretinoin, facial shaving, waxing, use of exfoliating scrubs or kissing a person with a heavy beard for prolonged periods, are more susceptible to superficial chemical peels extending deeper than intended (**Fig. 24-2**). Consequently,

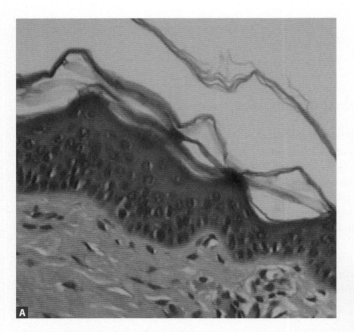

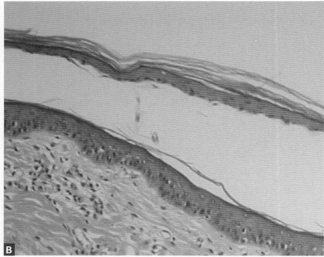

FIGURE 24-1. Hematoxylin and eosin (H&E) stain of **A.** untreated normal bovine skin and **B.** bovine skin treated with a superficial chemical peel (two coats of the Pigment Peel Plus). This biopsy demonstrates a split in the spinous layer of the epidermis.

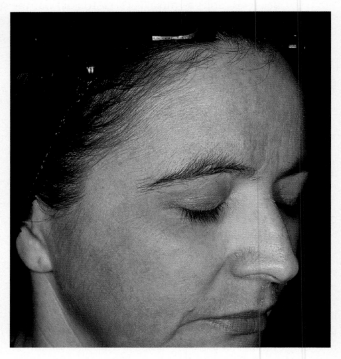

FIGURE 24-2. Patient on Retin A with retinoid dermatitis. Peeling this patient will result in excessive redness and scaling. It is best to wait 1 week prior to proceeding with chemical peeling.

it is necessary to closely examine the condition of the skin, obtain a good history from the patient prior to performing the first peel, and have follow-up visits planned ahead of time (Box 24-1). Chemical peels should also be avoided in patients with the stigmata of skin picking or severe mental illness. Absolute contraindications include active infections.

Patient's expectations and lifestyle must be evaluated. Downtime from chemical peels can be significant and this needs to be discussed at length in order to set correct expectations. The longer the recovery, the more prolonged the results, and vice versa. Results from deep peels have been found to last 15–20 years clinically and histologically.[6] However, one must clearly set expectations on the 2 weeks of serious downtime, erythema that can last up to 3 months, skin sensitivity that can last up to 6 months, and the risk of failure to eradicate rhytids at the vermillion border. Conversely, with superficial

peels one needs to set the expectation that multiple sessions are required for effect and that peels are part of a maintenance program (Box 24-1). Each superficial chemical peel is only able to produce subtle changes in the skin. It is the cumulative benefits of the peels that yield the most noticeable changes in the skin. At least four superficial peels are usually necessary before patients can begin to see amelioration of photodamage, solar lentigines, and melasma. Those with more severe damage may require eight or more. If this is not explained to patients, they will become discouraged after one or two chemical peels and will not be compliant with the prescribed regimen. For medium depth peels one must set expectations that there is significant downtime of 7–10 days and that deep wrinkles will persist; however, texture, color, and skin vitality will be significantly improved.

Setup

Each chemical peel may be set up differently, but one always needs to set up with four main concepts before beginning. These are 1) comfort measures such as ice water with towels, fan, ice packs, Zimmer, nerve blocks, etc. 2) correct labeling and placement when multiple different acids are being used 3) eye wash safety protocol and 4) multiple applicators for options to ensure even application of solutions (**Fig. 24-3**).

Chemical peels can be applied with a sable or goat hair brush, gauze, cotton balls, cotton-tipped applicators (CTA), or a wooden skewer with 1–2 cotton balls wound around one end into a uniform cylinder shape (**Fig. 24-4**). For superficial peels, brushes allow for quick application with little waste of solution, and can be cleansed with soap and water. Gauze or cotton can absorb more material therefore more solution is wasted. A wooden skewer with cotton wound around one end is used for pressured rolling motions and not rubbing and is useful for even application and avoiding streaking.[5] A single CTA is

BOX 24-1	How to Use Chemical Peels in First 3 Visits—Dr. Baumann's Perspective

1. At the first visit, assess the patient's skin using a UV or Wood's light to determine the extent of pigmentation abnormalities. This will help convince the patient of the necessity of sunscreen use. Discuss skincare, sunscreen use and the importance of topical retinoid treatments and offer product recommendations based on the patient's skin type. Also at this juncture, it is imperative to caution patients to refrain from using at-home topical AHAs, BHA, and other irritating ingredients such as vitamin C in order to avoid excessive skin irritation. It is important at each visit, but particularly so at the first visit, to find out if the patient has any significant forthcoming social obligations that might be compromised or made embarrassing owing to erythema or conspicuous skin flaking.
2. At the second visit, the practitioner can go to the next level in peel strength if the patient experienced minimal or no peeling after the initial peel. Most patients are started on a topical retinoid on the first visit so care must be taken to avoid peeling skin that exhibits "retinoid dermatitis" (**Fig. 24-2**). In such a case, the practitioner should refrain from performing a peel until the retinoid dermatitis resolves. On this visit, it is also important to assess how well the patient tolerates the social/psychological impact of peeling. If the patient complains about flaking skin or erythema, the physician should titrate the peels more slowly. If the patient feels that significant erythema and/or flaking are the sine qua non of an adequate peel, the physician may want to proceed more rapidly.
3. Visit three and beyond—Manufacturers of most superficial chemical peel brands recommend treatments at 10- to 14-day intervals. One may continue the peelings until the initial presenting symptoms have resolved and, thereafter, perform peels at 4-week intervals for maintenance. One should occasionally inquire about retinoid and sunscreen use to ensure patient compliance. After the third peel, patients should be consistently using the retinoids with no skin irritation. If this is the case, it is a good time to add an at-home AHA or BHA preparation.

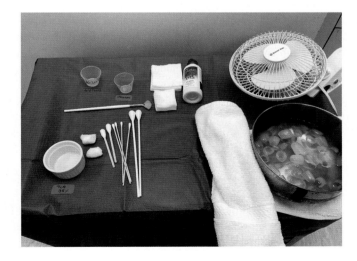

FIGURE 24-3. Set up for a medium depth Jessner's and TCA 35% peel with clearly labeled acetone, Jessner's and TCA 35%, with multiple applicators, eye wash, and comfort measures such as a bowl of ice water with a face towel, fan, etc. Not seen here that is often used as well are ice packs, nerve blocks, or a Zimmer cooling device, etc.

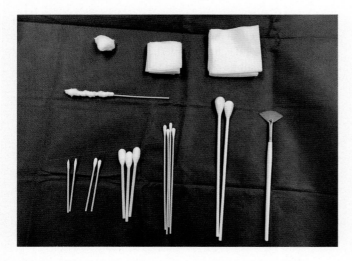

FIGURE 24-4. Applicator choices from top left to right: cotton ball, 2 × 2 gauze, 4 × 4 gauze, wooden skewer with cotton wound uniformly on one end to form a cylinder, mini tapered tip cotton applicators, 3" CTA, large CTA 4" plastic stick, 6" CTA, 8" OB/GYN rayon tipped applicators, and sable brush. In general, the dryer the applicator, the safer the procedure, whichever one is selected by personal preference.

ideal for application of TCA under the eyes while the patient is temporarily looking up, whereas a moist 4 × 4 gauze is ideal for rapid and pressured application of TCA to the rest of the face in medium depth peels.[2] Deep chemical peels are applied with CTAs because they can withstand significant pressure with application. In addition, one can control how wet each CTA is. Any excess solution can be removed by squeezing out the CTA on the rim of the glass or metal container.

Patients should be positioned with their heads slightly elevated recumbent on the table. It is important to have an assistant standing by with dry CTAs to look for tearing at the lacrimal puncta and lateral canthi. It has been shown that rubbing alcohol, chlorhexidine gluconate, and acetone are equally effective in the prepeel skin preparation. Vigorous prepeel scrubbing is recommended for sebaceous skin or advanced photoaging. The nose and glabellar area may frost slower than the central cheek if it is not sufficiently degreased. Conversely, a wipe is sufficient preparation for patients with acne, seborrhea, or thin translucent skin,[4] and when performing glycolic acid peels.

Pre-treatment

Pre-treatment refers to the 2 to 4 week period before the office-based chemical peel where actions are taken for epidermal thinning, reduced post-inflammatory hyperpigmentation, and enhanced healing. The products usually used to prepare the skin are sunscreens, tretinoin, AHAs, and tyrosinase inhibitors. Waxing or dermabrasion should be avoided 3–4 weeks before a peel. Medium and deep peels into the reticular dermis often use prophylactic antivirals, antibiotics, and anti-yeast oral medications to prevent complications. It is necessary to take measures to prevent herpes infections for all medium and deep peels, and some superficial peels (patients with a

history of herpes simplex infection). Acyclovir or Valacyclovir are given for 7–10 days as prophylaxis.

Patients with darker skin types (III and higher) should use hydroquinone beforehand for 4 weeks and after peels to lower the incidence of hyperpigmentation.[7] Prevention of expected pigmentary changes in skin types > III include using the tyrosinase inhibitors such as hydroquinone, kojic acid, azelaic acid, arbutin, licorice, etc. and are recommended to begin 4 weeks prior to peels. Tretinoin should be discontinued 1 week prior to peels in Fitzpatrick Skin Types IV–VI.[8] Retinoids or AHAs (such as glycolic acid 10%) are used to thin the epidermis in order to allow even penetration of the chemical peels, but should be avoided in patients with visible telangiectasias suggesting rosacea or thin skin. The risk of thinning the skin is that the chemical peel could go deeper than expected. Tretinoin has the added benefit of accelerating healing, regardless of the body region, even after only 2 weeks of use.[9] It is also important to have patients apply a daily moisturizer in the pre-treatment stage as dryness can increase the risk for overpenetration or complications.

Post-treatment

Following all chemical peels, it is important for patients to use sunscreen and to practice sun avoidance. During the healing stages, patients must have clear instructions to avoid picking their skin, taking baths, swimming in pools or jacuzzis, exercise, heat, sunlight, and pets coming into contact with their face or pillow.

Although superficial chemical peels are very safe when used properly, they can all cause erythema, itching, peeling, increased skin sensitivity, and even epidermolysis. Allergic contact dermatitis has been reported to occur with resorcinol, salicylic acid, kojic acid, lactic acid, and hydroquinone. Irritant contact dermatitis has been linked to glycolic acid. Any peel can cause irritant dermatitis when used with excessive frequency, inappropriately high concentrations, or with a vigorous skin preparation using acetone or another "degreasing" solution.

Post care for most medium peels entails gentle soaking and cleansing followed by ointment for at least 3–5 days. Occlusive ointments enhance wound healing and are recommended to allow for reepithelialization. For medium and deep peels, acetic acid or white distilled vinegar is diluted and can be formulated into an ice bath or a spritzer spray bottle (dilution of one tablespoon vinegar in one cup of water) to be used for its anti-inflammatory, anti-yeast, anti-bacterial, and soothing properties. Acne-prone patients are likely to have an acne flare after a medium to deep peel and should be prepared ahead of time; they can use oral antibiotics as soon as the flare begins.

Complications of medium and deep depth peels include scarring, hyper- or hypopigmentation, and infections. Pain is a hallmark of infection, the most common of which include *Candida albicans*, *Staphylococcus aureus*, *Pseudomonas aeruginosa*, and herpes simplex virus. Therefore, if there is postpeel pain, malaise, or pustules, then prophylaxis with fluconazole 200 mg single dose, trimethoprim-sulfamethoxozole twice daily, and gentamycin 0.1% cream three times daily for 7 days is indicated.[8] Postpeel erythema for medium depth peels usually lasts 2–3 weeks. Prolonged erythema is defined as lasting longer than 3 weeks and can occur as a result of infection, overpenetration of TCA (seen by a frost that lasts > 30 minutes) or due to irritant or allergic contact dermatitis.[4,10] Postpeel erythema for deep peels is normal up to 1–3 months.

SUPERFICIAL PEELS

Although a wide variety of agents have been shown to be effective for superficial peeling, alpha hydroxy acids (AHAs), beta hydroxy acid (BHA), Jessner's solution, modified Jessner's solution, resorcinol, and trichloroacetic acid (TCA) are the most commonly used in-office peel compounds. All of these compounds produce effects on the skin by inducing desquamation with resultant hastening of the cell cycle, yielding skin that is smoother in texture and more evenly pigmented. The individual ingredients of these peels will be discussed but, notably, these ingredients are often used in combination as seen in the numerous commercial combination chemical peels (**Table 24-2**).[11] Most superficial peels are being performed by aestheticians with or without physician supervision.

EVALUATING AND COMPARING SUPERFICIAL ACID PREPARATIONS

The most important aspect of superficial chemical peel strength is the amount of available free acid. The amount of free acid itself is affected by the following: concentration of the peel, the pK_a of the acid preparation, the pH of the solution (which is also affected by the type of vehicle used), and whether or not the peel is buffered. The pK_a of a substance measures its capacity to donate protons. The pK_a is the pH at which the level of free acid is the same as the level of the salt form of the acid (**Table 24-3**). Some chemical peel formulations are "buffered," or made to be more tolerable, by adding a base such as sodium bicarbonate or sodium hydroxide to the solution. This produces an increased amount of the salt form, which results in less free acid and a higher pH. Buffered solutions are resistant to pH changes but may also have a decrease in efficacy. These formulations are safer for use by beginners and nonphysicians, which may account for their popularity. It is important to remember that the vehicle can also cause irritation and affect clinical response. In fact, studies indicate that irritation associated with AHA products is usually related to the formulation of the product and not to the AHA itself.[12] AHAs have actually been demonstrated to reduce the irritation experienced when known irritants are placed on the skin without compromising the barrier function.[12–14]

AHAs AND BHA

AHAs and BHA are naturally occurring organic acids that contribute to inducing exfoliation and accelerating the cell cycle. Research in the 1970s demonstrated that topical preparations that contain AHAs exert profound influence on epidermal keratinization.[13] When AHAs and BHA are applied to the skin in high concentrations, the result is detachment of keratinocytes and epidermolysis; application at lower concentrations reduces corneocyte cohesion directly above the granular layer, advancing desquamation and thinning of the SC.[12] AHAs are beneficial in dry skin because they function as humectants (see Chapter 32, Cosmetic and Drug Regulations), causing the skin to hold onto water. Once the desquamation is enhanced, the skin is more flexible and better able to reflect light.

A major difference between AHAs and BHA is that BHA is lipophilic, which enables it to penetrate the sebaceous material in the hair follicle and exfoliate the pores. Secondly, unlike some AHAs, BHA does not need neutralizing.[15] AHAs, which are water-soluble, do not exhibit BHA's comedolytic characteristic (**Table 24-4**).[16]

AHAs

Glycolic Acid

Glycolic acid (**Fig. 24-5**) is the AHA most commonly used in chemical peels in the offices of dermatologists and aestheticians. It is popularly known as "the lunchtime peel" because it can be completed during the patient's lunch hour and the patient can return to work without any telltale signs. GA is water-soluble and comes in four different delivery systems: free acid (non-neutralized), partially neutralized (combined with a base like ammonium hydroxide), buffered (no practical benefit in peeling), and esterified (glycol-citrate solution).[17] Partially neutralized formulas or lower concentrations of free glycolic acid should be used for patients with atopic dermatitis, dry skin or if inflamed or sensitive skin. Glycolic acid peels should be avoided if taking oral isotretinoin or if using a topical retinoid due to high risk of overpenetration. **Table 24-5** provides a list of commonly used glycolic acid peels. Glycolic acid peels must be neutralized to avoid overpenetration as soon as the clinical endpoint of significant erythema or burning is seen or felt, or after 2–5 minutes, whichever comes first (**Table 24-6**). GA is safe at lower concentrations such as 35–50% but has higher risks at 70% of focal irritation or hot spots, which can lead to rapid blistering also known as epidermolysis. Unlike many other peels, glycolic acid must be neutralized after use so as to prevent burning. For this reason, it is difficult to use on large areas of the body. It is best used in a small area on which it can be quickly applied and quickly neutralized.

Well-designed studies have demonstrated the efficacy of AHA peels as a treatment for photoaging. In 1996, Ditre showed that application of AHAs resulted histologically in a 25% increase in skin thickness, increased acid mucopolysaccharides in the dermis, improved quality of the elastic fibers, and increased collagen density.[18] In fact, in a study by Kim et al., glycolic acid treatments increased fibroblast proliferation in vitro as well as collagen production.[19] It is for this reason that when superficial chemical peels, such as glycolic acid, are combined with a physical injury, they can be used to treat acne scars (**Table 24-7**). In a study by Sharad, 60 patients (FST III–V) with acne scars were treated with five sessions of either microneedling alone (group 1, n = 30) or microneedling combined with 35% glycolic acid peels on the same day

TABLE 24-2 Examples of Combination Peels Currently on the Market

Peel	TCA	SA	Phenol	CO	HQ	Retinol	RA	Resorcinol	Citric Acid	LA	AA	MA	KA	Other
Jessner's		14%						14%		14%				ethanol (95%)
Modified Jessner's		17%							8%	17%				
PCA Enhanced Jessner's		14%						14%	yes	14%			Yes	isopropyl alcohol
VI Peel	<12%	<12%	<12%				<0.1% pad							Vitamin C 4% pad
VI Precision Boosters	<12%	<12%	<30%				<0.1% pad							
Vi Precision Plus Boosters	<12%	<12%	<30%		4%		<0.1% pad							HQ 4%, vitamin C and HC pads
Z.O. 3-step stimulation peel	17%	10%					6% cream ×2 app			5%				
Pro Peel Extra Strength (vivant)	20%	8%	2%			10%								
Apeele Light (3 steps)	10%	20%	3.5%		8%	3% in red	0.5% in black			15%		10%		
Apeele Medium	15%	20%	5%		8%	3%	0.5%			15%		10%		
Apeele Forte	20%	20%	7.5%		8%		0.5%			15%		10%		
Melanage HP Masque (Young)					14%									Arbutin 20%, HQ from precursor
RevePeel Medium Depth	10–14%	10–14%	<10%	<0.1%						10–14%				
RevePeel Enlighten Rx		6%			8%	3%							yes	Arbutin, Vit B3, THD Ascorbate, Silver
Biomedic Pigment Peel Plus	30%	20%												La Roche-Posay glycerin base

Product										Other
PCA Ultra Peel I	10%			20%				yes		
PCA Ultra Peel Forte (MD's)	20%			10%				yes		
PCA Sensi Peel	6%			12%				yes		In glycerin base, ascorbic acid, chaste tree extract
PCA w/o HQ	15%			15%	10%			3%		Ethanol 57%
PCA w/HQ	15%		2%	15%	10%			3%		
PCA w/ HQ & Resorcinol	14%		2%	14%	1%		14%	3%		
Replenix MD Perfect 10	yes			yes		yes	yes			Glycolic acid, pyruvic acid
Skin Medica Vitalize Peel	10%			10%		10%	Yes			
Skin Medica Rejuvenize	15%			15%		15%	Yes			Panthenol, iso-ceteth-20
Skin Medica Illuminize	Yes					Yes	Yes			Phytic acid, malic acid
Melanage Gloss	17%			17%			2 pads			
Universal Peel	Yes	30%		10%				yes	0.05%	Phytic acid
Radiant Peel	>5%	>5%		26%			1% BID days 2–4		~0.1%	

AA, azelaic acid; CO, croton oil; HQ, hydroquinone; KA, kojic acid; MA, mandelic acid; RA, retinoic acid; SA, salicylic acid

TABLE 24-3	Understanding the acidity and strengths of chemical peels* 3,5 (citation)	
pH > pK$_a$	AHAs are essentially moisturizers	Neutralized AHA creates the salt form with more moisturizing and less caustic effects - the higher the pH, the less efficacious and less irritating
pH < or = to pK$_a$	AHAs increase skin exfoliation and cell replacement	Acid form predominates which is more absorbent and penetrates better (acid form is active form) - the lower the pH, the more irritation and efficacy
TCA	pK$_a$ = 0.53	*lowest pK$_a$ of all acids for peels therefore is the most aggressive acid
Salicylic acid	pK$_a$ = 2.97	→ if you mix AHA+BHA in pH of 3.5, the AHA acid form would predominate and salt form of BHA, and BHA would be rendered suboptimal.
AHA	pK$_a$ = 3.83	
*pKa is the pH at which level of free acid is the same as the level of the salt form		

TABLE 24-4	Comparison of AHAs and BHA	
	AHAs	BHA
S Used in rosacea	No	Yes
Useful in acne	Yes	Yes
Useful in melasma	Yes	Yes
Useful for dry skin	Yes	Yes
S Speeds cell cycle	Yes	Yes
Enhances exfoliation	Yes	Yes
Lipophilic	No	Yes
Inhibits arachidonic acid	No	Yes
Anesthetic properties	No	Yes
Anti-inflammatory properties	Maybe	Yes
Must be neutralized	Yes	No
Visible frost	No	Yes
Variety of available concentrations	Yes	Yes
Shown to increase collagen synthesis	Yes	No
Useful in pregnancy/breast feeding	Yes	No

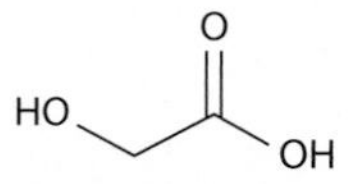

Glycolic Acid

(2-Hydroxyethanoic acid)

FIGURE 24-5. Chemical structure of glycolic acid. The OH group is in the alpha position; therefore, this is in the alpha hydroxy acid family.

(group 2, n = 30). At 3-month follow-up, mean improvement was 31% in group 1, compared with 62% in group 2.[20] The safest combination approach for darker skin types is to alternate microneedling and peels every 3–4 weeks, rather than performing them on the same day.

GA Application Techniques

The skin should not be degreased or scrubbed, just lightly wiped down or gently washed prior to the peel. The GA should be applied quickly over 20 seconds maximum so that the contact time is the same, starting with the most resistant areas of the face first (lateral face or forehead) and the midface last. The contact time is the time the AHA is left to act before being neutralized, which stops its effects. The contact time is relative and the end point depends more on the appearance of erythema and the patient's reported sensation of burning. AHAs in aqueous solutions do not penetrate evenly and erythema does not appear evenly either; therefore, one must remain beside the patient and not take eyes off the treated area. The contact time should end as soon as erythema begins because it can progress to a frost very quickly, especially when using higher concentrations like 70%. It is important to continuously receive feedback from the patient with this peel. One must neutralize areas with severe burning first, as oftentimes erythema is difficult to visualize. In addition, upon neutralization, there may occur a fizzing on the face associated with more burning. Care must be taken to ensure all of the GA is neutralized and therefore all burning has ceased. Frosting should not occur. The presence of frost signifies dermal injury and potential pending epidermolysis.

Pyruvic Acid

Pyruvic acid is an alpha ketoacid that is physiologically converted to lactic acid; however, it is rarely used by dermatologists due to its disadvantages. Pyruvic acid's disadvantages include the need for neutralization, like glycolic acid, and intense stinging and burning sensation during application. The safest strength to use is 40%, because, like glycolic acid, it must be neutralized as soon as the time endpoint or clinical endpoint of erythema is reached so as to avoid complications from overpenetration.[8] The pyruvic acid peel has been used with success in the treatment of inflammatory acne, photoaging, post-inflammatory hyperpigmentation and melasma.[21,22] It is important to note that pyruvic acid must not be used in high (50%) or full-strength concentrations since there is the potential for scarring. Concentrations above 50% should only be used for focal hyperkeratotic lesions, such as actinic keratosis and seborrheic keratoses (**Table 24-8**).[23] It has been used successfully in combination with 5-fluouracil for the treatment of actinic keratoses and warts, and when used at 70% can be comparable to salicylic acid for warts.[24-26] Pyruvic acid, if left in place for an extended period of time, converts into CO_2 and acetaldehyde, and the CO_2 buildup may cause the bottle to explode.[27]

TABLE 24-5	Commonly Used Glycolic Acid Peel Brands*a*							
Product name	Company	Percent Glycolic Acid	Percent Free Acid	pH	Neutralized	Buffered	Additives
GA 35%	Delasco	35%	35	1.63	No	No	
GA 70%	Delasco	70%	70	1.17	No	No	
Refinity Skin Solution	Cosmederm Technologies	70%	70%	>1	No	No	Strontium Nitrate
Gly Derm—20% GA swab	ICN	20%	Free acid is esterified	1.4			Citric alcohol 5%
MicroPeel 20	BioMedic	20	20	1.3	No	No	Glycerin
MicroPeel 30	BioMedic	30	30	1.3	No	No	Glycerin
MicroPeel 50	BioMedic	50	50	0.8	No	No	Glycerin

*a*The amount of free acid determines the strength of the peel. Esterified free fatty acid must be hydrolyzed to the free acid by the skin's natural esterases to be active.

TABLE 24-6	Endpoints		
Peel Depth	**Skin types**	**Peel**	**Endpoints**
Superficial	all	Jessner's Peel	Speckled pseudofrost & erythema
		Modified Jessner's	Speckled pseudofrost & erythema
		20–30% SA-HA	White Pseudofrost +/− erythema
		20–30% SA-PEG	Clear even coat with or without erythema
		Lactic Acid	Clear coat with mild erythema
		TCA 10–25%	*Epidermis* *Level I frost:* a light reticular frost with background erythema *Papillary Dermis* *Level II frost:* a confluent light white frost with background erythema *Epidermal Sliding:* exaggerated skin wrinkling when pinching the skin occurs transiently
		Pyruvic acid < 40%	Erythema and burning
		Solid CO2 (dry ice)	Transient white congelation (or thickening from freezing) with residual erythema **Fig. 24-16**
Medium	I–III	CO2 + TCA 35% Jessner's + TCA 35% Glycolic + TCA 35% CROSS Phenol 88%	*Upper Reticular Dermis* *Edema:* epidermal sliding fades and edema can be observed by pinching the skin Level III: a solid white frosting without erythema
Deep	I–II	Modified Croton Oil/Phenol Peels	*Papillary Dermis* *Pink White Frost:* For Thin Skin of Eyelids, Forehead or Temples should see background erythema *Upper Reticular Dermis* *Solid White Frost:* a solid white frosting without erythema to jawline or cheeks *Mid Reticular Dermis* *Grey-White Opaque Frost (that persists):* for thicker skin on chin, perioral area, glabella. *Fine Grey Cast:* is a delayed visual change that occurs due to dermal edema which causes the white frost to turn greyish as seen in Fig. – *Red-Brown Vesicles (epidermolysis):* delayed endpoint seen after 10 minutes defrosting **Fig. 24-23**

TABLE 24-7	Recommended Full Face Peels for Common Skin Conditions	
Depth	Skin Condition	Chemical Peel
Superficial	Acne	20–30% Salicylic Acid Jessner's Solution
	Post-Inflammatory Hyperpigmentation	20–30% Salicylic Acid
	Melasma	Hydroquinone/Retinol Combination Masks 20–30% Salicylic Acid TCA 10–15% (1 pass) Jessner's Solution Glycolic Acid 35%
	Acne Scars	35% Glycolic Acid alternating with microneedling (MN) TCA combined or alternating with MN TCA 20% combined with MN and fractional laser alternating (Ieheta)
Medium	Actinic Keratoses	any of the combination TCA 35% peels
	Acne Scars	any of the combination TCA 35% peels Medium-depth chemical peels using solid CO_2 slush with focal 50% TCA to efface scar rims[2]
	Glougau 1–II	any of the combination TCA 35% peels
Deep	Acne Scars	Modified Phenol-Croton Oil Peel (enhanced resulted when combined with 2nd day debridement, chemabrasion and/or subcision)
	Glougau III–IV	Modified Phenol-Croton Oil Peel

TABLE 24-8	Common Focal Chemical Destruction
Actinic Keratoses	Pyruvic acid 40% TCA 50% Phenol-croton oil peels
Seborrheic Keratoses	Pyruvic Acid 40–70%
Acne Scars (ice pick and box scars)	CROSS Carboxyl Acid 88% (phenol) CROSS TCA 30–90%
Verruca Vulgaris	TCA 50–100% Pyruvic acid 40–70%

Lactic Acid

Lactic acid (**Fig. 24-6**) is a popular AHA among aestheticians that is also found in many at-home products and prescription moisturizers. Lactic acid decreases corneocyte cohesion, leading to a thinner stratum corneum. It also moisturizes and brightens the skin and improves the appearance of scars.[18] Lactic acid is hypothesized to be part of the skin's natural moisturizing factor which plays a role in hydration. Several studies on the activity of buffered 12% ammonium lactate lotion (LacHydrin™) have documented its moisturizing ability.[28] Recently, lactic acid was also found to inhibit melanogenesis by suppressing the formation of tyrosinase, irrespective of its acidity.[29] It has been found to be effective for frictional dermal melanosis,[30] for melasma when used every 2 weeks in its full-strength lactic acid 92% concentration (pH 3.5),[31] and infraorbital melanosis at 15%.[32] Dayal et al. compared once weekly infraorbital peels (x 3 weeks) using lactic acid with GA for periorbital melanosis. Lactic acid 15% had statistically significant improvement on global assessment, although GA was found to have most improvement at 12 weeks (GA also had the most adverse reactions). Lactic acid 15 % weekly for 3 weeks was better than daily vitamin C 20%.[32] Additional studies are needed as lactic acid is a growing area of clinical application.

BHA

Also known as salicylic acid (SA), BHA is another commonly used chemical peel, used most often for acne due to its lipophilic, comedolytic, anti-inflammatory, and antimicrobial properties. Derived from willow bark, wintergreen leaves, and sweet birch, SA is the only member of the BHA family, so named because the aromatic carboxylic acid has a hydroxy group in the beta position (**Fig. 24-7**).

Most physicians use preparations of 20% or 30% SA for in-office peels. Such peels have been shown to fade pigment spots and decrease surface roughness with similar results to those seen with AHAs[16]. However, unlike AHAs, BHA affects the arachidonic acid cascade and, therefore, exhibits anti-inflammatory capabilities. These properties may allow SA peels to be effective while inducing less irritation than AHA peels. The anti-inflammatory effects of BHA make it a very useful peel in patients with acne and rosacea (**Table 24-4**). It can be combined with traditional acne therapy to speed the resolution of comedones and red inflamed papules. SA peels also has a whitening effect in patients with darker skin types. In a study of 24 Asian women who were treated with bi-weekly facial peeling with 30% SA in absolute ethanol for 3 months, some lightening of skin color was seen.[15]

SA comes in two different vehicles: hydroalcoholic (HA) or polyethylene glycol (PEG).[33] SA in ethanol or HA produces the classic white pseudofrost that can be wiped off the skin

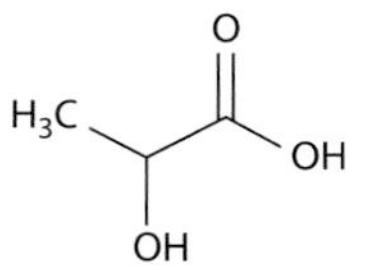

O
‖
H₃C   C
           OH

OH

Lactic Acid
(2-Hydroxypropanoic acid)

FIGURE 24-6. Chemical structure of lactic acid.

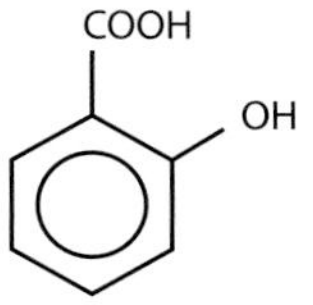

COOH
        OH

Salicylic Acid

FIGURE 24-7. Chemical structure of salicylic acid.

BOX 24-2

It is important to note that the frost seen in a BHA peel represents precipitated SA as ethanol evaporates, while the frost in a TCA peel represents precipitated skin proteins. These "skipped" areas in salicylic areas can and should be easily touched up, whereas those seen in a TCA peel should not be touched up as they can be with a BHA peel, because the TCA peel frosting time depends on the concentration used and takes around 5 minutes to develop. Lower concentrations take longer to frost.

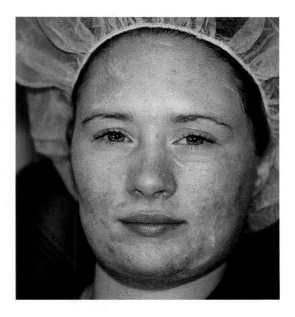

FIGURE 24-8. Beta hydroxy acid peels can be used to treat acne, rosacea, and photoaging on any part of the body. The salicylic acid in ethanol or hydroalcoholic vehicle produces a classic white pseudofrost upon alcohol evaporation.

with a wet cloth (**Fig. 24-8**). Pseudofrost represents the SA crystals that cannot penetrate the skin and appear as the ethanol evaporates. By definition, a pseudofrost can be wiped off. However, any superficial peel that over-penetrates, can lead to a deeper peel or an endpoint beyond that which is intended. For example, a salicylic acid peel can also produce a level I frost, where after the pseudofrost is wiped off, there remains a reticulated irregular white frost as seen in **Fig. 24-9**.

The HA vehicle is best for hyperpigmentation or oily skin with acne, but has slightly higher risk of over-penetration that can result in post-inflammatory hyperpigmentation (PIH),

despite the fact that it is used to treat PIH (**Table 24-7**). The risks of skin lightening or darkening should be explained to patients with darker skin types prior to their use. The goal is to use a strong enough peel to be effective but not strong enough to induce inflammation. If in doubt use a lower strength peel and titrate to stronger peels in future sequential treatments. Burning upon application of the SA-HA usually fades within 3 minutes, and can be left on or washed off once the burning has ended. For oily skin with significant acne leaving the pseudofrost on provides more of a drying effect. Any areas that have been inadequately peeled can be easily identified and then treated by reapplying the BHA solution (**Box 24-2**). It is important to immediately use the chemical peel liquid once the cap has been taken off the bottle, otherwise it will evaporate and crystalize upon ethanol evaporation. In addition, do not use a fan when you use this peel because it will increase the rate at which the vehicle becomes volatile and will lessen the effect of the peel.

In contrast, the PEG vehicle does not produce a pseudofrost. Instead its endpoint is a clear, even coat with some possible mild erythema (**Table 24-6**). Dainichi et al. found the PEG SA to be superior to the HA vehicle for acne due to increased follicular penetration, with milder desquamation. However, the benefits of leaving the crystalized salicylic acid on the face in comparison to a 5-minute wash with SA-PEG have not been studied. PEG SA is best used for larger surfaces areas, such as for back acne or when applied to the face, chest and back due to less systemic absorption, but it needs to be rinsed off after 5 minutes due to the occlusive nature of PEG.[33] Although toxic levels of salicylates have not been reported in association with the concentrations currently used for SA peels,[3] there have been case reports of children with multiple excoriations and elderly patients with ichthyosis developing salicylism after topical SA treatment.[34] The International Peel Society consensus is that salicylism is very rare (the signs of which include nausea, disorientation, and tinnitus). However, when treating large body surface areas such as the face, chest, arms and legs, the PEG vehicle should be used because there is no systemic absorption and no risk of salicylism. Of course, BHA, whether in concentrations developed for in-office peels or in at-home products, is contraindicated in patients who are pregnant, breastfeeding, or allergic to aspirin.

OTHER PEELS

Resorcinol

Resorcinol (meta-dihydroxybenzene) has been used as a chemical peeling agent since Unna described its use in 1882.[35] It acts similarly to hydroquinone (para-dihydroxybenzene). It is mainly used as a treatment for pigmentary disorders and acne, but is also a common component of combination chemical peels, including Jessner's peel. Resorcinol paste (Unna's paste) comes in 30% and 50%. After an allergy test, it is applied for 10–25 minutes, for up to 3 days consecutively (**Fig. 24-10**). However, due to complexity of the procedure, risks, and downtime, this procedure is not accepted by most patients.

Prolonged use of resorcinol has been associated with myxedema and hypothyroidism; the drug has an antithyroid action thought to be due to the hydroxy group in the meta position blocking the metabolism of iodine.[36] Although resorcinol is very useful in the treatment of disorders of hyperpigmentation, it can cause hyperpigmentation in patients with a Fitzpatrick Skin Type greater than IV, and is therefore is contraindicated in skin types IV–VI.[37]

Jessner's Solution

This popular peel is a combination of resorcinol 14 g, salicylic acid 14 g, and lactic acid 14 g in a sufficient quantity of ethanol (95%) to make 100 cc of solution. Dr. Max Jessner originally formulated this peel to reduce the concentration and toxicity of each of the individual ingredients while increasing efficacy.[38] The strength of the peel is determined by how many layers are applied and if it is used in combination with other peeling formulas. Jessner's peel is commonly used with other peels because it does not have to be neutralized. Once the peel frosts, a second type of peel such as TCA can be applied on top of the Jessner's peel to increase the depth of the overall peel. Although this peel is very safe, it should be used with caution on patients with darker skin types because resorcinol is associated with an increased risk of post-inflammatory

hyperpigmentation, redness, and swelling. In order to avoid systemic absorption and the combined effects of the resorcinol and salicylic acid, this peel should not be used on multiple body areas at once. Cases of salicylism have been reported only when it is applied to the face, chest, arms and legs.[36,38]

Use of the Jessner's Peel

For only a couple days of exfoliation, one to three coats should be applied until the endpoint of mild erythema and whitish-powdery appearance (mild pseudofrost) (**Table 24-6**). For 2 to 4 days of red-brown exfoliation and a week of noticeable flaking, 4 to 10 coats are applied until pinpoints of white frost occur (speckled) over an erythematous base. The first coat is complete once frosting occurs (usually in 4 to 6 minutes). When using this peel on patients with a tendency to develop dyschromias (e.g., patients with melasma, post-inflammatory hyperpigmentation, etc.), it is a good idea to proceed slowly with one coat of the solution every 1 to 3 weeks to avoid exacerbating the hyperpigmentation. Jessner's peel is a well-known effective treatment for acne, especially back acne. It is also effective in rosacea patients because it contains salicylic acid.

Modified Jessner's Solution

The modified Jessner's solution (which includes lactic acid 17%, salicylic acid 17%, and citric acid 8% in ethanol 95%) was created to avoid possible allergic reactions and hyperpigmentation, which may be created by resorcinol, especially in skin types V and VI (**Fig. 24-11**).[39] The modified Jessner's solution has been found to be effective for melasma when added to a TCA 15–20% peel. With modified Jessner's solution as a pre-treatment keratolytic, the epidermal barrier is altered prior to TCA peeling, to assist in a more rapid and uniform uptake and avoid side effects that commonly occur in darker skin types following TCA peels.[40,41]

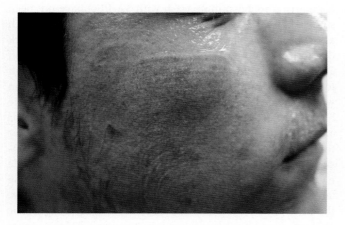

FIGURE 24-9. Overpenetration of a salicylic acid 30% peel can result in a level I frost. After the pseudofrost was wiped off and aloe vera was applied, the irregular white frost remains. The patient experienced 3–5 days of fine flaking or peeling.

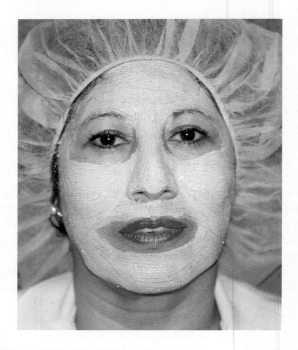

FIGURE 24-10. Resorcinal paste mask.

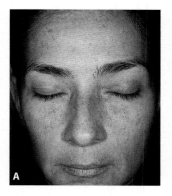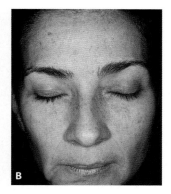

FIGURE 24-11. Superficial modified Jessner's peel. **A.** Note the solar lentigos prior to modified Jessner's peel. **B.** After one modified Jessner's peel. The solar lentigos are mildly improved, but it will take at least three more peels for the patient to note a significant difference in these pigmented lesions.

Tretinoin Peel

Tretinoin peels are non-acidic and have an intranuclear mechanism, which makes them painless. Healing consists of mild erythema or a sunburned appearance with fine desquamation on postpeel days 2 to 3. A randomized trial showed that tretinoin 0.05% cream nightly was comparable to a 5% tretinoin peel every 2 weeks.[42] The peeling solution is orange in color, preserved in brown containers, and painted on the desired treatment site. The patient is advised to wash off the solution after 4 to 6 hours of treatment. The peeling may be variable and usually begins after 2 days. Kligman et al. studied tretinoin 0.25% in a solution of 50% ethanol and 50% polyethylene glycol 400 in 50 women between 30 and 60 years of age with diagnoses of photoaging, rosacea, and acne. The solution was applied to the face by the patients every other night for 2 weeks and later, on a nightly basis. Patients showed clinical improvements as manifested by a smoother appearance of the epidermis, reduction of fine lines, and improvement of hyperpigmentation. Histologic examination of the skin revealed increased thickness of the basal layer and fibroblasts in the papillary dermis, decreased numbers of melanosomes, diminished SC thickness, and better organized rete ridges. Kligman and colleagues proposed that the effects of using low-strength tretinoin for 6 to 12 months may be achieved by higher strengths in 4 to 6 weeks.[43]

Trichloroacetic Acid Peels 10% to 35%

TCA is a caustic peeling solution that induces protein coagulation. The higher the concentration, the more acidic it is and the faster and deeper it penetrates. TCA peels are very versatile, ranging from superficial to medium to deep peels. It is incorrect to refer to the depth of the peel solely on the concentration of TCA, because higher volumes (more passes) drive the peel deeper. Low-strength TCA (10–15%) is often used, as it helps to ameliorate fine wrinkles, dyschromias such as melasma, acne scars and to provide the skin with a smooth, healthy appearance.[44] TCA is often combined with Jessner's solution for enhanced results (**Fig. 24-12**). It is also combined with microneedling for acne scarring on the same day, in either

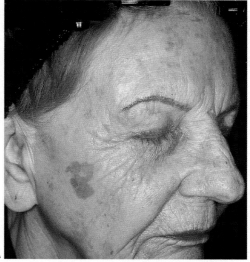

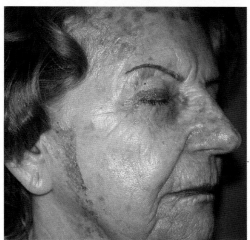

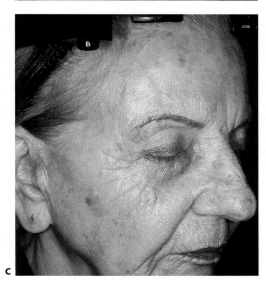

FIGURE 24-12. A. Patient with photodamage prior to one coat of a Jessner's peel followed immediately by a commercial TCA 16% peel (Accupeel 16%). **B.** Same patient 4 days later. The peeling has begun. The solar lentigo on the right cheek is much improved. **C.** Eight days later. The solar lentigo on the right cheek is beginning to reappear, which is often the case with larger lesions and only superficial depth peels.

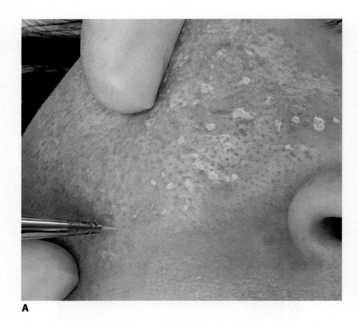

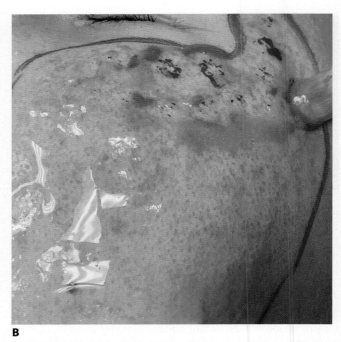

FIGURE 24-13. A. TCA 20% was applied to atrophic acne scars on the cheeks, then CROSS using carbolic acid 88% with a fine paint brush was applied inside the ice pick scars, **B.** then microneedling was performed last in a stamping pattern to achieve punctate bleeding.

order, or performed on alternating weeks (**Fig. 24-13**).[45] In a study by El-Domyati et al., 24 subjects received six biweekly treatments and demonstrated that the combined use of dermaroller and TCA 15% was more effective in post-acne atrophic scars than the use of dermaroller and PRP or dermaroller only.[46] In a study by Leheta et al., 39 subjects with post-acne atrophic scars were randomly divided into three groups; group 1 was subjected to six sessions of percutaneous collagen induction (PCI), also known as microneedling, combined with TCA 20% in the same session, group 2 was subjected to six sessions of 1540 nm fractional laser, and group 2 was subjected to combined alternating sessions of the previously mentioned two modalities. Scar severity scores improved by the highest mean of 78.27% in group 3, and were statistically significant,[47] but group 1 had about 60% improvement and group 2 62%. TCA peels are often used in combination with laser resurfacing or microneedling for acne scars (**Table 24-7**).

The currently accepted standard preparation of TCA is weight to volume (wt/vol) (**Table 24-9**). Unfortunately, not all authors use this form of measuring. One must understand how the peel strength was calculated when reading the literature to avoid underestimating the strength of the peel. This precaution reduces the risk of inducing scarring.[39] **Table 24-10** lists commonly used TCA peels on the market.

Unique to TCA is that the visual changes or frosting, represent the degree of protein coagulation. These are completely coat dependent (i.e., dependent on the number of layers applied), whereas the results with alpha-hydroxy acids are time dependent. With TCA, the physician has control over the depth of the peel based on technique and endpoints. The more coats that are used, the deeper the peel; therefore, multiple coats of

TABLE 24-9	**Standard Preparation of TCA Is Weight to Volume (wt/vol)**
TCA 50% (wt/vol) = TCA 35% (wt/wt)	
TCA 50% (wt/vol) = 50 g TCA in 100 ml water	
TCA 50% (wt/wt) = 50 g TCA in 50 g water	
wt/volume is less strong that equal % wt/wt, therefore wt/wt has higher risks of complications	

a 15% TCA can mimic the results of one or two coats of 35% TCA. The weaker strengths of trichloroacetic acid allow more time to observe the frosting changes in the skin. In addition, a wet coat where more solution is applied also goes deeper. TCA is hydrophilic, which often is evidenced by the patchy frost that develops. This can be mitigated by using topical retinoids prior to application which thins the stratum corneum and therefore allows a more even penetration of the peeling solution. This also means that if dripping occurs in the eye, safety measures of rinsing with water or saline should be readily available. TCA peels are straightforward, but what is often underemphasized, is that TCA penetrates slowly. Therefore, it is imperative to wait 3 to 6 minutes between coats.

There are three levels of frosting (**Table 24-6**) that indicate how deep the epidermal and dermal protein denaturation have occurred. For superficial peels to achieve a level I frost, only one to two thin coats should be applied so that there is minimal to no frost. A level I frost is a light reticular frost with erythema (epidermal penetration). Another important endpoint for superficial peels is called "epidermal sliding," which is seen in **Fig. 24-14** and shows exaggerated skin wrinkling

Name	Company	Strength (wt/vol)	TCA Included	How Supplied	Cost	Cost per Patient	Ease of Use	Other
TCA 30% liquid	Delasco	30%	Yes	2 oz bottle	$45	$1.50	Fast	Clear, so can drip
TCA 35% liquid	Delasco	35%	Yes	2 oz bottle	$49	$1.50	Fast	Clear, so can drip
Obagi Blue Peel	Obagi	15% 20% 22.5% 24%	No	Box of 6 kits	$740	$123	Slower and more even penetration, time consuming but more control	Blue, even coats
ZO Controlled Depth Peel	ZO	20% 26%	No	Yields 12 treatments	$300	$25	Slower and more even penetration, time consuming but more control	Blue, even coats

TABLE 24-10 Comparison of Costs and Properties of Available TCA Peels

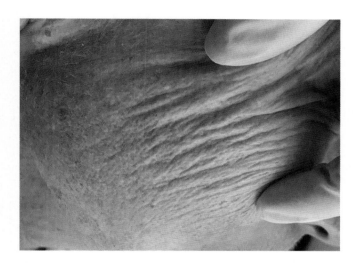

FIGURE 24-14. Exaggerated skin wrinkling when the skin in pinched is referred to as "epidermal sliding" and occurs as a result of disruption of the anchoring fibrils between the epidermis and dermis upon papillary dermis injury.

when the skin in pinched. This occurs as a result of disruption of the anchoring fibrils between the epidermis and dermis and indicates papillary dermal penetration. Level II frost (confluent white frost with background erythema) correlates with papillary dermal penetration. Superficial peels as evidenced by a level I or II frost should always see background erythema. The chest and neck should also only have a speckled frost and a pink background (level I frost); the hands and forearms can tolerate a deeper peel with a uniform frost and background erythema (level II frost). In addition, TCA > 35% should not be used on the entire face or larger areas, but rather only for focal treatment of individual lesions (such as ice pick scars) due to risks of pigmentary complications and scarring.

MEDIUM DEPTH PEELS

The three most commonly used medium depth modified TCA peels are the Jessner's solution-35% TCA peel ("Monheit

Peel"),[48] 70% glycolic acid-35% TCA peel ("Coleman Peel"),[49] and the dry ice-35% TCA peel ("Brody Peel").[50] The combination peels include a first step that is a physical or chemical agent to decrease and even out the SC by reducing the cohesion of the epidermal cells (epidermolysis), allowing enhanced penetration of the subsequent 35% TCA solution. These combination peels are effective treatments for upper dermal or epidermal pathology: photodamage, actinic keratoses (AK), lentigines, ephelides, fine rhytides, and very superficial acne scars.[48,50] The combination peels were developed to enhance safety and allow for even penetration. Medium depth peels by definition achieve a level III solid white frost with penetration to the upper reticular dermis. Medium depth peels should only be performed on the face and scalp and avoided on the body due to the limited sebaceous glands.

TCA 35% is the standard TCA used for combination medium depth peels, but a medium depth peel can be achieved with TCA 20% as well (for thin, dry or sensitive skin or for the novice peeler), to afford more control. There are five techniques to enhance the TCA peel depth: degrease with acetone, apply firm pressure when applying the peel solution, apply more volume, use higher concentrations, or use different forms of exfoliation before the peel. Thinner skin requires fewer coats and thicker skin requires more coats. Even though TCA between 35 and 50% can be a medium depth peel, it is not recommended for use due to the risk of uneven penetration, erosions, PIH, and scars. Similarly, pure phenol 88% solution (carboxylic acid) is merely a medium depth peel without the addition of croton oil but it should not be used on a full face due to the risk of cardiotoxicity and hypopigmentation.[51,52]

In a split-face comparison using one application of JS plus TCA 35% versus topical 5-flurouracil twice daily for 3 weeks, both groups achieved a 75% reduction in AKs and biopsies showed a decrease in keratinocyte atypia.[53] The sustained efficacy at 12 months was similar between the two groups as well.[54] The solid CO_2 plus TCA is histologically the deepest peel, improving wrinkles when performed to a solid white frost (level III). Unless a medium depth peel penetrates the entire papillary dermis, it cannot maximize its potential results and improve wrinkles.[50] There is unlikely to be static wrinkle effacement with a level II frost injury.

The second step for combination medium depth peels is application of TCA 35% (however, 20% can also be used with higher volumes or more passes to drive the peel deeper and achieve the same depth as TCA 35%). The strength of acid signifies the speed of penetration, and not the depth. Thin skin should have fewer wet applications or lower TCA strength. Comfort measures, such as cold air or ice compresses, may be applied at any time, as they do not neutralize the peel. After a single coat and after waiting 3 to 6 minutes for the frost to develop, one begins to see a level I frost developing, which is patchy white (non-organized speckled) with background erythema. With more coats and after waiting another 3 to 6 minutes, a level II frost will develop. This is characterized by a confluent white frost with background erythema, and correlates to penetration to the papillary dermis. Epidermal sliding is a visual clue to also confirm papillary dermal penetration. The endpoint goal of a true medium depth peel is a level III solid white frost without erythema which correlates to upper reticular dermis penetration (**Fig. 24-15**). The loss of erythema correlates with the superficial vascular plexus being obliterated by protein coagulation. Pay attention to the areas that have correctly achieved endpoint frost so as to not reapply TCA to those areas when they begin to defrost. The frost should "defrost" over 20 minutes. A persistent frost over 20 minutes can signify overpenetration and risk of persistent erythema and scarring.

The scalp, which is often peeled for actinic keratoses, however, should only achieve a level II frost as alopecia or a thin skin can predispose to scarring. Other important bony prominences prone to scarring include the zygomatic arch and mandible. Although by definition, a level III frost is the endpoint goal for medium depth peels, one will often achieve areas with a level II frost in riskier areas (e.g., thin skin, balding scalps, and bony prominences). **Table 24-11** differentiates the common medium depth peels.

BLUE TCA PEELS

The Obagi Blue Peel™ and the ZO Controlled Depth Peel™ are modified TCA peels designed to peel between the papillary dermis to the most superficial aspect of the reticular dermis. They both contain glycerin, saponins, and a blue dye color which helps to ensure a more uniform application. Instead of the conventional clear coat, a color sensitive reaction indicates the amount of peel applied, thus ensuring a more uniform application. In addition, saponins decelerate the peel to provide greater control over the depth of penetration. The saponin is an emulsifying agent allowing for more even and slow penetration, and is less patchy than the conventional clear TCA solutions. These peels are safer because the saponins allows for more controlled penetration of TCA.[55] These commercial blue peels are therefore good options for neck, chest, or hand peeling (**Fig. 24-17**).

HEALING STAGES IN MEDIUM DEPTH PEELS

A solid white frost without erythema to the upper reticular dermis results in 10 days of peeling and up to 3 weeks of healing. Papillary dermal peels (solid frost with erythema) will take 7 days to heal.[54] There should be no pain or discomfort after 24 hours. Peak edema is expected at 24–48 hours. Edema results in the skin having a "greyish" discoloration, superimposed on the brown darkening (**Fig. 24-18**). Edema can be minimized by sleeping with the head elevated and icing the face for 10 minutes per hour for the first 24 hours.[54] The grey-brown skin discoloration progressively darkens and tightens. After 48 hours, the grey-brown discoloration becomes red-brown as the edema resolves. Peak erythema is seen on post-peel days 3 and 4 as the pre-existing brown spots on the face darken. Lastly, the cracked pottery appearance of skin peeling off in sheets begins from areas of movement (around the mouth) extending centrifugally between postpeel days 4 and 10 (**Fig. 24-19**).

DEEP DEPTH PEELS

Phenol-croton oil peels have been used since the 1920s in Europe by the non-medical community. In 1960, Brown published on the formulas of lay-peeler, noting that phenol was an active ingredient. In 1961, Baker published a reproducible formula that popularized the peel; however, in 1962 he modified the formula with dramatic consequences. He decreased the phenol and water quantity because he did not want too much solution, but he left the three drops of croton oil unchanged. This increased the croton oil strength from 1.2% to 2.1%. The Baker peel was excellent for deep rhytides but had common risks of hypopigmentation, scars, prolonged erythema, and long healing times, not to mention

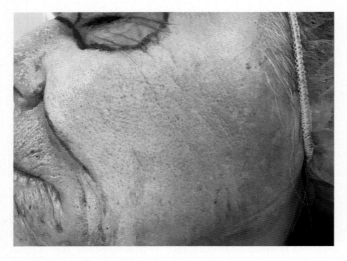

FIGURE 24-15. Monheit peel performed with Jessner's Solution and then TCA 35% until Level III solid white frost without erythema endpoint achieved for medium depth chemical peel to the upper reticular dermis.

TABLE 24-11	Medium Depth Peels	
Agent	Procedure	Comments
Solid CO2 and 35% TCA (Brody)	Buy a block of dry ice (CO2) at a local supermarket, and break a small piece so you can hold it with a towel. Degrease the skin, dip the ice in a 3:1 solution of acetone to alcohol to decrease friction on the skin, and apply it to the skin with mild pressure (3–5 sec), moderate pressure (5–8 sec), or hard pressure (8–15 sec). The endpoint is congelation **Fig. 24-16**. For best technique, the skin should be stretched taut, and the dry ice rubbed as follows: hard pressure for deeper rhytides, rims of acne scars, static rhytides or keratoses; less pressure to the scar-prone bony prominences, such as the zygomatic arch and mandible. The skin is wiped dry and then 35% TCA is applied with 5 minutes between coats. Dr. Brody recommends applying TCA in this order: eyelids, nose, cheeks perioral, then forehead. Then apply ice packs for 2-5 minutes, then ointment.	- Advantage: strongest combination (when dry ice is applied with pressure for 12–15 seconds) and more effective for acne scarring or thicker epidermal lesions - disadvantage is difficulty storing CO2, inconvenience of going to grocery store to pick up CO2, and learning the technique-dependent congelation endpoints.
Jessner's and 35% TCA (Monheit)	After degreasing vigorously with acetone, Jessner's solution is applied with 2×2 gauze, applying several coats until an even speckled white frost with erythema develops. Wait 6 minutes, then apply TCA 35% is applied with gauze or CTA's waiting 3-6 minutes between coats, similar to Brody's peel. Set-up seen in **Fig. 24-3**.	- Most popular combination because of ease of application of Jessner's solution - Jessners is lipophilic unlike glycolic acid, and preferred for oily skin or acne
70% Glycolic acid and 35% TCA (Coleman)	Wash face with gentle soap, but no further degreasing. 70% unbuffered glycolic acid is applied with large cotton swab or 2×2 inch gauze and left on the skin for 2 minutes contact time, unless severe burning or erythema ensues before this timed endpoint. Then the skin is rinsed with water or 10% sodium. Bicarbonate until all burning has subsided and all glycolic has been removed from the skin. 35% TCA is then applied same as above.	- Effective combination with more neoelastogenesis than Jessner's and 35% TCA[62] - disadvantages is that glycolic acid may have more absorption in inflamed or abraded areas of the skin and neutralization is needed.
CROSS Using 88% Phenol (carbolic acid) or TCA 50–90%	Using a toothpick, a sharpened wooden applicator or a fine tip paint brush, the applicator is placed in a small cup containing carbolic acid 88% or TCA. Stretch out the ice pick or box scars, and carefully apply the solution into the scar avoiding spillage outside the scar itself, also known as shouldering. Apply until a solid white frost is seen (Fig. 24-13A). At least 5 sessions are needed every 2–6 weeks to achieve clinical improvement.	- Carbolic acid has less adverse reactions than TCA 90% while being as effective[67] - safe in darker skin types, with manageable PIH

risks of cardiotoxicity. It wasn't until 2000 that Hetter published four comprehensive studies that evaluated the ingredients and strengths and their effects, proving that croton oil was the active ingredient. He named his new formulas the Hetter Heresy Formulas, having croton oil ranges from 0.1 to 1.1%.[56] Stone also published studies that showed histological depth of injury based on numerous factors including technique and number of passes with multiple different formulations, including the "lay-peelers" formulas.[58] The standard phenol-croton oil peels used today and since the year 2000, are known as Hetter's formulas.[53] However, there are many formulas (**Table 24-12**) that have existed since the 1920s and have been used safely by the "lay-peelers," some of which are still used by expert peelers around the world today.[57]

Ingredients

Croton oil (CO) is the active ingredient and determines the depth of penetration. CO is an oil extracted from the seed of the Croton tiglium plant. It is insoluble in water and highly

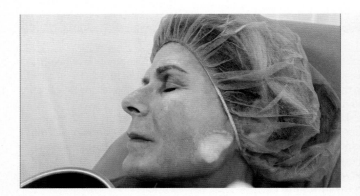

FIGURE 24-16. White congelation (or thickening from freezing) is the endpoint for dry ice (solid CO₂) part of the Brody medium depth peel.

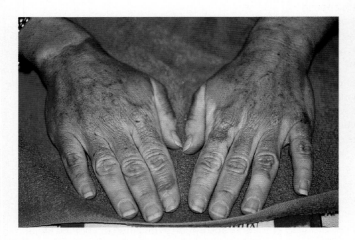

FIGURE 24-17. Obagi Blue Peel applied to hands. Advantages of the ZO or Obagi modified TCA peels that include the blue dyes, are that they also include saponins which emulsify the acid and allow for more even and less patchy penetration of the TCA, at a slower rate, therefore, allowing more control and safety to easily see where the solution is based on the blue color.

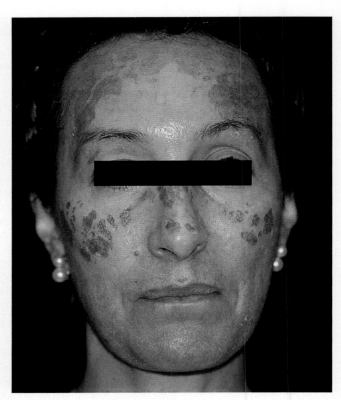

FIGURE 24-18. Patient 4 days after four coats of the Obagi Blue Peel. Patient should be told not to peel off the dark skin, but to let it peel naturally. The dark brown peeling in sheets is characteristic of TCA peels past the papillary dermis.

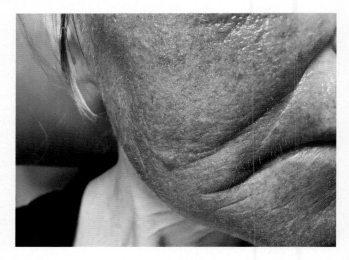

FIGURE 24-19. At 24 hours after hard pressure dry ice and TCA 35% (Brody peel), peak edema and classic grey-brown darkening of skin are seen in a medium depth peel. Edema imparts a grey color. Therefore, grey-brown discoloration with edema is seen for 2 days, and then becomes red-brown upon resolution of edema.

soluble in alcohol and phenol. CO > 2% is associated with hypopigmentation. Varying the concentration of croton oil in phenol enables tailoring of appropriate formulas to the degree of sun damage requiring treatment. Light croton oils such as 0.1% are used in thin skin around the eyes. Stronger concentrations such as 1.1% are used for lip lines.[53] Phenol (also known as carbolic acid or hydroxybenzene) 88–89% is hydrophobic. It is melanotoxic, antiseptic, cytotoxic, and analgesic. It disrupts sulfide bonds and induces protein coagulation. A full strength, unoccluded 88% phenol peel gives a result comparable to any medium depth peel. Septisol (also known as hexachlorophene) is an antiseptic with surfactant properties (basically a soap or detergent) to reduce the surface tension. Reducing the surface tension promotes emulsification of the oil in water solution, allowing for more uniform and deeper penetration.[59] Septisol is no longer being manufactured, therefore there are current studies examining other soaps and emulsifiers such as Chlorhexidine and Novisol (PEG-80 Sorbitan Laurate).[60] Humectants are also alternatives to detergents such as glycerin or olive oil, which are found in popularized "lay-peeler" formulas by Grade, Stone, and Exoderm™. Olive and sesame oil slow the cutaneous absorption rate to reduce toxicity, whereas glycerin keeps water in solution to prevent evaporation. **Fig. 24-20** shows the clear pure phenol (a clear

TABLE 24-12

Formula Name	Croton Oil	Phenol USP 88%	Water	Septisol*	Glycerin	Olive Oil
Stone Venner-Kellson	3 drops (0.16%)	60 ml (62.5%)	8 ml	None	None	5 ml
Stone II	12 drops (0.2%)	159 ml (60%)	73.5 ml	None	None	3 drops
Grade II	12 drops (0.2%)	159 ml (60%)	73.5 ml	None	None	3 drops
Hetter Heresy Very Light 1996	3 ml of 0.35% (0.10%)	2 ml (27.5%)	5 cc	0 drops	None	None
Hetter Heresy Medium Light	1 drop (0.35%0	4 cc (33%)	6 cc	16 drops	None	None
Hetter Heresy Heavy	3 drops (1.1%)	4 cc (33%)	6 cc	16 drops	None	None
Hetter Heresy Medium Heavy	2 drops (0.7%)	4 cc (33%)	6 cc	16 drops	None	None
Bakers (classic) 1962	3 drops (2.08%)	3 cc (49.25%)	2 cc	8 drops	None	None
Bakers 1961	3 drops (1.2%)	5 cc (47.48%)	4 cc	5 drops	None	None

*Septisol is no longer commercially available.

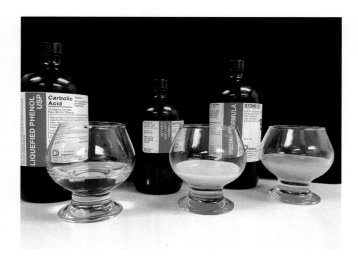

FIGURE 24-20. Solutions from Delasco, showing the difference in appearance, where the pure phenol 88% solution is clear on the left, Hetter's solution has a milky white color in the center from the septisol, and the Stone Formula has an orange-brown discoloration on the right from the glycerin and olive oil.

TABLE 24-13

Medium Peel Histology	Deep Peel Histology
- Thickened neocollagen bundles in dermis and a Grenz zone overlying a reticular elastotic band[62] - Coleman's Peel produced greater neoelastogenesis than Monheit's Peel[63] - Phenol 35% alone shows minimal neocollagensis after a medium depth lyphocytic infiltrate[64]	- Dense dermal neocollagenesis zone(61) - Pig model, an average of 600 µm (0.6 mm) band of neocollagenesis with an unoccluded 1.6% Hetter Peel in 2020 after band of neutrophils (Fig. 24-21B)[64]

solution) beside the milky white Hetter's phenol-croton oil mixtures (center) in contrast to the orange-tinged Stone formulas that do not have emulsifying detergents (right).

Histology

Kligman et al. evaluated the long-term histologic effects of deep peels and found changes resulted in a wide band of healthy dermis sharply demarcated from the deeper, untreated sun-damaged dermis. Changes consisted of a parallel arrangement of collagen and elastic fibers and persisted for 15 to 20 years.[6] Histological studies consistently show a dense dermal zone of neocollagenesis (**Table 24-13**).[61–64] More recent histological studies in a porcine model showed an average thickness of 600 µm (0.6 mm) band of neocollagenesis with an unoccluded 1.6% Hetter's peel at 21 days (Fig. 24-21). The authors postulated that the phorbol esters in croton oil have

a direct effect inducing neutrophilic inflammation (pus-like appearance during healing) which leads to the increased neocollagenesis when compared to the 35% phenol alone vehicle without CO.[65]

At 3-month follow-up, the neocollagenesis zone measured 350 µm in occluded Baker-Gordon peels compared with 260 µm without occlusion and 150–200 µm with CO_2 lasers.[65,66] The clearance of deep solar elastosis with phenol-croton oil peels is unmatched.

FOCAL DEEP PEELS

Focal deep peels are best used for AKs, lentigines, and acne scars. The pathology for AKs and lentigines is in the basal layer of the skin. Therefore, to effectively treat this, the peel must reach the papillary dermis. The endpoint would be a solid white frost with or without erythema. Any strength of the phenol-croton oil solutions can be applied focally, depending on the thickness of the skin. The author frequently uses this in-office procedure for AK of the face due to ease of application, less pain and hypopigmentation when compared with cryotherapy, and more effectiveness for sensitive areas such as the nose and periorbitally. Atrophic acne scars, including ice

A

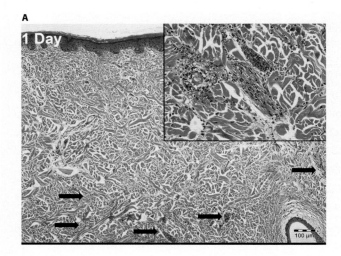

B

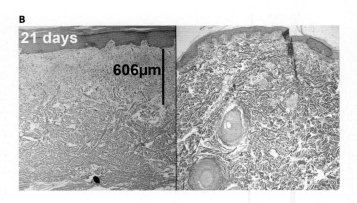

FIGURE 24-21. Courtesy of Dr. Carlos Wambier, MD, PhD, Alpert Medical School of Brown University, RI and Prof. Flavio Beltrame, PharmD, PhD – State University of Ponta Grossa, Brazil. **A.** 1st post-operative day of 1.6% Croton oil in 35% phenol (Hetter's very heavy peel): edema and deep coagulative necrosis with vascular ectasia and intense pericoagulative neutrophilic inflammatory band (black arrows), inset. Hematoxylin-eosin x100, inset x 400. **B.** 21st post-operative day, neocollagenesis (type III collagen, stained in blue) was only evident in samples of 1.6% croton oil in 35% phenol. 35% phenol showed minimal neocollagenesis, similar to a superficial to medium-depth chemical peel. Herovici stain, x 20.[65]

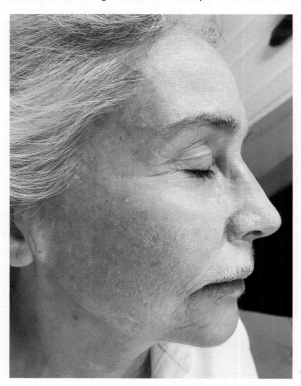

FIGURE 24-22. The patient was peeled with a perioral segmental deep phenol peel using the Rullan Rormula (phenol 35%, CO 0.7%) without occlusion and a medium depth Monheit peel on the rest of the face until a level III frost was achieved. Some defrosting has occurred in the photo therefore frost of face appears to be almost a level II frost and the upper lip is a solid grey white frost.

pick and box scars, are treated focally with either high concentration TCA or pure phenol, known as carboxylic acid 88%, with CROSS (Chemical Reconstitution Of Skin Scars). Both acids are effective, although more severe adverse reactions have been reported in those treated by TCA, such as depigmentation and widening of scars.[67,68]

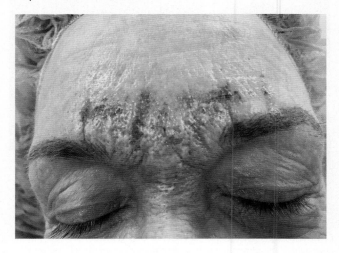

FIGURE 24-23. Focal deep 1.1% CO/phenol 33% peel to Glougau IV deep rhytides and solar elastosis of the glabellar showing adequate delayed endpoints of grey cast from dermal edema as frost defrosts and red-brown overtones known as epidermolysis in deep rhytides.

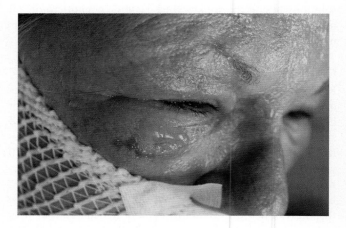

FIGURE 24-24. Honey crusting with significant edema and exudate is the ideal endpoint at 24 hours for deep peels. The honey crusting should be gently debrided with hydrogen peroxide daily to promote healing.

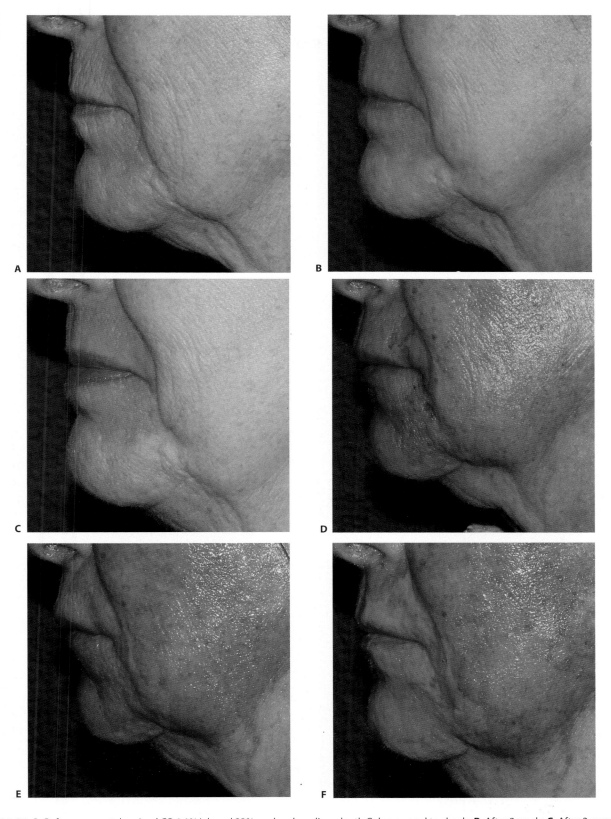

FIGURE 24-25. A. Before segmental perioral CO 1.1%/phenol 33% peel and medium depth Coleman peel to cheeks **B.** After 2 weeks **C.** After 3 months **D.** 24 hours: perioral (deep) brownish erosions and honey crusting (epidermolysis) with significant edema; cheek (medium) grey-brown darkening with edema **E.** 48 hours: perioral yellow green purulent coagulum (necrotic epidermis and papillary dermis with neutrophils); cheeks gray-brown darkening, prexisting brown darkening **F.** postpeel day 3: perioral peak creamy yellow color of purulent coagulum; cheek red-brown darkening with early sloughing

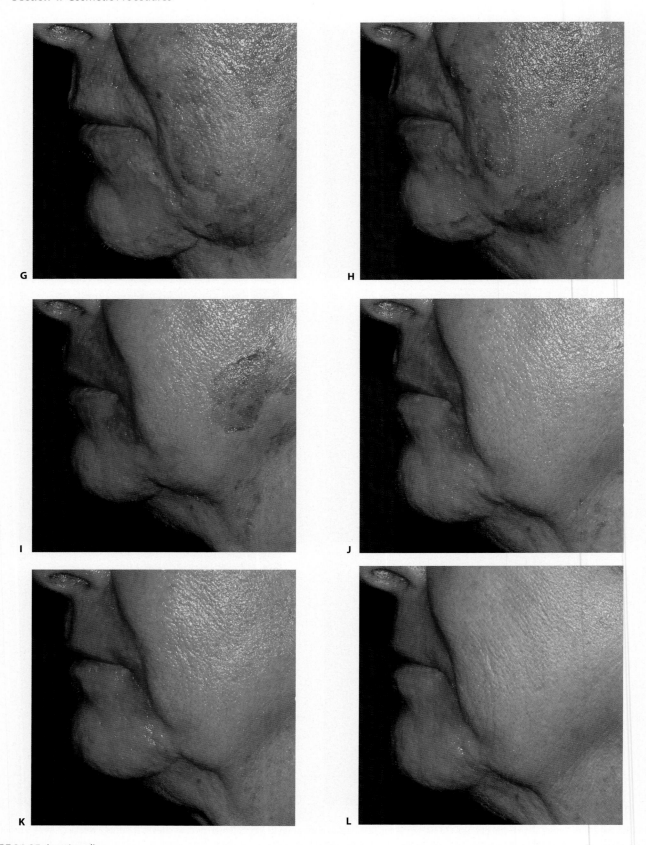

FIGURE 24-25. (*continued*)
G. postpeel day 4 **H.** postpeel day 5 **I.** postpeel day 6: perioral coagulum resolving, peak erythema; cheeks reepithelialized and peeling in brown sheets like cracked pottery **J.** postpeel day 7: perioral erythema; cheek faint pink healed, medium depth healed as is usual **K.** postpeel day 8: perioral deep almost completely re-epithelized except for marionette line **L.** postpeel day 9: perioral deep 99% re-epitheliazed as expected, residual erythema expected to last 1–3 months.

CROSS was first described by Lee et al. in 2002 using a sharp wooden-tipped applicator with TCA 65% or 100%, even in darker skin types IV–V.[67] In 2007, Lee et al. changed the applicator to a 1 ml syringe filled with 0.1–0.2 ml with a 31 G needle. The downtime for makeup or creams is about 5 days or until the crusts fall off. TCA 50% is usually the strongest strength for darker skin types. Darker skin types should also reinitiate hydroquinone as soon as the crusts fall off.

Atrophic acne scars can also be treated with a "chemabrasion" technique which is a chemical injury followed by abrasion. When one combines a physical injury and a deep peel, the results are even greater. Chemabrasion was introduced by Fintsi as a procedure that includes occlusion for 24 hours, debridement and then reapplication of phenol/CO on the second day.[69,70] There has since been further modifications and changes in techniques published by Rullan et al.[71] Chemabrasion has been shown to be more effective than dermabrasion or a deep chemical peel alone.[69–71]

SEGMENTAL DEEP PEELS

For many dermatologists, doing a full-face phenol is not an option due to the need for cardiac monitoring, sedation and analgesia. However, performing a segmental deep peel and an ablative laser or medium depth peel to the rest of the face is a real option. A segmental peel uses different peeling agents on different cosmetic units to tailor the wounding agent to the degree of photodamage. Not uncommonly, the perioral or the periorbital area exhibits Glogau III or IV wrinkles while the remainder of the face exhibits only mild sun damage and can be peeled with a medium depth peel (**Fig. 24-22** and **Fig. 24-25**) or an ablative laser. When combining modalities, the medium depth peel is performed first, or if combined with an ablative resurfacing laser, it would be used second after the peel is finished and fully dry (overlapping the laser by 1 cm over the peel to feather results).[72] When you apply phenol to less than 2% body surface area (which correlates to one to two cosmetic subunits), cardiac monitoring is not necessary. Full face phenol peels need cardiac monitoring since there exists a 7% change of transient cardiac arrhythmias, which tend to occur more often in patients taking QT-prolonging medications (e.g., antidepressants, narcotics) or with inadequate pain control.[64,72,73] Such deep peels must also be applied at a rate of 10–15 minutes per cosmetic unit with good hydration.

Healing Stages

The phenol/CO peel endpoints are seen in **Table 24-6**. Whatever technique or concentration is used, one must always judge the depth of the peel by the visual clues and frost described. The three main frosts include a pink white frost (papillary dermis), a solid white frost (upper reticular dermis), and then after multiple rubbings with pressure and the skin stretched taut, a more solid, dense, even opaque grey-white frost develops which indicates reaching the upper to mid-reticular dermis (**Fig. 24-22**). Thin skin around the eyes or temples, should be peeled less deeply to the papillary

dermis, whereas thick skin on the vermillion border, should be peeled to the grey-white frost using higher concentrations of croton oil. Without further peeling, the frost is gradually lost in about 15–20 minutes, and during that time, two delayed endpoints will appear. First occurs the grey-cast due to dermal edema which is seen around 5 to 10 minutes (Fig. 24-23). Another delayed endpoint of red-brown crusts or vesicles, called epidermolysis should be appreciated to confirm adequate depth penetration to the mid-reticular dermis (Fig. 24-23).[74] Honey crusting with substantial edema and exudate is the ideal endpoint at 24 hours for deep peels (Fig. 24-24). The honey crusting should be gently debrided with hydrogen peroxide daily to promote healing.[71,72] Refer to **Fig. 24-25 A–K** for stages of healing of perioral deep peels and medium depth cheek peels.

CONCLUSION

Superficial and medium depth peels are dynamic tools when used as part of office procedures for the treatment of acne, pigmentary disorders, and photoaging. They should be used in combination with sun avoidance, sunscreen, retinoids, and home care products to achieve maximum efficacy. Phenol-croton oil peeling effects have greater longevity than many other resurfacing procedures.[65,66] The improved safety profile of phenol-croton oil peels has launched new momentum in chemical peeling with significant wrinkle improvement, skin tightening, and natural results without the "alabaster white" depigmentation associated with the classical Baker-Gordon peel. The "Phenol-Croton Oil" peel is the most effective modality for facial resurfacing because it has the greatest ability to correct deep wrinkles and provide long term tightening of the skin. Unfortunately, deep peels are limited in use because of inadequate training in dermatology residency programs. Supervised hands-on training is irreplaceable, either in training programs or in continuing medical education. The International Peeling Society offers several workshops annually. The cost-effectiveness of medium and deep chemical peeling is unmatched when compared with other resurfacing methods. Successful outcomes in all chemical peels depend on a balance of art and technique, patient education, and safety standards.

References

1. Brody HJ, Monheit GD, Resnik SS, Alt TH. A history of chemical peeling. *Dermatol Surg.* 2000;26:405–409.

2. Brody HJ. *Chemical Peeling and Resurfacing.* 2nd ed. St. Louis, Missouri: Mosby-Year Book, Inc.; 1997.

3. Rubin MG. What are skin peels? In: *Manual of Chemical Peels: Superficial and Medium Depth.* Philadelphia, PA: Lippincott Williams & Wilkins; 1995:19–20.

4. Fabbrocini G, Padova M, Tosti A. Superficial to Medium-Depth Peels: A Personal Experience. In: Tung R, Rubin M, eds. *Procedures in Cosmetic Dermatology Series: Chemical Peels.* 2nd ed. London: Elsevier Health Sciences; 2010: 123–129.

5. Deprez P. *Textbook of Chemical Peels: Superficial, Medium and Deep Peels in Cosmetic Practice.* 2nd ed. CRC Press; 2017: 29–44.

6. Kligman AM, Baker TJ, Gordon HL. Long-term histologic follow-up of phenol face peels. *Plast Reconstr Surg.* 1985;75:652–659.

7. Silpa-archa N, Kohli I, Chaowattanapanit S, Lim HW, Hamzavi I. Postinflammatory hyperpigmentation: a comprehensive overview. *J Am Acad Dermatol.* 2017;77:591–605.

8. Lee KC, Wambier CG, Soon SL, et al; International Peeling Society. Basic chemical peeling: Superficial and medium-depth peels. *J Am Acad Dermatol.* 2019 Aug;81(2):313–324.

9. Hevia O, Nemeth AJ, Taylor JR. Tretinoin accelerates healing after trichloroacetic acid chemical peel. *Arch Dermatol.* 1991;127:678–682.

10. Maloney BP, Millman B, Monheit G, et al. The etiology of prolonged erythema after chemical peel. *Dermatol Surg.* 1998;24:337–341.

11. Rullan PP, Karam AM. *Rejuvenation of the Aging Face; Chemical peels for the aging faces of all skin types.* Amir Karam, Mitchel Goldman, eds. London: JP Medical LTD; 2015: 81–82.

12. Berardesca E, Distante F, Vignoli GP, et al. Alpha hydroxyacids modulate stratum corneum barrier function. *Br J Dermatol.* 1997;137:934.

13. Van Scott EJ, Yu RJ. Control of keratinization with alpha-hydroxy acids and related compounds. I. Topical treatment of ichthyotic disorders. *Arch Dermatol.* 1974;110:586.

14. Yu R, Van Scott E. Bioavailability of alpha-hydroxyacids in topical formulations. *Cosmet Dermatol.* 1996;9:54.

15. Ahn HH, Kim IH. Whitening effect of salicylic acid peels in Asian patients. *Dermatol Surg.* 2006;32:372.

16. Davies M, Marks R. Studies on the effect of salicylic acid on normal skin. *Br J Dermatol.* 1976;95:187.

17. Fabbrocini G, Padova M, Tosti A. Superficial to Medium-Depth Peels: A Personal Experience. In: Tung R, Rubin M, eds. *Procedures in Cosmetic Dermatology Series: Chemical Peels.* 2nd ed. London: Elsevier Health Sciences; 2010: 7–16.

18. Ditre CM, Griffin TD, Murphy GF, et al. Effects of alpha-hydroxy acids on photoaged skin: a pilot clinical, histologic, and ultrastructural study. *J Am Acad Dermatol.* 1996;34:187.

19. Kim SJ, Park JH, Kim DH, et al. Increased in vivo collagen synthesis and in vitro cell proliferative effect of glycolic acid. *Dermatol Surg.* 1998;24:1054.

20. Sharad J. Combination of microneedling and glycolic acid peels for the treatment of acne scars in dark skin. *J Cosmet Dermatol.* 2011 Dec;10(4):317–23.

21. Cotellessa C, Manunta T, Ghersetich I, et al. The use of pyruvic acid in the treatment of acne. *J Eur Acad Dermatol Venereol.* 2004;18:275.

22. Ghersetich I, Brazzini B, Peris K, et al. Pyruvic acid peels for the treatment of photoaging. *Dermatol Surg.* 2004;30:32.

23. Caperton C, Valencia O, Romanelli P, Fulton J. Pyruvic acid facilitates the removal of actinic keratoses and seborrheic keratoses. *Dermatol Surg.* 2012 Oct;38(10):1710–5.

24. Griffin TD, Van Scott EJ. Use of pyruvic acid in the treatment of actinic keratoses: a clinical and histopathologic study. *Cutis.* 1991;47:325.

25. Shahmoradi Z, Assaf F, Al Said H, Khosravani P, Hosseini SM. Topical pyruvic acid (70%) versus topical salicylic acid (16.7%) compound in treatment of plantar warts: A randomized controlled trial. *Adv Biomed Res.* 2015;4:113.

26. Halasz CL. Treatment of warts with topical pyruvic acid: with and without added 5-fluorouracil. *Cutis.* 1998;62:283.

27. Milstein E. Is pyruvic acid potentially explosive? *Schoch Lett.* 1990;40:41.

28. Wehr R, Krochmal L, Bagatell F, et al. Controlled two-center study of lactate 12 percent lotion and a petrolatum-based cream in patients with xerosis. *Cutis.* 1986;37:205.

29. Usuki A, Ohashi A, Sato H, Ochiai Y, Ichihashi M, Funasaka Y. The inhibitory effect of glycolic acid and lactic acid on melanin synthesis in melanoma cells. *Exp Dermatol.* 2003;12(Suppl 2):43–50. doi:10.1034/j.1600-0625.12.s2.7.x. PMID: 14756523.

30. Sharquie KE, Al-Dhalimi MA, Noaimi AA, Al-Sultany HA. Lactic Acid as a new therapeutic peeling agent in the treatment of lifa disease (frictional dermal melanosis). *Indian J Dermatol.* 2012;57(6):444–448.

31. Sharquie KE, Al-Tikreety MM, Al-Mashhadani SA. Lactic acid as a new therapeutic peeling agent in melasma. *Dermatol Surg.* 2005 Feb;31(2):149–54.

32. Dayal S, Sahu P, Jain VK, Khetri S. Clinical efficacy and safety of 20% glycolic peel, 15% lactic peel, and topical 20% vitamin C in constitutional type of periorbital melanosis: a comparative study. *J Cosmet Dermatol.* 2016 Dec;15(4):367–373.

33. Dainichi T, Ueda S, Imayama S, Furue M. Excellent clinical results with a new preparation for chemical peeling in acne: 30% salicylic acid in polyethylene glycol vehicle. *Dermatol Surg.* 2008;34:891–899.

34. Brubacher JR, Hoffman RS. Salicylism from topical salicylates: review of the literature. *J Toxicol Clin Toxicol.* 1996;34:431.

35. Unna PG. Therapeutiques generales des maladies de la peau. 1882.

36. Deprez P. *Textbook of Chemical Peels: Superficial, Medium and Deep Peels in Cosmetic Practice.* 2nd ed. CRC Press; 2017: 211.

37. Karam PG. 50% resorcinol peel. *Int J Dermatol.* 1993;32:569.

38. Rubin MG. Jessner's peels. In: *Manual of Chemical Peels: Superficial and Medium Depth.* Philadelphia, PA: Lippincott Williams & Wilkins; 1995:88.

39. Bridenstine JB, Dolezal JF. Standardizing chemical peel solution formulations to avoid mishaps. Great fluctuations in actual concentrations of trichloroacetic acid. *J Dermatol Surg Oncol.* 1994;20:813.

40. Safoury OS, Zaki NM, El Nabarawy EA, Farag EA. A study comparing chemical peeling using modified Jessner's solution and 15% trichloroacetic Acid versus 15% trichloroacetic acid in the treatment of melasma. *Indian J Dermatol.* 2009;54(1):41–45.

41. Abdel-Meguid A.M., Taha E.A., Ismail S.A. Combined Jessner solution and trichloroacetic acid versus trichloroacetic acid alone in the treatment of melasma in dark-skinned patients. *Dermatol Surg.* 2017; 43: 651–656.

42. Sumita J, Soares J, Tannus F, Miot H, Bagatin E. Tretinoin 5% peeling versus 0.05% cream for advanced photoaging of the forearms: an open, randomized, evaluator-blinded and comparative study. *J Am Acad Dermatol.* 2017;76(6 suppl 1):AB269.

43. Kligman DE, Sadiq I, Pagnoni A, et al. High-strength tretinoin: a method for rapid retinization of facial skin. *J Am Acad Dermatol.* 1998;39:S93.

44. Dinner MI, Artz JS. The art of the trichloroacetic acid chemical peel. *Clin Plast Surg.* 1998;25:53.

45. Sharad, J. Treatment of Acne Scars with a Combination of Chemical Peels and Microneedling, in Procedures in Cosmetic

Dermatology Chemical Peels 3rd ed, edited by Obagi, S. St. Louis, Elsevier, 2021 p 137–143.

46. El-Domyati M, Abdel-Wahab H, Hossam A. Microneedling combined with platelet-rich plasma or trichloroacetic acid peeling for management of acne scarring: A split-face clinical and histologic comparison. *J Cosmet Dermatol.* 2018 Feb;17(1):73–83.

47. Leheta TM, Abdel Hay RM, El Garem YF. Deep peeling using phenol versus percutaneous collagen induction combined with trichloroacetic acid 20% in atrophic post-acne scars; a randomized controlled trial. *J Dermatolog Treat.* 2014;25: 130–136.

48. Monheit GD. Medium-depth chemical peels. *Dermatol Clin.* 2001;19:413.

49. Coleman WP III, Futrell JM. The glycolic acid trichloroacetic acid peel. *J Dermatol Surg Oncol.* 1994;20:76.

50. Brody HJ. *Chemical Peeling and Resurfacing.* St. Louis, MO: Mosby; 1997:109–110.

51. Hetter GP. An examination of the phenol-croton oil peel: part I. Dissecting the formula. *Plast Reconstr Surg.* 2000;105:227–239.

52. Hetter GP. An examination of the phenol-croton oil peel: part IV. Face peel results with different concentrations of phenol and croton oil. *Plast Reconstr Surg.* 2000;105:1061–1083.

53. Lawrence N, Cox SE, Cockerell CJ, Freeman RG, Cruz PD Jr. A comparison of the efficacy and safety of Jessner's solution and 35% trichloroacetic acid vs 5% fluorouracil in the treatment of widespread facial actinic keratoses. *Arch Dermatol.* 1995;131: 176–181.

54. Witheiler DD, Lawrence N, Cox SE, Cruz C, Cockerell CJ, Freemen RG. Long-term efficacy and safety of Jessner's solution and 35% trichloroacetic acid vs 5% fluorouracil in the treatment of widespread facial actinic keratoses. *Dermatol Surg.* 1997;23:191–196.

55. Obagi S. Medium-Depth Peels and TCA Blue Peel, in *Procedures in Cosmetic Dermatology Chemical Peels* 3rd ed. Obagi, S. St. Louis ed. Elsevier; 2021: 52–63

56. Hetter GP. An examination of the phenol-croton oil peel: part III. The plastic surgeons' role. *Plast Reconstr Surg.* 2000;105: 752–763.

57. Stone PA. The use of modified phenol chemical face peels: recognizing the role of application technique. *Clin Plast Surg.* 2001;28:13–36.

58. Larson DL, Karmo F, Hetter GP. Phenol-croton oil peel: establishing an animal model for scientific investigation. *Aesthet Surg J.* 2009 Jan–Feb;29(1):47–53.

59. Justo ADS, Lemes BM, Nunes B, et al. Depth of injury of Hetter's phenol-croton oil chemical peel formula using 2 different emulsifying agents. *J Am Acad Dermatol.* 2020 Jun;82(6):1544–1546.

60. Behin F, Feuerstein SS, Marovitz WF. Comparative histological study of mini pig skin after chemical peel and dermabrasion. *Arch Otolaryngol.* 1977;103:271–277.

61. Coleman WP 3rd, Futrell JM. The glycolic acid trichloroacetic acid peel. *J Dermatol Surg Oncol.* 1994; 20: 76–80

62. Tse Y, Ostad A, Lee HS, et al. A clinical and histologic evaluation of two medium-depth peels. Glycolic acid versus Jessner's trichloroacetic acid. *Dermatol Surg.* 1996;22:781–786

63. Wambier CG, Lee KC, Soon SL, et al. Advanced chemical peels: phenol-croton oil peel. *J Am Acad Dermatol.* 2019;81(2): 327–336.

64. Justo AS, Lemes BM, Nunes B, et al. Characterization of the activity of Croton tiglium oil in Hetter's very heavy phenol-croton oil chemical peels. *Dermatol Surg.* 2020;in press.

65. Moy LS, Kotler R, Lesser T. The histologic evaluation of pulsed carbon dioxide laser resurfacing versus phenol chemical peels in vivo. *Dermatol Surg.* 1999;25:597–600.

66. Lee JB, Chung WG, Kwahck H, Lee KH. Focal treatment of acne scars with trichloroacetic acid: Chemical reconstruction of skin scars method. *Dermatol Surg.* 2002;28:1017–21.

67. Dalpizzol M, Weber MB, Mattiazzi AP, et al. Comparative study of the use of trichloroacetic acid and phenolic acid in the treatment of atrophic-type acne scars. *Dermatol Surg.* 2016;42:377–383.

68. Fintsi Y. Exoderma novel, phenol-based peeling method resulting in improved safety. *Int J Cosmet Surg.* 2001a;1:40–44.

69. Fintsi Y. Exoderm chemoabrasion original method for the treatment of facial acne scars. *Int J Cosmet Surg.* 2001b;1:45–52.

70. Rullan PP, Lemon J, Rullan J. The 2-day light phenol chemabrasion for deep wrinkles and acne scars: a presentation of face and neck peels. *Am J Cosm Surg.* 2004;21:199–210.

71. Lee KC, Sterling JB, Wambier CG, et al. Segmental phenolecroton oil chemical peels for treatment of periorbital or perioral rhytides. *J Am Acad Dermatol.* 2019;81(6):e165–e166.

72. Wambier CG, Wambier SPDF, Pilatti LEP, et al. Prolongation of rate-corrected QT interval during phenol-croton oil peels. *J Am Acad Dermatol.* 2018;78:810–812.

73. Landau M. Cardiac complications in deep chemical peels. *Dermatol Surg.* 2007;33:190–193.

74. Bensimon R. Croton Oil Peels. *Aesthe Surg J.* 2008;28:33–45.

CHAPTER 25

Dermal Fillers

Kerry Heitmiller, MD
Nazanin Saedi, MD

SUMMARY POINTS

1. The dermal filler market is rapidly growing worldwide, and several innovations have led to a parallel expansion in product variety.
2. Currently, a variety of dermal fillers are available for use including temporary fillers (i.e., hyaluronic acid fillers), semi-permanent fillers (i.e., calcium hydroxylapatite and poly-L-lactic acid), and permanent fillers (i.e., polymethylmethacrylate, silicone, autologous fat). Hyaluronic acid fillers are the most frequently used for soft tissue augmentation.
3. It is important for the aesthetic practitioner to understand the unique physicochemical and rheological properties of the available dermal fillers to achieve optimal cosmetic outcomes. Additionally, the aesthetic practitioner should be well educated on any potential adverse effects and complications associated with soft tissue filler injection, so that they can be prevented or treated appropriately should they arise.
4. Pre-procedural patient assessment including a discussion of appropriate expectations and potential adverse events is critical prior to treatment with dermal fillers.
5. Newer hyaluronic acid products have been developed recently, specifically, a collection of fillers uniquely designed to be more flexible and to more closely resemble naturally occurring hyaluronic acid, indicated for dynamic wrinkles and folds with less reactivity.
6. Research is ongoing to develop filler products that address the shortcomings of the earlier products while incorporating and expanding on their advantages. Additional hyaluronic acid products, combination hyaluronic acid-calcium hydroxylapatite products, and a number of novel filler products are currently in development.
7. To keep astride with the rapidly changing cosmetic dermatology arena, it behooves the aesthetic practitioner to be aware of the current availability, application, and future potential of dermal fillers.

INTRODUCTION

The dermal filler market is rapidly growing worldwide, and several innovations have led to a parallel expansion in product variety. According to the 2018 American Society of Dermatologic Surgery physician survey, there has been a 78% increase in soft tissue filler treatments since 2012.[1] Similarly, based on the 2018 International Society of Aesthetic Plastic Surgery survey, injection of hyaluronic acid (HA) fillers was the second most performed non-surgical procedure with 3 729 833 procedures worldwide (**Table 25-1**).[2] The actual number is likely much higher when factoring in procedures performed by dermatologists and other aesthetically oriented physicians and physician extenders. Although collagen products (Zyplast and Zyderm) were the first dermal fillers to become widely available, collagen fillers have largely been replaced by HA fillers.

The ultimate goal of dermal fillers is to smooth out wrinkles and folds, even out scars, volumize furrows and sunken valleys, contour unevenness and laxity, and sculpt skin into a 360-degree, rejuvenated look. Over the last quarter century, several kinds of products suitable for soft tissue augmentation have become available, with intense industry research yielding more and more filler options with increasing regularity. Different regulatory mechanisms usually leave the United States (US) a few years behind other developed countries in making the latest products available to patients.

TABLE 25-1	Soft Tissue Augmentation Procedures Performed in 2018 by Members of the Academy of Aesthetic Plastic Surgeons in the United States
Procedures	**Number Performed in 2018**
Fat injections	49 413
Calcium hydroxylapatite (Radiesse/Radiance)	30 349
Hyaluronic acid	763 000
Poly-L-Lactic Acid (Sculptra)	21 798

HISTORY

In 1893, by transplanting fat from the arms into facial defects, Neuber became the first physician to practice soft tissue augmentation.[3] In the middle of the 20th century, soft tissue augmentation could best be characterized by the use of silicone. Although popular in the 1940s and 1950s, silicone use was associated with the development of foreign body granulomas, which ultimately prompted the banning of silicone in 1992 until a new form of the substance (intended for ophthalmologic use) was approved by the United States Food and Drug Administration (FDA) in the late 1990s. In the meantime, though, the field of soft tissue augmentation had come into its own, in the 1970s, with the introduction by Stanford University researchers of animal-derived collagen implants.[4] By the 1980s, the use of collagen injections for wrinkles had entered the mainstream. While Americans were enjoying the benefits of bovine collagen fillers (i.e., Zyderm and Zyplast), other countries began to experiment with dermal HA fillers such as Hylaform and later Restylane in the mid to late 1990s. The beginning of the 21st century ushered in the introduction of newer nonbovine collagen fillers, CosmoDerm and CosmoPlast, and HA fillers, such as Captique and Juvéderm, as well as other synthetic fillers, Sculptra, Radiesse, and Artefill into the US market. With different forms of soft tissue augmentation agents currently available in the US and others in the pipeline, selecting the appropriate filler is challenging for physicians and patients alike. In order to achieve optimal results, it is incumbent upon dermatologists to obtain thorough comprehension of the characteristics of available fillers, their indications, contraindications, benefits and drawbacks, and ways to resolve potential complications. In this chapter, we will review the basics behind the art and science of the broad array of dermal fillers on the market in the US. This will be preceded by a brief discussion of regulatory issues and the patient evaluation and consultation.

REGULATION

In the US, dermal fillers are regulated as medical devices. In order to obtain FDA approval, the company applying for approval for a dermal filler must satisfy the intense safety and efficacy criteria including non-teratogenicity, non-migration, non-carcinogenesis, biocompatibility, and optimal purity, as well as reproducible and durable efficacy in correcting skin defects. Unfortunately, some physicians and physician extenders choose to use dermal filler products that have not yet received FDA approval for any indication. This is not advisable for several reasons including the fact that it is illegal and that the safety of these products has not been established. With the multitude of safe, efficacious, and durable fillers on the market, there is no need or justifiable reason to use unapproved dermal fillers in the US.

PATIENT EVALUATION AND CONSULTATION

When embarking on soft tissue augmentation, proper patient evaluation is essential. An initial consultation should include distant and close evaluation of the patient's facial structure and discussion of the cosmetic treatment options. The patient's history is taken to assess contraindications including allergy to filler components, history of herpes simplex or cold sores, pregnancy/lactation, keloid predisposition, and autoimmune diseases. In addition, use of medications that inhibit clotting such as aspirin and ibuprofen should be reviewed. The ideal cosmetic outcome is achieved through a combination of various cosmetic procedures in order to attain an even tone, smooth texture, and adequate facial volume and shape. The discussion of the sequence and description of each proposed procedure, alternatives, risks and benefits, financial cost, and recovery period prepares the patient for realistic expectations and informed decision-making. After the treatment procedures are selected and informed consent is signed and witnessed, the patient should undergo pretreatment photography for the purpose of documentation; posttreatment photography is scheduled immediately after and on the follow-up visits. For novice patients, it may be optimal to start with temporary and predictable fillers (e.g., HA fillers), and then gradually advance with more lasting fillers (e.g., Sculptra and Radiesse) based on patient comfort level and desire.

The best approach to minimizing the side effects of soft tissue augmentation is, first, to prevent them. To reduce bruising, patients should avoid anticoagulant medications (i.e., aspirin) or supplements (i.e., vitamin E, fish oil, etc.) for 10 days prior and several days after the procedure (see Chapter 21). The utility of *Arnica montana* oral tablets or topical gel or postprocedure oral bromelain supplements to decrease ecchymoses is anecdotal but these are often used in clinical practice. The pain associated with injection can be diminished with topical (e.g., lidocaine cream, ice), regional (e.g., infraorbital, dental nerve block), or intraprocedural anesthesia (e.g., fillers that contain lidocaine). Patients prone to regional herpes outbreaks should receive antiviral prophylaxis with systemic medications (e.g., valacyclovir 1 g twice daily for 3 days, starting a day before the procedure). The procedure should be conducted in a clean, safe, well-lit, and soothing environment that is prepared to address any potential complications. Vasovagal responses are not uncommon; therefore, orange or apple juice should be available in the event that the patient feels dizzy or faint. Topical steroids may be needed in case of a contact allergy to lidocaine cream. Most importantly, for physicians using HA fillers, hyaluronidase should be easily and immediately available in the case of intra-arterial injection (see discussion below).

TYPES OF FILLERS

Dermal fillers can be classified based on various criteria: depth of implantation (superficial upper and middermis, deep dermis, and subcutaneous levels); longevity of correction (temporary, semipermanent, and permanent); allergenicity (whether pre-procedure allergic testing is required); composition of the agent (xenografts, allografts, or autologous, semi/fully synthetic); and stimulatory behavior (capacity to drive physiologic processes of endogenous tissue proliferation) versus replacement fillers (space-replacing effect). Safety and efficacy studies of the available fillers are required by the FDA; however, studies looking at the durability of the filler are not required and, therefore, subject to disagreement and frequent citing of anecdotal evidence. The lasting effect of the filler is dependent on the composition, amount used, depth injected, and carrier of the agent. Our discussion of fillers will proceed by dividing them according to composition: temporary HA fillers will be discussed first, followed by semipermanent and permanent agents. Collagen fillers will be mentioned for historical purposes.

TEMPORARY FILLERS

Injectable fillers such as collagen and HA are biodegradable and last from 4 to 12 months. These fillers commonly serve an important role as the initial step for new patients interested in soft tissue augmentation. Because of their transient effect, the potential patient dissatisfaction and side effects are also short-lived. Therefore, temporary fillers are often ideal as the first line of therapy, saving the longer-lasting fillers for future patient visits.

Prior to the use of HA fillers, collagen was used for temporary fillers. Collagen is a major structural component of the dermis, the most abundant protein in the human body as well as the skin, and confers strength and support to the skin. Collagen is also one of the strongest natural proteins, imparting durability and resilience to the skin, comprising 70% of dry skin mass (see Chapter 2, Basic Science of the Dermis).[5] Bovine collagen and human collagen were both used but a limitation was the need for skin testing to assess any hypersensitivity or allergic reaction. Two skin tests, performed at 6 and 2 weeks before the scheduled treatment, are required before the use of bovine collagen agents to reduce the risk of inducing hypersensitivity or allergic reactions (**Fig. 25-1**).

Hyaluronic Acid

In the last several years, HA fillers have become the new gold standard, far outpacing in usage the other soft tissue

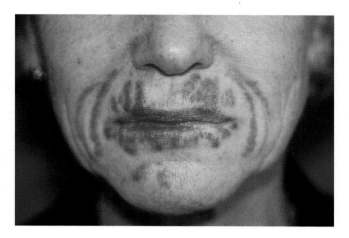

FIGURE 25-1. Collagen hypersensitivity reaction in a patient treated by another physician after only one skin test.

augmentation agents.[6] HA is a nonsulfated glycosaminoglycan (GAG) that occurs naturally in the skin and other tissues (specifically, connective, epithelial, and neural tissues) as space-occupiers of the extracellular matrix. HA is also ubiquitous across animal species, which makes it nonimmunogenic. This polysaccharide has the capacity to bind water up to 1000 times its mass. The biologic behavior of HA is predictable; it creates lubrication and volume with an aqueous and pliable framework that suspends and adheres to collagen, elastin, and cells. With age, the concentration of HA in skin decreases, translating to more lax, sallow, and dull skin. The viscoelastic qualities of HA serve to plump up the skin, yielding a more youthful appearance. Naturally occurring, unmodified, or uncross-linked HA has a half-life of about 24 hours. For this reason, HA is cross-linked when formulated into a dermal filler product. Higher concentrations and moderate cross-linking of the HA in a product impart greater longevity. There exists a certain threshold where beyond that value additional cross-linking can cause biocompatibility issues. In effect, cross-linking has to be in the right balance to maintain duration and biocompatibility of the HA filler. HA is readily metabolized by the liver into by-products, water, and carbon dioxide. In the skin, HA is broken down by hyaluronidase, mechanical degradation caused by facial movement, and by free radicals. Supplementation with oral antioxidants theoretically may increase the duration of HA fillers, but this has not been proven (see Chapter 34, Skincare Retail in a Medical Setting).

There are two main categories of HA fillers: animal-derived (e.g., Hylaform) and bacteria-derived (e.g., Restylane, Juvéderm, Revanesse Versa, Belotero Balance, RHA Collection). Due to the increased expense of animal-derived products, the vast majority of HA products are now bacteria derived. Multiple products are now manufactured to contain lidocaine which has made injection of these products far less uncomfortable and has been shown in several randomized trials to reduce patient discomfort without affecting product efficacy.[7–12] Because of their nonallergenic nature and manufacturing, HA fillers do not require prior testing and can be stored at room temperature. Their advantages over collagen products are longer duration (6–12 months), better pliability, and decreased risk of immunogenic and allergic side effects. On the whole, side effects of various HA fillers are similar, mild, and rare; these include bruising (**Fig. 25-2**), temporary swelling, lumps, acneiform eruptions, and, rarely, acute hypersensitivity.[13] In addition, vascular occlusion, thought to be due to swelling of the HA implant or intravascular injection causing vascular compromise, can rarely occur (**Fig. 25-3**).

A major advantage of HA fillers is that if skin nodules or vascular compromise do arise, these reactions can be easily dissolved with intralesional hyaluronidase (**Fig. 25-4**).

Considerations in choosing an HA filler

HA fillers do not require skin testing and the risk of allergy with all products that are FDA approved is minimal. Cost, availability, duration of correction, and size of the required needle for injection all play a role in product selection and manufacturers all strive to create an affordable, long-lasting product that can be injected with a 30-gauge or smaller needle. However, there are other, less obvious, scientific considerations to be taken into account when choosing a filler, including the rheologic properties of a given filler (**Table 25-2**). The stiffness or G′ (G prime) of a product is one of the most important considerations. G′ is a measurement of gel hardness. It is obtained when a gel is placed on a plate. A second plate is placed over the gel and a lateral force is applied. The measurement of resistance to deformation is known as the elastic modulus or the G′ (**Fig. 23-5**). Together with the cohesivity of the product, G′ values could be used to determine the appropriate placement of an HA dermal filler. For example, more robust products (higher G′ values and higher cohesivities) such as Juvéderm Ultra Plus and Restylane Lyft should be used in deeper lines

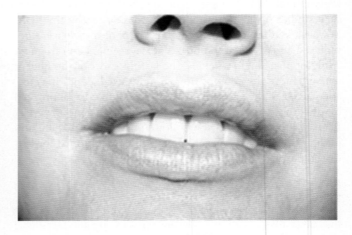

FIGURE 25-4. Visible lumps of Hylaform in the upper lip.

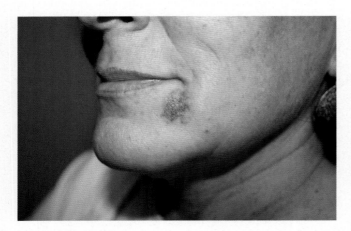

FIGURE 25-2. This is a common site at which bruises occur after a dermal filler is injected.

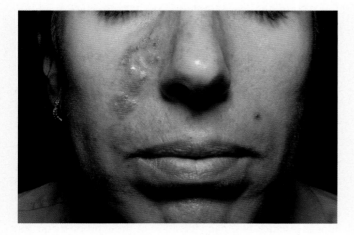

FIGURE 25-3. This patient developed redness, blisters, and lumps after receiving an HA injection. The most likely cause was vascular compromise due to swelling of the implant. All cultures were negative, other treated sites were normal and the lesions resolved without scarring.

TABLE 25-2	Factors to Consider When Choosing a Hyaluronic Acid Filler
Concentration of HA	
Cost	
Cross-linking	
Degree of cross-linking	
Quantity of HA cross-linked versus uncross-linked	
Type of cross-linking technology used	
Duration of correction	
G′ (elastic modulus)	
Hydration level of product in the syringe	
Presence of lidocaine	
Required needle size for injection	
Sizing technology	
Syringe	
Design of syringe	
Size	

Data obtained from www.surgery.org.

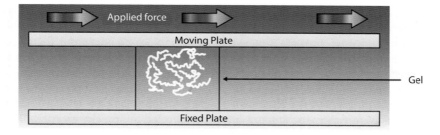

FIGURE 25-5. Measurement of G′. A force is applied laterally on the top plate. The more the gel resists the movement, the harder the gel, the higher the G′.

TABLE 25-3	Hyaluronic Acid Fillers: Cross-Linking Technology and Concentration of HA	
Product	Cross-Linking Technology	Concentration (Mg/Ml)
Captique	Bacterial-sourced HA	4.5–6.5
Hylaform	Avian-sourced HA	4.5–6.5
Prevelle Dura	Bacterial-sourced HA	20
Prevelle Silk	Bacterial-sourced HA	4.5–6.5
Restylane	NASHA	20
Restylane Lyft	NASHA	20
Restylane Silk	NASHA	20
Restylane Refyne	XpresHAn	20
Restylane Defyne	XpresHAn	20
Restylane Kysse	XpresHAn	20
Juvederm Ultra XC	Hylacross	24
Juvederm Ultra Plus XC	Hylacross	24
Juvederm Voluma XC	VyCross	20
Juvederma Vollure XC	VyCross	17.5
Juvederm Volbella XC	VyCross	15
Revanesse Versa	Thiofix	22–28
RHA 2	Resilient	23
RHA 3	Resilient	23
RHA 4	Resilient	23

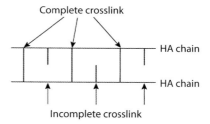

FIGURE 25-6. Cross-links that occur during the cross-linking process may be complete or incomplete.

like the nasolabial folds and marionette lines, as well as to lift the lateral brow, to correct the nasal bridge, to give the ear lobe youthful volume, to evert the nipples, and to raise the nasal tip. More fluid products such as Juvéderm Ultra and Restylane are better suited to be used over large areas such as the cheekbones and cheeks. Low G′ products such as Restylane Silk, Juvéderm Ultra, and Juvéderm Volbella are necessary in areas that require a softer agent, such as the body of the lip or the tear trough. As new products reach the market, knowing the G′ will allow practitioners to select the appropriate filler for a given indication and anatomical location for optimal cosmetic outcomes.

The concentration of HA in a product is important to consider as well (**Table 25-3**). Many authorities believe that the higher the concentration of HA, the stiffer the product and

the longer its duration. This is true in general when comparing products within a brand. However, this does not hold true across brands because not all of the HA in the dermal fillers is cross-linked. Many HA fillers contain uncross-linked HA and lightly cross-linked chains and fragments. The uncross-linked HA, fragments of HA, and lightly cross-linked HA are included in the overall concentration measurement but only remain in the skin for a limited time and minimally contribute to the longevity of the filler. The uncross-linked HA helps to decrease extrusion force and make injection easier, which is the main reason it is included. Therefore, the fact that Restylane contains 20 mg of HA/ml and Juvéderm contains 15 to 24 mg of HA/ml does not give a physician enough information to decide which filler will have longer duration. It is actually the amount of modified HA that plays the primary role in duration.

The type of modification (cross-linking) and the cross-linking agent used is also important (**Table 25-3**). Cross-linking can be best visualized by imagining a ladder (**Fig. 25-6**). Each side of the ladder is an HA chain. The "rungs" of the ladder are the cross-links. When the rungs of the ladder attach to both sides of the ladder, the agent is considered completely modified. However, the cross-linking agent used may incompletely cross-link the chains of HA, leaving the sides of the rungs unattached and resulting in incomplete modification. Such a product might not be as durable as a completely modified product. In addition, there are two types of rungs in the HA ladder. One is called an ether linkage and the other is called an ester linkage. Ether linkages are formed by 1,4-butanediol diglycidyl ether (BDDE, the cross-linking agent in Restylane, Juvéderm, and Revanesse Versa) and divinyl sulfone (DVS, the agent used in Prevelle Silk, Captique, and Hylaform). The cross-linking agent used in Prevelle Dura, 1,2,7,8-diepoxyoctane (DEO), forms both ether and ester linkages (known as "double cross-linking"). It is unknown at this time what advantages, if any, ether linkages impart to a dermal filler.

The hydration status of the filler once it is packaged in the syringe also affects filler performance. HA is well known to bind up to 1000 times its weight in water. The amount of water bound to the HA prior to its packaging in the syringe determines how much more water the filler can absorb once it is injected into the skin. In other words, fillers that are completely hydrated in the syringe will bind less water on injection and the volume will expand less upon injection as compared to fillers that are not completely hydrated in the syringe. Fillers that are not completely hydrated in the syringe will swell somewhat within 24 hours after correction; therefore, it is prudent to slightly undercorrect with these substances. In addition, patients can be told that they will "look even better" 24 hours after the injection. Restylane and Juvéderm are not completely hydrated in the syringe while Captique and Hylaform are close to being fully hydrated (**Table 23-4**).

HA fillers were originally believed to volumize through their water-binding and space-filling properties. However, studies have demonstrated that HA fillers also stimulate neocollagenesis.[14–16] The injected HA provides structural support to the extracellular matrix in the dermis, which then promotes fibroblast activation and initiates production and deposition of collagen.[14,15] Increased levels of type I collagen have been observed in skin biopsies up to at least 3 months after injection of an HA filler.[14,15] Therefore, the soft tissue augmentation that occurs with HA fillers appears to be due to the effects of hydration, direct fill, and new collagen synthesis.

Another process that may affect the performance of the filler is referred to as "sizing technology." This term is used by Allergan to differentiate Juvéderm from the other HA fillers. When an HA filler is cross-linked, the chains of modified sugars form a gel. In the process of manufacturing Restylane family products, this gel is extruded through a screen. This produces various sizes of the gel that are considered "sized." The large pieces become Restylane Lyft (previously Perlane), while the small pieces are marketed as Restylane Silk. The medium-sized pieces are Restylane. The larger pieces yield products that are best used in the mid to lower dermis while the small pieces such as Restylane Silk can be used more

superficially. The Juvéderm family of products is not sized. In other words, Juvéderm is not pushed through a screen and broken into sized pieces and, therefore, it consists of randomly sized and shaped pieces.[17] It is unknown at this time what role sizing technology plays, if any, in the performance of a filler.

There are many factors that must be understood in order to make the most suitable choice of HA filler. More data need to be collected to properly ascertain if, for example, sizing technology makes a difference or if ester bonds last longer than ether bonds. These distinctions will become clearer and more important as more HA fillers are introduced in the market and more data are collected. A discussion of the individual HA brands follows.

Restylane
Overview

Restylane (Galderma Laboratories, Fort Worth, TX) was the first nonanimal HA product approved in the US. It is a nonanimal derived synthetic hyaluronic acid (NASHA) gel formulated through fermentation, with sugar present, in bacterial cultures of equine streptococci. Restylane has a higher concentration of HA compared with Hylaform and Captique and the highest G' of the fillers currently on the market, denoting that it is a slightly stiffer product. It is the most popular of the HA fillers in the US because of its safety profile, brand recognition, and ease of injection. Restylane is composed of approximately 100 000 particles/ml (approximately 250 μm on average, range 350–450 μm) and contains 20 mg/ml of HA.[18] Restylane was the first HA filler approved in the US in 2003 and is currently FDA approved for lip augmentation and correction of moderate to severe facial wrinkles (FDA).[19–21] Restylane Lyft, another product in the Restylane family, is also FDA approved for significantly deeper folds and furrows of the face as well as dorsal hand augmentation. Of note, this product was renamed to Restylane Lyft in the US in 2016. These products are made up of suspensions of equally sized particles in a gel base. Restylane is made of medium-sized particles of HA gel, while Restylane Lyft is composed of larger HA gel particles (approximately 750–1000 μm),[18] but with the same HA concentration. Restylane has a smaller particle size, a lower degree of cross-linking, and demonstrates less spreading given a lower cohesivity compared with other HA products. The Restylane family of products also includes Restylane-L, Restylane Lyft, Restylane Refyne, Restylane Defyne, and Restylane Kysse. These products have the same formulation as Restylane and differ primarily in particle size and that they contain 0.3% lidocaine. Restylane-L and Restylane Silk are produced using NASHA technology, with similar rheologic properties and clinical effects and indications as Restylane.[22,23] However, Restylane Silk has a slightly smaller particle size and is associated with a slightly lower G' compared with Restylane-L, resulting in a softer gel, ideal for finer wrinkles and lip augmentation.[22,23] Restylane Lyft, as mentioned earlier, contains a larger gel particle size and fewer number of gel beads compared to Restylane products. In a study comparing the physicochemical characteristics of the various HA fillers, Restylane Lyft demonstrated the highest G'.[22] The larger particle size theoretically

TABLE 25-4	Hyaluronic Acid Filler Hydration in the Syringe
Almost Completely Hydrated in the Syringe[a]	**Not Completely Hydrated in the Syringe[b]**
Captique	Restylane
Hylaform	Juvéderm
Prevelle Silk	Prevelle Dura

[a]No need to undercorrect.
[b]Slightly undercorrect.

decreases the rate of degradation and increases the duration of effects.[22,24,25] However, Restylane and Restylane Lyft appear to have similar durations of correction based on prior studies.[26] Restylane Refyne, Restylane Defyne and Restylane Kysse are designed with XpresHAn cross-linking technology. Each product has its own unique properties leading to differences in clinical performance.[27–29] Restylane Refyne is a softer gel with a lower G', making it more appropriate for mild to moderate facial wrinkles and folds. In comparison, Restylane Defyne is a firmer gel, associated with a higher G', making it more ideal for correction of prominent, deeper wrinkles and folds.[22,30] Restylane Kysse is the most recent addition to the Restylane family, specifically formulated for use in the lips and is FDA approved for lip augmentation and perioral rhytides. It has rheological properties that fall between Restylane Refyne and Defyne, creating an elastic product ideal for mobile areas such as the perioral region and lips.[31]

Restylane products are packaged as transparent gels, with a shelf life of 18 months, and stored at room temperature. Restylane products are enclosed in 1.0 ml syringes and injected via a 29-gauge or 30-gauge needle. Restylane is the only Restylane product that does not contain lidocaine. Restylane is implanted using serial puncture, linear threading anterograde or retrograde techniques and cross-hatching technique. A fanning threading technique can also be employed with Restylane at the nasolabial fold or lip commissures. It is important to avoid injecting at withdrawal of the needle, which can result in superficial injection, creating blue-colored nodules.

Benefits

Overall, given the higher G', increased stiffness and lower cohesivity with decreased spreading, Restylane is optimal for subdermal placement to correct moderate to severe facial rhytides. Restylane Lyft may be preferable over Restylane in the setting of deeper facial defects given its larger particle size. The cosmetic effects of Restylane and Restylane Lyft are thought to last over 6 months with some studies showing up to 18 months. Similarly, the effects of Restylane Refyne and Restylane Defyne have been shown to last up to 12 months. Product stiffness makes Restylane, Restylane Lyft, and Restylane Defyne more suitable for moderate and deep wrinkles than for use in the body of the lips or the tear trough. Restylane is ideal to fill nasolabial and marionette lines, chin and jowl depressions, nasal deformities, and for nasal tip-lift as well as acne scars and other defects. Restylane Kysse is the first filler designed specifically for use in the lips for flexible movement and natural-looking volume shown to last up to 12 months based on current studies.[31,32] It has also been shown to require a smaller volume of product for lip augmentation compared to Juvéderm Volbella with comparable aesthetic improvement.[32]

Drawbacks

Bruising is associated with all HA fillers. However, the stiffness is a downside if the product is used by a poorly skilled physician, with bumps and blue nodules possibly arising from improper injection technique. Injection into the tear trough may result in visible nodules or blebs. Slower injection of any HA filler will limit the risk of inflammation. Restylane can be used in the vermilion border to augment the shape of the lip. However, Restylane and Restylane Lyft are a poor choice for the body of the lips due to the moderate stiffness of the products. On the other hand, Restylane Kysse was formulated and approved by the FDA specifically for use in this area. Restylane may be associated with more injection-related pain compared with the other Restylane products that are premixed with lidocaine. The use of topical anesthetics and/or dental nerve blocks can be adjunctively used to reduce the pain on injection. In general, Restylane tends to sting less after injection when compared to Juvéderm. It is unknown why this occurs as they are both the same pH of approximately 7.0.

Juvéderm™

Overview

Juvéderm (Allergan, Irvine, CA), is manufactured by a bacterial fermentation process similar to that used for other stabilized bacteria-based HA fillers and was approved by the FDA in late 2006. There are many products in the Juvéderm line including Juvéderm Ultra XC, Juvéderm Ultra Plus XC, Juvéderm Voluma XC, Juvéderm Volbella XC, and Juvéderm Vollure XC. Juvéderm family products are composed of suspensions of variably sized particles in a gel base, unlike Restylane which consists of a fairly narrow range of particle sizes. These products are designed using Hylacross (Juvéderm Ultra, Juvéderm Ultra Plus) or VyCross technology (Juvéderm Voluma XC, Juvéderm Vollure XC, Juvéderm Vobella XC).[20] Overall, these products rely on a higher cohesivity to achieve a high lift capacity despite a lower G'.[22,33] All the products in the line vary by the amount of HA concentration, the amount of cross-linking, and the regularity of the cross-linking. Therefore, there are slight differences in rheologic properties between individual products based on unique manufacturing properties, ultimately translating into differences in clinical outcomes and performance. Both Juvéderm Ultra and Ultra Plus consist of 24 mg/ml of HA, but Juvéderm Ultra Plus has a higher degree of cross-linking than Juvéderm Ultra, which makes Ultra Plus more suitable for the deepest facial grooves and furrows. Juvéderm Voluma has the highest G' and greatest lift capacity of all the Juvéderm products, although its G' is still lower than that of Restylane products. Juvéderm Volbella XC has the lowest G' and cohesivity of the fillers in the VyCross family and Juvéderm Vollure XC has a G' and cohesivity between those of Volbella XC and Voluma XC.[34] These products are manufactured with VyCross technology using high and low molecular weight HA particles, which improves cross-linking efficiency, creating a highly cohesive, stiffer gel with longer lasting clinical effects.[22,25]

Juvéderm products are packaged as a clear gel in 1.0 ml syringes premixed with 0.3% lidocaine. They are stored at room temperature. Juvéderm Ultra, Juvéderm Volbella, and Juvéderm Vollure are injected into the middermis via a 30-gauge needle while Juvéderm Ultra Plus and Juvéderm Voluma are implanted deeper via a 27-gauge needle.[35] The needles must be tightly attached to the Luer-lock syringe to prevent detachment during injections. Various techniques of injection can be used with Juvéderm, including serial puncture and tunneling.

Benefits

Juvéderm Ultra and Ultra Plus are in the medium range of stiffness; therefore, they can be used in any wrinkles, moderate or deep, and to correct scars. The high concentration of HA in Juvéderm Ultra and Ultra Plus and the high degree of cross-linking results in longer-lasting aesthetic effects as compared to products such as Hylaform. Similar to Restylane, the longevity of Juvéderm Ultra is about 6 to 9 months and Ultra Plus may last up to 12 months. Juvéderm Voluma has the greatest lift capacity of the Juvéderm products and is optimal for long-term correction of deep volume loss. The increased cross-linking efficiency also prolongs the clinical effects of Juvéderm Voluma, with studies demonstrating effects lasting up to 24 months,[20,36,37] while most other HA fillers last about 6 to 12 months.[33,34,38] Juvéderm Ultra and Juvéderm Volbella are easily placed in the vermilion border or the body of the lips. As with other HA products, these agents have an overall low, mild, and transient adverse event profile. Juvéderm is not completely hydrated in the syringe,[35] so it will slightly expand after injection as it absorbs more water. This is important to remember when injecting the body of the lips, which should be slightly undercorrected to allow for the expansion.

Drawbacks

All HA products can cause erythema, swelling, and bruising after implantation (see Chapter 21). Pain during injection is alleviated to an extent as all Juvéderm products are pre-mixed with 0.3% lidocaine. Additional use of topical or regional anesthesia can make the procedure more tolerable. While HA fillers have been rarely associated with the formation of hypersensitivity reactions or delayed-onset nodules, recent studies suggest that the VyCross line of Juvéderm products may be associated with greater immunogenicity and increased incidence of delayed nodules.[39] Since the introduction and increased use of HA fillers manufactured with VyCross technology, the incidence of delayed nodules associated with HA fillers, which was previously considered zero to less than 1%, has increased ranging from 1 to 4.25%. It is speculated that the presence of low molecular weight fragments of HA may be more immunogenic and pro-inflammatory, stimulating an immune response, which increases the risk of delayed-onset nodule formation. These low molecular weight HA chains are unique to the VyCross family fillers. A recent retrospective review by Humphrey and colleagues evaluated delayed adverse events following treatment with Juvéderm Voluma in 4500 patients.[40] The rate of delayed adverse events was 0.98% per patient and 0.23% per syringe with delayed swelling and nodule formation being the most common reactions, which occurred within a median of 4 months after treatment. Patients who experienced delayed adverse events received a slightly greater cumulative amount of Juvéderm Voluma compared with those who did not. An increased frequency of events was noted to occur between October and January with about one

third of reactions preceded by an identifiable immunologic stimulus (i.e., dental procedure, sinus infection). Therefore, the authors postulated that an increase in fragmentation during the degradation of the filler may incite an inflammatory response after an immunologic trigger. Various treatment modalities were used including systemic or intralesional steroids, hyaluronidase, and oral antibiotics with oral prednisone demonstrating the greatest efficacy. Most of the swelling and nodules resolved without recurrence and did not appear to increase risk of adverse events with subsequent treatment with Juvéderm Voluma or other HA fillers.[40] Further long-term studies will continue to elucidate the exact etiology and nature of these reactions. Current recommendations favor the use of systemic steroids with or without hyaluronidase for management and the utility of oral antibiotics in this setting remains unclear.[41]

Juvéderm can be placed with care in the tear trough area, but the proximity to the eye is unnerving with the risk of the needle popping off, so injections should be very slow with only moderate extrusion force. The needle is more likely to pop off when the syringe is almost empty; therefore, the tear trough area should be injected with a new syringe and the last part of the syringe can be saved for less dangerous areas such as the nasolabial folds. As with all fillers, the skill and experience of the physician is crucial for optimal outcome. If Juvéderm is injected too superficially, it can create a bluish hue due to the Tyndall effect, especially in the tear trough area. Blue nodules and unwanted bulges can be corrected with the use of hyaluronidase. Caution should be taken in over-injecting the vermilion border and creating an unnatural "duckbill" appearance.

Belotero Balance®

Overview

Belotero Balance® is sold by Merz Aesthetics (Merz North America, Inc., Raleigh, NC) and is another HA dermal filler FDA approved for the correction of moderate to severe wrinkles, especially around the nose and the mouth.[20,21,42] It is manufactured with a unique cohesive poly-densified matrix technology that creates a homogenous gel without individual particles, made up of HA chains with zones of different degrees of cross-linking. The variably cross-linked zones ensure optimal spreading of the gel, allowing larger deficits to be filled with denser parts of the gel and finer deficits to be filled with the lower density parts of the gel. The gel contains an HA concentration of 22.5 mg/ml. Integration of this filler is often more homogenous and appears more natural compared to other fillers. Belotero is packaged in a 1.0 ml pre-filled syringe with two sterile 30-gauge needles.

Benefits

Compared to the other HA fillers, Belotero has a lower G', less lift capacity, and higher cohesivity, allowing it to integrate into the skin easily and making it ideal for superficial injection to correct softer, finer facial rhytides.[22,24,25] While it is indicated for injection into the mid to deep dermis, it can be injected more superficially compared with many of the other

HA products without increased risk of nodule formation or of Tyndall effect. It is ideal for superficial injection to correct softer, finer facial rhytides, including perioral rhytides, creating a natural appearance.

Drawbacks

Belotero is one of the only dermal fillers on the market that is not pre-mixed with lidocaine, and therefore, may be more painful on injection compared to many of the Restylane and Juvéderm products that contain lidocaine. However, the authors of this chapter often mix the product with 0.3 to 0.5 ml of lidocaine without epinephrine prior to injection to decrease pain associated with injection.

Revanesse® Versa™

Overview

Revanesse® Versa™ is manufactured by Prollenium Medical Technologies (Aurora, Canada) and was recently FDA approved in 2017 for the injection into the mid to deep dermis for correction of moderate to severe facial wrinkles and folds, such as the nasolabial folds.[20,43] This product is created using Thiofix technology and is made up of spherical particles of monophasic HA that is slightly less hydrophilic than other HA fillers. Revanesse® Versa™ appears to have a G' between that of Restylane and Juvéderm Ultra Plus, although there is currently limited data on the true rheologic properties of this product. The concentration of HA ranges from 22–28 mg/ml. Two products are available, Versa™ and Versa™+, which is premixed with 0.3% of lidocaine. The gel is delivered in a pre-filled disposable glass syringe and each box of Revanesse® Versa™ contains two 1.0 ml or 1.2 ml syringes of product along with two sterile 27-gauge needles.

Benefits

Revanesse® Versa™ is an HA filler with a medium stiffness and lift capacity making it optimal for the correction of moderate to deep rhytides as well as lipoatrophy and facial wasting, with cosmetic effects lasting 6 to 12 months. This product is less ideal for areas with greater mobility such as the lips and perioral area.

Drawbacks

Similar to other HA products, the most frequent treatment-related adverse events are transient and mild including bruising, swelling, pain, and injection site erythema based on prior studies. Revanesse Versa+ has been shown to be associated with less pain, likely due to the incorporation of lidocaine within the product. Currently, there are no reports of delayed onset nodule formation following implantation of Revanesse® Versa™. However, given that this product has been recently introduced into the market, long-term studies evaluating treatment-related adverse events are limited.

RHA® Collection

Overview

The RHA® collection of resilient HA dermal fillers is sold by Revance (Newark, CA) and TEOXANE SA (Geneve,

Switzerland) and includes RHA®2, RHA®3 and RHA®4. These are the newest HA fillers on the market introduced in 2017 and the first and only HA fillers FDA approved for dynamic wrinkles and folds.[20] RHA®2 and RHA®3 are indicated for injection into the mid to deep dermis for correction of moderate to severe dynamic facial wrinkles and folds, and RHA®4 is indicated for injection into the deep dermis to superficial subcutaneous tissue for the correction of moderate to severe dynamic facial wrinkles and folds such as the nasolabial folds. This line of HA fillers is unique due to the Preserved Network Technology (PNT) creating filler products with longer HA chains, a lower degree of chemical modifications, more preserved covalent bonds, and less BDDE bonds required for stabilization. Therefore, these products are more flexible, less rigid, and more closely resemble naturally occurring HA in the skin. The products contain the same concentration of HA (23 mg/ml) but each product differs in the degree of cross-linking with RHA®2 having the lowest degree of cross-linking (3.1%) and RHA®4 having the highest (4.0%). The degree of cross-linking correlates with the strength and lift capacity of the filler. Studies have compared the strength and stretch of the RHA fillers to the current HA fillers on the market.[44] RHA®2 demonstrated greater stretch but less strength compared to Juvederm Ultra but had more stretch and strength compared to Juvederm Volbella. RHA®3 was found to have greater dynamic strength and stretch compared to Juvéderm Ultra and Juvéderm Vollure. RHA®4 demonstrated a high degree of dynamic stretch and strength, although its lift capacity was not as much as Juvéderm Voluma.[44]

All products are premixed with 0.3% lidocaine and each box contains a 1.0 ml syringe of product with two sterile 30-gauge needles. Multiple injection techniques can be used to deliver the filler into the mid to deep dermis (RHA®2, RHA®3) or deep dermis to superficial subcutaneous tissue (RHA®4) including serial puncture, linear threading and fanning technique. It is important to inject this product slowly as with other HA fillers to prevent post-procedural edema and bruising.

Benefits

These fillers are uniquely designed to look natural both in motion and at rest. The little cross-linking and longer HA chains maintains flexibility, stretch, and strength while allowing the product to move with the tissue rather than resisting it, creating a natural appearance with movement. This is unlike the other HA filler products on the market that have a greater degree of cross-linking and are slightly more rigid. Therefore, the RHA products can be used for dynamic areas of the face and can even be injected more superficially. RHA products deliver long lasting aesthetic improvements comparable to competitor products with results lasting up to 15 months.[44,45] The unique design, increased stretch, and flexibility make these products easier to inject compared to other HA filler products. Additionally, as these products more closely resemble naturally occurring HA, they are theoretically less reactive with a decreased risk of adverse events. Current studies have corroborated the favorable safety profile of these products with only transient and mild associated adverse events reported. At the time of writing this chapter, there have been no reports of delayed-onset nodules following injection of these fillers. Injection site pain is also minimal with these products as they are premixed with lidocaine.

Drawbacks

Like other HA fillers, the RHA collection has been associated with transient and mild adverse events including bruising, pain, swelling, tenderness, erythema, pruritus, lumps, and bumps. Pain is minimized with the incorporation of lidocaine premixed into the product and risk of edema and bruising can be decreased with slow injection.

Hyaluronidase

Hyaluronidase is a soluble enzyme that hydrolyzes HA, other GAGs, and other connective tissue components in the skin and vitreous humor of the eye.[46] It has been approved by the FDA as Vitrase, Hylenex, Amphadase, and Hydase for enhancement of injectable drug absorption and resorption of radiopaque agents. However, effective off-label uses include wound care, postsurgical flap care, reversal of HA fillers, among other uses.

Several reports have indicated the usefulness of hyaluronidase to dissolve HA filler overcorrection for symmetric contouring, as well as to manage complications associated with HA fillers including bluish discoloration or nodules, retinal artery occlusion, impending tissue necrosis, and HA filler-induced granulomatous reactions.[32,40,47-52] Specifically, Hirsch and colleagues published two cases of imminent tissue necrosis caused by intra-arterial injection of HA and surrounding tissue compression of vital vessels, which resolved with employment of hyaluronidase. After using other appropriate techniques to manage impending tissue necrosis including systemic aspirin, nitroglycerin paste twice daily under occlusion, and hot compresses with massage without significant response, the authors injected 30 units of hyaluronidase into deep dermal tissue and subcutis using a serial puncture method along the distribution of affected arteries, which led to the resolution of symptoms within a day.[46,47] Although early reports have recommended the utility of hyaluronidase only within 16 minutes of the critical event, Hirsch and colleagues reported successful responses after several days.[46] The optimal dose of hyaluronidase has not yet been established and doses reported in the literature range from less than 5 units to 75 units per injection site. Effective doses may vary depending on the problem or complication being treated (i.e., vascular occlusion or granulomatous reaction) as well as the specific HA filler requiring dissolution. In the setting of vascular occlusion, doses of 450 to 1500 units have been effectively used. Furthermore, the effectiveness of hyaluronidase for bluish (Tyndall) manifestations and asymmetric lumpiness from HA overcorrection has also been reported at various concentrations.[48,49,53] Recent studies suggest that different doses of hyaluronidase are required to dissolve certain HA filler products, with VyCross HA fillers showing greater resistance to hyaluronidase likely due to the greater degree of cross-linking making them more resistant to degradation. Approximately 30 units of hyaluronidase is suggested to dissolve 0.1 ml of Juvéderm Voluma compared to 10 units of hyaluronidase for 0.1 ml of Juvéderm Ultra and 5 units for 0.1 ml of Restylane.[54] Similarly, Ryu and colleagues evaluated the response of 12 different HA filler gels to varying doses of hyaluronidase.[52] Restylane-L and Lyft were most easily dissolved with a good response to 2.5 units/0.2 ml filler. Juvéderm Ultra, Belotero, Restylane Silk, and Restylane Defyne had moderate resistance to hyaluronidase and Restylane Refyne, Juvéderm Ultra Plus, Juvéderm Volbella, Juvéderm Vollure, Juvéderm Voluma, and Renavesse Versa were most resistant requiring 20 units/0.2 ml.

Recent consensus recommendations for management of HA filler-induced vascular occlusion includes (a) immediately inject hyaluronidase, (b) apply warm compresses and vigorously massage the affected area, (c) apply nitroglycerin paste, (d) start oral aspirin (e.g. 650 mg/day).[55] Many recommend high dose pulse therapy of hyaluronidase which involves injection every hour until capillary refill is observed.[56] Some even recommend injecting hyaluronidase even if a non-HA filler is used since it reduces tissue edema and vessel-occluding pressure.[57] If no improvement is seen despite hyaluronidase use, alternative and adjunctive therapies shown to be effective in anecdotal reports includes nitroglycerin, low molecular weight heparin, prostaglandin E, sildenafil, and hyperbaric oxygen.[57]

Hyaluronidase is imperative for a cosmetic dermatologist to have on hand in the office if treating patients with HA fillers.[58] Hyaluronidase is a clear liquid that is stored in the refrigerator and reconstituted with 1 ml of normal saline to generate 150 units. Very rare, adverse, acute, and delayed-type hypersensitivity reactions to hyaluronidase have been reported, so it may be prudent to perform a skin test prior to the use of this agent. Injection of hyaluronidase into patients with an allergy to hymenoptera stings and thimerosal is contraindicated.[47]

Semipermanent Fillers

Calcium hydroxylapatite and poly-L-lactic acid are considered semipermanent fillers because they are partly biostimulatory and partially biodegradable; this balance allows them to last approximately 1 to 3 years.[59] The adverse events associated with semipermanent fillers include rare granuloma formations. The aesthetic effects of these fillers are best preserved with annual touch-up sessions.

Calcium Hydroxylapatite

Overview

Calcium hydroxylapatite (CaHA), referred to by the brand name of Radiesse (Merz North America Inc., Franksville, WI), was approved by the FDA in 2006 and is now indicated for the correction of moderate to severe folds and wrinkles, HIV-associated facial lipoatrophy, and dorsal hand augmentation.[20,60] Hyperdilute formulations are also used off-label for tightening and rejuvenation of the lower face and areas off the face including the neck, the chest, upper arms and thighs. It is composed of 30% CaHA microspheres (25–45 μm) suspended in an aqueous gel carrier (1.3% sodium carboxymethyl cellulose, 6.4% glycerin, and 36.6% sterile water). New collagen synthesis appears to be responsible for most of the clinical results seen with CaHA. Immediate fill and lift are seen at the time of injection from the gel carrier, which then decreases over several weeks leaving the CaHA at the site of injection. As the gel carrier dissipates in several months, the microspheres subsequently stimulate a subclinical inflammatory response and act as a scaffold for fibroplasia and new collagen formation.[60–64] This leads to envelopment of the microspheres by fibrin, collagen, and fibroblasts, and slows the degradation by macrophages and metabolism into calcium and phosphate ions. Because of a similar mineral constitution as human bones, and no foreign antigenic properties, CaHA is particularly biocompatible. It is critical for patients to be aware that Radiesse is a radiopaque material that can be visualized and misinterpreted on facial radiographs, but importantly, it does not radiographically mask surrounding tissues.

Radiesse is a white material packaged in a 0.8 ml or 1.5 ml syringe and injected via a 25- to 27-gauge needle into the deep dermis or subcutis without overcorrection.[60] Radiesse+ is packaged similarly but is premixed with 0.3% lidocaine. The product should be stored at room temperature.[60] A reasonable injection method for Radiesse is tunneling or crisscross threading techniques.[60] Placement of Radiesse in the supraperiosteal plane yields better control and ability to contour skin with this stiffer filler.[65]

Benefits

Since Radiesse is immunologically inert, it does not require skin testing. With more than 20 years of use as implantable devices for otolaryngology and orthopedic specialties, CaHA possesses an excellent safety record. The average duration of Radiesse is 9 to 18 months. The proper locations of injection include the malar eminence, zygomatic arch, nasolabial folds, marionette lines, prejowl sulcus, and chin. Radiesse is ideal for areas requiring more robust lift with less spread and offers better lift in individuals with thicker skin. Interestingly, although Radiesse induces foreign body reaction, it is not known to cause granuloma formation. In its gel form, the device is also quite pliable, permitting timely manipulation and appropriate modification. In addition, it can be combined with other fillers, such as Sculptra, HA, and collagen.

Drawbacks

Similar to Sculptra, the true benefits of Radiesse are often not seen until about 6 months after treatment. Patients should be counseled that results are not immediate as with HA fillers and appropriate expectations should be established for optimal patient satisfaction. The main drawback of Radiesse is that it is not completely reversible like HA fillers. However, recent case reports and animal model studies have demonstrated the efficacy of dissolving CaHA nodules with the use of intralesional sodium thiosulfate.[66,67] Additionally, animal studies and a few anecdotal reports have described the successful dispersion of CaHA nodules with intralesional saline or sterile water via a suspected dilutional effect.[68,69] Minimal side effects such as ecchymoses, edema,

and erythema appear soon after Radiesse injection and are transitory. Rare nodules have also been associated with Radiesse and can be managed with intralesional steroids or excision. Similar to Sculptra, an implantation of Radiesse in the superficial and mobile wrinkles (e.g., lips and periorbital area) and the body of the lips is discouraged because of the palpable and visible, white papules that can develop (also known as "popcorn lips"). Radiesse should not be performed in the nose of a patient anticipating rhinoplasty. Several facial plastic surgeons have given anecdotal reports in lectures suggesting that this complicates rhinoplasty surgery. An HA or collagen filler would be a more appropriate choice in preoperative rhinoplasty patients.

Poly-L-Lactic Acid

Overview

Poly-L-lactic acid (PLLA) is a synthetic, biodegradable, biocompatible, immunologically inert, peptide polymer, known by the trade name of Sculptra.[20,70–72] Sculptra (Galderma Laboratories, Fort Worth, TX) is composed of poly-L-lactic acid (PLLA) microspheres, sodium carboxymethylcellulose, and nonpyrogenic mannitol and is manufactured from powdered, absorbable suture material. It is the only filler that requires reconstitution prior to administration. This agent is not a true dermal filler because it does not fill the dermis the way collagen and HA do but, rather, it promotes the production of new and organized collagen in the dermis. Therefore, it is considered to be a biostimulatory filler, similar to CaHA. Sculptra stimulates a subclinical inflammatory response followed by new collagen synthesis, which volumizes the tissue and results in the desired cosmetic outcome.[62,73–75] Sculptra is eventually cleared from the skin via phagocytic digestion. In the US, it is FDA approved for the treatment of HIV-associated facial lipoatrophy and severe wrinkles in immunocompetent individuals. However, it has been used off-label for pan-facial rejuvenation and off the face (i.e., chest, buttocks) for body volumetric correction and tightening. When it was first introduced, it was diluted with a lower amount of saline and many granules and nodules were reported. This led to new recommendations to dilute one bottle with 5 to 10 ml of sterile water and massage after application. Some recommend dilution with 9 ml of sterile water for the face and 18 ml of sterile water for off-the-face injections. With the new recommendations, adverse events have been minimal.

Freeze-dried Sculptra powder is stored at room temperature and reconstituted with sterile water with or without lidocaine prior to injection. The package label states that the product should be used within 72 hours. It is often preferable to use Sculptra that has been reconstituted for at least 2 days because the solution is easy to work with and results in less needle clogging. Longer rehydration times also appear to be associated with decreased risk of complications (i.e., nodule formation). Sculptra is reconstituted and kept in the refrigerator for 2 days to 2 weeks. Although the package label recommends that the formulation be reconstituted with 5 ml of sterile water, many physicians reconstitute with 4 ml of sterile water and 1 ml of 2% lidocaine with epinephrine. The lidocaine decreases pain while the epinephrine reduces bruising. Strong agitation of the filled syringes is recommended directly before injection to homogenize the white suspension (Sculptra tends to settle in the bottom of the syringe). By means of tunneling and threading techniques in a grid pattern (cross hatch), a 26-gauge needle is utilized to implant Sculptra into overlapping deep dermal and subcutaneous layers of the skin.

The mechanism of action and proper technique of injecting Sculptra require practitioners to restore volume to a selected treatment plane rather than a specific wrinkle.[76] Indeed, injecting Sculptra is more similar to fat injection procedures than collagen or HA injections, because it serves to sculpt the prominent hollows and deep grooves associated with loss of deep soft tissue. In addition, specialized training to use Sculptra is required prior to injections. Small and exact aliquots of Sculptra are injected in the correct tissue plane without overcorrection. Injections should be performed supraperiosteally directly onto bone. In general, 2 to 3 ml of the product are used for patients in their thirties, 4 ml for patients in their forties, and 5 ml or more for older patients.

Once Sculptra is injected, there is a transient period lasting about 1 hour during which the patient can see a slight effect because of the volume of fluid injected. Once this resolves, results are not seen until about 4 weeks after treatment when results *may* begin to appear. Injections are performed on a monthly basis until desired results have been obtained. The number of injection sessions required varies greatly from person to person and it is difficult to predict the total number of sessions needed. In general, the degree of volume loss determines the number of sessions required for desired results. Injections are performed 4 to 8 weeks apart. Anecdotal reports state that premenopausal women and postmenopausal women on hormone replacement therapy (HRT) require fewer sessions than postmenopausal women not on HRT. Postmenopausal women not on HRT may require up to 8 sessions. Men tend to correct more quickly than women for unknown reasons. After the procedure, the patient's skin is strenuously massaged with topical arnica (for its anticoagulant properties) for about 5 minutes to reduce bruising, pain, and nodule formation. Patients should be told to massage the treated area for 5 minutes every night for 5 nights.

Sculptra treatments can be combined with other fillers for instant gratification. In this case, Sculptra is injected first, then massage with arnica is performed, and then the HA or collagen filler is applied in the treatment area. Sculptra is often used in the cheeks and cheekbone area while an HA filler is used in the nasolabial folds, marionette lines, and the lips. Alternatively, a course of 3 to 4 Sculptra treatments is performed and then an HA filler is used after Sculptra at the last visit. Sculptra should always be used first, then massaged, before the HA is injected so that massaging will not affect the placement of the HA filler.

Benefits

Sculptra does not require prior skin testing. It is ideal for treating volume loss in the cheeks, nasolabial folds, and the malar area. It is also effective for volumetric and textural correction of the body (i.e., buttocks, arms, cellulite dimples).

Once the desired result is achieved, results last about 18 to 24 months.[70,75,77] The correction is very natural looking. Having been used successfully in various medical devices for more than 30 years, PLLA has an established safety record.[78] Moreover, new product guidelines and injection techniques (e.g., using a more dilute product, avoiding overcorrection, not injecting too superficially, and postinjection massage) have reduced the incidence of side effects (i.e., formation of granulomas and nodules) as compared to when the product was originally packaged as NewFill.[79]

Drawbacks

Sculptra injection results are not immediate and multiple courses are required to achieve the optimal cosmetic effect, with the number of treatments depending on the volume of the defect being treated.[71] Preinjection reconstitution can contribute to scheduling limitations because it must be made at least 2 hours in advance. Injecting suspension can be slightly difficult because of recurrent clogging of the needles, which leads to frequent needle changes. Adverse events are rare, but PLLA can cause postinjection site pain, bruising, and swelling, as compared to other products, partly because of the larger needle used. Adding lidocaine to the diluent mitigates injection pain. Ecchymoses can be reduced by mixing epinephrine into the PLLA suspension and taking bromelain supplements (500 mg twice daily) *after* injection (see Chapter 21) Hyperkinetic areas (e.g., crow's feet and the corner of the mouth) and regions with thin skin (e.g., around the eyes, smoker's lines above the lips) should not be treated with Sculptra because of irregular papules that can emerge. Most lumps that do arise are from superficial administration of Sculptra and are not visible, although they are palpable by the patient. Reassuring patients that these lumps are transient in nature is important. Intralesional steroids or 5-fluorouracil are other adjunctive methods of management. Nodule and hematoma formation are the other rare adverse effects that have been reported but are less likely if the new injection guidelines are followed.[80,81] Sculptra injection technique is very different than that of HA fillers and the learning curve is higher. In addition, there is lack of reversibility as with HA fillers, which is extremely problematic in the setting of accidental intra-arterial injection or vascular occlusion. Specialized training is required by the manufacturers of Sculptra before they will sell the product to a physician.

Permanent Fillers

Although the current momentum in the cosmetic market is toward the more temporary filler products which are safer, permanent fillers are very popular outside the US because of the lower cost. Many of these products are used by unskilled practitioners and lead to disfiguring results. If practitioners are to use a permanent filler, they should be skilled in the technique and certain of the patient's expectations. In the primary author's opinion, it is best to use a temporary filler first, to make sure that a patient is pleased, before proceeding to a permanent or semipermanent option. These nonbiodegradable fillers stay enclosed by the skin for an indeterminate and lasting period of time. However, these fillers are not to be used for and by the lighthearted. They are associated with rare, significant side effects such as granulomas, migration, and asymmetry and are best implanted into a patient experienced with prior soft tissue augmentations and by a proficient physician. Remember, as with anything enduring, if one is not pleased with the results, one has to live with long-term consequences.

Polymethylmethacrylate

Overview

In October 2006, the FDA approved the novel permanent filler polymethylmethacrylate (PMMA), known as Artefill (Suneva Medical, Inc., San Diego, CA) for the correction of nasolabial folds.[82] Artefill is a third generation PMMA and is constituted with 20% homogenous PMMA microspheres suspended in equilibrium with partly denatured 3.5% bovine collagen (from enclosed US cattle herds) and 0.3% lidocaine. In the US, Artefill was rebranded as Bellafill (Suneva Medical, Inc., San Diego, CA, USA) in 2014.[83] It is currently FDA approved for the correction of nasolabial folds and moderate to severe, atrophic facial acne scars,[83,84] but has been used successfully to correct malar atrophy and infraorbital rhytides and for nonsurgical rhinoplasty.[85–89] It is currently the only permanent filler FDA approved in the US. As opposed to the original European product, Artecoll, which contained different sized microspheres of PMMA that potentially contributed to a higher risk of granulomas, Bellafill is composed of uniformly sized PMMA microspheres (30–50 μm) that are less likely to result in the formation of granulomas. Small size, uniformity, and smoothness are refined characteristics of Bellafill that promote biocompatibility and resistance to phagocytic degradation and migration as well as ensure encapsulation by collagen leading to lasting nonimmunogenic results.

Similar to CaHA and PLLA, the volumizing effects of PMMA can be explained by its ability to stimulate collagen synthesis. PMMA relies on the host response for its ultimate cosmetic effects as opposed to direct fill at the time of treatment, although subtle effects from immediate fill can be seen at the time of treatment. After injection, a subclinical inflammatory response occurs leading to collagen production and formation of a network of fibroplasia encapsulating the PMMA microspheres.[90] The viscosity of the collagen carrier appears to be important in ensuring even distribution of the microspheres, which facilitates tissue ingrowth between the microspheres.[90–92] These microspheres then remain in place, acting as a scaffold for new collagen and tissue synthesis as the bovine collagen carrier is metabolized.[90] Unlike CaHA and PLLA, PMMA microspheres are too large to be degraded by phagocytosis and, therefore, are permanent after injection into the skin.[90]

Bellafill is packaged in a kit of three 0.8 ml and two 0.4 ml syringes that are injected through a 26-gauge needle into the deep dermis and subdermal plane via a linear technique without overcorrection.[93] Atrophic scars can be treated using both a retrograde linear threading and serial puncture technique. After injection, gentle massage is recommended to evenly distribute material in the skin and prevent clumping. Bellafill must be stored via refrigeration (2–10 °C) and warmed before use. In order to achieve optimal correction of rhytides, two to three treatment sessions, a few months apart, are suggested. Like Sculptra, specific injection training for Bellafill is required.

Benefits

Bellafill offers the dual action of immediate wrinkle correction from collagen (lasting about 1–3 months) and permanent deep-fold ablation from PMMA (lasting for more than 5 years).[82,94] The stimulatory influence of PMMA on the surrounding skin, causing fibroblast and collagen proliferation around the material starting at 1 month allows for sustained, long-term soft tissue augmentation not necessarily achieved with other biologic fillers that are completely metabolized within 6 months to 1 year.[90,92,93] Bellafill is ideal for atrophic acne scars and significant volume loss or unsatisfactory results or duration with other filler products. Lidocaine content eliminates the necessity for alternative anesthesia and alleviates intrainjection discomfort. As compared to the standard of bovine collagen, PMMA filler has been found to be superior in efficacy with a comparable safety profile.[90,95] Widely used in implantable medical devices for more than 50 years, PMMA has a long safety record.

Drawbacks

Bellafill contains bovine collagen; therefore, skin testing prior to injections is strongly advised 4 weeks prior to treatment to reduce the incidence of hypersensitivity. This means that patients cannot be treated on the initial office visit. Furthermore, because of Bellafill's higher viscosity, more administration pressure is required by the clinician, and the product is more difficult to inject than collagen and HA fillers. Although the majority of side effects caused by Bellafill are mild and transient (e.g., swelling, redness, hypersensitivity, and temporary lumpiness, which is amenable to massage), rare moderate to severe effects have been reported including granuloma and inflamed nodule formation developing months to years after injection.[90,95] The rate of granuloma formation following PMMA implantation is about 1.9% based on the current literature.[95] While granuloma formation is often treated using systemic or intralesional steroids with or without 5-fluorouracil, management can be difficult. Surgical excision can be used but not favorable as the typical location of these granulomas or nodules is often in cosmetically sensitive areas on the face. A recent anecdotal report demonstrated the success of the long-pulsed 1064 nm neodymium-doped yttrium aluminum garnet (Nd:YAG) laser in decreasing the size of nodules following PMMA injection in seven patients. While this appears to be a promising additional modality for management of this undesirable delayed complication of PMMA, the true efficacy of laser therapy in this setting remains unknown. Due to the reported lumpiness with this product, it is currently discouraged for lip augmentation, perioral or periocular areas, or any superficial wrinkle correction. Having to inject through a larger bore needle may induce more posttreatment edema and ecchymoses, which require slightly longer downtime. The disadvantage of implanting permanent fillers such as Bellafill is the inability to foretell the long-term appearance of the patient; since the skin changes with age, the natural look may be altered. Time will tell the exact risk-to-benefit ratio of this filler.

Silicone
Overview

Silicone is composed of dimethylsiloxane chains linked by oxygen with varied viscosity based on the length of the polymer. Used in patients since the 1940s, the liquid form of this product is one of the oldest soft tissue augmentation materials.[96] The use of this injectable filler is fraught with controversy because the initial unpurified product was associated with long-term disfiguring side effects, including migration and granuloma formation. It was illegal to perform silicone injections in the US in some states until recently. However, because of the purification of liquid silicone and honing of the injection technique, this soft tissue filler has returned and is very popular in Brazil. At the turn of the 21st century, the FDA approved two forms of medical-grade silicone oils: ADATO (or Sil-ol 5000, Bausch & Lomb Surgical, Inc., San Dimas, CA) with 5000 centistoke (cs) viscosity and Silikon 1000 (Alcon Laboratories, Inc., Fort Worth, TX) with 1000 cs viscosity. These are both indicated for the ophthalmologic uses of retinal tamponade and detachment. Although neither of these products have been approved by the FDA as skin injectables, they are used off-label. Furthermore, there are ongoing studies in the US assessing the safety and efficacy of SilSkin (a 1000 cs, highly purified polydimethylsiloxane, OFAS-Therapeutic Silicone Technologies, Inc., New York, NY) for the correction of nasolabial folds and HIV-associated lipoatrophy. Pilot studies in patients with HIV-lipoatrophy have revealed satisfactory results with minimal side effects.[97]

Similar to PMMA, PLLA, and CaHA, silicone oil biostimulates the surrounding skin to slowly generate a focal fibro-granulomatous reaction that leads to a permanent volumizing. Zappi and colleagues analyzed the microscopic biologic behavior of liquid silicone and concluded that it was an effective, durable (up to 23 years), and immunologically compatible filler.[98] Silikon 1000 is the preferred injectable filler over ADATO because of its lower viscosity and therefore easier injectability. It is stored at room temperature and packaged as clear oil. The proficiency in the injection technique is the crucial variable in achieving successful soft tissue augmentation with silicone. The favored technique is a serial puncture of microdroplets and subdermal implantation of 0.01 to 0.02 ml silicone aliquots at 2 to 4 mm intervals using a glass syringe with a 30-gauge needle. The key is not to overcorrect. Instead, patients should anticipate steady changes with multiple treatment sessions, 1 to 2 months apart, in order to achieve the most natural and safe outcome in several months.

Benefits

Since it is immunologically inert, no prior skin testing is required. Practitioners with experience in using Silikon have reported its value in correcting wrinkles and scars, augmenting lips, and pan-facial contouring of deeper folds and valleys.[99] Its low cost and longevity are obvious benefits.

Drawbacks

As with any temporary filler, potential long-term consequences should be broached when discussing this treatment option with patients. Most side effects associated with medical-grade silicone injectables are minimal and include anticipated temporary pain, edema, bruising, and redness.[100,101] The pain is likely because of the absence of anesthetic as part of the product formulation, so appropriate preprocedure anesthesia should be provided. However, it is important to keep in mind that rare reports of appropriately injected, purified silicone causing significant nodules, granulomas, cellulitis, and ulceration also exist.[102–107] The skill of the physician is crucial as this is a permanent filler. The primary author has seen myriad unhappy patients who have lumps and asymmetry after treatment by other physicians (**Figs. 25-7** and **25-8**). In addition,

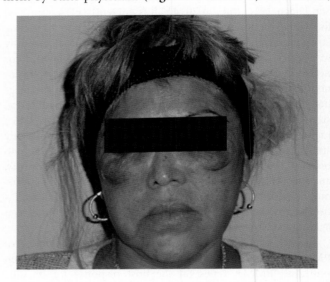

FIGURE 25-7. Patient who had an unknown substance injected by an aesthetician in a hotel room in Miami. Analysis of biopsy material showed silicone. No treatments have been effective long-term in this patient.

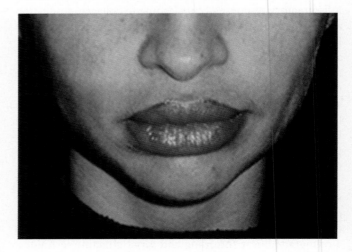

FIGURE 25-8. Patient who had silicone injections to the lips. She is unhappy with the large size of her lips.

many patients who are treated by nonphysicians are treated with impure silicone. This results in disfiguring edema and long-term complications. Reported management strategies to treat complications of silicone injections by nonphysicians have included intralesional steroids, tacrolimus, cyclosporine, and imiquimod with minimal and short-term improvement. Surgical excision has remained the only effective long-term treatment.

Autologous Fat

Overview

Originating in the 1890s, transplantation of fat from a patient's excess adipose areas to other skin defects is the oldest soft tissue augmentation method.[3] Fat injection filling has gained recognition for several reasons. Naturally, the patient's own cells are unlikely to cause sensitivity or inflammation and are therefore considered supremely biocompatible. Furthermore, the technique of fat implantation has undergone remarkable polishing over many years, especially with the advent of harvesting subcutis through liposuction. The procedure is a multistep process, whereby the fat cells are obtained from the buttock, thigh, and abdominal regions, then segregated, stored (refrigerated up to 18 months), and injected back into the patient's subcutis on the face, hands, and any other areas requiring volume enhancement. As anticipated, this process is more invasive, time-consuming, both for the clinician to prepare and perform as well as the patient to recover from, as well as more costly. In effect, the optimal efficacy with minimal adverse effects is mainly achieved in the hands of a qualified dermatologic surgeon. Approximately 0.1 ml aliquots of fat are inserted into subcutis through a 17- to 18-gauge needle via a tunneling technique, without overcorrection.[108] Post procedure massage is recommended for proper shaping of contours.

Benefits

Because of its autologous character, lipotransfer is unlikely to cause sensitivity and reactivity of the tissue, minimizing potential long-term side effects and obviating prior testing. Nasolabial folds, sunken cheeks, tear troughs, marionette lines, scars, and lips are the most appropriate areas of correction with fat. Furthermore, fat transfer provides a reported duration of about 12 months; although the concrete duration is controversial.[109] Because the injectable material used is the patient's own tissue, its use decreases the amount of money spent on the actual filler. The procedure also has an attractive double gain, where two cosmetic areas can be simultaneously addressed, lipoexcess and lipodystrophy. Stem cells have been isolated from fat cells. It is believed that the stem cells found in fat lead to increased skin rejuvenation (see Chapter 3). When performed by a skilled physician, the results of lipotransfer are remarkable.[110]

Drawbacks

Fat injections require prophylactic local or regional anesthesia. Because of the fact that the procedure is more surgically invasive, more complex preparations and settings are required with longer and more frequent office visits. Although the harvesting portion can cause a longer recovery time and an increased risk of side effects (e.g., infection, scarring), the actual injection has a similar adverse event profile to the other fillers (e.g., edema, redness, bruising, and discomfort lasting a few days).[48] Another variable to consider when selecting candidates for this procedure is to ensure that the patient has a sufficient graft supply. In some patients, the fat injections last several years and in other patients the injections last merely months. Many tricks are employed to try and increase longevity, but at this time there are no guarantees.

HOW TO SELECT A FILLER

There are many filler options available, so deciding on which filler to use is difficult. The A, B, C, D approach can help (**Table 25-5**). "A" stands for *assess* the patient. Determine which areas can be treated with the greatest potential for improvement. Look at the entire face and decide where to get the "best bang for the buck." For example, if the patient has prominent nasolabial folds, there are two main options: treating the nasolabial folds, or treating the cheek or cheekbone area to add volume that will improve the fold by pulling the skin back. A patient with large round cheeks would do better to have the nasolabial fold treated (**Fig. 25-9**), while a patient with thin cheeks and facial volume loss would have a better result if the cheeks were treated (**Figs. 25-10** and **25-11**). As a practitioner, it is important to form your own impression first before the patient tells you his or her thoughts. In some

TABLE 25-5	The A, B, C, D Approach to Choosing the Appropriate Filler
A—Assess the patient	a. Which areas show aging or asymmetry?
	b. Which areas can be easily corrected?
	c. Imagine how the patient will look if various areas are corrected.
	d. Determine the best areas of injection and proceed to next step.
B—Budget	a. Determine the patient's financial budget.
	b. Determine the patient's time budget.
	c. Refine plan in your mind about which areas are most important to treat.
C—Considerations	a. Learn more about the patient.
	b. What bothers the patient most?
	c. Ask about prior experience with fillers.
	d. Are there any religious restrictions?
	e. Can the patient return for future treatments?
	f. Does the patient have an event coming up?
	g. Is the patient on anticoagulants?
	h. Are there any concerns about outcome?
	i. Are there any product promotions going on?
D—Device	a. Assess pros and cons of available fillers.
	b. Match attributes of fillers to what was learned in steps A, B, and C.
	c. Choose the appropriate device.
	d. Discuss the plan with the patient.

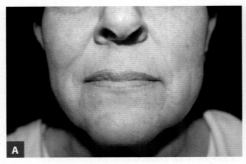 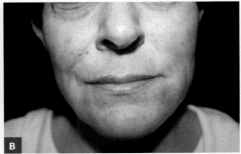

FIGURE 25-9. A. Those with a normal to large buccal fat pad are best treated with injections directly into the nasolabial folds and marionette lines. **B.** Immediately after treatment of nasolabial folds and marionette lines.

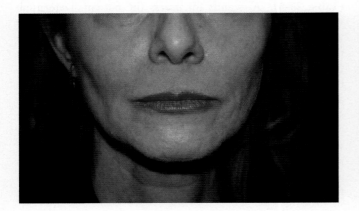

FIGURE 25-10. This patient has thin cheeks from buccal fat pad wasting; therefore, she is a good candidate for a filler such as Sculptra, Juvéderm Ultra, or Restylane to the cheek area below the cheekbones.

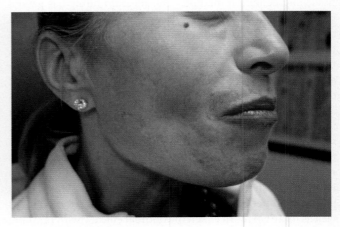

FIGURE 25-11. This patient appears to have buccal fat pad wasting, but actually is missing a tooth on this side, leading to the defect. A dental consult is more appropriate for this patient rather than a dermal filler.

cases, you may notice factors that the patient does not even realize are contributing to an aged appearance (**Figs. 25-12** and **25-13**). These observational skills are developed with experience. **Table 25-6** provides an overview of which fillers are best suited for each facial area. Once you have an idea of what areas would make the most significant impact if treated, then move to the "B" section, which is ***budget***. It is crucial to determine how much money the patient is willing to spend. It is often the case that the budget is lower than what is necessary, so the physician must determine what areas to treat to achieve the best cosmetic effect possible within the patient's budget. In addition, the practitioner must consider the patient's time budget or schedule. For example, if a patient is visiting from another country and planning to leave the following day, a course of Sculptra injections is not an option. Once the time and financial budgets have been determined, the practitioner should talk to the patient about other ***considerations***. The most important question is what facial feature bothers him or her the most. It is often different than what the physician sees. Patient happiness is contingent on improving what he or she sees as the problems, not what bothers the physician. The following or similar questions may be appropriate to frame such a discussion, then, in the

attempt to identify the most suitable filler for a patient: What have you tried before? Were you satisfied with the results? Why or why not? What concerns do you have? Are you a frequent bruiser? Are you worried that your lips will look too big? Do you hate it when your lipstick bleeds up into the lines on the top lip? Do you have any religious restrictions? Do you have any events coming up? What amount of downtime can you tolerate? These are all critical issues in determining the most appropriate filler. Once all this information has been gathered, the physician must choose a filling ***device*** that meets all the criteria. It is a relatively easy choice after the preceding questions have been answered. In addition, the physician should have many filler choices on hand to give the patient the best result.

Injection Technique

Injection technique varies from filler to filler. Most physicians use a threading (either an anterograde or retrograde), fanning, or serial puncture technique. Most collagen and HA fillers are injected at a 45-degree angle (**Fig. 25-14**). It is important to be individually trained on the injection techniques of each filler. Fillers can be used in combination with botulinum toxins and other cosmetic

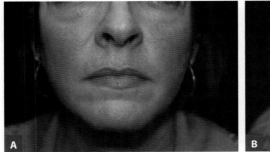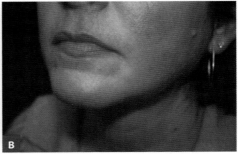

FIGURE 25-12. (A and **B)** Soft tissue loss around the mental area is often one of the first signs of facial aging. It is hard to capture on film and patients do not really notice it until it is pointed out to them.

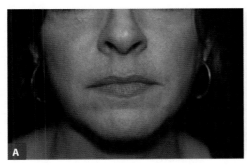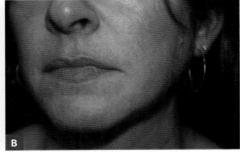

FIGURE 25-13. (A and **B)** Once the soft tissue around the mental bone has been filled, the face looks more youthful. An HA filler was used in this patient.

TABLE 25-6	Fillers by Region (Listed from the Top of the Face Down)
Forehead lines	
CosmoDerm I	
Restylane Fine Lines, Juvéderm[18], or Prevelle Silk	
Zyderm I	
Belotero Balance	
RHA2	
Raising lateral brows (almost any will work)	
CosmoPlast	
Evolence	
Juvéderm Ultra	
Juvéderm Ultra Plus	
Restylane Lyft	
Prevelle Silk	
Prevelle Dura	
Radiesse	
Restylane	
Zyplast	
Revanesse Versa	
RHA3	

Glabella (use with caution)
CosmoDerm I
Zyderm I
Belotero Balance
RHA2
Tear trough (soft fillers preferred)
Hylaform
Juvéderm Ultra
Prevelle Silk
Restylane
Restylane Refyne
Revanesse Versa
RHA2
RHA3
Crow's feet
CosmoDerm I
Juvéderm Ultra
Prevelle Silk
Restylane
Zyderm I
RHA2

(Continued)

TABLE 25-6	Fillers by Region (Listed from the Top of the Face Down) (*Continued*)
Cheek bones	
Juvéderm Ultra	
Juvéderm Ultra Plus	
Juvéderm Voluma	
Prevelle Dura	
Prevelle Silk	
Radiesse	
Restylane	
Restylane Lyft	
Restylane Defyne	
Sculptra	
RHA3	
RHA4	
Nasolabial folds	
CosmoPlast	
Evolence	
Juvéderm Ultra	
Juvéderm Ultra Plus	
Restylane Lyft	
Prevelle Silk	
Prevelle Dura	
Radiesse	
Restylane	
Sculptra	
Zyplast	
Revanesse Versa	
RHA3	
RHA4	
Vermilion border of the lip	
CosmoPlast	
Evolence	
Juvéderm Ultra	
Juvéderm Volbella	
Prevelle Silk	
Restylane	
Restylane Kysse	
RHA2	
Belotero Balance	
Zyplast	
Body of the lip	
Hylaform	
Prevelle Silk	
Restylane Silk	
Restylane Kysse	

Juvéderm Ultra	
Juvéderm Volbella	
Marionnette lines	
CosmoPlast	
Evolence	
Juvéderm Ultra	
Juvéderm Ultra Plus	
Restylane Lyft	
Prevelle Silk	
Prevelle Dura	
Radiesse	
Restylane	
Restylane Refyne	
Restylane Defyne	
Revanesse Versa	
Zyplast	
RHA3	
RHA4	
Pre-jowl sulcus	
CosmoPlast	
Evolence	
Juvéderm Ultra	
Juvéderm Ultra Plus	
Restylane Lyft	
Prevelle Silk	
Prevelle Dura	
Radiesse	
Restylane	
Sculptra	
Zyplast	
RHA4	

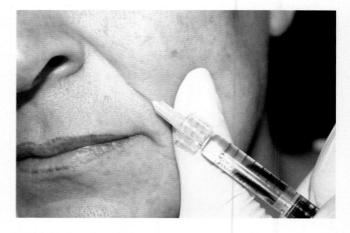

FIGURE 25-14. Most collagen and HA fillers are injected using a 45-degree angle. Injecting over the thumb can help ensure this angle.

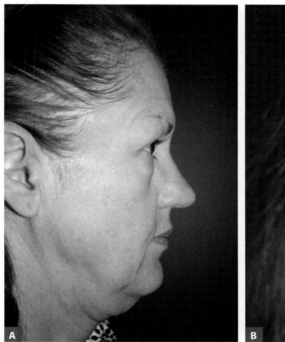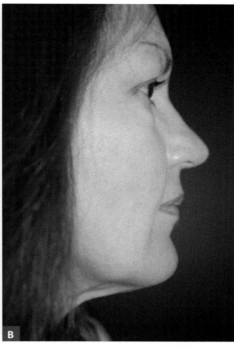

FIGURE 25-15. (A and **B)** A patient treated with Radiesse to several facial areas and with Botox to the platysma. (Photos courtesy of Lisa Grunebaum, MD.)

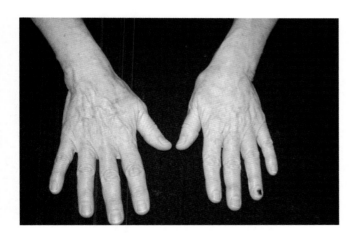

FIGURE 25-16. The hand on the left is before Radiesse treatment. The image with the dark nail is after Radiesse. (Photos courtesy of Lisa Grunebaum, MD.)

procedures (**Fig. 25-15**). Although this chapter focused on facial use, fillers can also be injected in other areas of the body such as the hands, and some fillers are now FDA approved for such use (i.e., Radiesse, Restylane Lyft) (**Fig. 25-16**). Many injection techniques can be used. However, it is difficult to teach various techniques without video and live demonstrations. The American Academy of Dermatology and the American Society of Dermatologic Surgeons offer training courses for dermatologists to develop the necessary skills required to provide optimal results for patients.

SUMMARY

Filling agents for soft issue augmentation are now widely available, based on the long-standing successful track records of the earliest products. Most agents in the soft tissue augmentation armamentarium can be safely used alone or in combination. The most frequently used agents are those that contain HA. Given the widespread popularity of soft tissue augmentation and the ever-present need to develop safer fillers that last longer than the current products, new fillers frequently enter the market. In short, the demand for soft tissue augmentation procedures has steadily increased since their inception and research is ongoing to develop products that address the shortcomings of the earlier products while incorporating and expanding on their advantages. Moreover, the "coupling" of fillers with other cosmetic interventions (e.g., botulinum toxin injections) enhances their longevity and efficacy, and creates an overall realistically aesthetic appearance.[111] To keep astride with the rapidly changing cosmetic dermatology arena, it behooves the aesthetic practitioner to be aware of the current availability, application, and future potential of dermal fillers.

References

1. ASDS survey on dermatologic procedures: report of 2018 procedures. http://www.asds.net/portals/0/PDF/procedures-survey-results-presentation-2018.pdf;2019. Accessed date December 6, 2020.
2. International Society of Aesthetic Plastic Surgery. ISAPS global statistics: ISAPS international survey on aesthetic/cosmetic procedures in 2018. Available at: https://www.isaps.org/wp-content/

uploads/2020/10/ISAPS-Global-Survey-Results-2018-1.pdf. Accessed December 6, 2020.

3. Neuber F. Fettransplantation. *Chir Kongr Verhandl Dsch Gesellch Chir.* 1893;22:66.

4. Klein A, Elson M. The history of substances for soft tissue augmentation. *Dermatol Surg.* 2000;26:1096.

5. Gniadecka M, Nielsen OF, Wessel S, et al. Water and protein structure in photoaged and chronically aged skin. *J Invest Dermatol.* 1998;111:1129.

6. Cosmetic Surgery National Data Bank 2005 Statistics (American Society of Aesthetic Plastic Surgery website). http://www.surgery.org/download/2005stats.pdf. Accessed June 7, 2006.

7. Levy PM, De Boulle K, Raspaldo H. Comparison of injection comfort of a new category of cohesive hyaluronic acid filler with preincorporated lidocaine and a hyaluronic acid filler alone. *Dermatol Surg.* 2009;35(Suppl 1):332–336.

8. Levy PM, De Boulle K, Raspaldo H. A split-face comparison of a new hyaluronic acid facial filler containing pre-incorporated lidocaine versus a standard hyaluronic acid facial filler in the treatment of naso-labial folds. *J Cosmet Laser Ther.* 2009;11:169–173.

9. Weinkle SH, Bank DE, Boyd CM, et al. A multi-center, double-blind, randomized controlled study of the safety and effectiveness of Juvéderm injectable gel with and without lidocaine. *J Cosmet Dermatol.* 2009;8:205–210.

10. Raspaldo H, De Boulle K, Levy PM. Longevity of effects of hyaluronic acid plus lidocaine facial filler. *J Cosmet Dermatol.* 2010;9:11–15.

11. Lupo MP, Swetman G, Waller W. The effect of lidocaine when mixed with large gel particle hyaluronic acid filler tolerability and longevity: a six-month trial. *J Drugs Dermatol.* 2010;9:1097–1100.

12. Monheit GD, Campbell RM, Neugent H, et al. Reduced pain with use of proprietary hyaluronic acid with lidocaine for correction of nasolabial folds: a patient-blinded, prospective, randomized controlled trial. *Dermatol Surg.* 2010;36: 94–101.

13. Lemperle G, Rullan PP, Gauthier-Hazan N. Avoiding and treating dermal filler complications. *Plast Reconstr Surg.* 2006;118:92S.

14. Wang F, Garza LA, Kang S, et al. In vivo stimulation of a de novo collagen production caused by cross-linked hyaluronic acid dermal filler injections in photodamaged human skin. *Arch Dermatol.* 2007;143:155–163.

15. Turlier V, Delalleau A, Casas C, et al. Association between collagen production and mechanical stretching in dermal extracellular matrix: in vivo effect of cross-linked hyaluronic acid filler. A randomised, placebo-controlled study. *J Dermatol Sci.* 2013;69:187–194.

16. Carruthers JDA, Carruthers JA, Humphrey S. Fillers and neocollagenesis. *Dermatol Surg.* 2014;40:S134–S136.

17. Baumann LS, Shamban AT, Lupo MP, et al. Comparison of smooth-gel hyaluronic acid dermal fillers with cross-linked bovine collagen: a multicenter, double-masked, randomized, within-subject study. *Dermatol Surg.* 2007;33:S128.

18. McCracken MS, Khan JA, Wulc AE, et al. Hyaluronic acid gel (Restylane) filler for facial rhytids: lessons learned from American Society of Ophthalmic Plastic and Reconstructive Surgery member treatment of 286 patients. *Ophthal Plast Reconstr Surg.* 2006;22:188.

19. Narins RS, Brandt F, Leyden J, et al. A randomized, double-blind multicenter comparison of the efficacy and tolerability of Restylane versus Zyplast for the correction of nasolabial folds. *Dermatol Surg.* 2003;29:588.

20. Jiang B, Ramirez M, Ranjit-Reeves R, et al. Noncollagen dermal fillers: a summary of the clinical trials used for their FDA approval. *Dermatol Surg.* 2019;45:1585–1596.

21. US Food and Drug Administration. Soft Tissue Fillers Approved by the Center for Devices and Radiological Health. 2020. Available from: https://www.fda.gov/MedicalDevices/ProductsandMedicalProcedures/CosmeticDevices/WrinkleFillers/ucm227749.htm. Accessed December 1, 2020.

22. Fagien S, Bertucci V, von Grote E, et al. Rheologic and Physicochemical Properties Used to Differentiate Injectable Hyaluronic Acid Filler Products. *Plast Reconstr Surg.* 2019;143: 707-720.

23. Wilson AJ, Taglienti AJ, Chang CS, et al. Current applications of facial volumization with fillers. *Plast Reconstr Surg.* 2016;137(5):872e–889e.

24. Herrmann JL, Hoffman RK, Ward CE, et al. Biochemistry, physiology, and tissue interactions of contemporary biodegradable injectable dermal fillers. *Dermatol Surg.* 2018;44:S19–S31.

25. Sundaram H, Rohrich RJ, Liew S, et al. Cohesivity of hyaluronic acid fillers: development and clinical implications of a novel assay, pilot validation with a five-point grading scale, and evaluation of six U.S. Food and Drug Administration-approved fillers. *Plast Reconstr Surg.* 2015;136:678–86.

26. Jones D, Flynn T. Hyaluronic acids: clinical applications. In: Jones D, ed. *Injectable fillers: principles and practice.* Chichester, UK: Wiley-Blackwell; 2010: 158–174.

27. Segura S, Anthonioz L, Fuchez F, et al. A complete range of hyaluronic acid filler with distinctive physical properties specifically designed for optimal tissue adaptations. *J Drugs Dermatol.* 2012;11(1 Suppl):s5-s8.

28. Rzany B, Bayerl C, Bodokh I, et al. Efficacy and safety of a new hyaluronic acid dermal filler in the treatment of moderate nasolabial folds: 6-month interim results of a randomized, evaluator- blinded, intra-individual comparison study. *J Cosmet Laser Ther.* 2011;13:107–112.

29. Solish N, Bertucci V, Percec I, et al. Dynamics of hyaluronic acid fillers formulated to maintain natural facial expression. *J Cosmet Dermatol.* 2019;18:738–746.

30. Swift A, von Grote E, Jonas B, et al. Minimal recovery time needed to return to social engagement following nasolabial fold correction with hyaluronic acid fillers produced with XpresHAn technology. *Clin Cosmet Investig Dermatol.* 2017;10:229–238.

31. Restylane Kysse. [Product and Safety Information]. Galderma Laboratories, L.P.; 2020.

32. Hilton S, Sattler G, Berg A-K, et al. Randomized, evaluator-blinded study comparing safety and effect of two hyaluronic acid gels for lips enhancement. *Dermatol Surg.* 2018;44: 261–269.

33. Kablik J, Monheit GD, Yu L, et al. Comparative physical properties of hyaluronic acid dermal fillers. *Dermatol Surg.* 2009;35(Suppl 1):302–312.

34. Fallacara A, Manfredini S, Durini E, et al. Hyaluronic acid fillers in soft tissue regeneration. *Facial Plast Surg.* 2017;33:87–96.

35. Monheit GD, Prather CL. Juvéderm: a hyaluronic acid dermal filler. *J Drugs Dermatol.* 2007;6:1091.

36. Sundaram H, Cassuto D. Biophysical characteristics of hyaluronic acid soft-tissue fillers and their relevance to aesthetic applications. *Plast Reconstr Surg.* 2013;132:5S–21S.

37. Carruthers J, Carruthers A, Tezel A, et al. Volumizing with a 20-mg/mL smooth, highly cohesive, viscous hyaluronic acid filler and its role in facial rejuvenation therapy. *Dermatol Surg.* 2010;36(Suppl 3):1886–92.

38. Sundaram H, Voigts B, Beer K, et al. Comparison of the rheological properties of viscosity and elasticity in two tissue fillers: calcium hydroxylapatite and hyaluronic acid. *Dermatol Surg.* 2010;36:1859–65.

39. Sadeghpour M, Quatrano NA, Bonati LM, et al. Delayed-onset nodules to differentially crosslinked hyaluronic acids: comparative incidence and risk assessment. *Dermatol Surg.* 2019;45:1085–1094.

40. Humphrey S, Jones DH, Carruthers JD, et al. Retrospective review of delayed adverse events secondary to treatment with a smooth, cohesive 20-mg/ml hyaluronic acid filler in 4500 patients. *J Am Acad Dermatol.* 2020;83:86–95.

41. Artzi O, Loizides C, Verner I, et al. Resistant and recurrent late reaction to hyaluronic acid-based gel. *Dermatol Surg.* 2016;42:31–7.

42. BELOTERO BALANCE®. [Instructions for use]. EM00494. Merz North America, Inc.; 2016.

43. Akinbiyi T, Othman S, Familusi O, et al. Better results in facial rejuvenation with fillers. *Plast Reconstr Surg Glov Open.* 2020;8:e2763. doi:10.1097/GOX.0000000000002763.

44. Rzany B, Converset-Viethel S, Hartmann M, et al. Efficacy and safety of 3 new resilient hyaluronic acid fillers, crosslinked with decreased BDDE, for the treatment of dynamic wrinkles: results of an 18-month, randomized controlled trial versus already available comparators. *Dermatol Surg.* 2019;45:1304–1314.

45. Monheit G, Kaufman-Janette J, Joseph JH, et al. Efficacy and safety of two resilient hyaluronic acid fillers in the treatment of moderate-to-severe nasolabial folds: a 64-week, prostepctive, multicenter, controlled, randomized, double-blinded, and within-subject study. *Dermatol Surg.* 2020;46:1521–1529.

46. Hirsch RJ, Lupo M, Cohen JL, et al. Delayed presentation of impending necrosis following soft tissue augmentation with hyaluronic acid and successful management with hyaluronidase. *J Drugs Dermatol.* 2007;6:325.

47. Hirsch RJ, Cohen JL, Carruthers JD. Successful management of an unusual presentation of impending necrosis following a hyaluronic acid injection embolus and a proposed algorithm for management with hyaluronidase. *Dermatol Surg.* 2007;33:357.

48. Goldberg RA, Fiaschetti D. Filling the periorbital hollows with hyaluronic acid gel: initial experience with 244 injections. *Ophthal Plast Reconstr Surg.* 2006;22:335.

49. Lambros V. The use of hyaluronidase to reverse the effects of hyaluronic acid filler. *Plast Reconstr Surg.* 2004;114:277.

50. Alsaad SM, Fabi SG, Goldman MP. Granulomatous reaction to hyaluronic acid: a case series and review of the literature. *Dermatol Surg.* 2012;38:271.

51. Brody HJ. Use of hyaluronidase in the treatment of granulomatous hyaluronic acid reactions or unwanted hyaluronic acid misplacement. *Dermatol Surg.* 2005;31:893.

52. Ryu C, Lu JE, Zhang-Nunes S. Response of twelve different hyaluronic acid gels to varying doses of recombinant human hyaluronidase. *J Plast Reconstr Aesthet Surg.* 2020. https://doi.org/10.1016/j.bjps.2020.10.051.

53. Pierre A, Levy PM. Hyaluronidase offers an efficacious treatment for inaesthetic hyaluronic acid overcorrection. *J Cosmet Dermatol.* 2007;6:159.

54. Jones, DH. Update on emergency and nonemergency use of hyaluronidase in aesthetic dermatology. *JAMA Dermatol.* 2018;154:763–764.

55. Cohen JL, Biesman BS, Dayan SH, et al. Treatment of hyaluronic acid fil- ler-induced impending necrosis with hyaluronidase: consensus recommendations. *Aesthet Surg J.* 2015;35:844–849.

56. Chesnut C. Restoration of visual loss with retrobulbar hyaluronidase injection after hyaluronic acid filler. *Dermatol Surg.* 2018;44(3):435–437.

57. Chiang YZ, Pierone G, Al-Niaimi F. Dermal fillers: pathophysiology, prevention and treatment of complications. JEADV. 2017;31:405–413.

58. Hirsch RJ, Brody HJ, Carruthers JD. Hyaluronidase in the office: a necessity for every dermasurgeon that injects hyaluronic acid. *J Cosmet Laser Ther.* 2007;9:182.

59. Goldman MP. Optimizing the use of fillers for facial rejuvenation: the right tools for the right job. *Cosmetic Dermatology.* 2007;20(7S):14.

60. RADIESSE injectable implant. [Instructions for use]. Franksville, WI: Merz North America, Inc.; 2013.

61. Hee CK, Shumate GT, Narurkar V, et al. Rheologic properties and in vivo performance characteristics of soft tissue fillers. *Dermatol Surg.* 2015;41: S373–S381.

62. Breithaupt A, Fitzgerald R. Collagen stimulators: poly-L-lactic acid and calcium hydroxyl apatite. *Facial Plast Surg Clin N Am.* 2015;23:459–469.

63. Berlin AL, Hussain M, Goldberg DJ. Calcium hydroxylapatite filler for facial rejuvenation: a histologic and immunohistochemical analysis. *Dermatol Surg.* 2008;34(Suppl 1):S64–S67.

64. Moers-Carpi M, Vogt S, Santos BM, et al. A multicenter, randomized trial comparing calcium hydroxylapatite to two hyaluronic acids for treatment of nasolabial folds. *Dermatol Surg.* 2007;33(Suppl 2):S144–S151.

65. Baumann L, Narins R, Werschler P. Dermal filling agents: evaluating more choices for your patients. Part 2. *Skin Aging.* 2007;15(6):50.

66. Rullan PP, Olson R, Lee KC. The use of intralesional sodium thiosulfate to dissolve facial nodules from calcium hydroxylapatite. *Dermatol Surg.* 2020;46(10):1366–1368.

67. Robinson DM. In vitro analysis of the degradation of calcium hydroxylapatite dermal filler: a proof-of-concept study. *Dermatol Surg.* 2018;44:S5–S9.

68. Robinson DM. Commentary on the use of intralesional sodium thiosulfate to dissolve facial nodules from calcium hydroxylapatite. *Dermatol Surg.* 2020;46(10):1368–1370.

69. Voigts R, DeVore DP, Grazer JM. Dispersion of calcium hydroxylapatite accumulations in the skin: animal studies and clinical practices. *Dermatol Surg*. 2010;36:798–803.

70. Majola A, Vainionpää S, Vihtonen K, et al. Absorption, biocompatibility, and fixation properties of polylactic acid in bone tissue: an experimental study in rats. *Clin Orthop Relat Res*. 1991;268:260.

71. Gogolewski S, Jovanovic M, Perren SM, et al. Tissue response and in vivo degradation of selected polyhydroxyacids: polylactides (PLA), poly(3-hydroxybutyrate) (PHB), and poly (3-hydroxybutyrate-co-3-hydroxyvalerate) (PHB/VA). *J Biomed Mater Res*. 1993;27:1135.

72. Viljanen JT, Pihlajamäki HK, Törmälä PO, et al. Comparison of the tissue response to absorbable self-reinforced polylactide screws and metallic screws in the fixation of cancellous bone osteotomies: an experimental study on the rabbit distal femur. *J Orthop Res*. 1997;15:398.

73. Fitzgerald R, Bass LM, Goldberg DJ, et al. Physiochemical characteristics of poly-l-lactic acid (PLLA). *Aesthet Surg J*. 2015;38(S1):S13–S17.

74. Vleggaar D, Fitzgerald R, Lorenc ZP. Composition and mechanism of action of poly-L-lactic acid in soft tissue augmentation. *J Drugs Dermatol*. 2014;13(4 Suppl):s29–s31.

75. Vleggaar D. Facial volumetric correction with injectable poly-L-lactic acid. *Dermatol Surg*. 2005;31:1511.

76. Vleggaar D, Bauer U. Facial enhancement and the European experience with poly-L-lactic acid. *J Drugs Dermatol*. 2004; 3:526.

77. Keni SP, Sidle DM. Sculptra (injectable poly-L-lactic acid). *Facial Plast Surg Clin North Am*. 2007;15:91.

78. Lowe NJ. Dispelling the myth: appropriate use of poly-L-lactic acid and clinical considerations. *JEADV*. 2006;20(Suppl 1):2.

79. Vleggaar D. Poly-L-lactic acid: consultation on the injection techniques. *JEADV*. 2006;20(Suppl 1):17.

80. Borelli C, Kunte C, Weisenseel P, et al. Deep subcutaneous application of poly-L-lactic acid as a filler for facial lipoatrophy in HIV-infected patients. *Skin Pharmacol Physiol*. 2005;18:273.

81. El-Beyrouty C, Huang V, Darnold CJ, et al. Poly-L-lactic acid for facial lipoatrophy in HIV. *Ann Pharmacother*. 2006;40:1602.

82. Cohen SR, Berner CF, Busso M, et al. Five-year safety and efficacy of a novel polymethylmethacrylate aesthetic soft tissue filler for the correction of nasolabial folds. *Dermatol Surg*. 2007;33:S222.

83. Gold MH, Sadick NS. Optimizing outcomes with polymethylmethacrylate fillers. *J Cosmet Dermatol*. 2018;17:298–304.

84. Karnik J, Baumann L, Bruce S, et al. A double-blind, randomized, multicenter, controlled trial of suspended polymethylmethacrylate microspheres for the correction of atrophic facial acne scars. *J Am Acad Dermatol*. 2014;71:77–83.

85. Mills DC, Camp S, Mosser S, et al. Malar augmentation with a polymethylmethacrylate-enhanced filler: assessment of a 12-month open-label pilot study. *Aesthet Surg J*. 2013;33:421–430.

86. Mani N, McLeod J, Sauder MB, et al. Novel use of polymethyl methacrylate (PMMA) microspheres in the treatment of infraorbital rhytids. *J Cosmet Dermatol*. 2013;12:275–280.

87. Rivkin A. A prospective study of non-surgical primary rhinoplasty using a polymethylmethacrylate injectable implant. *Dermatol Surg*. 2014;40:305–313.

88. Cohen S, Dover J, Monheit G, et al. Five-year safety and satisfaction study of PMMA-collagen in the correction of nasolabial folds. *Dermatol Surg*. 2015;41(Suppl 1):S302–S313.

89. Lemperle G, Romano JJ, Busso M. Soft tissue augmentation with artecoll: 10-year history, indications, techniques, and complications. *Dermatol Surg*. 2003;29(6):573–587.

90. Lemperle G, Knapp TR. Artefill permanent injectable for soft tissue augmentation: I. mechanism of action and injection techniques. *Aesth Plast Surg*. 2010;34:264–272.

91. Smith KC, Melnychuk M. Five percent lidocaine cream applied simultaneously to the skin and mucosa of the lips creates excellent anesthesia for filler injections. *Dermatol Surg*. 2005;31:1635–1637.

92. Murray CA, Zloty D, Warshawski L. The evolution of soft tissue fillers in clinical practice. *Dermatol Clin*. 2005;23:343–363.

93. Bellafill. [Instructions for Use]. Suneva Medical Inc.; 2021.

94. Cohen SR, Berner CF, Busso M, et al. ArteFill: a long-lasting injectable wrinkle filler material--summary of the U.S. Food and Drug Administration trials and a progress report on 4- to 5-year outcomes. *Plast Reconstr Surg*. 2006;118:64S.

95. Paulucci BP. PMMA Safety for facial filling: review of rates of granuloma occurrence and treatment methods. *Aesth Plast Surg*. 2020;44:148–159.

96. Narins RS, Beer K. Liquid injectable silicone: a review of its history, immunology, technical considerations, complications, and potential. *Plast Reconstr Surg*. 2006;118:77S.

97. Jones DH, Carruthers A, Orentreich D, et al. Highly purified 1000-cSt silicone oil for treatment of human immunodeficiency virus-associated facial lipoatrophy: an open pilot trial. *Dermatol Surg*. 2004;30:1279.

98. Zappi E, Barnett JG, Zappi M, et al. The long-term host response to liquid silicone injected during soft tissue augmentation procedures: a microscopic appraisal. *Dermatol Surg*. 2007;33:S186.

99. Hevia O, Cazzaniga A, Brandt F, et al. Liquid injectable silicone (polydimethylsiloxane): four years of clinical experience. [Abstract] *J Am Acad Dermatol*. 2007;56(2):AB1.

100. Hevia O. Six-year experience using 1,000-centistoke silicone oil in 916 patients for soft-tissue augmentation in a private practice setting. *Dermatol Surg*. 2009;35(Suppl 2):1646.

101. Jones DH, Carruthers A, Orentreich D, et al. Highly purified 1000-cSt silicone oil for treatment of human immunodeficiency virus-associated facial lipoatrophy: an open pilot trial. *Dermatol Surg*. 2004;30:1279.

102. Duffy DM. Liquid silicone for soft tissue augmentation. *Dermatol Surg*. 2005;31:1530.

103. Ficarra G, Mosqueda-Taylor A, Carlos R. Silicone granuloma of the facial tissues: a report of seven cases. *Oral Surg Oral Med Oral Pathol Oral Radiol Endod*. 2002;94:65.

104. Pimentel L, Barnadas M, Vidal D, et al. Simultaneous presentation of silicone and silica granuloma: a case report. *Dermatology*. 2002;205:162.

105. Poveda R, Bagán JV, Murillo J, et al. Granulomatous facial reaction to injected cosmetic fillers--a presentation of five cases. *Med Oral Patol Oral Cir Bucal*. 2006;11:E1.

106. Schwartzfarb EM, Hametti JM, Romanelli P, et al. Foreign body granuloma formation secondary to silicone injection. *Dermatol Online J.* 2008;14:20.

107. Altmeyer MD, Anderson LL, Wang AR. Silicone migration and granuloma formation. *J Cosmet Dermatol.* 2009;8:92.

108. Broder KW, Cohen SR. An overview of permanent and semipermanent fillers. *Plast Reconstr Surg.* 2007;118:7S.

109. Bucky LP, Kanchwala SK. The role of autologous fat and alternative fillers in the aging face. *Plast Reconstr Surg.* 2007;120:89S.

110. Stashower M, Smith K, Williams J, et al. Stromal progenitor cells present within liposuction and reduction abdominoplasty fat for autologous transfer to aged skin. *Dermatol Surg.* 1999;25:945.

111. Michaels J, Michaels B. Coupling advanced injection techniques for cosmetic enhancement. *Cosmetic Journal.* 2008;21:31.

CHAPTER 26

Lasers and Light Devices

Lisa Akintilo, MD, MPH
Evan A. Rieder, MD

SUMMARY POINTS

What's Important?

1. Lasers and light therapy are expanding areas of dermatology with increasing applications for conditions of skin, hair, and mucosa. The principle of selective photothermolysis has completely transformed methods of laser and light delivery to the skin, with increased focus on targeting specific chromophores (e.g., hemoglobin, melanin, water) to achieve a desired clinical result.

What's New?

1. Novel picosecond technology has transformed the utility and scope of laser therapy with increased safety for patients of many skin types. Picosecond lasers are particularly effective for tattoo removal and photorejuvenation.

What's Coming?

1. Skin tightening devices, particularly radiofrequency and ultrasound, are rapidly expanding on the horizon of medical devices with enhanced clinical effects and improved patient safety profiles.

Don't Forget

1. Lasers and light therapy are effective methods of treating various dermatological conditions.
2. Picosecond technology is relatively new and has been shown to be an excellent method of laser delivery with increased safety.
3. Laser and light therapy can be used in patients of all skin types; however, patients with skin of color warrant increased caution to avoid adverse events such as post-inflammatory pigment alteration.

Patient Education Points

1. Patients should be educated on pre- and post-laser and light therapy instructions to maximize the benefits and minimize the risks of these procedures.

Clinical Pearls

1. With appropriate knowledge of their functions and safety profile, laser and light therapy can be a highly effective tool for dermatologists to utilize in treating a wide variety of patients.

From Einstein's initial proposals regarding photons and quantum mechanics to the first laser being invented by T.H. Maiman at the Hughes Research Laboratory in 1960, research and development of lasers has steadily blossomed into a multibillion-dollar industry. Scientists, physicians, and laypeople alike have been especially fascinated by the capabilities and possibilities of laser light. Beginning with the ruby laser, these instruments have quickly become an integral part of dermatology. Lasers and light devices are now used in almost every medical specialty and our daily lives, including eye surgery, dentistry, barcode scanners, lighting displays, and even traffic lights.

LASER BASICS

To realize their usefulness in medicine and aesthetic medicine in particular, it is important to understand the basics of laser terminology (Box 26-1), which are based on the principles of electromagnetic radiation. Understanding the interactions of light with the skin is critically important for both patient/provider safety and to help make clinical treatments more successful. The word "laser" is actually an acronym for Light Amplification by Stimulated Emission of Radiation. A laser amplifies light by stimulating photons, storing them, and releasing them as identical photons in the form of a light beam. To accomplish this, the laser must have a source of energy, referred to as the pump. Energy from the pump is absorbed by atoms in the form of photons. The atoms then emit photons in the form of light. This light is amplified between mirrors to generate a high intensity beam. Of note, this entire process occurs in the lasing medium. Many lasers are named based on the type of lasing medium that they contain. Lasing mediums can be liquid (e.g., rhodamine dye), solid (e.g., crystals such as alexandrite, neodymium-doped yttrium aluminum garnet, or ruby; or semiconductors such as diode) or gas (e.g., argon, CO_2, or helium-neon).

Several of the instruments in the cosmetic armamentarium are not true lasers. This fact does not render them any less useful in treating patients, but is an important distinction. The importance lies in the nature of the interaction between light and skin. In 1983, Anderson and Parish introduced the theory of selective photothermolysis.[1] This theory states that the selectivity of a laser for its target relies on the fact that different wavelengths of light will be absorbed by different chromophores in the skin (Box 26-2). This allows for the selective destruction of these targets without damaging surrounding tissues. To accomplish this, the pulse duration (defined as the duration of active lasing, also known as pulse width) should be sufficiently long enough to heat tissue to the level of destruction, but not long enough for that heat to transfer out of the target to surrounding normal skin. The ideal pulse duration for selective destruction of a target is determined by the size of that target. The time it takes for the target to dissipate two-thirds of its heat to the surrounding tissue is directly proportional to its size and is termed the thermal relaxation time (Trt). The pulse duration should be equal to or shorter than this Trt in order to selectively destroy a target and not the normal surrounding tissue. If the laser pulse is longer than the Trt, there is risk of unwanted damage to other tissues.

It is important to note that lasers can emit light in a continuous fashion or in pulses. The theory of selective photothermolysis only applies to pulsed laser systems, as continuous lasing results in bulk heating of tissue, and hence little selectivity. Nearly all dermatologic lasers emit pulsed light.

When light of any wavelength or intensity hits the skin, four possible results ensue. One, the light can be directly *reflected* from the skin. This usually takes place at the stratum corneum and is the reason that practitioners wear protective eyewear even when not lasing near the eye. Light that passes through the stratum corneum can be *scattered* by collagen in the dermis or *transmitted* through the dermis to the subcutaneous tissues. Finally, light that results in actual work being done on the tissues is the light that is *absorbed*.

There are three main chromophores that can be absorbed in the skin. Each of these target chromophores absorbs light at a different wavelength (**Fig. 26-1**). By using these absorption spectra, we can specifically select a laser with a wavelength that will be absorbed by the chromophore. This allows us to treat the target and not the normal skin. When the target tissue is beneath the epidermis, treatment of the target without damage to the epidermis is difficult to achieve without epidermal protection. Such protection is achieved via cooling systems which are critical in many laser procedures. There are several modes of cooling used in lasers today, including contact (copper tips, sapphire tips, ice, aqueous gels) and non-contact (cryogen spray, forced refrigerated air) methods.[1] Employing these methods reduces injury to the epidermis. Conversely, employing too much cooling when the target is in the epidermis results in an ineffective treatment. Cooling systems are essential in laser hair removal, as high energies are needed to produce damage to the hair follicle. Applying this much energy to the skin without cooling the epidermis would result in catastrophic epidermal damage. Even with cooling, in some instances complete epidermal protection may still be unattainable, particularly in patients with darker skin types.

The energy of lasers is expressed in Joules. Fluence is the energy per area, expressed in Joules per centimeter squared (J/cm2). The power of a laser is expressed in Watts. When using lasers in clinical applications, it is important to remember all aspects of the laser, including wavelength, pulse duration, fluence, and cooling. Lasers are just machines; it is up to the operator to adjust and use them correctly to achieve desired clinical results and minimize risk of adverse effects.

In the next sections, the use of lasers by clinical diagnosis will be reviewed. Several lasers can be used for each type of lesion, some more effectively than others. The most effective lasers for each condition will be discussed.

BOX 26-1	A device is not deemed a true laser unless it fulfills three criteria:
Monochromicity: the device emits light of a single wavelength. Collimation: all waves travel in a single direction. Coherence: all waves are in phase with each other.	

BOX 26-2	The three main chromophores in the skin include:
Water Hemoglobin Melanin	

VASCULAR LASERS

There are many different vascular lesions that can be treated with lasers. This treatment modality first became popular with the advent of the argon laser in the 1970s. Since that

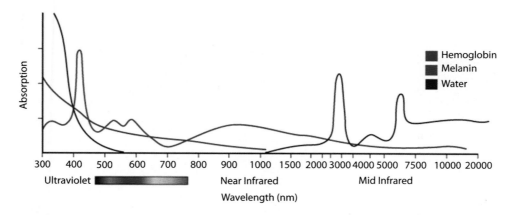

FIGURE 26-1. Absorption spectrum for the three primary skin chromophores. (Reproduced with permission from Dr. Joely Kaufman, MD.)

time, several laser systems targeting vascular lesions have been developed. The chromophore for vascular lesions is hemoglobin, which may be oxygenated or deoxygenated based on the type of lesion. The peak absorption by hemoglobin lies between 400 and 600 nm. It is for this reason that most lasers used for vascular lesions emit light with wavelengths within this range. However, because longer wavelengths penetrate deeper with less scattering by collagen, wavelengths outside the range of 400–600 nm can also be used for deeper vascular lesions. Lesions amenable to laser treatment with a vascular wavelength include hemangiomas, nevus flammeus (port-wine stains), rosacea, lymphangiomas, venous lakes, angiomas, telangiectasias, spider veins, and poikiloderma of Civatte. Vascular lasers can also successfully treat a variety of other dermatologic conditions including verruca vulgaris, keloids and hypertrophic scars, and striae.

Early vascular lasers were associated with a high incidence of dyspigmentation and scarring. Recognition of the importance of selective photothermolysis and pulse widths ultimately allowed for safe and effective treatment of vascular lesions without these adverse events. For optimal and safe results, the hemoglobin target must absorb light, generate heat, and coagulate the vessel all without damaging surrounding tissue. Because of the dermal location of vessels, the need for epidermal cooling when treating vascular lesions is critical when using wavelengths that are also within the melanin absorption spectrum. Longer wavelength vascular lasers can safely be operated without epidermal cooling.

The pulsed dye laser (PDL) was introduced in 1989 and remains the gold standard in laser treatment for hemangiomas. The original pulsed dye laser operated at a wavelength of 577 nm. Subsequent generations of PDLs have slightly longer wavelengths, corresponding to deeper penetration. Longer-wavelength lasers, however, operate further outside the peak absorption of hemoglobin, and therefore require more fluence for comparable results. Today, the most popular systems used for vascular lesions are the PDL (585 nm), long-pulsed dye laser (595 nm), the potassium titanyl phosphate (KTP, 532 nm), and the 1064 nm neodymium-doped yttrium aluminum garnet

TABLE 26-1	Vascular Laser and Light Devices	
Laser Type	**Wavelength (Nm)**	**Laser Devices**
Pulsed dye lasers	585, 595+1064	Candela Vbeam Cynosure Cynergy
Intense pulsed light	500–1200	Lumenis One, Lumenis IPL Quantum, Palomar StarLux, Palomar MediLux
Diodes	940	Dornier
KTP	532 (for cutaneous and endovenous)	
Long-pulsed Nd:YAG	1064	Cutera Xeo, Cutera Coolglide, Candela Gentle Yag, Laserscope Lyra, Wavelight Mydon, Cynosure Acclaim
Nd:YAG for endovenous	1320	Cooltouch CTEV

A 1064 nm handpiece for vascular lesions is also available on several IPL devices.

(Nd:YAG). There are also a few diode systems that are very effective for vascular lesions, including a 940 nm diode that functions very well for facial telangiectasias, spider veins on the body, and angiomas (Table 26-1).

PDL devices, with a target chromophore of oxyhemoglobin, are effective for telangiectasias on the face, neck, and chest, but perform less well on the body (**Fig. 26-2**). This is related to the short wavelength and superficial penetration of the laser. PDLs are also used for vascular malformations in adults and children, including hemangiomas, port-wine stains, and lymphangiomas. PDLs available today come equipped with cryogen cooling, various spot sizes, and adjustable pulse durations. The desired pulse duration should be adjusted to the vessel diameter and its thermal relaxation time. As previously mentioned, the larger the vessel diameter is, the longer the optimal pulse

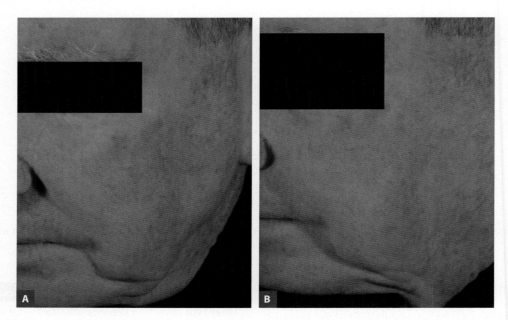

FIGURE 26-2. A. Before treatment with PDL for telangiectasia. **B.** After treatment with PDL for telangiectasia. (Reproduced with permission from Dr. Joely Kaufman, MD.)

width should be. Very short pulse widths lead to vessel rupture and resultant purpura. Historically, this common but aesthetically undesirable side effect made PDLs very unpopular with cosmetic patients. Recent use of longer pulse widths and double passes has resulted in comparable efficacy for telangiectasias, with little purpura. Still, for treatment of hemangiomas and port-wine stains, purpuric settings are often needed for adequate lesion clearing. Beyond purpura, PDL side effects include blistering, post-inflammatory pigment alteration (PIPA) from cryogen spray, as well as scarring from overly aggressive fluences. Lesions on the chest and neck should always be treated with lower energies than those on the face.

The potassium titanyl phosphate (KTP) laser, with a wavelength of 532 nm, is also highly absorbed by oxyhemoglobin. It has proven to be at least as effective for facial telangiectasias as PDLs.[2] Furthermore, it can also be used for port-wine stains and angiomas. KTP lasers can operate in a range of longer pulse durations, resulting in no purpura. Shortcomings are related to a short wavelength and lack of penetration. As such, treatment with the KTP is most effective for very superficial vessels. In addition, treatment of tanned or richly pigmented skin should be performed with caution (if at all), as the 532 nm wavelength is well absorbed by melanin and can cause epidermal injury even with contact cooling.

Longer-wavelength lasers such as the 1064 nm Nd:YAG or 940 nm diode can also be used effectively for vascular lesions such as facial telangiectasias, hemangiomas, or port-wine stains;[3] they are also useful for patients with skin of color, conferring an attenuated risk of dyspigmentation and bruising. The longer wavelengths allow for deeper penetration and hence are excellent choices for the lower extremities. In addition, they are particularly useful for spider veins or high flow vessels on the face.

LASERS FOR PIGMENTED LESIONS

When treating pigmented lesions, it is important to consider the laser physics and the properties of the chromophores of interest. Melanosomes are very small and hence have a very short thermal relaxation time at approximately 1 millisecond. In order to selectively target melanin without harming surrounding tissue, pulse durations equal to or shorter than the thermal relaxation time of melanin are used. Q-switched and picosecond lasers, with pulse widths in the nano second and picosecond ranges respectively, are ideal for selective destruction of epidermal and dermal melanin in conditions such as café-au-lait macules, nevi of Ito and Ota, lentigines, and melanocytic nevi.

The clinical endpoint of treating pigmented lesions with laser therapy is whitening of the lesion with preservation of surrounding skin. Choosing which laser to use largely depends on the color and depth of the lesion to be treated. Longer wavelengths are better for deeper pigment and pigment in dark-skinned patients, whereas shorter wavelengths are used in more superficial lesions and fair-skinned patients.

The ruby was both the first laser invented and also the first to be used for removal of pigment. The ruby laser emits a wavelength very well absorbed by melanin. Unfortunately, it cannot distinguish between normal pigment and unwanted pigment. Thus, it fell out of favor for pigment and hair removal because of the high incidence of hypopigmentation.

Today the most common Q-switched lasers used for pigmented lesions are the Q-switched alexandrite (755 nm), Q-switched Nd:YAG (1064 nm), and the frequency-doubled Nd:YAG (532 nm) (**Fig. 26-3**). As mentioned above, picosecond lasers have been commercially available since 2013 and are particularly effective in treating pigmented lesions

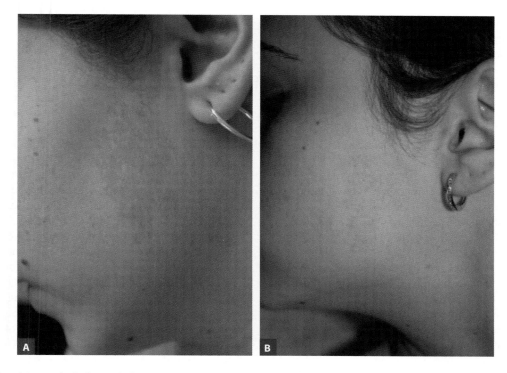

FIGURE 26-3. Café-au-lait macules before and after treatment with Q-switched laser. (Reproduced with permission from Dr. Joely Kaufman, MD.)

resistant to Q-switched laser therapy.[4-6] Picosecond lasers with wavelengths of 532, 755, and 1064 nm have been shown to be successful and safe in clearing pigmented lesions.[7,8]

Alternative approaches to treating pigmented lesions include intense pulsed light (IPL), KTP, and even PDL.[9-11] Lasers and light therapy have also been investigated in treating pigmented lesions recalcitrant to first- or even second-line therapy. For example, there is increasing evidence of benefit in melasma with use of Q-switched Nd:YAG, picosecond lasers, PDL, non-ablative fractional lasers, and IPL, in addition to a variety of devices used as vehicles for laser-assisted drug delivery.[12-16]

When using any laser with a wavelength absorbed by melanin, it is important to remember the laser does not distinguish between normal melanin in the skin and abnormal unwanted melanin. As such, the most common and significant complication with these lasers is pigment alterations. PIPA can occur as a direct result of the inflammation caused by high-peak energies or secondary to lasers ablating normal melanin. These complications are more common in darker skin types.

As a final point, physicians must be cautious in treating pigmented lesions with lasers. It is always best to be certain of a diagnosis before treating, as recurrent lesions may be evidence of malignancy such as melanoma.[17]

LASERS FOR TATTOOS

The prevalence of tattoos has continued to increase and they are inextricably linked to mainstream American culture. With continued improvement in color variety and ink quality, this upward trend should be expected to continue and with it, the subsequent rates of tattoo removal. In the past, laser tattoo removal involved the nonspecific ablation of skin overlying the tattoo, resulting in removal, but also pigment alterations and scarring. Nonselective removal procedures include the CO_2 laser, the argon laser, and dermabrasion. Currently, tattoo removal is performed primarily via selective photothermolysis, using tattoo ink as the target chromophore. Each ink color is absorbed by a different wavelength of light; hence the more ink colors in the tattoo, the more difficult it is to remove. Cosmetic tattoos are usually a blend of several different inks, rendering them extremely challenging to remove with laser. Professional tattoos typically place ink in the mid-dermis, requiring a device that can penetrate to this depth in order to achieve adequate treatment. Amateur tattoos typically use less ink and placement is more superficial, making them easier to remove.

Just like with removal of melanosomes from the skin, removal of tattoo ink must be achieved with a very short pulse-width system in the nanosecond (Q-switched) or picosecond range. Test spots are critically important to determine which laser is most optimal.

The ruby was the first Q-switched system available, and at a wavelength of 694 nm, it is good for removing black, blue, brown, green, and purple pigments.[18]

The alexandrite (755 nm) is also very effective at removing black, blue, brown, and green tattoo pigments.[19] This laser is the gold standard for removal of green tattoos as the other two Q-switched lasers tend to perform inadequately in this area.[20]

Prior to the development of picosecond lasers, the Nd:YAG (1064 nm) was the workhorse for professional tattoo removal because of its capacity for deep penetration. Q-switched Nd:YAG lasers are still used for the basic black ink seen in both amateur and professional tattoos, in addition to dark blue and brown pigments. The frequency-doubled Nd:YAG (532 nm) can be used for orange, red, and yellow pigments.

White pigment tattoos are best removed with fractional CO2 or Er:YAG lasers.

In recent years, picosecond lasers have emerged as the new gold standard in tattoo removal. These lasers deliver energy in shorter pulse durations and are more efficacious than previously used methods.[21-24] The first picosecond laser became commercially available in 2013 and required fewer treatments and lower fluence than Q-switched lasers.[25-28] A recently published study showed superiority of picosecond lasers to other tattoo removal laser devices for blue, green, and yellow tattoos.[7,8]

The most important aspect of tattoo removal is setting realistic expectations for the patient from the beginning. Laser tattoo removal is not an eraser, as many tattoos will not be completely removed no matter how many treatments are performed. In most cases, residual ink or a shadow of the tattoo may persist despite numerous treatment sessions. In addition, there are reports of some tattoo inks (particularly light/flesh-colored tattoos containing ferric oxides) actually darkening post-laser because of oxidation of the tattoo particles. This may result in an ink that requires an increased number of treatments. For the removal of professional tattoos, 6 to 10 treatments, spaced at least 6 weeks apart, may be required. For amateur tattoos, three to five treatments are generally effective.[29] In patients with darker skin types, tattoo removal may result in scarring or dyspigmentation. Many authors advocate the use of topical bleaching agents and sunscreen to reduce the number of competing chromophores (skin melanosomes) and decrease the risk of adverse events. With every patient, regular use of sunscreen in the treatment area is essential. Any patient with tanned skin in the area of interest should not be treated.

Wound healing and postoperative care are also essential parts of laser tattoo removal. Moist wound healing via topical emollient creams and dressings are recommended for all patients for 1 to 2 weeks after laser treatment. Straying from this regimen will increase the risk of post-inflammatory changes and scarring, in addition to delaying additional treatments.

LASERS FOR EPILATION

Hair removal is the most commonly performed cosmetic laser procedure. Countless salons, spas, and medical offices offer this service to their patients, all using a variety of different devices. Several methods of hair removal with lasers and light devices have been investigated in the literature. The most common of these is via selective photothermolysis, with melanin as the target chromophore in the hair shaft, outer root sheath, and hair bulb matrix. However, in order to permanently remove hair, one must eradicate not only the hair itself but also the reproducing cells of the follicle. Although the Trt of melanin is very short, simply destroying melanin would only result in hair fragmentation with temporary hair removal followed by subsequent regrowth. As such, the laser pulse duration will need to be longer than melanin's Trt so heat can diffuse from the melanin chromophore to the desired target of the follicular stem cells. It is important to note that about 15–30% long-term hair loss can be seen with each laser hair removal treatment, and often 3–12 treatment sessions are required to see optimal results.[30]

The choice of which laser to use for epilation should be based on three overarching factors: (1) the hair color (2) the hair caliber and (3) the patient's skin color. All of these factors must be adequately considered for successful hair removal. Light or fine hair can be treated at shorter wavelengths that absorb melanin well. In contrast, dark or coarse hair absorbs more light energy from laser devices and hence can be removed at longer wavelengths that typically are less absorbed by melanin. Melanin in the skin competes with melanin in the hair for laser absorption. Hence the darker the skin color, the more difficulty lasers have in distinguishing between these two melanin sources and the more challenging the treatment. As such, cooling is critical for protection of the epidermis and avoidance of burns and other adverse events. Hair with very little pigment (white, grey, or red/blonde) cannot be permanently removed due to the lack of an adequate laser target chromophore.

The alexandrite laser (755 nm) is currently the shortest wavelength hair removal system used and is often the laser of choice for light-skinned patients resulting in high efficacy, safety, and patient satisfaction.[31] One drawback of using the alexandrite, which has a wavelength that is highly absorbed by melanin, is that it needs to be used with extreme caution in darker skin types. Treatment of darker skin types with the alexandrite can result in PIPA; however, studies have shown safety and efficacy in using the alexandrite in Fitzpatrick Skin Types IV–VI.[32] In addition, use on recently tanned skin can also result in transient pigment abnormalities. There are also reports of paradoxical hypertrichosis after laser hair removal with the alexandrite, particularly in women with skin of color.[33]

The long-pulsed diode laser (800–810 nm) can be safely used on Fitzpatrick Skin Types I–V. Optimal results are achieved with coarse, dark hair. Studies have shown increased risk of side effects in patients with darker skin tones.[34]

The Nd:YAG (1064 nm) systems operate at a wavelength that is minimally absorbed by melanin. Consequently, this laser is effective for removal primarily of dark, coarse hairs. The introduction of this laser made laser hair removal widely and safely available to darker-skinned patients and it remains the gold standard for patients with Fitzpatrick Skin Types V–VI.

Comparisons of laser systems for hair removal have considered the clinical efficacy of the alexandrite, diode, and Nd:YAG. The alexandrite and the diode are comparable in efficacy and pain tolerability. The Nd:YAG was rated more painful and less efficacious in one study.[30,35] Other studies have shown comparable efficacy among all three laser systems.[36,37] See Table 26-2 for a list of lasers used for hair removal.

Intense pulsed light (IPL), discussed below, is not a laser but is widely utilized as a method of light-based hair removal.

TABLE 26-2	Hair Removal Light Devices
Wavelength	**Light Device**
694-nm ruby	Not currently used for hair removal
755-nm alexandrite	Candela GentleLASE, Cynosure Apogee
800–810-nm diode	Lumenis LightSheer, Opusmed F1 Diode, Syneron eLaser
1064-nm Nd:YAG	Candela GentleYag, Cutera Coolglide, Cynosure Apogee Elite

Several studies have shown IPL is inferior to other methods of photoepilation such as the Nd:YAG or alexandrite.[37]

Prior to full treatment, every patient should be evaluated by a physician trained in laser hair removal practices. Skin should not be tanned, damaged, or show any signs of infection. In darker-skinned patients, pretreatment with bleaching agents is often recommended to prevent PIPA. In addition to dyspigmentation, other risks of photoepilation that must be reviewed as part of the informed consent process include blisters, scar, folliculitis, infection, ulceration, or hives (**Figs. 26-5** and **26-6**).[30] For adequate removal, hair must have at least some pigment as melanin is the target chromophore for laser epilation. As such, patients must understand that white, grey, red/blonde, or very fine hairs will not be well removed by these devices. Prior to full treatment, test spots are generally performed. Full treatment can be carried out after 2 weeks provided there is a good response without adverse effects.

Immediately after therapy, treated areas should exhibit follicular edema and erythema (**Fig. 26-4**). This is the normal response to laser heating of the follicle. Postprocedural application of a class 5 or 6 topical steroid for 5 days is often used in darker skin types to avoid PIPA. Depending on the hair, treatment area, and skin type, complete removal can take anywhere from 3 to 12 sessions. These should be spaced approximately 1 month apart, longer for slower growing areas such as the legs and back. Sun protection is critical both before and after laser hair removal.

RESURFACING LASERS

Many lasers and light devices can be utilized for skin rejuvenation and treatment of rhytides. However, the most impressive results come from ablative resurfacing, which was first performed using the CO2 laser. Ablative lasers work by delivering a controlled wound to the skin: removing the epidermis while heating the underlying dermis. Eliminating of the outer layers of skin can help smooth contours, while deeper heating can stimulate the growth of collagen.

Since its introduction in 1968, the CO2 laser has been used for the treatment of scars, rhytides, and other signs of photoaging. At a wavelength of 10 600 nm, high water absorption from the CO2 laser results in rapid ablation of the epidermis. The erbium:YAG (Er:YAG), also used for ablative resurfacing,

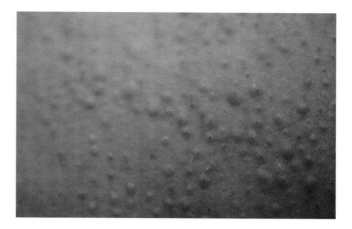

FIGURE 26-4. Follicular edema with laser hair removal. (Reproduced with permission from Dr. Joely Kaufman, MD.)

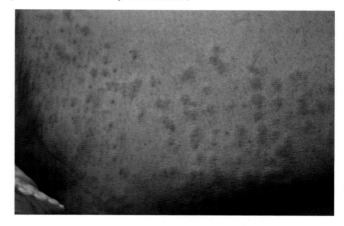

FIGURE 26-5. Hives after 1064 nm Nd:YAG laser hair removal. (Reproduced with permission from Dr. Joely Kaufman, MD.)

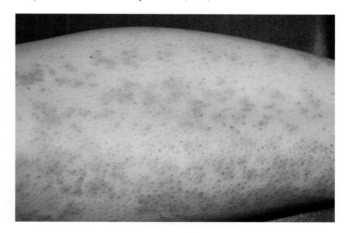

FIGURE 26-6. Urticaria after 755 nm alexandrite laser hair removal. (Reproduced with permission from Dr. Joely Kaufman, MD.)

emits a wavelength of 2940 nm and is even more highly absorbed by water. This intense absorption by water results in a more superficial depth with the Er:YAG when compared to the CO2 laser. With rapid vaporization of tissue from any ablative laser comes impressive tissue tightening and smoothing of the skin not achieved with most other non-ablative laser systems. Of all the existing ablative devices, tightening is most dramatic with the CO2 lasers. However, the possible complications, including scarring and hypopigmentation, and required downtime have resulted in a decrease in use of these systems. Recent technological updates have led to resurfacing devices that can achieve some of the tightening effects with lower risk of side effects.

Fractional Resurfacing

The concept of fractional resurfacing was introduced in 2004 by Manstein et al.[38] The term fractional refers to treating a portion or "fraction" of the skin. The definition does not specify laser type, spot size requirements, or wavelength; it just describes the manner of distribution of the treatment spots. By only treating microscopic areas in a single session, healing time is greatly reduced as each treated area is surrounded by normal viable skin from which migration of keratinocytes can occur. Each treatment spot is termed a microscopic treatment zone (MTZ). The MTZs heal via migration of the normal surrounding epidermis, as opposed to healing via differentiation.[39] Because of this unusual manner of spot placement, very high energies can be tolerated without bulk heating. Epidermal healing with a true microspot fractional device has been shown to be complete within 36 hours. This rapid healing time reduces incidence of infections, PIPA, and scarring.

Spot size is a critical part of fractional resurfacing. It is unclear how small the treatment spots must be to still obey the concept of fractional resurfacing. Fractional devices have energy adjustments just as with any other laser system. Additionally, they feature density adjustments which is also a critical part of treatment efficacy. The higher the density, the closer together the MTZs will be and the more aggressive the treatment. In addition, the higher the density, the greater the chance of PIPA. Ablative results can be obtained with very high energies at very high densities with any device.

Fractional devices come in two varieties: non-ablative and ablative. The first fractional non-ablative device, Fraxel Restore (Reliant Technologies), was introduced in 2004 as a 1550 nm non-ablative erbium-doped fiber fractionated laser. Since then, there has been development of many other fractional non-ablative devices targeting water as the chromophore. These lasers are termed non-ablative as they do not result in ablation, but rather coagulation of the epidermis. MTZs can be placed in a random or stamped pattern. Untreated skin surrounding each MTZ serves as a reservoir for epidermal cells which rapidly migrate to heal the treated areas. Higher energies translate to deeper penetration by the laser. Penetration well into the dermis results in better collagen production. MTZ diameters also increase as the energy is increased, so ideally each device should have density adjustments that would account for this change. To avoid bulk heating at very high energies the density of the treatment should be reduced with wider spacing of the MTZs. These non-ablative fractional devices are currently approved for treatment of periorbital rhytides, photoaging, and acne/surgical scars (**Fig. 26-7**). They have also been reported to be effective for striae, melasma, and lentigines. Fractional non-ablative lasers are safe for use off the face as well. Studies in darker-skin types indicate that fractional non-ablative lasers at wavelengths 1440, 1540, and 1550 nm are safe to use at adjusted energy and density settings.

Given the complication rates with fully ablative lasers, fractionally ablative devices have surpassed their fully

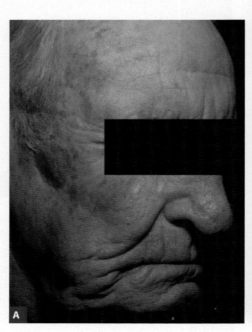
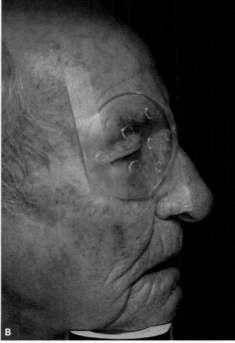

FIGURE 26-7. A. Surgical scar before fractional resurfacing with Fraxel. **B.** Surgical scar after fractional resurfacing with Fraxel. (Reproduced with permission from Dr. Joely Kaufman, MD.)

ablative counterparts. The reintroduction of CO2 devices with a fractional delivery system such as Fraxel Repair (Reliant Technologies) has changed conventional thought about the CO2 laser. Many other fractional ablative devices including the yttrium-scandium-gallium-garnet and Er: YAG can be used to achieve improvement in skin texture and tone with excellent results and minimal side effects.

More recently, picosecond lasers, both fractionated and unfractionated, have also been shown to be effective for photorejuvenation.[40] This is particularly true in skin of color patients given the increased safety profile of picosecond technology.[8,41]

NONLASER SYSTEMS

Intense Pulsed Light (IPL)

IPL devices are light instruments that may be utilized like lasers but are not true lasers because of their lack of coherent, monochromatic light. Some IPL systems are able to pump true laser devices in a separate handpiece, allowing for the purchase of one system for many indications. This has made these systems very popular since their introduction in 1995. The first system introduced, the Photoderm (Lumenis), was touted as the best modality for treating leg veins. It was only after early use of the system that its true capabilities of removing other skin lesions such as lentigines and telangiectasias were recognized.[42] IPLs have been used in several aforementioned conditions, including acne, facial telangiectasias, hair removal, lentigines, photodamage, poikiloderma, and spider veins.

IPL devices emit noncoherent polychromatic light with wavelengths between 400 and 1200 nm. These are flashlamp-based systems that contain an internal filter and several external cutoff filters. These external filters are used to block emission of light lower than the desired wavelengths. Many cutoff filters are available for each system and generally come in a handpiece that can be changed on the unit body. By using these filters, one can employ the theory of selective photothermolysis even with noncoherent, polychromatic light.

IPL devices also benefit from multiple adjustable pulse durations. Depending on the target and patient's skin type, pulse widths can be manipulated accordingly. Pulse widths can be shortened for treatment of targets with short Trts and lengthened for targets with longer Trts. This is important in treatment of telangiectasias; for example, when vessels seem to be resistant to treatment, simply changing the pulse width can result in an effective clinical response. Sequential pulsing, which allows time for cooling in between pulses, reduces the risk of bulk heating and scarring. Sequential pulsing is also thought to aid in the treatment of telangiectasias by generating deoxygenated hemoglobin with the first pulse and using this as the target for the second pulse.[12]

IPLs have also been favored over some lasers because of the large spot sizes available with these devices. This renders treatment of larger areas more feasible. Another important component of IPLs is the cooling apparatus. With cooling of the epidermis, complications such as blistering and dyspigmentation are kept to a minimum. Most IPL devices are now outfitted with a cooling device.

IPLs are one of the primary treatments for facial telangiectasias (**Figs. 26-8** and **26-9**), lentigines, poikiloderma, and photorejuvenation. Several IPLs also have interchangeable filter handpieces for hair removal, non-ablative skin tightening, and even fractional resurfacing. Preparation of a patient for IPL involves determining skin type and recent sun exposure. Treating a patient who is recently tanned may result in hypopigmentation caused by the absorption of melanin (**Fig. 26-10**). Patients should be instructed to use proper photoprotection both before and after treatments. Special care should be taken when using these devices to treat patients with darker skin types (Fitzpatrick Skin Types IV and V) due to risk of burning and PIPA (**Fig. 26-11**).[13,14] Pulse widths and delays between pulses should be lengthened when treating this population. Care should be taken to place pulses close together, as spacing pulses far apart can result in striping in patients with severe photodamage (**Fig. 26-12**). Striping can also occur in any patient when higher fluences are used and pulses are not

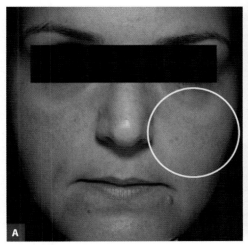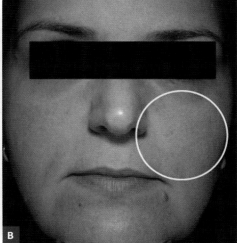

FIGURE 26-8. A. Rosacea before IPL treatment. **B.** Rosacea after one IPL treatment. For maximum results, two to three more will be needed. (Reproduced with permission from Dr. Joely Kaufman, MD.)

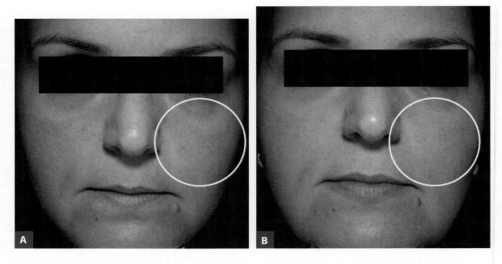

FIGURE 26-9. A. Rosacea before IPL. **B.** Rosacea after IPL. (Reproduced with permission from Dr. Joely Kaufman, MD.)

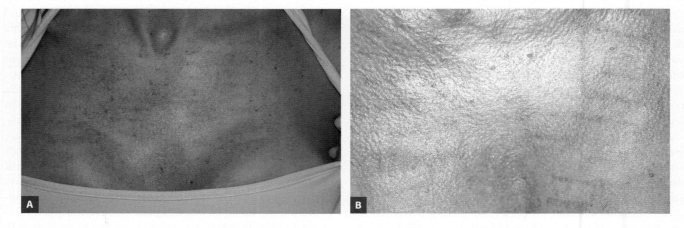

FIGURE 26-10. A. Undesired chest marks after IPL. **B.** Undesired red chest marks after IPL. (Reproduced with permission from Dr. Joely Kaufman, MD.)

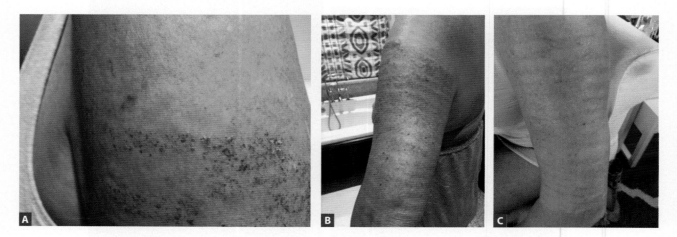

FIGURE 26-11. A. Burn after IPL performed on darkly pigmented skin. **B.** Close-up of burn after IPL performed on darkly pigmented skin. **C.** Post-inflammatory pigment alteration after IPL performed on darkly pigmented skin. (Reproduced with permission from Dr. Joely Kaufman, MD.)

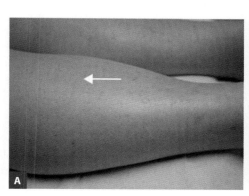
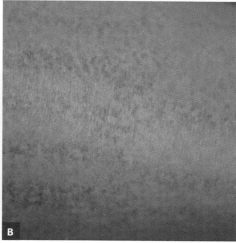

FIGURE 26-12. A. The IPL device can result in rectangular-shaped "striped" areas. These are treated by turning the handpiece 90 degrees for the next treatment. **B.** Closer view of striping from the IPL. This occurs most commonly on the legs and chest. (Reproduced with permission from Dr. Joely Kaufman, MD.)

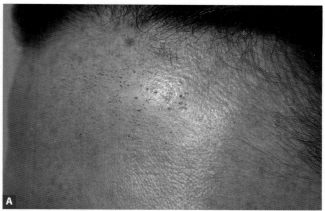

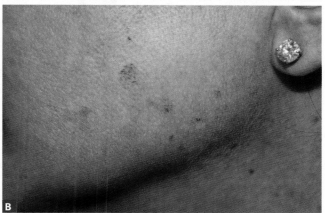

FIGURE 26-13. A. Normal forehead crusting after IPL. **B.** Normal jawline crusting after IPL. (Reproduced with permission from Dr. Joely Kaufman, MD.)

placed closely together. This complication is easily remedied by further treatment of the untreated areas.

When using IPLs, the laser is placed directly against a thin layer of ultrasound gel that has been placed on the skin surface. After treatment, treated areas are cleansed of all gel and sun protection is applied. A full-face treatment generally takes approximately 15 minutes. No topical anesthesia is required for most types of IPL treatment; however, some patients may require topical anesthesia for port-wine stains due to high fluences used. Three to five treatments at monthly intervals are recommended for clearing of photodamage.[43] More treatments are generally needed for port-wine stains and other vascular malformations. Downtime is minimal with mild darkening of treated lentigines and erythema of treated areas. Crusting and flaking can occur (**Fig. 26-13**). Patients can generally return to work immediately following the procedure, making IPLs very popular with patients. The ability to treat vascular and pigmented lesions with one instrument, as well as the rapid treatment times and consistent, reproducible results achieved when these devices are used properly have catapulted the IPL systems to the forefront of the industry.

Light Emitting Diodes

Light emitting diodes (LEDs) have garnered increased attention in recent years because of their ease of use and popularity as activation sources for aminolevulinic acid in photodynamic therapy. These devices emit non-coherent light of one primary wavelength or a short range of wavelengths. Unlike the previously mentioned instruments, LEDs do not operate by the theory of selective photothermolysis. LEDs operate on the theory of photobiomodulation, which is the ability of light to alter cellular activity. This capacity to change cellular metabolism via light energy has been demonstrated in the laboratory setting.[44] In subsequent in vivo studies LEDs have altered fibroblast and immune cell activity[45] and resulted in increases in collagen production.[46]

LEDs are an essentially nonthermal manner of treating the skin, and have been shown to be effective for several conditions when used as low level laser therapy (LLLT).[47] The advent of LED systems introduced a method by which large areas could be easily and painlessly treated. These systems consist of panels of lights of a particular wavelength or range of wavelengths. Currently available LEDs include blue, yellow, red, near infrared, and infrared. LEDs are most commonly used for acne and photorejuvenation. Reports of LED use in wound healing, psoriasis, eczema, and rhytides also appear in the literature.[48] The primary advantage of LEDs over lasers is the ease of painless, rapid, and safe treatment for all skin types. The main disadvantage is that the clinical results may not be as dramatic as some other laser and light procedures. Adverse events are generally mild and include dryness, stinging, and pigmentary changes.

Several LEDs are currently available on the market in a range of wavelengths and pulse sequencing. To date, it has not been demonstrated that one particular pulsing sequence is superior to any other. Such studies, along with comparisons of different wavelengths, are warranted to hone the use of these devices and perhaps expand the range of indications.

PHOTODYNAMIC THERAPY

The notion of photodynamic therapy (PDT) has been around since the early 1900s, but it was not until Kennedy et al. re-introduced PDT that its true advantages could be realized in dermatology.[49] PDT represents the use of a photosensitizer activated by light to selectively treat the skin. Currently approved use of PDT in the United States is for non-hyperkeratotic actinic keratoses of the face using 5-aminolevulinic acid (ALA) (Levulan® Kerastick, DUSA Pharmaceuticals) activated by blue LED light. However, several off-label indications have received attention in the literature and are now commonly used in cosmetic practice, including photoaging and sebaceous hyperplasia.[50,51] PDT can also be utilized for treatment of malignancies such as basal cell carcinoma or squamous cell carcinoma in situ.[52]

5-ALA is a prodrug applied to target areas and selectively absorbed by proliferating cells and pilosebaceous units. 5-ALA is metabolized into protoporphyrin IX (PpIX), which is innately photosensitizing. PpIX is then activated by several different wavelengths of light, resulting in the production of free radicals and selective destruction of target cells. Currently approved drugs for PDT include 5-ALA and the methyl ester of ALA (mALA) (Metvix, Galderma). Commonly used activation sources include LEDs (red and blue), pulsed dye laser (585 nm, 595 nm), and IPL devices.

PDT has recently been used to enhance the effectiveness of commonly used photorejuvenation procedures. Split-face studies have shown that the addition of ALA to traditional IPL treatments results in enhanced clinical amelioration of photoaging than IPL alone.[50,53] One group even demonstrated a greater increase in collagen production from PDT + IPL when compared with IPL alone.[54] The addition of ALA to IPL photorejuvenation procedures is useful for patients looking for treatment of precancerous lesions in addition to aesthetic treatment of photodamage.

TIGHTENING DEVICES

A newer area of investigation regarding light devices is skin tightening. Although non-ablative fractional resurfacing has

been quite successful at rejuvenation, it has proven insufficient in actual skin tightening. Evaluation of the action of "tightening" can be difficult as there is no standardized quantitative measure. Photographic assessments are generally inadequate, as even a slight change in subject position can alter the perceived result. In addition, it is almost impossible to measure any subtle tightening that occurs, especially if it occurs over many months. Nevertheless, many practitioners who use these devices do believe in their efficacy in a subset of patients.

The practice of skin tightening is based on the idea that collagen will contract when heat is applied. Several light- and energy-based devices have been introduced with the goal of delivering heat to the dermis while leaving the epidermis unharmed. This heat presumably causes collagen contraction and hence lifting. The epidermis remains protected as a result of dynamic cooling. The procedure is painless with resultant mild erythema that resolves in a few minutes to hours. Collagen contraction is immediate, but in addition to this contraction collagen synthesis is also induced. Not all patients respond to these treatments. Patient selection, energies used, and overall skin quality may play a role in determining if a treatment will be successful.

Traditional and ablative laser treatments utilizing CO_2 or erbium:YAG lasers have been investigated as a means to achieve skin tightening via neocollagenesis and remodeling as part of the wound healing process.[55,56] Nonablative lasers have also been shown to lead to improvement in skin laxity, although results are mild.[57]

Some non-laser tightening products include monopolar, bipolar, and combination unipolar and bipolar radiofrequency devices (Table 26-3). The theory is the same: nonselective heat is applied to the dermis via direct contact with the skin. The epidermis must be protected with a cooling system. Radiofrequency devices tend to be somewhat more painful than the infrared devices; as such, some radiofrequency instruments require application of topical anesthesia prior to the procedure. Adverse events are limited and include transient erythema, depressions, and superficial burns. No cases of permanent scarring have been reported. Radiofrequency is safe to perform in all skin types.

Other non-laser tightening products include infrared light and high-intensity focused ultrasound. Infrared light has been shown to be effective in treating skin laxity by means of dermal heating and targeting water as a chromophore, leading to

TABLE 26-3	Skin Tightening Devices
Device	**Technology**
Titan (Cutera)	Infrared light
Aluma (Lumenis)	Radiofrequency: Bipolar
Accent (Alma)	Radiofrequency: Bipolar, unipolar
ReFirme (Syneron)	Radiofrequency
Lux Deep IR (Palomar)	Infrared light (850–1350 nm)
ThermaCool (Thermage)	Radiofrequency: Monopolar

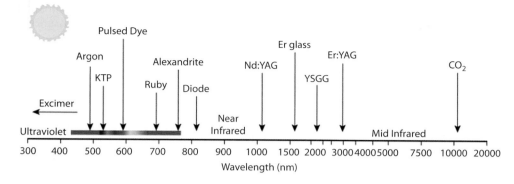

FIGURE 26-14. Wavelength diagram of available devices. KTP: potassium titanyl phosphate; Nd:YAG: neodymium-doped yttrium aluminium garnet; YSGG: yttrium scandium gallium garnet; CO_2: carbon dioxide. (Reproduced with permission from Dr. Joely Kaufman, MD.)

delayed collagen remodeling.[58] High-intensity focused ultrasound heats tissue with acoustic energy resulting in immediate tissue contraction and delayed collagen remodeling.[59-61] Both infrared and ultrasound systems can be safely used in all skin types.[62]

With nearly all laser and non-laser modalities, it is important to notify patients that improvements are gradual and may require 6 months to 1 year to appreciate final results.

SUMMARY

Since their introduction in 1960, lasers have continued to expand in popularity and availability (**Fig. 26-8**). Laser science was changed forever with the introduction of the theory of selective photothermolysis by Anderson and Parrish. Based on this theory, our understanding of how lasers can be used to treat numerous conditions has flourished. More recently, picosecond lasers have come to the forefront to effectively treat dermatologic conditions with minimized unwanted side effects. Paired with our continued understanding of wound healing, new developments in the laser industry have significantly increased the safety of these procedures while managing to improve efficacy. With each year comes the introduction of newer technologies with the goal of developing even safer and more effective devices (**Fig. 26-14**). It is recommended that practitioners start slow with any new device or new patient. Being too aggressive with any laser or light device can cause severe complications that unfortunately are sometimes permanent. Additional research in this area is ongoing, as are increased regulations in laser training and operation. Continued education, oversight, and refinement of laser technology and practice will ensure the safe and effective treatment of all patients.

References

1. Das A, Sarda A, De A. Cooling Devices in Laser therapy. *J Cutan Aesthet Surg.* 2016;9(4):215–219.

2. Uebelhoer NS, Bogle MA, Stewart B, Arndt KA, Dover JS. A split-face comparison study of pulsed 532-nm KTP laser and 595-nm pulsed dye laser in the treatment of facial telangiectasias and diffuse telangiectatic facial erythema. *Dermatol Surg.* 2007;33(4):441–448.

3. Tierney E, Hanke CW. Randomized controlled trial: Comparative efficacy for the treatment of facial telangiectasias with 532 nm versus 940 nm diode laser. *Lasers Surg Med.* 2009;41(8):555–562.

4. Cen Q, Gu Y, Luo L, et al. Comparative Effectiveness of 755-nm Picosecond Laser, 755- and 532-nm Nanosecond Lasers for Treatment of Café-au-Lait Macules (CALMs): A Randomized, Split-Lesion Clinical Trial. *Lasers Surg Med.* 2020.

5. Chan JC, Shek SY, Kono T, Yeung CK, Chan HH. A retrospective analysis on the management of pigmented lesions using a picosecond 755-nm alexandrite laser in Asians. *Lasers Surg Med.* 2016;48(1):23–29.

6. Ge Y, Yang Y, Guo L, et al. Comparison of a picosecond alexandrite laser versus a Q-switched alexandrite laser for the treatment of nevus of Ota: A randomized, split-lesion, controlled trial. *J Am Acad Dermatol.* 2020;83(2):397–403.

7. Torbeck RL, Schilling L, Khorasani H, Dover JS, Arndt KA, Saedi N. Evolution of the Picosecond Laser: A Review of Literature. *Dermatol Surg.* 2019;45(2):183–194.

8. Wu DC, Goldman MP, Wat H, Chan HHL. A Systematic Review of Picosecond Laser in Dermatology: Evidence and Recommendations. *Lasers Surg Med.* 2020.

9. Bjerring P, Christiansen K. Intense pulsed light source for treatment of small melanocytic nevi and solar lentigines. *J Cutan Laser Ther.* 2000;2(4):177–181.

10. Chern PL, Domankevitz Y, Ross EV. Pulsed dye laser treatment of pigmented lesions: a randomized clinical pilot study comparison of 607- and 595-nm wavelength lasers. *Lasers Surg Med.* 2010;42(10):705–709.

11. Friedmann DP, Peterson JD. Efficacy and safety of intense pulsed light with a KTP filter for the treatment of solar lentigines. *Lasers Surg Med.* 2019;51(6):500–508.

12. Zaleski-Larsen LA, Fabi SG. Laser-Assisted Drug Delivery. *Dermatol Surg.* 2016;42(8):919–931.

13. Zoccali G, Piccolo D, Allegra P, Giuliani M. Melasma treated with intense pulsed light. *Aesthetic Plast Surg.* 2010;34(4):486–493.

14. Choi YJ, Nam JH, Kim JY, et al. Efficacy and safety of a novel picosecond laser using combination of 1 064 and 595 nm on patients with melasma: A prospective, randomized, multicenter,

split-face, 2% hydroquinone cream-controlled clinical trial. *Lasers Surg Med.* 2017;49(10):899–907.

15. Passeron T. Long-lasting effect of vascular targeted therapy of melasma. *J Am Acad Dermatol.* 2013;69(3):e141–e142.

16. Katz TM, Glaich AS, Goldberg LH, Firoz BF, Dai T, Friedman PM. Treatment of melasma using fractional photothermolysis: a report of eight cases with long-term follow-up. *Dermatol Surg.* 2010;36(8):1273–1280.

17. Zipser MC, Mangana J, Oberholzer PA, French LE, Dummer R. Melanoma after laser therapy of pigmented lesions--circumstances and outcome. *Eur J Dermatol.* 2010;20(3):334–338.

18. Taylor CR, Gange RW, Dover JS, et al. Treatment of tattoos by Q-switched ruby laser. A dose-response study. *Arch Dermatol.* 1990;126(7):893–899.

19. Alster TS. Q-switched alexandrite laser treatment (755 nm) of professional and amateur tattoos. *J Am Acad Dermatol.* 1995;33(1):69–73.

20. Fitzpatrick RE, Goldman MP. Tattoo removal using the alexandrite laser. *Arch Dermatol.* 1994;130(12):1508–1514.

21. Bernstein EF, Schomacker KT, Shang X, Alessa D, Algzlan H, Paranjape A. The First Commercial 730 nm Picosecond-Domain Laser is Safe and Effective for Treating Multicolor Tattoos. *Lasers Surg Med.* 2020.

22. Herd RM, Alora MB, Smoller B, Arndt KA, Dover JS. A clinical and histologic prospective controlled comparative study of the picosecond titanium:sapphire (795 nm) laser versus the Q-switched alexandrite (752 nm) laser for removing tattoo pigment. *J Am Acad Dermatol.* 1999;40(4):603–606.

23. Izikson L, Farinelli W, Sakamoto F, Tannous Z, Anderson RR. Safety and effectiveness of black tattoo clearance in a pig model after a single treatment with a novel 758 nm 500 picosecond laser: a pilot study. *Lasers Surg Med.* 2010;42(7):640–646.

24. Ross V, Naseef G, Lin G, et al. Comparison of responses of tattoos to picosecond and nanosecond Q-switched neodymium: YAG lasers. *Arch Dermatol.* 1998;134(2):167–171.

25. Brauer JA, Reddy KK, Anolik R, et al. Successful and rapid treatment of blue and green tattoo pigment with a novel picosecond laser. *Arch Dermatol.* 2012;148(7):820–823.

26. Saedi N, Metelitsa A, Petrell K, Arndt KA, Dover JS. Treatment of tattoos with a picosecond alexandrite laser: a prospective trial. *Arch Dermatol.* 2012;148(12):1360–1363.

27. Reiter O, Atzmony L, Akerman L, et al. Picosecond lasers for tattoo removal: a systematic review. *Lasers Med Sci.* 2016;31(7):1397–1405.

28. Torbeck R, Bankowski R, Henize S, Saedi N. Lasers in tattoo and pigmentation control: role of the PicoSure(®) laser system. *Med Devices (Auckl).* 2016;9:63–67.

29. Bernstein EF. Laser treatment of tattoos. *Clin Dermatol.* 2006;24(1):43–55.

30. Ibrahimi OA, Avram MM, Hanke CW, Kilmer SL, Anderson RR. Laser hair removal. *Dermatolc Ther.* 2011;24(1):94–107.

31. Russe E, Purschke M, Herold M, Sakamoto FH, Wechselberger G, Russe-Wilflingseder K. Evaluation of Safety and Efficacy of Laser Hair Removal With the Long-Pulsed 755 nm Wavelength Laser: A Two-Center Study With 948 Patients. *Lasers Surg Med.* 2020;52(1):77–83.

32. Garcia C, Alamoudi H, Nakib M, Zimmo S. Alexandrite laser hair removal is safe for Fitzpatrick skin types IV-VI. *Dermatol Surg.* 2000;26(2):130–134.

33. Alajlan A, Shapiro J, Rivers JK, MacDonald N, Wiggin J, Lui H. Paradoxical hypertrichosis after laser epilation. *J Am Acad Dermatol.* 2005;53(1):85–88.

34. Atta-Motte M, Załęska I. Diode Laser 805 Hair Removal Side Effects in Groups of Various Ethnicities - Cohort Study Results. *J Lasers Med Sci.* 2020;11(2):132–137.

35. Rao J, Goldman MP. Prospective, comparative evaluation of three laser systems used individually and in combination for axillary hair removal. *Dermatol Surg.* 2005;31(12):1671–1676; discussion 1677.

36. Amin SP, Goldberg DJ. Clinical comparison of four hair removal lasers and light sources. *J Cosmet Laser Ther.* 2006;8(2):65–68.

37. Dorgham NA, Dorgham DA. Lasers for reduction of unwanted hair in skin of colour: a systematic review and meta-analysis. *J Eur Acad Dermatol Venereol.* 2020;34(5):948–955.

38. Manstein D, Herron GS, Sink RK, Tanner H, Anderson RR. Fractional photothermolysis: a new concept for cutaneous remodeling using microscopic patterns of thermal injury. *Lasers Surg Med.* 2004;34(5):426–438.

39. Hantash BM, Bedi VP, Chan KF, Zachary CB. Ex vivo histological characterization of a novel ablative fractional resurfacing device. *Lasers Surg Med.* 2007;39(2):87–95.

40. Wu DC, Fletcher L, Guiha I, Goldman MP. Evaluation of the safety and efficacy of the picosecond alexandrite laser with specialized lens array for treatment of the photoaging décolletage. *Lasers Surg Med.* 2016;48(2):188–192.

41. Wat H, Yee-Nam Shek S, Yeung CK, Chan HH. Efficacy and safety of picosecond 755-nm alexandrite laser with diffractive lens array for non-ablative rejuvenation in Chinese skin. *Lasers Surg Med.* 2019;51(1):8–13.

42. Goldman MP, Weiss RA, Weiss MA. Intense pulsed light as a nonablative approach to photoaging. *Dermatol Surg.* 2005;31(9 Pt 2):1179–1187; discussion 1187.

43. Bitter PH. Noninvasive rejuvenation of photodamaged skin using serial, full-face intense pulsed light treatments. *Dermatol Surg.* 2000;26(9):835–842; discussion 843.

44. Whelan HT, Buchmann EV, Dhokalia A, et al. Effect of NASA light-emitting diode irradiation on molecular changes for wound healing in diabetic mice. *J Clin Laser Med Surg.* 2003;21(2):67–74.

45. Takezaki S, Omi T, Sato S, Kawana S. Light-emitting diode phototherapy at 630 +/- 3 nm increases local levels of skin-homing T-cells in human subjects. *J Nippon Med Sch = Nippon Ika Daigaku zasshi.* 2006;73(2):75–81.

46. Rigau JT, Trelles MA, Calderhead, RG. Changes in fibroblast proliferation and metabolism following in vitro helium-neon laser irradiation. *Laser Ther.* 1991;3(25).

47. Enwemeka CS, Parker JC, Dowdy DS, Harkness EE, Sanford LE, Woodruff LD. The efficacy of low-power lasers in tissue repair and pain control: a meta-analysis study. *Photomed Laser Surg.* 2004;22(4):323–329.

48. Jagdeo J, Austin E, Mamalis A, Wong C, Ho D, Siegel DM. Light-emitting diodes in dermatology: A systematic review of randomized controlled trials. *Lasers Surg Med.* 2018;50(6):613–628.

49. Kennedy JC, Pottier RH, Pross DC. Photodynamic therapy with endogenous protoporphyrin IX: basic

principles and present clinical experience. *J Photochem Photobiol B.* 1990;6(1-2):143–148.

50. Dover JS, Bhatia AC, Stewart B, Arndt KA. Topical 5-aminolevulinic acid combined with intense pulsed light in the treatment of photoaging. *Arch Dermatol.* 2005;141(10):1247–1252.

51. Alster TS, Tanzi EL. Photodynamic therapy with topical aminolevulinic acid and pulsed dye laser irradiation for sebaceous hyperplasia. *J Drugs Dermatol.* 2003;2(5):501–504.

52. Ablon G. Phototherapy with Light Emitting Diodes: Treating a Broad Range of Medical and Aesthetic Conditions in Dermatology. *J Clin Aesthet Dermatol.* 2018;11(2):21–27.

53. Alster TS, Tanzi EL, Welsh EC. Photorejuvenation of facial skin with topical 20% 5-aminolevulinic acid and intense pulsed light treatment: a split-face comparison study. *J Drugs Dermatol.* 2005;4(1):35–38.

54. Marmur ES, Phelps R, Goldberg DJ. Ultrastructural changes seen after ALA-IPL photorejuvenation: a pilot study. *J Cosmet Laser Ther.* 2005;7(1):21–24.

55. Omi T, Numano K. The Role of the CO2 Laser and Fractional CO2 Laser in Dermatology. *Laser Ther.* 2014;23(1):49–60.

56. Tierney EP, Hanke CW, Petersen J. Ablative fractionated CO2 laser treatment of photoaging: a clinical and histologic study. *Dermatol Surg.* 2012;38(11):1777–1789.

57. Miller L, Mishra V, Alsaad S, et al. Clinical evaluation of a non-ablative 1940 nm fractional laser. *J Drugs Dermatol.* 2014;13(11):1324–1329.

58. Ruiz-Esparza J. Near [corrected] painless, nonablative, immediate skin contraction induced by low-fluence irradiation with new infrared device: a report of 25 patients. *Dermatol Surg.* 2006;32(5):601–610.

59. Alam M, White LE, Martin N, Witherspoon J, Yoo S, West DP. Ultrasound tightening of facial and neck skin: a rater-blinded prospective cohort study. *J Am Acad Dermatol.* 2010;62(2):262–269.

60. Suh DH, So BJ, Lee SJ, Song KY, Ryu HJ. Intense focused ultrasound for facial tightening: histologic changes in 11 Patients. *J Cosmet Laser Ther.* 2015;17(4):200–203.

61. Fabi SG. Noninvasive skin tightening: focus on new ultrasound techniques. *Clin Cosmet Investig Dermatol.* 2015;8:47–52.

62. Suh DH, Shin MK, Lee SJ, et al. Intense focused ultrasound tightening in Asian skin: clinical and pathologic results. *Dermatol Surg.* 2011;37(11):1595–1602.

CHAPTER 27

Microneedling and PRP

Paula Purpera, MSHS, PA-C
Gabrielle Pastorek
Mary D. Sun, MSCR, MA

SUMMARY POINTS

What's Important?

1. Microneedling is effective for acne scars, other cutaneous scars, stretch marks, and fine facial lines.

What's New?

1. Microneedling has been shown to be effective with and without platelet-rich plasma.

What We Don't Know

1. It is currently unknown which products are safe to apply after microneedling, so the current standard of care is to place nothing on the skin for the first 24 hours.

What's Coming?

1. Microneedling is an interesting way to deliver ingredients into the dermis.
2. Products developed for application over microchannels will help improve efficacy.
3. Studies evaluating peptides, stem cells, and growth factors to use after microneedling treatments are ongoing.

HISTORY OF MICRONEEDLING

In 1971, Martin S. Gerstel and Virgil A. Place submitted a US patent describing a new drug delivery device that would today be called a microneedle.[1] At that time, however, the technology to create this device did not yet exist. It was not until 1994 that Drs. Orentreich and Orentreich first introduced the concept of what they termed "subcision," which involved the use of needles to treat acne scars and wrinkles.[2,3] During this process, Orentreich and Orentreich punctured the skin with small hypodermic needles to release the fibers responsible for creating depressions like deep scars and wrinkles.

Camirand and Doucet followed suit, using a tattoo gun with needles but no ink to successfully treat surgical scars on two patients.[4] In 2002, plastic surgeon Desmond Fernandes applied these findings to create the first microneedling device—a dermaroller with tiny needles that is rolled along the skin to create microchannels and therefore stimulate collagen and elastin production. He called this process "percutaneous collagen induction," or PCI.[5]

While dermarollers became popular at-home devices among consumers, it was not until 2018 that the FDA approved a microneedling instrument, the SkinPen®. Currently, microneedling is very popular in the medical setting, and an increasing number of reports of its efficacy are being published.

CURRENT USE OF MICRONEEDLES

Microneedling is now used to treat a number of adverse skin conditions, including acne scars, burn and surgical scars, hair loss, wrinkles, skin laxity, and stretch marks. Modern devices, including rollers and hand-held, electric-powered pens, contain very fine needles that usually range from 0.5 to 1.5 mm in length.[6] Both types of devices work by creating several microwounds, also called microchannels, in the skin, without damaging the surface. By triggering natural wound healing within the skin, this process results in an increase of growth factors, collagen and elastin proteins, and glycosaminoglycans like hyaluronic acid.[2]

There are numerous advantages to electric-powered pen devices over dermarollers. Because the operating speeds and penetration depths of microneedling pens are adjustable, more precise results can be achieved using these instruments. They also contain disposable needle tips, which reduce the risk of infection in a medical setting.[2]

Needle Size

The optimal size and length of the needle depends on the location of the treatment area, as well as the specific skin concern being addressed. Singh and Yadav found that a needle length of 1.5 to 2 mm is ideal for treating acne scars, while 0.5 to 1 mm needles are better suited for aging skin and wrinkles.[7] Henry et al. reported that microneedles up to 0.75 mm are generally perceived as painless, making them ideal for drug delivery.[8,9]

Needle length varies according to the issue being treated and how thick the epidermis and dermis are in that area. (See **Fig. 27-1** and **Table 27-1.**)

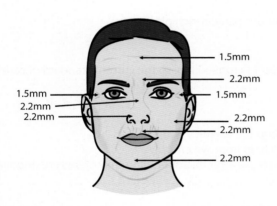

FIGURE 27-1. Length of needles to be used on various parts of the face to treat fine lines.

TABLE 27-1	Treatment Protocols by Area	
Indication	Number of Treatments	Treatment Spacing
Hair loss	4–6	Every 4–6 weeks
Crows' feet	4–6	Every 4–6 weeks
Bar code lines	4–6	Every 4–6 weeks
Mid-face	4–6	Every 4–6 weeks
Neck	4–6	Every 4–6 weeks
Chest	4–6	Every 4–6 weeks
Acne scars on face	At least 6 treatments	Every 4–6 weeks
Scars on body	At least 6 treatments	Every 4–6 weeks
Stretch marks	At least 6 treatments	Every 4–6 weeks

Microneedles for Drug Delivery

Because of the microchannels in the skin that microneedling creates, this technique is an effective method of drug delivery. Many treatment ingredients that would otherwise be too large to penetrate the skin, including various proteins, can be delivered via microchannels.[9] Microneedles used for drug delivery can be composed of steel, silicone, and polymers, and can also be hollow, solid, or dissolving.[1,10] While this is primarily an in-office treatment, microneedle patches or "arrays" that contain prescription medications may be applied to the skin at home like a bandage, as they are designed to be virtually painless and have been shown to increase the effectiveness of certain topical ingredients.[10]

PLATELET-RICH PLASMA

Microneedling is often combined with platelet-rich plasma (PRP). PRP contains high concentrations of growth factors and important proteins that occur naturally in human blood. Kim et al. found that PRP can effectively stimulate collagen and tissue remodeling, resulting in improved scarring, wrinkles, and hair loss, when properly prepared and injected or applied to the skin.[11]

To prepare PRP, a regular blood draw, similar to the process of blood donation, is performed. One tube of blood is typically used per treated area. Next, the blood is placed in a centrifuge to separate the PRP from the other blood components.[11] PRP is then injected directly into the treatment area, such as the face or neck, following microneedling, or it can be applied topically to the skin immediately after the needle channels are made.

EFFICACY STUDIES

Many studies have shown promising results when using microneedling on its own to treat skin concerns such as acne scars, wrinkles, and stretch marks. The attenuation of acne scars is one of the most often cited uses for this treatment. In a randomized clinical trial involving 20 adults, Alam et al. found that three microneedling treatments, each spaced 2 weeks apart, improved the appearance of acne scars by 41%.[12] During each treatment visit, study participants received microneedling on one side of their face, and only a topical anesthetic on the control side. For the microneedling treatment, a topical anesthetic containing 2.5% lidocaine and 2.5% prilocaine was applied. Next, a rolling device was used, with a needle length of either 1 or 2 mm, depending on skin thickness and the severity of acne scars. Following the treatment, a saline solution was applied to the skin.

In 2012, Fabbrocini et al. explored the effects of microneedling on 10 female participants with upper lip wrinkles, aged 50 to 65. After two treatment sessions, wrinkles were shown to improve by 2 points on the Wrinkle Severity Rating Scale.[13] Similarly, El-Domyati et al. administered six microneedling treatments spaced 2 weeks apart to 10 patients with class II or III wrinkles. Three months after the final treatment, the levels of collagen types I, III, and VII, newly synthesized collagen, and tropoelastin were quantified, revealing a significant increase.[14]

When combined with PRP, microneedling results may be enhanced. A 2014 split-face study involving 30 adults with acne scars found that microneedling with PRP was more effective at treating scars than topical vitamin C applications.[15] Prior to PRP treatment on the right side of the face, a topical anesthetic was applied to the skin. Investigators added 1 mL of calcium gluconate to 9 mL of PRP, and a microneedling roller with 1.5-mm-long needles was used. On the left side, 2 mL of 15% vitamin C was applied. Participants received this same treatment four times, each spaced 4 weeks apart. Following each procedure, participants were advised to take oral antibiotics for 2 to 3 days and wear sunscreen. After all four treatments, the improvement in acne scars on each patient was rated as "poor," "good," or "excellent." "Excellent" results were seen in 18.5% of PRP treatments, compared to 7% of the vitamin C treatments. Overall, patients reported being more satisfied with PRP treatments compared to vitamin C.[15]

A similar 2016 split-face study found that PRP combined with microneedling can enhance the results of microneedling alone. This study included 50 people, aged 17 to 32, with atrophic acne scars. Microneedling using a roller with 192 1.5-mm-long needles was performed on both sides of the face. The right side of the face received both PRP injections and a topical PRP application, consisting of a 1:5 ratio of calcium chloride to PRP. Distilled water was injected into the left side of the face, which did not receive any PRP. Results indicated a 62.2% improvement on the right side of the face, which was treated with both microneedling and PRP, and a 45.8% improvement on the left side of the face, which received only microneedling treatments. Moreover, 20 and 30 patients saw "excellent" and "good" improvements, respectively, to PRP-treated skin, based on Goodman's Qualitative scale. This was compared to 5 and 42 patients, respectively, observing "excellent" and "good" improvements to non-PRP treated skin.[16]

ADVERSE EVENTS

Infection, scarring, and skin sensitivity are always a risk of this type of procedure but properly prepping the skin and using the correct post-procedure skincare regimen can minimize the likelihood of such reactions. Hyperpigmentation is a chronic risk from procedures that engender inflammation of the skin. Exposure to sun, light, and heat increases the probability of post-inflammatory hyperpigmentation so it is important to educate patients about avoiding exposure to heat, light, and sun as much as possible.

PRE- AND POST-PROCEDURE SKINCARE WITH MICRONEEDLING

For about 10 days prior to microneedling treatments, it is recommended that patients avoid taking any aspirin-containing medications, non-steroidal anti-inflammatories (NSAIDs), or supplements like St. John's wort, vitamin E, and omega fatty acids. These products can increase the risk of bruising after microneedling, as well as decrease the effectiveness of PRP.[17] Retinoids and vitamin C should be used for at least 2 to 4 weeks prior to microneedling to increase collagen production.[18]

After microneedling, patients are advised to avoid touching their skin for at least 2 hours, and strenuous physical activity should be avoided for at least 24 hours. Additionally, patients should not apply anything to their skin, including SPF, for the first 24 hours following microneedling treatments. Sun avoidance is imperative, since the skin is not protected from the sun during this time. After the first 24 hours, the only products that should be placed on the skin are a gentle cleanser, a barrier repair moisturizer, and a physical sunscreen. Patients should also be instructed to avoid using chemical sunscreens and other topical products for the first 7 days. After that period, they can resume their normal skincare regimen.

TREATMENT PROTOCOLS

To achieve optimal results, multiple microneedling treatments are required (**Fig. 27-2**). The number of treatments needed can depend on the condition being treated, the area of the face or body addressed, and needle length.[7] Three to six treatments may be necessary to obtain the best results. The average amount of time between each session is 4 weeks, although some patients may be able to schedule treatments 2 weeks apart if on a tight timeline. A maintenance treatment can be performed every 6 months for optimal long-lasting outcomes (**Table 27-2**).

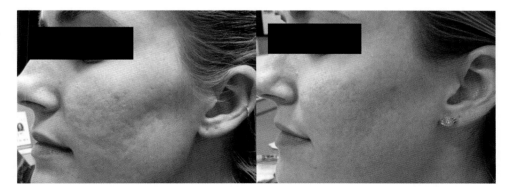

FIGURE 27-2. Patient with acne scars before and after five treatments with 1.5–1.75 mm needles on cheeks and 1 mm on forehead. Photo courtesy of Ilanit Samuels PA-C.

TABLE 27-2	Optimal Needle Length Varies by Indication
Needle Length	**Indication**
0.5–1 mm	Wrinkles
0.75 mm	Drug delivery
1.5 mm	Hair loss on scalp
1.5–2 mm	Scars

CONCLUSION

Microneedling and PRP are very popular procedures that can be performed by trained aestheticians, PAs, NPs, and doctors. There is no consensus on what products to apply post-PRP, although growth factors, hyaluronic acid, heparin sulfate, and defensins are currently being studied as adjuvants to microneedling and PRP.

References

1. Lev-Tov H. How microneedles can change cutaneous drug delivery—small needles make a big difference. *JAMA Dermatol.* 2017 Jul 1;153(7):631–632.

2. Alster TS, Graham PM. Microneedling: a review and practical guide. *Dermatol Surg.* 2018 Mar;44(3):397–404.

3. Orentreich DS, Orentreich N. Subcutaneous incisionless (subcision) surgery for the correction of depressed scars and wrinkles. *Dermatol Surg.* 1995 Jun;21(6):543–549.

4. Camirand A, Doucet J. Needle dermabrasion. *Aesthetic Plast Surg.* 1997 Jan–Feb;21(1):48–51.

5. Fernandes D. Percutaneous collagen induction: an alternative to laser resurfacing. *Aesthet Surg J.* 2002 May;22(3):307–309.

6. Vandervoort J, Ludwig A. Microneedles for transdermal drug delivery: a minireview. *Front Biosci.* 2008 Jan 1;13:1711–1715.

7. Singh A, Yadav S. Microneedling: Advances and widening horizons. *Indian Dermatol Online J.* 2016 Jul–Aug;7(4):244–254.

8. Henry S, McAllister DV, Allen MG, Prausnitz MR. Microfabricated microneedles: a novel approach to transdermal drug delivery. *J Pharm Sci.* 1998 Aug;87(8):922–925.

9. Kalluri H, Kolli CS, Banga AK. Characterization of microchannels created by metal microneedles: formation and closure. *AAPS J.* 2011 Sep;13(3):473–481.

10. Ita K. Transdermal delivery of drugs with microneedles—potential and challenges. *Pharmaceutics.* 2015 Jun 29;7(3):90–105.

11. Kim DH, Je YJ, Kim CD, et al. Can platelet-rich plasma be used for skin rejuvenation? Evaluation of effects of platelet-rich plasma on human dermal fibroblast. *Ann Dermatol.* 2011 Nov;23(4):424–431.

12. Alam M, Han S, Pongprutthipan M, et al. Efficacy of a needling device for the treatment of acne scars: a randomized clinical trial. *JAMA Dermatol.* 2014 Aug;150(8):844–849.

13. Fabbrocini G, De Vita V, Pastore F, et al. Collagen induction therapy for the treatment of upper lip wrinkles. *J Dermatolog Treat.* 2012 Apr;23(2):144–152.

14. El-Domyati M, Barakat M, Awad S, et al. Multiple microneedling sessions for minimally invasive facial rejuvenation: an objective assessment. *Int J Dermatol.* 2015 Dec;54(12):1361–1369.

15. Chawla S. Split face comparative study of microneedling with PRP versus microneedling with vitamin C in treating atrophic post acne scars. *J Cutan Aesthet Surg.* 2014 Oct–Dec;7(4):209–212.

16. Asif M, Kanodia S, Singh K. Combined autologous platelet-rich plasma with microneedling verses microneedling with distilled water in the treatment of atrophic acne scars: a concurrent split-face study. *J Cosmet Dermatol.* 2016 Dec;15(4):434–443.

17. Schippinger G, Prüller F, Divjak M, et al. Autologous platelet-rich plasma preparations: influence of nonsteroidal anti-inflammatory drugs on platelet function. *Orthop J Sports Med.* 2015 Jun 23;3(6):2325967115588896.

18. Mukherjee S, Date A, Patravale V, et al. Retinoids in the treatment of skin aging: an overview of clinical efficacy and safety. *Clin Interv Aging.* 2006;1(4):327–348.

CHAPTER 28

Sclerotherapy

Peter B. Chansky, MD
Evan A. Rieder, MD

SUMMARY POINTS

What's Important?

1. Telangiectasias, venulectasias, dilated reticular veins, and torturous varicose veins are common age-related manifestations of chronic venous hypertension and valvular incompetence. A multifactorial pathogenesis is implicated in the development of lower extremity venous disease, including hereditary, hormonal, gravitational, thrombotic, and sedentary factors.
2. Sclerosing agents produce their clinical effect through the permanent fibrosis and destruction of the vessel wall. Treatment guidelines include utilization of both the smallest quantity and lowest concentration of sclerosing agent to produce venous wall fibrosis and the treatment of larger, proximal veins before the treatment of smaller, distal veins.
3. Common complications following sclerotherapy include hyperpigmentation, telangiectatic matting, and cutaneous ulceration and necrosis. Implementation of graduated compression for 2–3 weeks after sclerotherapy is essential to reduce the risk of complications and endovascular recanalization.
4. Cosmetic treatment of superficial leg veins with sclerotherapy is an effective, safe, and satisfying treatment modality. Proper assessment, utilization of duplex ultrasonography, and knowledge of both sclerosing agents and injection techniques are critical to a successful outcome.

What's New?

1. Sclerotherapy combined with laser treatment has demonstrated enhanced clinical outcomes.
2. Duplex ultrasonography is a helpful resource to provide real-time guidance of sclerotherapy for the treatment of deep leg veins with a foamed sclerosant.

What's Coming?

1. Novel endovenous ablation devices and sclerosants are potential future advancements in the treatment of medical and cosmetic venous disease.

In addition to the face, neck, chest, and hands, the aesthetic appearance of the legs is a significant area of concern to patients. In 2018, according to statistics gathered by the American Society of Plastic Surgeons, sclerotherapy ranked as the 11th most common minimally invasive cosmetic procedure.[1] In order to maximize the successful treatment of leg veins with sclerotherapy, a thorough understanding of venous pathology, specifically venous hypertension and chronic venous insufficiency, is crucial for practitioners.

The aim of this chapter is to familiarize the reader with the underlying pathology, the diagnosis, and the treatment of venous hypertension, and to help the reader differentiate between the medical and the cosmetic sclerotherapy patient. The treatment section of this chapter will focus on sclerotherapy as it pertains to the cosmetic patient, specifically regarding the treatment of leg telangiectasias, venulectasias, and reticular veins. Treatment options for patients with clinically relevant venous disease will be briefly mentioned. Treatment of varicosities, while technically within the purview of the cosmetic dermatologist, will not be discussed in detail. And finally though much progress has been made in the use of sclerotherapy for the treatment of lymphatic malformations of the head and neck, this chapter will not discuss this novel procedure.

THE VENOUS SYSTEM AND VARICOSE VEINS

The venous system is a low-pressure system that functions as a blood reservoir and an avenue to return deoxygenated blood to the heart. Unlike arteries, which carry oxygenated blood and have a thick elastic muscular lining designed to withstand high pressures, veins carry deoxygenated blood, are thin-walled, and easily distend with increased pressure. The map of venous circulation is more variable than that of arterial circulation, and interconnected anastomoses between veins commonly occur. This multiplicity allows for surgical repair of the venous system as there are several routes for deoxygenated blood to return to the heart. Proper venous function relies on the heart and skeletal muscle contraction for forward circulation as well as a network of one-way valves to prevent retrograde flow. Contraction of skeletal muscle compresses the veins within them and helps to propel blood back to the heart. This is particularly important in the lower extremities where the force of gravity must be overcome to maintain proper circulation. The contractile action of the skeletal muscles, primarily the calf muscles, helps to transport blood upward.

The Venous System of the Leg

The venous system of the leg consists of an interconnected network with both a superficial and a deep component. The superficial component comprises less than 5% of venous blood and is located above the fascia, while the deep component comprises 95% of venous blood and is located below the fascia.

The principal superficial veins are the lesser saphenous vein, which runs from the ankle to the knee, and the greater saphenous vein, which runs from the ankle to the groin. The superficial veins of the leg connect and empty into the deep veins via perforating veins, which pierce through the fascia separating the compartments of the leg. Deep veins ultimately return deoxygenated blood to the right-side of the heart.

The skin surface of the leg may consist of superficial pink telangiectasias found in the papillary dermis that empty into blue-appearing reticular veins found in the reticular dermis, which empty into the superficial venous system located above the fascia. These superficial veins drain into the deep venous system that is located below the fascia and within the muscle.

Besides being identified according to their location, veins can also be categorized by size. Telangiectasias are flat red vessels that are up to 1 mm in diameter, venulectasias are bluish vessels that may distend above the skin surface and are usually 1 to 2 mm in diameter, and reticular veins are those that have a cyanotic hue and are 2 to 4 mm in diameter. Nonsaphenous varicose veins are 3 to 8 mm in diameter, and saphenous varicose trunks are usually greater than 5 mm in diameter. These larger vessels typically lie deep below the skin surface and are better visualized with duplex ultrasound.

Varicose Veins

Veins have one-way valves that occur every few inches along their course and are positioned to oppose back flow so deoxygenated blood can continue to flow forward in the direction of the heart. Contraction of leg and calf muscles aid in the forward flow of venous blood through the one-way valves. A varicose vein is a vein that has lost its elasticity. While any vein in the body may be affected, the superficial veins of the legs are by far the most frequently involved. These weakened veins dilate under the pressure of supporting a column of blood against the force of gravity. Varicose veins have a caliber greater than normal, and their valve cusps no longer meet. This results in valvular incompetence and reflux. Varicose veins impede proper circulation by permitting blood to flow away from the heart, decreasing the efficiency of the entire venous system, and leading to venous hypertension. The severity of venous hypertension is directly related to the skin changes seen in chronic venous insufficiency. The progression to chronic venous insufficiency follows the leaking of fluids out of the veins into the perivascular tissue. This leakage engenders symptoms of leg swelling, aching, and eventually dermatologic manifestations such as increased vascular markings, skin discoloration (hyper- or hypopigmentation and hemosiderin deposition), stasis dermatitis, lipodermatosclerosis, and possibly ulceration.

The etiology of varicose vein formation is multifactorial. There is a familial tendency to develop varicose veins, usually in patients who present with this disease early in life. Its relation to gender appears to be a more significant factor, as it is seen in approximately 26% of women versus 5% of men. In addition, advancing age appears to be involved, as those older than 35 almost triple their risk compared to those aged 24 to 35 years.[2] Physical states that increase the pressure on the venous system by physically compromising venous return, such as pregnancy, obesity, decreased mobility, and frequent constipation, are also associated with an increased risk of varicose vein formation.[2-4] Other exacerbating factors, such as the presence of estrogen in pregnancy, as well as estrogen and progesterone supplementation, have been shown to have an impact on the vascular system. While estrogen appears to protect against the formation of venous ulcers of the lower limbs,[5] it has been implicated in raising telangiectatic matting (the appearance of tiny vessels less than 0.2 mm in diameter), which occurs in women after undergoing sclerotherapy for the treatment of leg veins.[6]

Current research on the etiology and pathology of varicose veins and chronic venous insufficiency suggests that the underlying pathologic mechanism is an inflammatory response that is initiated by an increase in shear stress on the venous endothelium. Several studies suggest that an increase in venous pressure induces leukocyte accumulation and subsequent free radical production that leads to degradation of valve leaflets by metalloproteinases,[7-9] which are enzymes that degrade collagen, elastin, and other components of the extracellular matrix. Based on this free radical-driven model of venous damage, flavonoids (plant-derived free radical scavengers) have been shown to ameliorate the symptoms and progression of chronic venous insufficiency.[10-13]

EXAMINATION OF THE SCLEROTHERAPY PATIENT AND DIAGNOSIS OF CHRONIC VENOUS INSUFFICIENCY

The current test of choice to investigate blood flow in the superficial and deep venous systems is the duplex ultrasound. This test is indicated for symptomatic patients and for patients who have clinical evidence of chronic venous insufficiency (see paragraph below). Duplex ultrasound is more reliable and faster than Doppler (hand-held) ultrasound because it provides actual visualization of veins. It is recommended that duplex ultrasound be performed on the upper and lower leg (superficial and deep veins, and venous perforators) in order to accurately locate points of reflux that should be targeted for treatment.[14]

Most patients with chronic venous insufficiency have specific symptoms and clinical signs that reveal their disease state. Physical exam findings indicative of chronic venous insufficiency include the presence of hemosiderin deposition, visible venulectasias, livedoid vasculopathy, eczematous dermatitis, lipodermatosclerosis, and either previous or current ulceration. A detailed clinical examination is adequate to diagnose most patients suffering from primary varicose veins.[15] Doppler vascular studies have been shown to be useful in patients presenting with recurrent varicose veins or obese patients with signs and symptoms of chronic venous insufficiency with no clinically clear varicosity.[16] Not all patients with venous reflux have symptoms of chronic venous insufficiency, but patients with symptoms of chronic venous insufficiency are more likely to have venous reflux. Moreover, the degree of symptoms correlates with the degree of venous disease.[17,18] Pain and a sensation of heaviness are the most common symptoms of chronic venous insufficiency,[16,19] while edema is the most frequent and the first objective sign.[19-21] Vessel diameter greater than approximately 4 mm is directly related to the likelihood of venous incompetence,[22] and patients with corona phlebectatica (fan-shaped intradermal telangiectasias in the medial and sometimes lateral portions of the ankle and foot; **Fig. 28-1**) have a 4.4 times greater risk of incompetent leg or calf perforators by duplex ultrasound than patients without this clinical finding.[23]

Based on these current research findings, the recommended approach to the sclerotherapy patient is as follows: if the patient is symptomatic (reports symptoms of leg pain, heaviness, swelling, aching, cramping, itching, or any other symptoms attributable to venous dysfunction), vascular testing is indicated. Likewise, if the patient is asymptomatic, but upon physical examination has two or more signs, vascular testing is indicated. These signs include edema, vessel diameter

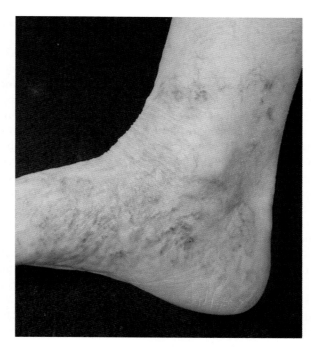

FIGURE 28-1. Corona phlebectatica around the medial malleolus. Presence of these fan-shaped vessels around the ankle is a clinical sign of underlying venous reflux. Patients with this finding should be examined by duplex ultrasound.

greater than 4 mm, corona of the lower extremities, hyper- or hypopigmentation, dermatitis, fibrosis, and current or healed ulcer. In addition, if there is a history of previous sclerotherapy with poor results, such as recurrence of vessels or appearance of new vessels in the previous treatment area after sclerotherapy, then vascular testing is indicated. Otherwise, patients who present with leg telangiectasias with or without reticular veins and without the previously listed features may be presumed to be cosmetic treatment candidates. In this case, the treating physician may decide that these patients do not need to undergo initial vascular studies. Sclerotherapy should not be performed on patients with current thromboembolism, migraine headache and patent foramen ovale (due to risk of embolism), diabetes, and peripheral arterial disease (due to risk of ulceration).[24,25] Of note, in a systematic review of the literature on the safety of cosmetic procedures during pregnancy and lactation, sclerotherapy was deemed safe after the first trimester but before week 36 of pregnancy.[26] That being said, the authors do not recommend the use of sclerotherapy during pregnancy.

SCLEROSING AGENTS

Many studies have reported the success of sclerotherapy in the treatment of both functional and cosmetic vein disorders. The ideal sclerosant produces complete destruction of the endothelial lining of the vessel wall and ultimately results in inflammation, fibrosis, and the eventual obliteration of the vessel. Removal of the endothelial lining is critical as the presence of thrombosis alone with intact endothelium will result in secretion of tissue plasminogen activator, dissolution of the thrombus, and patency of the vessel.

There are two classes of sclerosants based on their mechanism of action: hyperosmotic agents and detergents. Hyperosmotic agents, such as hypertonic saline and non-chromated glycerin, produce endothelial damage through dehydration. Detergents, such as sodium tetradecyl sulfate, sodium morrhuate, ethanolamine oleate, and polidocanol, cause vascular injury by altering the surface tension around endothelial cells, diminishing their ability to adhere to one another. Chromated glycerin and polyiodide iodide, may also produce chemical irritant properties, and can injure endothelial cells by acting as a corrosive secondary to the heavy metal component. Systematic reviews of sclerosants do not demonstrate superiority of one modality over another.[27,28]

Current practice includes the use of sclerosants in solution or those that are manually foamed. Liquid sclerotherapy is the gold standard for treating most lower extremity telangiectasias and reticular veins (<6 mm). Foamed sclerosants (either sodium tetradecyl sulfate or polidocanol mixed with air) are mainly used to treat larger veins (≥6 mm) and functional vein disorders, such as chronic venous insufficiency and venous ulceration under duplex-guided ultrasound.[29,30] This approach has been very successful for the medical sclerotherapy patient. However, a known risk of foam sclerotherapy includes transient vision disturbances.[31]

Other preparations include cyanoacrylate glue and mechanochemical ablation. Microbeads of cyanoacrylate glue obliterate the vein distal to the intersection of the saphenous and femoral vein. The technique involves injecting the product while simultaneously pulling back on the catheter from proximal to distal end. This technique is often facilitated with an ultrasound probe. Mechanochemical ablation is an endovenous technique that obliterates the vein through both an agitating wire to disrupt the vein proximally and injection of a sclerosant distally. Both polidocanol and sodium tetradecyl sulfate are potential sclerosants for this procedure.[32]

In the United States, the only agents approved by the FDA for sclerotherapy are sodium tetradecyl sulfate (Sotradecol®), polidocanol (Varithena™, Asclera®, Aethoxysklerol®), sodium morrhuate (Scleromate®), and ethanolamine oleate; the latter two have an extensive side effect profile and are used primarily for esophageal varices. While hypertonic saline is commonly used as a sclerosing agent, it is approved as an abortifacient rather than a sclerotherapy agent. Chromated glycerin is an agent recognized for superior treatment of leg telangiectasias. In the treatment of telangiectatic leg veins, chromated glycerin has been shown to clear vessels significantly better than polidocanol in solution or polidocanol foam.[33] Chromated glycerin is not FDA approved for sclerotherapy and is not available in the United States. Glycerin alone is a hyperosmotic agent and it is likely that its mechanism of action in sclerotherapy is dehydration of the vessel wall, similar to hypertonic saline. Another sclerosing solution that is not FDA approved is polyiodinated iodine. Overall, the major sclerosants used in the US include sodium tetradecyl sulfate, hypertonic saline, glycerin, and polidocanol.

It is important to know the risk profiles of commonly used sclerosants (**Table 28-1**). Hypertonic saline is associated with burning and cramping upon injection and an increased risk of ulcerative necrosis secondary to extravasation. Sodium tetradecyl sulfate has also been associated with hyperpigmentation, pain upon extravasation, and skin necrosis. Rarely, sodium tetradecyl sulfate and, even more rarely, polidocanol have been associated with allergic hypersensitivity reactions. While it has been suggested that allergic reactions to detergent sclerosants are often caused by solubilized latex products from the rubber plunger in the syringe into the sclerosant solution, this has not been substantiated and remains a subject of controversy. Overall, the estimated incidence of allergic reactions is 0.3% and may occur with the use of any sclerosing agent,[34] as allergic reactions to components found in gloves, syringes, and other supplies that come in contact with a patient through treatment can arise. As such, it may be prudent to take at least 20 minutes for in-office observation postprocedure after every sclerotherapy session, especially in patients with a history of asthma or a history of allergies. Likewise, it is imperative to have basic life support skills as well as subcutaneous epinephrine, corticosteroids, antihistamines, oxygen, and other resuscitative equipment readily available to treat this potentially life-threatening complication if it arises.

The optimal concentration of sclerosant may vary with the diameter of the vessel being treated, with a greater concentration of sclerosant being required for vessels of larger diameter.[35] If the sclerosant is too weak, insufficient damage to the endothelium results and a thrombus may form that eventually recanalizes and leaves the vessel patent. If the sclerosant is too strong, then extravasation may occur leading to exaggerated destruction of the endothelial lining and possibly deeper wall layers producing hyperpigmentation, telangiectatic matting, and ulceration.

Management of side effects can be a challenge. While pain and cramping are acute and quickly resolve, hyperpigmentation, telangiectatic matting, and ulceration are more chronic.

Hyperpigmentation after sclerotherapy is delayed and can take several months to a year to resolve. It has been associated with high total body iron stores.[36] This type of hyperpigmentation is caused by extravascular hemosiderin deposition and is not melanocytic; therefore, it does not respond to topical bleaching agents as much as to tincture of time. The Q-switched ruby laser has demonstrated some efficacy in treatment of post-sclerotherapy hyperpigmentation.

Telangiectatic matting usually lasts between 3 and 12 months and is more common in hyperestrogenemic states, obese patients, and during pregnancy.[6,37] Such matting results from high injection pressure and administration of more than 1 mL of sclerosant per injection site. Telangiectatic matting may also be a sign of underlying venous reflux and should be investigated by duplex ultrasound. Both hyperpigmentation and telangiectatic matting may benefit from treatment with intense pulsed light as this modality has shown some success in treating vascular lesions, including telangiectasias,[38,39] as well as treatment of dyspigmentation.[39,40]

It is important to emphasize that necrosis with subsequent ulceration can potentially occur with extravasation of any of

TABLE 28-1	Characteristics of Common Sclerosing Solutions			
Solution	FDA Approval	Advantages	Risks/Disadvantages	Recommended Dose Limitations Per Treatment Session
Hypertonic saline (23.4%)[a]	Yes, as abortifacient	Nonallergenic	Off-label	10 mL
			Pain and cramping	
			Skin necrosis	
			Hyperpigmentation	
			Microthrombi formation	
Sodium tetradecyl sulfate (Sotradecol) (0.25%)[a]	Yes	Can be foamed to treat varicose veins under ultrasound guidance	Pain upon extravasation	10 mL of 3%
			Skin necrosis	
			Hyperpigmentation	
			Microthrombi formation	
			Rare anaphylaxis	
Polidocanol (0.25%)[a]	No	Painless	Hyperpigmentation	10 mL of 3%
		Can be foamed to treat varicose veins under ultrasound guidance	Microthrombi formation	
			Allergic reactions	
			Rare anaphylaxis	
Glycerin (72% glycerin mixed with 1% lidocaine and 1:100,000 epinephrine, combined 2:1)[b]	No	Rare hyperpigmentation	Pain and cramping	10 mL
			Rare allergy	
			Too weak for large veins	

[a]Average reported concentration used to treat veins from 1 to 4 mm in diameter.
[b]Best used for the treatment of fine telangiectasias (vessels up to 1 mm in diameter).

the sclerosants into the skin or by inadvertent intra-arterial or periarterial injection of sclerosants. The sclerosant with the least risk of inducing necrosis seems to be glycerin, effective only for the treatment of leg telangiectasias. When extravasation of sclerosant occurs in the skin it is generally secondary to the treatment of small vessels, such as telangiectasias or reticular veins. This complication presents as a small and painful slow-to-heal blister, erosion, or ulceration. Healing typically resolves with a skin-colored scar. If blanching occurs after injection, application of 2% nitroglycerin ointment can increase blood flow and decrease the likelihood of ulceration. In contrast, reports of intra-arterial injection occur when treating larger, deeper vessels. This risk is increased when targeting veins around the ankle, knee or when treating deeper veins. In all of these cases, the veins and their accompanying arteries are in close proximity to one another. When arteries are accidentally injected, the entire area supplied by the artery quickly becomes ischemic and pale, and is usually painful. In this situation, affected areas are large, involving a segment of the leg or foot. Injection of a sclerosing agent into

an artery is a vascular emergency as the sclerosing agent forms a sludge embolus and occludes part of the arterial circulation. Fortunately, intra-arterial injection is a very rare event, but the risk is not completely avoidable and can still occur even under ultrasound guidance.[41] Management in this case is emergent, and may result in possible amputation. To minimize the incidence of most complications, use of proper injection technique is critical. Using the minimal concentration of sclerosant for the vessel size, small volumes, and slow injection to maintain low pressure in the vessel will assure the best results. Cosmetic treatment of veins around the ankle with sclerotherapy should be avoided and, in this specific group of patients, the possibility of reflux should be explored.

SCLEROTHERAPY FOR THE COSMETIC PATIENT

When treating leg veins, it is important to treat proximal sites and larger vessels first, as treatment of these vessels may obliterate those vessels that are smaller and distally located. As

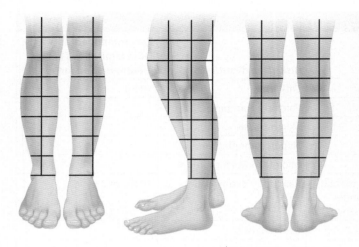

FIGURE 28-2. Sample flow sheet or map for recording sclerotherapy sessions.

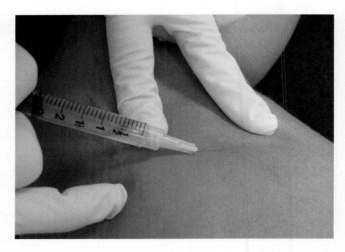

FIGURE 28-3. Injection of leg telangiectasias. Hand traction is employed to keep the skin taut. The needle is bent at a 30-degree angle and inserted just below the skin surface, bevel side up. Injections are performed slowly to maintain low pressure on the vessel wall to minimize extravasation of sclerosant.

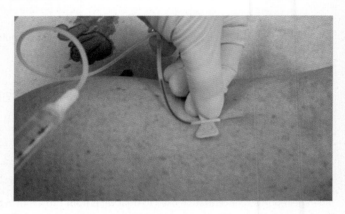

FIGURE 28-4. Injection of reticular veins. A 25-gauge butterfly needle is attached to a 3-cc syringe. Intraluminal vein placement is confirmed by pulling back on the plunger of the syringe prior to injection. Sclerosant is then slowly injected.

previously mentioned, cosmetic treatment is undertaken only if the patient does not have any clinical signs or symptoms of chronic venous insufficiency or has had all sources of reflux already treated. Preoperative photographs and fully informed consent outlining all possible risks and complications should be obtained prior to therapy. A discussion of postprocedure care is also essential.

A body map with segmental divisions of the legs is helpful in documenting each session (**Fig. 28-2**). Treatment is repeated at 6-week intervals to allow for complete resolution of previously treated sites as complete fibrosis of the endothelial lining may take up to 6 weeks. The number of treatment sessions may vary, usually from one to six, based on the aggressiveness of the physician as well as the clinical presentation and expectations of the patient.

There are four injection techniques commonly used in the treatment of cosmetic leg veins: (i) the puncture-fill technique, (ii) the aspiration technique, (iii) the empty vein technique, and (iv) the air-bolus technique. The *puncture-fill technique* relies on the feeling associated with perforating a vessel wall. It is probably the most common, but also the most difficult to grasp for beginners and better mastered over time while using the other listed approaches. The *aspiration technique* is most useful for the treatment of reticular veins, with the observation of the aspirated dark blood into the hub of the syringe or the tubing of a butterfly needle confirming correct needle placement. The *empty vein technique* involves leg elevation and kneading the vessel to remove as much blood as possible prior to injecting the sclerosant. Emptying the vein of blood before injection allows for maximum exposure of the endothelium to the sclerosant and improved efficacy. The *air-bolus technique* uses the injection of a small amount of air (0.2 cc or less) prior to the introduction of sclerosant. The air in the tip of the syringe displaces the blood in the vessel confirming correct needle placement.

Alcohol is used to clean the skin as well as increase the refractile index of the skin, rendering vessels more visible upon the skin surface. A common approach is to use a combination of the aspiration and empty vein techniques for reticular veins, and puncture-fill for venulectasias and telangiectasias. It is also helpful when using the puncture-fill technique to target the most superficial portion of the vessel. For telangiectasias less than 1 mm in size, where cannulating the vessel is a challenge, it is necessary to start injecting with the tip of the needle just barely underneath the skin surface, bevel side facing up (**Fig. 28-3**). When treating reticular veins, the use of a butterfly needle helps to secure venous access; however, prior to injecting these vessels it is essential to pull back on the plunger to visualize dark blue blood in the tubing and ensure location inside the lumen of the vein (**Fig. 28-4**). Injection can then proceed slowly. In all cases, when resistance is encountered, injection should be stopped or extravasation can occur.

Prior to injecting, the needle may be bent at an angle of 20 to 45 degrees. Upward hand traction is employed by the sclerotherapist using the nondominant hand or by an assistant to keep the skin taut. Sclerosant is injected slowly to allow adequate time for contact with the endothelium as well as to prevent vascular distention and rupture. A small amount of sclerosant is used at each puncture site (approximately 0.1 to 0.3 cc for telangiectasias and 0.5 to 1 cc for reticular veins) in order to minimize side effects such as ulceration caused by extravasation, telangiectatic matting, and hyperpigmentation. Reticular veins are treated at intervals of approximately 3 to 6 cm along the length of the vessel, proximal to distal. Larger vessels, such as reticular veins, are injected before smaller vessels, such as venulectasias and telangiectasias, and areas of arborization are treated before isolated linear areas.

Immediately upon withdrawal of the needle, the treatment areas should be compressed manually. Then each area is taped with either dry cotton balls or dental rolls, and wrapped with Coban or an elastic wrap (Box 28-1). The patient is instructed to keep this in place for a minimum of 4 hours, after which time graduated compression stockings are substituted for an average of 2 to 3 weeks. The garment should have a pressure of at least 15 mm Hg and should be worn 24 hours a day to prevent any venous dilation. Compression therapy is known to tighten the paracellular barrier by elevating the expression of specific tight junctions, inhibiting permeability of fluid into the perivascular tissue, and thereby preventing progression of chronic venous insufficiency.[42] It also decreases symptoms of chronic venous insufficiency,[43] such as pain and discomfort,[44] as well as edema.[45] Finally, following sclerotherapy, compression also maximizes contact between the sclerosant and the venous wall further enhancing lumen occlusion while simultaneously reducing the risk of telangiectatic matting, hyperpigmentation, and canalization of the vein. While graduated compression garments are not favorably accepted by most patients, especially cosmetic patients in warm climates, it should be emphasized that the use of these garments is associated with greater clinical resolution and decreased risk of hyperpigmentation.[45] Lastly, patients should refrain from exercise while wearing compression stockings in the 2–3 week post-procedure period.

Lasers for Cosmetic Leg Veins

Laser leg vein treatment has been explored with a variety of wavelengths, and the long-pulsed 1064-nm Nd:YAG laser has shown the most promising results.[46,47] However, when compared with sclerotherapy in the treatment of lower extremity telangiectasias, sclerotherapy continues to offer superior clinical results.[46] Notably, laser therapy should only be an option for patients who have avoided sun exposure to the intended treatment areas for several weeks prior to the procedure and who have Fitzpatrick Skin Types I to III. Primary indications for laser or intense pulsed light treatment of leg veins include ankle telangiectasias, needle phobia, telangiectatic matting, allergic reaction to sclerosants, poor outcome from sclerotherapy, or vessels too small to cannulate (< 0.3 mm). As with sclerotherapy, optimal results are achieved with lasers when larger feeding vessels are treated first.

Treatment of Varicose Veins

Varicose veins, an eventual complication of venous hypertension and chronic venous insufficiency, may be managed in several ways. Daily graduated compression is of paramount importance in slowing the progression of venous disease, controlling the associated pain and swelling, and reducing the risk of thrombosis and venous ulcer development. Compression therapy works by decreasing the diameter of veins which ultimately increases flow velocity, minimizes stasis and extravasation of blood into surrounding tissues, and decreases the risk of venous thrombosis. Oral agents, like flavonoids (found in such foods as citrus fruits, berries, green tea, red wine, and dark chocolate with cocoa content of at least 70%), have also proven to be beneficial. Similarly, daily intake of vitamin C, while not directly investigated, may also be helpful. Maintaining an active lifestyle and avoiding obesity are additional recommended measures.

Treatment options are best explored after duplex ultrasound examination once all points of reflux have been determined. Besides sclerotherapy, mainly using the foamed method,[29,30,48,49] other types of procedures that can be used to treat leg varicosities include ambulatory phlebectomy, vein stripping and/or ligation, or endovenous vein ablation techniques.

SUMMARY

Sclerotherapy remains the gold standard for treatment of cosmetic leg veins. Optimal results occur when individual patient characteristics are evaluated, thus separating the cosmetic sclerotherapy patient from the medical sclerotherapy patient. Sclerotherapy is a technique that is mastered with practice. By understanding venous pathology and etiology, and by being able to choose the right sclerosant and right technique for the vein in question, a successful outcome will surely be achieved.

References

1. Surgeons ASoP. Plastic Surgery Statistics Report 2018. Accessed January 9, 2021, Available at https://www.plasticsurgery.org/documents/News/Statistics/2018/plastic-surgery-statistics-full-report-2018.pdf
2. Ahumada M, Vioque J. [Prevalence and risk factors of varicose veins in adults]. *Med Clin (Barc)*. Nov 13 2004;123(17):647–651.

	Materials Used for Sclerotherapy for Cosmetic Patients
BOX 28-1	

1. Cotton balls or swabs soaked with 70% isopropyl alcohol
2. Protective gloves
3. Protective eyewear
4. 3-cc disposable syringes
5. 32-gauge needles
6. Light source
7. 25- or 27-gauge butterfly needle
8. Dental rolls (or dry cotton balls)
9. Paper tape
10. Coban® or elastic bandage

Prevalencia de varices en adultos y factores asociados. doi:10.1016/s0025-7753(04)74632-1

3. Fowkes FG, Lee AJ, Evans CJ, Allan PL, Bradbury AW, Ruckley CV. Lifestyle risk factors for lower limb venous reflux in the general population: Edinburgh Vein Study. *Int J Epidemiol.* Aug 2001;30(4):846-852. doi:10.1093/ije/30.4.846

4. Jawien A. The influence of environmental factors in chronic venous insufficiency. *Angiology.* Jul-Aug 2003;54(Suppl 1):S19-S31. doi:10.1177/0003319703054001S04

5. Berard A, Kahn SR, Abenhaim L. Is hormone replacement therapy protective for venous ulcer of the lower limbs? *Pharmacoepidemiol Drug Saf.* May 2001;10(3):245-251. doi:10.1002/pds.582

6. Davis LT, Duffy DM. Determination of incidence and risk factors for postsclerotherapy telangiectatic matting of the lower extremity: a retrospective analysis. *J Dermatol Surg Oncol.* Apr 1990;16(4):327-330. doi:10.1111/j.1524-4725.1990.tb00043.x

7. Pascarella L, Penn A, Schmid-Schonbein GW. Venous hypertension and the inflammatory cascade: major manifestations and trigger mechanisms. *Angiology.* Sep-Oct 2005;56(Suppl 1):S3-S10. doi:10.1177/00033197050560i102

8. Kosugi I, Urayama H, Kasashima F, Ohtake H, Watanabe Y. Matrix metalloproteinase-9 and urokinase-type plasminogen activator in varicose veins. *Ann Vasc Surg.* May 2003;17(3):234-238. doi:10.1007/s10016-003-0005-2

9. Gillespie DL, Patel A, Fileta B, et al. Varicose veins possess greater quantities of MMP-1 than normal veins and demonstrate regional variation in MMP-1 and MMP-13. *J Surg Res.* Aug 2002;106(2):233-238. doi:10.1006/jsre.2002.6455

10. Bergan JJ. Chronic venous insufficiency and the therapeutic effects of Daflon 500 mg. *Angiology.* Sep-Oct 2005;56(Suppl 1):S21-S24. doi:10.1177/00033197050560i104

11. Cesarone MR, Belcaro G, Pellegrini L, et al. Venoruton vs Daflon: evaluation of effects on quality of life in chronic venous insufficiency. *Angiology.* Mar-Apr 2006;57(2):131-138. doi:10.1177/000331970605700201

12. Smith PC. Daflon 500 mg and venous leg ulcer: new results from a meta-analysis. *Angiology.* Sep-Oct 2005;56(Suppl 1):S33-S39. doi:10.1177/00033197050560i106

13. Cesarone MR, Belcaro G, Rohdewald P, et al. Comparison of Pycnogenol and Daflon in treating chronic venous insufficiency: a prospective, controlled study. *Clin Appl Thromb Hemost.* Apr 2006;12(2):205-212. doi:10.1177/107602960601200209

14. Wong JK, Duncan JL, Nichols DM. Whole-leg duplex mapping for varicose veins: observations on patterns of reflux in recurrent and primary legs, with clinical correlation. *Eur J Vasc Endovasc Surg.* Mar 2003;25(3):267-275. doi:10.1053/ejvs.2002.1830

15. Classification and grading of chronic venous disease in the lower limbs. A consensus statement. Ad Hoc Committee, American Venous Forum. *J Cardiovasc Surg (Torino).* Oct 1997;38(5):437-441.

16. Safar H, Shawa N, Al-Ali J, Al-Nassar M, Dashti H, Asfar S. Is there a need for Doppler vascular examination for the diagnosis of varicose vein? A prospective study. *Med Princ Pract.* Jan-Feb 2004;13(1):43-46. doi:10.1159/000074051

17. Jantet G. Chronic venous insufficiency: worldwide results of the RELIEF study. Reflux assEssment and quaLity of lIfe improvEment with micronized Flavonoids. *Angiology.* May-Jun 2002;53(3):245-256. doi:10.1177/000331970205300301

18. Ruckley CV, Evans CJ, Allan PL, Lee AJ, Fowkes FG. Chronic venous insufficiency: clinical and duplex correlations. The Edinburgh Vein Study of venous disorders in the general population. *J Vasc Surg.* Sep 2002;36(3):520-525. doi:10.1067/mva.2002.126547

19. Callejas JM, Manasanch J, Group E. Epidemiology of chronic venous insufficiency of the lower limbs in the primary care setting. *Int Angiol.* Jun 2004;23(2):154-163.

20. Boccalon H, Janbon C, Saumet JL, Tafani A, Roux T, Vilain C. Characteristics of chronic venous insufficiency in 895 patients followed in general practice. *Int Angiol.* Dec 1997;16(4):226-234.

21. Langer RD, Ho E, Denenberg JO, Fronek A, Allison M, Criqui MH. Relationships between symptoms and venous disease: the San Diego population study. *Arch Intern Med.* Jun 27 2005;165(12):1420-1424. doi:10.1001/archinte.165.12.1420

22. Kurt A, Unlu UL, Ipek A, et al. Short saphenous vein incompetence and chronic lower extremity venous disease. *J Ultrasound Med.* Feb 2007;26(2):163-167. doi:10.7863/jum.2007.26.2.163

23. Uhl JF, Cornu-Thenard A, Carpentier PH, Widmer MT, Partsch H, Antignani PL. Clinical and hemodynamic significance of corona phlebectatica in chronic venous disorders. *J Vasc Surg.* Dec 2005;42(6):1163-1168. doi:10.1016/j.jvs.2005.08.031

24. Gillet JL, Guedes JM, Guex JJ, et al. Side-effects and complications of foam sclerotherapy of the great and small saphenous veins: a controlled multicentre prospective study including 1,025 patients. *Phlebology.* Jun 2009;24(3):131-138. doi:10.1258/phleb.2008.008063

25. Hartmann K, Harms L, Simon M. Reversible neurological deficit after foam sclerotherapy. *Eur J Vasc Endovasc Surg.* Nov 2009;38(5):648-649. doi:10.1016/j.ejvs.2009.06.022

26. Trivedi MK, Kroumpouzos G, Murase JE. A review of the safety of cosmetic procedures during pregnancy and lactation. *Int J Womens Dermatol.* Mar 2017;3(1):6-10. doi:10.1016/j.ijwd.2017.01.005

27. Schwartz L, Maxwell H. Sclerotherapy for lower limb telangiectasias. *Cochrane Database Syst Rev.* Dec 7 2011;(12):CD008826. doi:10.1002/14651858.CD008826.pub2

28. Tisi PV, Beverley C, Rees A. Injection sclerotherapy for varicose veins. *Cochrane Database Syst Rev.* Oct 18 2006;(4):CD001732. doi:10.1002/14651858.CD001732.pub2

29. Pascarella L, Bergan JJ, Mekenas LV. Severe chronic venous insufficiency treated by foamed sclerosant. *Ann Vasc Surg.* Jan 2006;20(1):83-91. doi:10.1007/s10016-005-9381-0

30. Barrett JM, Allen B, Ockelford A, Goldman MP. Microfoam ultrasound-guided sclerotherapy of varicose veins in 100 legs. *Dermatol Surg.* Jan 2004;30(1):6-12. doi:10.1111/j.1524-4725.2004.30008.x

31. Coleridge Smith P. Saphenous ablation: sclerosant or sclerofoam? *Semin Vasc Surg.* Mar 2005;18(1):19-24. doi:10.1053/j.semvascsurg.2004.12.007

32. Scovell S, Eidt J, Mills J, Dover J, Collins K. Liquid, foam, and glue sclerotherapy techniques for the treatment of lower extremity veins. Accessed January 9, 2021, Available at https://www.uptodate.com/contents/liquid-foam-and-glue-sclerotherapy-techniques-for-the-treatment-of-lower-extremity-veins?-search=sclerotherapy&source=search_result&selectedTitle=1~96&usage_type=default&display_rank=1

33. Kern P, Ramelet AA, Wutschert R, Bounameaux H, Hayoz D. Single-blind, randomized study comparing chromated glycerin,

polidocanol solution, and polidocanol foam for treatment of telangiectatic leg veins. *Dermatol Surg.* Mar 2004;30(3):367–372; discussion 372. doi:10.1111/j.1524-4725.2004.30102.x

34. Ramelet AA, Monti M. *Phlebology: The Guide.* Elsevier; 1999.

35. Sadick NS. Sclerotherapy of varicose and telangiectatic leg veins. Minimal sclerosant concentration of hypertonic saline and its relationship to vessel diameter. *J Dermatol Surg Oncol.* Jan 1991;17(1):65–70. doi:10.1111/j.1524-4725.1991.tb01595.x

36. Thibault PK, Wlodarczyk J. Correlation of serum ferritin levels and postsclerotherapy pigmentation. A prospective study. *J Dermatol Surg Oncol.* Oct 1994;20(10):684–686. doi:10.1111/j.1524-4725.1994.tb00453.x

37. Sadick NS. Predisposing factors of varicose and telangiectatic leg veins. *J Dermatol Surg Oncol.* Oct 1992;18(10):883–886. doi:10.1111/j.1524-4725.1992.tb02921.x

38. Fodor L, Ramon Y, Fodor A, Carmi N, Peled IJ, Ullmann Y. A side-by-side prospective study of intense pulsed light and Nd:YAG laser treatment for vascular lesions. *Ann Plast Surg.* Feb 2006;56(2):164–170. doi:10.1097/01.sap.0000196579.14954.d6

39. Ross EV, Smirnov M, Pankratov M, Altshuler G. Intense pulsed light and laser treatment of facial telangiectasias and dyspigmentation: some theoretical and practical comparisons. *Dermatol Surg.* Sep 2005;31(9 Pt 2):1188–1198. doi:10.1111/j.1524-4725.2005.31925

40. Gupta AK, Gover MD, Nouri K, Taylor S. The treatment of melasma: a review of clinical trials. *J Am Acad Dermatol.* Dec 2006;55(6):1048–1065. doi:10.1016/j.jaad.2006.02.009

41. Trinh-Khac JP, Roux A, Djandji A, Aractingi S. [Nicolau livedoid dermatitis after sclerotherapy of varicose veins]. *Ann Dermatol Venereol.* May 2004;131(5):481–485. Dermite livedoide de Nicolau apres sclerotherapie de varices. doi:10.1016/s0151-9638(04)93645-9.

42. Herouy Y, Kahle B, Idzko M, et al. Tight junctions and compression therapy in chronic venous insufficiency. *Int J Mol Med.* Jul 2006;18(1):215–219.

43. Vayssairat M, Ziani E, Houot B. [Placebo controlled efficacy of class 1 elastic stockings in chronic venous insufficiency of the lower limbs]. *J Mal Vasc.* Oct 2000;25(4):256–262. Efficacite versus placebo de la contention classe 1 dans l'insuffisance veineuse chronique des membres inferieurs.

44. Weiss RA, Weiss MA. Resolution of pain associated with varicose and telangiectatic leg veins after compression sclerotherapy. *J Dermatol Surg Oncol.* Apr 1990;16(4):333–336. doi:10.1111/j.1524-4725.1990.tb00044.x

45. Goldman MP, Beaudoing D, Marley W, Lopez L, Butie A. Compression in the treatment of leg telangiectasia: a preliminary report. *J Dermatol Surg Oncol.* Apr 1990;16(4):322–325. doi:10.1111/j.1524-4725.1990.tb00042.x

46. Lupton JR, Alster TS, Romero P. Clinical comparison of sclerotherapy versus long-pulsed Nd:YAG laser treatment for lower extremity telangiectases. *Dermatol Surg.* Aug 2002;28(8):694–697. doi:10.1046/j.1524-4725.2002.02029.x

47. Eremia S, Li C, Umar SH. A side-by-side comparative study of 1064 nm Nd:YAG, 810 nm diode and 755 nm alexandrite lasers for treatment of 0.3-3 mm leg veins. *Dermatol Surg.* Mar 2002;28(3):224–230. doi:10.1046/j.1524-4725.2002.01162.x

48. Kakkos SK, Bountouroglou DG, Azzam M, Kalodiki E, Daskalopoulos M, Geroulakos G. Effectiveness and safety of ultrasound-guided foam sclerotherapy for recurrent varicose veins: immediate results. *J Endovasc Ther.* Jun 2006;13(3):357–364. doi:10.1583/05-1781.1

49. Darke SG, Baker SJ. Ultrasound-guided foam sclerotherapy for the treatment of varicose veins. *Br J Surg.* Aug 2006;93(8):969–974. doi:10.1002/bjs.5423

CHAPTER 29

Thread Lifts

Lana X. Tong, MD, MPH
Evan A. Rieder, MD

SUMMARY POINTS

What's Important?

1. Suspension sutures combat the aging process by anchoring the soft tissue to the periosteum.
2. In contrast to traditional cosmetic surgery, thread lifts carry the advantages of decreased downtime and cost, lack of a need for general anesthesia, and less procedural invasiveness.
3. Conversely, thread lifting results are thought to have less dramatic results that are temporary.

What's New?

1. Thread lifting has gained in popularity with the advent of other minimally invasive techniques.
2. The development of absorbable barbed sutures has accelerated the popularity of this technique, as opposed to non-absorbable sutures, which have had a higher complication rate in the past.

What's Coming?

1. Absorbable suture materials, such as polydioxanone and poly-L-lactic acid, are favored due to their properties of collagen stimulation, although the long-term effects from the placement of threads composed of these materials are unknown.
2. Threads composed of poly-L-lactic acid in combination with other suture materials with collagen stimulation properties are continuing to be developed, as the popularity of thread lifting further grows.

INTRODUCTION

History

Although surgical facelifts have long been considered the gold standard for facial rejuvenation, the development of and interest in minimally invasive techniques have grown dramatically. Surgical lifting of the superficial musculoaponeurotic system (SMAS) along with general anesthesia is a highly invasive procedure carrying numerous potential perioperative complications in addition to prolonged postprocedural downtime and scarring.[1] As our understanding of the mechanism behind the aging process and the mechanical anatomic vectors involved—particularly loosening of the SMAS—continues to advance, less invasive procedures have been developed and become increasingly popular. Although noninvasive neurotoxins, injectable fillers, radiofrequency, and ablative resurfacing tools play a significant role in facial rejuvenation, they do not address the need to lift the laxity of the underlying ptotic tissues.[2] Recently introduced minimally invasive procedures include quick-recovery and limited-incision face-lifting, micro-focused ultrasound with high-resolution ultrasound visualization (MFU-V), in addition to barbed-suture lifting. The advantages these techniques purport to carry include a shorter downtime, lack of need for general anesthesia, faster procedure time, and fewer complications, which bestow increased convenience for both the patient and physician.[3]

Injectable fillers, skin resurfacing, and MFU-V play a major role in minimally invasive facial rejuvenation; however, fillers

TABLE 29-1	Summary of Barbed Suture Characteristics and Current Availability	
Suture Name	Suture Design	Current FDA Approval
Nonabsorbable Threads		
Aptos Threads		
Aptos Thread 2G	25 cm prolene or polylactic acid suture with multidirectional barbs	No
Aptos Needle 2G	60 cm 2-0 prolene or polylactic acid suture with multidirectional barbs	No
Isse Endo Progressive Face Lift Suture	25 cm polyprolene suture with 50 barbs along the distal 10 cm; smooth 15 cm proximal segment attaches to fascia and is reinforced with surgical mesh.	No
Multianchor Suspension Suture	2-0 polydioxanone or Maxon suture with 5–7 anchors placed 15 cm from the distal end	No
Contour Threads	25 cm polyprolene suture with unidirectional barbs centrally	Yes, for suture materials only
Silhouette Sutures		
Featherlift Silhouette Sutures	25 cm 3-0 polypropylene suture with 11 polylactide/glycolide copolymer cones (PLGA)	Yes
Silhouette Lift	26.8–30 cm 3-0 polypropylene suture with 9 PLGA cones located centrally	Yes
Absorbable Threads		
Polydioxanone Threads	17–43 cm 1-0 polydioxanone suture with unidirectional, bidirectional or multidirectional barbs	Yes, for suture materials only
Poly-L-Lactic Acid Threads		
Silhouette Instalift	Poly-L-lactic acid suture with 8–16 bidirectional PLGA bidirectional cones	Yes
Aptos Threads	7–25 cm poly-L-lactide and caprolactone suture with multidirectional barbs	No

can result in unnatural contours, and resurfacing and MFU-V may not always sufficiently address the degree of tissue ptosis present.[4] Suture suspension, also referred to as thread lifting, was first pioneered by Sulamanidze et al. in the 1990s[5] and has gained popularity among dermatologists, plastic surgeons, and other cosmetic surgery practitioners. Although thread lifting initially employed conventional polypropylene, polyglactin, and polytetrafluoroethylene sutures, long-term efficacy was poor.[6] Thread lifts with barbed sutures were then introduced, known as anti-ptosis (Aptos) threads, along with the development of absorbable threads.[7] Other variations have since been developed including Xtosis,[8] Isse Endo Progressive Face Lift Sutures, Silhouette sutures, and Contour Threads (**Table 29-1**).[9]

Significance

Thread lifting works via placement of barbed sutures underneath sagging tissue along a specific trajectory to address ptosis.[10] Threads are first implanted in the dermis; when tugged in the opposite direction, the barbs anchor in adipose tissue, thereby increasing tensile strength while suspended in the dermis and overlying tissue. Barbed sutures were initially used in tendon repair,[11] and are also thought to produce a fibrous adhesion capsule that helps to solidify anchorage of the suture long-term.[4] Fibrosis has been shown to increase local collagen production.[12] Suspension techniques either lift the SMAS or rearrange facial structures at the supraperiosteal level.[13,14] Sutures can also be placed endoscopically, allowing anchorage

to the fascia or periosteum. Additionally, threads made with polydioxanone (PDO) and poly-L-lactic acid (PLLA) are theorized to stimulate collagen production.[15,16] In comparison to traditional surgical face-lifting, thread lifting possesses the advantages of decreased downtime and cost, lack of a need for general anesthesia, and less procedural invasiveness; conversely, thread lifting results also are thought to have less dramatic results that are usually temporary.

THREAD LIFTING CATEGORIZED BY SUTURE TYPE

Non-Absorbable Threads

Aptos, Isse Endo, and Multianchor Suspension Threads

Initial thread lifts were performed with non-absorbable barbed sutures, such as Aptos threads. These were the first commercially available barbed sutures, using 2-0 polyprolene and bidirectional barbs with free floating suture placement.[5,19] In studies published by Sulamanidze et al. (Aptos Ltd., Moscow, Russia)[5] and Lycka et al.,[20] adverse events included thread disruption, suture extrusion, asymmetry, visible threads with pain, thread migrations, infections or granulomas, and skin dimpling or irregularities.[9,12] More serious complications such as Stensen's duct rupture, nerve damage, chronic foreign body sensation, and scarring appearing as late as 2 years following the procedure have been reported by other investigators.[21–25] A continued high complication rate described in subsequent reports, including suture migration and expulsion, resulted in a decrease in popularity of Aptos thread usage [21,26,27] Aptos threads do not currently have FDA clearance.

In 2005, Lee and Isse modified the Aptos suture with distal barbs in order to proximally anchor the suture in the temporalis fascia to target the midface.[28] Adverse events were transient with the exception of one case of submalar dimpling. The Isse Endo Progressive Face Lift suture (KMI Inc, Anaheim, CA) does not currently have FDA clearance.

Eremia et al. described thread suspension of the midface with a 2-0 absorbable monofilament suture with large multi-anchoring threads using the same absorbable monofilament sutures.[29] These threads were made from commercially available 2-0 polydioxanone and polyglyconate sutures, and were thus not submitted for FDA clearance. Positive outcomes at 100% were reported in the midface, jowls, and neck. As the sutures were absorbable, reversal of results was noted at 6-month follow-up. At 1-year follow-up, 100% of jowl and 80–100% of midface corrections were lost. No adverse events were reported.

Contour Threads

Contour Threads, which were patented as Featherlift Extended Aptos Length Threads (Surgical Specialties Corp., Reading, PA) but are unique from the original Aptos threads, are 2-0 polyprolene sutures with a central segment of unidirectional barbs that are anchored proximally. They were cleared by the Food and Drug Administration (FDA) in October 2004 for mid and lower facial rejuvenation.

A retrospective study was performed in 2009 by Abraham et al. on 33 subjects: 10 underwent thread lifts alone with Contour Threads and 23 underwent thread lifting with additional rejuvenation procedures. Results were compared with 10 patients who underwent non-thread lift rejuvenation only.[3] Subjects were followed from 12–31 months (average 21 months) and postoperative results were graded by blinded physicians. The thread only group received an average score of 0.2–0.5 (0 = no improvement, 3 = considerable improvement), in comparison with 0.5–1.4 and 1.8–2.3 for thread lifting with additional procedures and non-thread lift rejuvenation, respectively. Skin dimpling and visible knots were reported, with three subjects requiring postprocedural thread removal.

Another retrospective study published by Garvey et al. in 2009 investigated the outcomes of Contour Threads in 72 female subjects.[30] Complications were reported in 64.8%, although adverse events described were mostly minor. Furthermore, 42.3% underwent revisional surgery at an average of 8.4 months, and 11.3% required thread removal due to palpable knots or suture extrusion.

In 2010, Rachel et al. conducted a retrospective study of 29 subjects who underwent barbed Contour thread lifts (Angiotech Pharmaceuticals, Vancouver, BC).[31] Recurrence of laxity was reported within 8 weeks in 14% and within 6 months in 45%. Approximately 69% described adverse effects, and 59% required additional surgery during follow-up.

As with Aptos threads, the increasing number of reports detailing complications resulting from Contour Threads

resulted in their discontinuation. In the United States, Contour Threads lost FDA clearance regarding the technique utilized in the thread lift; however, the sutures themselves still have FDA clearance for midface suspension surgery, specifically the Featherlift Extended Aptos Length Threads (Surgical Specialties Corp., Reading, PA) and the Featherlift Extended Aptos Threads (Kim Kolster Methods, Inc., Corona, CA).

Silhouette Sutures

Featherlift Silhouette Sutures (Kolster Methods, Inc., Corona, CA) are 3-0 polypropylene sutures with absorbable cones cleared by the FDA for midface rejuvenation and jawline definition by fixating the cheek subdermis in an elevated position.[32] They are anchored proximally in the temporal fascia and then reinforced with polyprolene mesh. de Benito et al. treated 316 subjects over 2 years with an 18-month follow-up period, 294 of which underwent thread lifts only. Minor adverse events were reported, although two individuals required revisional surgery for asymmetry and one patient required thread removal.[32]

In 2008, Gamboa et al. studied thread lift outcomes using Silhouette Lifts (Silhouette Lift Inc, Irvine, CA) in 17 subjects; these threads also currently have FDA clearance for midface suspension surgery.[33] At 9 months, 90% reported they were very satisfied and 10% reported they were moderately satisfied. About 5.6% required a revisional procedure. Only minor adverse events were reported.

Absorbable Threads

Polydioxanone Threads

Given the complications reported with non-absorbable barbed sutures, absorbable thread lifts have gained in popularity. Several studies in Asia have been published using PDO threads. In the United States, the Quill Knotless Tissue-Closure Device and Synthetic Absorbable Barbed Suture (Quill Medical Inc., Research Triangle Park, NC) are absorbable barbed PDO threads cleared by the FDA for soft tissue closure.

Since 2015 there have been five published studies of PDO threads, containing 31–39 subjects in each trial. Each study demonstrated high patient satisfaction rates (> 80% in each) with results lasting 6–12 months.[34,36] Those which also measured physician-rated metrics scored well too. Adverse events were transient and mild, with the exception of one case of thread extrusion.[6]

Of note, one study of 1-0 to 2-0 unidirectional barbed PDO threads (Youngs Lift, Y. Jacobs Medical, Seoul, Korea)[35] used ultrasonography and a three-dimensional scanner to evaluate postprocedural changes in mean dermal thickness and midfacial volume, respectively. Approximately 86.3% of patients reported at least moderate satisfaction with the procedure after 3 months. At 3-month follow-up, midfacial volume decreased by 7.6 and dermal thickness increased from 1.30 to 1.87 mm; at 7 months, average volume decreased by 8.7 and dermal thickness was stable at 1.89 mm.

Lee et al. published a study in 2017 with similarly high patient satisfaction scores and limited adverse events.[37]

In this study, 35 subjects underwent thread lifts with PDO sutures followed by oral antibiotics, and 94.3% were satisfied with their outcomes with a mean follow-up period of 1 year. Independent physicians evaluated pre- and postprocedural photos and rated 100% of subjects as improved.

Other PDO barbed sutures currently available in the United States include PDS™ Barbed Sutures (Ethicon, Inc., Somerville, NJ) and the Contour Thread Synthetic Absorbable PDO Barbed Suture (Surgical Specialties Corp., Reading, PA); however, these, including the Quill Synthetic Absorbable Barbed Suture, have FDA clearance for soft tissue approximation and not specifically for midface suspension.

Poly-L-Lactic Acid Threads

Recently, interest has grown in PLLA threads, in particular due to their potential collagen-stimulating properties.[38] However, a known complication with PLLA injections is the formation of subcutaneous nodules and late-onset granulomas.[39] Other devices made of PLLA such as screws and pins have been described to have delayed inflammatory reactions.[38] The Silhouette Instalift (Silhouette Lift, Inc., Westwood, MA), also known as Silhouette Soft or Lift is a PLLA suture with bidirectional poly Lactide/Glycolide (PLGA) copolymer cones designed for lifting the eyebrows, lower neck, jaw, and cheek.[40] These threads differ from prior iterations of thread lifts in that they utilize cones rather than barbs, and are cleared by the FDA for temporary midface suspension targeting the elevation of the cheek subdermis, in contrast to PDO threads. In one study, 148 subjects underwent thread lifts with these PLLA/PLGA threads with the goal of lifting the cheeks, cheekbones, eyebrows, neck, and lower jaw. Mostly transient adverse outcomes were reported over a median of 22 months; one subject experienced persistent skin dimpling, requiring subsequent subcision.

A subsequent pilot study was performed using Silhouette Instalift threads in 20 women for improving jawline contour.[41] At 6-month follow-up, 75% of subjects were considered to be improved by blinded physicians, and 55% were rated as improved at 1-year follow-up. Seventy percent of patients reported high or medium satisfaction while 55% achieved results lasting over 6 months. Only transient adverse events were reported.

Goldberg conducted a prospective study using Instalift threads targeting the midface on 17 patients.[42] Patient satisfaction consistently improved over 9 months of follow-up. Moreover, punch biopsies were collected adjacent to the suture insertion site. These were assessed with a type I polyclonal collagen antibody to determine collagen and elastin content, and demonstrated a significant increase in collagen between baseline and day 270 ($P = 0.0015$). Only transient adverse events were reported, including erythema and edema.

Recently, Aptos has released absorbable barbed sutures composed of poly-L-lactide and caprolactone. Khiabanloo et al. published a study with these threads to target the midface, neck, mandible, and nose in 58 patients.[43] Patients were assessed by both the surgeon performing the procedure and an independent surgeon using the GAIS at the first week, third

month, and sixth month: 81%, 88.7%, and 79.3% of patients reported satisfaction, respectively. Complications included ecchymosis (30%), pain (17.2%), tumefaction (6.9%), and dimpling (1.7%). Aptos threads are not currently approved for use by the FDA.

FUTURE DIRECTIONS

Thread lifting is one of many minimally invasive rejuvenation procedures that have been growing in popularity. As interest in specific cosmetic procedures is often driven by patient demand and company marketing rather than supportive objective clinical data, it is crucial for healthcare providers to critically analyze novel materials and techniques to provide cutting-edge care that is also safe and beneficial to patients.[44,45]

Suture suspensions performed with non-absorbable sutures are fraught with many drawbacks.[46,47] High complication and revision rates were reported, although revisions are not necessarily an anomaly for cosmetic procedures. Just as importantly, it has been postulated that the transient initial improvement in outcomes may be due to local inflammation and edema rather than the thread lift itself.[9,48,49] An additional concern regarding non-absorbable barbs is that their removal can be difficult, often leaving residual fragments that continue to be symptomatic. Finally, the long-term ramifications of SMAS scarring are uncertain.[50]

Although the physicians who patented Aptos threads argued that the complication rate is significantly operator-dependent, a necessary goal in the development of a successful minimally invasive technique is ease of implementation and widespread adoption. As several barbed sutures were initially FDA cleared and then withdrawn from the market due to adverse effects, it is important to always exercise appropriate skepticism and caution when adopting any early techniques.

Recently, interest in thread lifts has again increased with absorbable threads. Numerous studies have been published demonstrating positive outcomes and rare complications using PDO thread, which is degraded in the body approximately within 4–6 months. PDO as well as PLLA are known to be collagen stimulants and are postulated to stimulate a long-term benefit in rejuvenation.[15,38] Thread lifting with barbed PDO threads can be complemented by the MESH technique, where smooth PDO threads are inserted subcutaneously in areas of hollowing to stimulate collagen growth and serve as a structure to support the efficacy of suspension threads.[56] However, the published studies have had short follow-up times and have yet to provide much objective data regarding long-term benefit, though Kim et al. did use 3D scanners and ultrasonography to evaluate skin thickness and lifting, and Goldberg performed histologic confirmation.[35,42] As with non-absorbable sutures, it has also been argued that short-term improvement observed may be the result of local edema and inflammation rather than structural change, particularly as laboratory studies investigating the long-term persistence of increased fibrous tissue following suture placement have not been conclusive.[1,9,24,47,50-52]

The overall evidence regarding thread lifts is weak. Studies have had short follow-up periods and no standardized protocol, with most studies following subjects for less than a year and no studies with longer than a 3-year follow-up. Many studies also investigated outcomes of thread lifts in combination with other rejuvenation procedures without a control group. With regard to outcomes, few studies reported objective procedural outcomes or utilized widely accepted patient reported outcome measures. Though subjects reported high satisfaction rates with thread lifting, more granular data using psychometrically validated outcome measures could help physicians better evaluate and tailor future iterations of devices for maximum subject satisfaction.[53]

There will likely remain a role for thread lifting in facial rejuvenation as technology continues to improve. Suture suspensions with barbed threads can be a very effective technique in the appropriate patient. New suture materials promoting collagen growth and better understanding of the vectors of aging will likely lead to additional improvements in efficacy. Thread lifting may also be a helpful tool for other cosmetic concerns, such as acne scarring. While there exist several barbed PDO sutures on the market, they are only cleared by the FDA for soft tissue approximation, versus the Silhouette Instalift PLLA/PLGA sutures which are cleared for midface suspension. A recently completed clinical trial investigated the use of 3-0 V-Loc 180 barbed sutures (Surgical Devices, Tycho Healthcare Group LP, New Haven, CT), composed of an absorbable copolymer of glycolic acid and trimethylene carbonate, in anchoring retaining ligaments to the temporal fascia as a different approach to the thread lift.[55]

At this point, it is prudent to fully inform patients of the limited supportive evidence for thread lifts, realistic expectations of outcomes, and potential adverse events. Thread lifting is generally regarded as an appropriate treatment for patients with signs of mild aging who are not interested in facial rejuvenation surgery.[56] Additionally, patients who are significantly overweight, patients with thick skin, and those having excess skin laxity are not considered to be ideal candidates. Additionally, while soft tissue fillers are considered to benefit those desiring a fuller midface, particularly in patients wishing to address pronouncement of the nasolabial fold, thread lifts may be more helpful to patients desiring a more oval face shape.[57] While the future of non-absorbable thread lifting appears promising, we must take caution and learn from our experience with previously marketed but subsequently failed cosmetic interventions before widely adopting novel techniques.

CONCLUSION

Thread lifting has been a commonly practiced aesthetic procedure for facial rejuvenation over the past few decades, although protocols vary widely. Robust data do not currently exist for thread lifting outcomes, although smaller scale studies have been published and indicate promise. While initial methods utilizing non-absorbable suture possessed a frequent complication and revision rate, newer published methods utilizing absorbable sutures have shown positive preliminary data regarding safety and efficacy. Further multicenter studies

with standardized protocols, including suture type and number of sutures, larger sample sizes, extended follow-up times, and outcome measures, are needed to better evaluate efficacy, safety, and optimal treatment regimens.

References

1. Kaminer MS, Bogart M, Choi C, et al. Long-term efficacy of anchored barbed sutures in the face and neck. *Derm Surg.* 2008;34(8):1041–1047.

2. Rachel JD, Jamora JJ. Skin rejuvenation regimens: a profilometry and histopathologic study. *Arch Facial Plast Surg.* 2003;5(2):145–149.

3. Abraham RF, DeFatta RJ, Williams EFIII. Thread-lift for facial rejuvenation: assessment of long-term results. *Arch Facial Plast Surg.* 2009;11(3):178–183.

4. Sulamanidze MA, Paikidze TG, Sulamanidze GM, et al. Facial lifting with "APTOS" threads: featherlift. *Otolaryngol Clin North Am.* 2005;38(5):1109–1117.

5. Sulamanidze MA, Fournier PF, Paikidze TG, et al. Removal of facial soft tissue ptosis with special threads. *Derm Surgery.* 2002;28(5):367–371.

6. Sasaki GH, Cohen AT. Meloplication of the malar fat pads by percutaneous cable-suture technique for midface rejuvenation: outcome study (392 cases, 6 years' experience). *Plast Reconstr Surg.* 2002;110(2):635–654.

7. Sulamanidze M, Sulamanidze G. Facial lifting with Aptos Methods. *J Cutan Aesthet Surg.* 2008;1(1):7–11.

8. Fukaya M. Long-term effect of the insoluble thread-lifting technique. *Clin Cosmet Investig Dermatol.* 2017;10:483–491.

9. Villa MT, White LE, Alam M, et al. Barbed sutures: a review of the literature. *Plast Reconstr Surg.* 2008;121(3):102e–108e.

10. Tavares JP, Oliveira C, Torres RP, et al. Facial thread lifting with suture suspension. *Braz J Otorhinolaryngol.* 2017;83(6):712–719.

11. McKenzie AR. An experimental multiple barbed suture for the long flexor tendons of the palm and fingers. *J Bone Joint Surg Br.* 1967;49(3):440–447.

12. Wu WT. Barbed sutures in facial rejuvenation. *J Aesthet Surg.* 2004;24(6):582–587.

13. Berry MG, Davies D. Platysma-SMAS plication facelift. *J Plast Reconstr Aesthet Surg.* 2010;63(5):793–800.

14. Verpaele A, Tonnard P. Lower third of the face: indications and limitations of the minimal access cranial suspension lift. *Clin Plast Surg.* 2008;35(4):645–659.

15. Kim J, Zheng Z, Kim H, et al. Investigation on the Cutaneous Change Induced by Face-Lifting Monodirectional Barbed Polydioxanone Thread. *Derm Surg.* 2017;43(1):74–80.

16. Tajirian AL, Goldberg DJ. A review of sutures and other skin closure materials. *J Cosmet Laser Ther.* 2010;12(6):296–302.

17. Medicine OCfE-B. Levels of Evidence. 2009; Available at https://www.cebm.net/2009/06/oxford-centre-evidence-based-medicine-levels-evidence-march-2009/. Accessed May 28, 2018.

18. Grading of Recommendations Assessment DaEGWG. Grading of Recommendations Assessment, Development and Evaluation (GRADE). 2007; Available at http://www.essentialevidenceplus.com/product/ebm_loe.cfm?show=grade. Accessed May 28, 2018.

19. Sulamanidze M, Sulamanidze G, Sulamanidze C. Elimination of Aesthetic Deformations of the Midface Area Our Experience. *Aesthet Plastic Surg.* 2018.

20. Lycka B, Bazan C, Poletti E, et al. The emerging technique of the antiptosis subdermal suspension thread. *Derm Surg.* 2004;30(1):41–44.

21. Silva-Siwady JG, Diaz-Garza C, Ocampo-Candiani J. A case of Aptos thread migration and partial expulsion. *Derm Surg.* 2005;31(3):356–358.

22. Helling ER, Okpaku A, Wang PT, et al. Complications of facial suspension sutures. *J Aesthet Surg.* 2007;27(2):155–161.

23. Winkler E, Goldan O, Regev E, et al. Stensen duct rupture (sialocele) and other complications of the Aptos thread technique. *Plast Reconstr Surg.* 2006;118(6):1468–1471.

24. Beer K. Delayed complications from thread-lifting: report of a case, discussion of treatment options, and consideration of implications for future technology. *Derm Surg.* 2008;34(8):1120–1123.

25. Lee CJ, Park JH, You SH, et al. Dysesthesia and fasciculation: unusual complications following face-lift with cog threads. *Derm Surg.* 2007;33(2):253–255.

26. Ruff G. Technique and uses for absorbable barbed sutures. *J Aesthet Surg.* 2006;26(5):620–628.

27. Sulamanidze M, Sulamanidze G, Vozdvizhensky I, et al. Avoiding complications with Aptos sutures. *J Aesthetic Surg.* 2011;31(8):863–873.

28. Lee S, Isse N. Barbed polypropylene sutures for midface elevation: early results. *Arch Facial Plast Surg.* 2005;7(1):55–61.

29. Eremia S, Willoughby MA. Novel face-lift suspension suture and inserting instrument: use of large anchors knotted into a suture with attached needle and inserting device allowing for single entry point placement of suspension suture. Preliminary report of 20 cases with 6-to 12-month follow-up. *Derm Surg.* 2006;32(3):335–345.

30. Garvey PB, Ricciardelli EJ, Gampper T. Outcomes in threadlift for facial rejuvenation. *Annals Plast Surg.* 2009;62(5):482–485.

31. Rachel JD, Lack EB, Larson B. Incidence of complications and early recurrence in 29 patients after facial rejuvenation with barbed suture lifting. *Derm Surg.* 2010;36(3):348–354.

32. de Benito J, Pizzamiglio R, Theodorou D, et al. Facial rejuvenation and improvement of malar projection using sutures with absorbable cones: surgical technique and case series. *Aesthet Plast Surg.* 2011;35(2):248–253.

33. Gamboa GM, Vasconez LO. Suture suspension technique for midface and neck rejuvenation. *Annals Plast Surg.* 2009;62(5):478–481.

34. Suh DH, Jang HW, Lee SJ, et al. Outcomes of polydioxanone knotless thread lifting for facial rejuvenation. *Dermatol Surg.* 2015;41(6):720–725.

35. Kim J, Kim HS, Seo JM, et al. Evaluation of a novel thread-lift for the improvement of nasolabial folds and cheek laxity. *JEADV.* 2017;31(3):e136–e179.

36. Kang SH, Byun EJ, Kim HS. Vertical Lifting: A New Optimal Thread Lifting Technique for Asians. *Dermatol Surg.* 2017;43(10):1263–1270.

37. Lee H, Yoon K, Lee M. Outcome of facial rejuvenation with polydioxanone thread for Asians. *J Cosmet Laser Ther.* 2017;1–4.

38. Siemenow MZ, Eisenmann-Klein M. *Plastic and reconstructive surgery.* London: Springer Specialist Surgery Series; 2010.

39. Storer M, Euwer R, Calame A, et al. Late-onset granuloma formation after poly-l-lactic acid injection. *JAAD Case Rep.* 2016 Jan; 2(1):54–56.

40. Sarigul Guduk S, Karaca N. Safety and complications of absorbable threads made of poly-L-lactic acid and poly lactide/glycolide: Experience with 148 consecutive patients. *J Cosmet Dermatol.* 2018.

41. Guida S, Persechino F, Rubino G, et al. Improving mandibular contour: A pilot study for indication of PPLA traction thread use. *J Cosmet Laser Ther.* 2018;1–5.

42. Goldberg DJ. Stimulation of collagenesis by poly-L-lactic acid (PLLA) and -glycolide polymer (PLGA)-containing absorbable suspension suture and parallel sustained clinical benefit. *J Cosmet Dermatol.* 2020;19(5):1172–1178.

43. Khiabanloo SR, Nabie R, Aalipour E. Outcomes in thread lift for face, neck, and nose; A prospective chart review study with APTOS. *J Cosmet Dermatol.* 2020.

44. Atiyeh BS, Dibo SA, Costagliola M, et al. Barbed sutures "lunch time" lifting: evidence-based efficacy. *J Cosmet Dermatol.* 2010;9(2):132–141.

45. Teitelbaum S. Enthusiasm versus data: how does an aesthetic procedure become "hot"? *J Aesthet Surg.* 2006;26(1):51–53.

46. Yoo KH, Kim WS, Hong CK, et al. Chronic inflammatory reaction after thread lifting: delayed unusual complication of nonabsorbable thread. *Dermatol Surg.* 2015;41(4):510–513.

47. Shin JJ, Park JH, Lee JM, et al. Mycobacterium Massiliense Infection After Thread-Lift Insertion. *Dermatol Surg.* 2016;42(10):1219–1222.

48. Jang HJ, Lee WS, Hwang K, et al. Effect of cog threads under rat skin. *Dermatol Surg.* 2005;31(12):1639–1643.

49. Van Winkle WJr, Hastings JC, Barker E, et al. Effect of suture materials on healing skin wounds. *Surg Gynecol Obstet.* 1975;140(1):7–12.

50. Stark GB, Bannasch H. The "golden thread lift": radiologic findings. *Aesthet Plast Surg.* 2007;31(2):206–208.

51. Jeong S, Ma YR, Park YG. Histopathological study of frontalis suspension materials. *Jpn J Ophthal.* 2000;44(2):171–174.

52. Kirsch WM, Zhu YH, Steckel R, et al. In vivo remodeling of surgically constructed vascular anastomoses: nonpenetrating, arcuate-legged clips versus standard suture. *Ann N Y Acad Sci.* 2002;961:284–287.

53. Pusic AL, Klassen AF, Scott AM, et al. Development and psychometric evaluation of the FACE-Q satisfaction with appearance scale: a new patient-reported outcome instrument for facial aesthetics patients. *Clin Plast Surg.* 2013;40(2):249–260.

54. Oh CH, Jang SB, Kang CM, Shim JS. Buttock Lifting Using Elastic Thread (Elasticum((R))) with a New Classification of Gluteal Ptosis. *Aesthetic Plast Surg.* 2018.

55. Winners Clinic. Thread Lift by Use of Retaining Ligaments (TL). 2017; Available at https://clinicaltrials.gov/ct2/show/NCT02235363. Accessed September 9, 2018.

56. Cobo R. Use of Polydioxanone Threads as an Alternative in Nonsurgical Procedures in Facial Rejuvenation. *Facial Plast Surg.* 2020;36(4):447–452.

57. El-Mesidy MS, Alaklouk W, Azzam OA. Nasolabial fold correction through cheek volume loss restoration versus thread lifting: a comparative study. *Arch Dermatol Res.* 2020;312(7):473–480.

CHAPTER 30

Skin Tightening

Joseph N. Mehrabi, MD
Elizabeth J. Kream, MD
Jordan V. Wang, MD, MBE, MBA
Nazanin Saedi, MD

SUMMARY POINTS

What's Important?

1. Novel technologies in the aesthetic market continue to facilitate the growth of skin tightening procedures. This has led to improved patient experiences and clinical outcomes, while encouraging patients to further embrace cosmetic dermatology. Since skin tightening is a common cosmetic goal of many cosmetic patients, physicians should be familiar with the many devices and modalities available in order to optimize results.

What's New?

1. Newer RF devices have been equipped with subdermal probes and real-time monitoring to increase patient safety and reduce the potential for over-heating. Novel ultrasound devices have incorporated high-intensity, high-frequency, parallel ultrasound beams that bypass the epidermal layer and directs the thermal damage to depths of 0.5–2 mm, while avoiding injury to deeper anatomic structures. Patient interest in absorbable thread lifting is high, and newer absorbable threads have a favorable safety and efficacy profile compared to their predecessors.

What's Coming?

1. Thermomechanical fractional injury (TMFI) is a relatively new modality that combines thermal energy with motion. A current TMFI device focuses thermal energy on a titanium tip with a grid of pyramids, which, when heated, is pulsed to contact the skin surface and coagulate the tissue. The expansion of topical drug delivery via lasers and other energy-based devices may offer synergistic effects when combined with these skin tightening devices.

INTRODUCTION

Lax and sagging skin is an inevitable sign of cutaneous aging. The onset and severity of crepiness is influenced by several intrinsic factors, such as fibroblast senescence with age, genetics, and ethnicity, as well as various extrinsic factors, such as ultraviolet radiation, environmental toxins, diet, smoking, and stress. On histology, lax skin shows dermal atrophy due to loss of collagen and elastin and decreased hydration.[1] On the face, laxity can manifest as severe wrinkles, dermatochalasis or eyelid skin redundancy, and jowls. Areas on the body, such as the inner arms, abdomen, and upper thighs, may begin to show laxity in the mid to late thirties or even earlier in postpartum patients or those with a history of rapid weight loss. The gold standard for addressing skin laxity is rhytidectomy, which mechanically tightens the skin by excising redundant tissue and re-draping the underlying fascia and musculature. However, many patients find the risks associated with general anesthesia, extended recovery time, and unavoidable surgical scars unacceptable and instead opt for less invasive options.

Additionally, there has been a growing population of aesthetic patients who are younger individuals who exhibit mild laxity or desire preventive interventions. Young patients with mild to moderate laxity can be candidates for the less invasive modalities discussed below. Highlighting the demand for non-surgical approaches, in 2019, body-sculpting procedures, which include skin tightening procedures, saw a 62% increase, which was the largest increase of any cosmetic procedural category.[2] Non-surgical approaches to tighten and lift sagging skin include microneedling, collagen-stimulating-soft-tissue injectables, laser and light devices, radiofrequency, intense focused ultrasound, thread lifting, cold atmospheric plasma, and thermomechanical fractional injury devices. With an array of methods now available, providers can combine modalities to safely deliver a tailored result.

MECHANISM OF SKIN TIGHTENING

While there has been an increase in available skin tightening devices over the last few decades, their mechanisms hinge on reinforcing dermal and subdermal turgor. For skin tightening, an ideal device bypasses the epidermis and delivers energy to the dermis and fibroseptal network to induce an immediate collagen contraction and subsequent induction of neocollagenesis and neoelastogenesis. Collagen Types I and III represent 75% of the dry weight of the dermis and 20–30% of its volume.[3] In addition to providing support to the dermis, collagen is also found in the fibroseptal network, around adipocytes, and in fascial networks, such as the superficial musculoaponeurotic system (SMAS).

Upon heating, collagen fibrils undergo defined conformational changes. Fibrils begin to shrink around 58°C which heralds the start of denaturation. The main transition or denaturation occurs at 65°C, which involves breaking of intramolecular crosslinks and further collagen contraction to a shorter and thicker conformation.[4,5] The crosslinks that remain are heat-stable and confer a more elastic property to the contracted fibrils. Immediate collagen contraction leads to tissue contraction, which decreases laxity and provides a lifting effect.

Additionally, the heat and/or mechanical insult induces a wound healing cascade, which results in de novo collagen formation by activated fibroblasts. Unsurprisingly, the time required for maximal collagen denaturation and contraction is inversely related to temperature. These basic principles translate to the mechanisms and properties of the devices discussed below.

MEASURING SKIN LAXITY

During the patient consult, the degree of laxity must be assessed so that the appropriate treatment regimen can be selected and realistic expectations can be set. There are several objective and subjective approaches to assessing for skin laxity. Several validated scales have been proposed for sites such as the neck[6], knees[1], thighs[1], and buttocks[1]. Scales generally consist of photonumeric grades with 0 typically denoting absent laxity and the upper limit denoting severe laxity. Another simple and low-cost method is the skin distention test (SDT), where two points are marked and the distance between these two points is measured before and after stretching the skin until resistance limits further extension.

When more precise measurements are desired, such as in the setting of clinical trials, there are a handful of more objective and elegant tools. To reduce inter- and intra-rater measurement variation in the SDT, the placement of micro (1–2 mm) tattoos within treatment sites has been used.[7] The micro tattoos can serve as fixed landmarks throughout the study period and can be easily removed with laser treatments.[7] A cutometer probe uses a suction chamber to measure the vertical deformation of skin when negative pressure is applied and released. Results are generated as a dislocation/relaxation curve. Other studies have used dermal thickness as a proxy for elasticity and haved employed optical coherence tomography (OCT) to measure dermal thickness.[8]

TREATMENT OPTIONS

Microneedling

Percutaneous collagen induction (PCI) therapy, known more commonly as microneedling, has been utilized to treat a variety of cutaneous conditions, including skin laxity.[9,10] Depending on the condition and the site of treatment, the penetration depth, typically 0.5–2 mm, is set by the practitioner. The depths can also be layered to create larger and more specific regions of controlled injury. In automatic microneedling pens, the needles glide perpendicularly over the skin, penetrating the dermis to create hundreds of microchannels, which can stimulate a dermal wound healing cascade and subsequent collagen formation.[11] Traditional devices were designed as mechanical rollers, which are now suboptimal. Newer devices in the form of electric powered pens are now more frequent in practice.[12] This newer form permits rapid modifications of penetration depth and pulse frequency in addition to using more hygienic, disposable, single-use tips.

A recent study showed significant improvements in global wrinkle score, skin laxity, and skin texture at 150 days following a series of four microneedling treatments in 48 subjects.[13] Another study of 58 patients treated with microneedling for arm and abdominal laxity and striae, showed high patient satisfaction and increased epidermal thickness seen on histology at 1 year.[14] Typically, 3–5 treatments spaced 2–4 weeks apart are recommended. Results from microneedling are modest, but it remains an affordable option that can concurrently treat the epidermis. Although microneedling procedures are primarily used for enhancing skin texture, minimal skin tightening may also be observed. The treatment endpoint is typically transient pinpoint bleeding. Common side effects are mild pain, erythema, edema, and peeling, which resolve within days.

Collagen Stimulating Soft-Tissue Injectables

Collagen stimulating soft-tissue injectables, such as polylactic acid (PLLA) and calcium hydroxylapatite (CaHA) can be diluted or hyper-diluted to induce neocollagenesis and improve skin laxity without a volumization effect. The addition of these diluted fillers to an energy-based device treatment series can further improve lax skin. CaHA stimulates fibroblasts by acting as a scaffold, while PLLA particles stimulate fibroblasts through a subclinical foreign body response. By 2 months after injection of CaHA, the microspheres are seen encompassed by histiocytes and fibroblasts rich in endoplasmic reticulum and dilated with procollagen.[15,16] Significant increases in collagen and mRNA expression of TGF-beta and inhibitors of matrix metalloproteinases have been noted in treated skin after a series of diluted CaHA or PLLA injections.[17,18]

Global consensus panels of core-specialty physicians have offered guidelines for the use of both diluted CaHA[19] and PLLA[20] for skin tightening. Numerous studies have shown both safety and efficacy for addressing laxity on the arms,[21] abdomen,[21] face,[22] decolletage,[23] and knees and upper thighs.[24,25] A series of treatments spaced a few months apart is recommended for best results. To date, no complications of vascular compromise have been reported after diluted CaHA or PLLA treatment. Adverse events usually include mild edema or bruising that resolve over 2–3 weeks following treatment. Nodules or delayed granuloma formation could be a rare side effect that should be considered.

Ablative and Non-Ablative Lasers

Initially, ablative resurfacing was the gold standard non-surgical approach for skin tightening. Unlike newer skin tightening devices, which generally bypass the epidermis, ablative lasers stimulate the dermis while ablating the epidermis. Therefore, for patients also requiring textural improvement and epidermal rejuvenation, ablative resurfacing can be considered.

When skin tightening is the goal, the chromophore for selective photothermolysis is water. Following superficial epidermal vaporization and intraepidermal injury, a wound healing phase ensues, which involves dermal matrix remodeling. Fibroblasts begin to produce Types I and III collagen, resulting in full re-epithelialization over time. The first laser used for confluent ablative resurfacing was the short-pulsed high-peak power carbon dioxide (CO2) laser in the 1980s, followed by the 2940 nm erbium YAG. While both target intracellular and extracellular water as the chromophore, the wavelength of Er:YAG is closer to the 3000 nm absorptive peak of water and thus it was purported that Er:YAG would cause less collateral damage compared to CO2.[26] Early ablative Er:YAG was noted to provide less impressive results than CO2 and thus more treatments were needed. Because the entire epidermis is ablated, the recovery period is several weeks, and there is risk of scarring and dyspigmentation.

Non-ablative lasers and light devices used for skin tightening include mid-infrared lasers, visible lasers (pulsed dye laser, potassium titanyl phosphate), and intense pulsed light. Non-ablative lasers can reach and heat the dermis. while sparing the overlying epidermis. While these devices are better tolerated than their ablative counterparts, the reduced thermal energy delivered can result in more modest clinical outcomes. A small split-face study of 12 patients with facial laxity suggested that a non-ablative laser can be as effective in skin tightening as a single early radiofrequency treatment.[27] However, since this study, radiofrequency devices have been refined and newer devices have been introduced, so the significance of this study remains questionable. Due the limited depth of penetration of these devices, non-ablative lasers are best used for the treatment of mild skin laxity and/or the treatment of other epidermal skin conditions.

Fractional photothermolysis was introduced in 2004 and led to a paradigm shift in aesthetic dermatology.[28] In contrast to treating a confluent area, the laser beam delivers energy in a grid-like pattern to create small columns of thermal injury termed microthermal treatment zones (MTZs) interlaced with untargeted skin. With surrounding reservoirs of untreated skin, wound healing is much quicker, downtime is decreased, and the side effect profile is improved. The density, width, and depth of these MTZs can be set by the device operator. Ablative fractional resurfacing (AFR) has the ability to penetrate deeper into the dermis, allowing for greater improvement of skin laxity.[29] AFR, like its non-fractional counterparts, can offer more noticeable clinical outcomes compared to non-ablative fractional modalities. Following AFR, patients can expect transient post-procedure erythema and other mild temporary side effects. such as edema, dry skin, pruritus, and acneiform lesions. Because the chromophore for skin tightening is water, treatment is considered safe in skin of color; however, caution should still be taken and provider knowledge and skill are essential. Post-inflammatory hyperpigmentation following treatment is more common in skin of color.[30] While fully ablative laser resurfacing requires pre-operative pain control, such as sedatives, topical anesthesia, intramuscular analgesia, and/or nerve blocks, patients typically tolerate fractional laser treatments with topical anesthesia alone.[31]

Radiofrequency

Radiofrequency (RF) has been used cosmetically for skin tightening since 2001.[32] RF devices can typically cause deeper effects than the previously mentioned modalities. RF uses a controlled electric current to distribute energy to the dermis.[33] The tissue resistance to the movement of electrons within an RF field is exceptionally high in fat and fibrous tissues, which leads to thermogenesis. RF devices typically raise the temperature of the dermis, while the epidermis remains cool. A study in 2003 of 86 patients demonstrated that a single RF treatment was safe and effective to improve periorbital skin laxity.[34] Thicker collagen fibers have been found on electron microscopy after multiple RF treatments as well.[35]

RF energy can be delivered in different devices using various modes, including monopolar, bipolar, and multipolar. Monopolar RF (MRF) was one of the first of the RF devices to be employed in skin tightening. In MRF, energy flows from an electrode in the device handpiece to a passive electrode placed on the patient. It can be difficult to control the energy delivery from MRF, which may contribute to a greater risk of deep tissue damage than bipolar RF. MRF energy can be administered in a stamped mode, gliding movement, or subcutaneous fiber, and recent studies have shown that monopolar RF is effective and safe.[36,37] Recently, a new MRF device was evaluated in treating facial and neck laxity in 40 patients.[38] While the study showed that 73% of patients had improvement at 6 months, the average pain score during treatment was 6.9 out of 10. In theory, MRF fluence output should be titrated to patient comfort feedback, and thus, analgesia should be limited. However, in practice, most providers will pre-treat with topical anesthesia and/or intradermal or intramuscular analgesia. Importantly, Kist et al. showed that collagen induction following monopolar RF is most significant with protocols using multiple passes with lower fluences compared to single passes with higher and more painful fluences.[39] In addition to discomfort, common adverse events include transient erythema, edema, and bruising.

In comparison, bipolar and multipolar RF deliver the energy between two or more poles at the tip of the handpiece, and the penetration depth is determined by the distance between them. Since the currents have a controlled distribution that is limited to the volume between the electrodes, bipolar and multipolar devices can deliver RF energy to more superficial skin layers.[40] For this reason, these devices can be used for younger patients who desire prophylaxis for skin laxity or those with only mild laxity.[41] Subdermal RF devices deliver energy through subdermal cannulas that completely bypass the epidermis, which limits collateral tissue damage. These devices come equipped with a thermistor on the probe, which detects changes in tissue resistance and modulates the energy output accordingly. Additionally, an infrared camera can provide real-time temperature monitoring to increase patient safety and reduce the potential for overheating and unintended burns, blistering, necrosis, and scarring. Studies of subdermal RF devices have shown safety and efficacy in treating facial[42] and arm laxity.[5]

Radiofrequency Microneedling

The concept of fractionation, or creating small columns of injury encased by untreated reservoirs, is not limited to lasers. In recent years, RF has been combined with traditional microneedling, termed "RF microneedling." RF microneedling is by definition a fractional treatment, parallel to the concept of AFR laser therapy. RF microneedling devices utilize an array of small needles to penetrate the epidermis and dermis and deliver RF energy and heat through the needles to the dermis.[12,43] The needles can be either insulated or non-insulated.

Insulated needles deliver energy focused on their tips, while non-insulated needles deliver heat throughout the entire length of the needle to cause more dramatic thermal damage. Monopolar and bipolar modes can be applied to the tips to control the pattern of RF energy delivery. Monopolar modes combined with non-insulated tips are thought to deliver more thermal injury, but with greater risk for adverse events. Devices on the market vary in terms of needle length, needle coating, needle sharpness, and method of needle insertion. One study demonstrated improved wrinkle reduction, skin tightening, and lifting of the mid-to-lower face using a non-insulated RF microneedling system in 49 patients undergoing 3 monthly treatments.[44] Off the face, Alexiades and Munavalli found that one session of RF microneedling administered to a total of 62 treatment areas (22 upper arm, 34 suprapatellar, and

6 bra line) improved laxity, and outcomes were maintained for at least 6 months.[45]

The addition of RF energy can raise the amount and depth of controlled injury to the dermis compared to traditional microneedling. Treatments can be stacked to produce more dramatic results. It is vital to allow for full needle retraction before moving sites to avoid dragging and unintended damage to the skin. Thinner skin may respond to RF microneedling better than thicker, sebaceous skin. Mild to moderate skin laxity may respond to treatment better than severe skin laxity. Skin laxity and rhytides of the perioral area, mid cheeks, jawline, and neck were shown to respond better given their more "volume-depleted" nature in contrast to the skin in the periocular area and forehead rhytides, which are mostly the result of muscle movement over time.

Ultrasound

Ultrasound encompasses high-intensity focused ultrasound (HIFU), microfocused ultrasound with visualization (MFU-V), and synchronous ultrasound parallel beam (SUPERB) technology. An advantage of ultrasound modalities is that they can effectively bypass the superficial layers of the skin, allowing for generation of higher subepidermal skin temperatures and controlled damage.[46] Therefore, selective targeting of certain facial anatomic structures, such as the SMAS, at 4–5 mm of depth can be more easily achieved. Some drawbacks include the lack of precise temperature feedback and also that some clinicians find the predefined depths restrictive.

HIFU, classically used to ablate tumors, emits acoustic energy to target tissue, which forms cavitations and thermal energy, heating tissue to 55–70°C. This thermomechanical reaction leads to a coagulative necrosis in targeted zones. Both fat reduction and skin tightening can be achieved with HIFU. Skin tightening is achieved because the quick increase in temperature denatures and contracts collagen fibers and stimulates new collagen formation.[47] Compared to monopolar radiofrequency, the neocollagenesis and neoelastogenesis from HIFU are deeper in the dermis and more focal.[48] HIFU was first approved to lift the brow area in 2009. Given the deeper treatment depth and end result of both fat reduction and skin tightening, HIFU can be an option for thin postpartum patients who desire abdominal rejuvenation.

MFU-V is a proven and popular modality for skin tightening. In 2019, the number of MFU-V procedures performed increased by over 200%.[2] Compared to HIFU, MFU-V uses higher frequencies and decreased energy to briefly heat tissue above 60°C and form microthermal zones of coagulation, approximately 1 mm³ in size at predefined depths of 1.5, 3.0, and 4.5 mm. MFU-V incorporates high-resolution ultrasonography up to 8 mm in depth to ensure that the underlying dermis and fascia is targeted. MFU-V was first approved for lifting of the neck in 2012. An early study of MFU-V demonstrated the safety and effectiveness in rejuvenating facial and neck areas in 36 patients, including notable brow elevation at 90 days following a single treatment.[49] A 2019 randomized split-face blinded trial comparing MFU-V and MRF at treating facial and neck laxity found no significant differences in tightening effect, patient satisfaction, or rate of adverse events.[50]

Synchronous ultrasound parallel beam (SUPERB) technology was more recently developed. This device generates high-intensity, high-frequency ultrasonic pulses that increase dermal temperatures to cause controlled areas of thermal damage. The handpiece contains seven parallel transducers that come in direct skin contact, which can deliver energy to the mid dermis, with the coagulation zone depths ranging from 0.5–2 mm and centered at 1.5 mm. A recent study of 58 subjects following a single treatment to the face and neck demonstrated significant improvement of 1 to 3 Fitzpatrick Wrinkle and Elastosis Scale units in 86% of subjects.[51] There were also no device-related adverse events.

Ultrasound has proven to be generally safe in all skin types and can be effective at modestly tightening and lifting sagging skin.[52–54] The most common side effects are transient purpura, edema, and mild to moderate pain. Pain can be minimized by pre-treating with a combination of topical anesthesia, inhaled nitrous oxide, oral sedative, and/or intramuscular analgesia. Refined devices should continue to improve clinical outcomes.

Suture Suspension/Absorbable Thread Lifting

While the advent of thread lifting occurred in the 1990s, the original procedure utilized non-absorbable sutures, which were associated with many adverse events, such as palpable nodules, migration, extrusion, and granuloma formation. The introduction of absorbable polydioxanone (PDO) and polyglycolic acid/poly-L-lactic acid (PGA/PLLA) threads has led to a recent resurgence. Most threads used for lifting come pre-cannulated and are attached with cogs or cones that grasp tissue for a lifting effect. The arrangement of cones or barbs can categorize threads as unidirectional, bidirectional, or multidirectional. Depending on the site and end goal, threads are typically tunneled through the subdermal layer or superficial musculoaponeurotic system (SMAS). When threads are pulled in the opposite direction, the barbs adhere to the underlying tissue, which provides traction and subsequent lifting of overlying tissue. In addition to this initial mechanical suspension, it is purported that the suture material elicits a foreign body response with subsequent neocollagenesis that provides enduring lifting.[55] A 2018 animal study involving histologic analysis of various implanted threads found a similar amount of Type III collagen induction at 12 weeks for PDO and PLLA threads and also noted that none of the threads induced elastic fiber formation.[56] Current threads can undergo complete hydrolytic degradation over 6–8 months (PDO) or 14–18 months (PLLA).

In 2015, two different absorbable thread lifting systems were approved: a bidirectional cog PDO thread and a bidirectional PLLA suture with 82% PLLA/18% PGA cones. Several literature reviews[57–59] have similarly remarked on the lack of randomized controlled trials and thus conclude that while thread lifting appears to be safe and well tolerated, high-quality studies are still needed to evaluate their safety and efficacy and to strengthen the recommendation level. Small studies have suggested a favorable side effect profile, high patient satisfaction, and increased lifting on the face.[60,61] Ogilvie et al. evaluated a commercially available PLLA/PGA thread for facial and neck lifting in 100 patients.[62] Adverse events included mild and transient edema, pinpoint bleeding, pain, ecchymosis, and 83.6% of patients showed at least one degree of improvement on a 5-point scale. Of note, the face was considered much more responsive than the neck. A 2018 single-provider comparative study of 42 patients treated with facial thread lifting and followed for 24 months, reported no permanent or serious adverse events, and there was a durable lifting effect appreciated.[63] A thorough understanding of anatomy and judicious technique is imperative. Placing threads too superficially can lead to dimpling and visibility of the threads, while placing them too deep can damage neurovascular structures. Modern thread lifting has been associated with improved safety and efficacy compared to its predecessor.

Cold Atmospheric Plasma

Plasma, known as the "fourth state," is created by ionizing gas. Lasers and radiofrequency can be used to convert gas, such as helium or nitrogen, into plasma. Cold atmospheric plasma (CAP) is considered non-thermal plasma, because while the electrons are hot, the heavy particles (neutrons and ions) are at room temperature.[64] Plasma devices have been used for near damage-free surgical cutting and ablating tumors, and more recently, plasma technology has expanded to aesthetic procedures. In plasma skin rejuvenation, radiofrequency has been employed to ionize nitrogen or helium gas into plasma. The plasma heats target tissue in a bimodal fashion: first the plasma beam itself emits heat as it rapidly neutralizes, and secondly, the plasma conducts a portion of the radiofrequency to the tissue.[65,66]

A novel subdermal plasma device equipped with a probe that can be introduced to the subdermal layer through a small incision, has been employed for skin tightening. This subdermal device uses radiofrequency to energize an electrode, which ionizes helium gas. The probe emits a beam of plasma. The radiofrequency that is conducted has a much lower current than a monopolar radiofrequency device, which prevents overtreating or diffusion to unintended areas. Increased target tissue temperatures cause tissue coagulation and contraction. Because not all of the helium will be ionized, the remaining helium gas acts a cooling agent to assist with immediate cooling. Although more studies are needed, current studies appear promising.[64]

Thermomechanical Fractional Injury

Thermomechanical fractional injury (TMFI) is a relatively new non-ablative skin rejuvenation method that combines thermal energy with motion.[67] Unlike RF, ultrasound, or laser, which rely on transforming one form of energy to another, TMFI directly delivers heat through conduction.[68] A current TMFI device has a tip composed of a gold-plated copper base and a titanium cover composed of a grid of pyramids. The pyramids are blunt-tipped, which allows for the conduction of heat but prevents mechanical puncturing of the epidermis. The backplane of the tip is maintained at 400°C during treatment. When heated, the tip is pulsed to contact the skin surface, which causes micropores to form through the evaporation of water. On histology, the thermal effect is non-ablative and hemispherical in shape.[68] Thermal heat transfer using TMFI does not involve any mechanical penetration deeper than the epidermis. In one study, most patients experienced mild to moderate improvement in skin laxity and facial rhytides after 2–3 treatment sessions at 3–5-week intervals.[69] Topical anesthetic is recommended prior to treatment, and postprocedural downtime is minimal at 1–2 days. Transient postprocedural events include erythema and post-inflammatory hyperpigmentation.

COMBINING MODALITIES

In limited experiences, combinations of the modalities discussed above have so far been demonstrated to be safe and effective in their tightening and lifting effects. The latest novel devices may incorporate multiple modalities in one handpiece. Treatments with lasers and diluted fillers generally have a more superficial effect and lax skin can be further supported by adding an energy-based device that can reach the deeper dermis and fibroseptal network. Especially for sites like the abdomen, where the fascia is deep, devices that use RF or ultrasound can be used to achieve appreciable results. Examples of successful combinations for facial laxity include confluent and fractional ablative lasers,[70] radiofrequency microneedling and bipolar radiofrequency,[71] monopolar radiofrequency and ultrasound,[72] and MFU-V and fractional CO2 laser.[73] A combination of MFU-V and diluted CaHA can improve laxity of the upper thighs and buttocks[74] as well as the abdomen.[11] Equipped with the principles discussed above, the clinician can develop a systematic way of assessing patients and developing a regimen that is both safe and efficacious.

CONCLUSION

Skin laxity occurs with aging, as well as after changes in weight and pregnancy. Many patients are distressed by crepey skin both on and off the face. Providers should be familiar with the numerous treatment options available and follow emerging trends in order to individualize an approach for each patient. Realistic expectations must be set from the initial patient encounter, as skin tightening procedures will not provide the same dramatic results as surgical intervention. Knowledge of device principles, training, and technique are necessary to safely deliver effective outcomes and maximize patient satisfaction.

References

1. Kaminer MS, Casabona G, Peeters W, et al. Validated Assessment Scales for Skin Laxity on the Posterior Thighs, Buttocks, Anterior Thighs, and Knees in Female Patients. *Dermatol Surg.* 2019;45(Suppl 1):S12–S21.

2. American Society for Dermatologic Surgery (ASDS) Survey on Dermatologic Procedures. Data were collected for the 2019 experience and generalized to represent all ASDS members.

3. Bolognia J, Jorizzo JL, Schaffer JV. *Dermatology.* 3rd ed. Philadelphia: Elsevier Saunders; 2012.G

4. Fabi SG. Noninvasive skin tightening: focus on new ultrasound techniques. *Clin Cosmet Investig Dermatol.* 2015;8:47–52.

5. Wu DC, Liolios A, Mahoney L, Guiha I, Goldman MP. Subdermal Radiofrequency for Skin Tightening of the Posterior Upper Arms. *Dermatol Surg.* 2016;42:1089–1093.

6. Guida S, Spadafora M, Longhitano S, Pellacani G, Farnetani F. A Validated Photonumeric Scale for the Evaluation of Neck Skin Laxity. *Dermatol Surg.* 2021;47:e188–e190.

7. Alam M, Pongprutthipan M, Nanda S, et al. Quantitative evaluation of skin shrinkage associated with non-invasive skin tightening: a simple method for reproducible linear measurement using microtattoos. *Lasers Med Sci.* 2019;34:703–709.

8. Gawdat H, Allam RSHM, Hegazy R, Sameh B, Ragab N. Comparison of the efficacy of Fractional Radiofrequency Microneedling alone and in combination with platelet-rich plasma in neck rejuvenation: a clinical and optical coherence tomography study. *J Cosmet Dermatol.* 2021. https://doi.org/10.1111/jocd.14331.

9. Leal Silva HG. Facial Laxity Rating Scale Validation Study. *Dermatol Surg.* 2016;42(12):1370–1379.

10. Alexiades-Armenakas M, Rosenberg D, Renton B, Dover J, Arndt K. Blinded, randomized, quantitative grading comparison of minimally invasive, fractional radiofrequency and surgical face-lift to treat skin laxity. *Arch Dermatol.* 2010;146(4):396–405.

11. Kream E, Boen M, Fabi SG, Goldman MP. Nonsurgical Postpartum Abdominal Rejuvenation: A Review and Our Experience. *Dermatol Surg.* 2021;47:768–774.

12. Alster TS, Graham PM. Microneedling: A review and practical guide. *Dermatol Surg.* 2018;44(3):397–404.

13. Hou A, Cohen B, Haimovic A, Elbuluk N. Microneedling: A comprehensive review. *Dermatol Surg.* 2017;43(3):321–339.

14. Aust MC, Fernandes D, Kolokythas P, Kaplan HM, Vogt PM. Percutaneous collagen induction therapy: an alternative treatment for scars, wrinkles, and skin laxity. *Plast Reconstr Surg.* 2008;121:1421–1429.

15. Zerbinati N, D'Este E, Parodi PC, Calligaro A. Microscopic and ultrastructural evidences in human skin following calcium hydroxylapatite filler treatment. *Arch Dermatol Res.* 2017;309:389–396.

16. Berlin AL, Hussain M, Goldberg DJ. Calcium hydroxylapatite filler for facial rejuvenation: a histologic and immunohistochemical analysis. *Dermatol Surg.* 2008;34(Suppl 1):S64–S67.

17. Yutskovskaya Y, Kogan E. A randomized, split-face, histomorphologic study comparing a volumetric calcium hydroxylapatite and a hyaluronic acid-based dermal filler. *J Drugs Dermatol.* 2014.

18. Stein P, Vitavska O, Kind P, Hoppe W, Wieczorek H, Schürer NY. The biological basis for poly-L-lactic acid-induced augmentation. *J Dermatol Sci.* 2015;78:26–33.

19. Goldie K, Peeters W, Alghoul M, et al. Global Consensus Guidelines for the Injection of Diluted and Hyperdiluted Calcium Hydroxylapatite for Skin Tightening. *Dermatol Surg.* 2018;44(Suppl 1):S32–S41.

20. Haddad A, Menezes A, Guarnieri C, et al. Recommendations on the Use of Injectable Poly-L-Lactic Acid for Skin Laxity in Off-Face Areas. *J Drugs Dermatol.* 2019;9:929–935.

21. Lapatina NG, Pavlenko T. Diluted Calcium Hydroxylapatite for Skin Tightening of the Upper Arms and Abdomen. *J Drugs Dermatol.* 2017;16:900–906.

22. Hexsel D, Hexsel CL, Cotofana S. Introducing the L-Lift—A Novel Approach to Treat Age-Related Facial Skin Ptosis Using A Collagen Stimulator. *Dermatol Surg.* 2020;46:1122.

23. Yutskovskaya YA, Kogan EA. Improved Neocollagenesis and Skin Mechanical Properties After Injection of Diluted Calcium Hydroxylapatite in the Neck and Décolletage:A Pilot Study. *J Drugs Dermatol.* 2017;16:68–74.

24. Kollipara R, Hoss E, Boen M, Alhaddad M, Fabi SG. A Randomized, Split-Body, Placebo-Controlled Trial to Evaluate the Efficacy and Safety of Poly-L-lactic Acid for the Treatment of Upper Knee Skin Laxity. *Dermatol Surg.* 2020;46:1623–1627.

25. Guida S, Longhitano S, Shaniko K, et al. Hyperdiluted calcium hydroxylapatite for skin laxity and cellulite of the skin above the knee: A pilot study. *Dermatol Ther.* 2020;33:e14076.

26. Farshidi D, Hovenic W, Zachary C. Erbium:yttrium aluminum garnet ablative laser resurfacing for skin tightening. *Dermatol Surg.* 2014;40(Suppl 12):S152–S156.

27. Key DJ. Single-treatment skin tightening by radiofrequency and long-pulsed, 1064-nm Nd: YAG laser compared. *Lasers Surg Med.* 2007;39:169–175.

28. Manstein D, Herron GS, Sink RK, Tanner H, Anderson RR. Fractional photothermolysis: A new concept for cutaneous remodeling using microscopic patterns of thermal injury. *Lasers Surg Med.* 2004;34(5):426–438.

29. Ortiz AE, Goldman MP, Fitzpatrick RE. Ablative CO_2 lasers for skin tightening: Traditional versus fractional. *Dermatol Surg.* 2014;40(Suppl 12):S147–S151.

30. Graber EM, Tanzi EL, Alster TS. Side effects and complications of fractional laser photothermolysis: experience with 961 treatments. *Dermatol Surg.* 2008;34:301–305; discussion 305–7.

31. Alexiades-Armenakas MR, Dover JS, Arndt KA. The spectrum of laser skin resurfacing: nonablative, fractional, and ablative laser resurfacing. *J Am Acad Dermatol.* 2008;58:719–737; quiz 738–40.

32. Gold MH. Noninvasive Skin Tightening Treatment. *J Clin Aesthet Dermatol.* 2015;8(6):14–18.

33. Greene RM, Green JB. Skin tightening technologies. *Facial Plast Surg.* 2014;30(1):62–67.

34. Fitzpatrick R, Geronemus R, Goldberg D, Kaminer M, Kilmer S, Ruiz-Esparza J. Multicenter study of noninvasive radiofrequency for periorbital tissue tightening. *Lasers Surg Med.* 2003;33(4):232–242.

35. Kist D, Burns AJ, Sanner R, Counters J, Zelickson B. Ultrastructural evaluation of multiple pass low energy versus single pass high energy radio-frequency treatment. *Lasers Surg Med.* 2006;38(2):150–154.

36. Carruthers J, Fabi S, Weiss R. Monopolar radiofrequency for skin tightening: our experience and a review of the literature. *Dermatol Surg.* 2014;40(Suppl 12):S168–S173.

37. Weiss RA, Weiss MA, Munavalli G, Beasley KL. Monopolar radiofrequency facial tightening: A retrospective analysis of efficacy and safety in over 600 treatments. *J Drugs Dermatol.* 2006;5(8):707–712.

38. Angra K, Alhaddad M, Boen M, et al. Prospective Clinical Trial of the Latest Generation of Noninvasive Monopolar Radiofrequency for the Treatment of Facial and Upper Neck Skin Laxity. *Dermatol Surg.* 2021;47:762–766.

39. Kist D, Burns AJ, Sanner R, Counters J, Zelickson B. Ultrastructural evaluation of multiple pass low energy versus single pass high energy radio-frequency treatment. *Lasers Surg Med.* 2006;38:150–154.

40. Krueger N, Sadick NS. New-generation radiofrequency technology. *Cutis.* 2013;91(1):39

41. Gentile RD, Kinney BM, Sadick NS. Radiofrequency technology in face and neck rejuvenation. *Facial Plast Surg Clin North Am.* 2018;26(2):123–134.

42. Sanan A, Hjelm N, Tassone P, Krein H, Heffelfinger RN. Thermistor-controlled subdermal skin tightening for the aging face: Clinical outcomes and efficacy. *Laryngoscope Investig Otolaryngol.* 2019;4:18–23.

43. Weiner SF. Radiofrequency microneedling: Overview of technology, advantages, differences in devices, studies, and indications. *Facial Plast Surg Clin North Am.* 2019;27(3):291–303.

44. Gold M, Taylor M, Rothaus K, Tanaka Y. Non-insulated smooth motion, micro-needles RF fractional treatment for wrinkle reduction and lifting of the lower face: International study. *Lasers Surg Med.* 2016;48(8):727–733.

45. Alexiades M, Munavalli GS. Single Treatment Protocol With Microneedle Fractional Radiofrequency for Treatment of Body Skin Laxity and Fat Deposits. *Lasers Surg Med.* 2021. https://doi.org/10.1002/lsm.23397.

46. Gutowski KA. Microfocused ultrasound for skin tightening. *Clin Plast Surg.* 2016;43(3):577–582.

47. Fabi SG. Noninvasive skin tightening: Focus on new ultrasound techniques. *Clin Cosmet Investig Dermatol.* 2015;8:47–52.

48. Suh DH, Choi JH, Lee SJ, Jeong K-H, Song KY, Shin MK. Comparative histometric analysis of the effects of high-intensity focused ultrasound and radiofrequency on skin. *J Cosmet Laser Ther.* 2015;17:230–236.

49. Alam M, White LE, Martin N, Witherspoon J, Yoo S, West DP. Ultrasound tightening of facial and neck skin: A rater-blinded prospective cohort study. *J Am Acad Dermatol.* 2010;62(2):262–269.

50. Alhaddad M, Wu DC, Bolton J, Wilson MJ, Jones IT, Boen M, et al. A randomized, split-face, evaluator-blind clinical trial comparing monopolar radiofrequency versus microfocused ultrasound with visualization for lifting and tightening of the face and upper neck. *Dermatol Surg.* 2019;45:131–139.

51. Wang JV, Ferzli G, Jeon H, Geronemus RG, Kauvar A. Efficacy and Safety of High-Intensity, High-Frequency, Parallel Ultrasound Beams for Fine Lines and Wrinkles. *Dermatol Surg.* 2021. Epub ahead of print.

52. MacGregor JL, Tanzi EL. Microfocused ultrasound for skin tightening. *Semin Cutan Med Surg.* 2013;32(1):18–25.

53. Minkis K, Alam M. Ultrasound skin tightening. *Dermatol Clin.* 2014;32(1):71–77.

54. Juhász M, Korta D, Mesinkovska NA. A review of the use of ultrasound for skin tightening, body contouring, and cellulite reduction in dermatology. *Dermatol Surg.* 2018;44(7):949–963.

55. McClean ME, Boen M, Alhaddad M, Hoss E, Kollipara R, Butterwick K. Suture Lifting: A Review of the Literature and Our Experiences. *Dermatol Surg.* 2020;46:1068–1077.

56. Lee CG, Jung J, Hwang S, et al. Histological Evaluation of Bioresorbable Threads in Rats. *Korean Journal of Clinical Laboratory Science.* 2018;50:217–224.

57. Gülbitti HA, Colebunders B, Pirayesh A, Bertossi D, van der Lei B. Thread-Lift Sutures: Still in the Lift? A Systematic Review of the Literature. *Plast Reconstr Surg.* 2018;141:341e–347e.

58. Tong LX, Rieder EA. Thread-Lifts: A Double-Edged Suture? A Comprehensive Review of the Literature. *Dermatol Surg.* 2019;45:931–940.

59. McClean ME, Boen M, Alhaddad M, Hoss E, Kollipara R, Butterwick K. Suture Lifting: A Review of the Literature and Our Experiences. *Dermatol Surg.* 2020;46:1068–1077.

60. Kim J, Kim HS, Seo JM, Nam KA, Chung KY. Evaluation of a novel thread-lift for the improvement of nasolabial folds and cheek laxity. *J Eur Acad Dermatol Venereol.* 2017;31:e136–e179.

61. Lee H, Yoon K, Lee M. Outcome of facial rejuvenation with polydioxanone thread for Asians. *J Cosmet Laser Ther.* 2018;20:189–192.

62. Ogilvie MP, Few JW Jr, Tomur SS, et al. Rejuvenating the Face: An Analysis of 100 Absorbable Suture Suspension Patients. *Aesthet Surg J.* 2018;38:654–663.

63. Ali YH. Two years' outcome of thread lifting with absorbable barbed PDO threads: Innovative score for objective and subjective assessment. *J Cosmet Laser Ther.* 2018;20:41–49.

64. Gentile RD. Renuvion/J-Plasma for Subdermal Skin Tightening Facial Contouring and Skin Rejuvenation of the Face and Neck. *Facial Plast Surg Clin North Am.* 2019;27:273–290.

65. Kilmer S, Fitzpatrick R, Bernstein E, Brown D. Long Term Follow-up On The Use Of Plasma Skin Regeneration (psr) In Full Facial Rejuvenation Procedures: 70. *Lasers Surg Med.* 2005;36.

66. Bogle MA, Arndt KA, Dover JS. Evaluation of plasma skin regeneration technology in low-energy full-facial rejuvenation. *Arch Dermatol.* 2007;143:168–174.

67. Elman M, Fournier N, Barneon G, Bernstein EF, Lask G. Fractional treatment of aging skin with Tixel, a clinical and histological evaluation. *J Cosmet Laser Ther.* 2016;18(1):31–37. doi:10.3109/14764172.2015.1052513.

68. Shavit R, Dierickx C. A New Method for Percutaneous Drug Delivery by Thermo-Mechanical Fractional Injury. *Lasers Surg Med.* 2020;52:61–69.

69. Daniely D, Judodihardjo H, Rajpar SF, Mehrabi JN, Artzi O. Thermo-Mechanical Fractional Injury Therapy for Facial Skin Rejuvenation in Skin Types II to V: A Retrospective Double-Center Chart Review. *Lasers Surg Med.* Mar 30 2021; doi:10.1002/lsm.23400.

70. Munavalli GS, Turley A, Silapunt S, Biesman B. Combining confluent and fractionally ablative modalities of a novel 2790nm YSGG laser for facial resurfacing. *Lasers Surg Med.* 2011;43(4):273–282.

71. Dayan E, Chia C, Burns AJ, Theodorou S. Adjustable Depth Fractional Radiofrequency Combined With Bipolar Radiofrequency: A Minimally Invasive Combination Treatment for Skin Laxity. *Aesthet Surg J.* 2019;39:S112–S119.

72. Catinis CA, Chilukuri S. The benefit of combined radiofrequency and ultrasound to enhance surgical and nonsurgical outcomes for the face and neck. *Plast Aesthet Res.* 2020;7.

73. Woodward JA, Fabi SG, Alster T, Colón-Acevedo B. Safety and efficacy of combining microfocused ultrasound with fractional CO2 laser resurfacing for lifting and tightening the face and neck. *Dermatol Surg.* 2014;40(Suppl 12):S190–S193.

74. Casabona G, Pereira G. Microfocused Ultrasound with Visualization and Calcium Hydroxylapatite for Improving Skin Laxity and Cellulite Appearance. *Plast Reconstr Surg Glob Open.* 2017;5:e1388.

SECTION 5

Skin Care

CHAPTER 31

Psychosocial Challenges in Aesthetic Dermatology

Mary D. Sun, MSCR, MA
Helen Liu, BS
Evan A. Rieder, MD

SUMMARY POINTS

What's Important?

1. Aesthetic practitioners may encounter patients who present with cosmetic concerns secondary to psychological distress or psychiatric illness. Identifying and appropriately managing these patients is critical to protecting the interests of both patients and providers.
2. To address challenges and issues during the clinical visit, providers can utilize a variety of techniques to set personal boundaries, screen for psychiatric disorders, and effectively communicate with dissatisfied patients.

What's New?

1. The advent of various technological advancements and widespread social media use can adversely impact individuals seeking cosmetic treatment.
2. Individuals who seek out aesthetic dermatology practices may be more likely to meet substance-related disorder criteria for cosmetic interventions.

What's Coming?

1. Research is ongoing to better understand and manage aesthetic-related effects of social media use, racial morphing, and cosmetic addiction.

INTRODUCTION

Interpersonal dynamics are an important component of the aesthetic dermatology visit. Given the elective nature and societal complexities of many cosmetic procedures, the development of positive patient-provider relationships is foundational to conducting a successful clinical experience. Though the majority of the provider-patient encounters go smoothly, aesthetic providers should recognize that some patients present with cosmetic concerns secondary to psychiatric disorders. Dermatologists, plastic surgeons, and other clinicians may be forced to manage psychopathologies in patients with low insight and self-awareness. These patients can present a variety of psychosocial challenges that may affect clinical practice. Learning how to effectively set personal boundaries, screen for common psychiatric disorders, and recognize emerging technology-associated developments in aesthetic trends can improve outcomes for both patients and providers. This chapter provides an overview of psychosocial challenges in aesthetic dermatology and discusses techniques that aesthetic providers can utilize to address and manage these significant, yet underrecognized issues.

BOUNDARIES

Consistently high stress levels have a variety of physiological effects on the body, including poor skin health.[1] When compounded by the presence of mental health comorbidities, psychological stress may lead affected individuals to turn to aesthetic professionals to seek cosmetic solutions. Such patients can be very challenging as while they present for the treatment of a cosmetic concern, in reality, they may be suffering from a psychiatric disorder that requires a completely different line of treatment. In some cases, patients may self-perceive significant cosmetic imperfections despite the lack of recognition by others. This creates difficult situations in which patients hold unreasonable expectations of treatment outcomes, disregard time limitations during clinical visits, and violate personal boundaries between themselves and their aesthetic providers.

While the nature of the mental health appointment varies greatly from the average cosmetic appointment, the structured framework used by mental health professionals can be applied to aesthetic appointments. For patients who routinely arrive late, their appointments should still end at the scheduled time to not infringe upon the next patient's appointment time. Regardless of start time, it is crucial that the aesthetic clinician be as efficient and boundaried as possible. For initial consultations that become unnecessarily prolonged, we recommend two strategies for providers.[2] The first approach is to listen to the patient in an uninterrupted manner for a few minutes, then set expectations by inquiring if it is OK to interrupt. If in receipt of an affirmative response from the patient, throughout the consultation, interrupt again as necessary when the patient's narrative derails, wanders, or needs to be curtailed for the sake of time. Asking more binary or close-ended questions and if necessary, setting up follow-up meetings to allow for more time to address their concerns can be useful. The second approach is to explicitly describe the time expectations of the consultation at the start of the visit. This technique is often utilized for follow-up patients when there might be a concern about time.

Many aesthetic practitioners have recently developed presences on social medial platforms to promote their services.[2] These applications have boosted the dissemination of information about cosmetic services, but may also lead to challenges and misinterpretations regarding the patient-physician relationship. Many clinicians decline to set adequate boundaries by sharing personal information about their relationships, social lives, and other non-clinically related topics online. This can create an atmosphere in which patients feel freer to broach personal topics in interactions with their clinicians. While the vast majority of these interactions may be interpreted positively and offer patients a greater sense of their clinician outside of the office setting, there may be exceptions in which patients feel overly familiar or intimate with their clinicians in ways that are not based in reality. Given the need for autonomy online but also the potential for personal boundary violations, we advise providing patients a copy of your practice policies document for repeated inappropriate behavior. In more severe cases in which there are repeated boundary violations, a behavioral contract can be signed by both parties when care is established. Such a contract explicitly discusses expectations from the treatment team (including clinician) and patient if a beneficial treatment relationship is to continue.

DIFFICULT PATIENTS

Patient satisfaction is crucial to the success of any medical practice and is especially important in aesthetic dermatology.[3] Providers may encounter "difficult" patients who are not satisfied despite their best efforts, and sometimes despite excellent cosmetic results. Such patients include those with difficult personalities, personality disorders, and/or psychiatric disorders such as body dysmorphic disorder and obsessive-compulsive disorder.

These situations may be understandably frustrating to providers. However, making an effort to understand the patient's personality style and adjusting behaviors to accommodate his or her personality has been demonstrated to maintain a higher quality patient-provider relationship.[4] Recent evidence suggests that patients who feel they share the same personality style as their provider are more satisfied with their care.[4] In clinical practice, aesthetic providers should anticipate needing to adapt to noncompliant patient responses and behaviors in real time.

Personality Disorders

A personality disorder is defined as an impairment in personality functioning (self and interpersonal) and enduring patterns of maladaptive thinking and behavior that pervade in many aspects of one's life.[5] Such disorders disproportionately present in the patient populations that seek out dermatologists, plastic surgeons and other aesthetic providers.[6-10] Patients with personality disorders must be treated differently, because the approach for the average patient is likely inadequate. Evidence suggests that the etiology of personality disorders are complex and involve biologic, developmental, environmental, and social triggers.[11-14] Attempting to treat a personality disorder is therefore unrealistic in a nonpsychiatric setting.[15] We instead recommend focusing on building and maintaining the patient-physician relationship and, once the clinician-patient relationship has been established, referring such patients to mental health providers for additional care.[2] While the purpose of this chapter is not to give a detailed approach to the treatment of personality disorders, an overview of some of the most common types of personality challenges in cosmetic dermatology is useful to have in the back of mind for instances in which a clinical encounter seems to be going wrong for reasons removed from cosmetic intervention. Several practical tips for how to approach patients with commonly presented personality disorders are presented in **Table 31-1**.[2] Patient satisfaction can be maximized by understanding the underlying factors contributing to the patient's personality disorder and responding accordingly.

TABLE 31-1	Practical Tips for How to Approach Patients with Each Personality Disorder	
Personality Disorder	**Clinical Presentation**	**Approach**
Borderline	• Instability in interpersonal relationships, self-image, and affect • Intense fear of rejection and abandonment • Splitting • Self-destructive behaviors	• Do not give in to patient's strong emotionality • Avoid unnecessary treatments/procedures but provide options not simple rejection • Regular follow-up appointments • Be aware of splitting and potential self-harming behavior
Histrionic	• Dramatic and excessive emotionality • Attention-seeking, provocative, seductive behavior • Perceives relationships to be more intimate than they are • Easily influenced by others	• Another individual should be present at all times • Involve patient in decision-making but provide guidance, reassurance, and support • Avoid unnecessary treatment/procedures • Do not let patient's seductive behavior cloud judgment • Give appropriate attention and compliments focusing on patient as a person • Respond firmly to inappropriate seduction
Obsessive Compulsive	• Preoccupation with orderliness, perfectionism, and control • Fear of losing control • Excessive attention to detail • Focus on facts and knowledge to replace or subdue emotions	• Professional, structured encounters • Set realistic expectations, be explicit about unattainable outcomes, and document discussion • Detailed explanations and plans (written information and guide to appropriate resources) • Regular follow-up appointments
Narcissistic	• Grandiosity • Uncomfortable in vulnerable or inferior position • Need for admiration • Lack of empathy • Demanding and entitled	• Do not take patient's behaviors personally • Engage patient at a medical level (discuss in medical terminology, discuss journal article, etc.) • Allow patient to have a sense of power by engaging in medical decision-making • Discuss details and risks of procedure and document discussion in medical records

Note. Reproduced with permission from Rieder and Fried. Essential Psychiatry for the Aesthetic Practitioner. Wiley-Blackwell; 2021.

Body Dysmorphic Disorder

Body dysmorphic disorder (BDD), which falls on the obsessive compulsive disorder (OCD) spectrum, is defined as a preoccupation with a perceived or insignificant flaw or defect in appearance enough to cause impairment in functioning.[5] Patients with BDD disproportionally present to aesthetic practitioners, with a recent meta-analysis finding that this disorder occurs in 15% of plastic surgery patients and 13% of dermatology patients as compared to only 1–2% of the general population.[16] Remarkably, over three-quarters of BDD patients pursue cosmetic procedures.[17,18] Patients with psychiatric causes of cosmetic symptoms are likely to seek out non-psychiatric providers due to denial and fear of stigmatization.[19] Unfortunately, BDD is currently underdiagnosed and underrecognized by dermatologists, plastic surgeons, and other aesthetic professionals. To safeguard their patients, support staff, and themselves, aesthetic clinicians should learn to screen for and accurately identify these disorders.

Patients with BDD tend to be preoccupied with facial features, skin, and hair, and most commonly seek out dermatologists to correct their perceived deformities.[22] Gender and age play important roles in the manifestation of BDD symptoms. Younger, female patients tend to focus on facial hair, weight, and body areas such as the arms, chest, stomach, buttocks, thighs, and legs.[16,23] In contrast, men with BDD tend to be preoccupied with their hair, body build, and genitalia.[21,24] Though different genders results in different presentations, gender incidence is roughly equal and symptoms begin during childhood and adolescence. Unless treatment is administered early on, these conditions continue chronically into adulthood.[19,20,25,26] Therefore, BDD patients generally struggle with their conditions throughout their entire lives; it is crucial to develop a compassionate and structural approach in treating them.

Two screening protocols have been validated in dermatology settings for BDD: the [1] Dysmorphic Concern Questionnaire and [2] Body Dysmorphic Disorder Questionnaire —Dermatology Version.[18,27,28] These screening protocols can help providers recognize cases of potential BDD and provide appropriate treatment. In the case of a positive BDD screen, clinicians should ask additional questions about their appearance concerns regarding the degree of the concern, examine the concern together, and understand the concern in the context of their history of cosmetic procedures. If a patient is identified as having BDD, practitioners should inform them of their potential diagnosis respectfully and in a nonjudgmental manner. Providers should emphasize building rapport with patients and clearly communicating their recommendations.

Outside of procedures done to repair damage from BDD-related behaviors, psychiatric experts recommend avoid conducting cosmetic procedures for these patients.[23,29,30] Instead, most patients with BDD will benefit from referrals to mental health providers rather than referrals to other aesthetic providers.[31]

In many cases of BDD, aesthetic providers will determine that their patient would benefit from co-treatment with a mental health practitioner. We recommend developing relationships with local psychologists, psychiatrists, and social work therapists and having their contact information readily accessible. Before introducing a psychological referral, aesthetic clinicians should establish a trusting relationship with the patient and emphasize the importance of destigmatizing mental healthcare. Importantly, providers should recognize their own limits and respect their own comfort and safety; they have the right to resign from any patient's care.

SAYING NO

Often, aesthetic providers will have to reject their patients' wishes to protect themselves and their support staff from potential harm. This can be especially difficult with self-pay cosmetic patients who are demanding or have unreasonable expectations. To optimize patient satisfaction while still denying their requests, we describe two techniques that can be used in different situations—LEAP for conducting cosmetic consultations and BLAST for approaching dissatisfied patients.[32-34]

LEAP AND BLAST TECHNIQUES

The LEAP (Listen, Educate and Empower, Align, Perform) technique is an easy-to-remember mnemonic to help ensure patient satisfaction even if the provider must say "no" to a patient's requests.

L) Listen—uninterrupted, active listening is foundational for building the patient-provider relationship. In particular, aesthetic providers should devote time at the beginning of the consultation to understand the patient's perspective and identify potential unrealistic expectations. Emerging evidence supports a correlation between patient-centered care and communication and higher patient satisfaction.[35-37] In fact, "being listened to" is often rated as one of the most important factors contributing to patient satisfaction.[38] Therefore, it is important not only to listen, but to actively listen to patient concerns.

E) Educate and empower—providers should thoroughly discuss the benefits, risks, alternatives, and realistic outcomes of a proposed procedure to allow patients to feel more informed and active in their treatment.

A) Align—by educating the patient, the patient-provider relationship becomes one of shared decision-making and shared responsibility.[39] Studies show that this partner model relationship is favored by the majority of patients and improves patient-reported outcomes.[40,41] If the patient's view differs from that of their provider, the provider should suggest alternative options rather than simply rejecting their view. Clinicians should communicate with the intent of making the patient feel that their treatment is a common goal between patient and provider.

P) Perform—given the nature of aesthetic dermatology, cosmetic intervention is the primary determinant of patient satisfaction. However, if the provider must say "no" and believes the intervention would lead to more harm than good, the provider should explain the reasoning behind their decision. The debate on whether denial of a patient's request leads to reduced satisfaction is ongoing.[42-44] Regardless, data shows that patients are more satisfied when physicians display interest, reassurance, and provide alternative solutions even if they differ from their original expectations.[43]

If, for any reason, a patient is still unhappy, the BLAST technique can be used:

B) Believe—even if the clinician does not agree with the patient's complaint, the clinician should believe and acknowledge the patient's feelings to empathize with them and ensure a more productive conversation.

L) Listen—similarly to LEAP, focused, active listening helps strengthen the relationship. Determining the reason(s) for patient dissatisfaction is critical, as they can range from unrealistic expectations to physiologic side effects of treatment. Through active listening, practitioners can accurately discern the source of their patients' concerns and respond efficiently and appropriately.

A) Apologize—aesthetic providers should recognize their ethical responsibility to apologize when a medical error occurs. However, patients are more often unhappy because of unmet expectations rather than true medical errors.[45] In these cases, providers can express an apology that sympathizes with the patient's feelings but does not acknowledge fault or imply clinical error.

S) Satisfy—in many cases, there may be alternative options or treatment plans that can satisfy the patient. While it is important to allow the patient to voice their opinions, aesthetic providers should ensure that they provide relevant suggestions and direct the conversation.

T) Thank—providers should sincerely thank the patient for expressing their concerns at the visit, being open and candid, and for having the confidence to trust the practitioner to address their issue.

Providing positive patient experiences is the ultimate goal in aesthetic medicine.[2] Elegantly saying "no" using LEAP and BLAST techniques can help ensure patient satisfaction.

FRONTIER AREAS

The field of dermatology has experienced many changes in recent years. With these changes come many advancements but also areas of concern. We discuss a few of these topics of concern such as the effects of technology and social media, perceptions of the ideal beauty aesthetic, and the possible risk of cosmetic procedures as an addiction.

Effects of Social Media

Cosmetic treatments such as neurotoxins and dermal filler have become increasingly sought after, in large part because of the rising popularity of visual-based social media applications.[46] While these interventions can be appropriate, aesthetic professionals must acknowledge the psychological vulnerabilities of their patients and recognize that technology and social media may have influenced their cosmetic requests. In the 1990s, the beauty industry promoted the concept of supermodels and regularly utilized photo-editing software to airbrush away skin imperfections and to narrow body shapes to proportions that were often impossible to achieve.[46] The widespread use of these images in the mass media contributed to the development of unrealistic beauty standards in western society.

In today's technological landscape, nearly all smartphone owners have access to social media, mobile apps designed to enhance images, and sophisticated photo-editing software. While beneficial in many ways, these technological advancements also come at a cost. The use of these and other photo-editing tools are often used to generate individualized, but unrealistic images of beauty that are widely consumed across social networks. Recent studies suggest that the comparative nature of social media usage may result in anxiety and depression.[47] Furthermore, when patients present for consultations, it is often clear that social media has created a discrepancy and warping of people's perceptions of their bodies. Dermatologic evidence and anecdotal experience suggest that rapid, repeated exposures to imagery—conditions created through social media applications such as Instagram—may retrain our brains to redefine what is attractive through visual adaptation.[48] Thus, even though social media has advanced the field of dermatology by destigmatizing cosmetic procedures and has provided more accessible information and education, social media continues to exploit and perhaps even develop patient vulnerabilities. To advance the best interests of cosmetic patients, aesthetic clinicians must consider the effects of the online environment when providing care.

Racial Morphing

"Racial morphing" is a phenomenon in which aesthetically modified faces have trended towards a unifying appearance, largely due to an overexposure of celebrity imagery on social media.[46] This has created a canon of "sameness" regardless of culture or background. Aesthetic professionals should aim to respect the beauty of diverse human appearances and be mindful to avoid perpetuating this phenomenon.

Cosmetic Addiction

Several studies demonstrate a relationship between adverse psychosocial factors, including poor mental health, psychosocial stress, and intimate partner violence, and the likelihood of undergoing cosmetic procedures.[49] These findings underscore the importance of screening for psychiatric conditions such as BDD prior to developing a treatment plan.

Aesthetic clinicians should also be aware of addictive behaviors, which are a potential risk factor for undergoing repeated cosmetic procedures. The field of psychiatry commonly qualifies behavioral addictions as substance-related disorders because they activate similar brain reward pathways

and feelings of pleasure as drugs of abuse do. Indeed, researchers are beginning to explore the possibility of a substance-related disorder involving repeated cosmetic procedure use. A small questionnaire study found that individuals who seek out aesthetic dermatology practices are more likely to meet substance-related disorder criteria for cosmetic interventions.[50] To this end, aesthetic providers should attempt to understand their patients' motivations for seeking cosmetic treatment and determine whether an alternative type of treatment may be beneficial.

References

1. Sun MD, Rieder EA. Psychosocial Stress and Mechanisms of Skin Health: A Comprehensive Update. *J Drugs Dermatol.* 2021 Jan 1;20(1):62–69. doi:10.36849/JDD.5608. PMID: 33400410.

2. Rieder EA, Fried RG. *Essential Psychiatry for the Aesthetic Practitioner.* Wiley Blackwell; 2021.

3. Manary MP, Boulding W, Staelin R, et al. The patient experience and health outcomes. *N Engl J Med.* 2013;368:201–203.

4. Krupat E, Bell RA, Kravitz RL, et al. When physicians and patients think alike: patient-centered beliefs and their impact on satisfaction and trust. *J Fam Pract.* 2001;50:1057–1062.

5. American Psychiatric Association. *Diagnostic and statistical manual of mental disorders.* 5th ed. https://doi.org/10.1176/appi.books.9780890425596. 2013.

6. Edgerton MT, Jacobson WE, Meyer E. Surgical-psychiatric study of patients seeking plastic (cosmetic) surgery: ninety- eight consecutive patients with minimal deformity. *Br J Plast Surg.* 1960;13:136–145.

7. Webb WL, Slaughter R, Meyer E, Edgerton M. Mechanisms of psychosocial adjustment in patients seeking "face-lift" operation. *Psychosom Med.* 1965;27(2):183–192.

8. Marcus P. Psychological aspects of cosmetic rhinoplasty. *Br J Plast Surg.* 1984;37(3):313–318.

9. Edgerton MT, Langman MW, Pruzinsky T. Plastic surgery and psychotherapy in the treatment of 100 psychologically disturbed patients. *Plast Reconstr Surg.* 1991;88(4):594–608.

10. Hay GG. Psychiatric aspects of cosmetic nasal operations. *Br J Psychiatry.* 1970 Jan;116(530):85–97.

11. Nunes PM, Wenzel A, Borges KT, et al. Volumes of the hippocampus and amygdala in patients with borderline personality disorder: a meta-analysis. *J Personal Disord.* 2009;23:333–345.

12. Schulze L, Dziobek I, Vater A, et al. Gray matter abnormalities in patients with narcissistic personality disorder. *J Psychiatr Res.* 2013;47:1363–1369.

13. Zanarini MC, Frankenburg FR, Reich DB, et al. Biparental failure in the childhood experiences of borderline patients. *J Personal Disord.* 2000;14:264–273.

14. Amad A, Ramoz N, Thomas P, et al. Genetics of borderline personality disorder: systematic review and proposal of an integrative model. *Neurosci Biobehav Rev.* 2014;40:6–19.

15. Combs G, Oshman L. Pearls for working with people who have personality disorder diagnoses. *Prim Care.* 2016;43:263–268.

16. Ribeiro RVE. Prevalence of Body Dysmorphic Disorder in Plastic Surgery and Dermatology Patients: A Systematic Review with Meta-Analysis. *Aesthetic Plast Surg.* 2017;41(4):964–970.

17. Koblenzer CS. Body dysmorphic disorder in the dermatology patient. *Clin Dermatol.* 2017;35(3):298–301.

18. Dey JK, Ishii M, Phillis M, et al. Body dysmorphic disorder in a facial plastic and reconstructive surgery clinic. *JAMA Facial Plast Surg.* 2015;17(2):137–143.

19. Sheikhmoonesi F, Hajheidari Z, Masoudzadeh A, Mozaffari, M. EPA-0054 – prevalence and severity of obsessive-compulsive disorder and its relationships with dermatological disease. *Eur Psychiatry.* 2014;29:1.

20. Mufaddel A, Osman OT, Almugaddam F, Jafferany M. A review of body dysmorphic disorder and its presentation in different clinical settings. *Prim Care Companion CNS Disord.* 2013;15(4): PCC.12r01464.

21. Möllmann A, Dietel FA, Hunger A, Buhlmann U. Prevalence of body dysmorphic disorder and associated features in German adolescents: a self-report survey. *Psychiatry Res.* 2017;254:263–267.

22. Zakhary L, Weingarden H, Sullivan A, Wilhelm S. Clincal Features, Assessment, and Treatment of Body Dysmorphic Disorder. *Oxford Medicine Online.* Oxford University Press; 2017.

23. Phillips KA, Didie ER, Menard W, et al. Clinical features of body dysmorphic disorder in adolescents and adults. *Psychiatry Res.* 2006;141(3):305–314.

24. Phillips KA, Menard W, Fay C. Gender similarities and differences in 200 individuals with body dysmorphic disorder. *Compr Psychiatry.* 2006;47(2):77–87.

25. Horwath E, Weissman MM. The epidemiology and cross-national presentation of obsessive-compulsive disorder. *Psychiatr Clin North Am.* 2000;23(3):493–507.

26. Bjornsson AS. Age at Onset and Clinical Course of Body Dysmorphic Disorder. Oxford Medicine Online. Oxford University Press; 2017.

27. Picavet V, Gabriëls L, Jorissen M, Hellings PW. Screening tools for body dysmorphic disorder in a cosmetic surgery setting. *The Laryngoscope.* 2011;121(12):2535–2541.

28. Dufresne RG, Phillips KA, Vittorio CC, Wilkel CS. A screening questionnaire for body dysmorphic disorder in a cosmetic dermatologic surgery practice. *Dermatologic Surgery.* 2001;27(5):457–462.

29. Phillips KA. Body Dysmorphic Disorder in Children and Adolescents. *Oxford Medicine Online.* Oxford University Press; 2017.

30. Wang Q, Cao C, Guo R, et al. Avoiding psychological pitfalls in aesthetic medical procedures. *Aesthetic Plast Surg.* 2016;40(6):954–961.

31. Crerand CE, Menard W, Phillips KA. Surgical and minimally invasive cosmetic procedures among persons with body dysmorphic disorder. *Ann Plast Surg.* 2010;65(1):11–16.

32. Watchmaker J, Kandula P, Kaminer MS. L.E.A.P.ing into the cosmetic consult. *J Cosmet Dermatol.* 2020;19(6):1499–1500.

33. Barneto, A. Dealing with Customer Complaints – B.L.A.S.T. Available at https://www. customerservicemanager.com/dealing-with-customers-complaints. Accessed 29 September 2019. Published 2009.

34. Steinman HK. A method for working with displeased patients – BLAST. *J Clin Aesthet Dermatol.* 2013;6(3):25–28.

35. Rathert C, Wyrwich MD, Boren SA. Patient-centered care and outcomes: a systematic review of the literature. *Med Care Res Rev.* 2013;70(4):351–379.

36. Stewart M, Brown JB, Donner A, et al. The impact of patient-centered care on outcomes. *J Fam Pract.* 2000;49(9):796–804.

37. Wanzer MB, Booth-Butterfield M, Gruber K. Perceptions of health care providers' communication: relationships between patient-centered communication and satisfaction. *Health Commun.* 2004; 16(3):363–383.

38. Wolf JA. The consumer has spoken: patient experience is now healthcare's core differentiator. *Patient Exp J.* 2018;5(1):1–4.

39. Stiggelbout AM, Pieterse AH, De Haes JC. Shared decision making: concepts, evidence, and practice. *Patient Educ Couns.* 2015;98(10):1172–1179.

40. Bailoor K, Valley T, Perumalswami C, et al. How acceptable is paternalism? A survey-based study of clinician and nonclinician opinions on paternalistic decision making. *AJOB Empir Bioeth.* 2018;9(2):91–98.

41. deBronkart D. From patient centred to people powered: autonomy on the rise. *BMJ: Br Med J.* 2015;350:h148.

42. Bell RA, Wilkes MS, Kravitz RL. Advertisement-induced prescription drug requests: patients' anticipated reactions to a physician who refuses. *J Fam Pract.* 1999;48(6):446–452.

43. Sanchez-Menegay C, Hudes ES, Cummings SR. Patient expectations and satisfaction with medical care for upper respiratory infections. *J Gen Intern Med.* 1992;7(4):432–434.

44. Peck BM, Ubel PA, Roter DL, et al. Do unmet expectations for specific tests, referrals, and new medications reduce patients' satisfaction? *J Gen Intern Med.* 2004;19(11):1080–1087.

45. Watchmaker LE, Watchmaker JD, Callaghan D, et al. The unhappy cosmetic patient: lessons from unfavorable online reviews of minimally and noninvasive cosmetic procedures. *Dermatol Surg.* 2020;46(9):1191–1194.

46. Sun MD, Rieder EA. How We Do It: Body Dysmorphic Disorder for the Cosmetic Dermatologist. *Dermatol Surg.* 2021 Apr 1;47(4): 585–586. doi:10.1097/DSS.0000000000002506. PMID: 33795577.

47. *Diagnostic and statistical manual of mental disorders: DSM-5.* Washington, DC: American Psychiatric Publishing; 2013.

48. Joseph AW, Ishii L, Joseph SS, et al. Prevalence of Body Dysmorphic Disorder and Surgeon Diagnostic Accuracy in Facial Plastic and Oculoplastic Surgery Clinics. *JAMA Facial Plast Surg.* 2017;19(4):269.

49. ASDS survey on dermatologic procedures: report of 2018 procedures. Available at https://www.asds.net/portals/0/PDF/procedures-survey-results-presentation-2018.pdf; 2019.

50. Shah P, Rangel LK, Geronemus RG, Rieder EA. Cosmetic procedure use as a type of substance-related disorder. *J Am Acad Dermatol.* 2021 Jan;84(1):86–91. doi:10.1016/j.jaad.2020.08.123. Epub 2020 Sep 10. PMID: 32920038.

CHAPTER 32

Cosmetic and Drug Regulations

Edmund M. Weisberg, MS, MBE
Leslie S. Baumann, MD

SUMMARY POINTS

What's Important?

1. "Cosmeceuticals" remains a popular but unofficial category for personal care product status despite its introduction nearly 40 years ago.
2. Current regulations discourage manufacturers from publishing supportive scientific clinical trials to evaluate the efficacy of their products.
3. There is no standard organic certification for skincare products used by all companies. Rather, there are several certification bodies, which is confusing for consumers.
4. The "dermatologist tested" term is used when one dermatologist has tried the formula but use of this expression does not require any official clinical research by that dermatologist.

What's New?

1. The ISO 16128 standard describes a nomenclature and process that should be used to define the presence and amount of natural ingredients in skincare products. It is being adopted by many reputable companies.
2. Medical grade skincare and professional grade skincare are descriptive terms but not legal categories.

What's Coming?

1. The Cosmetic Ingredient Review is constantly publishing new safety reports on ingredients.
2. New sunscreen claim rules are expected in the future but have been in a holding pattern for over a decade.

COSMECEUTICALS: DRUGS VERSUS COSMETICS

According to the US Food and Drug Administration (USFDA), a personal care product can be classified as a drug, an over-the-counter (OTC) drug, or a cosmetic, or in some cases more than one of these groups (see **Box 32-1**). The term "cosmeceutical" was introduced in 1984 by Albert Kligman, MD, at a meeting of the Society of Cosmetic Chemists because he felt that a new regulatory category should exist.[1,2] Although this topic has been debated for decades, the classification "cosmeceuticals" has still not been officially recognized. In other words, it has no legal meaning. The term, however, is increasingly a part of the mainstream vernacular and frequently used to describe products that are known to exert a biologic action but are regulated as cosmetics (e.g., products containing

retinol). Although it is well known that retinol stimulates retinoic acid receptors resulting in biologic activity, retinol is a popular ingredient contained in numerous cosmetic skincare products. Companies often list retinol as an inactive ingredient on product labels to avoid regulatory action by the FDA.

Which category a product fits in depends on its ingredients, how much of the ingredient is present, and what claim will be made (e.g., acne lotion vs. moisturizer).

The stage for the unforeseen regulatory loophole in which cosmeceuticals reside was set in 1938 when the US Congress passed a statute known as the Federal Food, Drug, and Cosmetic Act (FD&C Act), which outlined formal criteria for classification of drugs and cosmetics. In this document, cosmetics were defined as: "...*articles intended to be rubbed, poured, sprinkled, or sprayed on, introduced into, or otherwise applied to the human body or any part thereof for cleansing,*

- **Drug**: Must be FDA approved, extensive data show efficacy and safety
- **OTC**: Must follow monograph guidelines, has ingredients that have shown efficacy and safety to treat a certain condition
- **Cosmetic**: Voluntary registration

beautifying, promoting attractiveness, or altering the appearance…"[3] In contrast, a drug is defined as a substance "*intended to affect the structure and function of the body.*"[3] Based on these definitions, the actual *intent* of the product and not its actions governs how it is classified. This allows for the classification of retinol as a cosmetic because it is listed as an inactive ingredient on product labels; therefore, retinol is not *intended* to serve a biologic purpose.

As in several other realms of society during our era of rapidly propagating technology, numerous legal implications failed to anticipate future developments. In terms of the debate over classifying products as drugs, cosmetics, or cosmeceuticals, there are some salient points to consider. The first is that the current regulations discourage companies from publishing supportive scientific clinical trials to evaluate the efficacy of their products. For example, if a manufacturer establishes in a study that an ingredient increases collagen synthesis, the company is proving that its product affects the "function of the body." If they were then to market or sell that product as a cosmetic intended to increase collagen synthesis, as would be desirable in an anti-aging product or a wrinkle cream, they would be violating the 1938 statute. The only legal option for the manufacturer would be, instead, to market its product as a drug.

Before approval for marketing in the United States, every new drug must be clinically tested in accordance with FDA guidelines for a new drug application (NDA). The FDA process of drug approval can take more than 10 years and cost hundreds of millions of dollars. Obviously, the cosmetic companies are left with compelling incentives to avoid such long delays and exorbitant costs by following the guidelines to keep their products classified as cosmetics. In such cases, even if the companies perform extensive research on such products, their findings are considered proprietary and remain unpublished. This, too, has several implications. The first is that dermatologists and other physicians do not have access to this scientific evidence and are rendered poorly equipped to evaluate the efficacy of the numerous and varied products making it to market. Physicians are taught to practice evidence-based medicine, but without evidence, have little reason to believe that any of these products are efficacious or effective. Consequently, the medical establishment dismisses these products as useless when such formulations may, in fact, offer potential benefits to patients. The second problem is that consumers may often become confused by all the sleek, glitzy marketing. They rarely know how to tell the difference between a reputable company that conducts scientific research and a company of charlatans seeking to capitalize on consumers' dreams of younger and healthier skin. With little guidance given the medical community's lack of information regarding these personal care products, consumers try products and likely feel disappointed with the lack of results. Consumers are also left to operate under the false assumption that you get what you pay for—that is, the more expensive the product, the more likely it is to be effective. This can lead to a general distrust of the entire cosmetic industry. The third problem with cosmetic companies performing internal research and not publishing the results for general review is the circumvention of the peer review process. Peer review has long been considered essential to validate the research findings of scientists. It is difficult to believe or have confidence in the results of a study that has not been subjected to the peer review process.

Also beyond the peer review process, there are individuals outside of companies that attempt to perform research on cosmetic products and procedures without concern for product classification; however, it is often difficult for these individuals to raise the research funding necessary to perform such studies. There are research grants available from several companies that may help these researchers in their efforts, though. On the flip side, one must consider the dilemma confronting the cosmetic companies: if they support a research study and the product does not work, they lose money and risk their credibility or reputation. If the product does work, the company faces regulation of its product as a drug and the related time lag to market, or they will be unable to use the research findings in their marketing of the product as a cosmetic. Some of the savvier companies fund research of their products and inform dermatologists of the results with the hope that the dermatologists will, in turn, become convinced of the product's efficacy and recommend it to patients or other physicians. In this way, the entire marketing problem is avoided because the dermatologist, rather than the company, is promoting the product. The US Federal Trade Commission (FTC) has caught on to this strategy, however, and released guidelines about experts endorsing products. These guidelines are described at the end of this chapter.

Numerous skincare products are referred to as cosmeceuticals, medical grade skincare, or professional skincare products, but these terms have no legal definition. Many people believe that a legal category called "cosmeceuticals" that includes products shown to have a biologic function but not subjected to the expensive drug approval process would solve the dilemma. However, many companies and individuals oppose such an enactment because it would likely lead to the regulation of most cosmetic products. For example, in Europe, under the European Economic Cosmetic Directive of 1993, the requirements for cosmetic product labeling became formidable and complex.[4] In contrast, companies in the United States do not have to demonstrate either efficacy or safety prior to marketing their products. Of course, all reputable companies ensure the safety of their products before distributing them; however, astonishingly, they are technically not required to do so.

What should cosmetic dermatologists and medical providers do to protect patients and themselves in an atmosphere in which companies are not required to research, or to release their research on, the efficacy and safety of cosmetic products? Here are some suggestions:

- Data in peer-reviewed journals is the best source, but study design and statistical manipulation can make a product look efficacious when it is not (as discussed in Chapter 37, Anti-Aging Ingredients).
- Poster presentations at meetings are also a helpful source of information. Companies seem more likely to present their findings in a poster format; however, it is important to remember that these posters are not peer reviewed.
- Some companies will provide unpublished research data on request to interested physicians. These data are not peer reviewed. They are also often provided by the ingredient company and are not based on the final product formulation.
- The Cosmetic Ingredient Review (CIR) is a helpful guide on ingredient safety but does not analyze the efficacy of the final product. An expert scientific panel examines worldwide published and unpublished safety data in an independent and unbiased manner.
- Look for certification marks or data from unbiased sources. In some cases, certification marks are difficult to receive and require good data and proof; however, some certification marks are received in exchange for a fee with minimal data requirements.

All cosmetic dermatologists and medical providers who hope to preserve and enhance the integrity of the skincare industry should insist that manufacturers of cosmetic products supply well-controlled published studies to support their claims. If these dermatologists and, later, consumers refuse to buy products lacking an evidence-based medicine approach, the studies will eventually be performed and certainly lead to exciting new developments in the field of cosmeceuticals.

CERTIFICATION MARKS FOR SKINCARE PRODUCTS

A certification mark, which is a legal term, requires a testing process, a list of standards, and an ongoing quality certification program. There is no oversight as to how rigorous the testing methods or standards should be; it just requires that they exist. This means that certain certification marks are more reliable and difficult to achieve than others. There are certification marks for several categories including: (1) organic, (2) disease specific, (3) from professional organizations, (4) from independent organizations, and (5) from consumer publications such as *Good Housekeeping* magazine. Here are a few examples of popular certification marks in the skincare industry (also see **Table 32-1**):

Association and foundation certifications:

- Skin Cancer Foundation Seal of Recommendation: SPF products must meet criteria for safe and effective sun protection.
- National Eczema Association: NEA Seal of Acceptance certifies that the product does not contain ingredients that exacerbate eczema.

Other notable certifications:

- Carbon Neutral: Demonstrates that the company has achieved carbon neutrality.
- Leaping Bunny Certification: Free of animal testing at all stages of development.
- Skin Type Solutions-Approved Products: These products must have the correct ingredients for corresponding Baumann Skin Types and are tested in complete regimens consisting of multiple brands. This approval applies to doctors and medical providers such as aestheticians that are approved to use the system, products approved to be included in the system, and skincare regimens composed of multiple brands to be used on one of the 16 Baumann Skin Types.[1]

SELF-REGULATION: THE NATIONAL ADVERTISING DIVISION

The National Advertising Division (NAD) of the Council of Better Business Bureaus is a self-monitoring society to which companies can report other companies for making false claims about products. The NAD renders a decision with the intention of objectively, quickly, and privately reaching a settlement. The goal is to promote truth in advertising and, in the process, keep the government from getting involved in the process and avoid costly litigation. The FTC also can play a role and sanction companies that lack the data to support its claims. Of dermatologic interest, the NAD once recommended that Skin Doctors Cosmeceuticals alter its claims regarding its "Eyetuck Anti-Bag Technology," particularly its favorable comparisons to plastic surgery. The NAD deemed that it was inappropriate for manufacturers of a product that works only on the skin surface to compare, without substantiating evidence, their cream/serum to plastic surgery procedures that penetrate into the skin.[5]

SKINCARE INGREDIENTS

The Food Allergen Labeling and Consumer Protection Act of 2004 (FALCPA) requires that purveyors of food that contains allergens, such as nuts or gluten, label the products as such. It is important to understand that this act does not apply to skincare products. In other words, skincare can contain

---

[1] Dr. Baumann helped develop this seal. Please note her conflict-of-interest statement.

nuts, gluten, and other allergens without a notice such as "gluten-free" or "contains nuts" being listed on the label. Reading the label is the only way to know what the product contains. Skincare ingredient nomenclature can be confusing because one ingredient may go by several names (see the gluten section of Chapter 13, Sensitive Skin)

Though many chemical ingredients used in cosmetics are widely considered safe for use, some safety factors have not been fully studied. Now that skincare products contain growth factors and other ingredients with significant biologic activity, the safety of skincare becomes more of a concern (see the discussion on growth factor safety in Chapter 37).

It is virtually impossible to evaluate the *cumulative effects* of repeated exposures from multiple sources. This is important because consumers, especially women, use several skin, hair, and beauty products each day. The ingredients in these products can potentially interact or lead to a higher combined rate of exposure to certain ingredients than is usually assessed by studying the safety of a single ingredient in the laboratory. Further, to accurately establish the baseline of the chemical exposures people can safely tolerate, it is necessary to account for *all* chemical exposures from food, urban smog, industrial waste, and other sources.

Long-term safety testing of cosmetic products is not part of routine assessments at this time. It would take several years and control of diet, environment, and lifestyle factors to be able to accurately determine safety. Organizations like the Environmental Working Group (EWG) provide information on individual ingredients, but ingredients act differently when combined with other ingredients so knowing the risks of one ingredient alone is not enough. In addition, there are rumors, myths, and poor science that complicate the issue.

GRAS

Generally recognized as safe (GRAS) is an expression used in Sections 201(s) and 409 of the Federal Food, Drug, and Cosmetic Act. The GRAS designation is bestowed to ingredients associated with a general recognition of safety through scientific procedures as determined by experts. To achieve GRAS status, the same quantity and quality of scientific evidence is required as is needed to obtain approval of the substance as a food additive.[6]

The Expert Panel for Cosmetic Ingredient Safety and CIR

The Expert Panel for Cosmetic Ingredient Safety is an independent, nonprofit scientific body established in 1976 to assess the safety of cosmetic ingredients used in the United States through the CIR program. The Expert Panel consists of world-renowned scientists and physicians who have been publicly nominated by consumer, scientific, and medical groups; government agencies; and industry.[7]

This respected expert panel reviews the data on ingredients and provides a lengthy report on that ingredient or group of ingredients. The CIR is the most reliable and unbiased cosmetic ingredient safety data that exists. The Expert Panel for Cosmetic Ingredient Safety is overseen by a seven-member steering committee. The CIR was established by the industry trade association called the Cosmetic, Toiletry, and Fragrance Association (which is now known as the Personal Care Products Council) with the support of the USFDA and the Consumer Federation of America. The CIR steering committee is headed by the President and CEO of the Council and includes: a dermatologist representing the American Academy of Dermatology, a toxicologist representing the Society of Toxicology, a consumer representing the Consumer Federation of America, an industry cosmetic scientist, the Chair of the Expert Panel for Cosmetic Ingredient Safety, and the Council's Executive Vice President for Science.[8]

Although CIR receives funding from the Personal Care Products Council, the review process is independent from the Council and the cosmetics industry. CIR and the Expert Panel for Cosmetic Ingredient Safety operate under a set of procedures to eliminate bias. The CIR reports are thorough reviews of the safety data on cosmetic ingredients. They also provide suggestions on ingredient nomenclature to provide more clarity to consumers.

Monographs

Over-the-counter (OTC) or nonprescription drug products are classes of drugs that the FDA has reviewed as a group, such as acne treatment products or sunscreens. For each group, the FDA develops a monograph that is published in the *Federal Register*. A monograph is a statement detailing the kind and amount of active ingredients that, when used at the concentration range stipulated, can be included in product claims. Claim language pre-approved by the FDA is allowed on a product monograph without supplying additional data. Generally, manufacturers are required to follow the wording used in the monograph for its claims. Companies are not mandated to test the final formulation for efficacy as long as they meet the ingredient and dose requirements.[9] However, they are not permitted to combine acne actives or other monograph actives. In other words, a formulation may not contain benzoyl peroxide and ultraviolet screens and then claim that it treats acne and imparts an SPF factor without undergoing FDA review and approval.[10]

Ingredient Safety

While not all widely used synthetic ingredients are considered problematic, certain ones represent a source for special concern. For example, the parabens (alkyl esters of *p*-hydroxybenzoic acid) are used as preservatives in numerous cosmetics as well as skin, hair, and body care products, and can sometimes provoke allergic reactions (see Chapter 44, Preservatives).[11,12] Parabens can be absorbed via the skin and migrate into the bloodstream and bodily tissue. One controversial study even found high concentrations of parabens in breast cancer tissue.[13] Products containing parabens should be avoided by most people who know they are allergic to parabens. (This can be determined by patch testing.) There are no cogent data to indicate that parabens pose a risk to those not allergic to this group of compounds. Nevertheless, many people opt to abstain from using products containing this type of preservative ingredient.

Toluene, which is found in several nail polish brands, has been associated with deleterious effects on males *in utero*. Therefore, major companies such as L'Oréal and Revlon as well as manufacturers of natural and organic products have taken steps to eliminate toluene from their nail polishes. Toluene can also induce a skin rash, typically on the eyelids, in people who use toluene-containing nail polishes. There are various other ingredients that warrant caution, but it is important to know that even organic products can cause problems. For example, coconut oil, a popular organic ingredient, can foster acne. Allergies to many essential oils and botanicals can also develop. In addition, because companies were not able to label their products as organic until recently, there have not been sufficient clinical research trials on the organic products on the market. In fact, it is plausible, if not likely, that some of the manufacturers of organic brands are just using the label for marketing purposes without proof that their products are efficacious.

Summary of Ingredient Safety

It is important for each person to consider the particular health risks of their skincare products as it applies to their own medical issues. Patients should seek reliable sources such as their dermatologist or medical provider to determine what skincare ingredients, products, and skincare routine are both efficacious and safe for their skin type.

In response to uncertainty, many consumers choose organic skincare products and try to limit chemical exposures as a precaution whenever feasible. However, organic does not mean that the product is safe or efficacious for the person's skin type. Organic products may also include allergens. Patients with multiple allergies must be more cautious with skincare products, especially with natural products, organic products, and formulations that contain essential oils. Botanical-derived products can be more allergenic than synthetic ones. Knowing the source of the products and the ethics of the company that manufactures them is the best guide for finding the safest skincare products. For patients that are allergic, the only way to ensure safety is to patch test them to know exactly which allergens to avoid (see Chapter 19, Contact Dermatitis from Cosmetic Ingredients).

REGULATION OF SKINCARE CLAIMS

There are numerous skincare claims not covered by an FDA monograph, but are allowed to be made without FDA oversight because they are considered to be cosmetic claims. The use of some claims is covered by the OTC monograph such as "anti-acne" or "skin protectant" or "sun protection." Other terms have no official meaning. These terms are discussed below.

Ingredient Claims

Allergen-free

There is no standard definition of "allergen-free" and no testing is required of companies to use this expression. Typically, "allergen-free" indicates that the product includes no fragrances on the European Union's "List of Substances Which Cosmetic Products Must Not Contain Except Subject to Restrictions and Conditions Laid Down" or other compounds typically identified as allergens.[9] Some manufacturers use human repeated insult patch testing (HRIPT) to evaluate their formulations for allergenicity.

Hypoallergenic

Each manufacturer has its own definition for this term, often using it liberally, as there is no standard established definition of hypoallergenicity. HRIPT of about 100 to 200 subjects and cumulative irritation testing (using a smaller panel) are the common methods to evaluate hypoallergenicity.[9] Occasionally, photoreactivity testing is conducted, depending on the product type.

Unscented/Fragrance-free

A product that lacks common fragrance ingredients, particularly those most often linked to allergic sensitivity, or a traditional fragrance intended to impart scent to a product, can be labeled as fragrance-free by its manufacturer. However, the "fragrance-free" description on a product does not necessarily mean that a fragrance is excluded. Companies sometimes include fragrance subcomponents or botanicals to render a cosmetic or preservative effect that, concomitantly, delivers a scent or pleasant aroma to a formulation. If the primary reason for including the "fragrance" is unrelated to scent, such as acting as a preservative, then the manufacturer is not required to label the ingredient as a fragrance and can label the product as fragrance-free.[9]

Notably, some ingredients, including preservatives like phenoxyethanol (the most often used one in organic and natural products), background wax odors from long chain/paraffins, or unfragranced sunscreens, are not considered fragrances, but do confer an odor and can provoke reactions in individuals sensitive or allergic to fragrance.

Formulations labeled as "unscented" usually have no detectable odor, but the product may include a "masking" fragrance to disguise background odor. Therefore, "unscented" does not necessarily translate to no added fragrance. In an era in which companies were compelled into advertising the absence of the preservative parabens, consumers have come to expect that if an ingredient is said to be absent from a product, it really is excluded. This lack of clarity in advertising is likely not problematic for any but the most sensitive individuals. Nonetheless, it is important to understand how the process works.

Testing and Approval Claims

Clinically Tested

Such products are indeed usually investigated through some form of clinical testing, but the test could be a simple 48-hour patch test for irritancy. There are no rules governing how many subjects or the type of trial required for a formulation to be considered "clinically tested," and it is not always clear whether the finished formulation or only components were tested.[9] When a product is described as "clinically tested," each word is carefully chosen (e.g., clinically tested "technology" or clinically tested "formula") to offer clarity to the attentive reader and sidestep any inaccuracy.

Clinical testing is distinct from more ordinary "consumer" testing, which could include focus groups and simple patient use questionnaires. Clinical tests are often run with scientific/medical experts, using an approved protocol, specified statistical analysis, and enough subjects to provide statistical significance, based on the study design. The most recent sunscreen monograph allows for as few as 10 subjects per panel for SPF. Other types of assessments (moisturization, anti-acne, etc.) would normally use more subjects, perhaps from 30 to 100.

Clinically Proven

According to the National Advertising Division (NAD) of the Council of Better Business Bureaus, "proven" requires two similar well-controlled clinical studies to make this claim. This is the standard for the major television networks with regard to broadcast advertising of a product. The Office of Broadcast Standards and Practices reviews ads and the data to support any claims before accepting them for broadcast. If there has been just one study, the wording might be limited to clinically "shown" or "tested." Sometimes, one study on the "technology" and another study on the final formulation will satisfy the network's requirements for "clinically proven."[9]

Despite attempts at rigor, the "clinically proven" claim can be nebulous for consumers, as this label may refer only to an ingredient or the actual final formulation. Furthermore, the advertising regulation does not apply to package labeling. If only the ingredient rather than the final formulation was tested, often the wording is carefully crafted (e.g., "with an ingredient that has been clinically proven to X").

Dermatologist Tested

This claim conjures images of a dermatologist applying a lotion to the face, deeming it as cosmetically acceptable, and subsequently approving the formulation. While "dermatologist tested" generally means much more than this, the claim is highly variable. Often if a formulation is "dermatologist tested," a dermatologist has reviewed the clinical study and signed off on it, but s/he may have simply reviewed the formula or a study report. The doctor may or may not have been involved in the conduct of the study and/or analysis of results.

Nonetheless, this claim is normally based on a specific clinical trial with a protocol, and the final marketed formulation sold in stores has been tested. Panel size depends on the manufacturer, but the general rule is a minimum of 30 subjects for claims of efficacy.[9] In this case, a certified dermatologist signs off and supervises the testing. However, this is not required to make the claim "dermatologist tested."

Dermatologist Approved

This claim requires only one dermatologist to approve the product in some fashion, perhaps based on an assessment of safety, efficacy, or just a brief review of ingredients. A small company producing infomercials may just use one dermatologist, who may also be its consultant or a stockholder in the company. Larger companies often sample four or five independent dermatologists with data to be reviewed, depending on the claim and the size of the company. This wording is not as common as "dermatologist recommended," which is typically based on a questionnaire that is sent to many dermatologists.[9]

Appearance Claims

Each company has its own research standards and some companies do not conduct any research at all to support their claims because research trials are not required by the FDA or FTC.[9] Some cosmetic companies try the study product on five of their employees, all of whom know what is being tested and are obligated to their employers. This of course is not close to the ideal study design but is frequently used. Many companies perform their "research trials" in house, do not share the design and results of the trials, and do not attempt to publish the results. Other companies use an independent dermatologist to evaluate subjects in an open-label trial (the subject and the investigator know the identity of the study product). A double-blinded vehicle-controlled trial is the gold standard and much preferred.

Although some trusted manufacturers exist in the cosmeceutical realm and some formulations have proven their clinical merit, the lack of official oversight, the proprietary nature of the formulations, and the disincentive for research data leave room for doubt about the efficacy claims of personal care products. Some reputable formulators test their main ingredients as well as finished products through *in vivo* (in living human skin) trials, but most rely on the ingredient manufacturers' *in vitro* (in test tubes or cell cultures) investigations of the individual ingredient and not the final formulation. It is nearly impossible for consumers to know the specifics of the research study design by reading a product label, but a few clues may reside in the language. The following terms and expressions are not regulated or legal definitions but are thought to convey the common connotations of the selected words.

Anti-Aging

Claims that a product confers an anti-aging benefit are often based on an ingredient claim. A grading by consumers or experts is usually included in this claim. SPF is known to gauge the ability of a product to prevent photodamage and premature photoaging, and new label revisions allow SPF products to make this claim. However, manufacturers of anti-aging products often tout the "anti-aging" benefits of their formulations based on ingredients other than ultraviolet screens.[9] For example, alpha hydroxy acids and vitamin A derivatives are popular ingredients in "anti-aging" products. There are no standard definitions or requirements for the use of the term "anti-aging."

"...Appearance of Wrinkles"

For cosmetic products, this claim is usually supported by a dermatologist's *in vivo* or photographic assessment of subjects at the end of a trial compared to baseline. Occasionally, bioinstruments (e.g., fringe projection, image analysis) or a consumer study with a questionnaire are used to support this claim. Normally, only a drug product (e.g., tretinoin) can make scientific claims of "increasing collagen production" or stimulating fibroblasts to produce collagen.[9] To skirt this issue, companies will instead claim their product "improves the appearance of wrinkles" and avoid the biological explanation of why the improvement occurs.

Brightening

The meaning of "brightening" is unclear, but it seems to pertain to light reflection off the skin's surface. This is also referred to as radiance or clarity.[9] Decreasing melanin levels in the skin leads to such an effect because melanin absorbs light. When there is less melanin, the skin reflects more light, making it appear brighter or more radiant. Visual elements are often placed in formulations to reflect light and cause brightening. For this reason, brightening can be noticed instantly upon application of the product. There are several approaches to assessing brightening effects. The assessment is usually performed via clinical evaluation, with dermatologists grading brightness on a scale (e.g., from very dull/not bright to very bright/no dullness) over the course of treatment. Results may also be obtained through measurement of luminosity image analysis such as photographs. This term is often used instead of "lightening" to evade regulatory hurdles.

Deep Cleaning

This claim is made but with no accompanying standard definition. Nevertheless, several approaches have been suggested. A standard compound can be applied to the skin and allowed to equilibrate, followed by a standardized washing procedure.[9] Normally, a new cleansing product (or device) is compared to either one or all of the following: a competitor, water alone, bar soap, or an older formulation (device). The amount of residual material can be quantified using laboratory instruments. For example, tape stripping is used to measure depth, and a sebumeter is used to demonstrate sebum reduction. Determining "cleanliness" may also be performed by consumers or expert graders. However, there is no proof required to state "deep cleaning" versus "cleansing."

Firming

Expert assessment and/or subject self-assessments are the foundation used to buttress a firming claim, but they are not on firm ground. Although some instrumental measurements have been applied (currently limited to ballistometry), few publications are available on this method and its validity is questionable.[9] Occasionally, a firming claim is based solely on the inclusion of a particular ingredient with no actual testing conducted. Firming is a nonsense claim with no underlying scientific basis, which is why companies use it.

Lifting

Three main methods are used to evaluate "lifting": bioinstruments (change in volume based on imaging software), expert graders, and consumer questionnaires.[9] Live grading can be performed split-face, if subjects are symmetrical, or 3D imaging can be used to grade lifting. Sometimes calculations can be managed on the images to measure in millimeters the appearance of visible lifting. "Lifting" is another nonsense term as lifting the skin with a topical skincare product is impossible.

Lightening

Lightening denotes reduced melanin or brown pigment in the skin. This can be assessed with any combination or single method of evaluation, including bioinstrumentation, clinical expert assessment, or consumer questionnaire.[9] Clinical studies typically include dermatologist assessments of overall skin fairness, overall evenness, and instrumental measurements such as $L^*a^*b^*$ values from chromameters. Image analysis for pigmented spots can be handled on high-resolution images, and dark marks can be followed for size and intensity compared to nearby skin. Photographic assessment is commonly used. Using the word "lightening" makes a biologic claim leading to FDA oversight so in many cases the term "brightening" is used instead.

Non-comedogenic

There is no standard definition associated with this claim. For years, this measurement was carried out on a rabbit ear model, but this model is no longer used. However, industry practice recommends implementing comedogenicity patch testing on the upper back in 10 to 20 subjects, based on the modified Kligman method in which cyanoacrylate follicular biopsies are then reviewed under a microscope.[9]

Plumping

Lip cosmetics often make this claim. Companies may use the assessments of lip volume, plumpness, color, or shape by one to three dermatologists. Subject self-assessment may also be used by product manufacturers, as subjects sometimes say they can "feel" the plumpness. This claim is also based on the use of digital imaging and grading by experts; advanced 3D imaging techniques can even allow quantification of volume changes.[9] Plumping may simply be a claim predicated on the incorporation of ingredients that engender increased blood flow, which temporarily expands the size of the lips.

Pore Reducing

The observation of a pore size reduction may be made by dermatologist reviewers/graders in person or through before/after photograph comparisons. Images can also be evaluated with bioinstrumentation (e.g., the software in the Canfield Visia system) that measures alterations in pore size.[9] More often, though, effects on pore size are self-assessed by subjects and graded using a questionnaire.

Smoothing

Smoothing can be measured using several methods. It may be as simple as a claim based on feedback from consumers or subjects.

A dermatologist may assess texture tactilely; improvements in tactile roughness would support a smoothing claim.[9] Rarely, 3D imaging or replicas are used to fortify this claim.

Tightening

Tightening claims are usually made to suggest that skin elasticity has increased. Measurements are often based on a Cutometer or other instrument that measures elasticity. However, these measurements are not very reliable for reasons that are beyond the scope of this chapter. It is impossible for the skin to increase elastin production after puberty (see Chapters 2, Basic Science of the Dermis, 5, Intrinsic Aging, and 6, Extrinsic Aging); therefore, any claims of increased elasticity are errant. In the case of peptides and saccharides on the skin, they make a movement-resistant layer on the top of the skin that resembles fondant on a cake. This can temporarily decrease skin pliability, which gives the sensation of skin tightening. Most skin-tightening claims are due to the presence of short-acting peptides that coat the skin's surface (see Chapter 37).

Volumizing

This is a common claim associated with eye cosmetics because any coating on the eyelash will expand the volume as measured in the volume equation $\pi r^2 h$. Thus, a doubling of the hair shaft radius will quadruple the volume (i.e., a 400% increase in lash volume). Photo assessments are usually completed, but there are no regulations on the number of subjects needed to claim that a product confers a plumping effect.[9]

ORGANIC SKINCARE

History

The term "organic" can be traced back to 1940. J.I. Rodale, who founded the Rodale book and magazine publishing empire with the modest publication *Organic Farming and Gardening*, coined the expression.[14] From then through 1992, when the US Department of Agriculture (USDA) approved the "organic" label and its accompanying standards, organic has mostly applied to agricultural foods and practices. Today, there are government-regulated standards only for organic food and topical products, but clothing and even pet food are now available in organic varieties. Currently, organic milk is far and away the most popular organic product.[15]

Organic plants are never grown with commercial pesticides or hormones, owing to concerns about human health and environmental impact. Although research has yet to prove that organics are healthier than nonorganic products, evidence has been uncovered to indicate why exposures to certain substances in nonorganic products could be harmful. For example, investigators found in a 2006 study that exposure to a compound derived from pesticides may be associated with male infertility since it lowered circulating testosterone levels in adult men.[16] Other studies have shown that pesticides in the soil, water, and air are harmful to wildlife. Environmentally conscious consumers take this kind of information into account in their product selections, and often opt for certified organic products when available.

Organic Certifications

There are myriad organic certifications worldwide as listed in **Table 32-1**. However, there is no one standard that everyone recognizes as *the* organic standard of choice. (In the food industry it is USDA Organic but that only applies to food.) The reputable organic and natural skincare brands are switching from organic certification marks and instead following the International Organization for Standardization (ISO) 16128: Guidelines on Technical Definitions and Criteria for Natural and Organic Cosmetic Ingredients and Products. The ISO 16128 standard is followed by several reputable companies and applies to cosmetic ingredients and finished skincare products. It does not offer a certification mark to be used on packaging; however, it describes a standard that should be used to define the presence and amount of natural ingredients in the product. The standard defines how to numerically determine the degree of natural and organic origin, making it easy to compare between individual raw materials and finished products. The ISO 16128 standard defines the following categories for cosmetic ingredients:

1. Natural ingredients
2. Derived natural ingredients
3. Organic ingredients
4. Derived organic ingredients

TABLE 32-1	Organic Certifications
• USDA Organic: Began in 2005. The strictest of organic standards because it is really a food standard. This is seen on individual ingredients. Requires 95% organic content to use logo. Disallows synthetic preservatives, and most chemical processing of ingredients.
• National Science Foundation (NSF): Began in 2009. NSF is one of the first US organic standards to emerge after USDA for cosmetic manufacturers. NSF requires a minimum of 70% of all ingredients (excluding water) to be organic to use its "made with organic" claim. Allows a broader array of preservatives and chemical processes than USDA.
• NaTrue: Began in 2008. NaTrue is a new non-profit standard from Europe started by German organic beauty manufacturers. It created a 3-star system to segregate "natural cosmetics" from "natural cosmetics with organic content" from "organic cosmetics." NaTrue 3-star requires 95% of all agricultural ingredients to be certified organic; 2-star requires 70%. A maximum of 5–15% (depending on the product category) of content can be from NaTrue's acceptable synthetic list.
• Cosmetics Organic Standard (COSMOS): Began in 2009. COSMOS is the first European Harmonized Standard for Organic beauty created by the first five EU organic beauty certifiers. COSMOS requires 95% of agricultural ingredients to be organic. Twenty percent of the total product by weight must be organic—including water. Allows a maximum of 5% synthetic content.

It also describes in a standardized manner for labels the degree of natural or organic origin of cosmetic ingredients. It provides the means to calculate the followed indices:

1. Natural index
2. Natural origin index
3. Organic index
4. Organic origin index

The index of the individual ingredients allows the degree of natural origin of finished cosmetic products to be calculated. If every company used this standard, it would be easier to compare products from one brand to another. However, it involves changing packaging that can be expensive and time consuming so it may take years for all skincare companies to adopt this standard.

Organic Skin and Body Products

Between 1998 and 2004, the use of natural and organic skin and body products rose by 51% according to "Packaged Facts" provided on www.MarketResearch.com. As recently as 2005, there were no rules regarding the use of terms such as organic or natural. Consequently, the use of these labels has typically caused significant confusion. For example, prior to regulation, manufacturers could call their product organic even if it had been composed of 90% water (a so-called organic ingredient), with no other organic active ingredients. To rectify this misleading situation (at the request of numerous manufacturers of natural and organic topical products), the USDA enacted new organic standards for skin and body care products in August 2005. Consumers can now purchase skin, body, and hair products with the USDA Organic Seal. A product that contains at least 95% organic ingredients can be legally labeled as organic. A product that contains at least 75% and up to 94% organic ingredients can be labeled as "made with organic ingredients."

The Rules of Organic Production

In the organic farming of food crops or those intended for topical products, farmers eschew synthetic pesticides, hormones, genetic modification of crops, and chemical products. Organic farming also follows traditional agricultural practices intended to enrich the soil, use resources in an environmentally sound manner, and treat livestock humanely. Specifically, a grower of organic ingredients must meet these basic criteria for the products to be certified as organic:

1. Abstain from the application of prohibited materials (including synthetic fertilizers, pesticides, and sewage sludge) for 3 years prior to certification and then continually throughout their organic license.
2. Prohibit the use of genetically modified organisms and irradiation.
3. Employ positive soil building, conservation, manure management, and crop rotation practices.
4. Avoid contamination during the processing of organic products.

5. Keep records of all operations [*courtesy of the Organic Consumers' Association*].

Organic Skincare Products

While there are no long-term studies documenting the effects of using topical organic products or ingredients, consumers of organic products are usually as interested in what products *do not* contain as in what they *do* contain. The organic label assures them that the key cleansing and conditioning ingredients are derived from organically grown plant products rather than conventionally grown plants, synthetic chemicals, or petroleum by-products. In addition, topical organic products exclude or minimize any ingredients that could be considered potentially harmful to people, animals, waterways, or the environment.

Natural Ingredients

It is important to note that a product touted as natural is not necessarily organic. The product may contain aloe, vitamin E, or other natural ingredients, but it may also contain chemicals intended to act as preservatives or to improve its texture. Only products that are truly organic are legally permitted to use the organic seal.

Of course, problems or allergic responses can be associated with ingredients that are natural and/or organic. For instance, many natural and organic brands contain certain fragrances and essential oils that can cause dermatitis. Oil of bergamot and balsam of Peru are both highly allergenic, so even an organic product containing them could irritate sensitive individuals. Organic products that include strong essential oils such as peppermint or rosemary can also irritate or inflame sensitive skin. Chamomile, generally considered a gentle and soothing herb, can induce allergies in some people (who may also tend to be allergic to wheat). Furthermore, conventional products as well as some natural ones contain a "perfume mix" to mask their odor. Components of the perfume mix are rarely listed on the product label since each company uses its own proprietary blend. Even a product listed as 95% organic could contain a perfume mix that might provoke allergic reactions in some people.

FTC GUIDELINES ON PRODUCT ENDORSEMENTS AND TESTIMONIALS

The FTC publishes "Guides Concerning the Use of Endorsements and Testimonials in Advertising," which covers endorsements by consumers, experts, organizations, doctors, and celebrities, as well as the disclosure of important connections between advertisers and endorsers.

The guide explains that payments or free products exchanged between advertisers and endorsers must be divulged (e.g., bloggers paid to write a review or celebrity endorsements on a talk show, or doctors posting on social media). Similarly, if a company refers in an advertisement to the findings of a research organization that conducted research sponsored by the company, the advertisement must reveal the connection between the advertiser and the research organization.

Doctors and their endorsement of skincare products is addressed in the 255.3 "Expert Endorsement" section of the guidance. If the endorser is referred to as "doctor," the advertisement must make clear the nature and limits of the endorser's expertise. The endorsement must be supported by an actual exercise of that expertise in evaluating product features or characteristics with respect to which s/he is expert, and which are relevant to an ordinary consumer's use of or experience with the product and are available to the ordinary consumer. An example the FTC provides is: A medical doctor states in an advertisement for a drug that the product will safely allow consumers to lower their cholesterol by 50 points. If the materials the doctor reviewed were merely letters from satisfied consumers or the results of a rodent study, the endorsement would likely be deceptive because those materials are not what others with the same degree of expertise would consider adequate to support this conclusion about the product's safety and efficacy. The FTC guidelines are nonbinding administrative interpretations of the law intended to help advertisers comply with the FTC Act.[17]

CONCLUSION

It is fair to say that skincare products that are considered to be cosmeceuticals fall through the regulatory loopholes in laws governing the testing and labeling of drugs and cosmetics. However, medical providers who have some understanding of certifications and claims can discern justifiable statements based on science versus inflated marketing claims. One of the goals of this textbook is to help medical providers navigate these opaque waters.

References

1. Kligman A. Cosmeceuticals: do we need a new category? In: Elsner P, Maibach H, eds. *Cosmeceuticals*. New York, NY: Marcel Dekker Inc.; 2000 1.

2. Kligman A. The future of cosmeceuticals: an interview with Albert Kligman, MD, PhD. Interview by Zoe Diana Draelos. *Dermatol Surg.* 2005;31(7 Pt 2):890–891.

3. The US Food and Drug Administration. FD&C Act Chapter VI: Cosmetics. Available at https://uscode.house.gov/browse/prelim@title21/chapter9&edition=prelim. Accessed March 29, 2021.

4. Rogiers V. Efficacy claims of cosmetics in Europe must be scientifically substantiated from 1997 on. *Skin Res Technol.* 1995;1(1):44–46.

5. National Advertising Division. Skin doctors cosmeceuticals participates in NAD forum. Skin Doctors Cosmeceuticals (Eyetuck Anti-Bag Technology), Report #4627, NAD/CARU Case Reports (February 2007). Available at https://case-report.bbbnp.org/Search/Results. Accessed March 31, 2021.

6. The US Food and Drug Administration. Available at https://www.fda.gov/food/food-ingredients-packaging/generally-recognized-safe-gras. Accessed January 17, 2021.

7. The Personal Care Council. Available at https://www.personalcarecouncil.org/science-safety/cosmetic-ingredient-review/. Accessed March 31, 2021.

8. Cosmetic Ingredient Review. Available at https://www.cir-safety.org/about. Accessed January 17, 2021.

9. Baumann LS. Cosmeceutical marketing claims. In *Cosmeceuticals and Cosmetic Ingredients*. New York: McGraw-Hill, 2014, pp. 11–15.

10. Baumann L. Inside Cosmeceutical Marketing Claims. *Pract Dermatol.* 2012:35–39.

11. Gilman AG, Goodman LS, Gilman A, eds. *Goodman and Gilman's The Pharmacological Basis of Therapeutics.* 6th ed. New York, NY: Macmillan Publishing Co. Inc.; 1980: 969.

12. Sax NI. The Butyl, Ethyl, Methy, and Propyl Esters have been found to promote allergic sensitization in humans. In: *Dangerous Properties of Industrial Materials.* 4th ed. New York, NY: Van Nostrand Reinhold; 1975: 929.

13. Vince G. Cosmetic chemicals found in breast tumours. *New Scientist.com news service*, January 12, 2004. Accessed March 22, 2021.

14. *Organic Gardening*. March 1998;22–25.

15. Severson K. An organic cash cow. *New York Times.* November 9, 2005. Available at https://www.nytimes.com/2005/11/09/dining/arts/an-organic-cash-cow.html. Accessed March 22, 2021.

16. Meeker JD, Ryan L, Barr DB, Hauser R. Exposure to non-persistent insecticides and male reproductive hormones. *Epidemiology.* 2006;17(1):61–68.

17. The US Federal Trade Commission. Available at https://www.ftc.gov/sites/default/files/attachments/press-releases/ftc-publishes-final-guides-governing-endorsements-testimonials/091005revisedendorsementguides.pdf. Accessed March 31, 2021.

CHAPTER 33

Choosing Skincare Products to Retail in Your Medical Practice

Leslie S. Baumann, MD

SUMMARY POINTS

What's Important?
1. Retail multiple brands, choosing the best from each.
2. Limit your inventory by knowing your patient demographic.
3. Offer the least expensive option when possible.

What's New?
1. Choose hero products from each brand and combine based on skin type.
2. Limit the number of anti-aging products to reduce inventory costs.

What's Coming?
1. Methods to analyze amounts of ingredients in products.
2. Methods to compare product efficacy.

INTRODUCTION

There is a plethora of cosmeceuticals from which to choose to retail in your medical practice. It is difficult to know how many and which products to carry. Inventory is expensive, particularly when considering that inventory may expire before it is sold. Knowing how many products to retail is just as important as choosing which skincare brands and products to offer to patients. This chapter discusses how many products to make available and how to choose the best skincare brands and products for patients.

CHOOSING A SKINCARE BRAND TO OFFER IN YOUR PRACTICE

Choosing a skincare brand to sell in your medical practice is challenging. Brands want you to exclusively sell their products. They will encourage you to sell entire regimens consisting of only their products. Also, they require minimum purchases that are often in the range of $2,500 to $3,000, which complicates carrying more than one brand. They offer discounts based on volume sales that entice you to sell only their brand. There are two main problems with only offering one skincare brand in your practice: efficacy and ethics.

Each brand is based on a core technology that serves as the "hero product." Once companies develop that product, for financial reasons they develop other products to sell to complement the original formulation. For example, if a brand has a serum with unique anti-aging ingredients, that is their hero product. They will develop other products to sell along with that product such as cleansers and moisturizers. The problem arises in that these "add on" or supporting products are not unique; often they are copycat products with no special technology. Although they are developed to be compatible with the hero product, they are usually not designed with various skin types in mind. Brands operate on the belief that there is one best product that works for everyone. They do not have the resources to develop individual formulations suited to all of the variations in the 16 Baumann Skin Types. Their product offerings and marketing strategies are developed to increase sales of the hero product and the supporting products, and not necessarily to improve the patient's skin. To offer the optimal and most efficacious cosmeceuticals for your patients, you should choose the hero products from the various brands and combine them in a scientific manner that increases the efficacy of each product (see Chapter 35, Skincare Regimen Design).

You can retail skincare products ethically following the steps discussed in Chapter 34 (Skincare Retail in a Medical Setting). You should be ethical when choosing what products to sell in your practice. The products you choose to sell in your practice should be:

- Proven to work
- Appropriate for the patient's skin issues and skin type
- Capable of providing comparable efficacy to prescription equivalents
- Limited so as to encompass the fewest number of products necessary
- Of lowest cost possible

Do Skincare Products Work Best When Only One Brand Is Used?

Brands will often claim that their products work best when used together because they were designed to be compatible. The problem with this statement is that it is impossible for the brand to have all of the most efficacious products for each skin type. Each brand has a core competency as discussed above. No one brand has the most advanced technologies across the board for all products. In some cases, a prescription medication would be more efficacious. You should be open to choosing the best hero products from each brand and combining them with prescription medications in an order that increases the efficacy of all of the products.

Developing Your Own Skincare Line

Some practitioners choose to develop their own skincare brand. In some cases, medical providers formulate their own products and in other cases they opt to sell private label products. If you choose the latter approach, you should make sure that you still offer prescription medications and other brands when they deliver superior efficacy for your patient's skin condition. Developing a skincare line is not easy. There are many issues to consider.

Anticipated volume

The number of products you sell in a set amount of time will significantly determine the costs of your product. Demand for your products, and the volume you will need, will be unpredictable. The required minimum order ranges across manufacturers. Unless you choose a private label company that offers the choice of small volumes, manufacturers will require

2,500+ pieces per product. As the order numbers rise, the prices decline. Ordering 5,000 pieces will cost less per piece than ordering 2,500 pieces; however, the discounts are not significant until you order around 100,000 pieces of one item. This makes it very difficult to develop your own skincare line for your patients at a cost that is comparable to larger brands. You should ask yourself, "Is the product I am developing worth the extra cost to my patients?"

Choosing product packaging

Manufacturing companies adjust minimum quantity requirements based on type of packaging. This pertains to how many units are included in a "run." It takes time for the manufacturer to set up the machine before each unique product run, so small quantities are not worth the effort for them. The set-up costs and number of items in the run are determined by the type of packaging.

Products are typically packaged in tubes, bottles, jars, and airless pump containers. Jars tend to be more expensive, particularly if gold tops are used. Some products require specific packaging: sunscreens must be in the exact same tubes that the SPF testing was conducted in, and some serums require airless pump bottles. Glass is more expensive, but better for the environment than plastic. Biodegradable packaging does not always protect products from heat and is easily damaged in shipping. Plastic containers confer several advantages such as reduced breakage, lighter shipping weight, and ease of labeling. It is important to note that the wrong grade of plastic, regardless of the packaging, can adversely affect the stability of a product. For example, the plastic used in sunscreen tubes is thicker than plastic used in cleanser tubes.

Product labeling

Product labeling is important and affects the final product cost. If your product is regulated as an over-the-counter (OTC) drug, the labels must have certain components. It is the intended use of the formulation that determines if it is considered a drug, an OTC drug, or a cosmetic. Each has different regulations to follow on the label and marketing materials. If an intended use of a product—to treat acne, for example—falls under the category of OTC it must follow regulations in the corresponding OTC monograph dictating which ingredients must be in the product, the amount of the ingredient, and the claims that can be made. Products that will be marketed for these indications must follow the corresponding FDA OTC monograph. Here are some examples of skin issues in the FDA OTC monographs (**Box 33-1**).

BOX 33-1

Acne
Anti-fungal
Dandruff
Hair growth
Psoriasis
Skin bleaching
Sunscreen
Wart removal

Once you finalize the text for your labels, hire a lawyer that specializes in cosmetic and OTC law to review your text. It is very expensive to replace labels once the products have already been made. Make sure you have it right the first time.

The cost of setting up printing plates for labeling can be exorbitant and you must create a separate one for each product. You will need a graphic artist to design the label for you based on the size and shape of the label. The cost of the product label will depend upon the type of label (e.g., sticker vs. silk screen) and the type of packaging. Be careful to limit the number of colors because each color will increase the cost. Remember that various label sizes would be needed if you choose to offer different product sizes such as a sample or travel size and a full-size product.

Stick-on labels by themselves are inexpensive but some companies require a minimum number of labels. Label material is another cost variable. Regular paper labels have nominal protective coating—neither waterproof nor sufficient to prevent creasing if the bottle is squeezed—and are the least expensive. Polylaminate or vinyl labels are water- and weatherproof and slightly elastic, thus retaining their form upon being squeezed. These are superior but more expensive.

Other costs

There are many other costs involved with starting your own skincare line such as shipping from the manufacturer, storage, design of materials, trademark, and advertising. You often need to hire someone to handle the process. All of these costs add up and increase the price that you need to charge for your products (known as cost of goods or COGS). You must ask yourself, "Am I giving the patient access to the best skincare technologies at the best price or am I just trying to make money?" How you answer that question should give you insight into your motivation and ethics.

CHOOSING WHAT PRODUCTS TO RETAIL IN YOUR PRACTICE

There are 16 Baumann Skin Types with subtypes of sensitive skin. When you analyze all of the different products needed to treat these skin types, you will need 20 different products (known as SKUs or "stock keeping units") to cover all the needs of the 16 Baumann Skin Types. In some cases you can find a product that will fulfill the needs of more than one of these and cut the SKU number down to 17 or 18, but for the sake of simplicity, we will discuss the 20 SKUs needed.

Four Cleanser Categories Cover All 16 Baumann Skin Types

You need at least four cleansers to target all 16 skin types. Cleansers are important because they prepare the skin for the products that follow and affect the efficacy and side effect profile of the other products. Oily skin types will need a foaming cleanser and maybe a salicylic acid cleanser, while dry types need a nonfoaming cleanser and maybe a hydroxy acid

cleanser. You may also choose to retail a benzoyl peroxide cleanser for your acne patients if you prefer that to salicylic acid cleansers. In general, oily types need foaming cleansers. If an oily skin type also has pigmentation problems or needs anti-aging benefits, a salicylic acid cleanser can be added. A salicylic acid cleanser should be used in the morning because the lower pH helps improve the efficacy of ascorbic acid and some other antioxidants used to protect the skin from light in the daytime. A foaming cleanser is best at night because it is superior at removing sunscreen, sweat, makeup, and dirt. Dry skin types need nonfoaming or creamy lipid-laden cleansers to help protect the skin barrier. If a dry skin type also has pigmentation problems or needs anti-aging benefits, a hydroxy acid cleanser can be added. The hydroxy acid cleanser should be used in the morning because the lower pH helps improve the efficacy of ascorbic acid and some other antioxidants used to protect the skin from light in the daytime.

Foaming cleansers

Foaming cleansers are used for oily skin types. Detergents, known as surfactants, provide the foam. Surfactants work by reducing the surface tension on the skin and emulsifying dirt.[1] These cleansers usually have a high pH of 8–10. There are various classes of surfactants found in cleansers. Anionic surfactants are negatively charged. These provide the most foam, but they remove lipids from the skin's surface and bilayer membrane barrier, thus injuring the skin barrier and increasing the risk of irritant dermatitis.[2] Anionic surfactants are often combined with other surfactants like amphoteric or nonionic surfactants to decrease irritation potential while preserving the ability to deliver a vigorous foam. Patients, especially oily skin types, like the clean feeling of the skin after an anionic surfactant but this must be balanced with protection of the skin barrier.

Many patients will request sulfate-free detergents. This trend emerged from the wide use of the compound sodium lauryl sulfate (SLS) that was found in cleansers and shampoos. SLS strips lipids from the skin, damages the skin barrier, and irritates the skin to such an extent that it is used in research labs to hinder the skin barrier to test "barrier repair products." Warnings to avoid SLS resulted in the "sulfate-free" trend. (Sulfates are also unpopular due to their petroleum-based origin.) Not all sulfates are as irritating to the skin as SLS. A much milder sulfate that serves as an alternative to SLS, sodium laureth sulfate (or sodium lauryl ether sulfate, also known as SLES) exhibits high foaming attributes but is less likely than SLS to cause irritation. Naturally derived surfactants like cocamidopropyl betaine and disodium cocoamphodiacetate from coconut oil or disodium laureth sulfosuccinate, which is often used in baby cleansing products, are gentle on the skin. Fatty acid esters of sucrose such as sucrose laurate are natural detergent options.[3]

Nonfoaming cleansers

Nonfoaming cleansers use lipids and oils to emulsify and remove dirt, makeup, and sunscreen from the skin. If they contain surfactants, they are very mild. Nonfoaming cleansers do not injure the skin barrier; in fact, they repair the skin barrier if they contain fatty acids such as stearic acid or stearic acid-derived surfactants such as glycol stearate and glycol distearate.[4] This class of cleansers includes superfatted soaps, combination bars (combars), syndet bars (bars composed of synthetic detergents), and compounds that deposit lipids on the skin such as oils. Cream and oil cleansers fall into this category. These cleansers usually have a neutral pH. If these cleansers contain surfactants, they are mild and usually nonionic like caprylyl/capryl glucoside, glyceryl stearate, caprylic/capric triglyceride, and monolaurin. Saponins are a large family of natural cleansing compounds derived from plants such as the soap nut and *Camellia oleifera*.[5,6] Nonfoaming cleansers are most appropriate for dry skin types. Oily skin types often report that they "do not feel clean" when they use these cleansers.

Alpha hydroxy acid cleansers

Alpha hydroxy acids (AHAs) are the best hydroxy acid cleansers for individuals with dry skin because they act as humectants with high water absorption capabilities. AHAs provide exfoliation, hydration, and help improve the penetration of subsequently applied ingredients especially ascorbic acid. The low pH causes an inhospitable environment for *Cutibacterium acnes*, making it harder for the bacteria to thrive. AHA cleansers do not dry out the skin the way that salicylic acid cleansers do because their hydrophilic nature renders them unable to penetrate through sebum. These formulations are ideal for dry skin types with acne, skin pigmentation, or cutaneous aging.

Salicylic acid cleansers

Salicylic acid (SA) cleansers are lipophilic and can penetrate through the sebum into pores, making these cleansers ideal for oily skin types. They are the most effective cleansers to unclog pores. SA is a member of the salicylate family, which includes aspirin, and displays anti-inflammatory properties. SA cleansers are ideal for use by individuals with oily, sensitive skin prone to acne, seborrheic dermatitis, rosacea, hyperpigmentation, and aging. See Chapter 40 to learn more about cleansers.

Four Moisturizer Categories Cover All 16 Baumann Skin Types

Moisturizers have several roles: hydrating, protecting, and increasing penetration of ingredients important to the skin. Four main types of moisturizers are necessary to effectively moisturize all types of skin: barrier repair moisturizer, soothing barrier repair moisturizer, noncomedogenic light moisturizer, and light anti-aging moisturizer. If you have all four of these, you will be able to design skincare regimens appropriate for each of the 16 Baumann Skin Types.

Dry skin types need barrier repair moisturizers. Barrier repair moisturizers should mimic the skin's natural barrier. An intact skin barrier shows a Maltese cross pattern when viewed under a cross polarized microscope. There are three technologies that have been demonstrated to repair the skin barrier and restore it to its natural shape and function:

1. An equal ratio of ceramides, fatty acids, and cholesterol[7]
2. MLE technology composed of myristoyl/palmitoyl oxostearamide/arachamide mea[8]
3. PSL repair technology with ceramide 3, stearic acid, and cholesterol
4. Ceramide dominant barrier repair technology containing ceramides, conjugated linoleic acid, and cholesterol in a 3:1:1 ratio[9]

These base formulas may be combined with anti-inflammatory ingredients in a soothing barrier repair moisturizer used to calm the side effects of acne medications and alleviate rosacea symptoms.

Oily skin types need a noncomedogenic light moisturizer if they are acne prone. If they have aging issues, a noncomedogenic light anti-aging moisturizer with ingredients such as heparan sulfate and hyaluronic acid can be used. Acne skincare and anti-aging skincare are discussed in Chapters 14, 19, 33, 34, and 35. To learn more about moisturizers see Chapter 43.

Six treatment product Categories to Cover All 16 Baumann Skin Types

At least five treatment products are needed to address all 16 Baumann Skin Types. These products include treatments for:

1. Acne (retinoid alternative)
2. Aging (retinoid alternative)
3. Acne and aging (retinoid)
4. Hyperpigmentation
5. Inflammation, rosacea

In many cases, a sixth product that contains vitamin C is necessary to boost anti-aging activity and to use when the patient is given a tyrosinase inhibitor holiday (see Chapter 41, Depigmenting Agents). Do not fall into the trap of carrying too many expensive anti-aging products. You can cover all skin types with three anti-aging products: a retinoid, an anti-aging retinol alternative with either growth factors, defensin, or other non-irritating anti-aging technologies, and an ascorbic acid product. See Chapter 35 for How to Design a Skincare Regimen.

One Eye Cream Category Can Cover All 16 Baumann Skin Types

A minimum of one eye cream is needed to hydrate the eye area and protect from acne medications and retinoids that transfer onto this area at night via the pillowcase. If you want to expand your product offerings, include a soothing eye product, an eye formulation to treat dark circles, and a product to diminish eye puffiness.

Two or more Sunscreen Categories Cover All 16 Baumann Skin Types

Sunscreen options include mineral and chemical, tinted and untinted, face and body, and noncomedogenic options. You may also wish to carry a hydrating facial SPF that eliminates the need for moisturizer. Before choosing which sunscreen options to carry, evaluate your patient demographic and decide which will be most likely used by your patients. The goal is to increase compliance with sunscreen. Many practices opt to sell four types of facial sunscreen:

1. Noncomedogenic chemical SPF for oily acne prone types, untinted
2. Noncomedogenic physical SPF for oily acne prone types, tinted
3. Hydrating chemical SPF for dry types, untinted
4. Hydrating physical SPF for dry types, tinted

Other options include:

5. Noncomedogenic physical SPF for oily acne prone types, untinted
6. Noncomedogenic chemical SPF for oily acne prone types, tinted
7. Hydrating chemical SPF for dry types, tinted
8. Hydrating physical SPF for dry types, untinted

You also may want to consider selling body SPF such as sprays, sticks, and lip balms. It depends on your patient population.

Two Hypoallergenic Categories Cover the 16 Baumann Skin Types

For patients with multiple allergies, it is ideal to offer a hypoallergic cleanser and moisturizer. In many cases patients will come to you with a long history of reactions to skincare products and patch testing that is non-conclusive. You will want to take them off everything except a hypoallergenic cleanser and moisturizer. Slowly, you will add back in products one at a time to find out which products they can tolerate. There are skincare formulations on the market that do not contain the 100+ most common allergens. These can be used to perform this wash out.

STAYING CURRENT WITH SKINCARE SCIENCE

These 20 products are the bare minimum you need to sell products in your practice. Many prefer to have two different soothing products: a soothing oil and a lotion or serum for anti-redness. You may choose to have two different skin-lightening products: one more moisturizing and one noncomedogenic. It all depends on how much space you have available to store inventory.

You should review the products that you sell in your practice every 6 months. Look at sales of each product, patient feedback, and the staff's opinions. Compare with new products on the market and see what you should update. Keep these 20 core products.

In summary, there are myriad products on the market. Do not be fooled by the marketing claims of manufacturers. For example, CBD is very popular but there are not yet methods to compare efficacy for the various CBD products. Methods are being developed to study ingredient amounts in each product and to compare antioxidant potential and other signs of efficacy. For now, our best bet to choose the most efficacious products are clinical trials. You will see the best efficacy if you choose the hero products from each brand and combine them in a skincare regimen suited to the patient's Baumann Skin Type. Chapter 35 will teach you how to design the individual skincare regimens.

References

1. Baumann LS. Overview of Cleansing Agents. In: *Cosmeceuticals and Cosmetic Ingredients*. New York, NY: McGraw-Hill; 2014:19–20.
2. Effendy I, Maibach HI. Surfactants and experimental irritant contact dermatitis. *Contact Dermatitis*. 1995;33(4):217–225.
3. Osipow L, Snell FD, Marra D, York WC. Surface activity of monoesters fatty acid esters of sucrose. *Ind Engineer Chem*. 1956; 48(9):1462–1464.
4. Bhadani A, Iwabata K, Sakai K, Koura S, Sakai H, Abe M. Sustainable oleic and stearic acid based biodegradable surfactants. *RSC Advances*. 2017;7(17):10433–10442.
5. Tmáková L, Sekretár S, Schmidt Š. Plant-derived surfactants as an alternative to synthetic surfactants: surface and antioxidant activities. *Chemical Papers*. 2016;70(2):188–196.
6. Chen YF, Yang CH, Chang MS, Ciou YP, Huang YC. Foam properties and detergent abilities of the saponins from Camellia oleifera. *Int J Mol Sci*. 2010;11(11):4417–4425.
7. Man MQ M, Feingold KR, Thornfeldt CR, Elias PM. Optimization of physiological lipid mixtures for barrier repair. *J Invest Dermatol*. 1996;106(5):1096–1101.
8. Park BD, Youm JK, Jeong SK, Choi EH, Ahn SK, Lee SH. The characterization of molecular organization of multilamellar emulsions containing pseudoceramide and type III synthetic ceramide. *J Invest Dermatol*. 2003;121(4):794–801.
9. Chamlin SL, Kao J, Frieden IJ, et al. Ceramide-dominant barrier repair lipids alleviate childhood atopic dermatitis: changes in barrier function provide a sensitive indicator of disease activity. *J Am Acad Dermatol*. 2002;47(2):198–208.

CHAPTER 34

Skincare Retail in a Medical Setting

Leslie S. Baumann, MD

SUMMARY POINTS

What's Important?
1. Patients should receive personalized skincare routines.
2. Customization of the skincare routine improves outcomes.
3. Proven skincare routines only work when patients are compliant.
4. Develop key performance indicators to track performance.

What's New?
1. Giving exact advice on how much product to use.
2. Product repurchase rates are directly tied to patient adherence.
3. Telemedicine consults are a great way to do follow-up visits.

What's Coming?
1. There are numerous evolving ecommerce options.
2. More people are purchasing skincare from their physicians.
3. Methods to engage patients to improve compliance are being devised.
4. Ways to electronically monitor compliance to topical treatments are being developed.

A report in July 2020 showed that physician-dispensed skincare is the largest growing segment of the skincare business with a projected compound annual growth rate (CAGR) of 9.9% from 2020 to 2027.[1] There are numerous reasons for this including that patients are confused by the plethora of choices on the market and want to obtain unbiased scientifically based skincare advice from someone they can trust. Although the number of skincare sales by doctors is rapidly increasing, most of these sales are completed by a few medical practices that are successful with skincare sales. Most doctors are unsuccessful at retailing skincare. This is usually because they feel conflicted or do not make it a priority. The doctors that are successful at selling skincare in their practice share some behaviors in common. The processes pursued by the medical providers who are successful at retailing skincare will be discussed in this chapter.

ETHICS OF SELLING SKINCARE IN A MEDICAL SETTING

There has been much debate over the years about the ethics of doctors selling skincare in medical practices.[2,3] The arguments against selling skincare include:

- Risking or potentially harming the physician-patient relationship
- Letting financial concerns override concerns for patient health
- Disclosing conflict of interest to the patient[4]
- Recommending products that are only available through physicians[5]

There is little doubt that when a physician tells a patient they should use certain skincare products, the patient feels compelled or strongly inclined to purchase and use them. The physician or medical provider should take great care not to take advantage of the power of the patient-physician relationship and recommend only products that are proven to work and necessary for the patient. Skincare should be thought of as prescription medications. They should be used for their efficacy, not to make a sale. The products should be the most efficacious available to treat the skin condition. The aggressive approach described in this chapter is ethical when the medical provider is absolutely certain that the products they are recommending are the best options to treat the patient's skin condition. There is much discussion about the ethics of selling skincare and it all comes down to these questions: "Is this the best option for the patient? Is it efficacious, accessible, likely to be used, at a fair price, and necessary?" If the answer is yes to all of these questions, then it is ethical.

Patients are bombarded by pseudoscience and are taken advantage of by false marketing claims. The plethora of products on the market is confusing. It has been said that 80% of people are using the wrong skincare for their skin type. It is clear that patients need guidance from someone who is knowledgeable and cares about health outcomes. The American Medical Association has stated that physicians can retail skincare but must disclose their financial interest in products being sold in their offices.[6] This means that physicians that sell private label products or develop their own skincare brand should disclose this to patients, especially if the exact same formulation is available in a less expensive product. It is much less complicated ethically to use products that are not the medical provider's own brand.

Offering products in the medical practice helps patients purchase the correct products and ensures the products are not counterfeit and have been stored correctly. The convenience of purchasing products in the medical office improves compliance, especially when combined with clear printed instructions. Any ethical pitfalls can easily be responsibly managed by a thoughtful and ethical physician.[7] When done properly, for the right reasons, and with good staff oversight, retailing skincare can strengthen the physician-patient relationship and improve outcomes.

Here are some steps to be used as a guide for how to ethically, scientifically, and successfully retail skincare.

CUSTOMIZED SKINCARE REGIMENS FOR EACH PATIENT

Diagnose Patient Skin Type

The first step to ethical skincare retail is to diagnose the patient's skin type and underlying skin issues. A correct diagnosis will lead to better skincare recommendations. Medical advice on skincare is valuable to the patient. They deserve to have a knowledgeable medical provider who cares about outcomes more than profit when giving them advice.

The traditional division of skin types into oily, dry, combination, and sensitive skin is not sufficient because it omits issues such as hyperpigmentation and aging. For this reason, the author has developed a skin typing system consisting of 16 Baumann Skin Types (BSTs), which is used in medical practices around the world[8] and discussed in multiple textbooks.[9-11] (See Chapter 10, The Baumann Skin Typing System.) The Skin Type Solutions System[9] uses a simple software-based questionnaire[12] that has been proven[13] to accurately determine a patient's BST within just a few minutes. The scientifically validated questionnaire[13] looks for the presence of barriers to skin health: dehydration, excessive sebum production, inflammation, dyspigmentation, and lifestyle habits that increase the risk of aging and skin cancer. This approach also provides the practitioner with the opportunity to screen for a history of contact dermatitis and diagnose skin conditions that may warrant prescription-based treatments, such as rosacea and melasma.

Using a valid questionnaire allows the physician to quickly obtain a thorough skincare history from the patient without increasing the amount of time spent in the exam room. Many dermatologists see 80–100 patients per day with an average of 3–5 minutes per patient. They do not have time to discuss skincare with patients. Using a standardized validated skin type questionnaire to determine the patient's barriers to skin health prior to seeing the patient serves multiple purposes:

- Allows for a more complete history of skin issues
- Gives the physician more insight into the patient's concerns
- Aids in diagnosis of skin disorders
- Facilitates designing a skincare routine including prescription medications
- Gives insights into patient's risk factors such as lack of sunscreen use or poor diet
- Improves patient communication and engages them in their own care
- Strengthens the physician-patient relationship
- Begins the skincare education process prior to seeing the physician
- Engages the patient and helps them see how their habits affect skin health
- Identifies cosmetic concerns that the patient is interested in discussing
- Helps set the goal of improving the skin type by targeting barriers to skin health.

Prescribe a Skincare Routine to Match the Baumann Skin Type

Giving medical advice on skincare and recommending exact skincare products in a step-by-step regimen helps improve compliance. This also discourages patients from wasting money on ineffective products or products that are not right for their skin type. When patients use the right skincare products to improve their barriers to skin health, the side effects that occur from the use of inappropriate products are eliminated or greatly reduced. Outcomes improve, patient satisfaction rises, and the patient-physician relationship is strengthened as trust builds. However, designing an efficacious skincare regimen is not easy (see Chapter 35, Skincare Regimen Design: Product Layering). This is why designing as much of the regimen prior to the patient visit is important to ensure your patients get a well-designed skincare routine. Software has been developed to generate skincare regimens based on the BST using products from brands the physician has decided to sell in the office. This saves time and effort and helps the physician keep current on skincare technologies and new science about how to order the products in the regimen. If a medical provider chooses not to use the software, they can develop all 32 skincare regimens themselves (16 skin types plus sensitive skin subtypes yield 32 skin types). However, there are over 40,000 different final regimen combinations when one considers patient preferences, lifestyle habits, and skincare needs. Whatever method is chosen, as much of the regimen as possible should be designed prior to the visit to account for the science of product layering discussed in Chapter 35.

Using a method to diagnose skin type in the waiting room or at home prior to the visit allows the medical provider to have these predesigned basic skincare regimens that can be swiftly adjusted and personalized for the patient during the office visit. For example, the BST DSNW (dry, sensitive, nonpigmented, wrinkle-prone) rosacea subtype will need a regimen designed to hydrate, reduce inflammation, and address wrinkles. The regimen should be devised to increase the efficacy of the rosacea medication. Products should include a nonfoaming cleanser, rosacea medication, barrier repair moisturizer, non-stinging sunscreen appropriate for sensitive skin, and an anti-aging retinoid alternative product. This skincare routine for rosacea can then be easily customized for the patient in the exam room. For example, retinoids are not usually prescribed to a rosacea patient on the first visit due to the increased risk of side effects. However, if a DSNW patient comes in already tolerating a topical retinoid, then the anti-aging retinoid alternative product can be switched to a retinoid. Most of the skincare consult can be performed by the staff when the regimens are designed and approved ahead of time. This allows the medical provider to review the regimen, personalize it for the patient, and prescribe any needed medications. The personalization of skincare routines with medical knowledge and advice is a crucial aspect of making skincare retail ethical.

Diagnosing the patient's skin type and using a standardized approach to regimen development solves the problem of the last-minute question at the end of the clinic visit that many dermatologists dread: "I have one last quick question."[14] Every patient deserves honest and thoughtful skincare advice, even if they are coming in for a general dermatology issue. Giving advice to every patient on daily sun protection, the use of the proper cleansers and moisturizers, and when and how to use their prescribed medications in the skincare routine is necessary to increase compliance. Training your entire staff on skincare science, as well as how to diagnose the skin type and develop a regimen will save time and improve patient communication.

Ensure Product Efficacy

Patients look to their medical provider to determine which marketing claims are valid vis-à-vis pseudoscience. It is impossible for someone who is not trained in skin science to discern hype from fact (see Chapter 33, Choosing Skincare Products).

In 1999, the American Medical Association (AMA) issued this statement about physicians selling skincare products: "Product claims must be scientifically valid and reinforced by unbiased scientific sources."[6] It is up to the medical provider to ensure that the products have the correct ingredients, are formulated and packaged properly, and are arranged in the appropriate order in the regimen to ensure efficacy.

Choose the Best Products from Various Brands

Skincare manufacturers typically display a core competency or specialty, such as antioxidant or sunscreen technology. Patients benefit when the best products from a variety of brands are selected for a regimen rather than relying on all the products of one particular brand (see Chapter 33). This improves outcomes as patients end up using the most effective formulation for each step in skincare. When products from various brands are combined in a regimen, this regimen should be tested on the various BSTs for efficacy.

Present the Proper Order of Product Application

The importance of product layering and how to decide at which step in the regimen a skincare product should be introduced is discussed in Chapter 35. The order in which products are applied to the skin influences efficacy. The physician must consider ingredient interactions, penetration times, and cross reactions along with skin type factors such as the condition of the skin barrier, sebum production, and thickness of the stratum corneum. Lifestyle factors like sun exposure, when patients exercise, and when they bathe factors into what time of day to apply the products.

Update the Skincare Regimen

The BST will often change. In fact, the goal is to change the skin type to the ideal skin type (ORNT Type 10). At each visit the patient's skin should be assessed and the regimen updated. It is important to manage the patient's expectations in the beginning so they know that the regimen will be adjusted every month as their skin changes and improves. It usually takes three or four visits spaced 1 month apart to get the skin into a stable long-term skincare regimen. The exception is patients with hyperpigmentation such as melasma who often need to be seen every month for at least 4 months. After 4 months they are placed on a tyrosinase inhibitor-free maintenance regimen. (See Chapter 20, Pigmentation Disorders, for more discussion on the treatment of melasma.)

Skin types can change seasonally, and with hormonal changes, a move to a new geographic location, increased stress, and changes in diet. Many patients who are on the border between dry and normal/oily skin will need a dry skin regimen in cold or dry months and an oily skin regimen in hot or humid months. Once the patient is placed on a skincare regimen, they should be re-evaluated in 4 weeks. At this visit the skincare regimen should be adjusted. Depending on the patient's issues, a retinoid can be added or increased in strength. If they are already on a higher dose of retinoid, a low-pH cleanser can be added. Many changes can be made at the follow-up visits to optimize the regimen and adjust to the patient's lifestyle changes and any issues affecting compliance.

Educate Patients

Using a skin typing system allows the medical provider to educate patients easily and systematically on their skin issues and personalized skincare routine. Prewritten information, categorized by skin type, can explain the thought process behind each selection, the significance of particular ingredients, and why the order of application in the regimen matters. Patients need to know exactly how much product to use, the ideal water temperature to use, as well as how and where to apply the product. They also need answers to the following questions: Do they need to rinse it off after a certain amount of time? How long will it take to see results? Will they get worse before they get better? What should they expect? How will they know if the products are working? Patients should be aware of potential side effects, how to handle the side effects, when to call the office, and how long it might take for such reactions to resolve before they resume therapy. Patients are more likely to comply with prescribed regimens when they have this information. Give patients written step-by-step instructions, information sheets on their underlying skin issues, and any other printed information that will help educate them.

Standardizing how much of each product to use is very helpful. Tell patients to use the following amounts of product for the face:

- Cleansers: ¼ teaspoon
- Creams: ¼ teaspoon
- Eye products: ⅛ teaspoon
- Lotions: ¼ teaspoon
- Oils: ⅛ teaspoon
- Ointments: ¼ teaspoon
- Serums: ⅛ teaspoon
- Sunscreen: ¼ teaspoon

Provide Products, Treatments, and Advice That Patients Cannot Obtain Elsewhere

Medical providers who retail skincare should understand the inner workings of the skin better than others and stay current on the latest skincare research, so they are always providing patients with the latest proven skincare technologies. Doctors have exclusive access to skincare products that patients cannot find in a department store or mass retailer. They can combine products with prescription medications in the regimen and track patient progress while monitoring potential side effects. Providing patients with skincare options they cannot obtain elsewhere differentiates the medical practice and is an ethical approach to skincare retail.[3] See Chapter 33 for advice on choosing skincare products from the various brands. Giving patients well thought out skincare regimens to use before and after medical procedures including skin cancer surgery will help improve outcomes as discussed in Chapter 36, Pre- and Post-Procedure Skincare.

PATIENT COMPLIANCE

The best skincare routine in the world only works when patients use the products regularly and properly. Adherence to topical medications in dermatology patients is notoriously poor, especially among acne and psoriasis patients.[15-17] Studies have shown that one in three prescriptions given to dermatology patients are never redeemed.[18] In fact, 95% of patients underdose their topical medications.[19] Barriers to compliance include lack of understanding and education, poor tolerance of side effects, confusing or complex treatment plans, extended length of time until noted improvement, high cost of treatment, and a treatment plan that does not match the patient's lifestyle.[20]

Most patients do not use sunscreen daily even though they know SPF use results in fewer wrinkles and reduced risk of skin cancer.[21] It is critical for medical providers to discuss sunscreen use with every patient. This reminds the patient of the importance of daily sunscreen and helps encourage its use. Patients that show the least compliance with daily SPF tend to be male and have lower household income, less education, and darker skin types.[22] Educating that SPF prevents skin sagging seen with aging is an important way to help increase sunscreen use in darker skin types who often believe they do not need SPF. Patients are much more likely to use sunscreen when it is suggested by their doctor. One study revealed that dermatologists only recommended sunscreen to their patients 56% of the time.[23] Another study in 2014 showed that dermatologists only discussed sunscreen use in 1.6% of visits.[24] Medical providers need a standardized approach to discuss skincare, especially sun protection, with every patient. They should have a system that allows the staff to help them recommend and encourage skincare routines that include a daily SPF. There are other methods to implement in your practice to help increase patient compliance with topical medications and skincare routines.[25]

Manage Patient Expectations

Patients have been programmed by social media and skincare companies' marketing campaigns to believe that their skin issues will resolve quickly. "Get rid of wrinkles in 24 hours!" is repeatedly marketed to patients and this affects their expectations. Patients should be educated that the cell cycle of the epidermis is 26 to 42 days, so it can take 4 or more weeks to see results from facial skincare products.[26] Acne usually takes 8 weeks to improve, melasma takes 12–16 weeks (maybe longer if there is a dermal component), and fine lines and wrinkles can take 6–12 months to improve with topical treatments. Of course, this can be accelerated by combining skincare with cosmetic procedures.

Educate patients that the skincare routine is organized in phases. Phase 1 includes the beginning products intended to soothe inflammation and hydrate skin so that it can tolerate the treatment products for skin issues such as acne, rosacea, pigmentation, or wrinkles. Phase 2 includes stronger products to target the skin issues. In some cases, the patient has too many issues to treat all at once. For example, they may suffer from rosacea, skin burning and stinging, aging, and skin pigmentation. They will not be able to tolerate skin lighteners and retinoids until their skin inflammation is under control. These patients will need multiple skincare routine phases to achieve the desired goals. The main point is to ensure that patients understand that the proper treatment of their skin will take at least two phases.

Remind patients that at the 1-month follow-up visit, the skincare routine will be readjusted based on their improvement. If they use the products as directed, they will be able to advance to the next level, or, if the products are too strong, some may be replaced. They need to understand that the skin's needs change as the skin type changes.

Raise Awareness of Adherence Issues

The medical staff should be taught that nonadherence is very common with topical skincare and medications and their role in educating and encouraging patients is as important as the medical provider's role. To be compliant with the treatment plan, the patient must understand how, when, and where to apply the treatment products.[25] The staff should make sure that the patient receives written instructions because patients do not remember much of what is told to them during the office visit.[27] At the follow-up visits, the staff should take the time to ascertain if the patients are using the products.

The medical provider should also stress the importance of a consistent skincare routine at the first visit and ask patients on the follow-up visit if they are using the products as prescribed. This should not be a yes or no question, because patients will often just say yes to please the doctor. The questions should be open-ended, such as, "Tell me what skincare products you are using in the morning," and "Then tell me what skincare products do you use at night." The way the patient responds to those questions/directions will give the medical provider insights into how regularly the patient is using the products. This is an extremely valuable tool to use for teenagers with acne. If they are using their products, they will know exactly what they are and can recite how they use them.

The best way to increase patient compliance is to measure it using electronic monitors and share the data with the patient.[28] Patients are often unaware of poor compliance until it is pointed out to them. There are mobile apps being developed to help improve compliance.[29] Research studies use chips in the lids of tubes to track how often the tubes are opened. This is unrealistic outside of a research trial but in the future, there may be more tracking options available. Physicians who sell skincare products in their practices have access to compliance data if they track product purchases and repurchases. If the patient buys all their skincare products from the physician's office or website, it is easier to monitor their compliance.

Hold Patients Accountable

Studies show that people are more likely to change a habit when they have a plan and are held accountable to that plan. Working with a patient to develop a skincare routine that fits their lifestyle and budget is only the first step but their involvement in the process helps motivate them. The role that the doctor plays is especially critical in motivating the patient. The power of the doctor's visit as a motivating factor is illustrated in a study that showed patients increased use of their medication for the 3 days before and 3 days after their dermatologist visit.[30] For this reason, it is recommended to have a staff member call, text, or email the patient 3 to 5 days after their first appointment to see if they have any questions. Texting and talking on the phone are the most successful methods because of the ease of a back-and-forth conversation. In this conversation, the patient should be specifically asked if they are using all the products as prescribed. If not, find out the reason and try and solve the issue. It is much better to solve the issue right away instead of waiting for their next office visit.

Track Product Volumes Used

Another way to hold patients accountable is to have them bring in the products they are using at every visit. In research studies, the bottles are weighed to ascertain compliance. This is not really feasible in the time limits of most medical practices; however, the weight of the tube or bottle and the appearance will often give an idea of usage. If the patient knows that the medical provider will be examining the bottles or tubes, they will be more likely to use the products to please the doctor. For example, if the patient says they are using a sunscreen daily but a 1 ounce tube is only 25% used, the medical provider knows that the patient is not using the SPF daily.

Track Product Repurchases

Tracking repurchases is another way to track compliance. In fact, this is one of the most important reasons to retail skincare in your practice—you will have a better sense about compliance. Of course, the patient may buy products elsewhere, but if the doctor offers a product for a cheaper price in the office than what is online, they will buy from the office and it is easier to track adherence and make certain that they are using the proper products.

Use Photography

Photography taken at the office visit can provide insights into compliance. The Canfield Visia camera system gives several views of the skin that can be used to gauge compliance. For example, if a skin lightener is prescribed for melasma, the "UV Spot" and "Brown Spot" images can be used to track compliance with the topical medication and sunscreen. Characteristically, the UV spot number will get worse in the first 4 weeks while the brown spot number will improve if they are using their products properly.

Taking the patient's photo at every visit helps encourage them and tracks their progress. Engage patients by showing them the numbers, explain what they mean and what the goals are for the numbers. Discuss their progress at each visit by looking at the images together. If they are on a retinoid, for example, you can review their images in 6–12 months and show them how their skin is improving. Anticipation of having the photo taken will increase compliance because patients want to see improvement. Most people perform better when they receive a score.

Change and Improve the Skin Type

The Baumann Skin Typing System (BSTS) identifies the underlying barrier(s) to skin health: dehydration, inflammation, dyspigmentation, and aging. If the patient is on the correct skincare products and is using them properly, their skin type should improve. Having the patient retake the quiz at standardized intervals will help track their progress. As the skin type changes, the regimen should be readjusted to address any of the barriers to skin health that are identified by the questionnaire. The goal is to get the patient as close as possible to the perfect skin type—ORNT (BST 10).

Provide a Caring and Supportive Environment

Patients need to feel they can ask questions and not be judged if their questions are "dumb." Calling the patient 3 to 5 days after the appointment gives them a way to ask questions. Offering a number that they can text for questions or an email is also very helpful. Medical practices are usually busy and may not have time to field questions in the daytime. Hiring an aesthetician to answer patients' skincare questions is beneficial.

Compliance requires an understanding of why following the instructions exactly as prescribed is important. Printed information about various issues such as acne or eczema is valuable. Younger patients, 13 and under, require their parents' participation in their care. Parents need to understand the benefits and risks of the treatment plans prescribed for their children or they will not be compliant.[31] Usually children 14 and older will be self-motivated to use their medications but only if: (1) they understand why, when, and how to use the medications, (2) the skincare routine makes sense for their lifestyle, and (3) they have some sort of accountability that is independent from their parents such as a follow-up visit to the doctor or aesthetician.

Skincare follow-up visits can be performed by aestheticians, or if prescription medications are used, physician assistants and nurse practitioners. Although live visits are preferred because photos can be taken, telemedicine visits are also an option, especially for college students who are away from their home city but need to be motivated to stay compliant.

Social media can be used to motivate patients. Educational posts about why to use various products and motivational content go a long way with patients under 40 years old. It is best to examine the demographics of the patient population and plan motivational strategies accordingly.

Help Patients Build Solid Habits

Engage patients in their care every way possible. Encourage communication. Offer some suggested "cue-routine-reward" strategies to help them build the habit of using the medications regularly.[25] For example, "put your sunscreen next to your toothbrush and apply every AM after brushing your teeth." Help patients identify their own cues such as before soccer practice, when bathing, or after working out. Choosing a regular activity to link to the use of the skincare routine will help boost compliance. The less the patient must try to remember to use the products, the more compliant they will be. Asking patients on follow-up visits to describe whether their compliance has been "poor, moderate, or excellent" is a helpful way to have them self-evaluate their adherence behavior. If they say "poor," ask, "What plan do you have to make it easier to remember?" Education, follow-up visits, electronic reminders, and interactive educational information have all been shown to help patients build good habits.[30,32,33]

DEVELOP THE SKINCARE RETAIL PROCESS

Assign a Staff Member to Supervise Skincare

Accountability is always important to improve performance. Assigning one person in the practice to oversee all skincare is critical to successful skincare retail. This should not be the medical provider because they need to concentrate on patient care. In a new practice that cannot hire a dedicated person right away, the medical provider may perform this role. However, set a goal that once met, a skincare director will be hired. For example, once the clinic is profiting at a selected level, then a skincare director will be hired. If this person is also an aesthetician, chances are their salary will pay for itself by increased revenue. This person should oversee implementing a skincare recommendation system throughout the office and educating everyone on their role in it. The skincare director will choose products to retail with the medical provider's supervision. They will be responsible for ordering products, inventory control, patient skincare consults, educating other staff members on skincare, setting financial goals, and tracking success. This should not be delegated to the office manager. It is much more effective when skincare is overseen by someone in direct contact with patients because they need to have the patient interactions for feedback about the products as well as to monitor success and patient outcomes. It is important to remember that although selling skincare is lucrative financially, the goal is improving patient outcomes. To approach skincare retail in an ethical manner, someone who is trained in skincare and patient consultations should manage this process rather than someone solely concerned with profit.

Divide the Skincare Retail Process into Segments

Analyze the patient journey through your practice starting at the introduction to your website when they first discovered you. Look at each step of the journey. Think about which staff member's role is critical at that step. What can you do at each step to optimize the journey? Every step is an opportunity for patient education and engagement. Using each step properly will help improve the patient experience, motivate them to be more compliant with the instructions, and give them a sense of comfort with the organization and professionalism of the practice. Consistency is the key to increasing skincare sales (**Fig. 34-1**).

Waiting Room and Front Desk

Patient education should begin before the office visit. Information can be emailed or texted to them prior to the visit or

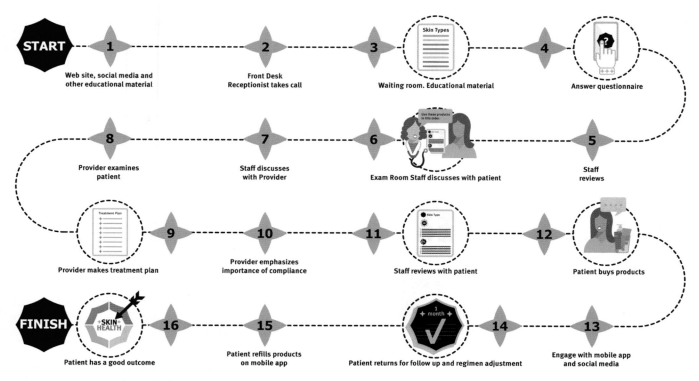

FIGURE 34-1. Divide the patient experience into steps in the office and optimize each step to improve the patient experience. Employees should be held accountable for KPIs at critical points.

they can be given links to the website or videos. Even if the patient is new and unknown to the practice, educational material about the importance of a daily skincare routine or daily sunscreen use can be given prior to the visit.

The waiting room is the perfect place to begin to educate patients. Instead of displaying popular magazines, consider having educational material, such as posters on the wall, videos, or brochures, that instruct patients about the importance of a correct and consistent daily skincare routine. Also consider posters, brochures, or videos that discuss the importance of sun protection to prevent skin aging and skin cancer. Educational material in the waiting room sets the tone for the office visit.

The receptionist at the front desk should have the patient complete an intake questionnaire to determine the skin type and disclose what issues they want to discuss with the medical provider. This questionnaire should ask about skincare history and what cosmetic concerns they have. This facilitates the conversation in the exam room. Also, this will not seem pushy or sales oriented if cosmetic concerns are addressed as part of a longer skincare history questionnaire. One option is to use an electronic questionnaire to diagnose the skin type and identify cosmetic concerns.

Taking a questionnaire prior to the patient consultation is important for many reasons as discussed in the beginning of this chapter. It sets the tone for the visit and leads the patient to consider how well they have been taking care of their skin and if they have been diligent with sunscreen use. Often the answer is "no," which makes them more likely to listen to their doctor's recommendations on sun protection and preventative skincare.

Exam Room

The exam room is where the conversation begins. A staff member will discuss the reason for the patient's visit to the clinic first, so that the patient feels comfortable that their most important concerns will be the focus of the visit. Then, once the history of the present issue has been discussed, the conversation can change to skincare. No matter the reason for the patient's visit, every patient should have skincare discussed. As mentioned above, studies show that patients will be more compliant with sunscreen if it is recommended by their doctor. This is the time to bring up the topic of preventative skincare and sunscreen use.

Usually, a staff member reviews the patient's skin type and produces a preliminary skincare regimen based on the patient's skin type and other answers to the questionnaire. In addition, the staff member will review the cosmetic concerns and ask the patient if they would like to discuss any of these issues. Once the staff member has learned as much as they can about the reasons for the visit, the patient's skincare needs, and any cosmetic procedures the patient is interested in, the staff member can present the background information to the medical provider.

Prior to entering the exam room, the staff member should tell the medical provider the skin type, chief complaint, recommended skincare regimen, and any cosmetic issues the patient wants to discuss. For example, the staff member might say, "Ms. Smith is a 40-year-old DSNW skin type who has been experiencing facial redness and burning of the skin after cleansing for 3 months. This is her first time to see a dermatologist. She has never been diagnosed with rosacea and is not on any rosacea therapies. Here is the basic skincare regimen for DSNW redness skin types. She is also interested in discussing the V beam laser to treat her facial redness to speed up the results because there is a family wedding in 3 months."

This kind of information will improve workflow so that the medical provider can use their limited time to probe deeper into the patient's concerns. In this example, the medical provider would examine the patient and determine if this is routine rosacea or another diagnosis. If the medical provider agrees with the diagnosis of rosacea, they can adjust the skincare regimen to include a rosacea medication. The medical provider should adjust the skincare regimen in front of the patient, so they see the medical provider's involvement in the process. The medical provider should state, "These are the exact steps to use on your facial skin. You should do them every day. In 1 month, I will assess your skin, and if you have used the products, we should be able to move to Phase 2 of the skincare treatment plan." This simple sentence will increase compliance and patient motivation.

Once the medical provider has discussed the plan with the patient, the staff member can review the instructions, answer questions, and distribute any information sheets. Patients should be given a way to contact the office if they have any questions or concerns. In addition, they should be told to follow up in 4 weeks.

Cashier

Although the medical assistant or aesthetician is usually the staff member that discusses the skincare regimen with the patient, the cashier is the one who sells the products to the patients. They will be asked questions about the products and their intended uses, so the cashier needs to be familiar with the products.

The cashier should not push patients to purchase products. It is best if they ask, "Do you need to purchase any products today?" If the patient chooses not to purchase the products, and states a reason, the cashier should note the reason. If there is a recurrent issue with a product (e.g., too expensive or the aroma is unappealing), the cashier should relay that information to the skincare director. The cashier can direct the patient to the online store for refills or have the patient ask for them directly when they need to make a purchase.

The cashier should help the patient make an appointment for the follow-up before they leave the office. This increases compliance with follow-up appointments because patients are more likely to return if they leave the office with a set appointment time. The cashier should play a role in tracking the inventory. Inventory is discussed later in this chapter.

MAKE BUSINESS DECISIONS

Taking time to think through the patient process and develop targeted business practices is critical. If this is not accomplished, time and money will be wasted and frustration will ensue. Selling skincare incorrectly and unethically can harm the physician-patient relationship. Every decision should be thought through as to how it will affect your practice. These are methods used by successful cosmetic dermatology practices to

retail skincare. **Table 34-1** lists retail nomenclature used in the industry.

Set Pricing

Profit is a goal in all types of retail, including the medical setting. It can be tempting to choose expensive products to retail to patients with the hope of making more money. There are many downsides to this approach. It is important to remember that the goal is to improve skin health by increasing patient compliance with scientifically developed skincare regimens. If products are expensive, patients will use less and replenish them less often. In the author's experience, products priced under $40 sell more than products priced over $40. There are several ways to keep the price down:

1. Team up with other doctors to order together and get volume discounts.
2. Choose less expensive brands that have the same efficacy.
3. Charge less than the manufacturer's suggested retail price (MSRP) for the products when sold in the office (keep the MSRP when sold online).

TABLE 34-1	**Basic Retail Nomenclature**

General Business Nomenclature
- COGs: Cost of goods or cost of skincare products
- Gross profit = sale price − cost of goods
- Gross sales: The sum of all sales during a set time period
- KPIs: Key performance indicators. A set of quantifiable measurements linked to goals (lead measures) that when met will predict success (lag measures).
- Net profit = Gross profit − commissions paid − lost, stolen, or expired product − money left over after all expenses including the cost of the products have been paid.
- Net sales = the gross sales − refunded and returned items

Product Pricing Nomenclature
- Wholesale price: The price at which products are sold to business buyers who purchase in bulk quantities.
- Retail price: The price of goods charged to the consumer
- MSRP: Manufacturer's suggested retail price

Commission Nomenclature
- Commission Rate: The percent of sales on which the commission rate is based. For example, the commission rate might be 10% or 20% of the commission basis.
- Commission Basis: The dollar amount on which the commission calculations will be based. For example, if the commission basis is based on net profits and the net profit is $5000, then the commission basis is $5000.
- Commission Period: The period over which the commission basis is calculated. Example is 1 month.
- Commission Split: The commission may be split among different teams or different people.

Ecommerce Nomenclature
- SKU: A Stock keeping unit
- OF: Outsourced fulfillment, when products are stored and shipped from a warehouse outside of the medical practice.
- FBM: Fulfillment by merchant (when the medical practice stores and ships the products to customers).

Skincare product manufacturers provide an MSRP, but they cannot legally require a selling price. Medical practices are free to charge any price for the products they sell. The MSRP is usually double the wholesale price of the product. For example, if a product costs the doctor or store $25, it is common practice to double the price to $50. When a product's wholesale cost is $100 and MSRP is $200, the medical provider can opt to mark up the cost only 50% and sell it at $150. It is good practice to sell products cheaper in your office than their price online. This resolves the ethical dilemma of charging more than other places and encourages compliance by having the patient leave with the product in hand. In the long run, the medical practice that offers less expensive products as compared to the same products on ecommerce sites will sell more overall and gain higher income than if they were to sell fewer high-priced products. This concept of "make more money selling products cheaper" is counterintuitive but has been borne out in the author's experience in mentoring over 150 medical practices in skincare retail.

To select products and set prices, evaluate your patient demographic. In some cases, patients will be more compliant with expensive products because they think they work better, while in other cases affordable products will be used more. Choose how much to charge for products based on what will motivate patients the most rather than by MSRP.

The difference between gross sales and net profit numbers will be greatly affected by how much you mark up the wholesale price of the products. If you sell the products at MSRP, the markup is 50%, so one half of the gross sales is the cost of goods. Keep in mind what percent markup was chosen when calculating commission structure discussed later in this chapter. The less you mark up the products, the lower your commission rates should be.

Product Return Policy

Develop a return policy that is printed on a visible sign in the cashier area and on any brochures or paperwork. There should be no mystery about the policy. If a product is defective, for example the pump is broken, most skincare brands will replace it with no issues. The problem arises when the patient uses the product and returns it saying it is "not right for their skin." The return rate is lowered when the BSTS is used to create the skincare regimen.[34]

A good practice is to allow skincare product returns for 2 weeks after purchase, even if they have been opened. Returned products should be returned to the skincare brand for replacement, if they allow this, or destroyed. Do not re-sell the product to another patient because it may have been adulterated.

Track Inventory

Invest in inventory tracking software if your electronic medical records system does not include it. Assign a staff member such as a "store manager" or "director of skincare" to manage the topical skincare inventory and follow the recommendations in this section. When products arrive and are unpacked, each item should be counted and matched to the invoice.

When possible, have two staff members count the received items together. This ensures that the correct number of products are received and discourages theft by the staff. Once all items have been matched to the invoice and it is confirmed that all items have been received, add them into the inventory software. Note the expiration dates that should then be tracked by the inventory software. If no inventory software is used, set a reminder 1 month before expiration to check inventory. If there is a large amount of the product left on the shelf at the expiration date, have a sale to clear items and consider switching to a different product that sells better. Develop a system to be altered when product numbers dwindle to a certain level so that a reminder will be triggered to reorder. The number that triggers replenishment can be anticipated by the number of patients seen in the practice with the skin type that corresponds to that product. Quarterly inventory assessments should be completed to identify best sellers as well as ones that attract little interest and consider replacing products for those with new technologies. Carry as little inventory as possible. Do not tie up your cash in a large unnecessary inventory. This is a big business mistake often made by new skincare retailers. It is to the skincare brand's advantage to sell large volumes of products to medical practices, and they often require minimum order amounts. Try and reduce the order volumes as much as you can.

ECOMMERCE

Skincare companies track repurchasing rates because ongoing replenishment of products results in an annuity (recurrent income) with minimal effort. For this reason, it should be easy and compelling for patients to repurchase products from the medical practice rather than purchasing elsewhere. Repurchasing products from the medical provider certainly increases income but is important for other reasons. When patients buy every skincare product from the medical practice, it is much easier to track adherence and ascertain when more motivation is needed.

Some doctors do not want to carry inventory and prefer to have the entire skincare process online with an ecommerce store. However, patients like to walk out of the office with products in hand so they can get started right away. Studies show clearly that patients are most compliant with their topical treatment regimens 3 days before and 3 days after a dermatology office visit.[30] This window will be missed if patients must wait for delivery of products. Offering products for sale in the office is an important part of increasing adherence to improve outcomes. It is always preferred that patients physically arrive at the office to buy products. This engages the patients and allows them to ask questions, and the interaction with the office helps increase patient adherence. For this reason, products should be offered at a lower price in the office than online.

Patients may prefer to call the office to order products, but this takes staff time to mail the products. You may choose to use a fulfillment center to ship products if volumes are high. A staff member can also take the patient's order on the phone and enter it into the online store for the patient, in the case of older patients who are not comfortable with technology.

Offering product sales online is more convenient for patients. There are many options as to how to accomplish this:

1. Partner with a company that caters to medical practices
   a. Software as a service company: Diagnoses the skin type, generates regimens, handles all ecommerce, stores inventory, and fulfills orders. Patients use a doctor's code to access. [Disclosure: the author is the owner of Skin Type Solutions, Inc.]
   b. Website management company: Manages the ecommerce website but the medical practice carries the inventory and does the fulfillment.
   c. Website management and fulfillment company: Handles ecommerce site; no inventory is carried by the doctor, products shipped directly from company's warehouse.
2. Use Shopify
   a. Fulfill items from your office yourself: Fulfillment by merchant or fulfill items yourself (FBM).
   b. Use Shopify Fulfillment Network.
3. Use Amazon
   a. FBM.
   b. Pay a fulfillment fee to have items mailed (fulfillment by Amazon or FBA).
4. Use your own website and hire a fulfillment company
   a. Charge will be for warehousing inventory.
   b. Charge per item shipped.

It is inexpensive to develop a website these days and there are many options. Ecommerce is rapidly growing and buying online is preferable for many people. In the author's opinion it is important to have both an in-office and an ecommerce option when retailing skincare.

TELEMEDICINE

During the COVID-19 pandemic, telemedicine consults became much easier. Numerous electronic medical records companies now offer telemedicine options. Skincare consults and follow-ups can easily be done online now. If no prescription medications are used, an aesthetician can complete the online skincare consults and follow-ups. If prescription medications will be prescribed, then follow the state laws on telemedicine. This frees up exam rooms, allows for more frequent patient interactions, and increases patient engagement.

Using a skin type quiz to determine skin type assists in the telemedicine setting when it is harder to see the patient's skin. Use a validated questionnaire to diagnose the skin type and ensure that skincare recommendations are correct for the patient's skin type.

View the online store with the patient when discussing skincare products. You can work with them to add the correct products to their cart while they are in the consult. Another option is to send the patient a link to the prescribed skincare regimen or products to make it easy for the patient to purchase the correct products. Schedule follow-ups 1 week after the initial skincare regimen and then every 4 weeks.

TRACK SUCCESS WITH KEY PERFORMANCE INDICATORS

Once the products have been chosen and the business processes have been developed, it is necessary to measure performance. Key performance indicators (KPIs) refer to a set of quantifiable measurements used to gauge a company's overall long-term performance. KPIs help define strategic initiatives and are used to develop operational processes. KPIs indicate performance of these processes and initiatives designed to affect the health of the company.

How to Identify KPIs

There are multiple business articles and sources to help a company develop KPIs. The important factor(s) should directly evaluate company success and be easily and accurately measurable. An easy method used to determine KPIs is to think of the concept of lead and lag measures.[35] A way to understand lead and lag measures is to use the example of weight loss. The number of pounds or kilograms on the scale is the lag measure because it is the goal that is reached later. The lead measures are the measures taken to get to the lag measure. In the example of weight loss, lead measures would be eating fewer calories and exercising more. The lag measure cannot happen if the lead measures do not happen. KPIs are lead measures. First identify the lag measures and then identify the lead measures.

In skincare retail, the lag measure is the net profit from skincare sales. **Net profit = sales revenues minus total costs.** Total costs should include cost of skincare products (known as cost of goods sold or COGS), employee salaries/commissions dedicated to skincare retail, shipping costs, marketing costs, and any other related costs. The skincare retail net profit is the "lag measure" and the goal is to increase this number.

Lead measures on skincare sales would include the number of:

- patients seen per day
- patients who have taken the skin type questionnaire
- patients that have received a printed skincare regimen

These lead measure events directly affect the amount of skincare that is sold. If skincare is not discussed, it is unlikely a sale will occur. Each of these KPI measurements can be linked to a point in the process and an employee's role. See **Fig. 34-2** for a form to use to track KPIs for skincare retail.

STAFF MOTIVATION

Hiring and Employee Retention

It is impossible to motivate staff members who do not understand the importance of an effective daily skincare routine. Skincare sales will not flourish if employees do not support the concept, have ethical concerns, or are too busy to be bothered. Examine the attitudes of the staff and only include staff

Key Performance Indicators are a set of quantifiable measures used to evaluate success in meeting target goals. These metrics are used to determine progress in achieving strategic and operational goals.

CHECK IN

On average we see _____ patients daily.	**COMMITMENTS**
	Give skin type questionnaire to all patients
Goal is to skin type at least **80% per day** which is	
_____ patients per day	

CONSULT

On average we skin type _____ daily.	**COMMITMENTS**
	Stress the importance of using sunscreen daily
Goal is to provide recommended skincare regimens to **100% of patients per day who were skin typed**	Give printed skincare regimen
Regimens for _____ patients per day	Give information sheets about skin issues

CHECK OUT

On average we consult _____ patients daily	**COMMITMENTS**
Goal is to ask 100% of skin typed patients if they need to purchase products	Ask question "Do you need to purchase any products today?"
Goal is to sell skincare to **30% of patients who were skin typed**	Schedule follow-up appointment
Checking out _____ patients per day	Give online store information after checkout is complete

FIGURE 34-2. Develop KPIs and assign to teams. This form can be used to give to staff members on each team and have them sign to commit to following the plan.

members in the skincare retail process and commission program who show enthusiasm. When hiring, ask about knowledge and attitudes about the skincare retail process. Employees with experience in sales are ideal.

It is not unusual for one employee to poison the well when a new process is implemented. Their negativity can spoil the attitude of the entire team. These employees should be identified early in the process. Discuss with them the importance of the standardized educational process to improve patient compliance and outcomes. Ask them if they support the concept and are willing to work to implement it and make sure they know that they will be held accountable. If the employee's attitude does not improve, replace them. The damage that one negative employee can cause is immense.

The director of skincare should be enthusiastic, willing to learn about skincare, able to understand the importance of the proper skincare for patient outcomes, and able to motivate the staff. They must have enough time to devote themselves to the role. An office manager does not have time to both manage the office and serve as the director of skincare. Hire a designated person. The income increase will easily cover the salary and will improve customer service and the patient experience. See **Table 34-2** for duties of the director of skincare. The director of skincare may also perform aesthetician duties. The ideal director has experience in sales and has an aesthetician license.

TABLE 34-2	**Job Description for Director of Skincare**

- Oversee product selection
- Watch for sales on products to manage costs
- Oversee inventory and perform quarterly inventory assessments
- Implement skin type questionnaire use or choose software
- Develop skin regimens for 16 skin types or use chosen software
- Divide the patient experience into segments (front desk, exam room, and cashier)
- Develop a process that includes skincare for each segment of the patient experience
- Arrange staff education on skin type, regimens, products, the patient experience, and commission plan
- Work with business owner to set KPIs and assign and weight the teams
- Motivate the staff and include their input in the process and products
- Call new patients within 3 to 5 days to see if they have any questions or concerns
- Re-evaluate skincare products quarterly and change brands or SKUs when needed
- Work with business owner to develop, calculate, and adjust commissions
- Oversee fulfillment of telephone orders
- Oversee online store
- Arrange office events to promote the practice and enhance patient engagement
- Depending on the number of staff members, this job may also include aesthetician activities that help cover salary cost
- Perform skincare consults in office
- Perform online telemedicine skincare consults
- Perform facials, microdermabrasion, and other aesthetic procedures
- Aid in cosmetic dermatology consults
- Handle social media
- Other marketing activities such as offering skin typing at events

Once employees have been trained to skin type patients, match them to a regimen, and educate patients about skincare, they should be able to implement the system in a way that provides a standardized, consistent approach. When every staff member is in sync, making the same recommendations, and giving the same answers to questions, this will give patients confidence and motivate them to be more compliant with prescription medications and skincare regimens. The harmony that results when the staff works together is powerful. Once this sweet spot is reached, make sure you are able to retain these valuable employees. Award them with prizes, public praise, and make sure they do not get burned out. Employees are most engaged when they feel they have input. Ask their opinions about products, marketing ideas, office events, and social media posts. Form marketing committees and let them give input. At the same time, be quick to eliminate any negative employees that refuse to follow the system and dampen the enthusiasm for others. Do not be held hostage by your employees. If you have standardized processes in place, it is easier to train new employees. If you have a generous commission plan, and your employees feel they have input and are contributing to improving patient health, it is easier to retain good employees. Most employees will excel when they understand the global purpose of improving skin health and have a set plan, clear instructions, a transparent commission structure, and feel their input is valued.

Staff Education

When possible, hire staff members who have an interest in skincare. The entire staff should then take the questionnaire and learn about their BST. If financially feasible, or if the skincare companies will provide sample products, give the staff their skincare regimen so they can see how the correct skincare products improve their skin health. If the staff is using the products, it is much easier for them to answer patient questions about products, especially when the patients have the same skin type as they do. They will be much more likely to be enthusiastic about products that they have seen work on their skin.

Set up an initial launch meeting with the staff. Review the patient process and what steps will be taken to educate and engage patients as discussed in this chapter. Review the KPIs with the staff and clearly explain how any bonus or commission structures will be calculated. Facilitate educational monthly staff meetings to keep staff engaged. Reveal the scores and prizes at these monthly meetings and make it fun. Work with skincare brands to provide educational lunches on the products. Make sure the staff has access to trusted educational materials and resources for when they have questions. Perform monthly educational activities to keep the staff educated and engaged.

Awarding Bonuses, Commissions, and Prizes

A consistent, well thought out, standardized process that allows for patient education and engagement is crucial to improve patient adherence to treatment plans. Although this chapter discusses business methods to increase income from skincare sales, one must never forget that the true goal is to improve the patient's skin health, which requires patients to comply with a topical treatment plan. The fact is that the more often patients use their skincare products, the healthier their skin will be (assuming the skincare regimen design guidelines are followed from Chapter 35 and efficacious products are chosen as described in Chapter 33).

Adherent patients will repurchase products more often than noncompliant patients and skincare retail sales will increase via adherent patients. It all boils down to patient education. For example, if you educate a patient to wear a sunscreen every day, suggest an affordably priced efficacious option and offer it for sale in your practice for convenience. Your sunscreen sales will rise. Assuming the patient is motivated to use the sunscreen every day, they will improve their skin health.

Patient education and motivation are directly tied to the medical provider's enthusiasm, but never underestimate the significant role that the entire staff plays in patient education and motivation. The whole office staff should be included in the process and should receive a "prize" for reaching the KPI goals. It is nice to believe that everyone will always perform their best just to do the right thing, but many studies have proven that people perform better when there is a prize.[36] In fact, employees perform best when divided into teams that compete against each other to reach set KPIs.[35] There are myriad prizes that can be awarded to staff including money, paid time off (PTO), cosmetic services, skincare products, gift cards, trophies, and verbal recognition such as being named employee of the month. Employees' needs differ. One may be motivated by a PTO day, while another prefers cash, and a third likes recognition. Keep the employees' needs in mind when designing an incentive plan. Some practices give points and let the employees redeem them for a PTO day, cash, services, or other items.

Commissions versus Bonuses

Prizes, including recognition, have been shown to motivate employees, especially when given soon after the behavior, occur frequently, and are awarded for an action or result in which the employee has a direct role. When the medical staff feels their behavior is recognized and appreciated, they will perform better. For example, the number of skin type questionnaires given has been shown to correlate with skincare sales.[37] The receptionists/front desk staff team can be compensated by the number of questionnaires administered, which is easily tracked with software. There should be a daily specific goal that at least 80% of patients take the skin type questionnaire. A bonus can be distributed when the 80% goal is reached. Another option to award the front desk staff for giving the questionnaire is a bonus of $1 per quiz given. If software is used to generate skincare regimens, medical assistants can receive a bonus based on the number of skincare regimens that have been generated and saved in the system. Bonuses can also be issued when a group goal has been met. For example, if $X of skincare is sold in 4 weeks, each staff member gets a $100 gift card. Bonuses can be awarded for milestones reached

or numbers or actions. Most importantly, the process must be communicated clearly to the staff, transparent, measurable, and directly tied to an employee's participation.

Many practices choose to commission employees on skincare sales. There are multiple models for achieving this, but the most effective models are linked to KPIs. Although the entire staff plays a role and should receive a commission, the author's experience has found that incentivizing the aesthetician or director of skincare at the same rate as the other employees is a disincentive. The staff member most directly involved with selling skincare to patients, such as the director of skincare, should receive the highest commission. This problem is solved by developing various teams as discussed below. Teams can receive one or a combination of the following: commissions, bonuses, or other prizes.

Develop Teams

Based on the size of the practice, split employees into different teams. Divide teams by how the employee links to a measurable KPI. One employee can be on several teams and can receive prizes in multiple ways. The director of skincare or aesthetician can be included on every team to increase their engagement with all the steps and to give them a higher compensation percentage.

Examples of teams include:

- Questionnaire Team (front desk)
- Patient Education Team (exam room)
- Sales Team (cashier or point of sale person)
- Store Management Team (inventory management, expenses)

Develop the best way to measure the success of each team

The KPIs are critical here. The goals for each team must be clear, measurable, and represent a KPI (**Table 34-2**). For example, the questionnaire team is measured by how many patients take the questionnaire. The target goal should be 80% of patients seen in the practice. This can be measured by software or by counting the number of printed questionnaires given. The patient education team can be measured by how many patients receive a printed step-by-step skincare regimen. Software can measure the number of printed regimens, a designated printer that keeps count can be used, or the cashier can ask each patient if they received a printed regimen and note when they say no. The sales team can be measured by the number of products sold or overall income. The store management team can be measured on inventory losses such as stolen and expired items as well as decreases in costs of goods (which encourages them to manage expenses), and how often various SKUs need to be reordered (which encourages them to discontinue SKUs that do not sell well).

Develop the best way to compensate each team

Once the KPIs and goals have been set, decide which compensation method works best for each team. The questionnaire team should receive bonuses based on the number of questionnaires given. There should be a daily specific goal of at least 80% of patients seen in the practice. One option is to offer a bonus of $1 per quiz given to the questionnaire team; however, they can also be included in the commission structure. Teams can receive bonuses when a target goal is met, receive commission as discussed below, or both. Each team can have different ways of being compensated. The easiest way, in the author's opinion, is to provide a bonus to the questionnaire team on questionnaires administered while the other teams receive commissions.

Develop a group commission structure

The first step in developing a commission structure is to establish the percent of profit the practice is willing to pay as commission to their employees after paying bonuses and other prizes. The amount of money to be paid out in commission is called the commission basis. A standard commission basis for a cosmetic dermatology practice ranges between 10–20% of net profits or 5–10% of gross sales.

Decide whether the commission basis will be based on gross sales, net sales, or net profit. Gross sales are easier to calculate but do not take costs into account. If costs are variable or unpredictable, net profit is a better choice. If time and staff resources are a factor, a gross sales calculation is easier. The commission recipient prefers commission based on gross sales because they will not be affected by theft, expired products, or returns.

Determine a commission period. This is the time over which you will calculate sales. Employees seem to prefer monthly commission periods rather than quarterly ones.[38] Establishing new goals every month enhances motivation.

Decide how much the team and corresponding KPI contribute to overall sales

Once teams have been chosen based on their role in the patient process and their link to a KPI, provide weights to each team based on how much that KPI contributes to the overall sales goal. For example, the number of printed regimens given to a patient by the education team will affect final sales numbers more than the number of inventory losses overseen by the store management team.

Here is an example of how to weight the teams and split the group commission basis:

- Store Management Team — 20%
- Education Team — 40%
- Sales Team — 40%

Calculating Group Commission Basis

The case example here is based on net profit and a commission basis of 20% with a commission period of 1 month. This model assumes no extra salary costs, nor stolen, lost, or expired items or other costs. This case example excludes the questionnaire team because the assumption is that the questionnaire team will be given bonuses on the number of questionnaires administered and will not participate in the commission split.

This case example is a generous commission model and shows how much commission each team will earn in 1 month.

Case example:

January had gross sales of $10,000. The cost of the skincare products sold (COGS) was $5,000. The net profit was $5,000.

The commission basis is 20% of net profits, which is $1,000. This $1,000 will be divided among teams as follows:

- Store Management Team — 20% of $1,000 = $200
- Education Team — 40% of $1,000 = $400
- Sales Team — 40% of $1,000 = $400

In this model, the commission paid to the teams is $1,000. If you choose to give a $1 bonus to the front desk staff for each questionnaire given, and assume 200 questionnaires were given, that is another $200 divided among the questionnaire team members.

There may be more than one member on each team. If so, divide the commission per team based on the number of team members.

- Store Management Team — $200 ÷ 1 Team Member = $200 per member
- Education Team — $400 ÷ 2 Team Members = $200 per member
- Sales Team — $400 ÷ 2 Team Members = $200 per member

Getting started with a bonus and commission plan

When beginning a compensation strategy, it is best to tell the staff that the percentage that determines the commission basis and the bonus plan will be adjusted after a 3-month trial period. Do not commit to an annual commission basis percentage and bonus plan until it is proven that the method is improving morale, employee motivation, and sales. If sales do not increase, look at the productivity of each team to pinpoint the problem. Team weights can be adjusted, and team members reassigned to other teams after 3 months.

VENDOR RELATIONSHIPS

Vendors such as skincare brands want the medical practice to succeed in skincare retail so they can sell more products. They can provide educational material, product training, and product brochures to help train the staff. Get to know the local representative and work closely with them to obtain resources such as product samples for the staff. They can help create practice promotion or product promotion ideas, social events, and provide product samples. In some cases, they will give the staff products to try and provide samples for patients.

CONCLUSION

There are several steps to carefully consider when planning to retail skincare in your office. **Table 34-3** is a checklist to facilitate the process. The advice in this chapter is based on mentoring over 150 medical practices on selling skincare. Skincare retail can be successful if the business owner does the following: make a plan, set goals, measure KPIs, train and motivate the staff, and re-evaluate quarterly.

Patient compliance with the appropriate skincare routine is critical for healthy skin. Using the proper process in the office will help improve compliance, but patient accountability is

TABLE 34-3	Skincare Retail in a Medical Setting Checklist

- Choose from:
  - In-office sales
  - Ecommerce sales
  - Both
- Choose or hire a director of skincare
- Analyze patient demographics: skin issues, skin types, age, gender, socioeconomic status
- Consider a consultant, find a partner like Skin Type Solutions, Inc., or educate yourself on skincare science.
- Choose products
- Design regimens for various skin types
- Determine KPIs
- Analyze patient process and divide into segments. Decide on approach.
  - Waiting room/front desk
    - Give skin type questionnaire
    - Begin education process
  - Exam Room
    - Who will discuss regimen with patient?
    - How to give printed regimen to patient?
  - Cashier
    - How to charge patient? Same transaction as other charges or separate transaction.
    - Ask patient if they need to buy any products today.
- Assign staff to teams based on the patient process steps and KPIs
- Choose product pricing (MSRP or lower in office)
- Decide on return policy
- Decide on commission policy
- Make a printed sign for cashier area
- Set up inventory tracking plan
- If ecommerce
  - Choose online store option and link website to online store
  - FBM or outsource fulfillment
  - Include in telemedicine process
- Educate the staff on the
  - System (skin type questionnaire, how to make a regimen, how to print the regimen, how to follow up)
  - Products
  - Patient nonadherence and how to improve compliance
  - Ethical approach to skincare retail
  - The KPIs
  - The teams
  - The commission policy
- Meet with vendors
- Plan a launch party
- Develop marketing and social media strategy

key. The skincare discussion must occur at every visit. New technologies are being developed to track product usage, how many times the tubes are opened, and weights of the tubes to track compliance. Electronic reminders, mobile apps, online video training, and other methods are being developed to motivate patients. Changes in photography findings, skin type, skin appearance, or symptoms are all indicators of compliance.

References

1. Globe News Wire. Global Physician Dispensed Cosmeceuticals Industry. July 13, 2020. Available at https://bit.ly/GlobeN. Accessed March 23, 2021.

2. Castanedo-Tardan MP, Baumann L. Ethics of selling skin care. *Clin Dermatol.* 2009;27(4):355–358.

3. Baumann L. Ethics in cosmetic dermatology. *Clin Dermatol.* 2012; 30(5):522–527.

4. Stoff BK. A case against in-office sales of skin care products. *J Am Acad Dermatol.* 2019:S0190-9622(19)32652-0.

5. Cantor J. Cosmetic dermatology and physicians' ethical obligations: more than just hope in a jar. *Semin Cutan Med Surg.* 2005;24(3):155–160.

6. AMA Council on Ethical and Judicial Affairs. AMA Code of Medical Ethics' Opinions on Physicians' Financial Interests. *AMA Journal of Ethics.* August 2015. Available at https:// journalofethics.ama-assn.org/article/ama-code-medical-ethics-opinions-physicians-financial-interests/2015-08. Accessed March 23, 2021.

7. Farris PK. Office dispensing: a responsible approach. *Semin Cutan Med Surg.* 2000;19(3):195–200.

8. Lee YB, Park SM, Bae JM, Yu DS, Kim HJ, Kim JW. Which Skin Type Is Prevalent in Korean Post-Adolescent Acne Patients?: A Pilot Study Using the Baumann Skin Type Indicator. *Ann Dermatol.* 2017;29(6):817–819.

9. Baumann L. Cosmetics and skin care in dermatology. In: *Fitzpatrick's Dermatology in General Medicine,* 7th ed. New York: McGraw-Hill; 2008: 1357–2363.

10. Baumann L. 14 A Scientific Approach to Cosmeceuticals. In: Nahai F, Nahai F, eds. *The Art of Aesthetic Surgery: Principles and Techniques, 3rd ed., Fundamentals and Minimally Invasive Surgery.* Vol. 1. London: Thieme; 2020.

11. Baumann LS. The Baumann Skin Typing System. In: Farage MA, et al., eds. *Textbook of Aging Skin Skin.* Berlin Heidelberg: Springer-Verlag; 2017; 1579–1594.

12. Baumann LS, Penfield RD, Clarke JL, Duque DK. A validated questionnaire for quantifying skin oiliness. *J Cosmet Dermatol Sci App.* 2014;4:78–84.

13. Baumann L. Validation of a questionnaire to diagnose the Baumann skin type in all ethnicities and in various geographic locations. *J Cosmet Dermatol Sci App.* 2016;6(1):34–40.

14. Slade K, Grant-Kels JM. Employing an aesthetician in a dermatology practice: facts and controversies. *Clin Dermatol.* 2013;31(6):777–779.

15. Furue M, Onozuka D, Takeuchi S, et al. Poor adherence to oral and topical medication in 3096 dermatological patients as assessed by the Morisky Medication Adherence Scale-8. *Br J Dermatol.* 2015;172(1):272–275.

16. Sevimli Dikicier B. Topical treatment of acne vulgaris: efficiency, side effects, and adherence rate. *J Int Med Res.* 2019;47(7): 2987–2992.

17. Svendsen MT, Feldmann S, Tiedemann SN, Sørensen ASS, Rivas CMR, Andersen KE. Improving psoriasis patients' adherence to topical drugs: a systematic review. *J Dermatolog Treat.* 2020;31(8):776–785.

18. Storm A, Andersen SE, Benfeldt E, Serup J. One in 3 prescriptions are never redeemed: primary nonadherence in an outpatient clinic. *J Am Acad Dermatol.* 2008;59(1):27–33.

19. Storm A, Benfeldt E, Andersen SE, Serup J. A prospective study of patient adherence to topical treatments: 95% of patients underdose. *J Am Acad Dermatol.* 2008;59(6):975–980.

20. Haidari W, Glines KR, Cline A, Feldman SR. Adherence in Acne. In: *Treatment Adherence in Dermatology.* Cham, Germany: Springer; 2020; 85–97.

21. Holman DM, Berkowitz Z, Guy GP Jr, Hawkins NA, Saraiya M, Watson M. Patterns of sunscreen use on the face and other exposed skin among US adults. *J Am Acad Dermatol.* 2015; 73(1):83–92.e1.

22. Weig EA, Tull R, Chung J, Brown-Joel ZO, Majee R, Ferguson NN. Assessing factors affecting sunscreen use and barriers to compliance: a cross-sectional survey-based study. *J Dermatolog Treat.* 2020;31(4):403–405.

23. Winkelmann RR, Rigel DS. Assessing frequency and quality of US dermatologist sunscreen recommendations to their patients. *J Am Acad Dermatol.* 2015;72(3):557–558.

24. Akamine KL, Gustafson CJ, Davis SA, Levender MM, Feldman SR. Trends in sunscreen recommendation among US physicians. *JAMA Dermatol.* 2014;150(1):51–55.

25. Feldman SR, Vrijens B, Gieler U, Piaserico S, Puig L, van de Kerkhof P. Treatment Adherence Intervention Studies in Dermatology and Guidance on How to Support Adherence. *Am J Clin Dermatol.* 2017;18(2):253–271.

26. Tortora GJ, Derrickson BH. *Principles of Anatomy and Physiology.* New York, NY: John Wiley & Sons; 2018: p. 149.

27. Ley P, Llewelyn S. Improving patients' understanding, recall, satisfaction and compliance. In: *Health Psychology.* Boston: Springer; 1995; 75–98.

28. Vrijens B, Urquhart J, White D. Electronically monitored dosing histories can be used to develop a medication-taking habit and manage patient adherence. *Expert Rev Clin Pharmacol.* 2014;7(5):633–644.

29. Svendsen MT, Andersen F, Andersen KH, et al. A smartphone application supporting patients with psoriasis improves adherence to topical treatment: a randomized controlled trial. *Br J Dermatol.* 2018;179(5):1062–1071.

30. Feldman SR, Camacho FT, Krejci-Manwaring J, Carroll CL, Balkrishnan R. Adherence to topical therapy increases around the time of office visits. *J Am Acad Dermatol.* 2007;57(1): 81–83.

31. Capozza K, Schwartz A. Does it work and is it safe? Parents' perspectives on adherence to medication for atopic dermatitis. *Pediatr Dermatol.* 2020;37(1):58–61.

32. Lee L, El-Den S, Horne R, Carter SR. Patient satisfaction with information, concerns, beliefs and adherence to topical corticosteroids. *Patient Educ Couns.* 2019;102(6):1203–1209.

33. Ramachandran V, Cline A, Hawkins S. Technological Advancements to Promote Adherence. In: *Treatment Adherence in Dermatology.* Cham, Germany: Springer; 2020: 99–112.

34. Data on file Skin Type Solutions, Inc.

35. McChesney C, Covey S, Huling J. *The 4 disciplines of execution: Achieving your wildly important goals.* New York: Simon and Schuster; 2012.

36. Navathe AS, Volpp KG, Caldarella KL, Bond A, Troxel AB, Zhu J, et al. Effect of Financial Bonus Size, Loss Aversion, and Increased Social Pressure on Physician Pay-for-Performance: A Randomized Clinical Trial and Cohort Study. *JAMA Netw Open.* 2019;2(2):e187950.

37. Data on file Skin Type Solutions franchise Systems, LLC.

38. Personal experience of the author.

CHAPTER 35

Skincare Regimen Design (Product Layering)

Leslie S. Baumann, MD

SUMMARY POINTS

What's Important?
1. Cleanser and moisturizer choices affect the efficacy of skincare regimens.
2. Product efficacy is affected by what products are used before and after application.
3. Incidence of side effects is influenced by the skincare routine order.

What's New?
1. Hyaluronic acid and fatty acids affect penetration of other ingredients.
2. There are three paths of penetration into the skin.
3. Identifying how much of each type of skincare product to use.

What's Coming?
1. Liposomes and other penetration enhancers are constantly being developed.
2. Software that can be used to generate science-based skincare regimens.

There are several factors to consider when designing a skincare routine for your patients. The goal is to achieve the greatest efficacy with the lowest level of side effects. The best skincare routines will not work if patients do not follow advice; therefore, it is critical to design a regimen that suits the patient's lifestyle and budget. Chapter 33 (Choosing Skincare Products) discusses how to choose which skincare products to retail in your practice and Chapter 34 (Skincare Retail in a Medical Setting) explains how best to retail them in your practice. This chapter will discuss what should be considered when designing a skincare routine for your patients.

Topical products should be applied in a particular order to maximize efficacy. This is necessary because cosmeceutical ingredients interact with each other thereby affecting stability, activity, solubility, and penetration. Environmental influences such as temperature, water type, presence of pollution, skin pH, humidity, and the microbiome will influence the efficacy of skincare products. Such chemical phenomena should be considered when developing the order of products for a skincare regimen. Some ingredients are more likely to interact with other ingredients, such as benzoyl peroxide,

retinoids, hydroxy acids, hydroquinone, vitamin C, and peptides. The most important issue to keep in mind when designing a skincare regimen is how much of the cosmeceutical ingredient will penetrate the skin without inactivating other important active components. The trick is to design the skincare regimen properly to maximize stability and penetration.

PATHWAYS TO PENETRATION

Most of the information we have on getting topical ingredients into the dermis is in the drug delivery literature. Topically applied cosmeceutical ingredients and drugs can penetrate the skin in three ways:

1. Transcellular route[1]: involves entering the skin by directly passing through the lamellar lipid layers and the cell membranes and moving across the hydrophilic keratin-enriched cytoplasm of stratum corneum (SC) keratinocytes. In this route, substances must cross both lipophilic and hydrophilic structures.[2]

2. Intracellular or paracellular route: involves passing between the intercellular spaces between keratinocytes.

3. Appendageal route: hydrophilic compounds and macromolecules may pass through the hair follicle and/or sweat gland to enter the dermis. This route is affected by anatomical location because of regional diversity in the number of hair follicles.[3]

Penetration of ingredients into the skin is based on multiple factors including whether they are hydrophilic or lipophilic as well as the size, polarity, charge, concentration, hydration, temperature, solubility, and presence of carrier molecules. Liposomes are often used to increase penetration of topical ingredients. The order of skincare products in the regimen will affect which route of penetration the ingredients take and how efficiently they can follow that route.

WATER AND FATTY ACIDS AFFECT PENETRATION

Hydration loosens the cell attachments in the SC and increases penetration.[4] Occlusion of the skin with occlusive ingredients, sebum, or occlusive patches will increase penetration. Hyaluronic acid (HA) is well known to increase absorption of topically applied drugs, most likely by increasing hydration of the surface layers of the skin and facilitating the retention of the drug within the more hydrated epidermal layers (possibly by exposure of potential drug-binding sites), thus decreasing drug diffusion into the lower skin layers.[5]

Fatty acids, found in cleansers and moisturizers, affect fluidization and cause disorganization of SC lipids.[6] Unsaturated fatty acids (e.g., oleic, linoleic, palmitoleic) increase skin penetration much more than saturated fatty acids (e.g., palmitic and stearic).[7] One of the most used fatty acids to enhance drug delivery is oleic acid, the predominant fatty acid in olive oil, because it interacts with the extracellular lipids in the SC.[8]

The efficacy of all cosmeceutical products is affected by which of these they are exposed to and when they are exposed to them in the regimen. The bottom line is the side effect profile of ingredients, such as benzoyl peroxide and retinoids, is greatly influenced by the presence of HA and fatty acids in cleansers and moisturizers.

Practitioners should carefully consider each step of the skincare routine in developing a regimen. Each regimen should be designed for the patient's skin type, lifestyle, and budget. To customize efficacious regimens for all Baumann Skin Types, lifestyle preferences, and specific needs, there are over 40,000 regimen options. Skin Type Solutions Software has been developed to generate regimens based on these issues. All regimens should follow this basic structure (**Fig. 35-1**).

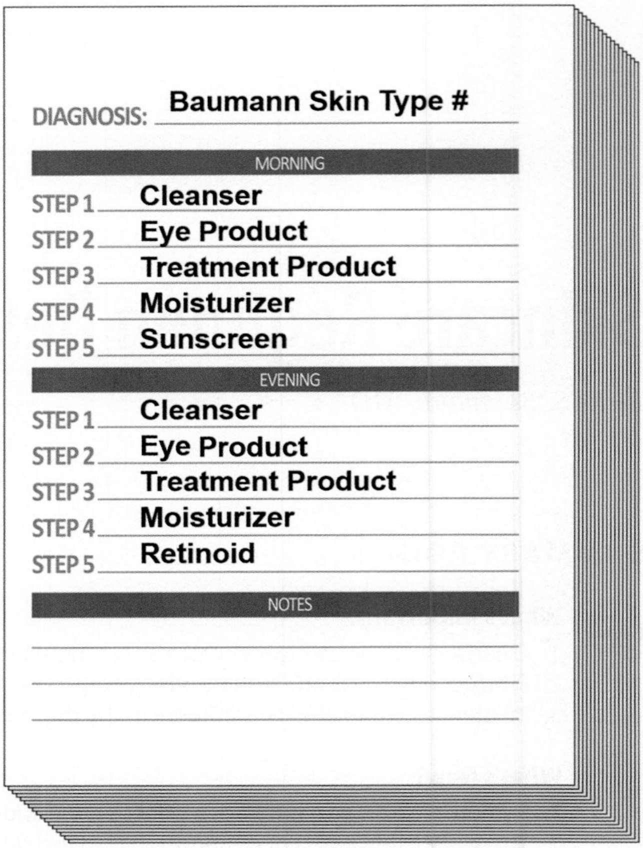

STEP 1: CLEANSERS

Cleansers can alter the pH of the skin, loosen attachments between cells, remove lipids from and disrupt the bilayer protective membrane, desquamate layers from the SC, and influence the penetrability of the skin for the next topical product

FIGURE 35-1. This is the basic structure of a skincare regimen. All five steps in the AM and PM are not always needed. It depends on the skin type's needs and ingredients in the available products.

that is applied. Therefore, cleansers should be selected based on the products that will follow them in the regimen. In addition, cleansers should be chosen according to the patient's Baumann Skin Type®.[9] For example, cleansers for use on oily skin should have the ability to remove excess sebum from the skin while cleansers designed for dry skin would not remove as many lipids from the skin. Washing with a foaming cleanser can disrupt the skin barrier allowing increased penetration of the treatment product that follows it (see Chapter 40, Cleansing Agents). Cleansers should be chosen to increase efficacy of the treatment product. For this reason, every ingredient and characteristic of the AM and PM cleansers is important. See Chapter 33 for how to choose a cleanser brand.

STEP 2: EYE PRODUCTS

Eye products treat issues such as dryness, puffiness, fine lines, and dark circles. However, they also play an overlooked role in protecting the thin delicate eye area from the treatment product. Using an eye product, especially one with protective ingredients such as barrier repair lipids, will help the patient tolerate the potentially irritating treatment product that follows the eye product. At night, treatment product ingredients can rub onto pillowcases and transfer to the upper and lower eyelids. Use of a protective eye product before bedtime can prevent the accompanying irritation. For example, acne patients often develop redness at the corners of the eyes when using benzoyl peroxide or a retinoid at night. Applying these medications after an eye cream can reduce this side effect. Eye products should be chosen independent of the skin type and targeted to any of the following issues the patient has: dryness, irritation, puffiness, fine lines, or dark circles. A different eye product can be used in the AM and PM. Use the antipuffiness products in the morning and the hydrating products in the evening.

STEP 3: TREATMENT PRODUCTS

Treatment products are defined as corrective formulations targeted to skin issues such as acne, rosacea, melasma, dryness, skin cancer, eczema, psoriasis, and photoaging. The entire skincare regimen should be designed to enhance efficacy and decrease side effects of the treatment products. Treatment products may be cosmeceuticals, OTC medications, or prescription medications. These formulations must be able to reach their target in the proper chemical structure to be effective. Each ingredient has various constraints and quirks that should be considered. One well known example is ascorbic acid (vitamin C). Ascorbic acid is a treatment product for skin pigmentation and skin aging that requires specific conditions to work properly. The maximum absorption of ascorbic acid occurs at a pH of 2–2.5.[10] However, applying these formulations on skin that has just been cleansed with a soap or foaming cleanser with a pH of 9 will raise the skin's pH and decrease the absorption of ascorbic acid. Having the patient cleanse with a low pH cleanser such as salicylic or glycolic acid cleanser (usually a pH of 2.5–3.5) will lower the pH of the skin and promote absorption of vitamin C. Each treatment product has specific requirements to improve penetration and efficacy that should be considered when designing the regimen.

STEP 4: MOISTURIZERS

Moisturizers perform many duties for the skin including hydration, protection, and delivery of important ingredients. However, moisturizers have a less discussed role of improving the efficacy of the previously applied treatment product. Moisturizers often contain oleic acid, HA, or other fatty acids that can increase penetration of other skincare ingredients. In addition, many moisturizers provide an occlusive effect that helps increase penetration (see Chapter 43, Moisturizers). Moisturizers help protect the underlying treatment product from getting wiped off on a pillowcase or into the environment. In other words, moisturizers "seal in" the treatment product. Some moisturizing ingredients such as heparan sulfate may affect how well the skin cells "hear" and respond to signals elicited by treatment formulations. For this reason, moisturizers should also be selected to improve the efficacy of the treatment product.

STEP 5 AM: SUNSCREEN

A daily sunscreen should be chosen based on the Baumann Skin Type and the patient's preferences. Several studies show that a low percentage of patients use sunscreen daily. Choosing an SPF that matches the patient's lifestyle and fits seamlessly into the skincare routine is important to boost compliance. Select the sunscreen based on the patient's preferences as follows:

- Tinted vs. Untinted
- Chemical vs. Mineral
- Delivery vehicle: stick, spray, lotion

STEP 5 PM: RETINOIDS

Most skin types should use a retinoid because retinoids control acne, improve pigmentation, and prevent and treat aging (see Chapter 45, Retinoids). Most skin types can tolerate retinoids when they are combined in the proper skincare regimen and started slowly. When using retinoids for the first time in a patient, apply them after the moisturizer to reduce the incidence of side effects and increase compliance. Retinoids, unlike other ingredients, penetrate easily into the deeper layer of the epidermis. Layering them on top of a moisturizer can help titrate retinoid absorption. The moisturizer can be chosen to slow or increase penetration of retinoids. Avoid moisturizers that contain HA and oleic acid when beginning retinoids in sensitive skin types because these ingredients speed absorption. Instead, select moisturizers with saturated fatty acids like stearic acid to slow penetration. Retinoids should always be used at night because many of them, especially retinol and tretinoin, are easily broken down by ultraviolet light exposure.

HOW MUCH PRODUCT TO USE

It is important to standardize how much skincare product to use so that patients can be properly coached on how much to use. This allows for predicting how much product they will apply in a set time period, and makes it easier to choose travel size needs and plan for product replacement. It also allows the practitioner to gauge compliance. There is a varied body of advice on how much product to use. A standardization of volume to use by product type has been developed to help improve communication and compliance. It is based on the fact that SPF testing uses 2 mg/cm^2. Using this amount as the basic volume for sunscreen, creams, and lotions is recommended to help train patients to use the proper amount. **Fig. 35-2** shows how much facial skincare product to use by product type.

CONCLUSION

There is much to consider when designing a skincare regimen. It is difficult to achieve at the time of the patient visit; therefore, the practitioner should be prepared before the visit and customize the regimen for the patient to save time. Software

Cleanser	Milks, Creams, Gels, Liquids	¼ teaspoon	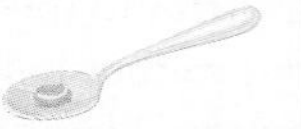
Eye Product	Serums, Lotions, or Creams	1/8 teaspoon	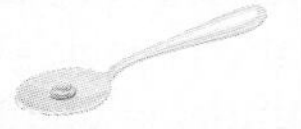
Moisturizer	Creams, Ointments, or Lotions	¼ teaspoon	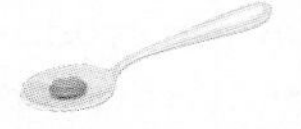
Sunscreen	Lotions, Creams, Gels	¼ teaspoon	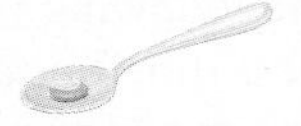
Oils and Serums		1/8 teaspoon	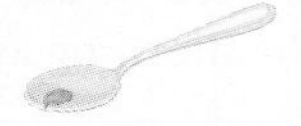

FIGURE 35-2. Cleanser - (milks, creams, gels, liquids) - ¼ teaspoon
Eye product - (serums, lotions, or creams) - $\frac{1}{8}$ teaspoon
Moisturizer (creams, ointments, or lotions) - ¼ teaspoon
Sunscreen (lotions, creams, gels) - ¼ teaspoon
Oils and serums - $\frac{1}{8}$ teaspoon

is available to make these decisions quickly and scientifically. Using software will allow the medical provider to delegate skincare recommendations to their staff with the confidence that the patient will receive the best skincare advice for their skin type.

Medical providers and their staffs can make a significant difference in their patients' long-term skin health by assisting them in identifying the proper skincare formulations for their individual skin type and guiding them as to how much, and in which order, to apply the products in their personalized skincare regimen. Patients will not remember what you told them and will confuse the order in which products should be used. For this reason, providing a written step-by-step skincare regimen is paramount to ensuring patient compliance.

References

1. Ghaffarian R, Muro S. Models and methods to evaluate transport of drug delivery systems across cellular barriers. *J Vis Exp.* 2013;(80):e50638.

2. Lopes CM, Silva J, Oliveira MECR, Lúcio M. Lipid-based colloidal carriers for topical application of antiviral drugs. In: *Design of Nanostructures for Versatile Therapeutic Applications.* Amsterdam, The Netherlands: William Andrew Publishing; 2018: 565–622.

3. Mohd F, Todo H, Yoshimoto M, Yusuf E, Sugibayashi K. Contribution of the Hair Follicular Pathway to Total Skin Permeation of Topically Applied and Exposed Chemicals. *Pharmaceutics.* 2016; 8(4):32.

4. Bucks D, Maibach HI. Occlusion does not uniformly enhance penetration in vivo. In: Bronaugh RL, Maibach HI, eds. *Percutaneous Absorption; Drugs, Cosmetics, Mechanisms, Methodology,* 3rd edition. New York: Marcel Dekker; 1999: 81–105.

5. Brown MB, Jones SA. Hyaluronic acid: a unique topical vehicle for the localized delivery of drugs to the skin. *J Eur Acad Dermatol Venereol.* 2005;19(3):308–318.

6. Barry BW. Mode of action of penetration enhancers in human skin. *J Control Release.* 1987;6(1):85–97.

7. Čižinauskas V, Elie N, Brunelle A, Briedis V. Fatty acids penetration into human skin ex vivo: A TOF-SIMS analysis approach. *Biointerphases.* 2017;12(1):011003.

8. Mak VH, Potts RO, Guy RH. Percutaneous penetration enhancement in vivo measured by attenuated total reflectance infrared spectroscopy. *Pharm Res.* 1990;7(8):835–841.

9. Baumann LS. The Baumann Skin Typing System. In: Farage MA, et al. eds. *Textbook of Aging Skin.* Berlin Heidelberg: Springer-Verlag; 2017: 1579–1594.

10. Pinnell SR, Yang H, Omar M, Monteiro-Riviere N, DeBuys HV, Walker LC, et al. Topical L-ascorbic acid: percutaneous absorption studies. *Dermatol Surg.* 2001;27(2):137–142.

CHAPTER 36

Pre- and Postprocedure Skincare Guide for Surgical Patients

Leslie S. Baumann, MD
Edmund M. Weisberg, MS, MBE

SUMMARY POINTS

What's Important?

1. Use retinoids, ascorbic acid, hydroxy acids, matrikines, and defensins topically 14 days before procedures.
2. Do not use retinoids, ascorbic acid, or hydroxy acids after procedures until complete re-epithelialization has occurred.
3. Avoiding foods, supplements, and topical products that increase bruising will improve filler outcomes.

What's New?

1. Matrikines used 14 days prior to procedures can speed healing.
2. Defensins used post procedure may speed healing.

What's Coming?

1. Identifying safe ingredients to use during and after microneedling.
2. Combining ingredients to maximize outcomes.

Cosmetic surgery outcomes are consistently enhanced when proper skincare is employed prior to and after the procedure, be it a biopsy, surgical excision, dermal filler injection, or Mohs surgery. This chapter should serve as a useful guide for how to best educate patients about pre- and postprocedure skincare needs before and after skin surgery.

PRE-SURGERY SKINCARE AND USE OF SUPPLEMENTS

The aim of the practitioner should be to accelerate healing while limiting infection, scarring, and hyperpigmentation. For the 2 weeks leading up to surgery, products that have been demonstrated to speed wound healing by increasing keratinization and/or collagen production should be recommended. Derived from vitamin A, the retinoid family includes compounds such as adapalene, β-carotene, carotenoids, retinol, tazarotene, and tretinoin. Retinoids such as tretinoin and

retinol are key ingredients that should be used *prior* to wounding. Multiple studies have cogently revealed that pretreatment with tretinoin accelerates wound healing.[1–3] Kligman assessed healing after punch biopsy in the mid-1990s and found that the wounds on arms pretreated with tretinoin cream 0.05% to 0.1% were significantly diminished by 35% to 37% on days 1 and 4, and 47% to 50% reduced on days 6, 8, and 11 as compared to the wounds on untreated arms.[4] A tretinoin pretreatment regimen of 2 to 4 weeks is supported by the preponderance of studies,[5] as peak epidermal hypertrophy emerges after 7 days of tretinoin application and normalizes after 14 days of continued treatment.[6] Such an approach gives the skin time to recover from any retinoid dermatitis before the scheduled surgery. Pretreatment with adapalene should be introduced 5 to 6 weeks before any procedure because it exhibits a longer half-life and requires an earlier initiation period.[7]

Although wound healing studies have not been conducted in this area, pretreating skin with topical ascorbic acid (vitamin C) and hydroxy acids might hasten wound healing by promoting collagen synthesis.[8,9] See **Table 36-1** for the range of products recommended leading up to a procedure.

INGREDIENTS AND ACTIVITIES TO AVOID PRE-SURGERY

To reduce bruising, patients should avoid aspirin, ibuprofen, naproxen, St. John's Wort, tocopherol (vitamin E), ω-3 fatty acids supplements, flax seed oil, ginseng, salmon, and alcohol. Most physicians agree that these ingredients should be avoided for 10 days prior to the procedure. Oral arnica supplements may prevent bruising. Smoking should be avoided 4 weeks prior to the procedure.

> Topical retinoids and hydroxy acids should be used prior to procedures but not immediately after procedures.

POST-SURGERY SKINCARE AND SUPPLEMENTS

Oral vitamin C and zinc supplements have been shown to speed wound healing in rats when taken immediately after a procedure.[10] Oral arnica tablets and tinctures are often used prior to and after surgery to reduce bruising and inflammation.

Topical products used after surgery play an important role in healing. The combination of topical *Arnica montana* and *Rhododendron tomentosum* (*Ledum palustre*) in a gel pad has been demonstrated to reduce postoperative ecchymosis and edema after oculofacial surgery.[11] Topical curcumin speeds wound healing in animals.[12] Another study has shown that an occlusive ointment containing a triad of antioxidants accelerated wound healing.[13]

A protein important in wound repair, defensin is available in a topical formulation. Defensin has exhibited the capacity to activate the leucine-rich repeat-containing G-protein–coupled receptors 5 and 6 (also known as LGR5 and LGR6) stem cells.[14] It speeds wound healing by increasing LGR stem cell migration into wound beds.

Wounds should be covered to provide protection from sun exposure until re-epithelialization occurs. Which occlusive ointments and wound repair products to use are beyond the scope of this chapter. Once epithelialized, zinc oxide

TABLE 36-1	Medications and Supplements Recommended at Least 2 Weeks Prior to Undergoing Cosmetic Procedures
Ascorbic Acid	
Defensin	
Growth Factors	
Hydroxy Acids	
Matrikines	
Retinoids	

sunscreens can be used. These have been shown to be safe with minimal penetration into the skin.[15]

INGREDIENTS TO AVOID POST-SURGERY

Topical retinoids should not be used post skin cancer surgery until epithelialization is complete. A study by Hung et al. in a porcine model used 0.05% tretinoin cream daily for 10 days prior to partial-thickness skin wounding. Tretinoin use accelerated re-epithelialization while use after the procedure slowed wound healing.[16]

Acidic products will sting wounded skin. For this reason, benzoic acid, hydroxy acids, and ascorbic acid should be avoided until the skin has completely re-epithelialized. Products with preservatives and fragrance should be avoided if possible.

Vitamin E derived from oral supplement capsules slowed healing after skin cancer surgery and had a high rate of contact dermatitis.[17] Chemical sunscreens are more likely to cause an allergic contact dermatitis and should be avoided for 4 weeks after skin surgery. Organic products with essential oils and botanical ingredients may present a higher risk of contact dermatitis due to allergen exposure.

RETINOID USE RECOMMENDATION SUMMARY

Use 2–3 weeks prior to procedures to speed healing.
Do not use after the procedure until re-epithelialization has occurred.
Vitamin C and zinc supplements taken after the procedure might speed wound healing.

BRUISING

Ecchymoses, or bruises, develop from damage to the capillaries, allowing blood to leak into the underlying tissue. This benign process resolves within a few days. Unfortunately, bruising is considered an inevitable side effect of injectable procedures. Certain techniques to mitigate and, ideally, prevent this outcome are employed in dermatologic practice. Nevertheless, patients should be made aware that bruises may take approximately 7 to 14 days to clear, so they can make appropriate accommodations in their lives.

Prevention and Treatment

It is beneficial to ask patients about any history of bleeding disorders or usage of anticoagulant medications when scheduling a cosmetic procedure that can cause bleeding. Patients should also be counseled to avoid certain medications 10 days before the procedure (**Table 36-2**). These medications and supplements should be reviewed over the phone and faxed or mailed to the patient when the appointment is made so that patients arrive for the procedure not having used any of these products. NSAIDs, including aspirin, are well recognized for imparting antiplatelet effects. Inhibitory effects on platelets are also induced by supplements such as garlic and ginkgo.[18] It is important to note that green tea enhances the tendency to bleed via antiplatelet activity, and vitamin E can contribute to bleeding by suppressing the intrinsic coagulation pathway.[19,20] The herbal supplements bromelain and arnica have been associated with the capacity to reduce the risk of bruising.[21]

Bromelain

Naturally present in mature pineapple stems (*Ananas comosus*), bromelain contains proteolytic enzymes, and has been used in medical settings for its antithrombotic, fibrinolytic, and anti-inflammatory activity.[22-24] Bromelain is thought to impart its anticoagulant activity via blocking of platelet aggregation.[25] For the treatment of osteoarthritis, bromelain has been used successfully in doses ranging from 540 to 1,890 mg/d.[26-28] The majority of cosmetic dermatology practices recommend the use of bromelain 500 mg twice daily for 1 day following a procedure to prevent bruising, or the same dose until bruising has cleared. Although bromelain is considered safe, the incidence of adverse events (e.g., headache, gastrointestinal symptoms, and cutaneous rash) is known to increase proportionately with higher doses.[29] Bromelain is contraindicated for patients on anticoagulant medications, such as warfarin and aspirin, pending a consultation with their primary care physicians. The author advises against the use of bromelain before the procedure because it appears to promote rather than prevent bruising.

Arnica

Arnice is derived from several mountain plants, including *Arnica montana*, *Arnica chamissonis*, *Arnica fulgens*, *Arnica cordifolia*, and *Arnica sororia*. Arnica, also known as leopard's bane or mountain tobacco, is widely used in homeopathic practice. Helenalin, a sesquiterpene lactone that is its major active ingredient, confers anti-inflammatory activity.[30] Arnica has influenced platelet function in vitro, though its mechanism of action in relation to bruising remains to be elucidated.[31] Clinical trials involving arnica to treat ecchymoses are inconclusive. A multicenter, randomized, double-blind, placebo-controlled study of 130 patients with phlebectomy failed to demonstrate a difference among patients treated with arnica before and after the procedure compared with the control group.[32] In a 2010 rater-blinded randomized controlled trial with 16 healthy patients, topical 20% arnica appeared to be more effective than placebo and a 1% vitamin K and 0.3% retinol formulation in reducing laser-induced bruising.[33]

In the author's experience, bruising seems to be prevented when patients take four homeopathic arnica pills labeled "with 30x dilution" 4 to 6 hours before a cosmetic procedure. Because high doses of oral arnica can lead to deleterious effects, patients should be cautioned not to exceed this dose. If patients develop a mild rash, it is likely that they are sensitive to helenalin and should discontinue the arnica regimen. In the author's practice, arnica gel is applied to the treated region following every cosmetic procedure. It is also used to massage patients after Sculptra treatments. Topical arnica is readily available in pharmacies. Patients are instructed to apply arnica creams three times daily at home until bruises clear. See **Table 36-3** for the range of products to consider post procedure.

Assessing Bruise Severity

Currently, there are no published scales rating the severity of bruises. Such ratings are important in assessing treatments aimed at preventing bruising or accelerating healing. The author co-developed the Baumann-Castanedo scale to rate bruises (see **Tables 36-4 and 36-5**). The Baumann-Castanedo scale aids the user in tracking the color and size of the bruise to gauge severity and improvement.

TABLE 36-2	Medications and Supplements to Avoid at Least 10 Days Prior to Undergoing Cosmetic Procedures
NSAIDs (Aspirin, Advil, Motrin, Ibuprofen)	
Vitamin E	
Green Tea	
Garlic	
Ginkgo	
Ginseng	
St. John's Wort	

TABLE 36-3	Post-Procedure Topical Product Selection Depends on Procedure and May Include:
Arnica	
Chamomile	
Defensin	
Green Tea	
Heparan Sulfate	
Mineral Sunscreen	
Panthenol	

TABLE 36-4	Bruise Dimension Scale
0 = no bruise	
1 = 0.1–0.4 cm	
2 = 0.5–1.0 cm	
3 = 1.1–2.0 cm	
4 = 2.1–3.0 cm	
5 = 3.1 cm or larger	

TABLE 36-5	Bruise Progression Scale (According to Changes in Color)
1 = Pink/Red	
2 = Purple/Dark Blue	
3 = Green/Dark Yellow	
4 = Pale Yellow/Brown	
5 = Hint of Color	

CONCLUSION

To ensure the best outcome from surgical treatments, patient education is a key step. The more that patients know and understand about the ways in which they can prepare for their procedure and treat their skin after the procedure, the better the outcomes will be. Providers should give this type of information in an easy-to-follow printed instruction sheet because studies show that patients cannot remember most of the oral instructions offered by practitioners. Patients should be encouraged to ask questions during their consultation and procedure and to express any concerns with the practitioner's office should any arise after they have returned home. These steps help improve patient compliance, satisfaction, and outcomes.

References

1. Vagotis FL, Brundage SR. Histologic study of dermabrasion and chemical peel in an animal model after pretreatment with Retin-A. *Aesthetic Plast Surg.* 1995 May-Jun;19(3):243–246.

2. Stuzin JM. Discussion. A randomized controlled trial of skin care protocols for facial resurfacing: lessons learned from the Plastic Surgery Educational Foundation's Skin Products Assessment Research study. *Plast Reconstr Surg.* 2011 Mar;127(3):1343–1345.

3. Elson ML. The role of retinoids in wound healing. *J Am Acad Dermatol.* 1998 Aug;39:S79–S81.

4. Popp C, Kligman AM, Stoudemayer TJ. Pretreatment of photoaged forearm skin with topical tretinoin accelerates healing of full-thickness wounds. *Br J Dermatol.* 1995 Jan;132(1):46–53.

5. Orringer JS, Kang S, Johnson TM, et al. Tretinoin treatment before carbon-dioxide laser resurfacing: a clinical and biochemical analysis. *J Am Acad Dermatol.* 2004 Dec;51(6):940–946.

6. Kim IH, Kim HK, Kye YC. Effects of tretinoin pretreatment on TCA chemical peel in guinea pig skin. *J Korean Med Sci.* 1996 Aug;11(4):335–341.

7. Basak PY, Eroglu E, Altuntas I, et al. Comparison of the effects of tretinoin, adapalene and collagenase in an experimental model of wound healing. *Eur J Dermatol.* 2002 Mar-Apr;12(2):145–148.

8. Murad S, Grove D, Lindberg KA, et al. Regulation of collagen synthesis by ascorbic acid. *Proc Natl Acad Sci U S A.* 1981 May;78(5):2879–2882.

9. Okano Y, Abe Y, Masaki H, et al. Biological effects of glycolic acid on dermal matrix metabolism mediated by dermal fibroblasts and epidermal keratinocytes. *Exp Dermatol.* 2003;12(Suppl 2):57–63.

10. Kaplan B, Gönül B, Dincer S, et al. Relationships between tensile strength, ascorbic acid, hydroxyproline, and zinc levels of rabbit full-thickness incision wound healing. *Surg Today.* 2004;34(9):747–751.

11. Kang JY, Tran KD, Seiff SR, et al. Assessing the effectiveness of Arnica montana and Rhododendron tomentosum (Ledum palustre) in the reduction of ecchymosis and edema after oculofacial surgery: preliminary results. *Ophthal Plast Reconstr Surg.* 2017 Jan/Feb;33(1):47–52.

12. Sidhu GS, Singh AK, Thaloor D, et al. Enhancement of wound healing by curcumin in animals. *Wound Repair Regen.* 1998 Mar-Apr;6(2):167–177.

13. McDaniel DH, Ash K, Lord J, et al. Accelerated laser resurfacing wound healing using a triad of topical antioxidants. *Dermatol Surg.* 1998 Jun;24(6):661–664.

14. Lough D, Dai H, Yang M, et al. Stimulation of the follicular bulge LGR5+ and LGR6+ stem cells with the gut-derived human alpha defensin 5 results in decreased bacterial presence, enhanced wound healing, and hair growth from tissues devoid of adnexal structures. *Plast Reconstr Surg.* 2013 Nov;132(5):1159–1171.

15. Holmes AM, Song Z, Moghimi HR, et al. Relative penetration of zinc oxide and zinc ions into human skin after application of different zinc oxide formulations. *ACS Nano.* 2016 Feb 23;10(2):1810–1819.

16. Hung VC, Lee JY, Zitelli JA, et al. Topical tretinoin and epithelial wound healing. *Arch Dermatol.* 1989 Jan;125(1):65–69.

17. Baumann LS, Spencer J. The effects of topical vitamin E on the cosmetic appearance of scars. *Dermatol Surg.* 1999 Apr;25(4):311–315.

18. Ang-Lee MK, Moss J, Yuan CS. Herbal medicines and perioperative care. *JAMA.* 2001 Jul 11;286(2):208–216.

19. Kang WS, Lim IH, Yuk DY, et al. Antithrombotic activities of green tea catechins and (−)-epigallocatechin gallate. *Thromb Res.* 1999 Nov 1;96(3):229–237.

20. Marsh SA, Coombes JS. Vitamin E and alpha-lipoic acid supplementation increase bleeding tendency via an intrinsic coagulation pathway. *Clin Appl Thromb Hemost.* 2006 Apr;12(2):169–173.

21. Weinkle S, Saco M. Approach to the mature cosmetic patient: aging gracefully. *J Drugs Dermatol.* 2017 Jun 1;16(6):s84–s86.

22. Rowan AD, Buttle DJ, Barrett AJ. The cysteine proteinases of the pineapple plant. *Biochem J.* 1990 Mar 15;266(3):869–875.

23. Rowan AD, Buttle DJ. Pineapple cysteine endopeptidases. *Methods Enzymol.* 1994;244:555–568.

24. Maurer HR. Bromelain: biochemistry, pharmacology and medical use. *Cell Mol Life Sci.* 2001 Aug;58(9):1234–1245.

25. Gläser D, Hilberg T. The influence of bromelain on platelet count and platelet activity *in vitro*. *Platelets.* 2006 Feb;17(1):37–41.

26. Singer F, Singer C, Oberleitner H. Phlyoenzyme versus diclofenac in the treatment of activated osteoarthritis of the knee. *Int J Immunother.* 2001;17:135.

27. Singer F, Oberleitner H. Drug therapy of activated arthrosis. On the effectiveness of an enzyme mixture versus diclofenac. *Wien Med Wochenschr.* 1996;146(3):55–58.

28. Tilwe GH, Beria S, Turakhia NH, et al. Efficacy and tolerability of oral enzyme therapy as compared to diclofenac in active osteoarthritis of knee joint: an open randomized controlled clinical trial. *J Assoc Physicians India.* 2001 Jun;49:617–621.

29. Brien S, Lewith G, Walker A, et al. Bromelain as a treatment for osteoarthritis: a review of clinical studies. *Evid Based Complement Alternat Med.* 2004 Dec;1(3):251–257.

30. Lyss G, Schmidt TJ, Merfort I, et al. Helenalin, an anti-inflammatory sesquiterpene lactone from *Arnica*, selectively inhibits transcription factor NF-κB. *Biol Chem.* 1997 Sep;378(9):951–961.

31. Schröder H, Lösche W, Strobach H, et al. Helenalin and 11α, 13-dihydrohelenalin, two constituents from *Arnica montana* L., inhibit human platelet function via thiol-dependent pathways. *Thromb Res.* 1990 Mar 15;57(6):839–845.

32. Ramelet AA, Buchheim G, Lorenz P, et al. Homeopathic arnica in postoperative haematomas: a double-blind study. *Dermatology.* 2000;201(4):347–348.

33. Leu S, Havey J, White LE, et al. Accelerated resolution of laser-induced bruising with topical 20% arnica: a rater-blinded randomized controlled trial. *Br J Dermatol.* 2010;163(3):557–563.

CHAPTER 37

Anti-Aging Ingredients

Leslie S. Baumann, MD
Edmund M. Weisberg, MS, MBE

SUMMARY POINTS

What's Important?

1. Anti-aging therapies remain focused on inducing fibroblasts to produce collagen and ECM components and preventing the breakdown of these vital dermal constituents.
2. No topical products can enhance elastin synthesis in the skin; increased elasticity claims are more likely due to greater moisturization than increased elastin.
3. Retinoids, including retinol, are still the most proven topical anti-aging ingredients.
4. Ascorbic acid also has significant efficacy data to show it increases collagen synthesis.
5. Antioxidants help mitigate several aging processes such as mitochondrial damage, inflammation, DNA mutations, and glycation.
6. Peptides have poor penetration and stability and are highly reactive with other ingredients.
7. The efficacy and safety of growth factors depend on growth factor type.

What's New?

1. The abstracts of peptide anti-aging efficacy studies are misleading.
2. Look closely at study design and statistical significance when evaluating anti-aging ingredient research.
3. The growth factor TGF-β has the most data to support its use for skin rejuvenation.
4. Stem cells in pre-packaged topical creams have no proven efficacy.
5. Defensins activate the stem cell LGR6+ leading to new keratinocytes.
6. Heparan sulfate improves cell-to-cell communication in aged fibroblasts.

What's Coming?

1. Safety data on the use of peptides, stem cells, and growth factors after microneedling.
2. Improvements in peptide penetration may improve efficacy and possibly decrease safety.
3. More information on growth factor safety in the presence of skin cancer.

INTRODUCTION

Anti-aging skincare begins with sun avoidance but does not end there. In addition to the wise practice of avoiding prolonged direct sunlight between 10 AM and 4 PM, you should coach your patients to prevent photodamage with sunscreens, which limit the impact of ultraviolet (UV) radiation and reduce the formation of free radicals and inflammation. The aim of anti-aging skincare is to preserve the mitochondria and prevent the loss of collagen, elastin, and hyaluronic acid (HA) as well as promote the synthesis of collagen and HA. While sunscreens represent the optimal anti-aging skincare product category, there are several ingredients effective in lessening the signs of skin aging. Of course, the best anti-aging skincare products are sunscreens and the best skin-protective behavior, sun avoidance.

There are numerous anti-aging products on the market and it can be difficult to decide which ones to carry in your medical practice (see Chapter 33, Choosing Skincare Products). Many are expensive and the cost of carrying several products in an inventory, including various anti-aging stock keeping units (SKUs) can be cost prohibitive. It is best to choose one from each of these categories to sell in your practice: retinoids, anti-oxidants, an anti-aging product that excludes a retinoid and is gentle on sensitive skin such as a heparan sulfate, defensins, and growth factors or matrikine products. HA should be considered more of a moisturizer and an agent to increase penetration of other ingredients rather than an anti-aging product. This chapter will discuss various categories of anti-aging ingredients found in skincare products.

EVALUATING ANTI-AGING INGREDIENT RESEARCH

The anti-aging skincare market in the United States alone exceeded $42.5 billion dollars in 2020.[1] The stakes are high to develop products that are successful in the market. There is a plethora of new cosmeceutical ingredients every year with studies to support their use for anti-aging. The FDA not only does not require efficacy data for cosmeceutical products to be launched, but they dissuade studies by disallowing biologic activity claims (see Chapter 32, Cosmetics and Drug Regulations). For this reason, support data on cosmeceutical ingredients can be intentionally difficult to comprehend. The abstract of the publication that discusses the trial results is the section most reviewed by readers and is available on Google Scholar and PubMed without a fee. The statements in the abstracts can be misleading, though. It is always necessary to read the entire study and not accept the statements made in the abstract. In addition, the quality of publications ranges widely and the ability to publish incorrect hypotheses and data depends on the journal quality. The best studies are published in peer-reviewed journals that have a high impact factor (IF). The IF is a measure of the importance and credibility of a scientific journal based on the frequency with which the average article in a journal has been cited in the previous two years. Although the data published in these journals is considered more credible, this does not preclude carefully reading the entire article. The highest impact journals in science include *The New England Journal of Medicine*, *The Lancet*, *Nature*, and *Science*. The highest IF journals in dermatology are the *Journal of the American Academy of Dermatology*, *JAMA Dermatology*, *British Journal of Dermatology*, *Dermatologic Surgery*, and the *Journal of Investigative Dermatology*. Google Scholar displays the highest impact articles at the top of search results. The abstract of the article, if there is one, will appear but access to the entire content may require a fee. For this reason, the abstract is especially important, but it can be intentionally misleading in low-impact journals.

In other words, take anti-aging cosmeceutical data with a grain of salt unless there are multiple studies and sound science to support the claims. Retinoids are the most studied, most proven compounds for aged skin,[2] and have FDA drug approval to treat photoaging, yet they are under-prescribed, often replaced with the next new drug. Novel ingredients are enticing to consumers but their use may be a waste of time

and money and prevents consumers from using established treatments such as retinoids. Such a dynamic affects patient compliance and skin health. This chapter will attempt to guide the medical provider on how to evaluate these ingredients and choose which skincare products to prescribe to patients for photoaging. (See Chapters 33 and 35, Skincare Regimen Design, for advice on choosing anti-aging skincare products to retail and where to place them in the skincare regimen.)

The companies that sell ingredients to product manufacturers will have cell culture or bioengineered skin equivalent data on their ingredients. (Animal studies are not performed very often anymore.) These are the data upon which the claims are usually based. Less commonly, they may have human trial results. It is always important to ascertain if the studies were performed *in vivo* (on animals or humans), *in vitro* (cell cultures), or on bioengineered skin equivalents. If the data are on cell cultures, determine if they are keratinocytes, fibroblasts, or other types of cells. Cell culture studies are less informative because penetration into the dermis is not required for activity. Double-blind studies on human skin are best, but bioengineered skin equivalent studies are also informative. The Franz cell skin permeability assay uses excised skin to apply the ingredients on the epidermal side to discern if the ingredients can penetrate to the dermis.[3]

When evaluating human cosmeceutical studies, study design should be assessed. A double-blind controlled study in which the subject and the evaluator do not know who received the study cosmeceutical and who received the control or placebo is the most convincing design. Evaluate what the control or placebo is. In some trials a cosmeceutical is compared to using nothing, which makes it easy to reveal the cosmeceutical as superior to the control. For example, the moisturizing capabilities of the product will render the skin smoother as compared to unmoisturized skin. It is important to look at the washout period prior to the study and what products are used. In some cases, in the washout period the subjects are not allowed to use any skincare products on the face for 2 weeks. This dehydrates the skin and allows for buildup of dead stratum corneum (SC) cells, which makes the skin look rough and dull, poorly reflect light, and develop textural fine lines. These conditions are ideal for "before" photos. Any type of humectant, emollient, occlusive, or exfoliating ingredients will yield quick improvement in textural changes and light reflection. This study design is used often in cosmeceutical studies that appear to show improvement of wrinkles in hours to seven days. Wrinkles do not improve this quickly and the keratinization cycle is much longer (see Chapter 1, Basic Science of the Epidermis), so rapid improvement of wrinkles is impossible and should arouse suspicion of the study design. Moisturizers, peptides, and saccharides temporarily coat the skin's surface, filling in the spaces between the edges of keratinocytes in the SC. When the spaces between these keratinocytes are filled by a saccharide or peptide coating, smoothing effects can be observed that are similar to those seen when fondant smooths the surface of a cake. This will give the appearance of an instant, albeit temporary, improvement of wrinkles but has no correlation with long-term improvement of the skin or skin health.

Data is reported as "statistically significant" or "not statistically significant" based on P values. For statistical significance, the P value must be < 0.05. If not, it means that it cannot be concluded that a significant difference exists between the groups. Studies should always report the P value when giving data. Be suspicious if they do not because when there is a significant difference, it is proudly stated in the article's abstract. If the P value is not provided, it usually means it was >0.05. When this is the case, analyze the data carefully.

Any anti-aging skincare studies that evaluate fine lines and wrinkles would optimally last at least 4 months on human skin; however, 6 months to a year would be more convincing (most studies are 12 weeks). For example, the landmark studies on tretinoin for photoaged skin in 1993 evaluated photoaged skin treated with tretinoin for 10 to 12 months.[4] Studies often include biopsies before and after a product is applied to render a qualitative measure of collagen content.[5] This is problematic because the act of wounding with a biopsy triggers a wound healing response that increases collagen content. Better models would assess quantitative outcomes such as gene expression, RNA, or protein expression. Advances in genomics and proteomics have improved the quality of cosmeceutical research, but these methods are expensive.

ANTIOXIDANTS

Free radicals, also called reactive oxygen species (ROS) or oxidants, are compounds with an unpaired electron that cause damage by stealing electrons from important cellular components in a process known as oxidation. The skin has numerous endogenous antioxidants to protect itself from environmental exposure. Antioxidants reduce activation of mitogen-activated protein kinases (MAPK), chelate copper to inhibit tyrosinase, and suppress inflammatory factors such as nuclear factor (NF)-κB.[6] Antioxidants are best known for their ability to neutralize ROS and take away their oxidation abilities. Free radicals are major culprits in aging. They injure mitochondria, lysosomes and other organelles, and alter gene expression toward pathways that degrade collagen. Free radicals also play a role in glycation of collagen, elastin, and other cell proteins, and can turn on inflammatory pathways.

Antioxidants neutralize ROS by providing another electron, which gives the oxygen ion an electron pair thereby stabilizing it. Once the antioxidant has given up its electron, it can no longer function as an antioxidant. The result is that they are consumed quickly by the skin accounting for why exogenously applied or ingested antioxidants are necessary.

To prevent the aging of skin through various pathways, using antioxidants is essential.[7] Antioxidants, such as tocopherol (vitamin E) and ascorbic acid (vitamin C), are known to protect collagen and elastin from glycation and free radical-induced damage, which contribute to cutaneous aging.[8] Mitochondria benefit from the presence of antioxidants because free radicals damage mitochondrial membranes leading to mutations of mitochondrial DNA, a decrease in ATP energy production processes, and ultimately to skin aging. Antioxidants can be taken orally or used topically. Both modes

of administration are probably ideal because antioxidants are rapidly used by the skin when it is exposed to environmental insults as discussed in Chapter 6, Extrinsic Aging. It is best to combine different antioxidants together in a formulation, rather than using just one type. For example, topical application of vitamins C and E with ferulic acid has been shown to reduce thymine dimer formation.[9] The ferulic acid helps increase the stability of the vitamin C and the vitamin E adds increased antioxidant protection.

Several antioxidants confer effects beyond scavenging ROS that make them unique. Coenzyme Q_{10} protects the mitochondria and aids in ATP production, ascorbic acid (vitamin C) stimulates procollagen genes in fibroblasts to increase collagen production,[10] and phloretin prevents UV-induced pigmentation by affecting the p53 pigmentation pathway through the rate-limiting step of p53 phosphorylation at site 15.[11,12] There is no one perfect antioxidant; combining as many as possible both orally and topically seems to be the best approach.

Ascorbic Acid

Also known as vitamin C, this antioxidant imparts anti-aging and tyrosinase-inhibiting effects. Along with retinol and sunscreen, vitamin C is one of the most important cosmeceutical ingredients for skin rejuvenation. It is used in anti-aging skincare regimens to increase collagen production and to scavenge free radicals. In 1987, a paper in the *Archives of Dermatology* first demonstrated that collagen synthesis could be induced by ascorbic acid.[13] This is not surprising because collagen production requires the presence of ascorbic acid.[14] Since 1987, myraid studies in high-impact journals have convincingly shown that collagen synthesis is increased by ascorbic acid,[10,15,16] and both young and old fibroblasts are responsive to it.[17]

Topical ascorbic acid has been shown to penetrate into skin when the L-ascorbic acid form is formulated at a pH of 2.5 or lower and protect the skin from free radicals.[9,18] Topical ascorbic acid should be used in the daytime to shield skin from UV light.[9,19] Oral doses of 1 g of ascorbic acid and 500 IUs of vitamin E (D-α-tocopherol) twice daily for 3 months have been shown to reduce susceptibility to sunburn from UVB exposure.[20] However, it is difficult to achieve high levels of vitamin C in the skin; therefore, topical and oral preparations are often used together.

The use of topical ascorbic acid is affected by its requirement for a low pH to achieve topical absorption and the fact that it easily breaks down upon exposure to light, oxygen, and any oxidizing ingredients. Adding ferulic acid to vitamin C has been demonstrated to stabilize the ascorbic acid.[21] Proper manufacturing, storage, and packaging will help keep the products stable. Once opened they should be discarded when the serum solution darkens, which indicates oxidation. Using a low-pH cleanser prior to applying ascorbic acid may help penetration (see Chapter 35). Ascorbic acid is one of the most important and proven ingredients for skin rejuvenation and will be discussed at length in Chapters 39, Antioxidants, and 41, Depigmenting Ingredients.

Argan Oil

Derived from the fruit of *Argania spinosa*, argan oil has been used for several hundred years for multiple purposes in Morocco, and is now employed as a treatment for acne, dry skin, dry hair, hair loss, psoriasis, wrinkles, skin inflammation, and joint pain.[22,23] This phenolic-rich oil is thought to be effective in conferring barrier repair, anti-inflammatory, and wound healing effects.[24] Further, daily topical application of argan oil has been demonstrated to enhance skin elasticity and hydration by aiding barrier function and supporting its capacity for water retention.[24,25] Its copious supply of linoleic acid provides argan oil with hydrating and anti-inflammatory properties in addition to anti-aging properties.

Coenzyme Q$_{10}$

Ubiquinone or coenzyme Q$_{10}$ (CoQ$_{10}$) is a fat-soluble component of the mitochondrial respiratory chain present in all human cells that plays a role in ATP production. Levels of CoQ$_{10}$ are 10-fold higher in the epidermis as compared to the dermis.[26] CoQ$_{10}$ also acts as a lipophilic antioxidant that can protect cell membranes. It is available in oral and topical formulations. Among antioxidants depleted from the dermis and epidermis due to UV exposure (such as vitamins C and E, glutathione, and CoQ$_{10}$), CoQ$_{10}$ has been found to be the first to diminish and is also associated with age-related decline.[7] As an antioxidant, it has been shown to foster collagen synthesis.[27,28]

Cholesterol-lowering drugs in the statin family decrease levels of CoQ$_{10}$. It is thought that the lower levels of CoQ$_{10}$ account for oxidative stress and mitochondrial dysfunction leading to premature aging of skin fibroblast cells seen *in vitro*.[29] Many physicians recommend oral CoQ$_{10}$ to patients on statin drugs. Oral CoQ$_{10}$ should be taken only in the morning due to its caffeine-like effect. Topically applied CoQ10 has been shown to improve the appearance of aged skin.[30] Topical CoQ$_{10}$ has a dark yellow color and may not be desirable to some patients for this reason. Like niacinamide, CoQ$_{10}$ acts to deliver cellular energy and improve DNA repair. In small studies, topical CoQ$_{10}$ has been found to ameliorate the appearance of wrinkles and, *in vitro*, decrease matrix metalloproteinase (MMP)-1 expression.[31-33]

Green Tea

Green tea is popular as an anti-redness, anti-aging, and antioxidant ingredient. EpiGalloCatechin-3-O-Gallate (EGCG), the primary active component of green tea, induces IL-12 to promote the production of enzymes that repair UV-induced DNA damage.[34] The established photoprotective effects of topical and oral green tea include the reduction of UV-induced erythema, sunburn cell formation, and DNA damage.[35] In 2010, Reuter et al. determined that the oral administration and topical application of antioxidant plant extracts of green and black tea, among other botanicals, can protect skin against the deleterious effects of UV exposure, including erythema, premature aging, and cancer.[36] Anti-elastase and anti-collagenase activities have been associated with white tea.[37] Green tea

extracts in combination with other ingredients have since been shown in small human trials to exert anti-wrinkle effects,[38,39] and topical green tea has also been demonstrated to dose-dependently suppress the erythema response engendered by UV exposure.[35]

Resveratrol

Resveratrol (*trans*-3,5,4'-trihydroxystilbene), a polyphenolic phytoalexin synthesized in nearly 70 species and found notably in the skin and seeds of grapes, as well as berries, peanuts, red wine, purple grape juice, grapefruits, and other plant sources, is known to possess robust antioxidant, antiproliferative, and anti-inflammatory characteristics.[28,40-47] The topical application of resveratrol in a proprietary blend (1% resveratrol, 0.5% baicalin, 1% vitamin E) rendered a statistically significant improvement in fine lines and wrinkles, hyperpigmentation, radiance, as well as skin roughness, firmness, elasticity, and laxity in a small 12-week study.[48] In an earlier pre-clinical study, the use of resveratrol prevented UVB-induced skin edema.[45] This potent antioxidant is also known to facilitate the expression of sirtuin genes, thus extending cell life.[28,49] Resveratrol is popular in anti-aging preparations but does not penetrate well so it should be combined with penetration enhancers to maximize its effects.

ANTI-INFLAMMATORIES

Inflammation emerges from various etiologic pathways, with several inflammatory mediators potentially involved, including histamines, cytokines, eicosanoids (e.g., prostaglandins, thromboxanes, and leukotrienes), complement cascade components, kinins, fibrinopeptide enzymes, NF-κB, and free radicals. Once one of the inflammatory pathways is triggered, it is more likely that other inflammatory pathways will be activated leading to a vicious cycle well known to patients with sensitive skin. Inflammation contributes to cutaneous aging through multiple mechanisms such as increasing free radicals and activating the immune system. Skin inflammation has also been linked to systemic conditions such as heart disease, diabetes, and Alzheimer's (see Chapter 13, Sensitive Skin).[50]

Several ingredients confer anti-inflammatory activity and have been used successfully in topical skin formulations, including aloe, argan oil, caffeine, chamomile, feverfew, green tea, licorice extract, linoleic acid (present in high concentrations in argan oil and safflower oil), resveratrol, and others (see **Table 37-1**).

Anti-inflammatories can be taken orally or used topically. The addition of linoleic acid oils to the diet can increase inflammation (see Chapter 9, Nutrition and the Skin). Oral supplements have also been shown to help reduce inflammation, especially after sun exposure. For example, the effect of UV radiation on COX-2 expression has been demonstrated to be suppressed through the use of oral polypodium leucotomos.[51] Anti-inflammatories will be further discussed in Chapter 38, Anti-Inflammatory Ingredients.

TABLE 37-1	Anti-inflammatory Ingredients for the Skin

- 4-Ethoxybenzaldehyde
- 7-(1H-imidazol-4-ylmethyl)-5,6,7,8-tetrahydroquinoline
- Allantoin
- Aloe
- Argan oil
- Arnica
- Bisabolol
- Caffeine
- Caffeyl glucoside
- Chamomile
- Colloidal oatmeal
- Cucumber extract
- Feverfew
- Gallyl glucoside (Endothelyol™)
- Grape seed extract
- Green tea (epigallocatechin-3-gallate (EGCG); epigallocatechin gallatyl glucoside or Unisooth®)
- Inoveal EGCG
- Licorice extract
- Macadamia nut oil
- Niacinamide (nicotinamide)
- Portulaca oleracea extract
- Resveratrol
- Rosmarinyl glucoside
- Safflower oil
- Unimoist U-125

Glycosaminoglycans

Glycosaminoglycans (GAGs) are polysaccharide chains composed of repeating disaccharide units linked to a core protein. Together the GAGs and attached core protein form proteoglycans (PG). GAGs make up a large portion of the extracellular matrix (ECM). The ECM is like a large water- and gel-filled cushion that surrounds the skin cells, protecting them from compression and providing them shape while allowing cell signals to float and move between cells so they can communicate.

The ECM gives skin its volume, bulk, and resiliency (see Chapter 2, Basic Science of the Dermis). PGs and GAGs bind water molecules, dampening mechanical forces and cushioning tissues.[52] The ECM interacts with fibroblasts in a structural organization that allows fibroblasts to spread and exert mechanical forces. The fibroblast-ECM structure is disrupted in aging and becomes unbalanced. Once this aged phenotype occurs, fibroblasts begin producing fewer GAGs and more MMPs, which further hastens aging.[52] Increasing GAGs in aged skin improves its appearance (e.g., HA dermal fillers). GAGs avidly bind water, plumping up the skin, and contribute to the maintenance of salt and water balance, thus playing a role in skin hydration. The most abundant GAGs in the dermis are HA, which is the only nonsulfated GAG, and dermatan sulfate. The other GAGs include heparan sulfate, keratan sulfate, chondroitin-4, and chondroitin-6-sulfate.

Hyaluronic Acid

Hyaluronic acid (HA) is a vital component of the dermis responsible for attracting water and providing volume to this layer of the skin (see Chapter 2). The name reflects its glassy appearance (the Greek word for glass is *hyalos*) and the presence of a sugar known as uronic acid. HA is known to be important in cell growth, membrane receptor function, and adhesion. HA appears to also play a role in keratinocyte differentiation and formation of lamellar bodies via its interaction with CD44,[53] a cell surface glycoprotein receptor with HA binding sites.[54–56] Its structure is identical, whether it is derived from bacterial cultures, animals, or humans (**Fig. 37-1**). HA appears freely in the dermis and is more concentrated in areas where cells are less densely packed. In young skin, HA is found at the periphery of collagen and elastin fibers and at the interfaces of these types of fibers. Such connections with HA are absent in aged skin.[57] HA is available in many different injectable dermal fillers for the treatment of wrinkles (see Chapter 25, Dermal Fillers). When injected into the skin, HA increases in volume, promotes fibroblast production of collagen, enhances the structural support of the ECM, expands mechanical forces in the area(s) of injection, and mediates upregulation of TGF-β and connective tissue growth factor.[58] It is unknown if topically applied HA imparts these effects because the size and crosslinking of HA in topical products varies.

HA is a popular ingredient in cosmetic products because it acts as a humectant and increases the penetration of other ingredients.[59] It avidly binds water, affecting skin hydration, volume, and plumpness.[28] HA also influences cellular mobilization and communication, and may protect collagen from degradation through the activity of interleukin (IL)-1.[60] HA is extremely hydrophilic; therefore, it is surprising that it can penetrate into the skin.[59] Its unique structure seems to allow it to penetrate to all layers of the epidermis if the molecule size is less than 500 kDa. The humectant properties of HA allow it to bind 1000 times its weight in water, and such characteristics render it a useful addition to multiple skincare products because it plumps skin almost immediately. In fact, its topical use has been demonstrated to enhance skin hydration,[61] particularly in a humid environment. A significant decrease in wrinkle depth was observed in a study of 76 female patients with periocular wrinkles who were administered 0.1% cream containing low-molecular HA (50 and 130 kDa).[61]

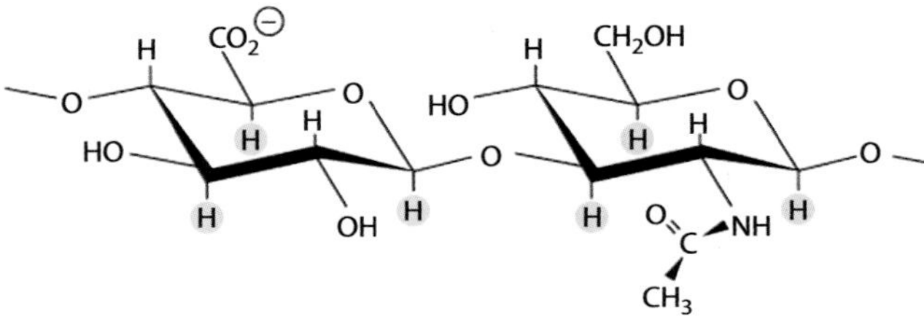

FIGURE 37-1. Hyaluronic acid is a nonsulfated glycosaminoglycan. It is a polymer of disaccharides made of alternating D-glucuronic acid and N-acetyl-D-glucosamine.

HA resides for a short time in the dermis before being broken down. The absorption of HA depends on the molecular weight and size of the HA chains in the formulation and if they are crosslinked or not. Larger and crosslinked HA will more likely remain on the skin's surface imparting humectant properties (uncrosslinked HA, when large, stays on the skin's surface and when small can enter the skin). HA is often used in topical drugs to increase skin penetration. It is important to remember that when combining HA with a retinol, increased side effects may be seen to increase absorption of the retinoid. Cosmeceutical products often combine various types of HA.

In a dry environment, HA can draw water from the skin, thus rendering it dehydrated. Therefore, in a dry environment, HA should be used in combination with moisturizers containing occlusive ingredients. Individuals with oily skin types can use HA in any environment because their sebum acts as an occlusive agent. Oily skin types seem to prefer moisturizers containing HA because such products hydrate without causing the stickiness associated with glycerin, oils, and occlusive ingredients.

Heparan Sulfate

Heparan sulfate (HS), another component of the ECM, increases cellular response to growth factors and plays a significant role in intercellular communications (**Fig. 37-2**). HS is an essential GAG, which enhances cellular response to growth factors by promoting the response of old, indolent fibroblasts to cellular signals. In other words, it helps old fibroblasts better hear and respond to cell signals. Old fibroblasts have glycated collagen, elastin fragments, and senescent cells between them in the ECM leaving it more difficult for the cell signals to pass from cell to cell. This clutter can block cytokines and growth factors from reaching their target receptors. HS ensures that the cell signals get to the receptor targets on the fibroblasts. Also, HS binds and stores growth factors and protects them until they arrive at their target receptors. Once at the receptor, they present the growth factor or cytokine to the appropriate binding site.[62] In a way, they chaperone the cell signals until they get to their destination. HS, in the form of a proprietary heparan sulfate analogue, has been found to rejuvenate photodamaged skin by improving skin hydration, firmness, elasticity, and barrier function.[63] As with other GAGs, the improvement of wrinkles is almost immediate as the HS binds water and pulls it to the skin's surface.

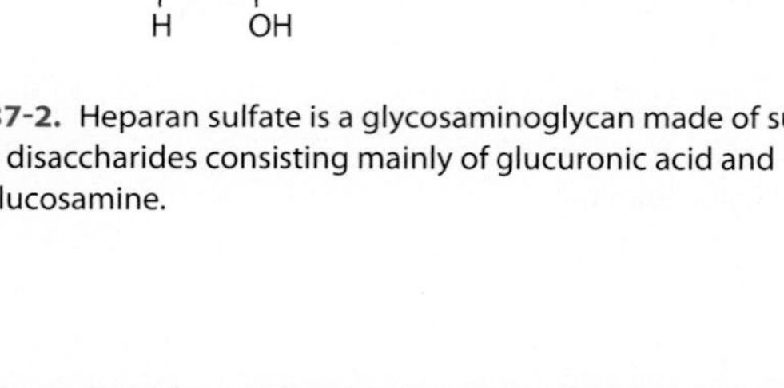

FIGURE 37-2. Heparan sulfate is a glycosaminoglycan made of sulfated repeating disaccharides consisting mainly of glucuronic acid and N-acetylglucosamine.

GAGs give wrinkled skin an almost immediate improvement in texture and appearance as all humectants do. However, they offer some long-lasting benefits as discussed above if they are small enough to enter the skin or if they are injected. GAGs should be combined with other anti-aging ingredients that have been shown to increase collagen production such as retinoids and ascorbic acid for maximum effects. HA and HS are great options for oily skin types who want a lighter, non-greasy product as a moisturizer.

Hydroxy Acids

Alpha hydroxy acids, with glycolic and lactic acids the most popular, have been known for decades to normalize SC keratinization and exfoliation.[64–66] Exfoliation triggers the epidermal stem cells to produce more keratinocytes to repopulate the epidermis. This, in turn, stimulates fibroblasts and spurs collagen genes to increase collagen and HA synthesis.[66–68] Other alpha hydroxy acids used to treat aging skin include citric, pyruvic, mandelic, and tartaric acids.[28,69] Alpha hydroxy acids are hydrophilic. Beta hydroxy acids, actually a misnomer adopted for marketing reasons (the side group is not actually in the beta position), are lipophilic. Salicylic acid is the beta hydroxy acid used in cosmeceuticals. It can penetrate through sebum and clear pores. Alpha hydroxy acids are humectants and display hydrating properties, while salicylic acid can dry skin by penetrating into pores and removing sebum. Both alpha hydroxy acids and salicylic acid increase desquamation and are effective adjuvants to any skincare routine because they improve penetration of other products and speed keratinization, thus achieving observable results more quickly.

Many studies have revealed success using alpha hydroxy acid and beta hydroxy acid products in the treatment of photoaging by ameliorating fine lines, ephelides (freckles), lentigines, mottled pigmentation, surface roughness, as well as actinic and seborrheic keratoses.[28,67,70] Topical formulations containing hydroxy acids affect epidermal keratinization by accelerating the cell cycle and reducing corneocyte cohesiveness, leading to increased desquamation.[64,71,72] Ascorbic acid, which also acts as an antioxidant, is known to exert the same activity, stimulating collagen genes yielding fibroblast augmentation of Type 1 collagen production.[10,17] (See Chapter 40, Cleansing Agents, for a discussion on hydroxy acids in cleansers and Chapter 24, Chemical Peels, for hydroxy acids in peels.)

Patient compliance is a significant problem in dermatology as discussed in Chapter 34, Skincare Retail in a Medical Setting. Most anti-aging products, with the exception of glycerin, GAGs, and defensins, take weeks to months to see results. Patients get impatient and adherence decreases. Adding hydroxy acids in the first or second phases of a skincare treatment plan will encourage compliance by offering faster results. Using hydroxy acids in pre-procedure regimens as discussed in Chapter 36, Pre- and Post-Procedure Skincare, will stimulate fibroblasts and speed healing. They should not be used until the skin has completely re-epithelialized after the procedure.

Niacinamide

Niacinamide, also known as nicotinamide or vitamin B_3, plays an essential role in the redox reactions involving the niacin coenzymes nicotinamide adenine dinucleotide (NAD+), nicotinamide adenine dinucleotide phosphate (NADP+), and their reduced forms NADH and NADPH. In turn, these coenzymes play a role in multiple cell reactions because they are involved in transferring electrons and the release of energy stored in oxygen bonds. These coenzymes are both oxidizing and reducing agents. They contribute to DNA production and repair among other cellular functions that require energy.

Niacinamide aids DNA repair by giving energy to DNA repair enzymes to unwind the DNA strand, replacing the nucleoside, and rewinding the strand.[73] Notably, niacinamide enhances DNA excision repair and correction of UVB-induced cyclobutane pyrimidine dimers and UVA-induced 8-oxo-7,8-dihydro-2′-deoxyguanosine[74] (**Figs. 37-3A–C**).

Niacinamide is used topically because oral forms of niacin are associated with flushing. Daily application of a 5% niacinamide cream has been demonstrated to reduce wrinkles and achieve other clinical improvements in skin texture and elasticity in several randomized, placebo-controlled trials.[28,75–77] Niacinamide also exhibits anti-inflammatory functions (see Chapter 38). It is used in skin-lightening regimens to treat pigmentation issues because it blocks the PAR-2 receptor preventing melanosome transfer into keratinocytes (see Chapter 41, Depigmenting Ingredients).

GROWTH FACTORS

In the skin, growth factors (GFs) are substances, usually proteins, secreted by keratinocytes, fibroblasts, platelets, and immune cells (mast cells and lymphocytes).[78] GFs have the capacity to directly stimulate genes or act as a signaling mechanism when presented to cell surface receptors by ECM components such as HS.

GFs affect cell migration, growth, proliferation, and differentiation. There are several kinds of GFs that can activate old keratinocytes and fibroblasts to enhance function.[79] GFs do not work in isolation; their presence affects the actions of other GFs. It is difficult to know the true effects of GFs when they are studied one at a time. In other words, GFs work as a team, each playing a specific role. When one is absent, the actions of other GFs may be affected.

GFs are formulated into topical skincare products with the intention that they will increase collagen, HA, or elastin production and help return skin cells to youthful function. However, there are many challenges to using GFs topically on the skin. GFs are unstable when subjected to higher temperatures that occur during product manufacturing. (Lipids and waxy substances like ceramides require higher temperatures during mixing.) High temperatures can also occur during storage and delivery of skincare products.[80] For GFs to deliver a biologic effect on the skin, the topically applied products must be able to penetrate into the target tissue (epidermis or

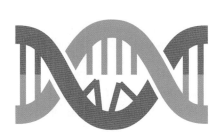

FIGURE 37-3A. Thymidine dimers form between nucleotides. These mutations cause aging and skin cancer.

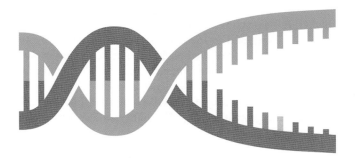

FIGURE 37-3B. Niacinamide gives the energy for DNA helicases to unwind the DNA helix.

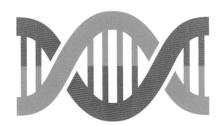

FIGURE 37-3C. The altered nucleotides are replaced with the correct ones, which also requires energy.

dermis), find the appropriate genes or receptors, and initiate a signal transduction cascade in order for the target cells to respond to their signals.[81] GFs are larger than the 500 kDa size that the epidermis allows to enter; therefore, ensuring that they arrive at the target tissue is difficult and requires special formulations. GFs break down rapidly and it is likely that few remain in the finished skincare product. The positive findings associated with some GF cosmeceutical studies may be due to the nutrient-rich media in which the GFs are cultured rather than the GFs themselves.

There are various types of GFs and each GF can bind to different types of receptors. In other words, all GFs are not the same. As mentioned above, GFs work together and affect each other and stimulate each other's receptors. Consequently, studying them in isolation may reveal different results than what is seen *in vivo*. The most common GFs found in anti-aging skincare products are discussed here but there are many more GFs and cytokines that can affect the skin.

Epidermal Growth Factor Family

The epidermal growth factor (EGF) family contains four proteins that are similar in structure, act on the same receptors, and have the same activity.[82] These GFs stimulate the proliferation and migration of keratinocytes, promote fibroblast motility, affect hair growth, spur the growth of sebaceous and sweat glands, increase HA production,[83] and play a role in wound healing. There are four types, but this discussion will focus on the epidermal growth factor receptor (EGFR).

Epidermal-derived Growth Factor

The EGFR is a glycoprotein on the cell surface membrane that is strongly expressed in the basal layer of the epidermis and the outer root sheath of the hair follicle. Its activation is modulated by ECM components, integrins, cytokine receptors, and ligands that bind the EGFR. The ligands include amphiregulin, betacellulin, epiregulin, EGF, TGF-α, heparin-binding EGF, and EGF-like growth factor.[84] UV light can also activate the EGFR.

When the EGFR is bound by EGF or a ligand, tyrosine kinase and other signal transduction pathways are activated that regulate cellular proliferation, differentiation, and survival. Once tyrosine kinase is activated, cellular calcium levels are increased, and DNA synthesis is induced.[85] EGFR activation stimulates proliferation and migration of keratinocytes, fosters fibroblast motility, and affects the skin barrier.[86] When UV light activates the EGFR, inhibition of apoptosis of keratinocytes results. EGF has been studied extensively and used in wound treatment products to speed wound healing.

The mitochondria convert ADP into ATP, producing energy; this is catalyzed by the enzyme creatine kinase. Phosphocreatine (PCR) is the molecule that stores energy in this reaction. The CPK/PCR system is important in helping protect the skin from ischemia and UV radiation.

EGF, when applied topically to murine skin, causes an over 50% decline in cytoplasmic creatinine kinase activity. The significance of this is not understood and there is no published follow-up to this 2008 study.[87]

EGF is found in cosmeceutical products as are GFs that upregulate production of EGF. Cosmeceutical ingredients such as phytosphingosine-1-phosphate (PhS1P), isolated from plants and fungi, stimulate the EGFR.[88] However, EGF is not justified for cosmetic use because EGF, or any substance that activates the EGFR, could increase proliferation of malignant cells,[89] such as skin cancer.[82,90] Plant- and fungal-derived EGF are no safer than human-derived EGFs.

EGFR inhibitors are used systemically to treat tumors such as small cell lung cancer. Systemic inhibition of the EGFR can decrease epidermal hyperproliferation, but can yield inflammation, folliculitis, acne, xerosis, altered hair growth, and nail abnormalities.[91] Topical EGFR inhibitors such as genistein, quercetin, daidzein, and glycitein are found in topical cosmeceuticals.[92] These have been shown to decrease keratinocyte proliferation and skin scaling due to increased levels of EGF that occur with overuse of detergents or when beginning retinoids.[84]

Transforming Growth Factor Alpha (TGF-α)

TGF-α is produced by keratinocytes. It shares the EGF receptor with EGF; therefore, the EGFR is often called the EGF/TGF α receptor. TGF-α binds the EGF/TGF receptor or it can directly stimulate keratinocytes.[93] TGF exhibits similar actions to EGF such as initiating proliferation of keratinocytes. Exogenously applied EGF or TGF-α increases the expression of TGF-α, which has been shown to play a role in angiogenesis. TGF-α upregulates production of angiogenic chemokines and is a well-established mediator of inflammation in psoriasis. Biologic medications to treat psoriasis block the binding of TGF-α to its receptor. TGF-α is expressed in squamous cell carcinoma cells,[93] and malignant tumors,[89,94] making it a poor choice for use in cosmeceuticals.

Fibroblast Growth Factor Family

Fibroblast Growth Factor (FGF)

There are at least 23 different growth factors in the FGF family that are essential for metabolism and development. Multiple cell types can secrete FGFs including fibroblasts, mast cells, and macrophages. FGF-1 and FGF-2 trigger proliferation of various cell types including keratinocytes and fibroblasts.[95] FGF binding to fibroblast growth factor receptors (FGFR) is assisted by heparan sulfate proteoglycans. Signaling from activated FGFR is important for controlling angiogenesis, metabolism, wound healing, and tissue repair among other activities. Basic fibroblast growth factor (bFGF) has been demostrated to increase the production of HA by human fibroblasts.[83] Abnormal activity of FGFR has been reported in a wide range of cancers. One study found FGFR involvement in 7% of cancers.[96] For this reason, use of FGFs in skincare products is not advised at this time.

Keratinocyte Growth Factor (KGF)

KGF is a member of the FGF family, but it appears to act only on epithelial cells.[97] In keratinocytes, KGF promotes early differentiation, inhibits terminal differentiation and apoptosis, induces cell migration, and reorganizes the skin's actin cytoskeleton. KGF helps transfer melanosomes into keratinocytes from melanocytes.[98] It may strengthen the skin by thickening the epidermis. As with other GFs, it is very difficult to introduce KGF into the skin when delivered topically.[99]

Insulin-like Growth Factor (IGF)-I

IGF-1 is produced by melanocytes and fibroblasts. It plays a critical role in the regulation of stress-induced apoptosis as well as keratinocyte and fibroblast survival.[100] The IGF-1 signaling pathway delays apoptosis and temporarily halts DNA replication giving the cells more time for DNA repair prior to replication.[101] As dermal fibroblasts age, they produce less IGF-1 and keratinocytes are more prone to damage and mutations. This is one reason why sun exposure is more damaging to older skin than younger skin. IGF-1 has been shown to protect mitochondria and restore mitochondrial function.[102] Increased levels of IGF have been associated with younger subjects as compared to older subjects.[103]

Transforming Growth Factor β (TGF-β)

TGF-β1 is an important GF used in skin rejuvenation and wound healing.[104] It is the major regulator in the production of ECM components. TGF-β stimulates dermal collagen remodeling, as well as the synthesis of collagen, elastin, and HA, and decreases MMPs.[83,105–107] When the TGF-β receptor is bound by a ligand and activated, Smad proteins help propagate the signal. This TGF-β/Smad pathway acts as a tumor suppressor pathway by inhibiting epithelial cell proliferation. UV radiation inhibits the TGF-β/Smad pathway, which contributes to photoaging and the development of skin cancer.[108] Because TGF-β confers such positive effects on skin rejuvenation, several methods have been used to coerce fibroblasts to secrete more TGF-β. 17β-estradiol increases TGF-β production and topically applied retinol increases TGF-β/Smad pathway activity.[109,110] Fibroblasts that are in hypoxic conditions produce more TGF-β.[111] TGF-β seems safe to use on skin; in fact, a *decrease* in TGF-β may predispose skin to cancer, but much more data are needed.[112,113]

Vascular Endothelial Growth Factor

VEGF contributes to the skin inflammation seen in atopic dermatitis and causes vessels to leak leading to swelling.[114] VEGF stimulates the growth of melanoma cells in cell cultures and may contribute to the pathogenesis of systemic sclerosis.[115,116] Its use is not suggested in cosmeceuticals.

Platelet-derived Growth Factors

PDGF levels are increased in hypoxic conditions, and with stimulation by various growth factors and cytokines. Activation of the platelet-derived growth factor receptor (PDGFR) leads to changes in cell shape and motility, reorganization of the actin filament system, and stimulation of chemotaxis. PDGF plays an important role in wound healing by affecting cell migration. It increases production of ECM components such as fibronectin, collagen, proteoglycans, and HA.[83] Production of PDGF is reduced in old fibroblasts.[117]

The use of PDGF is limited by the evidence that it can cause malignant tumors.[118]

Many different growth factors are found in cosmeceuticals although there is a paucity of research on which growth factors work best together to rejuvenate the skin.[119] TGF-β has the most data to support its use. However, GFs are characterized by temperature instability and have difficulty penetrating into the skin because they are larger than the 500 kDa size identified as the threshold for penetration into the epidermis.[120,121] GFs can be rapidly broken down by protease enzymes in the skin. For this reason, the way that the products are formulated and the position they are placed in the skin regimen is very important (see Chapter 35).

Topical Cosmeceuticals That Contain Growth Factors

Human Conditioned Fibroblast Media

Human conditioned fibroblast media, known commercially as TNS® (Tissue Nutrient Solution) and Nouri-Cel-MD® (both from SkinMedica®, Carlsbad, CA, USA), is extracted from cultured neonatal human dermal fibroblasts. The company website boasts that the TNS products contain 380 GFs, cytokines, and matrix proteins; however, they do not specify which ones.[122] Proprietary protein stabilization techniques are used to render the GFs temperature stable. An article by Mehta et al. used a RayBio® Human Cytokine Antibody Array G series 2000 assay to detect GFs in TNS and an ELISA assay to quantify GFs.[123] They found over 110 GFs and cytokines in the products that were stored in five different lots for varying amounts of time, which testifies to the fact that GFs survived the formulation process. Some of the GFs found in TNS are listed in **Table 37-2**.

TABLE 37-2	Growth Factors Isolated from Tissue Nutrient Solution (TNS)[123] (This is only a partial list as the substance contains over 300 growth factors according to SkinMedica®.)
Bone morphogenetic protein: BMP7	
Colony stimulating factors: GCSF, GM-CSF, M-CSF	
Fibroblast growth factors: bFGF (FGF-2), FGF-4, FGF-6, KGF (FGF-7), FGF-9	
Hepatocyte growth factors: HGF	
Insulin-like growth factors: IGF-1, IGF-BP1, IGF-BP2, IGF-BP3, IGF-BP6w	
Interleukin: IL-1a, IL-1B, IL-2, IL-3, IL-4, IL-6, IL-7, IL-8 IL-10, IL-13, IL-15	
Leptin	
Placenta growth factor: PLGF	
Platelet-derived growth factors: PDGF AA, PDGF BB, PDGF Rb	
Tissue inhibitor of metalloproteinases: TIMP1 (MPI1), TIMP2 (MPI2)	
Transforming growth factor: TGF-β1, TGF-β2, TGF-β3	
Vascular endothelial growth factor: VEGF	

In the Mehta study, 60 male and female subjects with mild to severe facial photodamage were treated with Nouri-Cel-MD versus a vehicle. Subjects underwent a 28-day washout period using only Cetaphil gentle skin cleanser and Cetaphil daily facial moisturizer with an SPF 15. The subjects were blinded and asked to apply the study products after cleansing and before moisturizing twice a day for 6 months. Optical profilometry measurements using silicone impressions of the crow's feet were performed at baseline, 3 months, and 6 months. Fine line and texture shadows showed statistically significant improvement in the subjects using the study products versus placebo only at month 3 and not at month 6 (the text of the article explains the results differently than it is displayed in **Table 37-2** of the data and P values are not given so this was difficult to interpret). There was no statistical difference in optical profilometry measurements between the active and the vehicle for major line R_a, fine line and texture R_a, or major line shadow at any time point. In spite of only one parameter (fine line and texture shadow) showing statistical significance (at month 3), the text reports: "The results provide evidence that treatment with the active gel for 3 months produces greater reduction in fine lines and wrinkles than the vehicle treatment," and these differences were "either significant or trending towards statistical significance," and, "The results confirm beneficial effects of active gel at 6 months." These statements are misleading. "Trending towards statistical significance" means it was *not* statistically significant and it is not correct to say that beneficial effects were seen at 6 months because statistical significance was *not* seen at 6 months. Photographs with a Canfield Visia® CR photography system were taken at baseline, 3 months, and 6 months and analyzed by three independent and blinded board-certified dermatologists using an 11-point photodamage scale. The only statistically significant finding was that subjects who had a baseline score of 4 (severe for photodamage) at baseline showed an improvement at 6 months (P = 0.014) but the data do not explain if this is an improvement from baseline or as compared to vehicle. (In other words, did the vehicle group also show improvement?) Blinded investigators evaluated the patients at each visit and assessed fine wrinkling, tactile roughness, telangiectasia, mottled pigmentation, and sallowness on a five-point scale. The paper states that a statistically significant reduction for fine wrinkles was seen in the active group but not the vehicle group. The data compare the active to baseline but not to the performance of the vehicle, so the significance is unclear. The subjects' assessment data did not report any statistically significant differences between active and vehicle. Despite the fact that the data showing efficacy are very slight, the abstract of the article states, "This study demonstrates that addition of a topical formulation of growth factors and cytokines to a basic skincare regimen reduces the signs of photoaging." Adverse events were mild. The safety of long-term use of the 110 GFs was not addressed in the article and there are no publications examining long-term use.

Processed Skin Proteins

Processed skin proteins (PSP®, Bio-restorative Skin Cream, Neocutis, Merz, Frankfurt, Germany) contains at least 16 GFs including IL-10 from fibroblasts grown in culture.[124] There are two studies quoted to support its use. The first was a double-blind, placebo-controlled, split-face trial comparing PSP to vehicle placebo in which 18 subjects applied the products to the face twice daily for 60 days.[125] Surface topography of the skin was tested using the PRIMO 3D device. The results revealed a statistical significance between active and placebo in some, but not all, roughness measures at 2 months; however, a P value was not given. Two independent blinded investigators using a five-point scale demonstrated that both the active and the placebo ameliorated crow's feet lines but there was no statistical difference between the active and placebo formulations.

In another study of PSP®, 37 females with fine lines and dark circles around the eyes underwent a 4-week washout period using SPF only.[124] (It does not specify if they were allowed to cleanse their face and what facial cleanser they used.) The subjects applied the study product to only one side of the face in the periorbital eye area for 6 weeks. There was no vehicle control. Investigators rated the appearance of skin color, texture, sagging, and wrinkles of the treated and untreated eye using a five-point scale. The data only looked at the treated side and did not compare to the untreated side. The baseline measurements of each parameter were averaged at baseline and at 6 weeks and compared. (The publication stated "6 months" but this is likely an error because it does not match the study design section that cited "6 weeks.") The investigators reported that the treated side, when compared only to itself at baseline, showed a 14–18% improvement in skin color, texture, sagging, and wrinkles. It should be remembered that the baseline scores were taken after 4 weeks of not using anything but sunscreen on the face so dehydration and an accumulation of keratinocytes in the SC were very likely present at baseline. In addition, the investigators knew which side had been treated. The study does not specify if the investigators knew which eye was the treated eye. Subjects completed a questionnaire asking about their eye area and reported improvement in all areas except eye puffiness. They knew which eye area was treated and were biased. In addition, the opposite eye area was untreated with any product so results may be due to hydration alone as the eye cream contained HA, a known humectant that hydrates skin. This study was very poorly designed, and the results do not provide any conclusive evidence at all except that an eye cream hydrates the eye area when compared to not using an eye cream. It provides no insights into the efficacy of GFs for the treatment of periorbital skin. There are no P values to be found and it is surprising that this study was accepted for publication. The abstract stated that "the clinical signs of wrinkles, sagging, dark circles and skin texture show significant improvement."

Plant-based Epidermal-derived Growth Factor

Bioeffect® EGF (Reykjavik, Iceland) is a 6 kDa polypeptide GF that was popular to treat wounds until it was found that human carcinomas express high levels of EGF receptors and its presence is associated with more aggressive tumors.[126] Despite the safety questions, a serum containing recombinant EGF produced from barley was developed to treat aged skin. This EGF-containing serum was examined in an open-label trial in 29 participants at least 30 years old with photoaging. The participants completed a survey in which they rated improvements in brown spots, red spots, age spots, and skin smoothness on a five-point scale, and differences were compared by paired t-tests. The study found that twice-daily application of EGF serum for 3 months significantly improved brown spotting, skin texture, pore size, red spotting, and wrinkles versus baseline ($P < 0.0002$ for all assessments). This open-label trial has inherent bias and did not contain a control group, so the data are not sufficient to claim efficacy for photoaging. In addition, the safety of this EGF gel has not been established.

CRS with Growth Factor

CRS Cell Rejuvenation System (Citrix®, Topix Pharmaceuticals, Amityville, NY, USA) contains TGF-β1, L-ascorbic acid, and extract from the plant *Cimicifuga racemose* in a liposome delivery vehicle to increase stability. This product was examined in a split-face, blinded, randomized study in women with facial wrinkling.[127] The study product was TGF-β1 and ascorbic acid and the vehicle contained just ascorbic acid. Twelve females applied the study cream to one side of the face and the vehicle to the other twice a day. In a second study published confusingly in the same publication, the identical study product was compared to SkinMedica TNS®. In this case, 20 females applied the study cream to one side of the face and the TNS product to the other twice daily for 3 months. Photos were taken with a Canfield Visia camera system and were assessed by four independent blinded dermatologists using a five-point wrinkle severity scale. Patients completed questionnaires. Treatment was considered successful if wrinkles were improved or stable from baseline. The data are confusing because the two studies are discussed together and it is hard to discern if the patients and live investigators were blinded. Also, it is difficult to understand which data are derived from the blinded dermatologist's assessments of the photos and which come from live investigator assessments. In the case of the CRS study, the effect of the cytokine TGF-β1 on photoaging was not clear. The paper concluded that the CRC and the TNS products improved wrinkles, but the sample size was too small to reach statistical significance.

Snail-derived Cryptomphalus aspersa (SCA)

Secretions from the snail *Cryptomphalus aspersa* (SCA) are a glycoprotein compound often included in GF discussions, although it is not a GF. A double-blind, split-face, placebo-controlled trial comparing morning application of 8% SCA emulsion and an evening application of 40% liquid serum (active group) to a placebo vehicle emulsion in the morning and a placebo serum in the evening (placebo group) included 25 subjects randomized to use the two active products on one side of the face and the placebo products on the other for 12 weeks.[128] Evaluations were made by the subjects and investigators at baseline and Weeks 8 and 12. Two weeks after the product was discontinued (14 weeks) the investigators performed another assessment. Silastic skin impressions were taken at baseline and 12 weeks. At 12 weeks, when compared to baseline, the investigator ratings of the active group demonstrated a statistically significant improvement ($P = 0.03$) of wrinkles around the eyes while the placebo did not. There were no other statistically significant findings at Week 12. The paper stated that the silicone replica cast of the crow's feet showed statistically significant improvement at Week 12; however, the P value was cited as ≤ 0.05 and a P value of 0.05 is not considered significant so that conclusion is invalid. This study claimed that SCA exhibits antioxidant properties, increases fibroblast proliferation, reduces MMPs, and plays a role in fibronectin assembly, but there are sparse data to support this conclusion.[129] At this time, there is not enough evidence to recommend the use of these snail secretions for aging skin.

Safety of Growth Factors

To date, it is unknown which GFs or combinations of GFs in cosmeceuticals play a stimulatory or inhibitory role in skin cancer.[78] It is known that carcinomas exhibit EGF receptors and the presence of EGF worsens prognosis.[130] There is evidence to suggest that EGF, TGF-α, FGF, VEGF, and PDGF play a detrimental role in cancer as discussed previously. Skincare products containing GFs isolated from cultured fibroblast cells have been on the market for decades. The safety of these GFs remains poorly understood,[78] especially in the presence of skin cancer. There have not been any proven cases of skin cancer arising from their use, but a lawsuit filed in 2014 claimed that manufacturers failed to disclose the risks to consumers; it was dismissed in 2018.[131] The concern is that these GFs could cause undesirable skin cells to flourish.[96,115,132]

HORMONES

Loss of estrogen during menopause is associated with skin aging (see Chapter 5, Intrinsic Aging). Estrogens have been used for years to treat menopause and their use is associated with decreased skin aging.[133] Estradiol protects skin from oxidation, as well as increases keratinocyte proliferation, collagen production, and vascularization.[134–137] Skin treated with estrogen exhibits increased epidermal thickness, hydration, elasticity, and reduced wrinkles, as compared to post-menopausal skin not treated with estrogen.

Phytoestrogens, or plant-derived estrogens, have shown efficacy in improving the signs of skin aging by increasing collagen and HA production as well as ECM protein levels.[138–140] Phytoestrogens are classified into the categories seen in **Table 37-3**. There are multiple forms of estrogen including

TABLE 37-3	Phytoestrogens[141]						
Flavonoids					Nonflavonoids		
Isoflavones	Flavanones	Flavones	Flavonols	Coumestans	Lignans	Stilbenes	Sterols (Plant)
Daidzein	Naringenin	Apigenin	Kaempferol	Coumestrol	Matairesinol	*Trans*-resveratrol	β-sitosterol
Genistein		Luteolin	Quercetin		Secoisolariciresinol		

bioidentical estrogen used to treat menopausal symptoms. It is beyond the realm of this text to review all of them, but it is certain that estrogen plays a role in skin rejuvenation.[142]

PEPTIDES

Peptides are short chains of amino acids, the building blocks of proteins. The name peptide comes from the Greek word *peptos* for digested because these are what proteins are broken down into when digested by enzymes. Peptides perform multiple functions as proteins are ubiquitous throughout the human body. For example, they function as receptors in cell membranes, in cell signaling, and as structural components such as collagen.

One of the roles of the epidermis is to prevent penetration and entry of microbes and foreign substances. Consequently, it can be difficult for peptides larger than 500 Da to penetrate the epidermis and even more difficult to reach the dermis.[143] New advances in penetration technologies, such as attaching the peptide to a fatty acid, have helped improve penetration of peptides but there are still many challenges using peptides in cosmeceutical formulations and skincare routines.[144] The penetration of peptides into skin is affected by several factors such as pH, charge, molecular weight, concentration, background electrolytes, presence of lipids, thickness of the SC, and temperature. Penetration is always a consideration with the use of peptides, so numerous companies are impregnating them in patches with microneedles to improve penetration.[145]

If a peptide is successful at permeating the skin, it will be faced with attack by over 500 protease enzymes.[146] Stability of peptides is also a concern. Some amino acids oxidize when exposed to light and peroxides, such as hydrogen peroxide and benzoyl peroxide.

In addition to being unstable, peptides are very reactive and tend to affect other ingredients around them. They can inactivate other ingredients in a skincare formulation and reduce efficacy of other products in a skincare routine (see Chapter 35). Most studies of the effects on peptides on the skin are in fibroblast cell cultures, which precludes the need for penetration to the dermis and can be misleading to consumers and medical providers.

However, peptides give a spackling type feel to skincare products that consumers seem to appreciate. Peptides temporarily improve the appearance of the skin by "getting into the grooves" between keratinocytes, causing a smoother appearance. Saccharides work in a similar fashion. There are few efficacy studies of peptides *in vivo* and the studies that do show efficacy are most likely reflecting the temporary smoothness imparted on the skin by peptides. There are some peptides such as defensins that can enter the skin through the hair follicle, obviating the need for penetration through the epidermis.

Peptide Nomenclature

The naming of peptides is very confusing because each peptide has multiple names. The Personal Care Products Council has rules about how substances are named and the agreed upon name structure is called the INCI name or International Nomenclature Cosmetic Ingredient name. The INCI nomenclature for synthetic peptides works as follows[147]:

- Peptides with 2–10 amino acids are named with a prefix such as di-, tri-, tetra-, etc., followed by the word peptide and an arbitrary number. An example is tetrapeptide-21.
- Peptides with more than 10 amino acids are called oligopeptides (*oligo* is Greek for few or small) followed by an arbitrary number. An example is oligopeptide-13.
- Peptides with more than 100 amino acids are called polypeptides followed by an arbitrary number. An example is polypeptide 5.
- Some peptides that have been used for years are called by the amino acid name. These names were set prior to the development of this nomenclature system. An example is glutathione, which is also called glutamyl cysteinyl glycine or tripeptide-35.
- The monograph of the peptide ingredient will contain the list of "natural amino acid residues" of which the peptide is composed in alphabetical order. Natural amino acid residues are alanine, arginine, asparagine, aspartic acid, cysteine, glutamic acid, glutamine, glycine, histidine, isoleucine, leucine, lysine, methionine, phenylalanine, proline, serine, threonine, tryptophan, tyrosine, and valine.
- If the peptide contains amino acids that are not considered a natural amino acid residue, then the amino acid is identified in the peptide name. An example is tripeptide-10-citrulline.
- Peptide derivatives are labeled utilizing the parent peptide name and the name of the modifying group as follows:
  - When the N-terminus is modified, the name of the modifying group precedes the peptide name, e.g., myristoyl hexapeptide-5.

- When the C-terminus is modified, the name of the modifying group is identified after the peptide name according to its composition. Examples include tripeptide-9 citrulline, caffeoyl tetrapeptide-19 caffeamide, tetrapeptide-29 argininamide, acetyl octapeptide-17 amide.

In addition to these complex rules, peptides are given trademarked names as well, such as TriHex technology. In other words, a cosmeceutical peptide can be referred to by several different names. There are five primary types of peptides used in topical or cosmeceutical products: signal or matrikine peptides, enzyme-inhibitor peptides, neurotransmitter-inhibitor peptides (or neuropeptides), antimicrobial peptides, and carrier peptides.[148,149]

There are multiple types of peptides on the market. This chapter will focus on the most popular peptides used to treat skin aging. The primary author has no financial conflict with any of these peptide technologies and has tried to decipher these studies in an unbiased manner. She encourages the reader to delve into the complete individual studies (not just the abstracts) with an attention to detail because peptide cosmeceutical studies tend to be intentionally misleading and the abstracts often omit the most important data.

Signal Peptides

Signal peptides act as messengers that give cells instructions as to how to function. In the case of cosmeceuticals, they entice cells to produce collagen, extracellular components, or elastin precursors. Matrikine peptides are a type of signal peptide made from constituents of the ECM. Elastin- and collagen-derived peptides can be considered as matrikines but are sometimes classified separately. In this chapter, they will be discussed separately at the end of the peptide section, unless they were included in formations with other types of peptides.

Defensins

Alpha- and β-defensins are natural immune molecules that structurally fall under the category of peptides.[150] Defensins are small cationic peptides that exhibit antimicrobial activities and enhance proliferation and migration of epithelial cells through intracellular mobilization of Ca^{2+}. They can be considered antimicrobial peptides but in the context of their anti-aging abilities, they are properly placed in the signal peptide portion of this chapter. Epithelial skin produces β-defensins while α-defensins are found in the intestines. In addition to antimicrobial properties, defensins are cytotoxic to tumor cells, activate immature dendritic cells, and improve the function of the epithelial tight junction barrier in human keratinocytes. The most interesting function in the area of anti-aging activity is their ability to turn on the leucine-rich repeat-containing G-protein–coupled receptors 5 and 6 (LGR5+ and LGR6+).[151]

Skin injury increases the expression of defensins, initiates an immune response to protect the skin from microbes, and stimulates LGR stem cells leading to repopulation of the epidermal keratinocytes. LGR6+ stem cells give rise to the entire epidermis and skin appendages, but they remain dormant until wounded.[152] After wounding LGR6+ cells create new epidermal basal cells, an action that is mediated by defensins.

Any time stem cells are stimulated, there is always the underlying potential of increased growth of skin cancer cells. LGR6+ cells are quiescent compared to basal stem cells and reside in the isthmus of the hair follicle, which is not as directly exposed to UV radiation and less likely to have mutations and damage than actively proliferating basal stem cells.[153] In fact, defensins seem to suppress cancer growth as evidenced by the observation that some tissues respond to tumor growth by increasing expression of defensins as a natural protective immune response.[154] Studies also demonsrate the ability of defensins to inhibit tumor growth both *in vitro* and *in vivo*.[155–157]

One of the advantages of defensins is that the target for anti-aging purposes, the LGR6+ stem cell, resides in the hair follicle. When applied topically in a liposome vehicle, it easily traverses the hair follicle and arrives at the target tissue. Thus, penetration is not an issue with defensins as it is with other peptides. Stability is always a challenge in relation to peptides, including defensins, so formulations must contain ingredients to stabilize defensins; however, defensins are not exposed to the same epidermal and dermal proteases as they would be if they had to traverse the epidermis and dermis. Topical defensin is used in cosmeceuticals to hasten the keratinization cycle (see Chapter 1), rejuvenate aged skin, and speed the results of skincare routines, thereby increasing compliance by allowing the patients to see changes sooner. The products that contain this defensin peptide are used in anti-aging skincare routines and as an adjunctive therapy for skin-lightening regimens. They can be used in sensitive skin types because they rarely cause inflammation.

The topical synthetic defensin known as DefenAge® (Carlsbad, CA, USA) uses a combination of α-defensin 5 and β-defensin 3 bound to plant-derived albumin; this defensin-albumin complex is very stable. It is formulated inside a liposome to improve the ability to enter the hair follicle and reach the LGR6+ stem cells, and contains antioxidants to help stabilize the formula. A three-product topical skincare regimen of DefenAge® formulations that contains synthetically produced α- and β-defensins incorporated in liposomes has been shown to convincingly improve the appearance of photoaged skin.[150] It is important to note that three of the investigators in this study are owners of MediCell Technologies LLC, which produces the defensin-containing products. However, the study was managed appropriately to avoid bias and was overseen by an IRB. The clinical staff who randomly assigned groups (placebo regimen vs. active study regimen) had no ownership and randomly assigned participants to study groups. The doctors and staff who performed assessments and collected data were blinded. This double-blind, 12-week study evaluated patients that used this three-product study regimen consisting of a serum, cream, and mask applied to the face, neck, and behind the ear. The control group used the same three products containing vehicle only (with no defensins). The subjects underwent a 1-week washout period from any products containing anti-aging ingredients, but continued cleansers, moisturizers, and sunscreens as needed. Forty-six subjects were enrolled (31 received the study regimen and 15 received the vehicle control regimen), and seven received postauricular biopsies (three from the study regimen group and four from the vehicle regimen group). Fifteen participants underwent bioengineering testing including transepidermal water loss (TEWL) measurements and high-resolution skin ultrasound as measured by the Skin Lab Combo Suite. All participants who were biopsied and received the study regimen had a histopathological increase in epidermal thickness while those who received the vehicle regimen did not (P = 0.027). Dermal thickness as measured by high-resolution ultrasound showed some increased dermal thickness in the study regimen group, but this was not statistically significant when compared to the placebo study group. Visual assessment using the Griffiths scale demonstrated a statistically significant improvement of pore size in the study regimen group (P = 0.036) and of superficial wrinkles (P = 0.048) as compared to the vehicle regimen group. A statistically significant improvement (P = 0.016) of pigmentation was seen in the study regimen treated group as compared to the vehicle regimen group (measured by the Skin Lab Combo Suite). A statistically significant difference was not seen in ultrasound measured dermal thickness, skin hydration, or elasticity. Inflammation was not noted in the study; however, the commercially available product has a form of niacinamide that can cause inflammation in niacinamide-sensitive patients.

Matrikine Peptides

Matrikines (from the Greek suffix -*kine* that means motion) are peptides made from ECM components,[33,158,159] and are known to modulate ECM remodeling. (Although these compounds are sometimes spelled as "matricines" this can be confusing because matricin is the name of a sesquiterpene in chamomile. "Matrikine" is preferred.) Matrikines interact with receptors on cell surfaces, activate intracellular signaling pathways, and lead to cellular events as diverse as cell adhesion, migration, proliferation, protein synthesis, apoptosis, or matrix degradation.

Matrikine peptides found in cosmeceuticals include carnosine, copper tripeptide, trifluoroacetyl-tripeptide-2, tripeptide-10-citrulline, acetyl tetrapeptide-5, acetyl tetrapeptide-9, acetyl tetrapeptide-11, tetrapeptide PKEK, tetrapeptide-21, hexapeptide, hexapeptide-11, palmitoyl pentapeptide-4, palmitoyl tripeptide-3/5, palmitoyl tetrapeptide-7, palmitoyl hexapeptide-12, palmitoyl tripeptide-1, and pentamide-6.[149]

Tripeptides and Hexapeptides (also known as Trihexide and TriHex Technology)

Tripeptide and hexapeptide matrikines are used to prepare the wound bed for cosmetic procedures. They are believed to remove senescent cells, glycated collagen, elastin fragments, and other debris from the ECM to make room for newly formed collagen and ECM components. Commercially available TriHex® technology contains palmitoyl tripeptide-1 and palmitoyl hexapeptide-12. Palmitoyl tripeptide-1 is also called pal-GHK or Pal-Gly-His-Lys (and was previously referred to

as palmitoyl oligopeptide but that name has been discontinued by the CIR to avoid confusion).[160] Pal-Gly-His-Lys is a messenger peptide used to stimulate production of collagen and glycosaminoglycans. This peptide is thought to act on TGF-β, which is known to play a role in collagen synthesis (see Chapter 2). These products are typically used in wound healing, 2 weeks prior to laser or peel procedures.

In 2017, Vanaman Wilson et al. conducted a randomized, single-blinded trial to ascertain the healing effects of the tripeptide and hexapeptide (TriHex Technology™, Alastin Skincare, Carlsbad, CA, USA) topical healing system after facial laser resurfacing on 15 female subjects between the ages of 45 and 70 years old. Ten participants were randomized to use the tripeptide/hexapeptide treatment and five participants to a dimethicone-based ointment and petrolatum-based cream between 3 weeks before and 12 weeks after the procedure. Less erythema and exudation during the week after procedure was observed in the TriHex group, blinded investigator ratings were better for the TriHex group, and subjects reported fewer side effects on Day 3 and greater satisfaction on Day 84 in the TriHex group.[161] Reivitis et al. also found, in a 2018 single-center pilot study of 10 patients, that a novel eye treatment containing TriHex peptides and botanical ingredients was effective in ameliorating the periocular skin, with overall improvement observed in fine lines or crow's feet, under eye hollowing, under eye bags, and dark circles.[162]

More recently, Nelson and Ortiz conducted a small single-center randomized trial in five subjects to compare the effects of an anhydrous gel with TriHex peptides (a proprietary tripeptide and hexapeptide blend) on healing after hybrid laser facial resurfacing. In this split-face protocol, use of the skin regimen, with and without the peptide formulation, started approximately 2 weeks prior to the hybrid laser resurfacing and concluded 7 days after the procedure. Evaluations by physicians revealed significant improvements in mean redness on Days 1 and 4 after the procedure and mean roughness on Days 3 and 4 post-procedure were on the side of the face treated with TriHex compared with the standard regimen side. These observations were supported by four out of five subjects in skin and complexion self-assessments.[163] A 2019 single-center clinical trial by Dr. Alan Widgerow, the Chief Medical Officer of Alastin Skincare, and other authors, studied the efficacy of a tripeptide and hexapeptide anti-aging regimen over 12 weeks in 22 female subjects with mild to moderate wrinkles and sagging facial skin. A statistically significant improvement in all measurements was associated with the regimen. Among five biopsied patients, elastin stimulation was noted in three of them, and improvement in solar elastosis, collagen production, and cornified layers was observed in all five. Self-assessments revealed patient satisfaction in a statistically significant proportion of participants.[164]

The concept of removing debris from the ECM to improve cell signaling and make room for new collagen and other matrix components is compelling. This concept was not proven in these studies because they were not designed to evaluate this on a basic science level. Instead, these studies focused on clinical signs. There is evidence that this technology speeds healing and rejuvenates the skin's appearance, but the scientific reasons for such observations remain unproven.

Pentapeptide – 4 (KTTKS) and Palmitoyl Pentapeptide-4 (Pal-KTTKS)

Collagen pentapeptide, also known as pentapeptide-4 (Pal)-KTTKS or Lys-Thr-Thr-Lys-Ser, is a synthetic peptide fragment of the C-terminal propeptide of Type I collagen, which has been shown to increase collagen synthesis and promote the production of fibronectin, a component of the ECM, by human foreskin-derived fibroblasts.[165,166] The KTTKS peptide seems to help augment TGF-β's ability to increase ECM production in human fibroblasts. KTTKS is unstable and breaks down rapidly when exposed to proteases in the skin. KTTKS does not penetrate well into the skin because it has a molecular weight of 563.64 Da, which exceeds the 500 Da threshold that can penetrate into the SC. KTTKS's use has largely been replaced by the lipoylated peptide Pal-KTTKS.

The fatty acid palmitic acid is attached to KTTKS to augment lipophilicity in order to increase skin penetration. This lipated peptide is called palmitoyl pentapeptide-4, palmitoyl-KTTKS, Pal-KTTKS, or palmitoylated Lys-Thr-Thr-Lys-Ser-OH.[167] It was formerly referred to under the broad expression palmitoyl oligopeptide, but, as mentioned above, this label is no longer allowed.[160] The commercial name of Pal-KTTKS is Matrixyl® (Sederma, Paris, France). This longer peptide Pal-KTTKS has a molecular weight of 802.05 Da, so penetration into the skin is still a challenge. Matrixyl is one of the most used peptides in cosmeceuticals because it has been deployed by large skincare companies and backed by commensurate marketing efforts. In addition, consumers like the feel of these peptides on their skin. Although there are no *in vivo* trials that convincingly demonstrate Matrixyl's efficacy, the study's abstracts as reviewed below misrepresent the data and are frequently quoted as proof of efficacy.

It is important to understand that there is no peer-reviewed study demonstrating efficacy of Matrixyl on facial wrinkles because skin penetration is difficult to achieve as shown by a Franz cell assay.[167,168] A study by Choi et al. revealed that KTTKS and Pal-KTTKS were not able to penetrate full-thickness mouse skin in a Franz cell assay.[167] In fact, KTTKS was not found in any of the skin layers. Although Pal-KTTKS did not penetrate the full skin thickness, low levels were found in the SC, epidermis, and dermis. Even if the peptide could enter the skin, it must be in a large enough concentration to be effective. Peptide stability also affects the ability to deliver significant levels of peptides to the target dermal tissue. Choi showed that in skin extracts, KTTKS was rapidly degraded and almost depleted within 30 minutes. Small levels of Pal-KTTKS remained in the dermis after 120 minutes. Although there are numerous challenges to using topical peptides due to these concerns, efforts continue because of the cell culture findings that make this a promising anti-aging ingredient should these hurdles be overcome.

Robust studies in human fibroblast cultures clearly demonstrate that a high concentration of Pal-KTTKS increases collagen production in fibroblasts.[168] In human fibroblast cell cultures, Pal-KTTKS inhibits fibroblast proliferation and greatly enhances collagen synthesis, which means that the rise in collagen production cannot be accounted for by an increase in fibroblasts, which is often the case in these fibroblast culture trials. While these data are promising evidence of the ability of Pal-KTTKS to rejuvenate skin by increasing collagen production, it is evident that a large concentration must be able to penetrate through the epidermis, resist the endogenous protease enzymes, and travel to the fibroblasts in the dermis to achieve these effects.

A Review of In Vivo Studies on Pal-KTTKS

A double-blind, placebo-controlled, split-face study on 93 women conducted by Proctor and Gamble had subjects undergo a 2-week washout period in which they used facial cleanser and an oil-in-water moisturizer with SPF.[169] The two study products were the same oil-in-water moisturizer used in the washout with and without 3 ppm of Pal-KTTKS. These were packaged in blind coded tubes. Subjects were instructed to use a pea size of the one marked "left" on the left side of the face and a pea-sized amount (approx. 0.4 grams) of the one marked "right" on the right side of the face twice daily for 12 weeks. (The evening application was at least one hour before bedtime to reduce movement of the product from one side of the face to the other via a pillowcase.) Photographs were taken at each visit and evaluated with a computer-based wrinkle image analysis system. The photos were also assessed by expert graders who were blinded as to whether the visits were at baseline, 4, 8, or 12 weeks. Graders chose which side was better with options being right image, left image, or neither. They also rated "how much better" with a -4 to +4 scale. Subjects completed a self-assessment score and TEWL measurements were taken at each with a DermaLab TEWL instrument. The results compared the study drug data versus the placebo data and are clearly presented in the publication. The quantitative image analysis demonstrated a small but significant difference in fine lines and wrinkles at Weeks 8 and 12. Expert grader analysis of the photos using the -4 to +4 scale revealed improvement in the Pal-KTTKS group as compared to placebo, most notably at 8 weeks ($P < 0.20$) and 12 weeks ($P < 0.10$), but these findings were not statistically significant. (A P value less than 0.05 is statistically significant.) It is interesting that the paper does not note that the expert graders' findings were not statistically significant, but this can be deduced by the supplied P values that are greater than 0.05.

Subject self-assessments for fine lines and wrinkles did not reveal a significant difference but they did note a significant improvement in age spots, dark circles, and skin firmness at 12 weeks. No difference in TEWL measurements was seen between the two groups. This well-designed study unfortunately did not achieve convincing results upon close data analysis, which did not prevent the abstract from claiming: "Pal-KTTKS provided significant improvement vs. placebo control for reduction in wrinkles/fine lines by both quantitative technical and expert grader image analysis. In self-assessments, subjects also reported significant fine line/wrinkle improvements and noted directional effects for other facial improvement parameters." A paper on peptides by Schagen[149] cited several other studies that support the use of Pal-KTTKS; however, these are based not on peer-reviewed publications but rather a patent,[170] and an interview in *Dermatology Times*.[171] In 2019, a report on attempts to improve upon Pal-KTTKS with a series of novel peptides made by adding acetyl and lipoyl residues revealed that no improvements on the original palmitoyl residues were observed.[172] These studies demonstrate that when a large concentration of Pal-KTTKS reaches fibroblasts, collagen production and ECM components are increased. However, topical application has not successfully delivered large concentrations to the dermis. For this reason, applications of this peptide after microneedling or injections of this peptide might be the answer; however, efficacy and safety has not been studied.

Other Signal Peptides

There are numerous other signal peptides used in cosmeceutical skincare products. For example, palmitoyl tripeptide-3/5 (Pal-Lys-Val-Lys bistrifluoracetate salt), which is known by the tradename SYN®-COLL (DSM, Basel, Switzerland). In cell cultures, it exerts similar effects as thrombospondin-1 (TSP-1), an ECM protein that increases TGF-β activity. *In vitro* studies show that palmitoyl tripeptide-3/5 prevents collagen breakdown by interfering with MMP-1 and MMP-3 collagen degradation.[173] Many of the peptides on the following list have similar cell culture data with poor *in vivo* data. All of these products are said to improve wrinkles or increase firmness to improve skin appearance. Short descriptions are available in these references,[149,174] but the author recommends reading the actual *in vivo* studies that do not support the exaggerated claims. Each of these would have the same stability and penetration issues as discussed above. Signal peptides used to treat aged skin include:

- Acetyl sh-heptapeptide-1 (Acetyl-DEETGEF-OH), known by the tradename Perfection Peptide™
- Acetyl tetrapeptide-11 (N-Acetyl-Pro-Pro-Tyr-Leu), known by the tradename Syniorage™
- Acetyl tetrapeptide-9 (N-Acetyl-Gln-Asp-Val-His), known by the tradename Dermican™
- GEGK (H-Gly-Glu-Lys-Gly-OH)
- Hexapeptide-11 (Phe-Val-Ala-Pro-Phe-Pro), also called pentamide-6
- Hexapeptide-14 (Pal-Val-Gly-Val-Ala-Pro-Gly-OH), also called palmitoyl hexapeptide-14
- Lipospondin (Elaidyl-Lys-Phe-Lys-OH)
- Palmitoyl tripeptide-1 (Pal-Gly-His-Lys-OH), known by the tradename Biopeptide CL™
- Palmitoyl hexapeptide-12 (Pal-Val-Gly-Val-Ala-Pro-Gly), which is the peptide in Biopeptide-EL
- Palmitoyl tetrapeptide-7 (Pal-Gly-Gln-Pro-Arg or pal-GQPR), known by the tradename Rigin™
- SA1-III (Ac-Met-Gly-Lys-Val-Val-Asn-Prp-Thr-Gln-Lys-NH2), also called KP1
- Tetrapeptide-21 (Gly-Glu-Lys-Gly), also named GEKG
- Trifluoroacetyl-tripeptide-2 (TFA-Val-Try-Val-OH)
- Tripeptide-10-citrulline (Lys-α-Asp-Ile-Citrulline), known by the tradename Decorinyl™
- Tripeptide-38 (Pal-Lys-Met(O2)-Lys-OH)

Enzyme Inhibitor Peptides

Enzyme-inhibiting peptides used for anti-aging should suppress the MMPs that break down elastin and collagen, the hyaluronidase that breaks down HA, or block proteases or other enzymes involved in aging. The following are a few of the enzyme-inhibiting peptides found in anti-aging skincare products and their purported activities. Their relevance is unclear and very few *in vitro* studies have been conducted.

- Silk fibroin peptide, derived from silkworms, may have anti-inflammatory and antioxidant activity.[175]
- Black rice oligopeptides inhibit MMPs and may increase HA production.[176]

Carrier Peptides

Carrier peptides stabilize and deliver important trace elements such as copper and manganese into skin cells. Copper is an essential cofactor that the enzyme lysyl oxidase needs to produce collagen.

Copper Tripeptide-1

Copper tripeptide-1 (Copper Gly-L-His-L-Lys) is known as Cu-GHK or GHK-Cu. This compound, in which copper is bound to a matrikine tripeptide called glycyl-histidyl-lysine (GHK), modulates new connective tissue formation.[158] GHK is naturally found in human plasma, saliva, and urine. Blood levels of GHK decline with age.[177] The synthetic peptide Cu-GHK was developed in 1973 by Loren Pickard who showed that GHK significantly increases the expression of DNA repair genes, modulates collagen and glycosaminoglycan remodeling, and affects MMPs,[178,179] playing an important role in wound healing and aging. Cu-GHK has been shown to increase collagen, dermatan sulfate, chondroitin sulfate, and decorin in cell cultures.[180] There have been *in vivo* studies using Cu-GHK in facial creams, but these were reported in poster presentations at meetings rather than in peer-reviewed publications and were sponsored by a cosmetic company.[177,181] A lipoylated form of the peptide in which a palmitoyl moiety was added (Pal-GHK) exists, as does a biotin complex derivative, an oligoarginine derivative, and manganese tripeptide-1, which has manganese bound to GHK.

Cu-GHK is found in numerous brands of anti-aging facial creams. It appears to easily penetrate through the SC, especially if the pH is higher, as when soap cleansers are used (see Chapters 35 and 40).[177] However, the peptide is most stable at a pH of 4.5–7.4. Therefore, it should not be used in conjunction with hydroxy acids, ascorbic acid, or other ingredients at a low pH. As with any peptide, the proteolytic enzymes will quickly break this down when it enters the skin. It seems particularly susceptible to degradation in the presence of oxidative stress as induced by hydrogen peroxide and benzoyl peroxide. Although the anti-aging data for Cu-GHK is sparse, it is a popular ingredient in wound healing products in which penetration is not an issue.

Antimicrobial Peptides

The only anti-aging antimicrobial peptide is defensin. It is discussed in the matrikine category because it is used in anti-aging formulations for its effects on LGR6+ stem cells and not for its antimicrobial properties.

Neurotransmitter-inhibiting Peptides

Neurotransmitter-inhibiting peptides became popular in early 2000 when awareness and understanding of the mechanism of action of botulinum toxin type A (Botox®, Allergan, Dublin, Ireland) rapidly increased. It is well established that botulinum toxin type A cleaves a protein called synaptosomal-associated protein 25 or SNAP-25 (part of the SNARE complex). This action blocks acetylcholine release, which is necessary for muscle contraction. Relaxed muscles lead to less wrinkle formation in areas of muscle movement. Cosmeceutical peptides were developed to hinder portions of the SNARE complex such as SNAP-25 and purportedly inhibit muscle contraction in the same way that botulinum toxin type A does (see Chapter 23, Botulinum Toxins). The advertising campaign that claimed that a skincare product was "Better than Botox" led to widespread popularity of these ingredients. However, it should be remembered that the peptide affects the SNARE complex in cell cultures, usually muscle cells, and penetration into muscle tissue after application to the epidermis is unlikely. This section will examine the trials of the most popular cosmeceutical neurotransmitter-inhibiting peptides.

Acetyl Hexapeptide-3

Acetyl hexapeptide-3, known by the trademarked name Argiriline®, is composed of Ac-Glu-Glu-Met-Gln-Arg-Arg-NH2.[182] It is sometimes listed as Acetyl-Glu-Glu-Met-Gln-Arg-Arg-NH2 or referred to as Ac-EEMQRR-NH$_2$, but is also known as acetyl hexapeptide-8. This peptide functions as a copy of SNAP-25 and destabilizes the SNARE complex. Companies that utilize this peptide habitually compare it to botulinum toxin type A. Close examination of the studies that are cited to support this claim follow.

A small placebo-controlled study of 10 women compared 10% acetyl hexapeptide-3 to a vehicle cream, both of which were applied twice daily in the lateral periorbital area for 30 days.[183] It is unknown if the investigators and subjects were blinded. Skin topography analysis data were used to support this claim in the abstract that "acetyl hexapeptide-3-treated skin areas showed a 30% improvement in wrinkles as compared to baseline while the control had a 10% improvement." With close examination of the data, the statistical significance of the comparison between the two data points is confusing. The study does not state if there is a statistical significance between the control product vs. the treatment product. Results indicated that acetyl hexapeptide-3 could pass through excised

epidermis. However, to reach the neuromuscular endplate where the SNARE complex plays a role in muscle contraction, the study product would also need to penetrate the dermis and subcutaneous fat to arrive at muscle, which was not evaluated.

In 2015, a study of acetyl hexapeptide-3 in 40 female subjects was conducted.[184] The publication did not state if the subjects and the investigators were blinded. A 2-week washout period occurred in which all subjects were asked not to use any skincare products in the test area (the ventral forearm and face). Subjects applied the study cream or vehicle twice daily. Both groups demonsrated increased hydration as measured by a corneometer, illustrating the contributions to hydrating the skin of the vehicle and a 2-week washout period with no moisturizing products. Measurements of shear wave propagation with a reviscometer showed a decrease in skin anisotropy (variations in physical properties in this case meaning the ability to be deformed or moved) only on the face (not on the forearm). This increase in skin firmness implies that the peptides increased skin rigidity of the face, which coincides with the cake fondant metaphor mentioned earlier. There were no changes seen in skin elasticity as measured with a cutometer. From these meager findings, the authors concluded that "acetyl hexapeptide-3 is an effective anti-aging compound as already mentioned by Blanes-Mira et al." They did not acknowledge the possibility that accumulated peptides on the skin's surface could affect firmness without affecting the skin's biology.

A study in 2017 examined a combination of tripeptide-10-citrulline and acetyl hexapeptide-3 on 24 women.[185] Skin Visioscan VC98 was used to evaluate skin roughness. The subjects were assigned to four groups as follows: Group 1 used both peptides, group 2 used only tripeptide-10-citrulline, group 3 used only acetyl hexapeptide-3, and group 4 was the vehicle alone (placebo). The cR3 measurements (also known as the cyclic average roughness, or the Rz parameter) showed no significant difference in roughness between the placebo group (group 4) and the group with both peptides (group 1). The lack of a significant difference between the control group and the two peptide groups is not mentioned in the abstract, which is the section most available to the public. R2 is the cyclic maximum roughness (also called the Rmax). At 20 days and 40 days, no significant differences between groups were seen in the Rmax measurements. On Day 60, a statistical difference between the placebo group and the group that contained both peptides was seen (P = .025). The confusing presentation of the data and the lack of transparency in the abstract regarding absence of significance makes one question this article's assertion that "our results are in agreement with the study reported by Blanes-Mira et al. when acetyl hexapeptide-3 at a 10% concentration reduced the depth of wrinkles up to 30% after 30 days of use." Firstly, this study did not consider wrinkle depth; rather, it studied only skin roughness. Secondly, the only significance difference between the placebo group and the other groups on skin roughness was at 60 days when the placebo was compared to the study product with both peptides. This study did provide evidence that peptides can reduce TEWL, but this is not surprising as they form a protective film on the skin's surface.

Pentapeptide-3

Vialox is a pentapeptide derived from snake venom (H-Gly-Pro-Arg-Pro-Ala-NH$_2$) that serves as an antagonist to acetyl choline, disabling the function of nerves and preventing the induction of muscle relaxation.[186] This peptide acts in a manner similar to that of tubocurarine, the main active compound of curare.[186] As with curare, Vialox operates at the postsynaptic membrane where it functions as a competitive antagonist at the acetylcholine membrane receptor. As the acetylcholine receptors are blocked, sodium ions (Na$^+$) are not released and muscles do not contract. *In vivo* and *in vitro* studies performed by the manufacturer claim that this product softened wrinkles and reduced skin roughness, but these data are not published in any scientific journals. At the time of publication of this text, there had been no further investigations examining the anti-wrinkle properties of Vialox. The only available data are provided by the manufacturer, which reports that *in vitro* and *in vivo* studies demonstrate the efficacy of Vialox because of reductions in wrinkle size and skin roughness. These data are no longer available online.

Other Peptides

Collagen Peptides

Collagen is found in bone, cartilage, tendons, skin, and skeletal muscle. There are 28 distinct types of collagen all of which contain hydroxyproline. Increased levels of Type I collagen in the skin are associated with a youthful skin appearance. Topical collagen does not penetrate into the skin, accounting for its loss in popularity, and has largely been replaced by topical ascorbic acid, which augments the cutaneous synthesis of collagen. Oral supplementation of collagen is popular for anti-aging treatment because consumers have learned the importance of collagen for youthful skin. There are a few reasons why the supplementation with collagen peptide improves skin appearance.[187] The amino acid proline makes up 10% of the total amino acids in collagen. Proline, which is hydroxylated to hydroxyproline and requires the presence of ascorbic acid, is necessary for collagen production. The endogenous synthesis of proline is insufficient to meet the body's needs, so it must be obtained by diet, supplementation, or topical administration.[188] Humans can synthesize proline from arginine, glutamine, glutamate, and ornithine. The presence of glutamine (or glutamate) and ascorbic acid are important for hydroxyproline production and the subsequent synthesis of collagen (**Fig. 37-4**). Arginine and ornithine supplementation have been shown to promote collagen production in the absence of supplemented proline, glutamine, glutamate, and ascorbic acid, perhaps by increasing proline production, independent of proline production, or related to the fact that arginine and ornithine augment growth hormone secretion.[189] Collagen peptides that enter fibroblasts exert antioxidant effects that reduce oxidative damage and inflammation. They also regulate cytokines and activate TGF-β/Smad or other signaling pathways, and inhibit collagen-dissolving enzymes such as nuclear transcription factor activating protein-1 (AP-1), MMP-1, and MMP-3.[187]

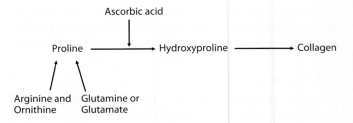

FIGURE 37-4. Proline and ascorbic acid are required to synthesize collagen.[189]

Collagen peptides contained in drinks and supplements include combinations of the following: hydroxyproline, glycine, and proline. These are usually extracted enzymatically from animal connective tissues and packaged as capsules, tablets, powders, or beverages. Once orally ingested, they are digested by stomach acids into di- and tripeptides that are absorbed into the blood stream via the intestines.[190,191] In rats, oral hydroxyproline reaches the bloodstream within an hour of ingestion. Gelatin is a heat-denatured form of collagen. Orally ingested gelatin is used to strengthen hair and nails. Hydrolyzed gelatin is called collagen hydrolysate. Oral collagen hydrolysate has been associated with positive skin changes as discussed above; however, there is no evidence that orally ingested collagen preferentially deposits in the dermis as opposed to other body tissues.[192]

Collagen peptides are typically extracted from fish, cattle, pigs, and sometimes plants. Formulations can also be made with recombinant protein production systems such as yeast. It is unknown which source is best for skin rejuvenation.[193,194] Studies have shown that cod-derived collagen hydrolysate taken orally at 154 mg per kg of body weight increased plasma levels of hydroxyproline while 30 mg did not.[191] Proline-hydroxyproline dipeptides have been demonstrated to enhance both collagen and HA synthesis.[195] Research has also shown that the absorbed peptides reach the skin and are retained in the tissue for up to 2 weeks.[196,197] Non-animal sources of collagen such as whey protein and walnut protein have been studied.[198] A review of the literature on oral collagen supplementation established no agreement about how much and what types of collagen should be taken to treat skin aging.[194] A thorough review by Jhawar described which studies have been performed and concluded that there may be benefits of oral collagen but much more data are needed.[199]

Collagen supplements and beverages are expensive, and must be taken in large quantities to achieve results. The various amino acids that compose collagen can be obtained through diet but, again, this mode may not be sufficient to achieve an observable effect. Bone broth is a good source of collagen, but homemade broth contains more of the key amino acids (i.e., glycine, lysine, proline, leucine, hydroxyproline, and hydroxylysine) than store-bought preparations.[200] It is currently unknown if collagen supplements are helpful in those who eat meat and other collagen-containing foods along with vitamin C. Dietary sources of L-arginine, such as fish, red meat, poultry, soy, whole grains, brans, and dairy products, along with dietary sources of ornithine, such as freshwater clams, fish, and cheese, should also help increase cutaneous collagen.

Elastin-derived Peptides

Tropoelastin, one of the precursors to elastin, has many functions beyond forming the elastin matrix. Elastin-derived peptides (EDPs) are found in numerous cell types, including fibroblasts, and have been shown to display diverse activities such as regulating MMP expression and stimulating the growth of fibroblasts in culture.[201] They can be considered matrikine peptides.[202]

EDPs can be physiologically beneficial or can contribute to pathology such as cancer.[203] In skin, EDP may influence photoaging of the skin by diminishing elastase, inhibiting fibroblast apoptosis, and augmenting the hydroxyproline and water content of skin.[204] EDPs have been found to play an important role in cancer progression, diabetes, and atherosclerosis. Interaction between EDPs and various cell types can trigger several biologic responses in cancer cells.[205,206] Therefore, it is suggested that these products not be used in cosmeceutical preparations, unless they have specifically been proven as safe.[205] EDPs play a role in the production of advanced glycation end products (AGEs) and increased EDP levels are seen in aging and considered markers of aging.[207]

An example of an EDP used in cosmeceuticals is hexapeptide-12 or valine-glycine-valine-alanine-proline-glycine (VGVAPG). VGVAPG is a repeating sequence found in elastin that allows elastin to bind to the elastin complex receptor. It used to be referred to as palmitoyl oligopeptide. This hexapeptide attracts fibroblasts and stimulates them to produce collagen.[208,209] Palmitic acid may be added to VGVAPG to enhance penetration with the resulting peptide palmitoyl hexapeptide-12. Myristoyl hexapeptide-12 is another lipolated form of VGVAPG. These three peptides were evaluated by the Cosmetic Ingredient Review (CIR) panel and found to be safe.[160] However, they specifically state that the safety assessment only applies to hexapeptides with the peptide sequence of Val-Gly-Val-Ala-Pro-Gly. (There is another "hexapeptide-12" with different amino acid residues, Ala-Pro-Gly-Val-Gly-Val, which they did not declare as safe.) The CIR panel also declared that the expression "palmitoyl oligopeptide" will no longer be used to avoid confusion. ("Palmitoyl oligopeptide" was used for both hexapeptide-12 and palmitoyl tripeptide-1 (Gly-His-Lys [GHK]). Now it can be used for neither.)

Keratin-based Peptides

Keratin is a key component of hair, wool, feathers, nails, and horns, as well as human skin. It is a protein that endows these structures with strength and insolubility and helps them retain moisture. Keratin plays a very important role in skin as discussed in Chapter 1. When exogenous keratin is applied to the skin, it forms a protective colloidal layer on the keratinocytes that shields the cells from the denaturing effects of detergents and other ingredients encountered by the skin.[210] Studies have demonstrated that keratins derived from wool can help skin

retain moisture. Moisturized skin is more elastic; therefore, these studies revealed an increase in elasticity as well.[211] A placebo-controlled study on nine women with dry skin tested wool-derived keratin peptides vs. deionized water in a hand cream. The keratin-containing hand cream-treated skin was better hydrated than the control group and it was surmised that the keratin-based peptide cream treatment prevented some of the damaging effects of detergents.[211] Keratin derived from chicken feathers has been shown to suppress UVB-induced MMPs in human dermal fibroblasts.[212,213] There are no plant sources of keratin.

Safety of Peptides

The safety of tripeptide-1, hexapeptide-12, their metal salts and fatty acyl derivatives, and palmitoyl tetrapeptide-7, palmitoyl tripeptide-1, palmitoyl hexapeptide-12, tripeptide-1, copper tripeptide-1, and palmitoyl tetrapeptide-7 used topically in cosmetics was reviewed by the CIR Expert Panel.[160] The authors stated that the typical dose used was a low concentration and that safety tests did not show any negative data. They concluded that these peptides are safe when used topically at concentrations < 10 ppm. The panel did caution about the use of EDP. The safety assessments about peptides from the FDA are based on the fact that these do not penetrate well and are rapidly digested upon entry into the SC. As new peptide formulations are developed to improve penetration and longevity this may change the safety parameters so peptides should be used with caution. It is unknown if these peptides are safe when applied to disrupted skin such as after microneedling or when injected into the skin (see Chapter 27, Microneedling and PRP). These uses should be discouraged until safety studies are performed.

Peptide Summary

Peptides are popular ingredients in anti-aging skincare formulations because consumers recognize the term and like the feel of these products. Unfortunately, few peptides can penetrate the skin and peptides present challenges in formulating because they are reactive and tend to interfere with other product ingredients, thus diminishing shelf-life. Consequently, several topical peptide-containing creams will display minimal effectiveness in treating cutaneous aging. Recent advances in penetration technology, such as attaching a fatty acid to create a lipoylated peptide, have improved the penetration of some peptide products, but not at a high enough concentration to demonstrate efficacy. To achieve significant concentrations of peptides to reach the epidermis, the SC would need to be disrupted.[168] Current studies are looking at disrupting the SC with chemical or mechanical exfoliation or microneedles. In addition, peptides could be injected into the skin, but this has not been studied and safety is undetermined. It is important to understand that there are myriad different peptide ingredients and the efficacy depends on which peptide is used, what other ingredients are in the formulation, and what other products are used with the peptide product.[28] The abstracts of efficacy *in vivo* studies of peptides are often misleading and efficacy claims exaggerated. The anti-aging studies should be read in their entirety, rather than just focusing on the abstract, and should be interpreted with a discerning eye. There is no doubt that peptides have biologic activity when studied in cell cultures. For this reason, the safety should be re-evaluated once the penetration and persistence issues have been overcome.

RETINOIDS

In the 1970s, female acne patients being treated with tretinoin observed that their wrinkles had diminished and skin texture had improved.[214] A subsequent clinical trial demonstrated that patients with photodamaged skin treated with tretinoin exhibited improvement.[215] Several clinical trials have since confirmed these early observations and retinoids are now well established as the most efficacious ingredients to address photodamaged skin,[216] with all-*trans* retinoic acid (tretinoin), a biologically active form of vitamin A, the first to be approved by the FDA for treating photoaged skin.[217] Tazarotene was also proven to be efficacious in treating wrinkles as judged by an FDA panel, which led to its approval as a drug to treat skin aging. Although only two retinoids (tretinoin and tazarotene) have undergone the FDA drug approval process to confirm that they ameliorate photoaged skin, retinol, once absorbed, turns into retinoic acid in the skin and therefore confers the same rejuvenating effects.

Retinol, retinal, and retinoic acid share the same structure and are all vitamin A derivatives grouped in a class of molecules called retinoids (which means "retinol like"). Retinol, the most effective retinoid available without a prescription, is lipophilic and easily penetrates the epidermis and the keratinocyte and fibroblast cell membranes.[110] Retinol is converted to retinoic acid in the skin, which binds the cytosolic retinol-binding protein (CRBP) receptors and retinoic acid receptors (RAR), thus promoting keratinocyte proliferation as well as collagen and HA synthesis by fibroblasts, reduction of degrading MMPs, and stimulation of the growth of new blood vessels in the papillary layer of the dermis while enhancing remodeling of fibers in the reticular dermis.[218,219]

Retinoids are best known to mitigate the breakdown of collagen by decreasing MMP levels and increasing collagen production. Working on intrinsically aged skin as well as photodamage, retinoids essentially hinder the production of collagenase and MMPs and stimulate the synthesis of collagen and HA. It is important to note that while retinol penetrates the skin well, esters such as retinyl palmitate and retinyl linoleate do not. The number of studies that demonstrate the efficacy of retinoids, including retinol, on aged skin is so abundant that an entire chapter of this book has been devoted to the topic (see Chapter 45, Retinoids).

The main disadvantage of retinoids is that with the exception of tazarotene and adapalene, retinoids are very susceptible to degradation by air and light and must be packaged in either small-mouthed aluminum tubes or airless pumps. They can be used in conjunction with hydroxy acids and ascorbic acid, but it is difficult to formulate these in the same product. The instability seen with light exposure is the reason it is recommended that retinoids be used at night, in conjunction with the skin circadian rhythm that performs nocturnal repair activities (see Chapter 1). Retinoids are the most proven ingredients to treat skin aging.

STEM CELLS

Stem cells packaged in cosmeceutical products are mostly useless, because these often plant-derived substances are too large to penetrate the SC, have short shelf lives, and do not act as human stem cells would. Stem cells isolated from human fat, known as adipose-derived stem cells, have shown promise in skin rejuvenation. Fat is harvested from the patient and the stem cells are isolated and reinjected into the patient. This topic is beyond the scope of this chapter.[220] The promise of human-derived stem cells should not be used to promote the use of apple stem cells and other plant-derived stem cells in cosmeceuticals.

ANTI-CANCER DRUGS FOR SKIN REJUVENATION

Imiquimod

Imiquimod is a topical immunomodulator approved as a drug by the FDA for the treatment of superficial basal cell carcinoma, actinic keratosis (AK), and genital warts. It binds the toll-like receptor 7 (TLR7), leading to an upregulation of cytokines such as IFN-α and IFN-ω,[221] which play a role in collagen synthesis. Imiquimod also upregulates IL-1α, which improves skin barrier homeostasis.[222] Aging leads to a decrease in TLR7 function.[223]

Several studies have reported that skin treated with imiquimod manifests enhanced appearance.[224–226] One unblinded, uncontrolled study had 10 women apply the imiquimod 5% study drug twice daily 5 days a week for 4 weeks. Global assessments by a dermatologist and subjects' assessments indicated an improvement in wrinkles and evenness of skin pigmentation.[227] Histology suggested normalization of the epidermis but no dermal changes. In 2007, histological assessment of 26 patients who had been treated with imiquimod 5% daily for 3 months for lentigo maligna evinced an increase in papillary dermal fibroplasia and a reduction in solar elastosis demonstrating that imiquimod can affect the dermis. The histological effects are more pronounced with longer use.

In 2018, a meta-analysis of four identical double-blind vehicle-controlled trials examining the effects of imiquimod on aging skin was conducted.[228] The studies included a total of 969 subjects with AK. Subjects received either imiquimod 2.5%, 3.75%, or vehicle, which was applied once daily for a 2-week treatment cycle, followed by a 2-week no-treatment period, culminating in a second 2-week treatment cycle. Data were collected at the Week 14 visit, which was 8 weeks after the last treatment. Investigators compared the Week 14 visit to the baseline visit using a seven-point IGIP scale that ranged from -3 (significantly worse than baseline) to +3 (significantly improved from baseline). At Week 14 the IGIP scores were 1.67 for imiquimod 2.5%, 1.98 for imiquimod 3.75%, and 0.73 for vehicle. (The differences in the imiquimod groups each compared to the vehicle group were statistically significant with P values = 0.0001 versus vehicle.) Severe erythema was reported in 21.4% of the imiquimod 2.5% group, 35% of the imiquimod 3.75% group, and 0% of the vehicle group but resolved in all before the end of the study. The data within the large sample size yield sufficient proof that imiquimod improves the appearance of photoaged skin, but its use is limited by side effects.

In a 2019 open-label study, 11 subjects applied a pea-sized amount of imiquimod 5% to the periorbital area 3 consecutive days per Week for 8 weeks.[225] Photographs were assessed at baseline and 8 weeks. Live assessments using a facial wrinkle scale (FWS) were conducted by investigators, which revealed that the post-treatment FWS scores were significantly improved from the baseline scores (P < 0.005). Seventy-three percent of subjects rated the improvement at 8 weeks compared to baseline as "fair" or "good" on the Likert five-point scale. Six patients of the 11 experienced mild itching, stinging, or irritation.

Although many studies have shown that imiquimod improves fine lines and causes histological changes in the dermis, its use is complicated by side effects. TLR7 plays multiple roles as an activator of the immune system and the long-term safety of its topical use has not been established. If the user has underlying AK or skin cancer, a vigorous reaction resulting in erosions and scabbing is not uncommon. If imiquimod is used for anti-aging purposes, care should be taken to begin very slowly on small segments to gauge the severity of the reaction. Some patients experience flu-like symptoms when using this medication topically.

Ingenol Mebutate

Ingenol mebutate is an agonist of protein kinase C (PKC), which is involved in several cellular functions including cell proliferation, differentiation, and senescence. Activation of PKC induces apoptosis of dysplastic keratinocyte cells but not normal differentiating keratinocytes.[229] It results rapid cell death by disrupting the plasma membrane and causing the mitochondria to swell. Several reports of its ability to improve the appearance of aged skin have been published in dermatology journals.[230,231]

In 2017, an unblinded prospective trial looked at the efficacy of ingenol mebutate 0.015% used for three consecutive days on facial aging in patients treated with biopsy proven AK. Twenty-three subjects completed the study. Investigators rated photoaging with a cutaneous photoaging scale that showed 21 subjects (84%) had improvement at the 60-day visit. All six parameters (AK appearance, overall skin appearance, wrinkling, dyschromia, erythema, and texture) showed statistically significant improvement on both Day 30 and Day 60 as compared to baseline (P< 0.01). Wrinkling specifically improved in 80% with a mean improvement score of 1.8 points. Eighty-eight percent of subjects showed improvement in visible skin texture with a mean improvement score of 1.97 in subjects' self-assessments.

In 2018, 19 patients were treated in an open-label study with topical ingenol mebutate for AK on the face once daily for three days in a row.[232] Two investigators rated overall skin appearance, wrinkles, pigmentation, and texture on a five-point scale. All 19 patients manifested a >50% improvement in pigmentation and 92% showed >50% improvement of wrinkles and skin texture. Biopsies taken at baseline and 8 weeks demonstrated that post-treatment skin was characterized by increased collagen and reduced elastosis. It appeared that elastotic skin had been replaced with bundles of collagen. Evaluation of RNA demonstrated statistically significant changes in mRNA levels: increased expression of mRNA for Type 1 collagen (P = 0.003) and TGF-β (P = 0.004) and decreased expression of MMP-1 mRNA (P = 0.012). In this study, 3 of 19 patients developed blisters and erythema.

Ingenol mebutate was used as an anti-skin cancer drug but reports that it may increase development of skin cancers led to its withdrawal from the UK market and others in October 2020 pending the satisfactory completion of more safety studies.[233] The high incidence of side effects such as blisters and the chance of increasing the risk of skin cancer limit the use of this drug for photoaging. It was included in this chapter to illustrate the scientific knowledge we have learned from this topical product's effects on aging skin, but its use is not recommended until more safety data are available.

CONCLUSION

There is a plethora of anti-aging skincare ingredients, but few have the rigorous scientific proof to justify their use. Some ingredients like epidermal-derived growth factor and ingenol mebutate have the efficacy data but should not be used to treat skin aging due to safety concerns. It is critical to closely read the studies supporting the claims of anti-aging ingredients because they are often meant to confuse. When possible, double-blind placebo-controlled trials should be performed. Studies should clearly display the P values to present the statistical significance of the findings. Objective information such as mRNA and gene expression data should be given priority over subjective data such as subjects' opinions. Biopsy data are helpful put it is important to remember that if a follow-up biopsy is taken from the same area as the first biopsy, the wound healing process will have turned on many cytokines, defensins, and collagen synthesis, so a beneficial effect will always be seen. Companies with robust study designs and statistically significant data will want to publish that information in the highest impact journal they can, so take the journal into account when reviewing data.

The most proven anti-aging cosmeceutical ingredients remain retinoids, including retinol. Ascorbic acid and hydroxy acids are next. Imiquimod has compelling data but its use is limited by side effects. Peptides, which target dermal fibroblasts or muscle cells, do not penetrate and are unstable; therefore, these compounds do not reach the target in sufficient volume to confer an effect. Growth factors have difficulty penetrating the dermis and have not been established as safe, especially epidermal-derived growth factors.

Even the most proven anti-aging ingredients are worthless if they are mixed with other ingredients and products that inactivate them or block their ability to penetrate into the dermis. Barrier repair moisturizers, saturated fatty acids such as stearic acid, and occlusive ingredients such as oils can decrease ingredient penetration, while HA and unsaturated fatty acids like oleic acid can increase ingredient penetration. Take care to consider ingredient interactions when designing a skincare regimen so that every product in the regimen improves the efficacy of the other products (see Chapter 35). Incorporating cleansers, moisturizers, antioxidants, retinoids, and anti-aging serums should be based on the Baumann Skin Type and the underlying barriers to skin health, notably dryness, inflammation, and melanocyte activity.

Preventing aging involves measures to protect cellular organelles and DNA from damage, as well as lowering levels of enzymes such as MMPs that break down important components such as collagen. Sunscreen remains the most important skin aging *prevention* ingredient followed by retinoids, ascorbic acid, and antioxidants. The basic goal of *treating* aged skin is to stimulate keratinocyte stem cells to accelerate the keratinization cycle and fibroblasts to produce more collagen, HA, and ECM components. This is achieved through wounding procedures (e.g., peels, laser treatments), exfoliation (using hydroxy acids, retinoids, mechanical means), and stimulating stem cell production.

References

1. Market Data Forecast. Global Anti-Aging Market Size, Share, Trends, Growth Analysis Report - Segmented By Products, Demographics, Services, Devices and Region - Industry Forecast | 2020 to 2025. February 2020. https://www.marketdataforecast.com/market-reports/anti-aging-market. Accessed December 23, 2020.
2. Fisher GJ, Talwar HS, Lin J, Voorhees JJ. Molecular mechanisms of photoaging in human skin in vivo and their prevention by all-trans retinoic acid. *Photochem Photobiol.* 1999;69(2):154–157.
3. Franz TJ, Lehman PA, Raney SG. Use of excised human skin to assess the bioequivalence of topical products. *Skin Pharmacol Physiol.* 2009;22(5):276–286.
4. Griffiths CE, Russman AN, Majmudar G, Singer RS, Hamilton TA, Voorhees JJ. Restoration of collagen formation in photodamaged human skin by tretinoin (retinoic acid). *N Engl J Med.* 1993;329(8):530–535.
5. Osman OS, Selway JL, Harikumar PE, et al. A novel method to assess collagen architecture in skin. *BMC Bioinformatics.* 2013;14:260.
6. Muthusamy V, Piva TJ. The UV response of the skin: a review of the MAPK, NFkappaB and TNFalpha signal transduction pathways. *Arch Dermatol Res.* 2010;302(1):5–17.
7. Baumann L. How to prevent photoaging? *J Invest Dermatol.* 2005;125(4):xii–xiii.
8. Pillai S, Oresajo C, Hayward J. Ultraviolet radiation and skin aging: roles of reactive oxygen species, inflammation and protease activation, and strategies for prevention of inflammation-induced matrix degradation – a review. *In: Int J Cosmet Sci.* 2005;27(1):17–34.
9. Murray JC, Burch JA, Streilein RD, Iannacchione MA, Hall RP, Pinnell SR. A topical antioxidant solution containing vitamins C and E stabilized by ferulic acid provides protection for human skin against damage caused by ultraviolet irradiation. *J Am Acad Dermatol.* 2008;59(3):418–425.
10. Geesin JC, Darr D, Kaufman R, Murad S, Pinnell SR. Ascorbic acid specifically increases type I and type III procollagen messenger RNA levels in human skin fibroblast. *J Invest Dermatol.* 1988;90(4):420–424.
11. Cui R, Widlund HR, Feige E, et al. Central role of p53 in the suntan response and pathologic hyperpigmentation. *Cell.* 2007;128(5):853–864.
12. Oresajo C, Stephens T, Hino PD, et al. Protective effects of a topical antioxidant mixture containing vitamin C, ferulic acid, and phloretin against ultraviolet-induced photodamage in human skin. *J Cosmet Dermatol.* 2008;7(4):290–297.
13. Pinnell SR, Murad S, Darr D. Induction of collagen synthesis by ascorbic acid. A possible mechanism. *Arch Dermatol.* 1987;123(12):1684–1686.
14. Peterkofsky B. Ascorbate requirement for hydroxylation and secretion of procollagen: relationship to inhibition of collagen synthesis in scurvy. *Am J Clin Nutr.* 1991;54(6 Suppl):1135S–1140S.
15. Murad S, Tajima S, Johnson GR, Sivarajah S, Pinnell SR. Collagen synthesis in cultured human skin fibroblasts: effect of ascorbic acid and its analogs. *J Invest Dermatol.* 1983;81(2):158–162.
16. Tajima S, Pinnell SR. Regulation of collagen synthesis by ascorbic acid. Ascorbic acid increases type I procollagen mRNA. *Biochem Biophys Res Commun.* 1982;106(2):632–637.
17. Phillips CL, Combs SB, Pinnell SR. Effects of ascorbic acid on proliferation and collagen synthesis in relation to the donor age of human dermal fibroblasts. *J Invest Dermatol.* 1994;103(2):228–232.
18. Pinnell SR, Yang H, Omar M, et al. Topical L-ascorbic acid: percutaneous absorption studies. *Dermatol Surg.* 2001;27(2):137–142.
19. Lin JY, Selim MA, Shea CR, et al. UV photoprotection by combination topical antioxidants vitamin C and vitamin E. *J Am Acad Dermatol.* 2003;48(6):866–874.
20. Placzek M, Gaube S, Kerkmann U, et al. Ultraviolet B-induced DNA damage in human epidermis is modified by the antioxidants ascorbic acid and D-alpha-tocopherol. *J Invest Dermatol.* 2005;124(2):304–307.
21. Lin FH, Lin JY, Gupta RD, et al. Ferulic acid stabilizes a solution of vitamins C and E and doubles its photoprotection of skin. *J Invest Dermatol.* 2005;125(4):826–832.
22. Charrouf Z, Guillaume D. Ethnoeconomical, ethnomedical, and phytochemical study of Argania spinosa (L.) Skeels. *J Ethnopharmacol.* 1999;67(1):7–14.
23. El Babili F, Bouajila J, Fouraste I, Valentin A, Mauret S, Moulis C. Chemical study, antimalarial and antioxidant activities, and cytotoxicity to human breast cancer cells (MCF7) of Argania spinosa. *Phytomedicine.* 2010;17(2):157–160.
24. Lin TK, Zhong L, Santiago JL. Anti-inflammatory and Skin Barrier Repair Effects of Topical Application of Some Plant Oils. *Int J Mol Sci.* 2017;19(1). pii: E70.
25. Boucetta KQ, Charrouf Z, Aguenaou H, Derouiche A, Bensouda Y. The effect of dietary and/or cosmetic argan oil on postmenopausal skin elasticity. *Clin Interv Aging.* 2015;10:339–349.

26. Sreedhar A, Aguilera-Aguirre L, Singh KK. Mitochondria in skin health, aging, and disease. *Cell Death Dis.* 2020;11(6):444.

27. Bhagavan HN, Chopra RK. Coenzyme Q10: absorption, tissue uptake, metabolism and pharmacokinetics. *Free Radic Res.* 2006;40(5):445–453.

28. Imhof L, Leuthard D. Topical Over-the-Counter Antiaging Agents: An Update and Systematic Review. *Dermatology.* 2020 Sep 3:1–13.

29. Marcheggiani F, Cirilli I, Orlando P, et al. Modulation of Coenzyme Q_{10} content and oxidative status in human dermal fibroblasts using HMG-CoA reductase inhibitor over a broad range of concentrations. From mitohormesis to mitochondrial dysfunction and accelerated aging. *Aging (Albany NY).* 2019;11(9):2565–2582.

30. Blatt T, Littarru GP. Biochemical rationale and experimental data on the antiaging properties of CoQ(10) at skin level. *Biofactors.* 2011;37(5):381–385.

31. Hoppe U, Bergemann J, Diembeck W, et al. Coenzyme Q10, a cutaneous antioxidant and energizer. *Biofactors.* 1999; 9(2-4):371–378.

32. Inui M, Ooe M, Fujii K, Matsunaka H, Yoshida M, Ichihashi M. Mechanisms of inhibitory effects of CoQ10 on UVB-induced wrinkle formation in vitro and in vivo. *Biofactors.* 2008;32(1-4):237–243.

33. Bradley EJ, Griffiths CE, Sherratt MJ, Bell M, Watson RE. Over-the-counter anti-ageing topical agents and their ability to protect and repair photoaged skin. *Maturitas.* 2015;80(3):265–272.

34. Meeran SM, Mantena SK, Elmets CA, Katiyar SK. (-)-Epigallocatechin-3-gallate prevents photocarcinogenesis in mice through interleukin-12-dependent DNA repair. *Cancer Res.* 2006;66(10):5512–5520.

35. Elmets CA, Singh D, Tubesing K, Matsui M, Katiyar S, Mukhtar H. Cutaneous photoprotection from ultraviolet injury by green tea polyphenols. *J Am Acad Dermatol.* 2001;44(3):425–432.

36. Reuter J, Merfort I, Schempp CM. Botanicals in dermatology: an evidence-based review. *Am J Clin Dermatol.* 2010;11(4):247–267.

37. Thring TS, Hili P, Naughton DP. Anti-collagenase, anti-elastase and anti-oxidant activities of extracts from 21 plants. *BMC Complement Altern Med.* 2009;9(1):27.

38. Hong YH, Jung EY, Shin KS, Yu KW, Chang UJ, Suh HJ. Tannase-converted green tea catechins and their anti-wrinkle activity in humans. *J Cosmet Dermatol.* 2013;12(2):137–143.

39. Mahmood T, Akhtar N. Combined topical application of lotus and green tea improves facial skin surface parameters. *Rejuvenation Res.* 2013;16(2):91–97.

40. Afaq F, Adhami VM, Admad N. Prevention of short-term ultraviolet B radiation-mediated damages by resveratrol in SKH-1 hairless mice. *Toxicol Appl Pharmacol.* 2003;186(1):28–37.

41. Adhami VM, Afaq F, Ahmad N. Suppression of ultraviolet B exposure-mediated activation of NF-kappaB in normal human keratinocytes by resveratrol. *Neoplasia.* 2003;5(1):74–82.

42. Foster S. *101 Medicinal Herbs: An Illustrated Guide.* Loveland, CO: Interweave Press; 1998: 108–109.

43. Hoffmann D. *Medical Herbalism: The Science and Practice of Herbal Medicine.* Rochester, VT: Healing Arts Press; 2003: 99–100.

44. Jang M, Cai L, Udeani GO, et al. Cancer chemopreventive activity of resveratrol, a natural product derived from grapes. *Science.* 1997;275(5297):218–220.

45. Baxter RA. Anti-aging properties of resveratrol: review and report of a potent new antioxidant skin care formulation. *J Cosmet Dermatol.* 2008;7(1):2–7.

46. Boyer JZ, Jandova J, Janda J, Vleugels FR, Elliott DA, Sligh JE. Resveratrol-sensitized UVA induced apoptosis in human keratinocytes through mitochondrial oxidative stress and pore opening. *J Photochem Photobiol B.* 2012;113:42–50.

47. Athar M, Back JH, Tang X, et al. Resveratrol: a review of preclinical studies for human cancer prevention. *Toxicol Appl Pharmacol.* 2007;224(3):274–283.

48. Farris P, Yatskayer M, Chen N, Krol Y, Oresajo C. Evaluation of efficacy and tolerance of a nighttime topical antioxidant containing resveratrol, baicalin, and vitamin E for treatment of mild to moderately photodamaged skin. *J Drugs Dermatol.* 2014;13(12):1467–1472.

49. Singh UP, Singh NP, Singh B, et al. Resveratrol (trans-3,5,4′-trihydroxystilbene) induces silent mating type information regulation-1 and down-regulates nuclear transcription factor-kappaB activation to abrogate dextran sulfate sodium-induced colitis. *J Pharmacol Exp Ther.* 2010;332(3):829–839.

50. Ye L, Mauro TM, Dang E, et al. Topical applications of an emollient reduce circulating pro-inflammatory cytokine levels in chronically aged humans: a pilot clinical study. *J Eur Acad Dermatol Venereol.* 2019;33(11):2197–2201.

51. Zattra E, Coleman C, Arad S, et al. Polypodium leucotomos extract decreases UV-induced Cox-2 expression and inflammation, enhances DNA repair, and decreases mutagenesis in hairless mice. *Am J Pathol.* 2009;175(5):1952–1961.

52. Cole MA, Quan T, Voorhees JJ, Fisher GJ. Extracellular matrix regulation of fibroblast function: redefining our perspective on skin aging. *J Cell Commun Signal.* 2018;12(1):35–43.

53. Bourguignon LY, Ramez M, Gilad E, et al. Hyaluronan-CD44 interaction stimulates keratinocyte differentiation, lamellar body formation/secretion, and permeability barrier homeostasis. *J Invest Dermatol.* 2006;126(6):1356–1365.

54. Aruffo A, Stamenkovic I, Melnick M, Underhill CB, Seed B. CD44 is the principal cell surface receptor for hyaluronate. *Cell.* 1990;61(7):1303–1313.

55. Culty M, Miyake K, Kincade PW, Sikorski E, Butcher EC, Underhill C. The hyaluronate receptor is a member of the CD44 (H-CAM) family of cell surface glycoproteins. *J Cell Biol.* 1990;111(6 Pt 1):2765–2774.

56. Underhill C. CD44: the hyaluronan receptor. *J Cell Sci.* 1992;103 (Pt 2):293–298.

57. Ghersetich I, Lotti T, Campanile G, Grappone C, Dini G. Hyaluronic acid in cutaneous intrinsic aging. *Int J Dermatol.* 1994;33(2):119–122.

58. Quan T, Wang F, Shao Y, et al. Enhancing structural support of the dermal microenvironment activates fibroblasts, endothelial cells, and keratinocytes in aged human skin in vivo. *J Invest Dermatol.* 2013;133(3):658–667.

59. Brown MB, Jones SA. Hyaluronic acid: a unique topical vehicle for the localized delivery of drugs to the skin. *J Eur Acad Dermatol Venereol.* 2005;19(3):308–318.

60. Nawrat P, Surazyński A, Karna E, Pałka JA. The effect of hyaluronic acid on interleukin-1-induced deregulation of collagen metabolism in cultured human skin fibroblasts. *Pharmacol Res.* 2005;51(5):473–477.

61. Pavicic T, Gauglitz GG, Lersch P, et al. Efficacy of cream-based novel formulations of hyaluronic acid of different molecular weights in anti-wrinkle treatment. *J Drugs Dermatol.* 2011;10(9):990–1000.

62. Simon Davis DA, Parish CR. Heparan sulfate: a ubiquitous glycosaminoglycan with multiple roles in immunity. *Front Immunol.* 2013;4:470.

63. Gallo RL, Bucay VW, Shamban AT, et al. The Potential Role of Topically Applied Heparan Sulfate in the Treatment of Photodamage. *J Drugs Dermatol.* 2015;14(7):669–674.

64. Berardesca E, Distante F, Vignoli GP, Oresajo C, Green B. Alpha hydroxyacids modulate stratum corneum barrier function. *Br J Dermatol.* 1997;137(6):934–938.

65. Newman N, Newman A, Moy LS, Babapour R, Harris AG, Moy RL. Clinical improvement of photoaged skin with 50% glycolic acid. A double-blind vehicle-controlled study. *Dermatol Surg.* 1996;22(5):455–460.

66. Smith WP. Epidermal and dermal effects of topical lactic acid. *J Am Acad Dermatol.* 1996;35(3 Pt 1):388–391.

67. Ditre CM, Griffin TD, Murphy GF, et al. Effects of alpha-hydroxy acids on photoaged skin: a pilot clinical, histologic, and ultrastructural study. *J Am Acad Dermatol.* 1996;34(2 Pt 1):187–195.

68. Bernstein EF, Lee J, Brown DB, Yu R, Van Scott E. Glycolic acid treatment increases type I collagen mRNA and hyaluronic acid content of human skin. *Dermatol Surg.* 2001;27(5):429–433.

69. Ramos-e-Silva M, Celem LR, Ramos-e-Silva S, Fucci-da-Costa AP. Anti-aging cosmetics: facts and controversies. *Clin Dermatol.* 2013;31(6):750–758.

70. Baumann L, Saghari S. Chemical Peels, In: Baumann L, Saghari S, Weisberg E, eds. *Cosmetic Dermatology: Principles and Practice.* 2nd edition. New York: McGraw-Hill; 2009: 148–162.

71. Van Scott EJ, Yu RJ. Control of keratinization with alpha-hydroxy acids and related compounds. I. Topical treatment of ichthyotic disorders. *Arch Dermatol.* 1974;110(4):586–590.

72. Van Scott EJ, Yu RJ. Hyperkeratinization, corneocyte cohesion, and alpha hydroxy acids. *J Am Acad Dermatol.* 1984;11(5 Pt 1):867–879.

73. Thompson BC, Halliday GM, Damian DL. Nicotinamide enhances repair of arsenic and ultraviolet radiation-induced DNA damage in HaCaT keratinocytes and ex vivo human skin. *PLoS One.* 2015;10(2):e0117491.

74. Surjana D, Halliday GM, Damian DL. Nicotinamide enhances repair of ultraviolet radiation-induced DNA damage in human keratinocytes and ex vivo skin. *Carcinogenesis.* 2013;34(5):1144–1149.

75. Kawada A, Konishi N, Oiso N, Kawara S, Date A. Evaluation of anti-wrinkle effects of a novel cosmetic containing niacinamide. *J Dermatol.* 2008;35(10):637–642.

76. Bissett DL, Oblong JE, Berge CA. Niacinamide: A B vitamin that improves aging facial skin appearance. *Dermatol Surg.* 2005;31(7 Pt 2):860–865.

77. Bissett DL, Miyamoto K, Sun P, Li J, Berge CA. Topical niacinamide reduces yellowing, wrinkling, red blotchiness, and hyperpigmented spots in aging facial skin. *Int J Cosmet Sci.* 2004;26(5):231–238.

78. Fabi S, Sundaram H. The potential of topical and injectable growth factors and cytokines for skin rejuvenation. *Facial Plast Surg.* 2014;30(2):157–171.

79. Aldag C, Nogueira Teixeira D, Leventhal PS. Skin rejuvenation using cosmetic products containing growth factors, cytokines, and matrikines: a review of the literature. *Clin Cosmet Investig Dermatol.* 2016;9:411–419.

80. Buchtova M, Chaloupkova R, Zakrzewska M, et al. Instability restricts signaling of multiple fibroblast growth factors. *Cell Mol Life Sci.* 2015;72(12):2445–2459.

81. Gandhi NS, Mancera RL. The structure of glycosaminoglycans and their interactions with proteins. *Chem Biol Drug Des.* 2008;72(6):455–482.

82. Hardwicke J, Schmaljohann D, Boyce D, Thomas D. Epidermal growth factor therapy and wound healing--past, present and future perspectives. *Surgeon.* 2008;6(3):172–177.

83. Heldin P, Laurent TC, Heldin CH. Effect of growth factors on hyaluronan synthesis in cultured human fibroblasts. *Biochem J.* 1989;258(3):919–922.

84. Rittié L, Varani J, Kang S, Voorhees JJ, Fisher GJ. Retinoid-induced epidermal hyperplasia is mediated by epidermal growth factor receptor activation via specific induction of its ligands heparin-binding EGF and amphiregulin in human skin in vivo. *J Invest Dermatol.* 2006;126(4):732–739.

85. King LE Jr, Gates RE, Stoscheck CM, Nanney LB. The EGF/TGF alpha receptor in skin. *J Invest Dermatol.* 1990;94(6 Suppl):164S–170S.

86. Franzke CW, Cobzaru C, Triantafyllopoulou A, et al. Epidermal ADAM17 maintains the skin barrier by regulating EGFR ligand-dependent terminal keratinocyte differentiation. *J Exp Med.* 2012;209(6):1105–1119.

87. Zemtsov A, Montalvo-Lugo V. Topically applied growth factors change skin cytoplasmic creatine kinase activity and distribution and produce abnormal keratinocyte differentiation in murine skin. *Skin Res Technol.* 2008;14(3):370–375.

88. Kwon SB, An S, Kim MJ, et al. Phytosphingosine-1-phosphate and epidermal growth factor synergistically restore extracellular matrix in human dermal fibroblasts in vitro and in vivo. *Int J Mol Med.* 2017;39(3):741–748.

89. Derynck R, Goeddel DV, Ullrich A, et al. Synthesis of messenger RNAs for transforming growth factors alpha and beta and the epidermal growth factor receptor by human tumors. *Cancer Res.* 1987;47(3):707–712.

90. Messing EM, Hanson P, Ulrich P, Erturk E. Epidermal growth factor--interactions with normal and malignant urothelium: in vivo and in situ studies. *J Urol.* 1987;138(5):1329–1335.

91. Chen J, Zeng F, Forrester SJ, Eguchi S, Zhang MZ, Harris RC. Expression and Function of the Epidermal Growth Factor Receptor in Physiology and Disease. *Physiol Rev.* 2016;96(3):1025–1069.

92. Kang S, Chung JH, Lee JH, et al. Topical N-acetyl cysteine and genistein prevent ultraviolet-light-induced signaling that leads to photoaging in human skin in vivo. *J Invest Dermatol.* 2003;120(5):835–841.

93. Coffey RJ Jr, Derynck R, Wilcox JN, et al. Production and auto-induction of transforming growth factor-alpha in human keratinocytes. *Nature.* 1987;328(6133):817–820.

94. Rosenthal A, Lindquist PB, Bringman TS, Goeddel DV, Derynck R. Expression in rat fibroblasts of a human transforming growth factor-alpha cDNA results in transformation. *Cell.* 1986;46(2):301–309.

95. de Araújo R, Lôbo M, Trindade K, Silva DF, Pereira N. Fibroblast Growth Factors: A Controlling Mechanism of Skin Aging. *Skin Pharmacol Physiol*. 2019;32(5):275–282.

96. Czyz M. Fibroblast Growth Factor Receptor Signaling in Skin Cancers. *Cells*. 2019;8(6):540.

97. Werner S. Keratinocyte growth factor: a unique player in epithelial repair processes. *Cytokine Growth Factor Rev*. 1998;9(2):153–165.

98. Cardinali G, Ceccarelli S, Kovacs D, et al. Keratinocyte growth factor promotes melanosome transfer to keratinocytes. *J Invest Dermatol*. 2005;125(6):1190–1199.

99. Dou C, Lay F, Ansari AM, et al. Strengthening the skin with topical delivery of keratinocyte growth factor-1 using a novel DNA plasmid. *Mol Ther*. 2014;22(4):752–761.

100. Kulik G, Klippel A, Weber MJ. Antiapoptotic signalling by the insulin-like growth factor I receptor, phosphatidylinositol 3-kinase, and Akt. *Mol Cell Biol*. 1997;17(3):1595–1606.

101. Decraene D, Agostinis P, Bouillon R, Degreef H, Garmyn M. Insulin-like growth factor-1-mediated AKT activation postpones the onset of ultraviolet B-induced apoptosis, providing more time for cyclobutane thymine dimer removal in primary human keratinocytes. *J Biol Chem*. 2002;277(36):32587–32595.

102. Puche JE, García-Fernández M, Muntané J, Rioja J, González-Barón S, Castilla Cortazar I. Low doses of insulin-like growth factor-I induce mitochondrial protection in aging rats. *Endocrinology*. 2008;149(5):2620–2627.

103. Noordam R, Gunn DA, Tomlin CC, et al. Serum insulin-like growth factor 1 and facial ageing: high levels associate with reduced skin wrinkling in a cross-sectional study. *Br J Dermatol*. 2013;168(3):533–538.

104. Pakyari M, Farrokhi A, Maharlooei MK, Ghahary A. Critical Role of Transforming Growth Factor Beta in Different Phases of Wound Healing. *Adv Wound Care (New Rochelle)*. 2013;2(5):215–224.

105. Murata H, Zhou L, Ochoa S, Hasan A, Badiavas E, Falanga V. TGF-beta3 stimulates and regulates collagen synthesis through TGF-beta1-dependent and independent mechanisms. *J Invest Dermatol*. 1997;108(3):258–262.

106. Kähäri VM, Olsen DR, Rhudy RW, Carrillo P, Chen YQ, Uitto J. Transforming growth factor-beta up-regulates elastin gene expression in human skin fibroblasts. Evidence for post-transcriptional modulation. *Lab Invest*. 1992;66(5):580–588.

107. Wisdom R, Huynh L, Hsia D, Kim S. RAS and TGF-beta exert antagonistic effects on extracellular matrix gene expression and fibroblast transformation. *Oncogene*. 2005;24(47):7043–7054.

108. Quan T, He T, Kang S, Voorhees JJ, Fisher GJ. Ultraviolet irradiation alters transforming growth factor beta/smad pathway in human skin in vivo. *J Invest Dermatol*. 2002;119(2):499–506.

109. Son ED, Lee JY, Lee S, et al. Topical application of 17beta-estradiol increases extracellular matrix protein synthesis by stimulating tgf-Beta signaling in aged human skin in vivo. *J Invest Dermatol*. 2005;124(6):1149–1161.

110. Shao Y, He T, Fisher GJ, Voorhees JJ, Quan T. Molecular basis of retinol anti-ageing properties in naturally aged human skin in vivo. *Int J Cosmet Sci*. 2017;39(1):56–65.

111. Falanga V, Qian SW, Danielpour D, Katz MH, Roberts AB, Sporn MB. Hypoxia upregulates the synthesis of TGF-beta 1 by human dermal fibroblasts. *J Invest Dermatol*. 1991;97(4):634–637.

112. Fabregat I, Fernando J, Mainez J, Sancho P. TGF-beta signaling in cancer treatment. *Curr Pharm Des*. 2014;20(17):2934–2947.

113. Glick AB, Kulkarni AB, Tennenbaum T, et al. Loss of expression of transforming growth factor beta in skin and skin tumors is associated with hyperproliferation and a high risk for malignant conversion. *Proc Natl Acad Sci U S A*. 1993;90(13):6076–6080.

114. Gousopoulos E, Proulx ST, Bachmann SB, et al. An Important Role of VEGF-C in Promoting Lymphedema Development. *J Invest Dermatol*. 2017;137(9):1995–2004.

115. Liu B, Earl HM, Baban D, et al. Melanoma cell lines express VEGF receptor KDR and respond to exogenously added VEGF. *Biochem Biophys Res Commun*. 1995;217(3):721–727.

116. Gerlicz-Kowalczuk Z, Zalewska-Janowska A, Dziankowska-Bartkowiak B. 434 Serum concentration of VEGF in systemic sclerosis patients with arthritis. *J Invest Dermatol*. 2016;136(9):S234.

117. Karlsson C, Paulsson Y. Age related induction of platelet-derived growth factor A-chain mRNA in normal human fibroblasts. *J Cell Physiol*. 1994;158(2):256–262.

118. Heldin CH, Westermark B. Mechanism of action and in vivo role of platelet-derived growth factor. *Physiol Rev*. 1999;79(4):1283–1316.

119. Baumann L. How to Use Oral and Topical Cosmeceuticals to Prevent and Treat Skin Aging. *Facial Plast Surg Clin North Am*. 2018;26(4):407–413.

120. Cal K. Across the skin barrier: known methods, new performances. In: Caldwell GW, ur-Rahman A, Yan Z, Choundhary MI, eds. *Frontiers in Drug Design and Discovery*. Bentham Science Publishers; 2009; vol. 4:162–188.

121. Mehta RC, Fitzpatrick RE. Endogenous growth factors as cosmeceuticals. *Dermatol Ther*. 2007;20(5):350–359.

122. Skinmedica. Growth Factors Rejuvenate Skin. https://www.skinmedica.com/TNSCampaign. Accessed 12/12/2020.

123. Mehta RC, Smith SR, Grove GL, et al. Reduction in facial photodamage by a topical growth factor product. *J Drugs Dermatol*. 2008;7(9):864–871.

124. Lupo ML, Cohen JL, Rendon MI. Novel eye cream containing a mixture of human growth factors and cytokines for periorbital skin rejuvenation. *J Drugs Dermatol*. 2007;6(7):725–729.

125. Gold MH, Goldman MP, Biron J. Human growth factor and cytokine skin cream for facial skin rejuvenation as assessed by 3D in vivo optical skin imaging. *J Drugs Dermatol*. 2007;6(10):1018–1023.

126. Mendelsohn J, Baselga J. The EGF receptor family as targets for cancer therapy. *Oncogene*. 2000;19(56):6550–6565.

127. Ehrlich M, Rao J, Pabby A, Goldman MP. Improvement in the appearance of wrinkles with topical transforming growth factor beta(1) and l-ascorbic acid. *Dermatol Surg*. 2006;32(5):618–625.

128. Fabi SG, Cohen JL, Peterson JD, Kiripolsky MG, Goldman MP. The Effects of Filtrate of the Secretion of the Cryptomphalus Aspersa on Photoaged Skin. *J Drugs Dermatol*. 2013;12(4):453–457.

129. Brieva A, Philips N, Tejedor R, et al. Molecular basis for the regenerative properties of a secretion of the mollusk Cryptomphalus aspersa. *Skin Pharmacol Physiol*. 2008;21(1):15–22.

130. Stoscheck CM, King LE Jr. Role of epidermal growth factor in carcinogenesis. *Cancer Res*. 1986;46(3):1030–1037.

131. TruthinAdvertising.org. Skinmedicas' TNS products. https://www.truthinadvertising.org/skinmedicas-tns-products/. Accessed 1/15/2021.

132. Lazar-Molnar E, Hegyesi H, Toth S, Falus A. Autocrine and paracrine regulation by cytokines and growth factors in melanoma. *Cytokine*. 2000;12(6):547–554.

133. Brincat M, Moniz CJ, Studd JW, et al. Long-term effects of the menopause and sex hormones on skin thickness. *Br J Obstet Gynaecol*. 1985;92(3):256–259.

134. Bottai G, Mancina R, Muratori M, Di Gennaro P, Lotti T. 17β-estradiol protects human skin fibroblasts and keratinocytes against oxidative damage. *J Eur Acad Dermatol Venereol*. 2013;27(10):1236–1243.

135. Thornton MJ. Oestrogen functions in skin and skin appendages. *Expert Opin Ther Targets*. 2005;9(3):617–629.

136. Stevenson S, Thornton J. Effect of estrogens on skin aging and the potential role of SERMs. *Clin Interv Aging*. 2007;2(3):283–297.

137. Thornton MJ. The biological actions of estrogens on skin. *Exp Dermatol*. 2002;11(6):487–502.

138. Gopaul R, Knaggs HE, Lephart ED. Biochemical investigation and gene analysis of equol: a plant and soy-derived isoflavonoid with antiaging and antioxidant properties with potential human skin applications. *Biofactors*. 2012;38(1):44–52.

139. Chua LS, Lee SY, Abdullah N, Sarmidi MR. Review on Labisia pumila (Kacip Fatimah): bioactive phytochemicals and skin collagen synthesis promoting herb. *Fitoterapia*. 2012;83(8):1322–1335.

140. Patriarca MT, Barbosa de Moraes AR, Nader HB, et al. Hyaluronic acid concentration in postmenopausal facial skin after topical estradiol and genistein treatment: a double-blind, randomized clinical trial of efficacy. *Menopause*. 2013;20(3):336–341.

141. Mostrom M, Evans TJ. Chapter 52, Phytoestrogens. In: Gupta RC, ed. *Reproductive and Developmental Toxicology*. Cambridge, MA: Academic Press; 2011: 707–722.

142. Sator PG, Schmidt JB, Rabe T, Zouboulis CC. Skin aging and sex hormones in women -- clinical perspectives for intervention by hormone replacement therapy. *Exp Dermatol*. 2004;13 (Suppl 4):36–40.

143. Bos JD, Meinardi MM. The 500 Dalton rule for the skin penetration of chemical compounds and drugs. *Exp Dermatol*. 2000;9(3):165–169.

144. Benson HA, Namjoshi S. Proteins and peptides: strategies for delivery to and across the skin. *J Pharm Sci*. 2008;97 (9):3591–3610.

145. Lim SH, Tiew WJ, Zhang J, Ho PC, Kachouie NN, Kang L. Geometrical optimisation of a personalised microneedle eye patch for transdermal delivery of anti-wrinkle small peptide. *Biofabrication*. 2020;12(3):035003.

146. Errante F, Menicatti M, Pallecchi M, et al. Susceptibility of cosmeceutical peptides to proteases activity: Development of dermal stability test by LC-MS/MS analysis. *J Pharm Biomed Anal*. 2021;194:113775.

147. Personal Care Products Council. INCI Nomenclature Conventions. https://inci.personalcarecouncil.org/inci-app/html/INCINomenclatureConventions.pdf. Accessed 1/17/2021.

148. Gorouhi F, Maibach HI. Role of topical peptides in preventing or treating aged skin. *Int J Cosmet Sci*. 2009;31(5):327–345.

149. Schagen SK. Topical peptide treatments with effective anti-aging results. *Cosmetics*. 2017;4(2):16.

150. Taub A, Bucay V, Keller G, Williams J, Mehregan D. Multi-Center, Double-Blind, Vehicle-Controlled Clinical Trial of an Alpha and Beta Defensin-Containing Anti-Aging Skin Care Regimen With Clinical, Histopathologic, Immunohistochemical, Photographic, and Ultrasound Evaluation. *J Drugs Dermatol*. 2018;17(4):426–441.

151. Snippert HJ, Haegebarth A, Kasper M, et al. Lgr6 marks stem cells in the hair follicle that generate all cell lineages of the skin. *Science*. 2010;327(5971):1385–1389.

152. Lough D, Dai H, Yang M, et al. Stimulation of the follicular bulge LGR5+ and LGR6+ stem cells with the gut-derived human alpha defensin 5 results in decreased bacterial presence, enhanced wound healing, and hair growth from tissues devoid of adnexal structures. *Plast Reconstr Surg*. 2013;132(5):1159–1171.

153. Campisi J, d'Adda di Fagagna F. Cellular senescence: when bad things happen to good cells. *Nat Rev Mol Cell Biol*. 2007;8(9):729–740.

154. Semple F, Dorin JR. β-Defensins: multifunctional modulators of infection, inflammation and more? *J Innate Immun*. 2012;4(4):337–348.

155. Hanaoka Y, Yamaguchi Y, Yamamoto H, et al. In Vitro and In Vivo Anticancer Activity of Human β-Defensin-3 and Its Mouse Homolog. *Anticancer Res*. 2016;36(11):5999–6004.

156. Lichtenstein A, Ganz T, Selsted ME, Lehrer RI. In vitro tumor cell cytolysis mediated by peptide defensins of human and rabbit granulocytes. *Blood*. 1986;68(6):1407–1410.

157. Biragyn A, Ruffini PA, Leifer CA, et al. Toll-like receptor 4-dependent activation of dendritic cells by beta-defensin 2. *Science*. 2002;298(5595):1025–1029.

158. Maquart FX, Bellon G, Pasco S, Monboisse JC. Matrikines in the regulation of extracellular matrix degradation. *Biochimie*. 2005;87(3-4):353–360.

159. Maquart FX, Pasco S, Ramont L, Hornebeck W, Monboisse JC. An introduction to matrikines: extracellular matrix-derived peptides which regulate cell activity. Implication in tumor invasion. *Crit Rev Oncol Hematol*. 2004;49(3):199–202.

160. Johnson W Jr, Bergfeld WF, Belsito DV, et al. Safety Assessment of Tripeptide-1, Hexapeptide-12, Their Metal Salts and Fatty Acyl Derivatives, and Palmitoyl Tetrapeptide-7 as Used in Cosmetics. *Int J Toxicol*. 2018;37(3_suppl):90S–102S.

161. Vanaman Wilson MJ, Bolton J, Fabi SG. A randomized, single-blinded trial of a tripeptide/hexapeptide healing regimen following laser resurfacing of the face. *J Cosmet Dermatol*. 2017;16(2):217–222.

162. Reivitis A, Karimi K, Griffiths C, Banayan A. A single-center, pilot study evaluating a novel TriHex peptide- and botanical-containing eye treatment compared to baseline. *J Cosmet Dermatol*. 2018;17(3):467–470.

163. Nelson AM, Ortiz AE. Effects of anhydrous gel with TriHex peptides on healing after hybrid laser resurfacing. *J Cosmet Dermatol*. 2020;19(4):925–929.

164. Widgerow AD, Jiang LI, Calame A. A single-center clinical trial to evaluate the efficacy of a tripeptide/hexapeptide antiaging regimen. *J Cosmet Dermatol*. 2019;18(1):176–182.

165. Katayama K, Seyer JM, Raghow R, Kang AH. Regulation of extracellular matrix production by chemically synthesized

subfragments of type I collagen carboxy propeptide. *Biochemistry*. 1991;30(29):7097–7104.

166. Katayama K, Armendariz-Borunda J, Raghow R, Kang AH, Seyer JM. A pentapeptide from type I procollagen promotes extracellular matrix production. *J Biol Chem*. 1993;268(14):9941–9944.

167. Choi YL, Park EJ, Kim E, Na DH, Shin YH. Dermal Stability and In Vitro Skin Permeation of Collagen Pentapeptides (KTTKS and palmitoyl-KTTKS). *Biomol Ther (Seoul)*. 2014;22(4):321–327.

168. Jones RR, Castelletto V, Connon CJ, Hamley IW. Collagen stimulating effect of peptide amphiphile C16-KTTKS on human fibroblasts. *Mol Pharm*. 2013;10(3):1063–1069.

169. Robinson LR, Fitzgerald NC, Doughty DG, Dawes NC, Berge CA, Bissett DL. Topical palmitoyl pentapeptide provides improvement in photoaged human facial skin. *Int J Cosmet Sci*. 2005;27(3):155–160.

170. Lintner K. Cosmetic or Dermopharmaceutical Use of Peptides for Healing, Hydrating and Improving Skin Appearances during Natural or Induced Ageing (Heliodermia, Pollution). US Patent 6,620,419, 16 September, 2003.

171. Guttman C. Studies demonstrate value of procollagen fragment Pal-KTTKS. *Dermatology Times*. 2002;23(9).

172. Tałałaj U, Uścinowicz P, Bruzgo I, Surażyński A, Zaręba I, Markowska A. The Effects of a Novel Series of KTTKS Analogues on Cytotoxicity and Proteolytic Activity. *Molecules*. 2019;24(20):3698.

173. Lupo MP, Cole AL. Cosmeceutical peptides. *Dermatol Ther*. 2007;20(5):343–349.

174. Husein El Hadmed H, Castillo RF. Cosmeceuticals: peptides, proteins, and growth factors. *J Cosmet Dermatol*. 2016;15(4):514–519.

175. Kim DW, Hwang HS, Kim DS, et al. Effect of silk fibroin peptide derived from silkworm Bombyx mori on the anti-inflammatory effect of Tat-SOD in a mice edema model. *BMB Rep*. 2011;44(12):787–792.

176. Sim GS, Lee DH, Kim JH, et al. Black rice (Oryza sativa L. var. japonica) hydrolyzed peptides induce expression of hyaluronan synthase 2 gene in HaCaT keratinocytes. *J Microbiol Biotechnol*. 2007;17(2):271–279.

177. Pickart L, Vasquez-Soltero JM, Margolina A. GHK Peptide as a Natural Modulator of Multiple Cellular Pathways in Skin Regeneration. *Biomed Res Int*. 2015;2015:648108.

178. Wegrowski Y, Maquart FX, Borel JP. Stimulation of sulfated glycosaminoglycan synthesis by the tripeptide-copper complex glycyl-L-histidyl-L-lysine-Cu2+. *Life Sci*. 1992;51(13):1049–1056.

179. Siméon A, Emonard H, Hornebeck W, Maquart FX. The tripeptide-copper complex glycyl-L-histidyl-L-lysine-Cu2+ stimulates matrix metalloproteinase-2 expression by fibroblast cultures. *Life Sci*. 2000;67(18):2257–2265.

180. Siméon A, Wegrowski Y, Bontemps Y, Maquart FX. Expression of glycosaminoglycans and small proteoglycans in wounds: modulation by the tripeptide-copper complex glycyl-L-histidyl-L-lysine-Cu(2+). *J Invest Dermatol*. 2000;115(6):962–968.

181. Leyden JJ, Stevens T, Finkey MB, Barkovic S. Skin care benefits of copper peptide containing facial cream. In: American Academy of Dermatology 60th Annual Meeting 2002 Feb. 22 (p. 29). American Academy of Dermatology, New York, NY, USA.

182. JUSTIA Trademarks. https://trademarks.justia.com/783/06/argireline-78306043.html. Accessed 1/22/2021.

183. BlanesMira C, Clemente J, Jodas G, et al. A synthetic hexapeptide (Argireline) with antiwrinkle activity. *Int J Cosmet Sci*. 2002;24(5):303–310.

184. Tadini KA, Mercurio DG, Campos PM. Acetyl hexapeptide-3 in a cosmetic formulation acts on skin mechanical properties-clinical study. *Braz J Pharm Sci*. 2015;51(4):901–909.

185. Raikou V, Varvaresou A, Panderi I, Papageorgiou E. The efficacy study of the combination of tripeptide-10-citrulline and acetyl hexapeptide-3. A prospective, randomized controlled study. *J Cosmet Dermatol*. 2017;16(2):271–278.

186. Errante F, Ledwoń P, Latajka R, Rovero P, Papini AM. Cosmeceutical Peptides in the Framework of Sustainable Wellness Economy. *Front Chem*. 2020;8:572923.

187. Cao C, Xiao Z, Wu Y, Ge C. Diet and Skin Aging-From the Perspective of Food Nutrition. *Nutrients*. 2020;12(3):870.

188. Karna E, Szoka L, Huynh TYL, Palka JA. Proline-dependent regulation of collagen metabolism. *Cell Mol Life Sci*. 2020;77(10):1911–1918.

189. Albaugh VL, Mukherjee K, Barbul A. Proline Precursors and Collagen Synthesis: Biochemical Challenges of Nutrient Supplementation and Wound Healing. *J Nutr*. 2017;147(11): 2011–2017.

190. Aito-Inoue M, Lackeyram D, Fan MZ, Sato K, Mine Y. Transport of a tripeptide, Gly-Pro-Hyp, across the porcine intestinal brush-border membrane. *J Pept Sci*. 2007;13(7):468–474.

191. Shigemura Y, Kubomura D, Sato Y, Sato K. Dose-dependent changes in the levels of free and peptide forms of hydroxyproline in human plasma after collagen hydrolysate ingestion. *Food Chem*. 2014;159:328–332.

192. Spiro A, Lockyer S. Nutraceuticals and skin appearance: Is there any evidence to support this growing trend? *Nutrition Bulletin*. 2018;43(1):10–45.

193. León-López A, Morales-Peñaloza A, Martínez-Juárez VM, Vargas-Torres A, Zeugolis DI, Aguirre-Álvarez G. Hydrolyzed Collagen-Sources and Applications. *Molecules*. 2019;24(22):4031.

194. Choi FD, Sung CT, Juhasz ML, Mesinkovsk NA. Oral Collagen Supplementation: A Systematic Review of Dermatological Applications. *J Drugs Dermatol*. 2019;18(1):9–16.

195. Ohara H, Ichikawa S, Matsumoto H, et al. Collagen-derived dipeptide, proline-hydroxyproline, stimulates cell proliferation and hyaluronic acid synthesis in cultured human dermal fibroblasts. *J Dermatol*. 2010;37(4):330–338.

196. Kawaguchi T, Nanbu PN, Kurokawa M. Distribution of prolylhydroxyproline and its metabolites after oral administration in rats. *Biol Pharm Bull*. 2012;35(3):422–427.

197. Watanabe-Kamiyama M, Shimizu M, Kamiyama S, et al. Absorption and effectiveness of orally administered low molecular weight collagen hydrolysate in rats. *J Agric Food Chem*. 2010;58(2):835–841.

198. Xu D, Li D, Zhao Z, Wu J, Zhao M. Regulation by walnut protein hydrolysate on the components and structural degradation of photoaged skin in SD rats. *Food Funct*. 2019;10(10):6792–6802.

199. Jhawar N, Wang JV, Saedi N. Oral collagen supplementation for skin aging: A fad or the future? *J Cosmet Dermatol*. 2020;19(4):910–912.

200. Alcock RD. Dietary collagen intake and sources for support of dense connective tissues in athletes. Doctoral dissertation, ACU Research Bank, 2019.

201. Kamoun A, Landeau JM, Godeau G, et al. Growth stimulation of human skin fibroblasts by elastin-derived peptides. *Cell Adhes Commun*. 1995;3(4):273–281.

202. Duca L, Floquet N, Alix AJ, Haye B, Debelle L. Elastin as a matrikine. *Crit Rev Oncol Hematol*. 2004;49(3):235–244.

203. Le Page A, Khalil A, Vermette P, et al. The role of elastin-derived peptides in human physiology and diseases. *Matrix Biol*. 2019;84:81–96.

204. Liu Y, Su G, Zhou F, Zhang J, Zheng L, Zhao M. Protective Effect of Bovine Elastin Peptides against Photoaging in Mice and Identification of Novel Antiphotoaging Peptides. *J Agric Food Chem*. 2018;66(41):10760–10768.

205. Ntayi C, Labrousse AL, Debret R, et al. Elastin-derived peptides upregulate matrix metalloproteinase-2-mediated melanoma cell invasion through elastin-binding protein. *J Invest Dermatol*. 2004;122(2):256–265.

206. Lapis K, Tímár J. Role of elastin–matrix interactions in tumor progression. In: *Seminars in cancer biology*. Vol. 12, No. 3. Academic Press, 2002, pp. 209–217.

207. Jud P, Sourij H. Therapeutic options to reduce advanced glycation end products in patients with diabetes mellitus: A review. *Diabetes Res Clin Pract*. 2019;148:54–63.

208. Senior RM, Griffin GL, Mecham RP, Wrenn DS, Prasad KU, Urry DW. Val-Gly-Val-Ala-Pro-Gly, a repeating peptide in elastin, is chemotactic for fibroblasts and monocytes. *J Cell Biol*. 1984;99(3):870–874.

209. Tajima S, Wachi H, Uemura Y, Okamoto K. Modulation by elastin peptide VGVAPG of cell proliferation and elastin expression in human skin fibroblasts. *Arch Dermatol Res*. 1997;289(8):489–492.

210. Teglia A, Secchi G. New protein ingredients for skin detergency: native wheat protein-surfactant complexes. *Int J Cosmet Sci*. 1994;16(6):235–246.

211. Barba C, Méndez S, Roddick-Lanzilotta A, Kelly R, Parra JL, Coderch L. Wool peptide derivatives for hand care. *J Cosmet Sci*. 2007;58(2):99–107.

212. Yeo I, Lee YJ, Song K, et al. Low-molecular weight keratins with anti-skin aging activity produced by anaerobic digestion of poultry feathers with Fervidobacterium islandicum AW-1. *J Biotechnol*. 2018;271:17–25.

213. Fontoura R, Daroit DJ, Corrêa APF, Moresco KS, Santi L. Characterization of a novel antioxidant peptide from feather keratin hydrolysates. *N Biotechnol*. 2019;49:71–76.

214. Kligman L, Kligman AM. Photoaging - Retinoids, alpha hydroxy acids, and antioxidants. In: Gabard B, Elsner P, Surber C, Treffel P, eds. *Dermatopharmacology of Topical Preparations*. New York: Springer; 2000: 383.

215. Kligman AM, Grove GL, Hirose R, Leyden JJ. Topical tretinoin for photoaged skin. *J Am Acad Dermatol*. 1986;15(4 Pt 2):836–859.

216. Baumann L, Saghari S. Retinoids. In: Baumann L, Saghari S, Weisberg E, eds. *Cosmetic Dermatology: Principles and Practice*. 2nd edition. New York: McGraw-Hill; 2009: 256–262.

217. Weiss JS, Ellis CN, Headington JT, Tincoff T, Hamilton TA, Voorhees JJ. Topical tretinoin improves photoaged skin. A double-blind vehicle-controlled study. *JAMA*. 1988;259(4):527–532.

Erratum in: JAMA 1988 Aug 19;260(7):926. Erratum in: JAMA 1988 Jun 10;259(22):3274.

218. Zasada M, Budzisz E. Retinoids: active molecules influencing skin structure formation in cosmetic and dermatological treatments. *Postepy Dermatol Alergol*. 2019;36(4):392–397.

219. Sorg O, Kuenzli S, Kaya G, Saurat JH. Proposed mechanisms of action for retinoid derivatives in the treatment of skin aging. *J Cosmet Dermatol*. 2005;4(4):237–244.

220. Park BS, Jang KA, Sung JH, et al. Adipose-derived stem cells and their secretory factors as a promising therapy for skin aging. *Dermatol Surg*. 2008;34(10):1323–1326.

221. Gibson SJ, Lindh JM, Riter TR, et al. Plasmacytoid dendritic cells produce cytokines and mature in response to the TLR7 agonists, imiquimod and resiquimod. *Cell Immunol*. 2002;218(1-2):74–86.

222. Barland CO, Zettersten E, Brown BS, Ye J, Elias PM, Ghadially R. Imiquimod-induced interleukin-1 alpha stimulation improves barrier homeostasis in aged murine epidermis. *J Invest Dermatol*. 2004;122(2):330–336.

223. Shaw AC, Panda A, Joshi SR, Qian F, Allore HG, Montgomery RR. Dysregulation of human Toll-like receptor function in aging. *Ageing Res Rev*. 2011;10(3):346–353.

224. Metcalf S, Crowson AN, Naylor M, Haque R, Cornelison R. Imiquimod as an antiaging agent. *J Am Acad Dermatol*. 2007;56(3):422–425.

225. Altalhab S. The effectiveness of imiquimod 5% cream as an anti-wrinkle treatment: A pilot study. *J Cosmet Dermatol*. 2019;18(6):1729–1732.

226. Sachs DL, Voorhees JJ. Age-reversing drugs and devices in dermatology. *Clin Pharmacol Ther*. 2011;89(1):34–43.

227. Kligman AM, Zhen Y, Sadiq I, Stoudemayer T. Imiquimod 5% cream reverses histologic changes and improves appearance of photoaged facial skin. *Cosmet Dermatol*. 2006;19(11):704–711.

228. Del Rosso J, Swanson N, Berman B, Martin GM, Lin T, Rosen T. Imiquimod 2.5% and 3.75% Cream for the Treatment of Photodamage: A Meta-analysis of Efficacy and Tolerability in 969 Randomized Patients. *J Clin Aesthet Dermatol*. 2018;11(9):28–31.

229. Skroza N, Bernardini N, Proietti I, Potenza C. Clinical utility of ingenol mebutate in the management of actinic keratosis: perspectives from clinical practice. *Ther Clin Risk Manag*. 2018;14:1879–1885.

230. Braun SA, Gerber PA. Cosmetic Effects of Ingenol Mebutate Gel in the Treatment of Field-Cancerized Photodamaged Skin. *Dermatol Surg*. 2015;41(11):1328–1329.

231. Handler MZ, Bloom BS, Goldberg DJ. Clinical and Histologic Evaluation of Ingenol Mebutate 0.015% Gel for the Cosmetic Improvement of Photoaged Skin. *Dermatol Surg*. 2018;44(1):61–67.

232. Kim M, Jung Y, Kim J, Jeong SW, Woo YR, Park HJ. Anti-aging effects of ingenol mebutate for patients with actinic keratosis. *J Am Acad Dermatol*. 2018;79(6):1148–1150.

233. The Pharma Letter. Denmark's LEO Pharma initiates Picato phase-out. October 28, 2020. https://www.thepharmaletter.com/article/denmark-s-leo-pharma-initiates-picato-phase-out Accessed 12/21/2020.

CHAPTER 38

Anti-Inflammatory Agents

Leslie S. Baumann, MD
Edmund M. Weisberg, MS, MBE

SUMMARY POINTS

What's Important?
1. Inflammation contributes to skin aging.
2. Once one inflammatory pathway gets activated, others become activated and inflammation is difficult to stop.

What's New?
1. Legalization of cannabis has led to research about the anti-inflammatory effects of cannabinoids.
2. Diet, exercise, and lifestyle habits are being studied to learn how they affect inflammation.

What's Coming?
1. Several botanical ingredients have been shown to block various inflammatory pathways but formulations that can deliver the ingredients into the skin need to be improved to ensure penetration and stability.
2. More knowledge about the microbiome and its effects on inflammation is anticipated.

DEFINING INFLAMMATION

Inflammation, from the Latin word *inflammatio* ("to set on fire"), is a dynamic vascular and cellular reflexive response of living tissue to injury; such injury may present in the form of infection, chemical damage (e.g., toxins, irritants), physical damage (e.g., heat, cold, radiation, mechanical trauma), and the binding of antibodies to antigens within the body.[1] Inflammation is therefore a protective mechanism of the organism intended to remove such injurious stimuli as well as to initiate the healing process of the damaged tissue.

Localized vasodilation, increased vascular permeability, extravasation of plasmatic proteins, and migration of leukocytes into the affected tissue produce what Cornelius Celsius defined in the first century as the "cardinal signs" of acute inflammation: *calor* (heat), *dolor* (pain), *rubor* (redness), and *tumor* (swelling).[2] *Functio laesa* (loss of function) was later added to the definition of inflammation by Rudolf Virchow in the 19th century.[3]

A basic sequence of events characterizes virtually all types of inflammatory responses regardless of the provocative stimuli.[4] The initial reaction is vasodilation followed by transient vasoconstriction. The microvascular endothelium then becomes more permeable to plasma proteins that leak out into the extravascular compartment, establishing an inflammatory exudate. Inflammatory mediators released in the area induce the expression of selectin-type adhesion molecules on the endothelial cells. Recruited leukocytes then interact with such adhesion molecules, bind to the inflamed endothelium and extravasate into the tissue where they respond to the insult through phagocytosis and degranulation. Finally, the inflammatory response must be actively terminated when no longer essential to prevent unnecessary damage to tissue.

The process of inflammation, both vascular and cellular, is orchestrated by a large array of inflammatory mediators, which will be reviewed in this chapter. These mediators include: (1) cellular-derived products, such as vasoactive amines (e.g., histamine), cytokines, eicosanoids (e.g., prostaglandins, thromboxanes, and leukotrienes), enzymes, and oxygen radicals; and (2) plasma-derived mediators, which include complement cascade components, kinins, and fibrinopeptides.

CELL-DERIVED INFLAMMATORY MEDIATORS AND THEIR ROLES IN THE INFLAMMATORY PROCESS

Role of Eicosanoids

In reaction to inflammatory stimuli, molecular signaling, or cell destruction, phospholipids contained in the cellular membrane are hydrolyzed by phospholipase A2 (PLA2), releasing free arachidonic acid (AA). This fatty acid is the primary precursor of eicosanoids (**Fig. 38-1**), important inflammatory mediators that include prostaglandins (PGs), thromboxanes (TXs), and leukotrienes (LTs) among others (**Fig. 38-2**).[5] Eicosanoids are not stored. Once formed, they act locally at the site of synthesis to regulate autocrine and paracrine functions.[6] Different cell types have particular sets of enzymes for eicosanoid synthesis that determine their eicosanoid profile. Similarly, different stimuli also influence the eicosanoid profile produced by the cell.[6] There are two different pathways in the synthesis of eicosanoids from AA:

(1) Cyclooxygenase pathway: All eicosanoids with ring structures, that is, the PGs, TXs, and prostacyclins, are synthesized via the cyclooxygenase pathway. Two cyclooxygenases have been identified: COX-1 and COX-2. The former is ubiquitous and constitutive, whereas the latter is induced in response to inflammatory stimuli. The products of these and subsequent reactions in this pathway are summarized in **Fig. 38-2**.

(2) Lipoxygenase pathway: Several lipoxygenase enzymes can act on AA to form different peroxidated derivatives [the hydroperoxyeicosatetraenoic (HPETE) acids 5-HPETE, 12-HPETE, and 15-HPETE] depending on to which carbon of AA they insert or attach oxygen. HPETEs are then rapidly reduced to hydroxylated derivatives (HETEs), LTs, or lipoxins, depending on the tissue.

Role of Cytokines

Cytokines are intracellular signaling polypeptides produced by activated cells. Most cytokines have multiple sources, targets, and functions (Chapter 8, Immunology of Skin Aging).[7] The primary cytokines that are produced during, and participate in, inflammatory processes are mentioned in **Table 38-1**.[8-10] These inflammation-associated cytokines are produced by various cell types, but the most important sources are macrophages and monocytes at inflammatory areas.[7] Chemokines (chemotactic cytokines) are small proteins that direct the movement of circulating leukocytes toward inflamed regions,[11] an essential step for the host response to injury. Although numerous cytokines are found within sites of inflammation, two of these cytokines, namely interleukin-1 (IL-1) and tumor necrosis factor-α (TNF-α), play a key role in orchestrating the mechanisms responsible for inflammation. These two cytokines induce the production of lipid mediators, proteases, and free radicals, all of which play a direct role in the development of the deleterious effects of inflammation.[8] In fact, certain cytokines, including interferon-γ (INF-γ) and granulocyte colony-stimulating factor (G-CSF), amplify the inflammatory response by increasing the production of IL-1 and TNF-α by macrophages.[8]

Role of Mast Cells

Mast cells, derived from hematopoietic precursors, are found predominantly near blood vessels, nerves, and subepithelial sites, where local immediate hypersensitivity reactions tend to occur.[12,13] These cells can be activated during acute reactions such as allergies through their high-affinity receptors for the Fc portion of immunoglobulin E (IgE) and by several other stimuli including complement components C3a and C5a,

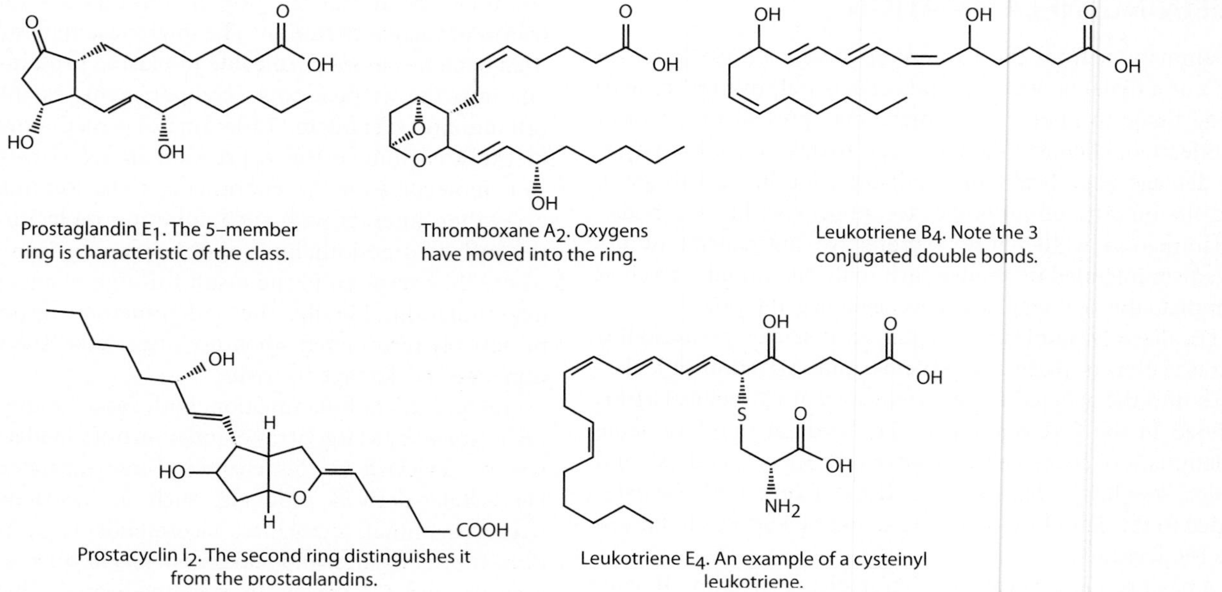

Prostaglandin E₁. The 5–member ring is characteristic of the class.

Thromboxane A₂. Oxygens have moved into the ring.

Leukotriene B₄. Note the 3 conjugated double bonds.

Prostacyclin I₂. The second ring distinguishes it from the prostaglandins.

Leukotriene E₄. An example of a cysteinyl leukotriene.

FIGURE 38-1. Eicosanoids are signaling molecules made by oxygenation of essential fatty acids. This figure shows the structure of several types of eicosanoids.

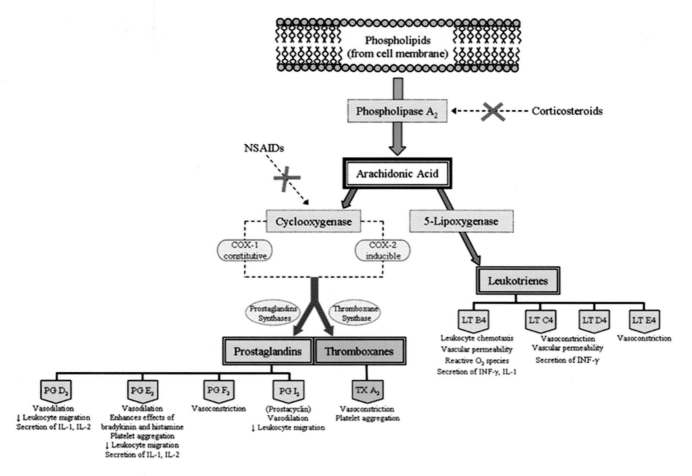

FIGURE 38-2. The arachidonic acid cascade that leads to inflammation.

which will be briefly explained later in this chapter. Other mast cell stimulators that promote the release of histamine include physical stimuli (e.g., heat, cold, and sunlight), macrophage-derived cytokines, bacterial toxins, venoms, trauma, and the presence of allergens. Mast cells are also present in chronic inflammatory reactions, and may produce cytokines that contribute to fibrosis.[14,15]

When a mast cell armed with IgE antibodies is re-exposed to the specific allergen, multiple responses occur, leading eventually to the release of various potent mediators responsible for the clinical expression of immediate inflammatory-hypersensitivity reactions. In the first step of this sequence, antigens bind to the IgE antibodies previously attached to the mast cells. The bridging of IgE molecules with the underlying IgE-Fc receptors activates signal transduction pathways that will translate into three outcomes[16]: (1) degranulation, with the secretion of preformed mediators like vasoactive amines (e.g., histamine), neutral proteases (e.g., chymase, tryptase, hydrolase), and proteoglycans (e.g., heparin, chondroitin sulfate); (2) *de novo* synthesis of pro-inflammatory lipid mediators (i.e., LTs C_4, D_4, and B_4, and PGD_2); and finally (3) synthesis and secretion of cytokines (i.e., TNF-α, IL-1, IL-3, IL-4, IL-5, IL-6, and GM-CSF), as well as chemokines, such as macrophage inflammatory protein (MIP)-1α and MIP-1β.[13]

Role of Histamine

Histamine is a naturally occurring low-molecular-weight amine synthesized by the decarboxylation of the amino acid L-histidine by the enzyme histidine decarboxylase. The synthesis of this important vasoactive amine occurs in sites where the former enzyme is expressed, such as basophils and mast cells found throughout the body (including lungs and skin), parietal cells of the gastric mucosa, and central nervous system neurons.[17,18]

Histamine plays a fundamental role in allergic inflammation,[18] which characterizes certain cutaneous diseases like allergic contact dermatitis (ACD) and immunologic contact urticaria (ICU). The diverse effects of histamine over human health depend upon four different types of receptors; however, its specific role in allergic inflammation mostly occurs through the H_1-receptor.[18,19] Through this receptor, histamine plays a pro-inflammatory role by inducing the release of cytokines and lysosomal enzymes from macrophages and the expression of cell-adhesion molecules.[18,19] Additionally, it influences the activity of basophils, eosinophils, and fibroblasts, causing smooth muscle contraction.[20] Although most of the effects of histamine in inflammatory allergic disease occur through the H_1-receptor, cutaneous itch may occur through both the H_1- and H_3-receptors.[21]

TABLE 38-1 Inflammation-Associated Cytokines

Inflammatory Cytokine	Secreted By	Target Cell or Tissue	Activity
IL-1 (α and β)	- Monocytes - Macrophages - B cells - Dendritic cells - Endothelial cells	- TH cells - B cells - Natural killer (NK) cells - Endothelial cells - Hepatocytes - Hypothalamus	Targets a wide variety of cells to induce many inflammatory reactions: activation of TH cells; maturation and clonal expansion of B cells; enhancement of the activity of NK cells; production of other cytokines; endothelial gene regulation (increasing the expression of adhesion molecules); chemotaxis of macrophages and neutrophils; leukocyte adherence, synthesis of acute-phase proteins by the liver; induction of fever.
IL-6	- Monocytes - Macrophages - TH2 cells	- B cells - Plasma cells - Hepatocytes	Promotes the terminal differentiation of B cells into plasma cells; stimulates antibody secretion by plasma cells; induces synthesis of acute-phase proteins.
IL-8	- Macrophages - Endothelial cells	Neutrophils	Potent chemokine, induces adherence to endothelium and extravasation to tissues.
IL-10	- TH2 cells	Macrophages	Also called cytokine synthesis inhibitory factor because it suppresses cytokine production by activated TH1 cells.
IL-11	- Bone marrow stromal cells - Some fibroblasts	- T cells - B cells - Hepatocytes	Stimulation of T cell-dependent B cell immunoglobulin secretion; increased platelet production; induction of IL-6; acute phase protein secretion.
Interferon (INF)-γ	- TH1 cells - Cytotoxic T cells - NK cells	- Macrophages - Inflammatory cells	Enhances the activity of macrophages, mediates effects important in delayed type hypersensitivity.
TNF-α	- Macrophages - NK cells	Inflammatory cells	Shares several pro-inflammatory properties with IL-1. Induces cytokine secretion. Important role in chronic inflammation.
Transforming growth factor-β	- Platelets - Macrophages - Lymphocytes - Mast cells	- B cells - T cells - NK cells	Inhibits T cell and NK cell proliferation and activation; attracts monocytes to the site of inflammation; enhances cell adhesion.
Granulocyte colony-stimulating factor (G-CSF)	- Macrophages - T cells	Neutrophils	Participates in acute inflammation.

Role of Free Radicals

Oxygen-derived free radicals may be released extracellularly from leukocytes after exposure to pathogens, chemokines, and immune complexes, or following a phagocytic challenge.[22] The physiologic function of these reactive oxygen intermediates is to destroy phagocytized microorganisms. Their production depends on the activation of the nicotinamide adenine dinucleotide phosphate (NADPH) oxidative system, which is a membrane-bound enzyme complex. This system can be found in the plasmatic membrane as well as in the membrane of phagosomes inside the cells. Superoxide anion (O_2^-), hydrogen peroxide (H_2O_2), and hydroxyl radical (OH) are the major species produced within the cell; these metabolites can combine with nitric oxide (NO) to

form other reactive nitrogen intermediates (Chapter 39, Antioxidants).[23] Extracellular release of low levels of these potent mediators can increase the expression of chemokines, cytokines, and endothelial leukocyte adhesion molecules, amplifying the cascade that elicits the inflammatory response. At higher levels, the release of these mediators can induce endothelial cell damage, which results in increased vascular permeability, neutrophil degranulation, and inactivation of antiproteases, such as α_1-antitrypsin, leading to increased destruction of the extracellular matrix.[24]

Serum, tissue fluids, and host cells all possess antioxidant mechanisms that protect against these potentially harmful oxygen-derived radicals. These include among others: (1) the copper-containing serum protein ceruloplasmin; (2) the iron-free fraction of serum, transferrin; (3) the enzyme superoxide dismutase, which is found or can be activated in various cell types; (4) the enzyme catalase, which detoxifies H_2O_2; and (5) glutathione peroxidase, another powerful H_2O_2 detoxifier.

The influence of oxygen-derived free radicals in any given inflammatory reaction always depends on the balance between the production and the inactivation of these metabolites by both cells and tissues.

PLASMA-DERIVED MEDIATORS AND THEIR ROLE IN THE INFLAMMATORY PROCESS

Role of Complement

A complete explanation of the complex complement system is beyond the scope of this chapter. However, when focusing on the inflammatory response, it is necessary to mention the important role of the complement components integral to the inflammatory process: C3a and C5a. Both C3a and C5a are plasma-derived mediators that stimulate histamine release by mast cells, thereby inducing vasodilation.[25] Additionally, C5a is able to act as a chemoattractant, directing cells via chemotaxis to the site of inflammation.[25]

Role of Kinins

The kinin-kallikrein system is a network of circulating proteins mainly known for its roles in inflammation, blood pressure control, coagulation, and pain. Several studies have concluded that this system plays broader roles than those classically described, for example, in rosacea, cancer, cardiovascular, renal, and central nervous system pathologies.[26]

The system consists of proteins, polypeptides, and a group of enzymes that activate and deactivate the compounds. Kinins [bradykinin (BK) and kallidin (KD)] are polypeptides produced from kininogen and broken down by kininases. They are rapidly generated after tissue injury and play a pivotal function in the development and maintenance of the inflammatory process, in which they cause dilation of blood vessels and increased vascular permeability. They act on PLA2 to increase AA release and thus eicosanoid production (**Fig. 38-1**).[27]

Kinins act by binding to two receptor types, namely B_1 and B_2, which belong to the G-protein coupled receptor family. B_2 receptors are constitutively expressed in various cells under physiological conditions. In contrast, B_1 receptors express rapidly under mainly pathological conditions.[26] Kinins (BK and KD) have a higher affinity to B_2 receptors, the activation of which leads to the release of cytokines and other inflammatory mediators (e.g., PG E_2).

Since its discovery, BK has been demonstrated to induce the four classical signs of inflammation—heat, redness, swelling, and pain,[28]—described at the beginning of this chapter. BK possesses vasoactive properties that enable it to induce vasodilation and increase vascular permeability. Additionally, it causes smooth muscle contraction, induces pain, and can activate nuclear factor-κB (NF-κB), further contributing to the inflammatory response.

Cutaneous Inflammation

The skin is the primary barrier between our bodies and the environment; therefore, the spectrum of insults to which it is exposed are numerous and diverse.[29] The translation of such insults, which include different pathogens and contact-sensitizing antigens, into cutaneous inflammation requires a complex interaction among multiple inflammatory mediators. Notably, NF-κB-mediated inflammation appears to be the final common pathway for the translation of environmental insults into inflammation of the skin. NF-κB, a potent cellular signaling pathway, can be activated by IL-1, TNF-α,[30] and as mentioned earlier, BK.[26] Interestingly, the epidermis is a "storehouse" of IL-1α and can produce considerable amounts of IL-1β and TNF-α.[31,32] It is known that ultraviolet (UV) radiation from sunlight induces activation of IL-1 and TNF-α,[33] leading to NF-κB-mediated inflammation. NF-κB regulates multiple genes in skin cells; however, those that are essential to the initiation of cutaneous inflammation include genes for E-selectin, cytokines, defensins (antibacterial peptides), and cell adhesion molecules.[30]

Of special importance for cutaneous immunity is a subgroup of memory T cells with the ability to circulate preferentially to the skin. These memory T cells are identified by a marker known as cutaneous lymphocyte antigen (CLA),[34] and are generated in the lymph nodes that drain the skin. They are then specifically recruited back to the skin during inflammation. These unique skin-associated lymphocytes may be positive for either CD4 or CD8 and, once activated, may be able to produce either type 1 T-cell cytokines (i.e., interferon-γ, IL-2, and lymphotoxin) or type 2 T-cell cytokines (i.e., IL-4, IL-5, IL-10, and IL-13).[29] It is the activation of the T cells and the subsequent release of cytokines and other effector molecules that result in clinically apparent T-cell-mediated inflammatory skin diseases.[29]

ANTI-INFLAMMATORY AGENTS FOR THE TREATMENT OF INFLAMMATORY SKIN DISEASES

Topical Corticosteroids

Not so long ago, dermatologic therapy was completely revolutionized with the introduction of corticosteroids in the early 1950s. Spies and Stone, two dermatologists from Alabama, were the first to use topical hydrocortisone to successfully treat a patient with chronic hand dermatitis.[35,36] After this therapeutic success, many dermatologists "seriously wondered if their specialty had come to its end."[37]

Corticosteroids are known to suppress pro-inflammatory genes that encode cytokines, cell adhesion molecules, and other mediators that interfere with the inflammatory response.[38] They selectively induce annexin I, an anti-inflammatory protein that physically interacts with and inhibits cytosolic phospholipase $A_2\alpha$ (c$PLA_2\alpha$).[39] By inhibiting this phospholipase they block the release of AA and its subsequent conversion to eicosanoids such as PGs, TXs, prostacyclins, and LTs.[40] A second anti-inflammatory protein induced by corticosteroids is MAPK phosphatase-1. Bacteria, viruses, cytokines, and, interestingly, UV radiation are all examples of inflammatory signals that activate the MAPK cascades.[41] Finally, glucocorticoids also induce and antagonize NF-κB, which is known to stimulate the transcription of COX-2, an enzyme essential for PG production.[42]

Since some of the anti-inflammatory mechanisms of glucocorticoids are also involved in physiologic signaling rather than inflammatory signaling, the therapeutic effects of these drugs in inflammation are often accompanied by clinically significant side effects.[40] Therefore, although topical corticosteroids are generally well tolerated for short-term use on inflammatory skin diseases, long-term widespread use can result in serious cutaneous adverse effects that include: acne, folliculitis, hirsutism, pigmentary changes, purpura, skin atrophy, striae, and telangiectasia.[43,44] Moreover, even more serious systemic side effects such as hypothalamic pituitary axis (HPA) suppression,[45] hyperglycemia,[46] avascular osteonecrosis,[47] glaucoma,[48] and posterior subcapsular cataracts[49] have also been reported in association with the long-term use of topical corticosteroids.

Topical Immune Modulators

Topical calcineurin inhibitors (TCIs) tacrolimus and pimecrolimus have been investigated in the past decade as treatment options for inflammatory skin disorders. These relatively new immunosuppressive drugs act by inhibiting the protein calcineurin, subsequently preventing T cell dephosphorylation of transcription factors. As a result of this inhibition, the signal transduction pathways in such cells are blocked, and inflammatory cytokine production is suppressed.[50]

Between December 2000 and December 2001, topical tacrolimus ointment and topical pimecrolimus cream received approval by the Food and Drug Administration (FDA) for the treatment of atopic dermatitis (AD).[51] Furthermore, topical tacrolimus has been proven to inhibit other inflammatory skin conditions such as nickel-induced ACD[52,53] as measured by a reduction in erythema, pruritus, vesiculation, induration,[53] and histopathological pattern.[54] Its inhibitory action has even been found by some researchers to be stronger than the steroid aclometasone dipropionate.[55]

Even though these medicaments are structurally very similar, pimecrolimus has a higher lipophilicity index than tacrolimus (20-fold more lipophilic). Although a higher lipophilicity index has been correlated with a higher affinity for the skin,[43] pimecrolimus is three-fold less potent an inhibitor of calcineurin than tacrolimus.[56]

In February 2005, the pediatric advisory committee of the Center for Drug Evaluation and Research of the FDA required that the labeling of tacrolimus and pimecrolimus include the placement of a "black box" warning about the potential cancer risks associated with the systemic administration of these medications.[57] However, although there is a theoretical concern, there has been no evidence to suggest an increased risk of cutaneous or visceral cancer associated with the use of these drugs in their topical form.[58]

Cyclooxygenase Inhibitors

An increasing number of anti-inflammatory agents specifically target bioactive lipids generated from AA, namely nonsteroidal anti-inflammatory drugs (NSAIDs). Although this group of medicaments is one of the most studied and used throughout medicine, their application for cutaneous disease is somewhat limited.[59] Ibuprofen, however, has been shown to be effective for the treatment of acne, since inflammatory acne lesions are infiltrated with neutrophils and ibuprofen is known to inhibit leukocyte chemotaxis.[60]

In 1984, Wong et al. conducted a double-blind study of 60 male and female patients 15 to 35 years old with acne vulgaris.[61] Patients were randomly assigned to one of four groups: 1) oral ibuprofen (600 mg) plus tetracycline (250 mg) four times daily (qid); 2) ibuprofen (600 mg) plus placebo qid; 3) tetracycline (250 mg) plus placebo qid; and 4) two placebos qid. Only the combination therapy had an effect statistically better than the placebo in the improvement of total lesion count. The administration of ibuprofen alone yielded beneficial results comparable to the ones of tetracycline alone but with fewer side effects.

As a follow-up to this study, 1 year later, Funt treated 22 male and female patients aged 14 to 25 with nodulocystic acne with a combination of minocycline (50 mg) plus oral ibuprofen (400 mg) three times daily. After 1 month, all patients apparently responded to the combination therapy with a percent improvement between 75% and 90%. Notably, all 22 patients had a history of unsuccessful oral antibiotic treatment (3-month course of minocycline, 50 mg three times daily).[62]

NSAIDs are also applied in dermatology to treat sunburn. Hughes et al. studied the ability to modify skin injury induced by UVB radiation by nonsteroidal drugs (i.e., oral ibuprofen or indomethacin) plus topical betamethasone dipropionate in 24 subjects.[63] Skin responses to UVB [erythema and increased skin blood flow (SBF)] were measured serially and showed a synergistic effect of oral NSAIDs in combination with topical corticosteroids in the reduction of UVB-induced skin injury. In addition, ibuprofen and placebo were compared in a randomized double-blind cross-over study of 19 psoriatic patients receiving UVB phototherapy. Signs and symptoms of UVB-induced inflammation were then assessed. Although a statistical difference was noted for only one variable (i.e., technician's assessment of erythema), results suggested that ibuprofen was more effective than placebo for the symptomatic relief of UVB-induced inflammation after high doses of UVB-phototherapy for psoriasis. The postulated biochemical basis for this result derives from the observation that dermal PGs are elevated after UVB irradiation.[64] Therefore, an NSAID agent that interferes with PG synthesis may reduce UVB-induced inflammation.

Salicylic Acid

Experimental and clinical data indicate that salicylates exhibit a spectrum of activities that include anti-inflammatory and antimicrobial functions.[65] As a member of the aspirin family, salicylic acid achieves its analgesic and anti-inflammatory properties by truncating the AA cascade. Salicylates are active in controlling inflammation by altering gene expressions. They suppress the expression of pro-inflammatory genes by inhibiting the DNA-binding activities of transcription activators such as NF-κB, activation protein-1 (AP-1) and CCAAT/enhancer-binding protein β (C/EBPβ).[65]

Salicylic acid is known to decrease the frequency and severity of acne eruptions by reducing acne-associated inflammation in addition to imparting an exfoliating action over the pores. It has therefore become a popular ingredient in over-the-counter acne products (Chapter 24, Chemical Peels). Salicylic acid is also used to treat rosacea and other superficial inflammatory disorders. In addition, it is found in products intended to treat photoaged skin. Topical salicylic acid in concentrations of up to 30% has been shown to fade age-related pigmented spots, decrease surface roughness, and reduce fine lines.[66] If used in high concentrations or too frequently, salicylic acid may lead to redness, pruritus, scaling, increased skin sensitivity, and even epidermolysis.

Sulfur/Sulfacetamide

The medicinal use of sulfur dates back to the time of Hippocrates, who is believed to have mentioned its use for the treatment of plague.[67] It is currently found in myriad products including the spa waters and elegant products from the Vichy spa in France. Most of what is known about sulfur was written decades ago, with moderate to little interest evinced in the recent literature. Nevertheless, sulfur continues to be used throughout the world mainly to treat acne, seborrheic dermatitis, rosacea, scabies, and tinea versicolor.[68] Elemental sulfur (a yellow, non-metallic element) and its various forms (e.g., sulfides, sulfites, and mercaptans) are believed to have antimicrobial, antifungal, and antiparasitic properties. Furthermore, sulfur-containing compounds have proven to be "excellent anti-inflammatory agents."[69] Interestingly, the action of sulfur in the skin depends on its direct interaction with the cutaneous surface: the smaller the particle size, the greater the area available for sulfur–skin interaction and the greater the efficacy.[70] Two sulfur preparations are found as official formulations in the United States Pharmacopoeia (USP): sublimed sulfur and precipitated sulfur. Precipitated sulfur has a smaller particle size and therefore is superior in efficacy to sublimed sulfur; in fact, this is the type of sulfur most widely used.

Sulfur was once the most common active ingredient incorporated in anti-acne formulations,[60] but has widely come into disuse mainly because of its malodorousness, resembling rotten eggs. The therapeutic effect of sulfur in acne and seborrheic dermatitis is thought to result from its keratolytic action.[71] The precise mechanism for this effect is unknown but probably depends on its interaction with the cysteine content of keratinocytes, allowing the formation of hydrogen sulfide, which in turn breaks down keratin.[70] In the treatment of acne and seborrheic dermatitis, sulfur is often combined with agents such as salicylic acid, the keratolytic action of which may be synergistic with that of sulfur.[72]

Sulfur is commonly combined with sodium sulfacetamide, a sulfonamide agent with antibacterial activity. It acts as a competitive antagonist to para-aminobenzoic acid (PABA), an essential component for bacterial growth.[73] In fact, sodium sulfacetamide has been demonstrated to be active against *Propionibacterium acnes*.[74] When mixed with sulfur in dermatologic preparations, the combined keratolytic and anti-inflammatory effect of sulfur with the antibacterial effect of sulfacetamide results in an effective topical formulation for the treatment of acne vulgaris, rosacea, and seborrheic dermatitis.[75] This combination is available as a cream, lotion, gel topical suspension, cleanser, and silica-based mask.

Botanicals and Other Natural Ingredients

Natural ingredients have been used in traditional medicine throughout the world for thousands of years; however, it is just since the early 1990s that botanically derived products have gained widespread usage and interest among the US population.[76] As a result, botanical products have become highly marketable. This increased popularity has occurred for several reasons: (1) concerns about the adverse effects of chemical drugs, (2) questions about the approaches and assumptions of allopathic medicine, (3) greater public access to health information, and (4) the growing popularity of organic products. All this translates into a broad array of botanical products now being used in different medical specialties including dermatology. Fortunately, we are now able to employ scientific methods to prove or question their efficacy and better understand their mechanisms of action. The following discussion focuses on some of the most important botanicals that confer anti-inflammatory properties. Of note, when looking for botanicals as ingredients of personal care products and cosmetics, it is important to consider the names given by the International Nomenclature for Cosmetic Ingredients (INCI), used for ingredient disclosures inside a product's list of ingredients.

Aloe Vera

Aloe vera is one of the most widely used herbal products in the world. It is native to northern Africa and the Arabian Peninsula. Through human trade, its use extended to most of the ancient civilizations (i.e., Egypt, Persia, Greece, Rome, India, and China) where it was used for the treatment of burns and wounds.[77] The Spanish later brought it to what is now the United States and parts of the Caribbean including Barbados (from which the alternate INCI name *Aloe barbadensis* is derived).[78]

A large body of anecdotal evidence attests to the efficacy of aloe for the treatment of several diseases; unfortunately, exaggerated claims are not uncommon and therefore caution is warranted in the interpretation of some of the available information.[79] Explanations of aloe gel efficacy are still varied because it has in fact several active constituents operating through different mechanisms.[80] Its action as a moisturizer, for example, is a popular use that may account for much of its effects.[81] Furthermore, aloe is reputed to exhibit potent anti-inflammatory effects, and the substances that have been proposed as its active anti-inflammatory constituents include salicylates (providing "aspirin-like effects"); magnesium lactate, which is believed to inhibit the production of histamine; BK and TX inhibitors, which provide pain reduction; and polysaccharides, particularly acemannan, which has reported immunomodulatory properties, as well as the constituents aloe-emodin, aloin, aloesin, and emodin.[82-86] Another substance isolated from aloe, C-glucosyl chromone, has exhibited topical anti-inflammatory activity equivalent to that of hydrocortisone (200 µg/mouse ear).[87]

A study by Habeeb et al.[88] explored reports of antimicrobial effects associated with aloe.[89] Using a simple *in vitro* assay, they determined the effect of the inner gel of aloe on bacterial-induced pro-inflammatory cytokine production (namely, TNF-α and IL-1β) from human leukocytes stimulated with *Shigella flexneri*. Results demonstrated the suppression of both bacterial-induced cytokines with the use of aloe inner gel.[88] Recent findings also suggest that topical *A. vera* facilitates wound healing by fostering the proliferation and migration of fibroblasts and keratinocytes,[90,91] and, in a small double-blind, randomized, controlled trial, accelerated split-thickness skin graft donor-site healing.[92] Aloe has also been shown to promote the production of hyaluronic acid and dermatan sulfate, contributing to wound healing by augmenting granulation tissue collagen and cross-linking.[77] Further studies are still needed for a deeper and more precise understanding of aloe constituents and their varied biological activities.

Calendula

Known as pot marigold, garden marigold, holligold/holigold, marigold, marybud, common marigold, maravilla, ruddles, and goldbloom, *Calendula officinalis* is a bright, flowering annual herb endemic to Asia, central and southern Europe, northern Africa, and the Mediterranean region.[93,94] Like many other members of the Asteraceae (or Compositae) family, which includes daisies, arnica, feverfew, chamomile, edelweiss, and yarrow, calendula is now cultivated worldwide. Calendula has long been considered a soothing herb in traditional medicine and used topically for its anti-inflammatory properties; in contemporary times, the herb has been found to exhibit anti-inflammatory, antibacterial, antioxidant, and wound-healing activity.[95-98] The German Commission E, European Scientific Co-operative on Phytotherapy, British Herbal Pharmacopoeia, and World Health Organization monographs recognize *C. officinalis* for wound healing and anti-inflammatory activity.[99] Its primary indications are cutaneous and inflammatory conditions, including eczema, scalds, bruises, boils, rashes, first-degree burns, and sunburns.[93,100] Topical calendula ointment, alone and in combination, has also been found effective in treating chronic venous leg ulcers.[101,102] Approximately 200 cosmetic creams, lotions, and shampoos are believed to contain *C. officinalis* extract.[94,99]

Calendula has been used as an antiseptic and anti-inflammatory agent, treating some skin disorders and pain.[103] Various calendula cream formulations have also been shown, in healthy volunteers, to protect against irritant contact dermatitis provoked by sodium lauryl sulfate.[104] In cosmetic or personal care products, it conditions the skin in concentrations ranging from 0.1% to 1.0%, and also contains salutary antioxidant activity and sun protection factor.[93,105] In recent years, the presence of several active ingredients, including flavonoids and phenolic acids, has spurred research further into the antioxidant activity of calendula and its potential role in conferring health benefits.

Cannabis

Despite its colorful legal history, marijuana—derived from *Cannabis sativa* and *Cannabis indica*—has long been used for medical purposes and is one of the most widely used drugs throughout the world.[106] Modern medicine deploys this dynamic plant to treat chronic pain, glaucoma, as well as nausea, while investigating its potential applications in a broad array of conditions including cutaneous disorders such as acne, eczema, lichen simplex, melanoma and nonmelanoma skin cancer, melasma, prurigo, pruritus, psoriasis, scleroderma and systemic sclerosis, as well as seborrheic dermatitis.[107-109]

Research during the last few decades has revealed that the cannabinoids present in *C. sativa* display anti-inflammatory activity and suppress the proliferation of multiple tumorigenic cell lines, some of which are moderated through cannabinoid (CB) receptors.[110-113] Notably, some CB receptors are present in human skin.[113] The endocannabinoid system features a pervasive network of endogenous ligands, enzymes, and receptors, which exogenous substances (including phytocannabinoids and synthetic cannabinoids) can activate.[114] Recent evidence suggests that the endocannabinoid system plays a significant role in cutaneous homeostasis, regulating proliferation, differentiation, and inflammatory mediator release.[114,115] Its dysregulation has been linked to AD, pruritus, inflammation, psoriasis, scleroderma, and skin cancer. Further, emerging data support the use of exogenous cannabinoids to treat inflammatory cutaneous conditions such as acne, AD, pruritus, psoriasis, seborrhea, and wounds, as several authors call for additional studies.[108,116-120] In a 2015 single-blinded, 12-week comparative study in healthy male volunteers to evaluate the effects of twice-daily application of 3% cannabis seed extract cream on human cheek skin, investigators found the base with 3% cannabis seed extract to be safe and effective, with skin sebum and erythema content on the treated side diminished significantly compared to the side treated only with the control (base). They concluded that this well-tolerated formulation would be indicated for the treatment of acne and seborrhea to ameliorate facial appearance.[121]

Exogenous and endogenous cannabinoids appear to influence the endocannabinoid system through cannabinoid receptors, transient receptor potential channels (TRPs), and peroxisome proliferator-activated receptors (PPARs).[120] Endogenous cannabinoids, including arachidonoyl ethanolamide and 2-arachidonoylglycerol, are believed to be significant mediators in the skin.[122] Also, endocannabinoids have been demonstrated to impart analgesia to the skin at the spinal and supraspinal levels.[123]

Oláh et al. have shown that the non-psychotropic phytocannabinoid ((-)-cannabidiol [CBD]) imparts anti-acne benefits by diminishing sebaceous lipid production, reducing proliferation, and easing inflammation in human SZ95 sebocytes.[117] In additional investigations of non-psychotropic phytocannabinoids and their effects on human sebocyte function, they reported in 2016 that the phytocannabinoids (-)-cannabigerol [CBG] and (-)-cannabigerovarin [CBGV] appear to display promise in treating xerotic and seborrheic skin, and ((-)-cannabichromene [CBC], (-)-cannabidivarin [CBDV], and (-)-Δ^9-tetrahydrocannabivarin [THCV]), in particular, exhibit potential as anti-acne ingredients. The investigators added that these compounds, due to their notable anti-inflammatory effects, warrant consideration for use in treating skin inflammation.

Attitudes about cannabinoid use in dermatology

In 2018, Robinson et al. developed a 20-question online survey about the knowledge, cognizance, and perceptions of cannabinoids among dermatologists, with a response rate of 21% (n = 531). Twenty-nine percent of respondents did not know that Δ^9-tetrahydrocannabinol (THC) is psychoactive and a significant majority (64%) did not know that CBD is not psychoactive. Nevertheless, most thought that cannabinoids should be legal for medical treatment (86%), and even more (94%) supported researching the cutaneous applications of cannabinoids. A robust majority (86%) supported prescribing an FDA-approved cannabinoid-containing topical formulation rather than an oral product (71%). In also noting that 55% of respondents revealed at least one conversation about cannabinoids initiated by a patient in the previous year while 48% expressed concern about a possible stigma associated with suggesting cannabinoid treatments to patients, Robinson et al. called for further education about the benefits and risks of cutaneous cannabinoids for dermatologists.[116]

Chamomile

Chamomile, a sweet-scented flower belonging to the Asteraceae (or Compositae) family, has been used as a medicinal herb worldwide for hundreds of years,[124] and remains one of the most widely used medicinal herbs. It has been recognized for its therapeutic properties since the age of Hippocrates (circa 500 BCE). The ancient Greeks and Egyptians used it to treat erythema and dry skin.[125]

There are two primary types of chamomile: Roman chamomile (INCI name: *Chamaemelum nobile*) and German chamomile (INCI name: *Matricaria recutita* or *Chamomilla recutita*). Although both plants have been used for therapeutic applications, the flowers of German chamomile contain a higher concentration of key active ingredients that have shown anti-inflammatory activity *in vivo*[126,127]: the terpenoids chamazulene and α-bisabolol. Consequently, the official medicinal chamomile is German chamomile. In an animal study in which inflammation was induced via the injection of carrageenan and PG E$_1$, German chamomile was found to suppress both the inflammatory effect and leukocyte infiltration.[128] Specifically, chamazulene decreases the inflammatory process by inhibiting LT synthesis.[126] It is believed that chamomile also confers significant beneficial effects to the skin, such as the improvement of texture and elasticity, ameliorating the signs of photodamage.

In addition to reports of anti-inflammatory effects, chamomile is said to possess some antioxidant properties,[129] which are mainly associated with other active ingredients, namely the terpenoid matricine and the flavonoids apigenin and luteolin, all of which have documented antioxidant activity.[130] As a result of its various beneficial functions, chamomile is now included in several cosmetic products intended to improve skin appearance. A chamomile gel has also been shown to be more effective in relieving acute radiation dermatitis in head and neck cancer patients while inducing fewer adverse side effects in a preliminary clinical trial.[131] Of note, chamomile has been reported to cause ACD in susceptible types.[132] Those with known allergies to the compositae plant family (e.g., ragweed) are at the greatest risk.

Cucumber Extract

Cucumber (INCI name: *Cucumis sativus*) is another botanical with a long history of use in ancient and folk medicine. Reputedly used by Cleopatra to preserve her skin,[133] cucumber extract has found regular usage in modern skincare, with most of its healthy characteristics observed when used topically. The ancient use of cucumber to treat cutaneous disorders also includes a place in Ayurvedic medicine, with its fruits deployed to address sunburn and other skin inflammations.[134]

Cucumber extract is known for its emollient and soothing properties, specifically. It contains high amounts of amino and organic acids that are beneficial to the skin's acid mantle, and it has been found to be safe in cosmetic formulations.[135] In addition, shikimate dehydrogenase, an enzyme extracted from cucumber pulp, has demonstrated anti-inflammatory properties when applied to the skin.[133] In 2018, Bernardini et al. demonstrated that a water/ethanol extract of *C. sativus* mitigated lipopolysaccharide-induced inflammatory response in endothelial cells.[134] Earlier that year, Trejo-Moreno et al. showed that aqueous fractions of *C. sativus* displayed anti-inflammatory and antioxidant activity *in vitro*.[136] More scientific studies are needed, though, to confirm and further expand the limited known cutaneous effects of treatment with cucumber extract.

Feverfew

Feverfew (FF) (INCI name: *Tanacetum parthenium*) is a rapidly growing small bush with citrus-scented leaves and daisy-like flowers (**Fig. 38-3**). It is part of the Asteraceae (or Compositae) family, characterized by the star-shaped flower head of its members. Since the first century, FF has been used to reduce fever and pain. The use of this herb as an antipyretic led to the appellation "feverfew," a corruption of the Latin word *febrifugia* (fever reducer).[137,138] FF acts as a PG antagonist,[139] and one of its extracts, parthenolide, has been reported to inhibit platelet aggregation. Additionally, it has been shown to bind to and inhibit IκB kinase β (IKKβ), the kinase subunit known to play a critical role in cytokine-mediated stimulation of genes involved in inflammation,[140,141] which may partly explain the anti-inflammatory properties attributed to this herb. Parthenolide is a type of sesquiterpene lactone, an essential oil commonly found in members of the Asteraceae family.

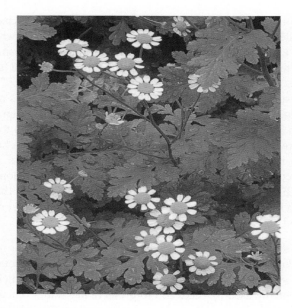

FIGURE 38-3. Feverfew.

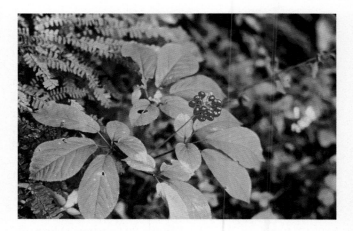

FIGURE 38-4. Ginseng.

Sesquiterpene lactones are known for their anti-inflammatory effects; nevertheless, they also exert the major allergenic effects of this plant family. In fact, FF-derived parthenolide forms part of the Compositae Mix (CM), a solution of extracts from five plant species that can be applied as a patch test to screen for Asteraceae allergy.[142] The Aveeno Ultra Calming line of skincare products contains FF that has had the parthenolide portion removed, thus yielding the anti-inflammatory properties of FF without posing the risk of contact dermatitis. The beneficial effects of this parthenolide-depleted extract of FF were demonstrated in a 2008 study.[143] In this research, *in vitro* FF was shown to attenuate the formation of UV-induced hydrogen peroxide and to reduce pro-inflammatory cytokine release; *in vivo*, topical FF reduced UV-induced epidermal hyperplasia, DNA damage, and apoptosis.[143]

Ginseng

Several types of ginseng are found throughout the world, and all belong to the Araliaceae family in the genus *Panax* (**Fig. 38-4**). The word *Panax* means "all healing," which describes the traditional belief that ginseng manifests characteristics that heal all the diseased aspects of the body. There are several different species of ginseng; two of the most commonly used are *P. ginseng* (Chinese ginseng), popular among Asian cultures, and *P. quinquefolius* (American ginseng), commonly used among Native Americans.[144]

Studies indicate that ginseng may exert chemopreventive properties against cancer. Mechanisms behind this assumption include inhibition of DNA damage,[145] induction of apoptosis,[146] and inhibition of cell proliferation.[147] There is also evidence that ginseng has potent effects on the inflammatory cascade and may inhibit the "inflammation-to-cancer sequence." For example, ginsan, a polysaccharide extracted from *P. ginseng*, has been shown to inhibit the release of pro-inflammatory cytokines *in vivo*.[148] Further, the ginsenoside

Rg3 has been demonstrated to inhibit the NF-κB-mediated induction of the inflammatory process.[149] Researchers have ascribed the preponderance of biological activities associated with ginseng to its constituent ginsenosides.[150] In addition, BST204, a fermented ginseng extract, can inhibit inducible nitric oxide synthase (NOS) expression and subsequent nitric oxide production in animal models. Ginseng has been proven to inhibit the production of TNF-α and other pro-inflammatory cytokines by cultured macrophages when exposed to bacterial lipopolysaccharides.[151] Potential applications for ginseng in dermatology include treatment for alopecia, cold hypersensitivity, dermatitis, hair loss, photoaging, skin cancer, as well as wound and injury.[150]

Horse Chestnut

Of the 15 known species of horse chestnut, which is found as both a tree and a shrub in all the temperate regions of Europe, Asia, and North America, the European horse chestnut, *Aesculus hippocastanum* (Hippocastanaceae family), is the one most often used in medical applications, traditionally for bronchitis, dysentery, hemorrhoids, and venous issues.[152] The use of topically applied horse chestnut in cosmetic formulations emerged in 1980, with authors describing treatment of the face, scalp, oral cavity, body, hands, feet, and legs, including uses for foot and bodily hygiene as well as hemorrhoids.[153] Anti-aging or anti-wrinkling applications have also been suggested, as Masaki et al. discovered in 1995 that *A. hippocastanum* extracts robustly scavenge active oxygen.[154]

Horse chestnut seed extract (HCSE) is found commonly in lotions, creams, massage oils, and sundry skincare products, often in combination with other herbal ingredients. Most such topical products are intended to treat varicose veins, swelling, and water retention, but some of the newer products attribute antioxidant potency to horse chestnut and purport to combat wrinkling.

The topical application of standardized HCSE balm with 2% aescin has been found to support healthy skin, blood vessels, and muscles, particularly in the legs and hemorrhoidal plexus.[155–157] One double-blind, randomized, single-dose study evaluating the effectiveness of a topically applied standardized HCSE balm (2% aescin) for localized swelling and blood accumulation revealed that the formulation significantly diminished tenderness in the affected area as compared to placebo.[155] Indeed, aescin has exhibited clinically significant activity in the treatment of hemorrhoids, chronic venous insufficiency (CVI), and post-operative edema.[152,158–161]

Topical and systemic HCSE products are popular in Europe for the treatment of CVI and varicose veins. The aescin featured in HCSE formulations displays anti-inflammatory properties and has been shown to ease edema after trauma, especially following head and sports injury, as well as surgery.[155,162] A topical aescin preparation is also popular during sporting events in Europe for treating acute sprains. Both oral and transdermal preparations are well tolerated and consistently demonstrate anti-inflammatory, anti-edematous, and venotonic activity.[163,164]

Lavandula

Native to the Mediterranean region, seeds of the shrub *Lavandula angustifolia* (better known as lavender), were transported to England and France through migration several hundred years ago. Now widely cultivated in southern Europe, the UK, Australia, and the US for its essential oil, lavender is a fragrant, hardy perennial shrub in the Labiatae (Lamiacieae), or mint, family.[165,166] Several species of *Lavandula* have been used for therapeutic, cosmetic, culinary, and commercial purposes for thousands of years. Though all 28 lavender species are thought to impart some therapeutic benefits to varying degrees, *L. angustifolia* (also known as English lavender or true lavender and previously known as *L. officinalis*) is the species included most often in medicinal formulations and is known to confer anti-inflammatory activity.[167,168] It is also a commercially important species in the lucrative perfume industry. *L. latifolia*, *L. stoechas* (known as French lavender in Europe and Spanish lavender in the US),[169] and *L. intermedia* (a sterile hybrid of *L. angustifolia* and *L. latifolia* and also known as lavandin) are also popular ingredients in cosmetic and therapeutic applications.[169–172] *L. stoechas*, with 1,8-Cineole as its main active constituent, is considered to have great potential for use in skincare products based on its anti-inflammatory and anticancer activity.[173] Traditional uses of lavender oil include relaxation, wound healing, and enhanced circulation to the skin.[165,174] Derived from the Latin word *lavare* ("to wash"), lavender was named for its practical antiseptic and disinfectant uses in ancient Arabia, Greece, and Rome.[165,166]

Lavender is an ingredient in a broad array of skincare products including soaps, moisturizers, lotions, bath gels, lip balms, hand creams, shampoos, and hair conditioners.[76] Current data on the uses of lavender bear out numerous traditional uses. Researchers studying perineal pain among women who had recently given birth found a link between use of lavender oil in baths and less discomfort.[175] Also, lavender has been used with moderate success for alopecia areata. In a randomized, double-blind, controlled trial over 7 months, 86 patients received daily scalp massage treatments with either essential oil in a mixture of carrier oils or carrier oil only. Nineteen

of 43 patients in the treatment group displayed significant improvement whereas 6 of 41 in the control group showed some improvement.[176]

Licorice Extract

Licorice (also known as *Liquiritae officinalis*) is best known in its popular confectionery form of black or red candy. Although it is not often thought of as a plant, it is a botanical source of systemic or topical medications that have been used in herbal medicine for approximately 4,000 years.[177] There are different species of licorice. *Glycyrrhiza glabra* (**Fig. 38-5**) and *Glycyrrhiza inflata* (**Fig. 38-6**) are the ones that have displayed the most therapeutic actions, including anti-inflammatory properties. *Glycyrrhiza inflata* is actually the Chinese licorice root, while *Glycyrrhiza glabra* grows around the Mediterranean Sea, the Middle East, as well as central and southern Russia.[178]

Glycyrrhiza glabra

Extracts from this more Western species of licorice are an increasingly common ingredient in anti-inflammatory products.[172] Glycyrrhizin is its primary active component, but it also contains polysaccharides and various polyphenols, such as the

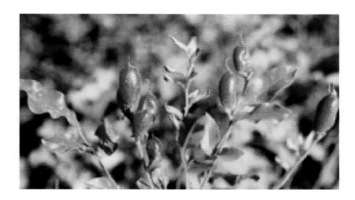

FIGURE 38-5. Glycyrrhizin is a main active ingredient of *Glycyrrhiza glabra*, one of the primary sources of licorice extract.

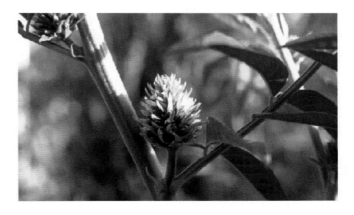

FIGURE 38-6. *Glycyrrhiza inflata* from NW China is the source of licochalone.

isoflavone formononetin, which exhibits antioxidant activity.[179] Glycyrrhetic acid (the biologically active metabolite of *G. glabra*) has been reported to display anti-inflammatory activity in subacute and chronic dermatoses; therefore, it has been used to treat eczema, pruritus, contact dermatitis, seborrheic dermatitis, and psoriasis.[180] In a double-blind study, Saeedi et al. evaluated the effect of 1% and 2% topical licorice extract preparations on AD in 60 patients. Results indicated that the 2% topical gel was effective in reducing erythema, edema, and pruritus, prompting the researchers to conclude that licorice extract might be effective in treating AD.[180] Studies have shown that glycyrrhetic acid is able to exert a cortisone-like effect, thus inhibiting pro-inflammatory PGs and LTs.[181] However, licorice (glycyrrhetic acid) has not been demonstrated to be superior to topical corticosteroids in treating acute inflammation, such as AD.[180] The combination of corticosteroids with glycyrrhetic acid has been proven to be effective, however. One study revealed effective potentiation of hydrocortisone activity in skin by the addition of 2% glycyrrhetic acid.[182] In a series of animal studies, Russian scientists found that glyderinine, a derivative of glycyrrhizic acid, exhibited anti-inflammatory, analgesic, as well as antipyretic properties, and concluded that glyderinine is an appropriate ingredient for the treatment of certain skin diseases.[183] Recent studies also suggest that glycyrrhizin has demonstrated efficacy in treating vitiligo and alopecia areata.[184]

Glycyrrhiza inflata

The primary active ingredient of Chinese licorice root is licochalcone A,[185] a compound that has exhibited anti-inflammatory activity against AA-induced mouse ear edema.[186] It is found in the Eucerin Redness Relief products. In a study assessing the effects of five different chalcones, researchers found that four of the five tested chalcones, including licochalcone A, inhibited the production of pro-inflammatory cytokines from monocytes and T cells. The investigators concluded that licochalcone A and some of its synthetic analogues may have immunomodulatory effects, potentially rendering them suitable agents for the treatment of infectious and other inflammatory diseases.[187] Chalcones also exhibit activity against oxidative stress. A study assessing their radical scavenging activity revealed that licochalcones B and D potently delay superoxide anion production.[188]

The long history of traditional uses of licorice root and the track record of positive research in the past few decades make licorice one of the most widely researched plants for medicinal purposes. The evidence supporting the medical use of *G. inflata* is slightly less extensive than that of the related species *G. glabra*, but it is similar in terms of the broad range of potential applications. Recent findings by Yang et al. suggest that licochalcone A lessens acne symptoms mediated by inhibiting the NLRP3 inflammasome.[189] In combination with 4-t-butylcyclohexanol (SymSitive®), licochalcone A has also been shown in a clinical trial to be well tolerated and effective in ameliorating the clinical grading for erythema, tactile roughness, and telangiectasia in patients with rosacea (subtype I).[190] The same combination was also found to be effective in a randomized, prospective, investigator-blinded study in reducing

facial dermatitis and was superior to triamcinolone acetonide in alleviating erythema and improving skin hydration.[191]

Mushrooms

Several mushroom species are believed to offer significant potential active ingredients in health-promoting pharmaceutical agents, since these have been used in traditional or folk medicine for thousands of years.[192] In particular, extracts from medicinal mushrooms such as *Ganoderma lucidum* (lingzhi in Chinese, reishi or mannentake in Japanese), *Lentinus edodes* (shiitake in Japanese), *Grifola frondosa* (maitake in Japanese), and *Cordyceps sinensis*, among others, have been used in China, Japan, and Korea to treat conditions including allergies, arthritis, bronchitis, gastric ulcer, hepatitis, hyperglycemia, hypertension, inflammation, insomnia, nephritis, neurasthenia, scleroderma, and cancer.[193] Furthermore, these various species have been used in topical dermatologic formulations designed for anti-aging purposes.

Ganoderma lucidum

Also known as reishi or lingzhi, *G. lucidum* has been used since ancient times in China in dried powder form to treat cancer,[193] and currently it continues to be used as a home remedy for the treatment of inflammation and wound healing.[194] Recent research using rats and mice has revealed that the ethanol extract of the mycelium of *G. lucidum* exhibits significant antiperoxidative, anti-inflammatory, antimutagenic,[195] and antioxidant properties.[196] Yin et al. have found that *G. lucidum* extracts have been effective in treating wounds and post-burn infections, achieving skin whitening, and useful in addressing photoaging, AD, and cutaneous sarcoidosis.[197] This mushroom species is one of the most studied botanical treatments in Asia and has become a popular ingredient in topical skincare products in the West. Also recognized for its anti-inflammatory, antioxidant, anticancer, and immunomodulatory activities, *G. lucidum* is considered the strongest adaptogen found in nature.[198]

Cordyceps sinensis

Mycelium extract of *C. sinensis* has been demonstrated to display immunomodulating activity and the capacity to decrease bacterial growth and dissemination, resulting in improved survival.[199] *C. sinensis* extracts have also been found to exert protective effects against UVB-induced damage.[200]

Grifola frondosa

The extract from *G. frondosa* has been shown to inhibit cutaneous photoaging in UVA-exposed human dermal fibroblasts.[201] During the last 30 years, evidence has emerged indicating that *G. frondosa* polysaccharides evince antioxidant, antitumor, and immunomodulatory activity, and may suppress AD-like lesions.[202]

Oatmeal

The skincare applications of oats (INCI name: *Avena sativa*) and oat-derived products date back to 2000 BCE in Egypt and the Arabian Peninsula. In the 19th and early 20th centuries, oatmeal baths were frequently used for the treatment of pruritic inflammatory skin conditions. Somewhat more recently, both Dick and Sompayrac reported in the late 1950s that colloidal oatmeal (CO) baths were demonstrably effective in the management of pediatric AD.[203,204] As a component of the modern dermatologic armamentarium, CO has replaced rolled oats and plain oatmeal. CO is composed of de-hulled oats ground to a fine powder that retains the moisturizing effects of the whole oat grain and disperses more easily in bath water. It can also be added to creams and lotions for use in topical products. CO has been characterized as exerting anti-inflammatory, antioxidant, antifungal, and antipruritic activities and is thought to have the capacity to contribute to barrier repair and skin pH stability.[205]

Polysaccharides (60%–64%), proteins (10%–18%), and lipids (3%–9%) are the primary components of CO. The remaining constituents include enzymes (such as superoxide dismutase), saponins, vitamins, flavonoids, and inhibitors of PG synthesis. Oat lipids contribute to the viscosity of CO and help decrease transepidermal water loss, a key factor in skin dryness. In addition, oatmeal proteins exhibit emulsification, hydration, and antioxidant activity. CO proteins and polysaccharides bind to skin and provide a protective barrier to external insults. The proteins further act as a buffer against strong acids and bases.[206]

The combination of components and properties of CO renders it suitable for various uses in the care of inflammatory skin conditions, such as cleaning, moisturizing, protecting (i.e., barrier preservation), and relieving pruritus in inflamed skin. In fact, oatmeal is one of the few natural products recognized by the FDA as an effective skin protectant.[207] As a consequence, CO is one of the few botanicals subject to FDA regulation.[207] The range of dermatologic applications for CO is extensive and includes adjunctive therapy in inflammatory and pruritic skin conditions such as AD; cercarial dermatitis; diaper dermatitis; ichthyosis; insect bites; irritant and allergic contact dermatitis including contact to poison ivy, oak and sumac; psoriasis; sunburn; urticaria; and xerosis .[203,206,208–210] CO also prevents and repairs damage caused by environmental insults such as bacteria, free radicals, smoke, and UV radiation.[172]

Published clinical studies of CO have generally yielded affirmative results that continue to support the therapeutic use of oatmeal. In a clinical model of skin irritation with sodium lauryl sulfate, two different types of CO products significantly reduced the amount of experimentally induced irritation and inflammation.[211] In a different clinical study, two shower gels were evaluated for relief of pruritus in burn patients.[212] Both gels contained liquid paraffin but only one also contained 5% CO. The oatmeal-containing compound was associated with significantly greater reduction in patient-reported pruritus and requests for antihistamines. Further, Boisnic et al. developed a clinical model of cutaneous inflammation involving the effects of an oatmeal extract on tissue fragments exposed to vasoactive intestinal peptide (VIP), a pro-inflammatory neuromediator.[213] The application of VIP increased inflammation,

which was significantly ameliorated by treatment with the oatmeal extract.

CO lotion has also been shown in clinical trials to confer significant improvements in skin dryness, moisturization, scaling, roughness, itch intensity, and barrier repair in patients with bilateral mild to moderate itch and moderate to severe lower leg xerosis.[214,215] In a double-blind study with 50 subjects conducted in 2020, CO cream 1% was found to be effective in managing chronic irritant hand eczema.[216] In addition, in two single-center, single-arm clinical trials 1% CO cream was effective in alleviating mild to moderate symptoms of AD, with the cream deemed well tolerated and clinically effective.[217]

The therapeutic and cosmetic uses of oatmeal have been enhanced by the isolation and identification of specific oat components. Specifically, avenanthramides, a newly discovered group of polypenolic alkaloids, have been found exclusively in oats.[218] As a group, phenolics display a broad range of biologic activities including prevention of inflammation and oxidation.[219] In fact, phenolics are the strongest antioxidants found in nature,[220] although within this class of compounds, individual substances exert varying levels of antioxidant activity. Oat phenolic compounds including avenanthramides have been identified as potent antioxidants that scavenge reactive oxygen and nitrogen species.[219] Furthermore, they have been reported to inhibit PG biosynthesis nearly as well as the synthetic anti-inflammatory agent indomethacin.[221] A 2007 study provided more evidence that avenanthramides evince potent anti-inflammatory activity.[222] In this research, keratinocytes were incubated with an inducer of pro-inflammatory IL-8 in the presence of vehicle or avenanthramides. The inclusion of avenanthramides reduced the release of the pro-inflammatory cytokine IL-8 by 10% to 25%. Various other preclinical and preliminary clinical studies have demonstrated a wide range of potential benefits from topical compounds that contain avenanthramides including the reduction of histamine-induced itch in humans; inhibition of NF-κB, thus inhibiting the activation of inflammatory pathways in the skin; and the improvement of skin irritation and erythema induced by exposure to UVB irradiation. Currently, CO is best known for its use in the arsenal against AD. Capone et al. showed in 2010 that 1% CO eczema cream also ameliorated microbiome composition in treating AD, significantly enhancing cutaneous pH as well as skin barrier function and hydration.[223]

Selenium

Selenium is an essential trace element present in the human body, and it is thought to have anticarcinogenic, anti-inflammatory, antioxidant, and therefore anti-aging properties. Water, soil, and plant foods are the major sources of selenium in most countries. Specifically, it is found in meat, fish, Brazil nuts, shellfish, dairy products, cereals, and cereal products. Selenium is a component of the water used in the La Roche-Posay spa in France that was founded to treat AD patients and psoriasis patients. Several La Roche-Posay products, including the thermal spring water, contain selenium. The anti-inflammatory role of selenium is very well expressed in one of the reductive metabolic pathways in humans: selenium is the vital antioxidant required to form glutathione peroxidase, one of our most important natural antioxidant defenses.[224] The function of this essential antioxidant enzyme (discussed above in the Role of Free Radicals section) is to protect cell membranes from oxidative deterioration, a role that it shares with vitamin E. In fact, studies have concluded that vitamin E and selenium act synergistically to deliver such protection.[225]

Selenium also exerts anti-inflammatory activity in preventing the production of inflammatory cytokines. One study showed that after damage to the skin from UV exposure, inflammatory cytokines inhibited the immune response, thus increasing the number of damaged skin cells.[226] These inflammatory cytokines also contribute to the formation of wrinkles and premature aging of the skin. Finally, selenium enhances both humoral and cellular immunity, increasing the host response to infection.[227]

As a result of its antioxidant and anti-inflammatory properties, selenium has been added to topical skincare products as well as natural spring water vaporizers for the skin. The current recommended daily allowance of oral selenium is 55 μg for both men and women. However, cancer researchers are currently considering daily doses as high as 400 μg. It must be noted that selenium toxicity, or selenosis, is possible. High doses of selenium are neurotoxic and can cause hair loss, nail loss, and dermatitis, as well as gastrointestinal upset. Despite advertising claims, most available topical formulations contain very low concentrations of selenium, which are not well absorbed by the skin. Formulated as selenium sulfide, selenium does not penetrate the skin. However, cutaneous selenium absorption can be achieved with L-selenomethionine. Recent animal and human studies have found that when taken orally or applied topically in the form of L-selenomethionine, selenium demonstrated protection against both daily and excessive UV damage. In its water-insoluble salt form, selenium sulfide has been used effectively to treat seborrheic dermatitis and tinea versicolor.[228]

In a 1996 study, treated patients experienced decreased skin inflammation and pigmentation, plus a delay in the onset and a decrease in the incidence of skin cancer.[229] In a different study performed in the 1990s, researchers at the University of Edinburgh (Scotland, UK) concluded that oral selenium resulted in significant protective effects against UV radiation-induced damage to skin cells. The researchers did not examine topical selenium.[227]

In 2018, Cohen and Anderson reported on the successful treatment of three patients with hyperkeratosis involving their palms and/or soles with the use of topical selenium sulfide in 2.5% lotion/shampoo or a 2.75% foam.[228] More double-blind, placebo-controlled trials are needed to support selenium as an adjunct to the anti-aging product market, but research is promising.

Turmeric/Curcumin

Turmeric (INCI name: *Curcuma longa*) is best known as a spice used primarily in Asian cuisine, particularly in curry and prepared mustard. It has a long history in both Chinese and Ayurvedic (Indian) medicine as an anti-inflammatory agent.[230] Curcumin (diferuloylmethane) is the yellow pigment that corresponds to the key biologically active component of turmeric and has been proven to have more acute anti-inflammatory effects when compared to the volatile oil fraction of turmeric.[231] When used orally, this herb inhibits LT formation as well as platelet aggregation and stabilizes neutrophilic lysosomal membranes, thus inhibiting inflammation at the cellular level.[232] A 1973 study by Srimal et al. showed that the anti-inflammatory activity of curcumin may even be superior to that of ibuprofen.[233] Moreover, it has been demonstrated to exhibit significant wound healing, antimicrobial, anticarcinogenic, and antioxidant activity.[234]

In 2018, Kumar et al. found that the essential oil from waste leaves of *C. longa* displayed anti-inflammatory activity *in vitro* and in animal models and warrants consideration for use in topical medications.[235] That same year, Bahraini et al. conducted a randomized, placebo-controlled clinical trial in 47 patients with mild to moderate scalp psoriasis, finding that turmeric tonic significantly diminished erythema, scaling, and induration of lesions compared to placebo. They concluded that the turmeric solution has potential as a scalp psoriasis treatment.[236] In a 2019 randomized, double-blind, placebo-controlled trial over an 8-week period, 47 healthy participants received daily intakes of water extract of *C. longa* with or without curcumin or a placebo. Results showed that the *C. longa* water extract exerted moisturizing effects on facial skin. Cell studies by the same group also supported the anti-inflammatory activity of *C. longa*.[237] In a systematic review of the literature completed in 2016, Vaughn et al. reported that 10 studies found a statistically significant improvement in skin disease severity imparted by turmeric in treatment groups as compared to control groups, with conditions such as acne, androgenetic alopecia, AD oral lichen planus, photoaging, pruritus, psoriasis, radiodermatitis, and vitiligo considered.[234] A more recent literature review of clinical trials specifically on the potential health benefits of curcumin also confirmed its anti-inflammatory properties and supported its use to treat inflammatory skin conditions.[238] Finally, curcumin produces different effects depending on the dosing level; at low dose it can be a PG inhibitor, while at higher levels it stimulates the adrenal glands to secrete cortisone.[239]

CONCLUSION

Inflammation is a multifactorial, convoluted process that plays a vital defensive role in protecting living tissues from an expansive variety of potentially deleterious injuries. However, protracted inflammation itself can pose danger to the very tissues and host organism that the cascading events of the inflammatory process were launched to protect. Indeed, this is the case in sensitive skin disorders in which inflammation plays a characteristic role, as discussed in Chapter 12, Dry Skin. In addition, inflammation is thought to play a role in skin aging. As such, anti-inflammatory agents have a crucial role to play in the practice of dermatology. Various modalities can help decrease cutaneous inflammation including topical skincare formulations, water used in spas, diet, supplements, as well as prescription and over-the-counter medications.

References

1. Gallin JI, Goldstein IM, Snyderman R. Overview. In: Gallin JI, Goldstein IM, Synderman R, eds. *Inflammation: Basic Principles and Clinical Correlates*. 2nd ed. New York: Raven Press; 1991:1–4.

2. Williams RH, Stedman TL. *Stedman's Medical Dictionary*. 25th ed. Philadelphia: Williams & Wilkins; 1990.

3. Cotran RS, Kumar V, Collins T, eds. *Robbins Pathological Basis of Disease*. Philadelphia: WB Saunders Co.; 1999: 7216–7335.

4. Kimball ES. *Cytokines and Inflammation*. Boca Raton, FL: CRC Press; 1991.

5. Needleman P, Turk J, Jakschik BA, Morrison AR, Lefkowith JB. Arachidonic acid metabolism. *Annu Rev Biochem*. 1986;55:69–102.

6. Smith WL. Prostanoid biosynthesis and mechanisms of action. *Am J Physiol*. 1992;263(2 Pt 2):F181–F191.

7. Gabay C, Kushner I. Acute-phase proteins and other systemic responses to inflammation. *N Engl J Med*. 1999;340(6):448–454.

8. Cavaillon JM. Contribution of cytokines to inflammatory mechanisms. *Pathol Biol (Paris)*. 1993;41(8 Pt 2):799–811.

9. Leirisalo-Repo M. The present knowledge of the inflammatory process and the inflammatory mediators. *Pharmacol Toxicol*. 1994;75(Suppl 2):1–3.

10. Feghali CA, Wright TM. Cytokines in acute and chronic inflammation. *Front Biosci*. 1997;2:d12–d26.

11. Charo IF, Ransohoff RM. The many roles of chemokines and chemokine receptors in inflammation. *N Engl J Med*. 2006;354(6):610–621.

12. Kitamura Y. Heterogeneity of mast cells and phenotypic change between subpopulations. *Annu Rev Immunol*. 1989;7:59–76.

13. Metcalfe DD, Baram D, Mekori YA. Mast cells. *Physiol Rev*. 1997;77(4):1033–1079.

14. Galli SJ. Mast cells and basophils. *Curr Opin Hematol*. 2000;7(1):32–39.

15. Sayama K, Diehn M, Matsuda K, et al. Transcriptional response of human mast cells stimulated via the Fc(epsilon)RI and identification of mast cells as a source of IL-11. *BMC Immunol*. 2002;3:5.

16. Kawakami T, Galli SJ. Regulation of mast-cell and basophil function and survival by IgE. *Nat Rev Immunol*. 2002;2(10):773–786.

17. Mycek MJ, Harvey RA, Champe PC. Autacoids and autacoid antagonists. In: Harvey RA, Champe PC, eds. *Lippincott's Illustrated Reviews: Pharmacology*. 2nd ed. Philadelphia: Lippincott Williams & Wilkins; 2000: 419–428.

18. Simons FE. Advances in H1-antihistamines. *N Engl J Med*. 2004;351(21):2203–2217.

19. Akdis CA, Blaser K. Histamine in the immune regulation of allergic inflammation. *J Allergy Clin Immunol*. 2003;112(1):15–22.

20. Simons FE, Simons KJ. The pharmacology and use of H1-receptor-antagonist drugs. *N Engl J Med*. 1994;330(23):1663–1670.

21. Sugimoto Y, Iba Y, Nakamura Y, Kayasuga R, Kamei C. Pruritus-associated response mediated by cutaneous histamine H3 receptors. *Clin Exp Allergy*. 2004;34(3):456–459.

22. Babior BM. Phagocytes and oxidative stress. *Am J Med*. 2000;109(1):33–44.

23. Beckman JS, Koppenol WH. Nitric oxide, superoxide, and peroxynitrite: the good, the bad, and ugly. *Am J Physiol*. 1996;271(5 Pt 1):C1424–C1437.

24. Guzik TJ, Korbut R, Adamek-Guzik T. Nitric oxide and superoxide in inflammation and immune regulation. *J Physiol Pharmacol*. 2003;54(4):469–487.

25. Barrington R, Zhang M, Fischer M, Carroll MC. The role of complement in inflammation and adaptive immunity. *Immunol Rev*. 2001;180:5–15.

26. Costa-Neto CM, Dillenburg-Pilla P, Heinrich TA, et al. Participation of kallikrein-kinin system in different pathologies. *Int Immunopharmacol*. 2008;8(2):135–142.

27. Randal A, Skidgel RA, Erdös EG. Histamine, bradykinin, and their antagonists. In: Brunton L, Lazo J, Parker K, eds. *Goodman & Gilman's The Pharmacological Basis of Therapeutics*. 11th ed. New York: McGraw-Hill; 2006: 629–652.

28. Elliott DF, Horton EW, Lewis GP. Actions of pure bradykinin. *J Physiol*. 1960;153(3):473–480.

29. Robert C, Kupper TS. Inflammatory skin diseases, T cells, and immune surveillance. *N Engl J Med*. 1999;341(24):1817–1828.

30. Barnes PJ, Karin M. Nuclear factor-kappaB: a pivotal transcription factor in chronic inflammatory diseases. *N Engl J Med*. 1997;336(15):1066–1071.

31. Kupper TS. Immune and inflammatory processes in cutaneous tissues. Mechanisms and speculations. *J Clin Invest*. 1990;86(6):1783–1789.

32. Lee RT, Briggs WH, Cheng GC, Rossiter HB, Libby P, Kupper T. Mechanical deformation promotes secretion of IL-1 alpha and IL-1 receptor antagonist. *J Immunol*. 1997;159(10):5084–5088.

33. Rosette C, Karin M. Ultraviolet light and osmotic stress: activation of the JNK cascade through multiple growth factor and cytokine receptors. *Science*. 1996;274(5290):1194–1197.

34. Picker LJ, Michie SA, Rott LS, Butcher EC. A unique phenotype of skin-associated lymphocytes in humans. Preferential expression of the HECA-452 epitope by benign and malignant T cells at cutaneous sites. *Am J Pathol*. 1990;136(5):1053–1068.

35. Steffen C. The introduction of topical corticosteroids. *Skinmed*. 2003;2(5):304–305.

36. Spies TD, Stone RE. Effect of local application of synthetic cortisone acetate on lesions of iritis and uveitis, of allergic contact dermatitis, and of psoriasis. *South Med J*. 1950;43:871.

37. Rasmussen N. Steroids in arms: science, government, industry, and the hormones of the adrenal cortex in the United States, 1930-1950. *Med Hist*. 2002;46(3):299–:324.

38. Tuckermann JP, Kleiman A, McPherson KG, Reichardt HM. Molecular mechanisms of glucocorticoids in the control of inflammation and lymphocyte apoptosis. *Crit Rev Clin Lab Sci*. 2005;42(1):71–104.

39. Kim SW, Rhee HJ, Ko J, Kim YJ, Kim HG, Yang JM, et al. Inhibition of cytosolic phospholipase A2 by annexin I. Specific interaction model and mapping of the interaction site. *J Biol Chem*. 2001;276(19):15712–15719.

40. Rhen T, Cidlowski JA. Antiinflammatory action of glucocorticoids--new mechanisms for old drugs. *N Engl J Med*. 2005;353(16):1711–1723.

41. De Bosscher K, Vanden Berghe W, Haegeman G. The interplay between the glucocorticoid receptor and nuclear factor-kappaB or activator protein-1: molecular mechanisms for gene repression. *Endocr Rev*. 2003;24(4):488–522.

42. Tanabe T, Tohnai N. Cyclooxygenase isozymes and their gene structures and expression. *Prostaglandins Other Lipid Mediat.* 2002;68-69:95–114.

43. Cohen DE, Heidary N. Treatment of irritant and allergic contact dermatitis. *Dermatol Ther.* 2004;17(4):334–340.

44. Marks R. Adverse side effects from the use of topical corticosteroids. In: Maibach HI, Surger C, eds. *Topical Corticosteroids.* Basel: Karger; 1992: 170–183.

45. Walsh P, Aeling JL, Huff L, Weston WL. Hypothalamus-pituitary-adrenal axis suppression by superpotent topical steroids. *J Am Acad Dermatol.* 1993;29(3):501–503.

46. Hengge UR, Ruzicka T, Schwartz RA, Cork MJ. Adverse effects of topical glucocorticosteroids. *J Am Acad Dermatol.* 2006;54(1):1–15.

47. Gebhard KL, Maibach HI. Relationship between systemic corticosteroids and osteonecrosis. *Am J Clin Dermatol.* 2001;2(6):377–388.

48. Becker B. The effect of topical corticosteroids in secondary glaucomas. *Arch Ophthalmol.* 1964;72:769–771.

49. Becker B. Cataracts and topical corticosteroids. *Am J Ophthalmol.* 1964;58:872–873.

50. Bornhövd E, Burgdorf WH, Wollenberg A. Macrolactam immunomodulators for topical treatment of inflammatory skin diseases. *J Am Acad Dermatol.* 2001;45(5):736–743.

51. FDA Public Health Advisory – Elidel (pimecrolimus) Cream and Protopic (tacrolimus) Ointment, March 10, 2005. Available at: ELIDEL® (pimecrolimus) Cream, 1% (fda.gov). Accessed on March 17, 2021.

52. Lauerma AI, Stein BD, Homey B, Lee CH, Bloom E, Maibach HI. Topical FK506: suppression of allergic and irritant contact dermatitis in the guinea pig. *Arch Dermatol Res.* 1994;286(6):337–340.

53. Saripalli YV, Gadzia JE, Belsito DV. Tacrolimus ointment 0.1% in the treatment of nickel-induced allergic contact dermatitis. *J Am Acad Dermatol.* 2003;49(3):477–482.

54. Lauerma AI, Maibach HI, Granlund H, Erkko P, Kartamaa M, Stubb S. Inhibition of contact allergy reactions by topical FK506. *Lancet.* 1992;340(8818):556.

55. Sengoku T, Morita K, Sakuma S, Motoyama Y, Goto T. Possible inhibitory mechanism of FK506 (tacrolimus hydrate) ointment for atopic dermatitis based on animal models. *Eur J Pharmacol.* 1999;379(2-3):183–189.

56. Gupta AK, Chow M. Pimecrolimus: a review. *J Eur Acad Dermatol Venereol.* 2003;17(5):493–503.

57. Ring J, Möhrenschlager M, Henkel V. The US FDA 'black box' warning for topical calcineurin inhibitors: an ongoing controversy. *Drug Saf.* 2008;31(3):185–198.

58. Eichenfield L. Therapeutics in pediatric dermatology. Program and abstracts of the 64th Annual Meeting of the American Academy of Dermatology, Symposium 325: Therapeutics Symposium. San Francisco, California, March 3–7, 2006.

59. Smith KJ, Skelton H. Arachidonic acid-derived bioactive lipids: their role and the role for their inhibitors in dermatology. *J Cutan Med Surg.* 2002;6(3):241–256.

60. Kaminsky A. Less common methods to treat acne. *Dermatology.* 2003;206(1):68–73.

61. Wong RC, Kang S, Heezen JL, Voorhees JJ, Ellis CN. Oral ibuprofen and tetracycline for the treatment of acne vulgaris. *J Am Acad Dermatol.* 1984;11(6):1076–1081.

62. Funt LS. Oral ibuprofen and minocycline for the treatment of resistant acne vulgaris. *J Am Acad Dermatol.* 1985;13(3):524–525.

63. Hughes GS, Francom SF, Means LK, Bohan DF, Caruana C, Holland M. Synergistic effects of oral nonsteroidal drugs and topical corticosteroids in the therapy of sunburn in humans. *Dermatology.* 1992;184(1):54–58.

64. Black AK, Fincham N, Greaves MW, Hensby CN. Time course changes in levels of arachidonic acid and prostaglandins D2, E2, F2 alpha in human skin following ultraviolet B irradiation. *Br J Clin Pharmacol.* 1980;10(5):453–457.

65. Wu KK. Salicylates and their spectrum of activity. *Anti-Inflammatory & Anti-Allergy Agents in Medicinal Chemistry (formerly Current Medicinal Chemistry – Anti-Inflammatory and Anti-Allergy Agents).* 2007;6(4):278–292.

66. Kligman D, Kligman AM. Salicylic acid peels for the treatment of photoaging. *Dermatol Surg.* 1998;24(3):325–328.

67. Harvey SC. Antiseptis and disinfectants; fungicides; ectoparasiticides. In: Gilman AG, Goodman LS, Rall TW, Murad F, eds. *Goodman and Gilman's The Pharmacological Basis of Therapeutics.* 7th ed. New York: MacMillan; 1985: 959–979.

68. Lin AN, Reimer RJ, Carter DM. Sulfur revisited. *J Am Acad Dermatol.* 1988;18(3):553–558.

69. Konaklieva MI, Plotkin BJ. Anti-inflammatory sulfur-containing agents with additional modes of action. *Anti-Inflammatory & Anti-Allergy Agents in Medicinal Chemistry (formerly Current Medicinal Chemistry – Anti-Inflammatory and Anti-Allergy Agents).* 2007;6(4):271–277.

70. Combes FC. Colloidal sulfur: some pharmacodynamic considerations and their therapeutic application in seborrheic dermatoses. *NY State J Med.* 1946;46:401–406.

71. McEvoy GK, McQuarrie GM, eds. Drug information 86, American Hospital Formulary Service. Bethesda: American Society of Hospital Pharmacists; 1986: 1800–1802.

72. Sheard C. *Treatment of Skin Diseases: A Manual.* Chicago: Year Book; 1978: 21–22.

73. Plexion SCT™ (sodium sulfacetamide 10% and sulfur 5%), [package insert]. Scottsdale, AZ, Medicis, The Dermatology Company, 2001.

74. Tarimci N, Sener S, Kilinç T. Topical sodium sulfacetamide/sulfur lotion. *J Clin Pharm Ther.* 1997;22(4):301.

75. Gupta AK, Nicol K. The use of sulfur in dermatology. *J Drugs Dermatol.* 2004;3(4):427–431.

76. Baumann LS. Less-known botanical cosmeceuticals. *Dermatol Ther.* 2007;20(5):330–342.

77. Long V. Aloe Vera in Dermatology—The Plant of Immortality. *JAMA Dermatol.* 2016;152(12):1364.

78. Baumann LS. Aloe vera. *Skin & Allergy News.* 2003;34:32.

79. Marshall JM. Aloe vera gel: What is the evidence. *Pharm J.* 1990;24:360–362.

80. Reynolds T, Dweck AC. Aloe vera leaf gel: a review update. *J Ethnopharmacol.* 1999;68(1-3):3–37.

81. Briggs C. Herbal medicine: aloe. *Can Pharm J.* 1995;128(2):48–50.

82. Talmadge J, Chavez J, Jacobs L, et al. Fractionation of Aloe vera L. inner gel, purification and molecular profiling of activity. *Int Immunopharmacol.* 2004;4(14):1757–1773.

83. Lee JK, Lee MK, Yun YP, et al. Acemannan purified from Aloe vera induces phenotypic and functional maturation of immature dendritic cells. *Int Immunopharmacol.* 2001;1(7):1275–1284.

84. Kumar R, Singh AK, Gupta A, Bishayee A, Pandey AK. Therapeutic potential of Aloe vera-A miracle gift of nature. *Phytomedicine.* 2019;60:152996.

85. Hęś M, Dziedzic K, Górecka D, Jędrusek-Golińska A, Gujska E. Aloe vera (L.) Webb.: Natural Sources of Antioxidants - A Review. *Plant Foods Hum Nutr.* 2019;74(3):255–265.

86. Sánchez M, González-Burgos E, Iglesias I, Gómez-Serranillos MP. Pharmacological Update Properties of *Aloe Vera* and its Major Active Constituents. *Molecules.* 2020;25(6):1324.

87. Hutter JA, Salman M, Stavinoha WB, et al. Antiinflammatory C-glucosyl chromone from Aloe barbadensis. *J Nat Prod.* 1996;59(5):541–543.

88. Habeeb F, Stables G, Bradbury F, et al. The inner gel component of Aloe vera suppresses bacterial-induced pro-inflammatory cytokines from human immune cells. *Methods.* 2007;42(4):388–393.

89. Klein AD, Penneys NS. Aloe vera. *J Am Acad Dermatol.* 1988;18(4 Pt 1):714–720.

90. Teplicki E, Ma Q, Castillo DE, et al. The Effects of Aloe vera on Wound Healing in Cell Proliferation, Migration, and Viability. *Wounds.* 2018;30(9):263–268.

91. Hekmatpou D, Mehrabi F, Rahzani K, Aminiyan A. The Effect of Aloe Vera Clinical Trials on Prevention and Healing of Skin Wound: A Systematic Review. *Iran J Med Sci.* 2019;44(1):1–9.

92. Burusapat C, Supawan M, Pruksapong C, Pitiseree A, Suwantemee C. Topical Aloe Vera Gel for Accelerated Wound Healing of Split-Thickness Skin Graft Donor Sites: A Double-Blind, Randomized, Controlled Trial and Systematic Review. *Plast Reconstr Surg.* 2018;142(1):217–226.

93. Re TA, Mooney D, Antignac E, et al. Application of the threshold of toxicological concern approach for the safety evaluation of calendula flower (Calendula officinalis) petals and extracts used in cosmetic and personal care products. *Food Chem Toxicol.* 2009;47(6):1246–1254.

94. Andersen FA. Final report on the safety assessment of Calendula officinalis extract and Calendula officinalis. *Int J Toxicol.* 2001;20:13–20.

95. Mills S, Bone K. *Principles and Practice of Phytotherapy: Modern Herbal Medicine.* London: Churchill Livingstone; 2000: 133.

96. Hoffmann D. *Medical Herbalism: The Science and Practice of Herbal Medicine.* Rochester: VT: Healing Arts Press; 2003: 458, 488, 491, 535.

97. Preethi KC, Kuttan G, Kuttan R. Anti-inflammatory activity of flower extract of Calendula officinalis Linn. And its possible mechanism of action. *Indian J Exp Biol.* 2009;47(2):113–120.

98. Nicolaus C, Junghanns S, Hartmann A, Murillo R, Ganzera M, Merfort I. In vitro studies to evaluate the wound healing properties of Calendula officinalis extracts. *J Ethnopharmacol.* 2017;196:94–103.

99. Arora D, Rani A, Sharma A. A review on phytochemistry and ethnopharmacological aspects of genus Calendula. *Pharmacogn Rev.* 2013;7(14):179–187.

100. Fonseca YM, Catini CD, Vicentini FT, Nomizo A, Gerlach RF, Fonseca MJ. Protective effect of Calendula officinalis extract against UVB-induced oxidative stress in skin: evaluation of reduced glutathione levels and matrix metalloproteinase secretion. *J Ethnopharmacol.* 2010;127(3):596–601.

101. Kundaković T, Milenković M, Zlatković S, Nikolić V, Nikolić G, Binić I. Treatment of venous ulcers with the herbal-based ointment Herbadermal®: a prospective non-randomized pilot study. *Forsch Komplementmed.* 2012;19(1):26–30.

102. Duran V, Matic M, Jovanović M, et al. Results of the clinical examination of an ointment with marigold (Calendula officinalis) extract in the treatment of venous leg ulcers. *Int J Tissue React.* 2005;27(3):101–106.

103. Cordova CA, Siqueira IR, Netto CA, et al. Protective properties of butanolic extract of the Calendula officinalis L. (marigold) against lipid peroxidation of rat liver microsomes and action as free radical scavenger. *Redox Rep.* 2002;7(2):95–102.

104. Fuchs SM, Schliemann-Willers S, Fischer TW, Elsner P. Protective effects of different marigold (Calendula officinalis L.) and rosemary cream preparations against sodium-lauryl-sulfate-induced irritant contact dermatitis. *Skin Pharmacol Physiol.* 2005;18(4):195–200.

105. Lohani A, Mishra AK, Verma A. Cosmeceutical potential of geranium and calendula essential oil: Determination of antioxidant activity and in vitro sun protection factor. *J Cosmet Dermatol.* 2019;18(2):550–557.

106. Russo EB. History of cannabis and its preparations in saga, science, and sobriquet. *Chem Biodivers.* 2007;4(8):161448.

107. Goldenberg M, Reid MW, IsHak WW, Danovitch I. The impact of cannabis and cannabinoids for medical conditions on health-related quality of life: A systematic review and meta-analysis. *Drug Alcohol Depend.* 2017;174:80–90.

108. Mounessa JS, Siegel JA, Dunnick CA, Dellavalle RP. The role of cannabinoids in dermatology. *J Am Acad Dermatol.* 2017;77(1):188–190.

109. Shalaby M, Yardley H, Lio PA. Stirring the pot: cannabinoids and atopic dermatitis. *Pract Dermatol.* 2018;68–70.

110. Sheriff T, Lin MJ, Dubin D, Khorasani H. The potential role of cannabinoids in dermatology. *J Dermatolog Treat.* 2020;31(8):839–845.

111. Sangiovanni E, Fumagalli M, Pacchetti B, et al. Cannabis sativa L. extract and cannabidiol inhibit in vitro mediators of skin inflammatioin and wound injury. *Phytother Res.* 2019;33(8):2083–2093.

112. Cintosum A, Lara-Corrales I, Pope E. Mechanisms of Cannabinoids and Potential Applicability to Skin Diseases. *Clin Drug Investig.* 2020;40(4):293–304.

113. Wilkinson JD, Williamson EM. Cannabinoids inhibit human keratinocyte proliferation through a non-CB1/CB2 mechanism and have a potential therapeutic value in the treatment of psoriasis. *J Dermatol Sci.* 2007;45(2):87–92.

114. Milando R, Friedman A. Cannabinoids: Potential role in inflammatory and neoplastic skin diseases. *Am J Clin Dermatol.* 2019;20(2):167–180.

115. Avila C, Massick S, Kaffenberger BH, Kwatra SG, Bechtel M. Cannabinoids for the treatment of chronic pruritus: A review. *J Am Acad Dermatol.* 2020;82(5):1205–1212.

116. Robinson E, Murphy E, Friedman A. Knowledge, attitudes, and perceptions of cannabinoids in the dermatology community. *J Drugs Dermatol.* 2018;17(12):1273–1278.

117. Oláh A, Markovics A, Szabó-Papp J, et al. Differential effectiveness of selected non-psychotropic phytocannabinoids on human sebocyte functions implicates their introduction in dry/seborrheic skin and acne treatment. *Exp Dermatol.* 2016;25(9):701–707.

118. Eagleston LRM, Kalani NK, Patel RR, Flaten HK, Dunnick CA, Dellavalle RP. Cannabinoids in dermatology: a scoping review. *Dermatol Online J.* 2018;24(6).

119. Marks DH, Friedman A. The therapeutic potential of cannabinoids in dermatology. *Skin Therapy Lett.* 2018;23(6):1–5.

120. Sunda F, Arowolo A. A molecular basis for the anti-inflammatory and anti-fibrosis properties of cannabidiol. *FASEB J.* 2020;34(11):14083–14092.

121. Ali A, Akhtar N. The safety and efficacy of 3% Cannabis seeds extract cream for reduction of human cheek skin sebum and erythema content. *Pak J Pharm Sci.* 2015 ;28(4):1389–1395.

122. Kupczyk P, Reich A, Szepietowski JC. Cannabinoid system in the skin – a possible target for future therapies in dermatology. *Exp Dermatol.* 2009;18(8):669–679.

123. Chuquilin M, Alghalith Y, Fernandez KH. Neurocutaneous disease: Cutaneous neuroanatomy and mechanisms of itch and pain. *J Am Acad Dermatol.* 2016;74(2):197–212.

124. O'Hara M, Kiefer D, Farrell K, Kemper K. A review of 12 commonly used medicinal herbs. *Arch Fam Med.* 1998;7(6):523–536.

125. Dockrell TR, Leever JS. An overview of herbal medications with implications for the school nurse. *J Sch Nurs.* 2000;16(3):53–58.

126. Safayhi H, Sabieraj J, Sailer ER, Ammon HP. Chamazulene: an antioxidant-type inhibitor of leukotriene B4 formation. *Planta Med.* 1994;60(5):410–413.

127. Lin TK, Zhong L, Santiago JL. Anti-Inflammatory and Skin Barrier Repair Effects of Topical Application of Some Plant Oils. *Int J Mol Sci.* 2017;19(1). pii: E70.

128. Shipochliev T, Dimitrov A, Aleksandrova E. Anti-inflammatory action of a group of plant extracts. *Vet Med Nauki.* 1981;18(6):87–94.

129. Lee KG, Shibamoto T. Determination of antioxidant potential of volatile extracts isolated from various herbs and spices. *J Agric Food Chem.* 2002;50(17):4947–4952.

130. Máday E, Szőke E, Muskáth Z, Lemberkovics E. A study of the production of essential oils in chamomile hairy root cultures. *Eur J Drug Metab Pharmacokinet.* 1999;24(4):303–308.

131. Ferreira EB, Ciol MA, de Meneses AG, et al. Chamomile Gel versus Urea Cream to Prevent Acute Radiation Dermatitis in Head and Neck Cancer Patients: Results from a Preliminary Clinical Trial. *Integr Cancer Ther.* 2020;19:1534735420962174.

132. Paulsen E, Chistensen LP, Andersen KE. Cosmetics and herbal remedies with Compositae plant extracts - are they tolerated by Compositae-allergic patients? *Contact Dermatitis.* 2008;58(1):15–23.

133. Borge GI, Vogt G, Nilsson A. Intermediates and products formed during fatty acid alpha-oxidation in cucumber (Cucumis sativus). *Lipids.* 1999;34(7):661–:673.

134. Bernardini C, Zannoni A, Bertocchi M, Tubon I, Fernandez M, Forni M. Water/ethanol extract of Cucumis sativus L. fruit attenuates lipopolysaccharide-induced inflammatory response in endothelial cells. *BMC Complement Altern Med.* 2018;18(1):194.

135. Fiume MM, Bergfeld WF, Belsito DV, et al. Safety Assessment of Cucumis sativus (Cucumber)-Derived Ingredients as Used in Cosmetics. *Int J Toxicol.* 2014;33(2 suppl):47S–64S.

136. Trejo-Moreno C, Méndez-Martinez M, Zamilpa A, et al. Cucumis sativus Aqueous Fraction Inhibits Angiotensin II-Induced Inflammation and Oxidative Stress In Vitro. *Nutrients.* 2018;10(3). pii: E276.

137. Isely D. *One Hundred and One Botanists.* Ames, IA: Iowa State University Press; 1994: 10–13.

138. Gunther RT, ed. *The Greek Herbal of Dioscorides.* Oxford, UK: Oxford University Press; 1933.

139. Vogler BK, Pittler MH, Ernst E. Feverfew as a preventive treatment for migraine: a systematic review. *Cephalalgia.* 1998;18(10):704–708.

140. Kwok BH, Koh B, Ndubuisi MI, Elofsson M, Crews CM. The anti-inflammatory natural product parthenolide from the medicinal herb Feverfew directly binds to and inhibits IκB kinase. *Chem Biol.* 2001;8(8):759–766.

141. Pareek A, Suthar M, Rathore GS, Bansal V. Feverfew (Tanacetum parthenium L.): A systematic review. *Pharmacogn Rev.* 2011;5(9):103–110.

142. Hausen BM. A 6-year experience with compositae mix. *Am J Contact Dermat.* 1996;7(2):94–99.

143. Martin K, Sur R, Liebel F, et al. Parthenolide-depleted Feverfew (Tanacetum parthenium) protects skin from UV irradiation and external aggression. *Arch Dermatol Res.* 2008;300(2):69–80.

144. Kitts DD, Wijewickreme AN, Hu C. Antioxidant properties of a North American ginseng extract. *Mol Cell Biochem.* 2000;203(1-2):1–10.

145. Park S, Yeo M, Jin JH, et al. Rescue of Helicobacter pylori-induced cytotoxicity by red ginseng. *Dig Dis Sci.* 2005;50(7):1218–1227.

146. Volate SR, Davenport DM, Muga SJ, Wargovich MJ. Modulation of aberrant crypt foci and apoptosis by dietary herbal supplements (quercetin, curcumin, silymarin, ginseng and rutin). *Carcinogenesis.* 2005;26(8):1450–1456.

147. Kang KA, Kim YW, Kim SU, et al. G1 phase arrest of the cell cycle by a ginseng metabolite, compound K, in U937 human monocytic leukamia cells. *Arch Pharm Res.* 2005;28(6):685–690.

148. Ahn JY, Choi IS, Shim JY, et al. The immunomodulator ginsan induces resistance to experimental sepsis by inhibiting Toll-like receptor-mediated inflammatory signals. *Eur J Immunol.* 2006;36(1):37–45.

149. Keum YS, Han SS, Chun KS, et al. Inhibitory effects of the ginsenoside Rg3 on phorbol ester-induced cyclooxygenase-2 expression, NF-kappaB activation and tumor promotion. *Mutat Res.* 2003;523-524:75–85.

150. Sabouri-Rad S, Sabouri-Rad S, Sahebkar A, Tayarani-Najaran Z. Ginseng in Dermatology: A Review. *Curr Pharm Des.* 2017;23(11):1649–1666.

151. Rhule A, Navarro S, Smith JR, Shepherd DM. Panax notoginseng attenuates LPS-induced pro-inflammatory mediators in RAW264.7 cells. *J Ethnopharmacol.* 2006;106(1):121–128.

152. Suter A, Bommer S, Rechner J. Treatment of patients with venous insufficiency with fresh plant horse chestnut seed extract: a review of 5 clinical studies. *Adv Ther.* 2006;23(1):179–190.

153. Wilkinson JA, Brown AM. Horse chestnut – Aesculus hippocastanum: potential applications in cosmetic skin-care products. *Int J Cosmet Sci.* 1999;21(6):437–447.

154. Masaki H, Sakaki S, Atsumi T, Sakurai H. Active-oxygen scavenging activity of plant extracts. *Biol Pharm Bull.* 1995;18(1):162–166.

155. Calabrese C, Preston P. Report of the results of a double-blind, randomized, single-dose trial of a topical 2% escin gel versus placebo in the acute treatment of experimentally-induced hematoma in volunteers. *Planta Med.* 1993;59(5):394–397.

156. Tozzi E, Scatena M, Castellacci E. Anti-inflammatory local frigotherapy with a combination of escin, heparin and polyunsaturated phosphatidylcholine (EPL). *Clin Ter.* 1981;98(5):517–524.

157. Desogus AI, D'Alia G. Venotropic therapy: results of clinical experimentation. *Clin Ter.* 1986;118(5):339–342.

158. Sirtori CR. Aescin: pharmacology, pharmacokinetics and therapeutic profile. *Pharmacol Res.* 2001;44(3):183–193.

159. Reuter J, Wölfle U, Korting HC, Schempp C. Which plant for which skin disease? Part 2: Dermatophytes, chronic venous insufficiency, photoprotection, actinic keratoses, vitiligo, hair loss, cosmetic indications. *J Dtsh Dermatol Ges.* 2010;8(11):866–873.

160. Leach MJ, Pincombe J, Foster G. Using horse chestnut seed extract in the treatment of venous leg ulcers: a cost-benefit analysis. *Ostomy Wound Manage.* 2006;52(4):68–70, 72–4, 76–8.

161. Pittler MH, Ernst E. Horse chestnut seed extract for chronic venous insufficiency. *Cochrane Database Syst Rev.* 2012;11:CD003230.

162. Guillaume M, Padioleau F. Veinotonic effect, vascular protection, anti-inflammatory and free radical scavenging properties of horse chestnut extract. *Arzneimittelforschung.* 1994;44(1):25–35.

163. Gallelli L. Escin: a review of its anti-edematous, anti-inflammatory, and venotonic properties. *Drug Des Devel Ther.* 2019;13:3425–3437.

164. Zhao SQ, Xu SQ, Cheng J, et al. Anti-inflammatory effect of external use of escin on cutaneous inflammation: possible involvement of glucocorticoids receptor. *Chin J Nat Med.* 2018;16(2):105–112.

165. Denner SS. Lavandula angustifolia Miller: English lavender. *Holist Nurs Pract.* 2009;23(1):57–64.

166. Basch E, Foppa I, Liebowitz R, et al. Lavender (Lavandula angustifolia Miller). *J Herb Pharmacother.* 2004;4(2):63–78.

167. Cardia GFE, Silva-Filho SE, Silva EL, et al. Effect of Lavender *(Lavandula angustifolia)* Essential Oil on Acute Inflammatory Response. *Evid Based Complement Alternat Med.* 2018;2018:1413940.

168. Hoffmann D. *Medical Herbalism: The Science and Practice of Herbal Medicine.* Rochester, VT: Healing Arts Press; 2003:489, 561–2.

169. Cavanagh HM, Wilkinson JM. Biological activities of lavender essential oil. *Phytother Res.* 2002;16(4):301–308.

170. Roller S, Ernest N, Buckle J. The antimicrobial activity of high-necrodane and other lavender oils on methicillin-sensitive and –resistant Staphylococcus aureus (MSSA and MRSA). *J Altern Complement Med.* 2009;15(3):275–279.

171. Wu J. Treatment of rosacea with herbal ingredients. *J Drugs Dermatol.* 2006;5(1):29–32.

172. Aburjai T, Natsheh FM. Plants used in cosmetics. *Phytother Res.* 2003;17(9):987–1000.

173. Boukhatem MN, Sudha T, Darwish NHE, et al. A New Eucalyptol-Rich Lavender (*Lavandula stoechas* L.) Essential Oil: Emerging Potential for Therapy against Inflammation and Cancer. *Molecules.* 2020;25(16):3671.

174. Prashar A, Locke IC, Evans CS. Cytotoxicity of lavender oil and its major components to human skin cells. *Cell Prolif.* 2004;37(3):221–229.

175. Cornwell S, Dale A. Lavender oil and perineal repair. *Mod Midwife.* 1995;5(3):31–33.

176. Hay IC, Jamieson M, Ormerod AD. Randomized trial of aromatherapy. Successful treatment for alopecia areata. *Arch Dermatol.* 1998;134(11):1349–1352.

177. Gibson MR. Glycyrrhiza in old and new perspectives. *Lloydia.* 1978;41(4):348–354.

178. Agarwal R, Wang ZY, Mukhtar H. Inhibition of mouse skin tumor-initiating activity of DMBA by chronic oral feeding of glycyrrhizin in drinking water. *Nutr Cancer.* 1991;15(3-4):187–193.

179. Wang ZY, Nixon DW. Licorice and cancer. *Nutr Cancer.* 2001;39(1):1–11.

180. Saeedi M, Morteza-Semnani K, Ghoreishi MR. The treatment of atopic dermatitis with licorice gel. *J Dermatolog Treat.* 2003;14(3):153–157.

181. Ohuchi K, Kamada Y, Levine L, Tsurufuji S. Glycyrrhizin inhibits prostaglandin E2 production by activated peritoneal macrophages from rats. *Prostaglandins Med.* 1981;7(5):457–463.

182. Teelucksingh S, Mackie AD, Burt D, McIntyre MA, Brett L, Edwards CR. Potentiation of hydrocortisone activity in skin by glycyrrhetinic acid. *Lancet.* 1990;335(8697):1060–1063.

183. Azimov MM, Zakirov UB, Radzhapova ShD. Pharmacological study of the anti-inflammatory agent glyderinine. *Farmakol Toksikol.* 1988;51(4):90–93.

184. Kwon YJ, Son DH, Chung TH, Lee YJ. A Review of the Pharmacological Efficacy and Safety of Licorice Root from Corroborative Clinical Trial Findings. *J Med Food.* 2020;23(1):12–20.

185. Friis-Møller A, Chen M, Fuursted K, Christensen SB, Kharazmi A. In vitro antimycobacterial and antilegionella activity of licochalcone A from Chinese licorice roots. *Planta Med.* 2002;68(5):416–419.

186. Shibata S, Inoue H, Iwata S, et al. Inhibitory effects of licochalcone A isolated from Glycyrrhiza inflata root on inflammatory ear edema and tumour promotion in mice. *Planta Med.* 1991;57(3):221–224.

187. Barfod L, Kemp K, Hansen M, Kharazmi A. Chalcones from Chinese liquorice inhibit proliferation of T cells and production of cytokines. *Int Immunopharmacol.* 2002;2(4):545–555.

188. Haraguchi H, Ishikawa H, Mizutani K, Tamura Y, Kinoshita T. Antioxidative and superoxide scavenging activities of retrochalcones in Glycyrrhiza inflata. *Bioorg Med Chem.* 1998;6(3):339–347.

189. Yang G, Lee HE, Yeon SH, et al. Licochalcone A attenuates acne symptoms mediated by suppression of NLRP3 inflammasome. *Phytother Res.* 2018;32(12):2551–2559.

190. Schoelermann AM, Weber TM, Arrowitz C, Rizer RL, Qian K, Babcock M. Skin compatibility and efficacy of a cosmetic skin care regimen with licochalcone A and 4-t-butylcyclohexanol in patients with rosacea subtype I. *J Eur Acad Dermatol Venereol.* 2016;30(Suppl 1):21–27.

191. Boonchai W, Varothai S, Winayanuwattikun W, Phaitoonvatanakij S, Chaweekulrat P, Kasemsarn P. Randomized investigator-blinded comparative study of moisturizer containing 4-t-butylcyclohexanol and licochalcone A versus 0.02% triamcinolone acetonide cream in facial dermatitis. *J Cosmet Dermatol.* 2018;17(6):1130–1135.

192. Wasser SP. Medicinal mushrooms as a source of antitumor and immunomodulating polysaccharides. *Appl Microbiol Biotechnol.* 2002;60(3):258–274.

193. Sliva D. Ganoderma lucidum (Reishi) in cancer treatment. *Integr Cancer Ther.* 2003;2(4):358–364.

194. Sliva D, Sedlak M, Slivova V, Valachovicova T, Lloyd FPJr, Ho NW. Biologic activity of spores and dried powder from Ganoderma lucidum for the inhibition of highly invasive human breast and prostate cancer cells. *J Altern Complement Med.* 2003;9(4):491–497.

195. Lakshmi B, Ajith TA, Sheena N, Gunapalan N, Janardhanan KK. Antiperoxidative, anti-inflammatory, and antimutagenic activities of ethanol extract of the mycelium of Ganoderma lucidum occurring in South India. *Teratog Carcinog Mutagen.* 2003;(Suppl 1):85–97.

196. Xie JT, Wang CZ, Wicks S, et al. Ganoderma lucidum extract inhibits proliferation of SW 480 human colorectal cancer cells. *Exp Oncol.* 2006;28(1):25–29.

197. Yin Z, Yang B, Ren H. Preventive and Therapeutic Effect of Ganoderma (Lingzhi) on Skin Diseases and Care. *Adv Exp Med Biol.* 2019;1182:311–321.

198. Abate M, Pepe G, Randino R, et al. *Ganoderma lucidum* Ethanol Extracts Enhance Re-Epithelialization and Prevent Keratinocytes from Free-Radical Injury. *Pharmaceuticals (Basel).* 2020;13(9):E224.

199. Kuo CF, Chen CC, Luo YH, et al. Cordyceps sinensis mycelium protects mice from group A streptococcal infection. *J Med Microbiol.* 2005;54(Pt 8):795–802.

200. He H, Tang J, Ru D, et al. Protective effects of Cordyceps extract against UVB-induced damage and prediction of application prospects in the topical administration: An experimental validation and network pharmacology study. *Biomed Pharmacother.* 2020;121:109600.

201. Bae JT, Sim GS, Lee DH, et al. Production of exopolysaccharide from mycelial culture of Grifola frondosa and its inhibitory effect on matrix metalloproteinase-1 expression in UV-irradiated human dermal fibroblasts. *FEMS Microbiol Lett.* 2005;251(2):347–354.

202. He X, Wang X, Fang J, et al. Polysaccharides in Grifola frondosa mushroom and their health promoting properties: A review. *Int J Biol Macromol.* 2017;101:910–921.

203. Dick LA. Colloidal emollient baths in pediatric dermatoses. *Arch Pediatr.* 1958;75(12):506–508.

204. Sompayrac LM, Ross C. Colloidal oatmeal in atopic dermatitis of the young. *J Fla Med Assoc.* 1959;45(12):1411–1412.

205. Allais B, Friedman A. ARTICLE: Colloidal Oatmeal Part I: History, Basic Science, Mechanism of Action, and Clinical Efficacy in the Treatment of Atopic Dermatitis. *J Drugs Dermatol.* 2020;19(10):s4–s7.

206. Grais ML. Role of colloidal oatmeal in dermatologic treatment of the aged. *AMA Arch Derm Syphilol.* 1953;68(4):402–407.

207. US Food and Drug Administration. Title 21: Food and Drugs, Chapter 1: Food and Drug Administration Department of Health and Humans Services, Subchapter D: Drugs for human use, Part 347: Skin protectant drug products for over-the-counter human use. US Dept of Health and Human Services, FDA;21 CFR347. April 1, 2007.

208. Smith GC. The treatment of various dermatoses associated with dry skin. *J S C Med Assoc.* 1958;54(8):282–283.

209. Dick LA. Colloidal emollient baths in pediatric dermatoses. *Skin (Los Angeles).* 1962;1:89–91.

210. Allais B, Friedman A. ARTICLE: Colloidal Oatmeal Part II: Atopic Dermatitis in Special Populations and Clinical Efficacy and Tolerance Beyond Eczema. *J Drugs Dermatol.* 2020;19(10):s8–s11.

211. Vié K, Cours-Darne S, Vienne MP, Boyer F, Fabre B, Dupuy P. Modulating effects of oatmeal extracts in the sodium lauryl sulfate skin irritancy model. *Skin Pharmacol Appl Skin Physiol.* 2002;15(2):120–124.

212. Matheson JD, Clayton J, Muller MJ. The reduction of itch during burn wound healing. *J Burn Care Rehabil.* 2001;22(1):76–81.

213. Boisnic S, Branchet-Gumila MC, Coutanceau C. Inhibitory effect of oatmeal extract oligomer on vasoactive intestinal peptide-induced inflammation in surviving human skin. *Int J Tissue React.* 2003;25(2):41–46.

214. Ilnytska O, Kaur S, Chon S, et al. Colloidal Oatmeal (Avena Sativa) Improves Skin Barrier Through Multi-Therapy Activity. *J Drugs Dermatol.* 2016;15(6):684–690.

215. Reynertson KA, Garay M, Nebus J, et al. Anti-inflammatory activities of colloidal oatmeal (Avena sativa) contribute to the effectiveness of oats in treatment of itch associated with dry, irritated skin. *J Drugs Dermatol.* 2015;14(1):43–48.

216. Mehrpooya M. The Efficacy of Colloidal Oatmeal Cream 1% as Add-on Therapy in the Management of Chronic Irritant Hand Eczema: A Double-Blind Study. *Clin Cosmet Investig Dermatol.* 2020;13:241–251.

217. Lisante TA, Nunez C, Zhang P, Mathes BM. A 1% Colloidal Oatmeal Cream Alone is Effective in Reducing Symptoms of Mild to Moderate Atopic Dermatitis: Results from Two Clinical Studies. *J Drugs Dermatol.* 2017;16(7):671–676.

218. Perrelli A, Goitre L, Salzano AM, Moglia A, Scaloni A, Retta SF. Biological Activities, Health Benefits, and Therapeutic Properties of Avenanthramides: From Skin Protection to Prevention and Treatment of Cerebrovascular Diseases. *Oxid Med Cell Longev.* 2018;2018:6015351.

219. Chen CY, Milbury PE, Kwak HK, Collins FW, Samuel P, Blumberg JB. Avenanthramides and phenolic acids from oats are bioavailable and act synergistically with vitamin C to enhance hamster and human LDL resistance to oxidation. *J Nutr.* 2004;134(6):1459–1466.

220. Tsao R, Akhtar MH. Neutraceuticals and functional foods: I. Current trend in phytochemicals, antioxidant research. *J Food Agric Environ.* 2005;3(1):10–17.

221. Saeed SA, Butt NM, McDonald-Gibson WJ, Collier HO. Inhibitors of prostaglandin biosynthesis in extracts of oat (Avena sativa) seeds. *Biochem Soc Trans.* 1981;9(444):144.

222. Wallo W, Nebus J, Nystrand G. Agents with adjunctive therapeutic potential in atopic dermatitis. *J Am Acad Dermatol.* 2007;56(Suppl 2):AB70.tract P712.

223. Capone K, Kirchner F, Klein SL, Tierney NK. Effects of Colloidal Oatmeal Topical Atopic Dermatitis Cream on Skin Microbiome and Skin Barrier Properties. *J Drugs Dermatol.* 2020;19(5):524–531.

224. Arbiser JL, Bonner MY, Ward N, Elsey J, Rao S. Selenium unmasks protective iron armor: A possible defense against cutaneous inflammation and cancer. *Biochim Biophys Acta Gen Subj.* 2018:S0304-4165(18)30150-8.

225. Vitoux D, Chappuis P, Arnaud J, Bost M, Accominotti M, Roussel AM. Selenium, glutathione peroxidase, peroxides and platelet functions. *Ann Biol Clin (Paris)*. 1996;54(5):181–187.

226. Leverkus M, Yaar M, Eller MS, Tang EH, Gilchrest BA. Post-transcriptional regulation of UV induced TNF-alpha expression. *J Invest Dermatol*. 1998;110(4):353–357.

227. McKenzie RC. Selenium, ultraviolet radiation and the skin. *Clin Exp Dermatol*. 2000;25(8):631–636.

228. Cohen PR, Anderson CA. Topical Selenium Sulfide for the Treatment of Hyperkeratosis. *Dermatol Ther (Heidelb)*. 2018;8(4):639–646.

229. Stewart MS, Cameron GS, Pence BC. Antioxidant nutrients protect against UVB-induced oxidative damage to DNA of mouse keratinocytes in culture. *J Invest Dermatol*. 1996;106(5):1086–1089.

230. Rico MJ. Rising drug costs: the impact on dermatology. *Skin Therapy Lett*. 2000;5(4):1–2, 5.

231. Arora RB, Kapoor V, Basu N, Jain AP. Anti-inflammatory studies on Curcuma longa (turmeric). *Indian J Med Res*. 1971;59(8):1289–1295.

232. Srivastava R. Inhibition of neutrophil response by curcumin. *Agents Actions*. 1989;28(3-4):298–303.

233. Srimal RC, Dhawan BN. Pharmacology of diferuloyl methane (curcumin), a non-steroidal anti-inflammatory agent. *J Pharm Pharmacol*. 1973;25(6):447–452.

234. Vaughn AR, Branum A, Sivamani RK. Effects of Turmeric (Curcuma longa) on Skin Health: A Systematic Review of the Clinical Evidence. *Phytother Res*. 2016;30(8):1243–1264.

235. Kumar A, Agarwal K, Singh M, et al. Essential oil from waste leaves of Curcuma longa L. alleviates skin inflammation. *Inflammopharmacology*. 2018;26(5):1245–1255.

236. Bahraini P, Rajabi M, Mansouri P, Sarafian G, Chalangari R, Azizian Z. Turmeric tonic as a treatment in scalp psoriasis: A randomized placebo-control clinical trial. *J Cosmet Dermatol*. 2018;17(3):461–466.

237. Asada K, Ohara T, Muroyama K, Yamamoto Y, Murosaki S. Effects of hot water extract of Curcuma longa on human epidermal keratinocytes in vitro and skin conditions in healthy participants: A randomized, double-blind, placebo-controlled trial. *J Cosmet Dermatol*. 2019;18(6):1866–1874.

238. Salehi B, Stojanović-Radić Z, Matejić J, et al. The therapeutic potential of curcumin: A review of clinical trials. *Eur J Med Chem*. 2019;163:527–545.

239. Srivastava R, Srimal RC. Modification of certain inflammation-induced biochemical changes by curcumin. *Indian J Med Res*. 1985;81:215–223.

CHAPTER 39

Antioxidants

Leslie S. Baumann, MD
Edmund M. Weisberg, MS, MBE

SUMMARY POINTS

What's Important?
1. Antioxidants protect against the ravages of free radicals by reducing and neutralizing them.
2. Antioxidants may be particularly useful in UVA-induced skin alterations that are believed to be determined, in large part, by oxidative processes.
3. Topical antioxidants are currently marketed for the prevention of aging and UV-mediated skin damage as well as the treatment of wrinkles and erythema due to inflammation, such as that induced by laser resurfacing.
4. The free radical theory of aging explains why antioxidants are thought to prevent wrinkles, but this theory does not justify the use of antioxidants to treat wrinkles that are already present.

What's New?
1. New antioxidants are being introduced into the market frequently.
2. Using combinations of antioxidant types is preferred rather than one antioxidant.
3. Antioxidants should be included in diet, beverages, and supplements in addition to topical skincare products.

What's Coming?
1. New methods are needed to quantify antioxidant strength so that efficacy between types can be compared. Current antioxidant quantitative measurements such as the ORAC value pertain to foods, not topical products.
2. Antioxidants are being evaluated to protect mitochondria and other cellular components.

THE FREE RADICAL THEORY OF AGING

The free radical theory of aging, proposed by Harman in 1956,[1] is one of the most widely accepted theories to explain the causes of aging.[2] Free radicals, also known as reactive oxygen species (ROS), are compounds formed when oxygen molecules combine with other molecules yielding an odd number of electrons. An oxygen molecule with paired electrons is stable; however, oxygen with an unpaired electron is "reactive" because it seeks and seizes electrons from vital components leaving them damaged.[3] DNA, cytoskeletal elements, cellular proteins, and cellular membranes may all be adversely affected by activated oxygen species.[4] ROS have not only been implicated in the overall aging process,[5] but are believed to be involved cutaneously in causing photoaging, carcinogenesis, and inflammation. It is known that ultraviolet (UV)-induced damage to the skin is in part mediated by reactive oxygen intermediates.[6] If antioxidants can absorb some of the resulting free radicals, they may be able to mitigate UV-induced damage to the skin. Free radicals may also lead to inflammation, which is believed to play a role in skin aging.[6] Lipid peroxidation, another sequela of free radical production, causes harm to cell membranes and can lead to skin aging, atherosclerosis, and other signs of aging. Free radicals are also thought to contribute to the development of skin cancer. There are multiple studies in the literature describing the role of free radicals and skin cancer. The exact mechanisms for all of the detrimental effects of free radicals have not been completely elucidated, however.

Free radicals also play an important role in intrinsic and extrinsic skin aging. They are formed naturally through normal human metabolism but can be produced via exogenous factors, such as UV exposure, air pollution, smoking, radiation, alcohol use, exercise, inflammation, and exposure to certain drugs or heavy metals such as iron. In fact, UV radiation, stress, cigarette smoke, pollution, drugs, and diet can be sources of ROS such as superoxide, hydroxyl anion, hydrogen peroxide (H_2O_2), and singlet oxygen. Free radicals can also induce various transcription factors, such as activator protein (AP)-1 and nuclear factor (NF)-κB.[7] Further, ROS increase the expression of matrix metalloproteinases (MMPs), specifically collagenase, which can degrade skin collagen.[8,9] Collagenase formation occurs due to the activation of transcription factors c-Jun and c-Fos, which combine to produce the AP-1 that, in turn, prompts the activity of the MMPs.[10] Additionally, the mitogen-activated protein kinase (MAPK) pathway is also a target of oxidative stress.[11]

ANTIOXIDANT THEORY

The human body has developed defense mechanisms, known as antioxidants, which protect against the ravages of free radicals by reducing and neutralizing them. Antioxidative enzymes that naturally occur in the skin include superoxide dismutase, catalase, and glutathione peroxidase (GPX); the nonenzymatic endogenous antioxidative molecules are α-tocopherol (vitamin E), ascorbic acid (vitamin C), glutathione, and ubiquinone.[12] As part of the natural aging process, our defense mechanisms diminish, while the production of ROS increases. This leads to an imbalance and an elevated number of unchecked free radicals that damage DNA, cytoskeletal elements, cellular proteins, and cellular membranes. Moreover, many of the body's antioxidant defense mechanisms are inhibited by UV and visible light.[13,14] Additionally, UV light exposure is known to cause an increase in free radical formation.[15] Researchers are currently studying the potential of using exogenous antioxidants to affect this process and mitigate the damage caused by free radicals. Many believe that topical application and oral consumption of combinations of antioxidants may result in a sustained antioxidant capacity of the skin due to synergistic actions of the combined antioxidants. Antioxidants may be particularly useful in UVA-induced skin alterations that are believed to be determined, in large part, by oxidative processes. In fact, topical application of antioxidants has been shown to raise the minimal UVA dose necessary to induce immediate pigment darkening and diminish the severity of UVA-induced photodermatoses.[15] Although antioxidants appear in vegetables and other foods in addition to the human body, many in research and development believe that higher levels can be achieved by supplementation. Consequently, the use of products touting antioxidants as protective ingredients in oral supplements and topically applied agents has become extremely popular.

Topical antioxidants are currently marketed for the prevention of aging and UV-mediated skin damage as well as the treatment of wrinkles and erythema due to inflammation, such as that induced by laser resurfacing. The free radical theory of aging explains why antioxidants are thought to prevent wrinkles, but this theory does not justify the use of antioxidants to treat wrinkles that are already present. Many companies claim that their antioxidant-containing products "treat" wrinkles; however, this is often an exaggeration. *At this time, vitamin C is the ONLY antioxidant that can treat wrinkles, but this capacity is due to its effects in promoting collagen formation, which is unrelated to its antioxidant effects.* When products such as the combination formulation studied by Cho et al. are associated with amelioration of wrinkles, such a result can be ascribed either to a swelling or hydrating effect of the product, or the vitamin C or retinol contained in the product.[16] It is important to stress to patients that antioxidants *prevent* wrinkles but do not *treat* wrinkles (with the exception of vitamin C).

In addition to their namesake antioxidant effects, all antioxidants exhibit anti-inflammatory properties, which are described in detail in Chapter 38, Anti-Inflammatory Agents. Some of the antioxidants depicted below also possess depigmenting activities, which are described in more detail in Chapter 41, Depigmenting Ingredients.

Although the theory of antioxidants is a sound one, there are several important factors to consider when evaluating the efficacy of antioxidants. In order to be considered biologically active, orally administered products must be absorbed and shown to raise antioxidant levels in the skin. Topically administered products must be absorbed into the skin and delivered to the target tissue in the active form and remain there long enough to confer the desired effects. Some antioxidants are very unstable; therefore, some ingredients such as vitamin C become oxidized and rendered inactive before reaching the target. Stabilizing ingredients in formulation and packaging them to minimize air and light exposure are challenging tasks. Absorption is also important and depends on several factors such as the molecular form of the compound, its pH, whether it is water soluble or fat soluble, and the vehicle that contains the product. This chapter will include a discussion of the most popular types of antioxidants found in cosmetic products or taken orally by cosmetic patients.

ANTIOXIDANT SYNERGY

Although there are hundreds of naturally occurring antioxidants, most of those currently used in the cosmetic industry are believed to work synergistically to regenerate and "enhance the power" of each other. The antioxidants that have been identified as working cooperatively have been referred to as network antioxidants.[17] For example, after an antioxidant "disarms" a free radical by eliminating the odd number of electrons (by either adding or removing an electron) it is unable to function further as an antioxidant unless it is recycled. The five antioxidants that have been labeled as network antioxidants are vitamins C and E, glutathione, lipoic acid, and coenzyme Q_{10} (CoQ$_{10}$). Vitamin C or CoQ$_{10}$ can recycle vitamin E, donating electrons to vitamin E to return the nutrient to its antioxidant state. Vitamin C and glutathione can be recycled by lipoic acid or vitamin C. These network antioxidants are being included in an increasing number of cosmetic preparations. It is likely that many antioxidants work synergistically, and that the term "network antioxidant" applies to many more antioxidants than the five identified as the "network."

FAT-SOLUBLE ANTIOXIDANTS

These are found in the lipophilic portion of the cell membrane and include vitamin E, carotenoids, and CoQ_{10}. Further, idebenone, the synthetic analog of CoQ_{10}, and food-derived lycopene are also fat-soluble antioxidants.

Vitamin E

Found in vegetables, oils, seeds, nuts, corn, soy, whole wheat flour, margarine, and in some meat and dairy products, vitamin E, or tocopherol, is actually a universal term for a group of compounds comprised of tocol and tocotrienol derivatives, specifically four pairs of racemic stereoisomers (**Fig. 39-1**). Of the four tocopherols (α-, β-, γ- and δ-), α-tocopherol (also known as AT) has the highest activity. Since the discovery that vitamin E is the primary lipid-soluble antioxidant in skin that protects cells from oxidative stress,[18] practitioners have used it to treat a wide variety of skin lesions. The general public has frequently looked to it for treatment of minor burns, surgical scars, and other wounds, even though its use for dermatoses has not been approved by the FDA. In addition, vitamin E is touted as beneficial in protecting against cardiovascular disease because lipid peroxidation is a major contributor to atherosclerosis and cardiovascular disease. Administration of vitamin E is thought to decrease the extent of lipid peroxidation and protect against cardiovascular disease.[19] In the same way that vitamin E protects the cells from lipid peroxidation in the arteries, it protects the cell membranes in the skin from peroxidation.

Authors have identified a correlation between dietary deficiency of vitamin E and an increase in oxidative stress and cell injury.[18] In 1993, Tanaka et al. reported that ROS induce changes in the biosynthesis of collagen and glycosaminoglycans (GAGs) in cultured human dermal fibroblasts.[20] This alteration was prevented with the addition of α-tocopherol to the fibroblasts. In addition, vitamin E has been shown to lower prostaglandin E_2 production,[21] and augment interleukin (IL)-2 production, leading to anti-inflammatory and immunostimulatory activity. It is believed that this stabilization effect may play a role in collagen biosynthesis.[22] Thus far, *in vivo* attempts to measure and link changes in collagen production with altered concentrations of vitamin E have proved inconclusive.

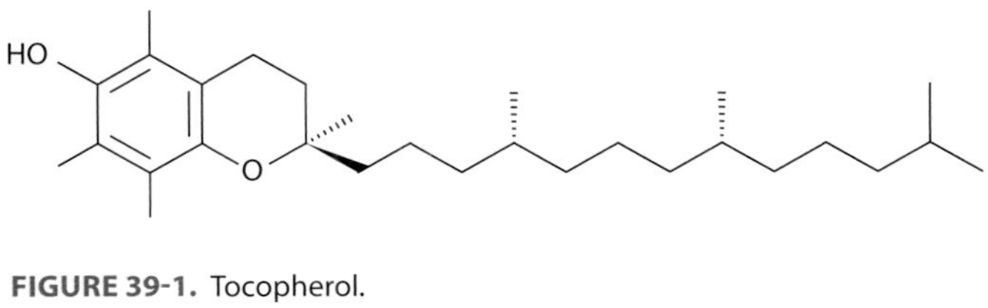

FIGURE 39-1. Tocopherol.

Depletion of cutaneous vitamin E is considered an early indication of extrinsically caused oxidative damage.[23,24] Studies on elderly subjects that exhibit high plasma tocopherol levels have revealed a lower incidence of infectious disease and cancer than in the age-matched population.[25–27] For this reason, vitamin E is considered by many to be a necessary and powerful antioxidant. In addition, vitamin E seems to offer photoprotection when taken orally and applied topically. Numerous reports indicate that the topical application of α-tocopherol to animal skin is effective in lowering the production of sunburn cells,[28,29] reducing the damage caused by chronic UVB exposure,[30,31] and inhibiting photocarcinogenesis.[32] Specifically, researchers have found that oral and topical vitamin E supplementation in certain animals diminishes the effects of photoaging, inhibits the development of skin cancer, and counteracts immunosuppression induced by UV radiation.[32–35] In 1992, Trevithick et al. noted that topical d-α-tocopherol acetate diminished erythema due to sunburn, edema, and skin sensitivity in mice when application occurred following exposure to UVB radiation.[36] In a study in which tocopherol 5% was applied to mice prior to UVB exposure, Bissett et al. observed a 75 percent decrease in skin wrinkling, a rise in tumor latency, and a reduction of cutaneous tumors; however, vitamin E failed to affect UVA-induced skin sagging.[37] In a different study in which subjects applied tocopherol 5% to 8% cream facially for 4 weeks, Mayer observed diminished skin roughness, shorter length of facial lines, and reduced wrinkle depth as compared to placebo.[38]

Oral administration and topical application of vitamin E have been demonstrated to inhibit UV-induced erythema and edema in animals.[39] In humans it has been shown that UV-induced expression of human macrophage metalloelastase, a member of the MMP family involved in degradation of elastin, could be inhibited by pre-treatment with vitamin E (5%). In this study, vitamin E was applied to the skin under light-tight occlusion 24 hours before UV treatment.[40]

A double-blind, placebo-controlled study examined the protective effects of orally administered vitamin E [400 international units (IU) per day] against UV-induced epidermal damage in humans. The subjects were followed for a 6-month period. Minimal erythema dose (MED) and histologic response were determined at baseline, 1 month, and 6 months. In this study, there was no significant difference between the placebo group and those treated with vitamin E and the investigators concluded that daily ingestion of 400 IU of oral α-tocopherol daily did not provide any meaningful photoprotection.[41] Other authors have suggested that if vitamin E provides any photoprotection at all, it may require interaction with other antioxidants, such as vitamin C, to do so.[42] This notion was supported by the study of Lin et al. who showed in Yorkshire pigs that the combined application of 1% α-tocopherol with 15% L-ascorbic acid provided superior protection against erythema and sunburn cell formation compared to either 1% α-tocopherol or 15% L-ascorbic acid alone.[43]

In 2008, a small study of nine patients conducted by Murray et al. demonstrated that a stable topical preparation of 15% L-ascorbic acid, 1% α-tocopherol, and 0.5% ferulic acid protected human skin *in vivo* from UV-induced damage, particularly erythema and apoptosis. The formulation also inhibited p53 activation and stymied thymine dimer mutations, which are linked to skin cancer.[44] The topical application of vitamin E is considered an effective approach for imparting skin protection and to treat atopic dermatitis.[24,45]

Wound Healing

Oxygen radicals form in response to injury and further inhibit recovery by attacking DNA, cellular membranes, proteins, and lipids. It is believed that antioxidants act to ameliorate wounds by reducing the damage induced by free oxygen radicals, which are released by neutrophils in the inflammatory phase of the healing process.[46] In the late 1960s, Kamimura et al. performed quantitative research demonstrating that topically applied vitamin E penetrates into the deep dermis and subcutaneous tissue.[47] Numerous scientists, as well as many laypersons, have interpreted this to mean that topically applied vitamin E may improve wound healing. Contradictory results have emerged from animal studies undertaken to evaluate the effects of vitamin E on wound healing, however. This may be explained by the fact that unlike other vitamins, tocopherols exhibit species-specific mechanisms of action.[48]

In a prospective, double-blind, randomized study on humans, Jenkins et al. tried to diminish scarring in burn patients following reconstructive surgery by applying topical vitamin E. The researchers observed no difference between the control and treatment groups, however, and nearly 20 percent of the patients reported local reactions to the vitamin E cream.[49] In another study,[50] the primary author and a collaborator assessed the cosmetic benefit resulting from the use of topically applied vitamin E to surgical scars. In a double-blind fashion, patients applied 320 IU of d-α tocopheryl/g of Aquaphor to one side of the scar and Aquaphor alone to the other side of the scar. The patients were followed for 6 months. At the conclusion of the study, the vitamin E preparation failed to improve the cosmetic appearance of surgical scars, and even exacerbated the scars in a few subjects.

Forms of Vitamin E

Vitamin E is a family of compounds called tocopherols, including, as mentioned above, α-, β-, γ-, and δ-tocopherol. Alpha-tocopherol is the most active form and the one on which the recommended daily allowance (RDA) is based. The names of all types of vitamin E begin with either "d" or "dl" designations that refer to differences in chemical structure. The "d" form is the natural form and "dl" is the synthetic form. The natural form is more active and better absorbed. Synthetic vitamin E supplements contain only α-tocopherol, while food sources contain several different tocopherols, including α -, δ -, and γ -tocopherol.

Vitamin E forms are listed as either "tocopherol" or the esterified "tocopheryl" followed by the name of the substance to which it is attached, as in "tocopheryl acetate." The two forms are very similar but tocopherol displays better absorption, while tocopheryl forms exhibit slightly better shelf life. In health food stores, the most common oral forms of vitamin E are d-α-tocopherol, d-α-tocopheryl acetate, and α-tocopheryl succinate. The vitamin E forms typically used in cosmetics are α-tocopheryl acetate and α-tocopheryl linoleate. These compounds are less likely to elicit contact dermatitis than d-α-tocopheryl and are more stable at room temperature. However, the tocopherol esters are also more poorly absorbed by the skin than the tocopherol forms,[51] and may not exert the same photoprotective effects. One study demonstrated that α-tocopheryl acetate or α-tocopheryl succinate not only failed to prevent photocarcinogenesis, but also may have enhanced it.[52] Because the α-tocopherol esters are included in many skin lotions, cosmetics, and sunscreens, further studies are needed to determine if the tocopherol esters indeed promote or contribute to photocarcinogenesis.

Side Effects

The primary author's study[50] as well as the one by Jenkins[49] suggest that the incidence of contact dermatitis due to topical vitamin E application may be relatively high for certain forms of tocopherol.[49] Tocopherol acetate seems to be the worst culprit,[53] but allergy to dl-α-tocopheryl nicotinate has also been reported.[54] In 1992, Swiss researchers evaluated 1,000 cases of an atypical papular and follicular contact dermatitis provoked by vitamin E linoleate that was an additive to cosmetics. The conclusion was that oxidized vitamin E derivatives can operate synergistically *in vivo* as haptens or as irritants.[55] The topical application of vitamin E has also been linked with contact urticaria, eczematous dermatitis, and erythema multiforme-like reactions.[56]

The recommended dose of oral vitamin E is 22 IU per day; however, many physicians recommend 400 IU twice per day. In 1988, a thorough literature review by Bendich and Machlin found extended use of oral vitamin E up to 3,000 mg/d to be safe.[57] A subsequent study by Kappus and Diplock established as absolutely safe vitamin E doses up to 400 mg/d, doses between 400 mg and 2,000 mg as unlikely to cause adverse reactions, and doses greater than 3,000 mg/d over an extended period as a potential source of side effects.[58] Because vitamin E can contribute to a blood-thinning effect, patients on anticoagulant therapy are advised to avoid high doses of vitamin E ($> 4,000$ IU).[59] Although there is likely no clinically significant reduction in platelet aggregation in those with normal platelets, patients are frequently advised to suspend vitamin E supplementation prior to surgery. This is essential for patients with abnormal platelets, vitamin K deficiency, or those taking anti-platelet agents.[60]

Summary

Vitamin E has been used to treat or protect against various dermatologic conditions including atopic dermatitis, discoid lupus erythematosus, dystrophic epidermolysis bullosa, granuloma annulare, lichen sclerosus et atrophicus, pemphigus, skin cancer, and yellow nail syndrome, among others.[39] Results have varied just as widely as the range of diseases treated. In fact, some authors have reported that the use of oral vitamin E will reduce the side effects of retinoids;[61] however, other studies have not shown this benefit.[62]

The most promising reason for research into the dermatologic use of vitamin E appears to be its antioxidant activity. The potency of vitamin E as an antioxidant can be increased through combination with other antioxidants. Vitamin E also appears to offer a ripe area for research into its potential for therapeutic benefit in the prevention and treatment of skin cancer and photoaging. In addition, vitamin E displays emollient properties and is stable, easy to formulate, and relatively inexpensive, rendering it a popular additive to anti-aging preparations. More research, in the form of controlled trials, is necessary to ascertain the role of vitamin E in treating various dermatoses.

Coenzyme Q_{10} (Ubiquinone)

Coenzyme Q_{10} (CoQ_{10}) is a naturally occurring nutrient available through food consumption. Fish and shellfish are good dietary sources of CoQ_{10}. The current recommended oral dose is 90–150 mg daily; however, many doctors are recommending 200–400 mg per day. CoQ_{10} is a fat-soluble compound found in all cells as part of the electron transfer chain responsible for energy production. It is estimated that CoQ_{10} provides 95% of the body's energy (adenosine triphosphate [ATP]) requirements.[63] CoQ_{10} has also been found to have antioxidant properties. The "Q" alludes to its membership in the quinone family; the "10" identifies the number of isoprenoid units on its side chain (**Fig. 39-2**). The biosynthesis of CoQ_{10} is a complex process that depends on a copious supply of essential amino acids, such as tyrosine, and several vitamins and trace elements. There are myriad studies on the use of CoQ_{10} in the cardiology literature.[64]

Researchers have identified an age-related decline of CoQ_{10} levels in animals and humans.[65] For this reason, many believe that the antioxidant activities of CoQ_{10} may make it useful as a treatment for aged skin. A study by Hoppe et al. demonstrated that CoQ_{10} penetrated into the viable layers of the skin and significantly suppressed the expression of collagenase in human dermal fibroblasts following UVA irradiation.[66] It was further shown that prolonged supplementation of CoQ_{10} in humans reduced wrinkle formation in the corner of the eye. In another study, the same group orally supplemented CoQ_{10} (0, 1, 100 mg/kg p.o.) daily for 2 weeks and noted that levels of CoQ_{10} significantly increased in the epidermis, but not in the dermis. They hypothesized that this might be a prerequisite to the reduction of wrinkles and other benefits related to the potent antioxidant and energizing effects of CoQ_{10} in skin.[67]

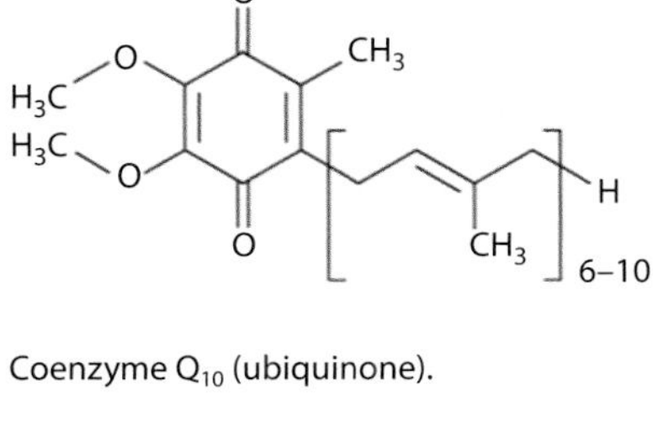

FIGURE 39-2. Coenzyme Q_{10} (ubiquinone).

Patients taking 3-hydroxy-3-methylglutaryl-coenzyme A (HMG-CoA) reductase inhibitors (statins) to lower their low-density lipoprotein cholesterol have been shown to have decreased mitochondrial CoQ_{10} levels. This is because statin drugs inhibit the conversion of HMG-CoA to mevalonate, a precursor for cholesterol and CoQ_{10}. In cell culture, decreased mitochondrial CoQ_{10} levels have been associated with a higher degree of cell death, increased DNA oxidative damage, and a reduction in ATP synthesis. Oral supplementation of CoQ_{10} has been demonstrated to reduce cell death and DNA oxidative stress, and increase ATP synthesis.[68] For this reason, many doctors recommend that patients taking statins should supplement CoQ_{10} orally. The most commonly prescribed dose is 200–400 mg/d, in the morning. CoQ_{10} exhibits caffeine-like effects and can lead to insomnia if taken at night.

Coenzyme Q_{10} Levels and Skin Cancer

Abnormally low plasma levels of CoQ_{10} have been found in patients with cancer of the breast, lung, and pancreas.[69] A 2006 study investigated the usefulness of CoQ_{10} plasma levels in predicting the risk of metastasis and the duration of the metastasis-free interval in melanoma patients. Rusciani et al. showed that CoQ_{10} levels were significantly lower in melanoma patients than in control subjects and in patients who developed metastases than in the metastasis-free subgroup. They suggested that baseline plasma CoQ_{10} levels could serve as a prognostic factor to estimate the risk for melanoma progression.[70]

In the adjuvant therapy of melanoma with interferon (IFN) it seems that large amounts of ATP are required for an immune response initiated by IFN to be effective. It has thus been hypothesized that the failure of some patients to respond to IFN therapy may be due to an inability to meet the excess demand for ATP induced by this medication. However, it is known that CoQ_{10} plays a key role in the mitochondrial respiratory cycle and production of ATP.[71,72] Therefore, Rusciani et al. conducted a clinical trial in stage I and II melanoma patients examining a post-surgical adjuvant therapy with recombinant IFN α-2b in combination with CoQ_{10} vs. IFN α-2b alone for the control group. In a 3-year trial they uninterruptedly treated the patients with low-dose recombinant IFN α-2b administered twice daily and CoQ_{10} (400 mg/day). The control group was treated with only low-dose recombinant IFN α-2b in the same dosage and administration. Treatment efficacy was evaluated as incidence of recurrences at 5 years. The group demonstrated that the risk of developing metastases was about 10 times lower in the IFN + CoQ_{10} patients compared with the IFN-alone group.[73] However, a 10-year follow-up will be needed to provide more significant results.

Anti-Aging Activity

In 2006, Fuller et al. found that CoQ_{10} can suppress the inflammatory response in dermal fibroblasts induced by UVR or IL-1. They also observed that CoQ_{10} hindered UVR-induced MMP-1 synthesis. In combination with the colorless carotenoids phytoene and phytofluene, CoQ_{10} enhanced inflammation inhibition. The investigators concluded that combining

CoQ_{10} and carotenoids in topical skincare formulations may render dual protection against photoaging and inflammation.[74]

In an *in vitro* study in 2012, Zhang et al. considered the effects of CoQ_{10} on primary human dermal fibroblasts. They demonstrated that CoQ_{10} spurred fibroblast proliferation, augmenting type IV collagen expression, and diminished the levels of MMPs induced by UV radiation. CoQ_{10} also dose-dependently fostered elastin gene expression in cultured fibroblasts and markedly decreased IL-1α production in keratinocytes induced by UVR. Further, they found that the antioxidant inhibited tyrosinase activity similarly to ascorbic acid, suggesting the potential for conferring depigmenting effects. They concluded that CoQ_{10} acted against intrinsic aging as well as photoaging.[75]

Thirteen years earlier, Blatt et al. showed through *in vivo* studies that the long-term application of CoQ_{10} could reduce crow's feet.[76] Subsequent *in vivo* studies have revealed reductions in the symptoms of photoaging through the use of topically applied CoQ_{10}, even though bioavailability of CoQ_{10} has remained poor.[77]

In 2012, Felippi et al. performed a pilot study on the safety and efficacy of a nanoparticle formulation encapsulating various active ingredients, including CoQ_{10}, retinyl palmitate, tocopheryl acetate, grape seed oil, and linseed oil. The nanoparticles displayed no irritating, sensitizing, or comedogenic characteristics and phototoxicity was not evident after exposure to UVA light. In the efficacy assessment with volunteers, significant reductions in wrinkles were noted as compared to controls after 21 days of treatment. The investigators concluded that the antioxidants-loaded nanoparticle formulation was safe for topical administration and merited consideration as a cosmetic anti-aging agent.[78]

In 2015, Knott et al. conducted a controlled, randomized study with 73 healthy, non-smoking, female volunteers between 20 and 66 years old and found that topical treatment with CoQ_{10} increased cutaneous levels of the nutrient and delivered antioxidant activity. They added that stressed skin was particularly improved with topical CoQ_{10} treatment.[79]

CoQ_{10} is stable in topical products. Penetration depends on the characteristics of the topical formulation due to the high molecular weight of this compound. Formulation with this ingredient may lead to a yellow tint in the product.

Side Effects

Oral CoQ_{10} supplementation has been associated with a caffeine-like side effect and may cause nervousness or a jittery feeling. So as not to induce insomnia, it is recommended that CoQ_{10} not be taken at night. Diarrhea, appetite loss, and mild nausea are among the other side effects reported.[80] No side effects have been reported with topical application. CoQ_{10} has not been reported to cause contact dermatitis.

Idebenone

Idebenone is the synthetic analog of CoQ_{10}, penetrating the skin more efficiently due to its lower molecular weight. Idebenone has been shown to possess superior antioxidant capacity compared to CoQ_{10}, tocopherol, kinetin, ascorbic acid, and lipoic acid in various *in vitro* and *in vivo* trials.[81]

Topical Application

McDaniel et al. examined the *in vivo* efficacy of idebenone in a topical skincare formulation for the treatment of photodamaged skin. In a randomized, blind-labeled, nonvehicle control study, 41 female subjects used either 0.5% or 1.0% idebenone formulations twice daily for 6 weeks.[82] Both user groups showed improvement of all examined parameters. A 26% reduction in skin roughness/dryness was measured in the 1.0% user group as was a 29% reduction in fine lines/wrinkles; this group also experienced a 33% improvement in overall global assessment of photodamaged skin. For users of the 0.5% idebenone formulation, reductions in skin roughness/dryness as well as fine lines/wrinkles were 23% and 27%, respectively, and improvement in overall global assessment of photodamaged skin was 30%. It is important to remember that the effects seen on wrinkles in these trials were likely due to hydration or skin irritation because antioxidants have exhibited no efficacy in treating wrinkles (with the exception of vitamin C) but can help prevent them. Skincare products containing idebenone are commercially available as Prevage MD® by Allergan (1% idebenone), and Prevage® and Prevage Eye Anti-Aging Moisturizing Treatment® by Elizabeth Arden and Allergan (0.5% idebenone).

It is important to note the poor water solubility and high lipophilicity of idebenone render it difficult to formulate for sufficient bioavailability. Various delivery systems (e.g., lipid-based nanoparticles, polymeric nanoparticles, liposomes, cyclodextrins, microemulsions, and others) have been investigated to ascertain how best to provide the benefits of this potent antioxidant.[83] The idebenone found in current topical products is unlikely to yield much added benefit.

Side Effects

A 2007 case report of contact dermatitis due to a facial treatment with an "anti-aging" cream in a beauty salon identified the allergen as idebenone 0.5% by patch testing.[84] As idebenone has become more popular, contact allergy to this compound has become more common.[84]

Lycopene

Lycopene is a natural pigment synthesized by plants and microorganisms. It is an open-chain unsaturated carotenoid found in red fruits and vegetables such as tomatoes, pink grapefruit, watermelon, and apricots. In fact, it is lycopene that is responsible for the red pigment we observe in those fruits and vegetables.[85,86] The dietary intake of tomatoes and tomato products containing lycopene is associated with decreased risk of chronic disorders such as cancer and cardiovascular diseases.[87–89]

Lycopene has been found to exhibit potent antioxidant properties. Due to its high number of conjugated double bonds, it demonstrates stronger singlet oxygen-quenching ability compared to α-tocopherol or β-carotene.[87] Clinical trials with tomato products suggest a synergistic action of lycopene with other nutrients in lowering biomarkers of oxidative stress and carcinogenesis.[90]

Further, lycopene has been shown to prevent carcinogenesis in various tumor models.[91–94] Reported mechanisms of action are arrest of tumor cell-cycle progression, insulin-like growth factor (IGF)-1 signaling transduction, and induction of apoptosis. A recent study suggested that part of the anti-tumor activity of lycopene might be due to the trapping activity of lycopene on platelet-derived growth factor (PDGF), suggesting that this antioxidant acts as an inhibitor on tumor stromal cells.[95] The chemopreventive effects of lycopene against photo-induced tumors have been demonstrated in mouse models.[96,97] Lycopene appears to have the potential to prevent skin cancer and warrants further investigation for such an indication.

Although the clinical data in humans are very limited, lycopene is included in various skincare products, including facial moisturizers, sunscreens, eye creams, and formulations touted for their "anti-aging" skincare. In a small study on 10 healthy volunteers, males and females aged 20 to 42 years (Fitzpatrick phototypes II and III), Andreassi et al. determined that a lycopene formulation exerted greater photoprotective effects against solar-simulated UV damage than did a product containing a mixture of vitamins C and E.[98] Further data in humans are needed to shed more light on the effects of lycopene on human skin.

Curcumin

Curcumin is a yellow pigment found in the root of the tropical turmeric plant *Curcuma longa,* which belongs to the Zingiberaceae family. Turmeric consists of a water-soluble component, turmerin, and a lipid-soluble component, curcumin.[99] Curcumin has been used for centuries in traditional medicine to treat inflammatory conditions and other diseases; in Indian cuisine it is used as a spice. Turmeric tubers contain curcuminoids, of which curcumin I (diferuloyl methane) is most abundant, followed by curcumin II (6%) and III (0.3%).[100] (**Fig. 39-3.**) Curcumin has been shown to exhibit a broad array of biologic activities, such as anti-inflammatory, anticarcinogenic, antioxidant, antimicrobial, and wound healing.[101–103] The molecular bases of these effects are mediated through the regulation of various transcription factors, growth factors, inflammatory cytokines, protein kinases, adhesion molecules, apoptotic genes, angiogenesis regulators, and other enzymes.[104,105]

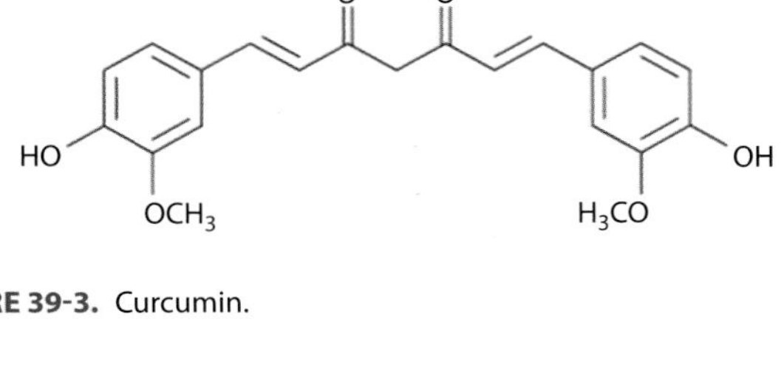

FIGURE 39-3. Curcumin.

Antioxidant and Anti-inflammatory Activities of Curcumin

Curcumin has been identified as a potent scavenger of various ROS, including superoxide anion radicals, hydroxyl radicals, and nitrogen dioxide radicals.[106] Also, curcumin has been shown to down-regulate the production of the pro-inflammatory cytokines IL-1 and tumor necrosis factor (TNF)-α, and to inhibit the activation of transcription factors NF-κB and AP-1, both regulating the genes for pro-inflammatory mediators and protective antioxidant genes.[107]

The antioxidant and anti-inflammatory properties of curcumin have been documented in mouse models, establishing that curcumin renders a beneficial effect against chemo- and photocarcinogenesis. Further studies are needed in order to determine whether topical applications or oral intake of curcumin can inhibit skin carcinogenesis in humans.[108–110] Oral intake of curcumin in humans has been shown to be nontoxic at doses up to 8 g/day when taken by mouth for 3 months.[111] These are promising developments; further studies are needed to elucidate the role of this antioxidant compound as a photo-chemopreventive agent.

A limited number of cosmetic products contain curcumin because its pungent aroma and distinct color render it especially challenging to formulate into a cosmetically elegant product. More clinical trials are required to assess the effects of topical curcumin on human skin. Bioavailability in topical products has also been problematic. A 2010 study of the inhibitory activity of encapsulated curcumin on UV-induced photoaging in mice represented the first clinical support for the topical delivery of curcumin to minimize the effects of photoaging.[112]

Three years later, Heng showed that the topical application of curcumin gel in the clinical setting yielded rapid healing of burns and nominal or no scarring, as well as ameliorated various signs of photodamage, including hyperpigmentation, solar elastosis, advanced solar lentigines, actinic poikiloderma, and actinic keratoses.[113] Curcumin is also believed to have potential in treating eczema and scleroderma.[114]

In 2014, Thongrakard et al. examined the protective effects on human keratinocytes of extracts of 15 Thai herb species against UVB-induced DNA damage and cytotoxicity. Their analysis revealed that the highest antioxidant activity was exhibited by the dichloromethane extract of turmeric. Further, the ethanol extract of turmeric and the dichloromethane extract of ginger demonstrated the maximum UV absorptions and stimulated the production of the antioxidant protein thioredoxin 1, and the capacity to protect human keratinocytes from the deleterious effects of UV exposure. They concluded that their findings suggest the viability of incorporating turmeric and ginger extracts into anti-UV cosmetic formulations.[115]

Wound Healing Effects of Curcumin

Sidhu et al. demonstrated that wound closure in curcumin-treated normal and genetically diabetic animals was significantly faster compared to controls. This enhanced healing effect was attributed to the improvement of neovascularization and re-epithelialization, the increase of expression and production of transforming growth factor (TGF)-β1 and fibronectin, and the reduction of cell death by curcumin.[116,117] Curcumin treatment has also improved collagen deposition and increased fibroblast and vascular density, enhancing both normal and impaired wound healing. The observed proangiogenic effect of curcumin in wound healing is believed to be based on inducing TGF-β1, which in turn induces angiogenesis and the accumulation of extracellular matrix.[118]

Curcumin and Skin Cancer

Curcumin has been demonstrated to inhibit carcinogenesis in several tumor model systems including skin neoplastic models.[108,109,119–121] Its mechanism of action is not precisely known, but it is thought to inhibit initiation, promotion, and progression of cancer.[122] Curcumin has been reported to inhibit UVA-induced metallothionein (MT) expression and ornithine decarboxylase (ODC) activity, and to induce p53-mediated apoptosis, as well as cell membrane-mediated apoptosis through Fas receptor induction and caspase-8 activation.[109,123,124]

Paradoxically, some studies have suggested that the anticancer activity of the antioxidant curcumin has actually promoted the generation of ROS.[125] In response, Chen et al. investigated the antioxidant and anticancer activity of curcumin in human myeloid leukemia (HL-60) cells. They determined that the anticancer activity of curcumin was effective in a concentration- and time-dependent manner in reducing the proliferation and viability of leukemia cells, but its effect on ROS was concentration dependent. That is, low concentrations of curcumin decreased ROS generation, but high concentrations had the opposite effect. In additional studies, Chen et al. found that the combination of water-soluble antioxidants amplified the antioxidant and anticancer activity of low curcumin concentrations.[125]

In 2013, Hwang et al. found in an *in vitro* investigation using human dermal fibroblasts that curcumin suppressed the UVB-induced expression of MMP-1 and MMP-3 as well as ROS generation, the activation of NF-κB and AP-1, and the phosphorylation of p38 and c-Jun N-terminal kinase. They concluded that the potent inhibitory anti-inflammatory activity of curcumin offers potential in the prevention and treat of photoaging.[126]

A 2016 systematic review by Vaughn et al. of the clinical evidence in PubMed and Embase databases identified 234 articles, with 18 studies meeting inclusion criteria, eight studies assessing the topical effects, as well as one article evaluating the oral and topical effects of turmeric/curcumin. Statistically significant improvement in skin disease (including acne, alopecia, atopic dermatitis, facial photoaging, oral lichen planus, pruritus, psoriasis, radiodermatitis, and vitiligo) severity was reported in 10 studies in treatment groups compared with controls.[127] Despite the limited, though affirmative, findings, Vollono et al. suggested that combining curcumin with other drugs in novel delivery systems looms as a likely target for harnessing this potent antioxidant.[128] Currently, there are only a few cosmetic products

containing curcumin because its distinct and pungent aroma and color make it difficult to formulate into a cosmetically elegant product. More clinical trials are needed to evaluate the effects of curcumin on human skin.

WATER-SOLUBLE ANTIOXIDANTS

These are found in hydrophobic areas of the cell and the serum and include glutathione and vitamin C.

Glutathione

Glutathione is the most abundant antioxidant in the "network." It is produced from the amino acids glutamic acid, cysteine, and glycine. Oral glutathione is not well absorbed into the body, so it is often used in IV form. Glutathione does not penetrate into skin; therefore, it would need to be formulated in a nanoparticle vehicle. At the time of publication, there were no glutathione-containing topical skincare products. Glutathione causes melanin production to convert from pheomelanin to the lighter eumelanin. For this reason, it would be a good ingredient to lighten skin if a topical formulation that could penetrate into skin is developed.

Vitamin C

Vitamin C is historically known for its role in the prevention of scurvy. By the 18th century, sailors knew that eating citrus fruits prevented this condition associated with dental abnormalities, bleeding disorders, characteristic purpuric skin lesions, and mental deterioration. In the 1930s, researchers confirmed that vitamin C is the key ingredient in citrus fruit that prevents scurvy.[129] In contrast to some animals, humans obtain vitamin C solely from food, such as citrus fruits, black currants, red peppers, and leafy green vegetables. Oral supplementation of vitamin C does unfortunately not increase the levels of vitamin C in the skin, as the transport from the gastrointestinal tract is limited. Moreover, sunlight and environmental pollution, such as ozone in city pollution, can deplete epidermal vitamin C.[130,131] Thus, enhancing the levels of vitamin C in the skin is an important goal, as vitamin C is known to be a potent antioxidant.

Today, vitamin C, also known as ascorbic acid, is being studied extensively for its impact as an antioxidant. Oral vitamin C has been associated with decreasing the risk of certain cancers, cardiovascular disease, and cataracts, as well as improving wound healing and immune modulation.[132,133] Topical vitamin C has been used to prevent sun damage, and for the treatment of melasma, striae albae, and post-operative erythema in laser patients.[28,134–136] Ascorbic acid is unique among antioxidants because of its ability to increase collagen production in addition to its free radical scavenging activity. It is also one of the most recognized antioxidants by consumers. Due to its capacity to interfere with the UV-induced generation of ROS by reacting with the superoxide anion or the hydroxyl radical, vitamin C has become a popular addition to "after-sun" products.[137,138]

Chemistry of Vitamin C

Vitamin C, or ascorbate, is an α-ketolactone that exists as a hydrophilic monovalent hydroxyl anion. Adding one electron to ascorbate creates the ascorbate free radical. This transient form is more stable than other free radicals and can accept other electrons, making it an effective free radical scavenger, and thus a great antioxidant. If the transient form cannot take an electron, it will cede the electron to an enzymatic reaction, thereby becoming an electron donor.

When two electrons are added to ascorbic acid (AA), the reaction forms a new substance called dehydro-L-ascorbic acid (DHAA). Under physiological conditions, vitamin C predominantly exists in its reduced form, ascorbic acid; it also exists in trace quantities in the oxidized form, DHAA (**Fig. 39-4**). This substance can be reduced back to ascorbate, but if the lactone ring irreversibly opens, forming diketogulonic acid, the compound is no longer active. Diketogulonic acid is often formed when vitamin C preparations are oxidized. When this occurs, these solutions are rendered ineffective and useless.[132,133] In other words, when vitamin C preparations are exposed to UV rays or to air, the molecule rapidly adds two electrons and converts to DHAA, which contains an aromatic ring. If further oxidized, the ring irreversibly opens and the vitamin C solution becomes permanently inactive.

Vitamin C as an Antioxidant

Vitamin C has become a popular addition to after-sun products because it has been shown to interfere with the UV-induced generation of ROS by reacting with the superoxide anion or the hydroxyl radical.[139,140] In fact, vitamin C is known to delay the incidence of UV-induced neoplasms in mice.[141] Topical vitamin C was studied as a photo-protectant first using a porcine skin model.[28] In this study, histological examination revealed that animals treated with topical ascorbic acid exhibited fewer sunburn cells than those treated with vehicle alone when exposed to both UVA and UVB irradiation. (Sunburn cells are basal keratinocytes undergoing programmed cell death due to irreparable DNA damage and represent a method of quantifying the damaging effects of UV irradiation.) Researchers also observed a significant decline in erythema in areas treated with vitamin C and decreases in the amount of vitamin C left on the skin after UV irradiation. In a subsequent study, Darr and colleagues discovered that topical vitamin C combined with either a UVA or UVB sunscreen improved sun protection as compared to the sunscreen alone.[142] Vitamins C and E, in combination, also provided notable protection from UVB insult, though the bulk of protection was attributable to vitamin E.

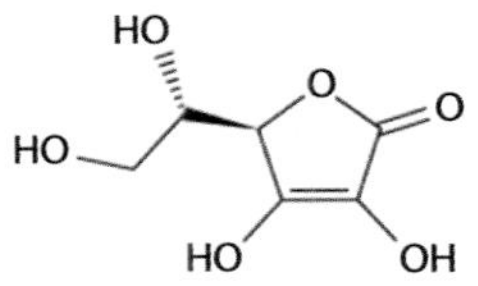

FIGURE 39-4. Ascorbic acid.

There are multiple studies that demonstrate that mice treated with topical vitamin C have less erythema, fewer sunburn cells, and decreased tumor formation seen in treated skin after UV exposure.[143] Vitamin C, a strong antioxidant itself, also reduces (and therefore recycles) oxidized vitamin E back into its active form so the antioxidant capabilities of vitamin E are amplified or regenerated in this way.[42]

In 2012, Xu et al. evaluated the efficacy and safety of topical 23.8% L-ascorbic acid on photoaged skin in a split-face study in 20 Chinese women. Significant improvements in fine lines, dyspigmentation, and surface roughness were observed, without adverse side effects.[144]

Also that year, Taniguchi et al. assessed a stable ascorbic acid derivative, 2-O-α-glucopyranosyl-L-ascorbic acid (AA-2G), and compared it with ascorbic acid for its protective activity on human dermal fibroblasts against cellular damage and senescence engendered by H_2O_2. Pre-treatment with AA-2G for 72 hours promoted the proliferation of normal human dermal fibroblasts and protected against H_2O_2-induced cell damage. The same results were achieved with ascorbic acid only when the culture medium was replenished every 24 hours. The derivative product was also found to be more robust than ascorbic acid in downregulating senescence-associated-β-galactosidase (SA-β-gal) activity, a cellular aging biomarker. Further, the expression of the anti-aging factor sirtuin 1 (SIRT1) was markedly diminished in H_2O_2-exposed normal fibroblasts compared to untreated cells. Pre-treatment with AA-2G prior to H_2O_2 exposure significantly limited the decrease in SIRT1 expression while ascorbic acid exerted no effect, however. Pre-treatment with AA-2G also prevented the increase of p53 and p21 expression levels due to H_2O_2 exposure. The investigators concluded that 2-O-α-glucopyranosyl-L-ascorbic acid protected against oxidative stress and cellular senescence, suggesting a potential role as an anti-aging agent.[145]

The Effects of Vitamin C on Collagen and Elastin Synthesis

Ascorbate is a cofactor for the enzymatic activity of prolyl hydroxylase, an enzyme that hydroxylates prolyl residues in procollagen, elastin, and other proteins with collagenous domains prior to triple helix formation, and thus is required for collagen synthesis.[146] Consequently, deficiency of ascorbic acid leads to impaired collagen production resulting in scurvy. Elastin also contains hydroxyproline; however, prolyl hydroxylation is not required for the biosynthesis and secretion of elastin,[147] and the role of vitamin C in elastin production is unclear.

The addition of ascorbic acid to fibroblast cultures has been reported to increase collagen production by increasing the transcription rate of procollagen genes and by elevating procollagen mRNA levels.[148] Although the increase of type I collagen production in cells cultured in the presence of ascorbic acid is well known, the effects of ascorbate on other extracellular matrix molecules are still poorly understood.[149]

In fact, studies by de Clerck et al. and Scott-Burden et al. have suggested that concentrations of ascorbic acid that maximally stimulate collagen biosynthesis act as an antagonist to elastin accumulation.[150] In a series of studies, Bergethon et al.[151] elaborated on these observations by showing that elastin accumulation was sharply diminished in cell cultures treated with vitamin C.[149] In other words, we know that the addition of ascorbic acid to fibroblast cultures increases production of collagen but may decrease production of elastin by an unknown mechanism.

Clinically the relevance of these effects on collagen and elastin are limited. One study examines the effects of topically applied vitamin C on wrinkles.[152] In this study, Cellex-C was shown to decrease wrinkles when applied topically for a period of 3 months. The patients were evaluated using photography assessments and optical profilometry. Unfortunately, this cannot be considered a blinded study because a large proportion of the patients experienced stinging on the side treated with vitamin C. However, there was a significant difference in the wrinkles on the treated side versus the untreated side. The mechanism of action of this difference is not understood. It might be explained by increased collagen synthesis or by inflammation and irritation induced by the product.

Humbert et al. evaluated the effects of topical vitamin C in healthy photoaged female volunteers in a double-blind randomized trial. They topically applied cream containing 5% vitamin C over a 6-month period, comparing the action of the vitamin C cream vs. excipient on photoaged skin. Clinically, a statistically significant improvement in hydration, wrinkles, glare, and brown spots was noted. A highly significant increase in the density of skin microrelief and a decrease of the deep furrows were also demonstrated. Ultrastructural evidence of the elastic tissue repair was documented. Tissue levels of the inhibitor of MMP-1 were increased, reducing UV-induced collagen breakdown. The mRNA levels of elastin and fibrillin remained unchanged. The topical application of 5% vitamin C cream was well tolerated.[153] However, more clinical trials are necessary to unravel all of the effects of vitamin C on skin and aging.

Vitamin C as an Anti-inflammatory Agent

Vitamin C has also been shown to possess anti-inflammatory activities. In various cell lines loaded with vitamin C by incubating them with DHA, Carcamo et al. were able to show a significant decrease in TNF-α-induced nuclear translocation of NF-κB, NF-κB-dependent reporter transcription, and IκBα phosphorylation, suggesting that intracellular vitamin C can influence inflammatory, neoplastic, and apoptotic processes via inhibition of NF-κB activation. The decrease of inflammation can lead to a reduction of post-inflammatory hyperpigmentation.

Topical Vitamin C

Most of the data available on the effects of vitamin C are derived from studies examining the effects of oral vitamin C or vitamin C applied to tissue cultures. Unfortunately, there are no studies that demonstrate that ingestion of oral vitamin C increases the levels of vitamin C in the skin. Consequently, topical vitamin C preparations have become popular. Ascorbic acid can be formulated into water- or lipid-soluble forms.[154] Topical ascorbyl palmitate, a lipid form, is non-irritating and reportedly photoprotective and anti-inflammatory.[155]

Unfortunately, many of the currently available topical preparations are unable to penetrate the stratum corneum and are, consequently, useless. Some manufacturers claim that their products are nonionic and less lipophobic, enhancing the opportunity for percutaneous absorption.[6,156] The aim of these topical products is to deliver higher amounts of vitamin C to a specific local area of the skin. Comparison of the absorption rate of various topical formulations has not yet been performed using human subjects.

Another problem with topically applied ascorbic acid is its lack of stability as described above in the chemistry section. Because few preparations of topical vitamin C are packaged in airtight containers that are protected from UV radiation, most preparations become inactive within hours of opening the bottle. Besides its combination with vitamin E and ferulic acid, prevailing evidence suggests that incorporation into a lipospheric delivery system may be the best way in the near future to provide topical vitamin C for cutaneous benefits.[157]

Other Cosmetic Applications

Melasma

As vitamin C inhibits the enzyme tyrosinase, through interaction at active tyrosinase locations,[158] it can be used as a depigmenting agent.[159] (See Chapter 41.) In the mid-1990s, Kameyama et al. found that a stable derivative of ascorbic acid produced a significant lightening effect in 19 of 34 patients treated for melasma and senile lentigos.[134] Among patients with normal skin, however, there was no significant lightening. Vitamin C combined with microneedling or iontophoresis has been found to be effective in reducing melasma or post-inflammatory hyperpigmentation (Chapter 27, Microneedling and PRP).[160]

Post-Laser Erythema

In a study of 10 patients who underwent skin resurfacing with a CO_2 laser, the application of topical vitamin C 2 or more weeks after surgery decreased the duration and degree of erythema.[136] In 2020, Kim et al. showed in a single-blinded, prospective, randomized split-face trial in 18 women and men (aged 26 to 53 years old) that a combination formulation of vitamins C and E and ferulic acid applied after Q-switched Nd:YAG laser treatment and twice daily for 2 weeks yielded significantly greater diminishment in melanin index but no appreciable difference in post-treatment erythema.[161]

Stretch Marks

In the late 1990s, Ash et al. compared topical vitamin C in combination with glycolic acid to tretinoin and glycolic acid for the treatment of striae alba.[135] Blinded and unblinded observers determined that both regimens produced an objective improvement in the striae. Although both regimens increased the epidermal thickness, only the tretinoin/glycolic combination augmented the elastin content of the striae. Notably, no topical products have yet been developed to eliminate or significantly improve the appearance of stretch marks.[162]

Side Effects

The administration of vitamin C, in either oral or topical form, appears to be safe for human use. In the studies reviewed, a small number of patients experienced minimal discomfort (stinging and mild irritation) from the topically applied formulations. The major disadvantages of the various formulations include high cost, questionable efficacy, and the possibility of an adverse effect on elastin production, the clinical significance of which is currently unclear. Ascorbic acid is a great addition to skincare particularly when patients insist on sun exposure, cigarette smoking, or other behavior that contributes to free radical production. The practitioner should advise patients, though, to take the oral form so that they will experience the same antioxidant benefits in the arteries, liver, and other amenable organs. If it really works, why limit its effects to the skin?

Summary

Vitamin C preparations are useful in preventing or lessening the harmful effects of UV radiation and ameliorating disorders of hyperpigmentation, striae, and post-laser erythema. Topical vitamin C products must be formulated properly and stored in airtight, light-resistant containers to be effective. Skinceuticals, Murad, and La Roche-Posay have formulated the most effective vitamin C-containing products.

Green Tea

Green tea has been consumed as a popular beverage in Asian countries, in particular, and throughout the world for many years. It has recently gained greater popularity in Western nations, though, because of its purported antioxidant and anticarcinogenic effects. There are numerous *in vitro* and *in vivo* studies on the effects of green tea on the skin; in fact, green tea is one of the most studied antioxidants.[163] Besides its antioxidant activity, green tea polyphenols possess anti-inflammatory and anticarcinogenic properties and modulate the biochemical pathways important in cell proliferation, when administered either topically or orally.[164,165] Indeed, a wide-ranging evidence-based review of the use of botanicals in dermatology by Reuter et al. concluded in 2010 that the oral administration and topical application of antioxidant plant extracts of green and black tea can protect human skin against the deleterious effects of UV exposure, including erythema, premature aging, and cancer.[166]

Polyphenols are a large, diverse family of thousands of chemical substances found in plants. Significantly, many of them are strong antioxidants (**Table 39-1**). There are four major polyphenolic catechins in green tea: ECG [(-) EpiCatechin-3-O-Gallate], GCG [(-)GalloCatechin-3-O-Gallate], EGCG [(-)EpiG-alloCatechin-3-O-Gallate], and EGC [(-)EpiGalloCatechin]. EGCG is the most abundant and biologically active component (**Fig. 39-5**). Special preparation of the tea plant ensures that the antioxidant activities of these polyphenols are preserved. White tea, like green tea, comes from the *Camellia sinensis* plant. However, white tea is more expensive because it is harder to obtain. White tea actually comes from the tips of the green tea leaves or from leaves that are not yet fully open, with the buds still covered by fine white hair. EGCG is the main compound in green and white tea responsible for antioxidant activity.[167,168] When evaluating the utility of a skincare product, it is necessary to know which polyphenols are in the product. EGCG is the most potent form of green tea polyphenols. In addition, it is necessary to know the concentration of polyphenols in the product. The most effective products contain 50–90% polyphenols. Such formulations are dark in color and look brown when they contain this high level of polyphenols. Replenix by Topix is an example of a product line with a high level of polyphenols.

Photoprotective Activity of Green Tea

In early studies, green tea polyphenols were shown to suppress chemical- and UV-induced carcinogenesis when fed orally or applied topically in hairless or Sencar mice.[169–171] Other studies have confirmed these results and shown EGCG to be a potent suppressor of photocarcinogenesis.[172] The profound photoprotective effects of topically applied green tea

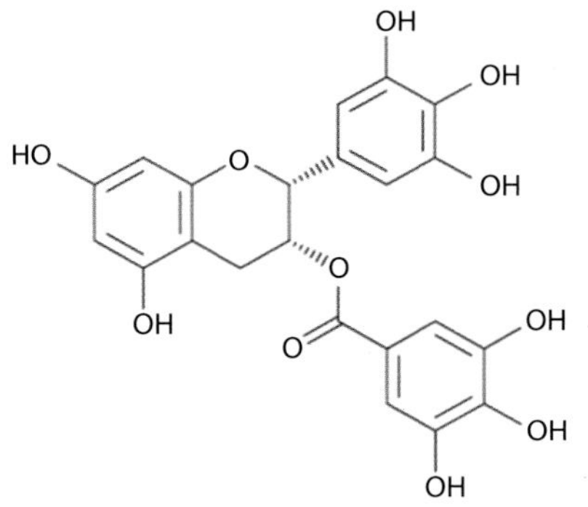

FIGURE 39-5. Epigallocatechin gallate (EGCG) is the most abundant catechin in tea.

TABLE 39-1	Polyphenols[a] Classed by Type and Number of Constituents. Examples Appear Below.				
Phenols	**Pyrocatechols**	**Pyrogallols**	**Resorcinol**	**Phloroglucinols**	**Hydroquinone**
Coumaric acid-derived lignins, kaempferol	Catechin, quercetin, caffeic acid- and ferulic acid-derived lignins, hydroxytyrosol esters	Gallocatechins (EGCG), tannins, myricetin, sinapyl alcohol-derived lignins	Resveratrol	Most flavonoids	Arbutin

[a]http://en.wikipedia.org/wiki/Polyphenol; accessed December 22, 2021.

polyphenols (GTPs) have also been observed in human skin, demonstrating a dose-dependent reduction of UV-induced erythema, decrease in the number of sunburn cells, protection of epidermal Langerhans cells, and limitation of DNA damage.[173] Recent studies have demonstrated that GTPs scavenge ROS, stabilizing GPX, catalase, and glutathione, as well as inhibiting nitric oxide synthase, lipoxygenase, COX and xanthine oxidase, and lipid peroxidase. In addition, they act as modulators of different gene groups and signal pathways.

In 2011, Katiyar elucidated aspects of the mechanisms of action of GTPs, topically applied or orally administered in the drinking water of mice, which resulted in the prevention of UVB-induced non-melanoma skin cancer development. The process was at least partly mediated through DNA repair.[174] Another study led by Katiyar showed that GTPs prevent UV-induced immunosuppression through a similar mechanism, rapid DNA damage repair, and amelioration of nucleotide excision repair genes. This may account for the chemopreventive effects of GTPs in warding off photocarcinogenesis.[175]

Molecular Mechanisms of Green Tea

Molecular targets of GTPs include among others Ras and AP-1, both of which are involved in the MAPK pathway.[176] The anti-apoptotic effects of EGCG on UVB-irradiated keratinocytes seem to be induced by an increase in the expression of the anti-apoptotic molecule Bcl-2 and a decrease in the pro-apoptotic protein Bax.[177] EGCG has further been shown to reduce UV-induced immunosuppression by limiting IL-10 production and increasing IL-12 production, two major cytokines that mediate UV-induced immunosupression.[178] In addition, the EGCG-induced IL-12 increase leads to an augmented synthesis of enzymes that repair UV-induced DNA damage.[179] Also, EGCG seems to reduce UVB-induced immunosuppression by decreasing CD11b, a cell surface marker for activated macrophages and neutrophils in animals treated with UVB.[180] In mice, EGCG has been shown to downregulate UV-induced expression of AP-1 and NF-κB and suppress MMPs, which are known to degrade collagen resulting in photodamage.[181] Prevention of UV-induced oxidative damage and induction of MMPs has been demonstrated *in vivo* in mouse skin. In this study, GTPs were administered in drinking water to SKH-1 hairless mice, which were thereafter exposed to multiple doses of UVB (90 mJ/cm², for 2 months on alternate days). Treatment with GTPs resulted in inhibition of UVB-induced protein oxidation *in vivo* in mouse skin, which could also be observed *in vitro* in human skin fibroblast HS68 cells. Further, oral administration of GTPs was shown to inhibit UVB-induced expression of matrix-degrading MMPs in hairless mouse skin, supporting the role of GTPs as anti-photoaging compounds.[181]

Green Tea Use in Humans

In contrast to the amount of scientific data on GTPs, there are limited studies in human skin examining the topical application of green tea-containing products. This is likely due to the difficulty of designing a study to measure the preventive effects of green tea on aging skin. Nevertheless, applying topical GTPs in the morning in combination with traditional sunscreens is thought to have the potential to protect the skin from UV-induced damage. In addition, topical green tea, as is the case with other antioxidants, may improve rosacea, prevent retinoid dermatitis, and play a role in managing pigmentation disorders. There are many products containing green tea that can be obtained over the counter. Most of the products, however, have not been tested in controlled clinical trials and the concentration of polyphenols in these products is too low to demonstrate efficacy. It is crucial to know the amount of GTPs in a formulation to judge its efficacy.

Green tea is included in several OTC skincare products. The formulations vary by the type of green tea polyphenol component (e.g., EGCG), and the amount of polyphenol, both of which are important to know when evaluating product efficacy. Green tea appears to attenuate skin inflammation and neutralize free radicals, which explains its popularity as an additive in rosacea and anti-aging skincare products. The anti-aging effects of green tea are difficult to measure because it functions as an antioxidant that prevents aging and cannot promote collagen synthesis or ameliorate already existing wrinkles. However, there is relatively good evidence (compared to other antioxidants) to indicate that topically applied green tea can help protect skin from UV radiation.

In a 2012 literature search, Pazyar et al. reviewed all *in vitro*, *in vivo*, and controlled clinical trials involving green tea formulations and their dermatologic applications. They evaluated 20 studies, with evidence suggesting that orally administered green tea exhibits a broad range of healthy activity, including quenching free radicals, cancer prevention, treating hair loss, slowing cutaneous aging, and protecting against the side effects of psoralen-UVA therapy. Further, they found supportive data for the use of topically applied green tea extract to treat several skin disorders, including acne, rosacea, atopic dermatitis, androgenetic alopecia, hirsutism, candidiasis, keloids, leishmaniasis, and genital warts.[182]

One particular green tea topical formulation, green tea sinecatechin polyphenon E (Veregen®) ointment, has been demonstrated to impart antioxidant, antiviral, and antitumor activity, and has evinced efficacy in treating condylomata acuminata (external anogenital warts).[183]

In 2013, Hong et al. conducted an 8-week study in 42 healthy Korean females (aged 30 to 59 years) to ascertain the anti-wrinkle effects of topically applied green tea extract displaying high antioxidant activity after tannase treatment, with increased levels of gallic acid, EGC, and EC. Randomly divided into two groups, subjects treated their crow's feet with tannase-converted green tea extract or normal green tea extract. Decreases in average roughness skin values were much greater in the tannase group as were the scavenging abilities against free radicals. Further, marked or moderate improvements in wrinkles were observed in the tannase group (63.6 percent) compared to the normal green tea group (36.3 percent). The researchers concluded that tannase treatment enhanced the antioxidant activity of green tea extract, rendering it more effective against wrinkles, adding that the tannase green tea formulation merits attention as an anti-wrinkle agent.[184]

Also in 2013, Gianeti performed clinical studies in 24 volunteers to evaluate the effects of a cosmetic formulation containing 6% *C. sinensis* glycolic leaf extracts. Skin moisture was enhanced after 30 days of topical application as was the viscoelastic-to-elastic ratio in comparison with vehicle and control (a forearm area left untreated). After 30 days, skin roughness was significantly diminished. The investigators concluded that the green tea topical cosmetic formulation yielded salient moisturizing and cutaneous microrelief benefits.[185] In a separate study in 10 healthy male volunteers over a 60-day period, Mahmood et al. found that a green tea extract cream exerted a significant impact on the viscoelastic properties of the skin.[186]

After previously demonstrating the efficacy of green tea and lotus extracts in skin disorders involving excess sebum, Mahmood and Akhtar conducted a 60-day, placebo-controlled, comparative split-face study in 33 healthy Asian men to assess the efficacy of two cosmetic formulations (green tea and lotus extract) in treating facial wrinkles. Subjects were divided into three groups, with one applying multiple emulsions with green tea, one applying multiple emulsions with lotus extract, and one applying a combination of both botanical agents. All of the once-daily applications (one active agent on one side of the face and placebo on the other) manifested in improvements in skin roughness, scaliness, smoothness, and wrinkling, with the greatest reduction in wrinkling delivered by the combination formulation. The investigators concluded that the synergistic activity of green tea and lotus extracts rendered significant improvement along several skin parameters, suggesting the potential for these ingredients in anti-aging products.[187]

Summary

Topically applying GTCs in the morning in combination with traditional sunscreens is thought to have the potential to protect the skin from UV-induced damage. Topical green tea may improve rosacea, prevent retinoid dermatitis, and warrant a role in managing pigmentation disorders. Few of the numerous OTC products that contain GTCs have been tested in controlled clinical trials and the concentration of polyphenols in these products is too low to demonstrate efficacy. Practitioners should know the amount of GTCs in a formulation to judge its efficacy and recommend based on a patient's Baumann Skin Type.

The antioxidant and other health benefits of green tea and its extracts have emerged in an increasing number of studies in recent years with evidence of inhibition of photocarcinogenesis, and delivering other photoprotective, anti-aging effects, as well as wound-healing functions, and activity against acne, rosacea, keloids, and hair disorders; however, few studies achieve the gold standard experimental status using double-blind, randomized structures in sufficiently large numbers of patients, suggesting promise but a need for much more research.[188]

Silymarin

Silymarin is a naturally occurring polyphenolic flavonoid compound derived from the seeds of the milk thistle plant *Silybum marianum*. Milk thistle has been used for medicinal purposes for over 2,000 years. Today, it is used in Europe and Asia as an antihepatotoxic agent and is available as a supplement in Europe and the US. Its primary active constituents are silybin, silydianin, and silychristine, of which silybin (also known as silibinin) is considered to be the most biologically active component in terms of its antioxidant, anti-inflammatory, and anticarcinogenic properties.[189,190] **(Fig. 39-6.)** Silymarin has been demonstrated to reduce lipid peroxidation through its scavenging of ROS and capacity to elevate the cellular content of glutathione; it has also exhibited scavenging activity against hydroxyl radicals and inhibitory activity in various steps in the NF-κB pathway.[190]

Photoprotection

Topical application of silybin prior to, or immediately after, UV irradiation has been found to confer strong protection against UV-induced damage in the epidermis by a reduction in thymine dimer-positive cells and an up-regulation of p53-p21/Cip1, which researchers believe may lead to inhibition of cell proliferation and apoptosis. This study suggests that mechanisms other than sunscreen effect are integral to silybin efficacy against UV-caused skin damage.[191] Researchers have also noted that silybin enhances UVB-induced apoptosis and speculated that it acts as a UVB damage sensor to impart its biological action.[192]

The antioxidant activity of silymarin is well established. Chemoprotective activity against skin cancer has also been reported and continues to be the subject of much investigation.[193-195] In a study to identify the mechanism of photocarcinogenesis prevention in mouse skin by the topical treatment of silymarin, prevention of UVB-induced immunosuppression and oxidative stress were found to be potentially related to the prevention of photocarcinogenesis in mice.[196] Authors concluded from this trial and related data from other recent studies that there are compelling arguments for the inclusion of silymarin in sunscreens or in other products in a skincare regimen.[197-199]

Mode of Administration

Most of the milk thistle or silymarin available in the US comes in the form of oral supplements. These may inactivate oral contraceptives. Topical formulations are available from SkinCeuticals. Silymarin has been used in topical formulations to treat rosacea.[200]

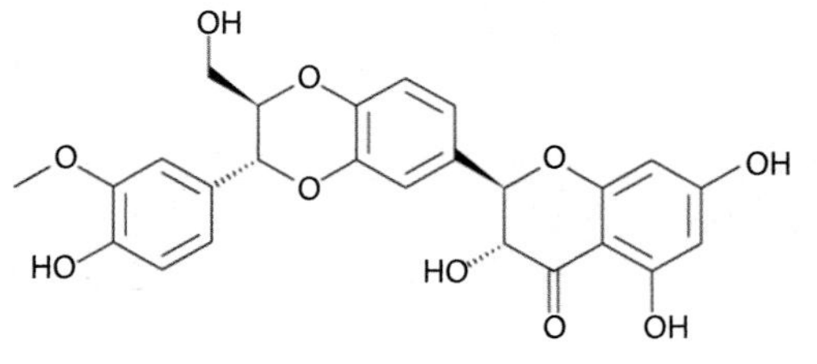

FIGURE 39-6. Silibinin (the active component of silymarin).

Coffea Arabica and Coffeeberry Extract

The coffee plant *Coffea arabica* is the source of the globally consumed coffee beverage, originating from Ethiopia and cultivated throughout the world. Extracts of the beans of the coffee plant have been shown to exhibit antioxidant activity after roasting.[201] (**Fig. 39-7.**) Besides the coffee beans, the fruit of the coffee plant, especially when harvested in a sub-ripened state, also possesses peak antioxidant activity, by dint of its constituent polyphenols, especially chlorogenic acid, condensed proanthocyanidins, quinic acid, and ferulic acid. Coffeeberry® is the proprietary name for the antioxidant that is extracted from the fruit of *C. arabica*. In the oxygen radical absorbance capacity assay (ORAC), Coffeeberry® has demonstrated higher antioxidant activity than green tea, pomegranate extract, as well as vitamins C and E.[202] It is worth noting that there is no standard way to measure antioxidant strength in topical preparations. The ORAC value is the standard for measuring antioxidant potency in food.

Polyphenols, which can be found in coffee beans, green and black tea, various fruits, vegetables, and grains, are known to provide multiple health benefits, mainly due to their anti-inflammatory and antioxidant properties.[203,204] In 2007, Stiefel Laboratories launched the product line RevaléSkin™, which contains 1% coffeeberry polyphenols. To build on some promising laboratory results, clinical studies assessing the antioxidant effects of topical preparations containing *C. arabica* and coffeeberry extract are needed.

C. arabica *in Skincare Research*

In 2009, green coffee oil was shown through *in vitro* studies and in *ex vivo* human skin models to dose-dependently promote the production of the key dermal constituents—collagen, elastin, and glycosaminoglycans—as well as stimulate a greater release of the growth factors TGF-β1 and granulocyte-macrophage colony-stimulating factor. In addition, green coffee oil spurred the expression of aquaporin (AQP)-3 mRNA, up to 6.5-fold higher than levels seen in control cultures. The

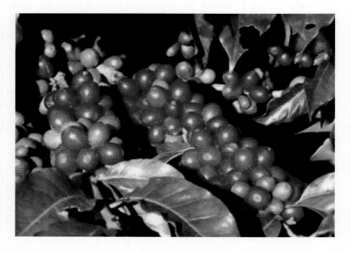

FIGURE 39-7. The coffee plant *Coffea arabica*. (Reproduced with permission from Leslie Baumann MD.)

investigators concluded that green coffee oil has potential to contribute to the formation of new connective tissue and to enhance cutaneous function by mitigating wrinkles and preventing xerosis by raising levels of AQP-3. Consequently, they suggested that including green coffee oil in cosmetic formulations merits consideration.[205]

Two years later, Chiang et al. reported on their investigation of the anti-photoaging effects of *C. arabica* leaf extract, its hydrolysates, chlorogenic acid, and caffeic acid. The various polyphenol-containing test compounds were subjected to MMP and elastase inhibition tests. They found that *C. arabica* extract stimulated type I procollagen expression, inhibited MMP-1, -3, and -9 expression, and suppressed the phosphorylation of JNK, ERK and p38. They concluded that the extract of *C. arabica* leaves can prevent photodamage by blocking MMP expression and the MAP kinase pathway.[206]

Human Studies

In 2008, Draelos performed a double-blind, randomized clinical trial in 50 subjects over age 30 with mild symptoms of photoaging to evaluate the cutaneous benefits of coffeeberry extract. Over the 12-week period, a coffeeberry facial cleanser was used twice daily by both groups. One group applied a coffeeberry day cream in the morning and a coffeeberry night cream in the evening to the whole face. The other group applied control creams. Significant improvements were seen in all study parameters (i.e., erythema, roughness, scaling, wrinkling, and global assessment) in the coffeeberry extract group compared to the control group. Transepidermal water loss declined from baseline in the coffeeberry group and rose in the control group. Draelos concluded that the coffeeberry extract system of facial cleanser and morning and evening creams was well tolerated and yielded significant reductions in multiple symptoms of photoaged skin.[207,208]

Led by McDaniel and sponsored by Stiefel Laboratories, a 6-week pilot study of 30 female patients (31 to 71 years old) with moderate actinic damage used an antioxidant system composed of 0.1% coffeeberry extract facial cleanser as well as 1% coffeeberry extract night and day creams (the latter of which contained octinate and oxybenzone with an SPF of 15).[202,209] Twenty subjects applied all three products to the whole face; 10 subjects applied each to half the face and vehicle on the other half. Split-face patients experienced significant improvements in fine lines and wrinkles, pigmentation, and overall appearance as compared to those using vehicle. Patients treated on the whole face exhibited improvements in all parameters (including fine lines and wrinkles, roughness and dryness, pigmentation, and overall appearance) compared to baseline, with pigmentation reduction as the most salient improvement. Skin biopsies revealed that the use of coffeeberry extract contributed to an increase in key structural dermal proteins (i.e., collagen I and collagen IV) as well as a decrease in collagenase and inflammatory mediators.[209]

In 2010, Palmer and Kitchin completed a 12-week, double-blind, randomized, controlled clinical usage study of the efficacy and tolerance of a *C. arabica*-containing topical, high antioxidant skincare system (facial wash, day lotion, night cream, and eye serum) to ameliorate photoaging in 40 Caucasian females. One group of participants used the test system, including twice daily facial wash, morning application of the antioxidant day lotion, and nightly application of the antioxidant night cream and eye serum; the other group used the control products according to the same protocol. The authors observed statistically significant improvements in the appearance of photodamaged skin in the subjects using the test regimen.[210] Coffeeberry extract has also been shown, in pre-clinical and small clinical trials, to protect skin from oxidative damage as well as UVB-induced pyrimidine dimer formation and inflammation, and to speed recovery from UVB exposure.[211]

Summary

The *C. arabica* plant is used in some botanical formulations intended to treat cellulite. The caffeine used in this context as an active ingredient is extracted from the leaves, however, not the berries.[212] Green *C. arabica* seed oil is also being broadly used as an ingredient in cosmetic formulations.[205] Therefore, multiple parts of the plant are now under investigation and active use in the dermatologic realm. Preliminary data on the use of the proprietary fruit suggest that coffeeberry extract has the potential to enhance overall appearance, hyperpigmentation, as well as fine lines and wrinkles.[213]

Polypodium Leucotomos

Polypodium leucotomos (PL) is an extract derived from the fern family. It is an oral photoprotectant with strong antioxidant properties. Its major phenolic components have been identified as 3,4-dihydroxybenzoic acid, 4-hydroxybenzoic acid, vanillic acid, caffeic acid, 4-hydroxycinnamic acid, 4-hydroxycinnamoyl-quinic acid, ferulic acid, and five chlorogenic acid isomers.[214] In traditional medicine, polypodium leucotomos extract (PLE) has been used for various indications, including psoriasis, atopic dermatitis, vitiligo, rheumatoid arthritis, as well as tumors and, 20 years ago, PLE was found to exhibit immunomodulatory activity *in vitro* and *in vivo*.[215]

Photoprotection

The photoprotective effect of PL has been shown for topical or oral administration in various studies.[216] In an investigation by Gonzáles et al., 21 healthy volunteers, either untreated or treated with oral psoralens (8-MOP or 5-MOP), were enrolled and exposed to solar radiation. Immediate pigment darkening (IPD), MED, minimal melanogenic dose (MMD), and minimal phototoxic dose (MPD) before and after topical or oral administration of PL were evaluated. PL was found to be photoprotective after topical application as well as oral administration revealing a prevention of acute sunburn and psoralen-induced phototoxic reactions. Immunohistochemistry revealed photoprotection of Langerhans cells by oral as well as topical PL.[217]

Antioxidant Effects

The antioxidant effects of PL have been demonstrated *in vitro* and *in vivo*, as well as for the prevention of photoaging.[218,219]

Gonzáles et al. showed that PL manifests photoprotective effects *in vivo* and *in vitro* by its ability to suppress free radical generation, prevent photodecomposition of both endogenous photoprotective molecules as well as DNA, and inhibit UV-induced cell death.[220] Oral administration of PLE has been proven to exert photoprotective effects in various studies. It has been shown to decrease sunburn and UV-induced mast cell infiltration in the skin, and reduce the loss of epidermal Langerhans cells of the skin associated with UV exposure.[221,222] Caccialanza et al. exposed 26 patients with polymorphic light eruption and two with solar urticaria to sunlight while directing them to consume 480 mg/day of PL orally through the study. The response of the skin to sunlight was compared with that occurring previously without administration of PL, and displayed statistically significant reduction of skin reaction and subjective symptoms.[223]

Molecular Mechanism

The molecular mechanisms of the photoprotective effects of PL have been investigated *in vitro* using a solar simulator as UV source in human keratinocytes. The results showed that the photoprotective effects of PL seem to involve inhibition of TNF-α, nitric oxide (NO) production, and inducible nitric oxide synthase (iNOS) up-regulation induced by UV light and the modulation of the transcriptional activation of AP-1 and NF-κB, two pro-inflammatory transcription factors induced by UV-radiation. Finally, it was demonstrated that PL prevents cytotoxic damage and apoptosis induced by UV light in HaCaT cells.[224]

Summary

It appears that the dermatologic potential of this tropical plant extract is being harnessed in clinical applications for the treatment of sunburn and the inhibition of the phototoxic reaction, as well as for the prevention of photoaging.[218,225,226] Experimental data support the inclusion of PL extract in sunscreen formulations.[227] This ingredient is available as an oral supplement in the US under the brand name Heliocare and is sold by the company OPKO Health Inc. One to two capsules of Heliocare should be taken one hour prior to sun exposure. It should be used in conjunction with a broad-spectrum sunscreen. A novel topical formulation, PL/Fernblock® (IFC Group, Spain) is available that is thought to provide photoprotection by shielding DNA integrity and promoting the immune response by virtue of the functions of its numerous phenolic constituents.[228,229]

Resveratrol

Resveratrol (trans-3,5,4′-trihydroxystilbene) is a polyphenolic phytoalexin compound found in the skin and seeds of grapes, berries (black currant, blueberry, cranberry, raspberry, strawberry), peanuts, red wine, as well as Japanese knotweed root, and has been reported to exhibit a wide range of biological and pharmacological properties.[230,231] It exists in two isoforms: *trans*-resveratrol and *cis*-resveratrol where the *trans*-isomer is the more stable form (**Fig. 39-8**). Resveratrol is a potent antioxidant with antiproliferative and anti-inflammatory

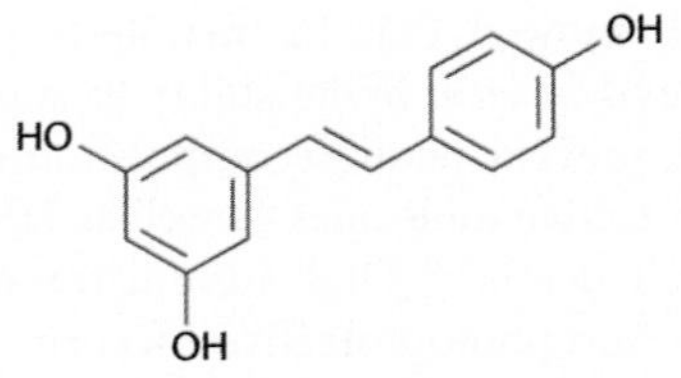

FIGURE 39-8. Resveratrol.

properties.[190,232,233] *In vitro* and *in vivo* studies have demonstrated that resveratrol exhibits chemopreventive and anti-proliferative activity against various cancers, including skin cancer, by exerting inhibitory effects on diverse cellular events associated with tumor initiation, promotion, as well as progression and triggering apoptosis in such tumor cells.[234–236]

Molecular Mechanisms of Photoprotection

Resveratrol has been shown to protect against UVB-mediated cutaneous damages in SKH-1 hairless mice. Topical application of resveratrol to SKH-1 hairless mice prior to UVB irradiation resulted in a significant decrease in UVB-mediated generation of H_2O_2 as well as infiltration of leukocytes and inhibition of skin edema. Also, topical application of resveratrol has been found to significantly inhibit UVB-mediated induction of COX-2 and ODC enzyme activities and protein expression of ODC, which are well-established markers for tumor promotion. Resveratrol further seems to inhibit the UVB-mediated increase of lipid peroxidation, a marker of oxidative stress.[232,237,238] In one study, pre-treatment of normal human epidermal keratinocytes (NHEK) with resveratrol inhibited UVB-induced activation of the NF-κB pathway.[233] This protective effect of resveratrol against the damage of multiple UVB-exposures was suggested to be associated with inhibition of the MAPK pathway and mediated via modulation in the expression and function of the cell cycle regulatory protein cki–cyclin–cdk network.[239] Further, in short-term experiments, the topical application of resveratrol to SKH-1 hairless mouse skin prior to UVB irradiation resulted in significant inhibition of cell proliferation and phosphorylation of survivin.[237] Long-term studies have demonstrated that topical application with resveratrol (both pre- and post-treatment) results in inhibition of UVB-induced tumor incidence and delay in the onset of skin tumorigenesis.[238] The post-treatment of resveratrol imparted equal protection to the pre-treatment, suggesting that resveratrol-mediated responses may not be sunscreen effects.

Evidence suggesting the photoprotective effects of resveratrol continues to be collected.[240,241] In a 2004 experiment, resveratrol was topically applied to SKH-1 hairless mice 30 minutes before exposure to UVB; 24 hours later, significant reductions were observed in bi-fold skin thickness, hyperplasia, and infiltration of leukocytes. Critical cell cycle regulatory proteins were substantially downregulated as a result of the resveratrol treatment. The researchers concluded that

this potent antioxidant may have the potential to help prevent UVB-mediated photodamage and carcinogenesis.[239]

In a small 2013 study by Ferzli et al., 16 subjects with erythema applied a formulation containing resveratrol, green tea polyphenols, and caffeine twice daily to the whole face. Clinical photographs and spectrally enhanced images taken before treatment and every 2 weeks through 3 months were assessed. The researchers reported that improvement was seen in 16 of 16 clinical images and 13 of 16 spectrally enhanced images. Erythema reduction was observable by 6 weeks of treatment.[242]

Anti-Aging Activity

In 2008, Baxter reported that in an ORAC comparison, a skin formulation with 1% resveratrol displayed 17 times the antioxidant activity of a 1% idebenone formulation.[243] Idebenone has been labeled by some as the most potent topical antioxidant.[244] In a 2010 *in vitro* study, Giardina et al. evaluated the tonic-trophic characteristics of resveratrol as well as resveratrol plus N-acetyl-cysteine on cultured skin fibroblasts. They found that both formulations dose-dependently led to an increase in cell proliferation and inhibition of collagenase activity.[245]

Two years later, Wu et al. studied the protective effects of resveratrate, a stable resveratrol derivative, against damage to human skin engendered by repetitive solar simulator UV radiation (ssUVR) in 15 healthy human volunteers. Six sites on non-exposed dorsal skin of each participant were studied, with four sites exposed to ssUVR and the remaining ones serving as positive control (ssUVR only) and baseline control (no treatment or exposure). The investigators observed minimal erythema on skin treated with resveratrate and the resveratrol derivative significantly inhibited sunburn cell formation. They concluded that resveratrate protects the skin against sunburn and suntan provoked by repetitive ssUVR.[246]

Summary

Currently, the preponderance of evidence suggests that resveratrol penetrates the skin barrier, delivers anti-aging activity, and its antioxidant characteristics protect the skin from UV and free radicals by attenuating the expression of AP-1 and NF-κB factors.[231] Resveratrol is suitable for inclusion in various product types (e.g., emollients, patches, sunscreens, and other skincare products) intended to prevent skin cancer and other conditions thought to be generated by the sun.

Grape Seed Extract

Grapes, also known as *Vitis vinifera,* are globally consumed fruits and the source of wine. The extract prepared from grape seeds is rich in proanthocyanidins, which belong to the polyphenolic flavonoid family. Specifically, grape seed proanthocyanidins are oligomers and polymers of polyhydroxy flavan-3-ol units, such as (+)-catechin and (-)-epicatechin, which are present in large amounts in the polyphenols of red wine and grape seeds. Sixty to seventy percent of the polyphenols are found in the seeds of the grapes.[247,248] Proanthocyanidins are believed to exhibit a wide range of biologic, pharmacologic, chemoprotective, and antioxidant activities.[249]

Antioxidant Activity

Various studies have reported on the potent antioxidative and free radical scavenging activities of proanthocyanidins.[250–254] Grape seed extract has been shown to be an even stronger scavenger of free radicals than vitamins C and E.[255] Dietary intake of grape seed proanthocyanidins (GSP) has been shown to inhibit UV-induced skin cancer in mice.[256] Mittal et al. demonstrated that oral intake of GSP in SKH-1 hairless mice resulted in prevention of photocarcinogenesis with reduced tumor incidence, multiplicity, and size compared with non-GSP–treated mice following a UVB-induced carcinogenesis protocol. Biochemical analysis revealed that treatment of GSP in *in vivo* and *in vitro* systems significantly inhibited UVB- or Fe^{3+}-induced lipid peroxidation, suggesting a possible antioxidant mechanism of photoprotection by GSP.[256]

In another study, investigators demonstrated that treatment of NHEK with GSP inhibited UV-induced oxidative stress by inhibiting UVB-induced H_2O_2, lipid peroxidation, protein oxidation, and DNA damage as well as scavenging hydroxyl radicals and superoxide anions in a cell-free system. Moreover, GSP also inhibited UVB-induced depletion of antioxidant defense components, such as GPX, catalase, superoxide dismutase, and glutathione. Treatment of NHEK with GSP further inhibited UVB-induced phosphorylation of ERK1/2, JNK, and p38 proteins of the MAPK family.[257] As UV-induced oxidative stress mediates activation of MAPK and NF-κB signaling pathways, the same group of investigators further examined the effect of dietary GSP on these pathways and proved that GSP exhibits the ability to protect the skin from the adverse effects of UVB radiation via modulation of the MAPK and NF-κB signaling pathways. This provides a molecular basis for the photoprotective effects of grape seed extract in an *in vivo* animal model.[258] Dietary GSP was also shown to modulate UVB-induced immunosuppression by reducing the immunosuppressive cytokine IL-10 while enhancing the production of the immunostimulatory cytokine IL-12, suggesting this to be one of the possible mechanisms by which grape seed extract prevents photocarcinogenesis in mice.[259] In 2021, Yarovaya et al. demonstrated that grape seed extract exerted photoprotective effects on human dermal fibroblasts exposed to UVA radiation and determined that the cream formulations containing grape seed extracts combined with octyl methoxycinnamate were photostable and may be suitable for use as a sunscreen to protect against premature cutaneous aging.[260]

Grape Seed Extract Applications in Humans

Grape seed extract is included in topical cosmetic formulations with the intention of imparting an anti-aging effect. It is a popular ingredient in "organic" products. However, additional studies are needed to further understand its effects on human skin when used topically. Currently, grape seed extract is thought to offer significant skin health potential because of its copious supply of antioxidant constituents including phenolic acids, phytosterols, flavonoids, tocopherols, carotenoids, tocopherols, and tocotrienols.[261,262]

Pomegranate

Pomegranate (*Punica granatum*) is an edible fruit native to northern India, Iran, Pakistan, as well as Afghanistan and cultivated in many countries. The fruits are widely consumed in fresh and beverage forms as juice. The pomegranate was one of the first known sources of medicines and has been used extensively in many cultures around the world for various diseases, such as skin inflammation, rheumatism, and sore throats.[263] In Ayurvedic medicine, pomegranates reputedly nourish and restore balance to the skin. The extract of the fruit contains two types of polyphenolic compounds: anthocyanins (such as delphinidin, cyanidin, and pelargonidin), as well as hydrolyzable tannins (such as punicalin, pedunculagin, punicalagin, as well as gallagic and ellagic acid esters of glucose).

Antioxidant Activity

Extracts can be obtained from various parts of the fruit, such as the juice, seed, and peel and have been reported to have strong antioxidant activity.[264–266] The phenolic components extracted from pomegranate have been shown to possess strong antioxidant properties in several instances.[267] One study compared the antioxidant potency of various beverages known to be rich in polyphenols, including pomegranate juice, applying four tests of antioxidant strength. Compared to various fruit juices (apple, açaí, black cherry, blueberry, cranberry, orange), red wines as well as black, green, and white tea, pomegranate juice displayed the greatest antioxidant potency and was at least 20% stronger than any of the other beverages tested.[268] (**Table 39-2**.) Also, other studies have reported that pomegranate imparts a more potent antioxidant effect than comparable quantities of green tea and red wine.[264,269] With regard to topical application, a methanolic extract of pomegranate peel followed by carbon tetrachloride was demonstrated to restore catalase, peroxidase, and superoxide dismutase enzyme activities in rats.[270]

Photoprotection

There have been numerous reports on the *in vitro* and *in vivo* anticancer properties of pomegranates.[271,272] Pomegranate fruit extract has been found to exert photochemopreventive properties, ameliorating UVA-mediated damages by modulating cellular pathways.[273] The seed oil of the pomegranate fruit has been shown to possess chemopreventive activity against skin cancer.[274] Afaq et al. demonstrated that topically applied pomegranate fruit extract (PFE) possesses anti-skin tumor-promoting effects in a CD-1 mouse model of chemical carcinogenesis.[267] They further studied the effect of PFE on UVB-induced adverse effects in NHEK and showed that PFE protects against the adverse effects of UVB radiation by inhibiting UVB-induced modulations of NF-κB and MAPK pathways.[275] The same group then investigated the effect of polyphenol-rich PFE on UVB-induced oxidative stress and photoaging in human immortalized HaCaT keratinocytes, showing that pre-treatment of HaCaT cells with PFE inhibited UVB-mediated reduction in cell viability and intracellular glutathione content as well as an increase in lipid

TABLE 39-2	Antioxidant Potency Composite Index[a], Based on the Ranking of Four Antioxidant Assays[b]
Beverage	**Antioxidant Potency Composite Index[a]**
Pomegranate juice	95.8
Red wine	68.3
Concord grape juice	61.7
Blueberry juice	50.9
Black cherry juice	46.5
Açaí juice	46.2
Cranberry juice	38.0
Iced green tea	24.2
Orange juice	19.1
Iced white tea	16.8
Apple juice	14.6
Iced black tea	12.2

[a]based on the ranking of all four antioxidant assays (free radical scavenging capacity by 2,2-diphenyl-1-picrylhydrazyl, DPPH; total oxygen radical absorbance capacity, ORAC; ferric reducing antioxidant power, FRAP; Trolox equivalent antioxidant capacity, TEAC) an overall antioxidant potency composite index was calculated by assigning each test equal weight. Antioxidant index score = (sample score/best score) × 100, averaged for all tests for all beverages.
[b]Seeram NP, Aviram M, Zhang Y, Henning SM, Feng L, Dreher M, Heber D. Comparison of Antioxidant Potency of Commonly Consumed Polyphenol-Rich Beverages in the United States. *J Agric Food Chem.* 2008;56(4):1415-1422.

peroxidation. It also inhibited the up-regulation of various MMPs and phosphorylation of MAPKs. These results suggest that PFE protects HaCaT cells against UVB-induced oxidative stress and markers of photoaging and could be a useful supplement in skincare products.[276] This is buttressed by further *in vitro* studies that suggest that pomegranate peel fractions may promote dermal regeneration while pomegranate seed oil fractions may foster epidermal regeneration, presenting potential additional dermatologic applications.[277] Pomegranate extract is already available over the counter in various skincare products. Other *in vitro* and animal studies have shown that topically applied pomegranate extract can exert antioxidant and hyperpigmentary effects potentially beneficial in human skin.[278] Specifically, such studies have shown pomegranate mitigating UVB-induced skin damage. In a randomized, controlled, parallel, three-arm, open-label study in 2019, Henning et al. evaluated the effects of oral pomegranate on 74 female subjects (30 to 45 years old) with Fitzpatrick skin types II to IV over 12 weeks, finding that daily consumption may have enhanced protection against UVB photodamage.[279]

THE FAT- AND WATER-SOLUBLE ANTIOXIDANT

The sole network antioxidant known to be both water and lipid soluble is lipoic acid.

Alpha-Lipoic Acid

Alpha-lipoic acid is an antioxidant agent used for the treatment and prevention of aging skin.[280] It differs from the other antioxidants insofar as it can be used as a superficial chemical peel to resurface the skin in a manner similar to glycolic acid. Alpha-lipoic acid is believed to have anti-inflammatory properties that may also make it useful in the treatment of post-laser erythema.[281] This discussion will focus on the science and potential therapeutic applications of α-lipoic acid in the cosmetic dermatology practice.

Chemical Composition

Formerly called thioctic acid, α-lipoic acid is an octanoic acid, which means an eight-carbon version of carboxylic acid combined with cysteine (**Fig. 39-9**). It is an essential cofactor in mitochondrial dehydrogenases.[282] In 1951, it was first discovered that α-lipoic acid acted as an antioxidant. It is both water and lipid soluble and, hence, has been termed the "universal" antioxidant.[283] Other popular antioxidants are either lipophilic, such as vitamin E, or hydrophilic, such as vitamin C.

Penetration into the Stratum Corneum

Dihydrolipoic acid (DHLA) is formed by reducing α-lipoic acid. It has a more powerful antioxidative effect than does its parent compound. DHLA is very unstable, however, and would get oxidized in a matter of minutes after application to the skin. Alpha-lipoic acid has become popular because it is absorbed in a stable form and after it enters the cells, it is immediately converted to DHLA.[284] Podda et al. studied the capacity of α-lipoic acid to penetrate the skin in anesthetized hairless mice after application of a 5% solution in propylene glycol for 0.5 to four hours. They showed the rate of α-lipoic acid absorption into the skin to be constant by 30 minutes after application, reaching the maximum concentration by the two-hour mark.[285]

Topical Application

Topical application of 3% α-lipoic acid in a lecithin base to human skin has been shown to decrease UVB-induced erythema in one-half the time of lesions treated with lecithin base alone.[285] This model indicated that topical application of α-lipoic acid could prevent free radical damage to skin, and thus prevent photoaging and carcinogenesis.[286] Although α-lipoic acid is available in topical cosmetic products and

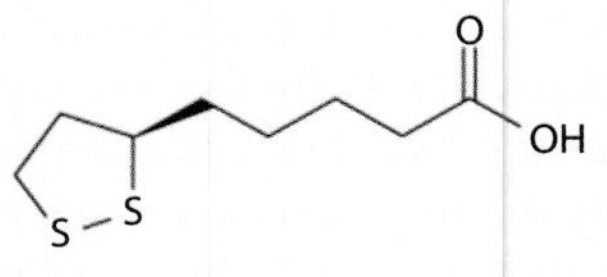

FIGURE 39-9. Lipoic acid.

in formulations used for office peels, there are no published peer-reviewed clinical trials examining the efficacy of these products.

In 2019, Kubota et al. developed a nanocapsule delivery system for α-lipoic acid and showed in murine skin that it effectively ameliorated UV-induced pigmentation and epidermal thickening, possibly paving the way for use as a topical preparation for humans.[287] The next year, Zhou et al. developed a w/o emulsion to deliver α-lipoic acid using different ionic liquids transdermally. In their *in vitro* experiments, they found notable anti-aging efficacy and concluded that research should commence on developing topical formulations.[288]

Systemic Administration

Alpha-lipoic acid can be used either topically or systemically. When systemically administered it has been used to influence glucose control and prevent chronic hyperglycemia-associated complications such as diabetes mellitus, Alzheimer's disease, cataracts, HIV activation, and radiation injury.[280,289] Alpha-lipoic acid has also been used as adjuvant therapy for glaucoma, ischemia-reperfusion injury, amanita mushroom poisoning, cellular oxidative damage,[290] and Chagas disease.[291] There is no currently established RDA but most proponents of α-lipoic acid supplementation suggest 25–500 mg daily.

Antioxidant Activity

There are four principal antioxidative properties of α-lipoic acid: metal chelating capacity, ability to scavenge ROS, capability of regnerating endogenous antioxidants,[292,293] and the ability to repair oxidative damage.[294]

In a 2017 experiment on the effects of α-lipoic acid on smoking-induced skin damage in Sprague-Dawley female rats, investigators observed improvement in treated animals according to all histological parameters (improvement in collagen bundles and hair follicle decline, sweat gland degradation). Biochemical measurements were also improved in the treated rats, as investigators concluded that the antioxidant and anti-inflammatory activity of α-lipoic acid was responsible for attenuating the cutaneous effects of smoke exposure.[295]

Alpha-lipoic acid is available in different forms and vehicles and currently marketed in cleansers, moisturizers, and oral supplements. When starting patients on α-lipoic acid-containing products, they should be warned that they may feel a slight tingling sensation, which decreases after a few seconds and disappears within minutes of application. Topical application of α-lipoic acid is recommended every other day for the first week, increasing to twice a day for the third week if no side effects occur. Alpha-lipoic acid can cause a significant amount of inflammation so these patients should be followed closely. Fine skin lines may improve after a few weeks; however, this may be due to the resultant inflammation. Contact dermatitis to α-lipoic acid has been reported.[296]

Summary

Alpha-lipoic acid is a potent antioxidant that also contains exfoliating properties that may render it a good choice for resistant skin types with a tendency to wrinkle (see Chapter 10, Baumann Skin Typing).

OTHER ANTIOXIDANTS

Genistein

Genistein (4',5,7-tri-hydroxyisoflavone), derived from and an active constituent in soybeans, is an isoflavone, thus a member of the polyphenol family. It was first isolated from soybeans in 1931. The recent heightened awareness of this potent compound can mostly be attributed to the fact that in Asia various positive beneficial health effects have been at least in part attributed to their increased soy consumption.[297] Most importantly, Asians show significantly lower incidences in breast, colon, and prostate cancers when compared to western populations.[298–301]

Although soybeans contain several ingredients with demonstrated anticancer activities, genistein is its most important component.[302] (**Fig. 39-10.**) Genistein is known to exert various biological activities, such as helping in the treatment and prevention of certain cardiovascular conditions and osteoporosis, as well as enhancing the effects of radiation in the treatment of prostate and breast cancers.[303] Its classification as a phytoestrogen accounts for additional health benefits including the modulation of peri-menopausal symptoms without the associated dangers of hormone replacement therapy.[304,305]

Biological Effects

Genistein is a potent antioxidant and its anticarcinogenic effects are well documented on several cancers, including the skin.[303,306–308] The capacity of genistein to inhibit UV-induced oxidative DNA damage as well as block UV-induced c-Fos and c-Jun proto-oncogene expression has been demonstrated *in vitro* and *in vivo*.[309–312] Genistein, either topically applied or orally supplemented, has been shown to inhibit UVB-induced skin carcinogenesis in mice and substantially hinder the subacute and chronic UVB-induced cutaneous damage and histological alterations related to photoaging. The possible mechanisms of the anticarcinogenic action include scavenging of ROS, thwarting oxidative and photodynamic damage to DNA, inhibition of tyrosine protein kinase, down-regulation of epidermal growth factor (EGF)-receptor phosphorylation and MAPK activation, and suppression of oncoprotein expression in UVB-irradiated cells and mouse skin.[303] In addition, the treatment of human keratinocyte cell line NCTC 2544 with genistein has been documented to limit lipid peroxidation and increases in ROS formation.[313] The potent chemopreventive effect of UVB-induced skin carcinogenesis in human skin was examined by assessing both cutaneous erythema and discomfort, which was significantly inhibited by pre-UVB

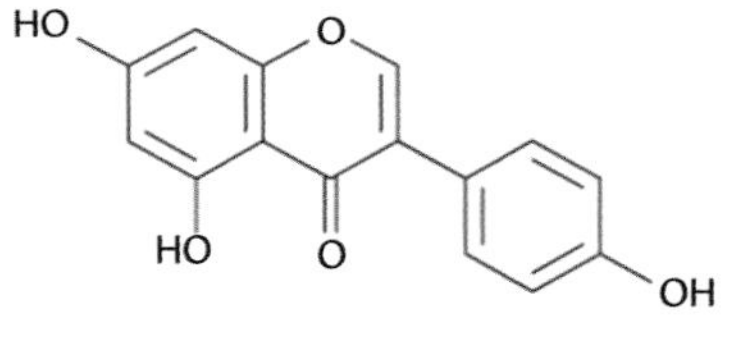

FIGURE 39-10. Genistein.

application of genistein, suggesting that genistein effectively protects human skin against UVB-induced skin photodamage. Genistein has also been demonstrated to protect mouse skin against photodamage induced by psoralen plus UVA (PUVA).

In 2017, Silva et al. reported on a prospective, double-blind, randomized, controlled clinical trial with 30 postmenopausal women between the ages of 45 to 55 years old in which the effects of topical estradiol and genistein on facial skin were compared over 24 weeks. Although the outcomes for the estrogen group were superior, both groups experienced increased levels of type I and type III facial collagen. The investigators suggested that more research was necessary to ascertain the prolonged effects of genistein.[314] Similar results were observed 4 years earlier in a 24-week prospective, randomized, double-blind trial of 30 postmenopausal women in which genistein was compared to estradiol. In this case, hyaluronic acid concentrations were found to be elevated by both topical treatments, with superior results seen with estradiol.[315]

Summary

Genistein substantially inhibits skin carcinogenesis and cutaneous aging induced by UV light in mice and photodamage in humans. Supported by extensive data, the soybean isoflavone genistein is thought to offer promising applications in preventing UV-induced skin cancer and photoaging. In fact, genistein is already included in various products such as facial moisturizers, sunscreens, and several skincare formulations claiming anti-aging effects.

Pycnogenol

Pycnogenol is the patented name for a standardized pine bark extract of the French maritime pine (*Pinus pinaster*). It is rich in condensed flavonoids and monomeric phenolic compounds, including catechin, epicatechin, taxifolin, and procyanidins, also called proanthocyanidins. Proanthocyanidins, as mentioned above (see Grape Seed Extract section), are potent free radical scavengers that can also be found in grape seed, grape skin, bilberry, cranberry, black currant, green tea, black tea, blueberry, blackberry, strawberry, black cherry, red wine, and red cabbage.[316] Pycnogenol is utilized as a nutritional supplement and a phytochemical remedy for various disorders, as it possesses potent antioxidant, anti-inflammatory, and anticarcinogenic properties.[317,318] A large body of literature on the free radical scavenging activity of pycnogenol exists.[319]

In an *in vitro* study in which the antioxidative effects of pycnogenol were again confirmed, researchers showed statistically significant antimutagenic properties with a correlation between the antioxidant and antimutagenic activities. They thus hypothesized that the antimutagenic effect of pycnogenol is most likely attributable to its antioxidant properties.[320] In humans it has been demonstrated that following oral supplementation with pycnogenol, the antioxidant capacity of plasma was significantly increased, as determined by ORAC.[321] The anticarcinogenic effect of pycnogenol was shown by topical application of 0.05–0.2% pycnogenol to the irradiated dorsal skin of Skh:hr hairless mice exposed daily to minimally inflammatory ssUVR. A reduction of the inflammatory sunburn reaction erythema and immunosuppression was observed. Further, tumor formation was delayed and prevalence reduced.[318] The potential of pycnogenol to confer photoprotection for humans has been investigated by Saliou et al. They showed in humans that by oral supplementation of pycnogenol the UV radiation level necessary to reach one MED was significantly elevated. They further suggested that inhibition of NF-κB-dependent gene expression by pycnogenol might contribute to the observed increase in MED.[322] Finally, pycnogenol exerts depigmenting effects, which are described in detail in Chapter 41. Thus, pycnogenol is a safe natural product included in various skincare products.

In 2012, Marini et al. performed a 12-week study to ascertain whether nutritional supplementation with Pycnogenol® could improve the cosmetic appearance of 20 healthy postmenopausal women. The skin condition of the volunteers was assessed before, during, and after supplementation using corneometry, cutometry, visioscan, and ultrasound analyses as well as biopsies and subsequent polymerase chain reaction (PCR) analyses. The investigators found that the well-tolerated supplementation improved skin hydration and elasticity. They also observed a significant increase in the mRNA expression of hyaluronic acid synthase (HAS)-1, an important enzyme involved in hyaluronic acid production, as well as marked increases in gene expression involved in collagen synthesis, to which the researchers ascribed the clinical improvements. The authors concluded that their results, including the first molecular evidence of the cutaneous benefits of improved hydration and elasticity, point to the potential for pycnogenol supplementation to mitigate the clinical signs of aging skin.[323] More recently, some of the same authors have reported that the oral consumption of pygnogenol provides photoprotection, diminishes hyperpigmentation, contributes to extracellular matrix homeostasis, and improves the function of the skin barrier.[324]

In 2017, Dogan et al. studied the effects of pygnogenol powder on wound healing in diabetic Sprague-Dawley rats, finding that collagen deposition and neovascularization were superior in wounds treated with pygnogenol as compared to cleanser (ethacridine lactate) and covered with silver sulfadiazine, and both reduced acute and chronic inflammation. The investigators concluded that pycnogenol presents potential as an agent to accelerate wound healing.[325] Further clinical studies are necessary to elucidate its efficacy when used in humans.

Dehydroepiandrosterone

Dehydroepiandrosterone (DHEA) is believed to be a powerful endogenous antioxidant.[326] However, its antioxidant abilities remain unproven. DHEA purportedly protects against aging and stimulates the immune system. The use of DHEA to combat aging is based on the fact that the secretion and blood levels of DHEA and its sulfate ester (DHEAS) decrease profoundly with age. Although the FDA noted in 1985 that the efficacy and safety of DHEA has never been confirmed, the agent continues to be sold over the counter and is discussed in many lay publications.

A study evaluating the safety of oral DHEA and its effects was published in April 2000.[327] In this double-blind, placebo-controlled study, 280 healthy individuals consumed 50 mg DHEA or placebo daily for a year. The subjects given DHEA had slightly elevated levels of testosterone and estradiol. Interestingly, the treated patients exhibited increases in sebum production, skin surface hydration, and epidermal thickness as well as decreased facial pigmentation. No harmful effects of DHEAS were noted. DHEA may protect cells from UV damage as well. A study by Coach et al. assessed whether pre-treatment of cells with various doses of DHEA could protect the cells from the damaging effects of UV radiation.[328] Cellular damage, cell counts, and cell morphology were evaluated. They found that the morphological evaluation of the cells treated with UV radiation showed an increase in degeneration of chromatin and a decrease in cell size as compared to non-treated groups, indicating that DHEA was efficient in protecting the cells from UV damage. Other reported effects of orally administered DHEA in healthy men include reduction of body fat, increase in muscle mass, and reduction of serum low-density lipoprotein cholesterol levels.[329]

A pilot study in 2008 included 20 postmenopausal women who applied topical DHEA (1%) or a vehicle for 4 months to facial and hand skin. The topical DHEA was shown to increase the rate of sebum production, which was well perceived by the patients.[330] Two years later, El-Alfy et al. conducted a placebo-controlled, randomized, prospective study in 75 postmenopausal women (from 60 to 65 years old) to assess cutaneous responses to topical DHEA treatment for 13 weeks. Patients received twice daily applications of 3.0 mL of placebo or 0.1%, 0.3%, 1%, or 2% DHEA cream on the face, arms, back of hands, upper chest, and right thigh. DHEA was found to have significantly increased androgen receptor expression as well as that of procollagen I and III mRNA. The investigators concluded that their results suggest the potential efficacy of topical DHEA as an anti-aging agent for the skin.[331]

Currently, DHEA is available in oral, injectable, and topical forms. It is important to understand that these products are considered nutritional supplements and are not regulated by the FDA. Further studies should be performed to evaluate the safety of DHEA and DHEAS before recommending their use.

Side Effects

DHEA is a relatively new product in the anti-aging armamentarium; therefore, little is known about the effects of long-term use. Endogenous DHEA concentrations peak at age 20–30 years. Consequently, the use of DHEA in those under age 35 may be risky. In fact, there has been a reported case of DHEA being suspected as a contributing factor in a manic episode of a young man.[332] The effects of long-term use of DHEA have not been studied.

Melatonin

Melatonin is a hormone secreted by the pineal gland; its discovery as a direct free radical scavenger is relatively recent. Besides its ability to directly neutralize various free radicals and reactive oxygen and nitrogen species, it stimulates several antioxidative enzymes including superoxide dismutase, GPX, and glutathione reductase. This increases its efficiency as an antioxidant.[333] Melatonin has been shown to markedly protect both membrane lipids and nuclear DNA from oxidative damage,[334] and has been demonstrated to reduce skin cancer formation in mice.[335] This may be due to its protective UV absorption effects.[336] Further, various studies in humans have revealed that topical melatonin reduces UV-induced erythema (sunburn).[337,338] However, controversial results were obtained in a small 2006 study with 16 subjects, with topical melatonin yielding no protection against immune suppression or sunburn.[339] With regard to photoprotection, melatonin has been shown to modulate the expression of apoptosis-related genes in UVB-irradiated HaCaT cells, resulting in increasing cell survival. This suggests that melatonin may be used as a sunscreen substance to reduce cell death of keratinocytes after excessive UVB irradiation.[340]

Melatonin is also used as a medication for sleep disturbance in depression and in people complaining of jet lag. It is currently available in an oral form and has also been added as an ingredient to various topical products, such as facial cleansers and moisturizers, eye creams, and skin lighteners. In recent years, melatonin has garnered attention in anti-aging medicine and dermatology because it has been found to exert potent antioxidant activity, particularly against hydroxyl radicals,[341,342] and melatonin levels are known to decline with age. In addition to its antioxidative and regulatory roles, including in seasonal reproduction control, melatonin is known to contribute to wound healing, modulating the immune system, and hindering inflammation.[343,344] Further, mounting evidence suggests its viability as an agent to prevent skin aging.[345] Topical application appears superior to oral administration for deriving cutaneous benefits because orally ingested melatonin is metabolized in the liver, yielding low levels in the blood and available to the skin.[345,346] Due to its potent lipophilicity, topical melatonin also can penetrate the stratum corneum and form a reservoir, from where it is continuously released to the rest of the skin and dermal vasculature potentially complementing and augmenting endogenous melatonin activity.[345,347,348]

Melatonin is an important hormone in the dermatologic realm insofar as it is known to inhibit UV-induced erythema, is implicated in skin functions such as hair growth, fur pigmentation/molting in various species, and melanoma control, and is thought to have potential in treating various human dermatoses (e.g., eczema, psoriasis, and malignant melanoma) as well as conditions such as androgenetic alopecia.[341,344,349] Notably, among the multiple plant species from which cutaneous applications are derived, feverfew is known to contain an appreciable level of melatonin.[350]

Androgenetic Alopecia

In 2012, Fischer et al. reported on one pharmacodynamic study and four clinical pre-post studies of topically applied melatonin to treat androgenetic alopecia. All five studies revealed significant reductions in hair loss seen in multiple tests all with good safety and tolerability. In a 3-month, multicenter (200 centers) study with over 1,800 participants—the largest of the five studies—the percentage of patients with a two- to three-fold positive hair-pull test decreased from 61.6 percent to 7.8 percent and those with a negative hair-pull test increased from 12.2 percent to 61.5 percent. Seborrheic dermatitis of the scalp declined significantly in these patients. The investigators concluded that topically applied cosmetic melatonin is a viable therapeutic choice for patients with androgenetic alopecia.[351]

Since then, Hatem et al. demonstrated in 2018 that melatonin combined with nanostructured lipid carriers displayed sustained release lasting six hours and yielded more clinically desirable outcomes in comparisons to melatonin solution in patients with androgenetic alopecia, increasing hair density and thickness and reducing hair loss.[352]

Antioxidant Activity

In 2013, Fischer et al. found that melatonin dose- and time-dependently protected against UVR-induced 8-hydroxy-2'-deoxyguanosine (8-OHdG) formation and antioxidant enzyme depletion (i.e., catalase, glutathione peroxidase, and superoxide dismutase) using *ex vivo* human full-thickness skin. They concluded that melatonin functioned as a robust antioxidant and protector of DNA against oxidative skin damage.[353] Previously, they had demonstrated that melatonin more potently scavenged UV-induced ROS in leukocytes than either vitamin C or the vitamin E analog trolox.[344,354]

Sierra et al. investigated the *in vivo* and *in vitro* protective effects of a melatonin-containing emulsion combined with UV filters against skin irradiation in 2013, finding sufficient physical stability and melatonin permeation in an emulsion with a mixture of three UV filters. The formulation exhibited significant radical scavenging activity and a photoprotective assay revealed that skin treated with the melatonin/UV filter formulation was statistically equivalent to nonirradiated control skin. The researchers concluded that melatonin was a strong antioxidant and activated endogenous enzymatic protection against oxidative stress.[355]

Human Studies

In one of the earliest studies of the effects of topically applied melatonin on UV-induced erythema, Bangha et al. led a double-blind, randomized study in 1996 with 20 healthy volunteers. Each subject was exposed to UVB (0.099 J/cm²) on the lower back and then treated with different concentrations of melatonin. The investigators observed a dose-response relationship between melatonin concentration and the degree of erythema, with significantly less redness appearing in the areas treated with 0.5% melatonin as compared to melatonin 0.05% or just the vehicle gel.[337]

The next year, Bangha et al. conducted another double-blind, randomized study in 20 volunteers to investigate the anti-erythema influence of topical melatonin and the role of the application time. Investigators treated small areas of the lower back with 0.6 mg/cm² melatonin 15 minutes before or 1, 30, or 240 minutes after simulated UVA and UVB irradiation at twice the individual MED. Post-treatment with melatonin delivered no protective effect but pre-treatment 15 minutes prior to irradiation yielded significant protective effects against erythema.[356] In a subsequent similar double-blind, randomized clinical trial with 20 healthy volunteers led by Fischer, the visual score indicated that melatonin application 15 minutes before irradiation significantly suppressed erythema as compared to vehicle control. Post-irradiation treatment with melatonin did not inhibit the effects of UV.[357]

In 1998, Dreher et al. conducted a randomized, double-blind study in 12 healthy adults (6 women and 6 men, all Caucasian, ranging from 29 to 49 years old) of the short-term photoprotective effects of topically applied melatonin as well as vitamins C and E, alone or in combination. Each formulation was applied 30 minutes after UV exposure. A dose-dependent photoprotective benefit was associated with melatonin, with modest effects observed with the vitamins alone. Photoprotection was clearly enhanced by the use of melatonin in combination with vitamins C and E. This is believed to be the first *in vivo* demonstration of a protective effect conferred by topical melatonin in combination with other antioxidants.[338] The next year, Dreher et al. assessed the short-term photoprotective effects of the same compounds in a randomized, double-blind, placebo-controlled human study. Each antioxidant was used alone or in combination after UV exposure in a single application (immediately or 30 minutes after UV exposure) or in multiple applications 30 minutes, one hour, and two hours after UV exposure (totaling three applications). No photoprotective effects were observed. The investigators concluded that given the speed of damage to skin from UV radiation, antioxidants likely must be applied at the appropriate site in sufficient concentrations at the outset of and during active oxidative insult.[358]

In 2004, Fischer et al. performed a clinical study in 15 healthy volunteers to consider the skin penetration activity of melatonin 0.01% in a cream and 0.01% and 0.03% in a solution. In a 24-hour time window, researchers collected blood samples for melatonin measurement before application at 9 AM as well as 1, 4, 8 and 24 hours after application. Pre-application serum melatonin levels ranged from 0.6 to 15.9 pg/mL. The mean serum value 24 hours after application of the 0.01% melatonin cream was 9.0 pg/mL. For the 0.01% solution group, the mean melatonin level was 12.7 pg/mL 24 hours after application. Melatonin levels also markedly rose just 1 and 8 hours after application in the 0.03% solution group, with cumulative melatonin recorded as 7.1 pg/mL in the 0.01% cream subjects, 8.6 pg/mL in the 0.01% solution participants, and 15.7 pg/mL in the 0.03% group. The investigators concluded that clearly lipophilic melatonin penetrates the skin with serum blood levels rising in a dose- and galenic-dependent manner without sparking increases above the physiological range.[347]

In 2012, Morganti et al. conducted a randomized, placebo-controlled, 12-week multicenter study with 70 healthy subjects to examine the combined activity of melatonin, vitamin E, and β-glucan complexed with chitin nano-crystals administered topically and orally. All skin parameters reviewed were significantly improved after treatment with the melatonin, vitamin E, β-glucan combination as compared to placebo, with better results observed when these ingredients were complexed with chitin nano-crystals. Specifically, the treatment diminished wrinkling and enhanced skin appearance.[359]

Four years later, Scheuer et al. conducted a randomized, placebo-controlled, double-blind study in 23 healthy volunteers (15 females, 8 males) to evaluate the protective effects of three doses of topical melatonin (0.5%, 2.5%, 12.5%) against erythema engendered by natural sunlight. The investigators observed a significant difference in erythema development between areas treated with 12.5% melatonin cream and those that received placebo or no treatment. They concluded that 12.5% melatonin cream protected against sun-induced erythema.[360]

Milani and Sparavigna reported in 2018 on their randomized, split-face, assessor-blinded proof-of-concept trial in which 22 women (mean age 55 years old) with moderate to severe cutaneous aging used day and night creams containing melatonin in liposomes (Nutriage day and night creams). Crow's feet were found to have been significantly reduced on the treated side after 3 months. Further, skin hydration and tonicity were markedly improved, with substantial diminishment in skin roughness seen. The researchers concluded that their results support the use of melatonin as a topical anti-aging agent.[361]

Summary

At the time of publication, the prevailing prediction is that melatonin, well established as a potent endogenous antioxidant, has a significant future role to play as a topical antioxidant agent against potential skin damage.[362-364]

Selenium

Selenium (Se) is an essential trace element found in Brazil nuts, kidney, shellfish, fish, and North American wheat. It is a frequent additive in anti-dandruff shampoos because it can inhibit proliferation of the yeast *Pityrosporum ovale*. The current RDA of selenium is 55 μg per day for both men and women. Selenium acts both as an antioxidant and anti-inflammatory agent. It is a component of the GPX family of enzymes, which break down peroxides. Therefore, it can deplete free radicals by reducing H_2O_2 and lipid and phospholipid hydroperoxides. Selenium can also reduce hydroperoxide intermediates in the cyclooxygenase and lipoxygenase pathways, thus resulting in a decrease in inflammation.[365] In addition, many studies have suggested that selenium confers an anticancer effect. Low levels of selenium have been associated with an increased incidence of cancer in several studies.[366] Selenium supplementation has been shown to prevent UVB-induced skin tumors in hairless mice.[367,368]

In addition to its antioxidant properties, the protective effects of selenium against skin cancer are enhanced because it prevents the production of inflammatory and immunosuppressive cytokines, which impair immune responses following UV exposure. In fact, selenium has been demonstrated to inhibit the UVB-induction of IL-6, IL-8, IL-10, and TNF-α in a dose-dependent manner.[369] Selenium has also been shown to boost both cellular and humoral immunity.[370] All of these actions work synergistically to give selenium its anticancer

properties. The anticancer activity was demonstrated in a large double-blind, placebo-controlled intervention trial that evaluated whether selenium supplementation could reduce the risk of cancer.[371] In this 1996 study, 1,312 individuals with a history of non-melanoma skin cancer were randomized to placebo or 200 μg selenium per day. Although there was no effect on the primary endpoint of non-melanoma skin cancer, those receiving selenium showed secondary endpoint effects of 50 percent lower total cancer mortality and 37 percent lower total cancer incidence with 63 percent fewer cancers of the prostate, 58 percent fewer cancers of the colon, and 46 percent fewer cancers of the lung.

Side Effects

The Institute of Medicine has set a tolerable upper intake level for selenium at 400 μg per day.[372] Selenium toxicity, or "selenosis," is associated with gastrointestinal upset, hair loss, white blotchy nails, and mild nerve damage.[373] Selenium and other antioxidants should always be taken as part of a balanced diet.[374] Otherwise, selenium can act as a pro-oxidant and cause DNA damage.[375]

CONCLUSION

Although there is much interest and enthusiasm regarding the use of antioxidants, there is a paucity of clinical trials examining the capacity of antioxidants to prevent or decelerate the aging of skin. One should remember that the theory behind the efficacy of these products is that they function by neutralizing free radicals, thus sparing the organs from the damage caused by these reactive oxygen species. There is no reason to believe that antioxidants treat already formed wrinkles unless it can occur by a different mechanism such as through increased collagen synthesis as seen with vitamin C. Current research suggests that combinations of various antioxidants might have synergistic effects and consequently more efficacy, as each antioxidant is endowed with various properties that distinguish it from other antioxidants.[16,376] Also, some data suggest a cumulative or additive benefit derived from using oral and topical antioxidant products in combination.[377,378] This has resulted in the entry of many antioxidant-containing beverages onto the market. It is unknown if these beverages help prevent aging and inflammation; however, they are harmless and may be beneficial. Further long-term studies in humans are needed to determine the efficacy of both the topical and oral products.

References

1. Harman D. Aging: a theory based on free radical and radiation chemistry. *J Gerontol.* 1956;11(3):298–300.
2. Pelle E, Maes D, Padulo GA, Kim EK, Smith WP. An in vitro model to test relative antioxidant potential: ultraviolet-induced lipid peroxidation in liposomes. *Arch Biochem Biophys.* 1990;283(2):234–240.
3. Werninghaus K. The role of antioxidants in reducing photodamage. In: Gilchrest B, ed. *Photodamage.* London: Blackwell Science Inc.; 1995: 249.

4. Greenstock CL. *Free Radicals, Aging, and Degenerative Diseases.* New York: Alan R. Liss, Inc.; 1986.

5. Rikans LE, Hornbrook KR. Lipid peroxidation, antioxidant protection and aging. *Biochim Biophys Acta.* 1997;1362(2-3): 116–127.

6. Black HS. Potential involvement of free radical reactions in ultraviolet light-mediated cutaneous damage. *Photochem Photobiol.* 1987;46(2):213–221.

7. Dhar A, Young MR, Colburn NH. The role of AP-1, NF-kappaB and ROS/NOS in skin carcinogenesis: the JB6 model is predictive. *Mol Cell Biochem.* 2002;234-235(1-2):185–193.

8. Kang S, Chung JH, Lee JH, et al. Topical N-acetyl cysteine and genistein prevent ultraviolet-light-induced signaling that leads to photoaging in human skin in vivo. *J Invest Dermatol.* 2003;120(5):835–841.

9. Fisher GJ, Wang ZQ, Datta SC, Varani J, Kang S, Voorhees JJ. Pathophysiology of premature skin aging induced by ultraviolet light. *N Engl J Med.* 1997;337(20):1419–1428.

10. Baumann L. Retinoids. In: *Cosmetic Dermatology: Principles & Practice.* New York: McGraw-Hill; 2002: 86–87.

11. Kim AL, Labasi JM, Zhu Y, et al. Role of p38 MAPK in UVB-induced inflammatory responses in the skin of SKH-1 hairless mice. *J Invest Dermatol.* 2005;124(6):1318–1325.

12. Shindo Y, Witt E, Han D, Epstein W, Packer L. Enzymic and non-enzymic antioxidants in epidermis and dermis of human skin. *J Invest Dermatol.* 1994;102(1):122–124.

13. Fuchs J, Huflejt ME, Rothfuss LM, Wilson DS, Carcamo G, Packer L. Acute effects of near ultraviolet and visible light on the cutaneous antioxidant defense system. *Photochem Photobiol.* 1989;50(6):739–744.

14. Fuchs J, Huflejt ME, Rothfuss LM, Wilson DS, Carcamo G, Packer L. Impairment of enzymic and nonenzymic antioxidants in skin by UVB irradiation. *J Invest Dermatol.* 1989;93(6):769–773.

15. Dreher F, Maibach H. Protective effects of topical antioxidants in humans. *Curr Probl Dermatol.* 2001;29:157–164.

16. Cho HS, Lee MH, Lee JW, et al. Anti-wrinkling effects of the mixture of vitamin C, vitamin E, pycnogenol and evening primrose oil, and molecular mechanisms on hairless mouse skin caused by chronic ultraviolet B irradiation. *Photodermatol Photoimmunol Photomed.* 2007;23(5):155–162.

17. Packer L, Colman C. *The Antioxidant Miracle.* New York: John Wiley & Sons, Inc.; 1999: 9.

18. Nachbar F, Korting HC. The role of vitamin E in normal and damaged skin. *J Mol Med (Berl).* 1995;73(1):7–17.

19. Halliwell B. The antioxidant paradox. *Lancet.* 2000;355(9210): 1179–1180.

20. Tanaka H, Okada T, Konishi H, Tsuji T. The effect of reactive oxygen species on the biosynthesis of collagen and glycosaminoglycans in cultured human dermal fibroblasts. *Arch Dermatol Res.* 1993;285(6):352–355.

21. Diplock AT, Xu GL, Yeow CL, Okikiola M. Relationship of tocopherol structure to biological activity, tissue uptake, and prostaglandin biosynthesis. *Ann N Y Acad Sci.* 1989;570:72–84.

22. Palmieri B, Gozzi G, Palmieri G. Vitamin E added silicone gel sheets for treatment of hypertrophic scars and keloids. *Int J Dermatol.* 1995;34(7):506–509.

23. Thiele JJ, Schroeter C, Hsieh SN, Podda M, Packer L. The antioxidant network of the stratum corneum. *Curr Probl Dermatol.* 2001;29:26–42.

24. Naidoo K, Birch-Machin MA. Oxidative stress and ageing: the influence of environmental pollution, sunlight and diet on skin. *Cosmetics.* 2017;4(1):4.

25. Knekt P, Aromaa A, Maatela J, Aaran RK, Nikkari T, Hakama M, et al. Vitamin E and cancer prevention. *Am J Clin Nutr.* 1991;53(1 Suppl):283S–286S.

26. Menkes MS, Comstock GW, Vuilleumier JP, Helsing KJ, Rider AA, Brookmeyer R. Serum beta-carotene, vitamins A and E, selenium, and the risk of lung cancer. *N Engl J Med.* 1986;315(20):1250–1254.

27. Chevance M, Brubacher G, Herbeth B, et al. Immunological and nutritional status among the elderly. In: Chandra RK, ed. *Nutrition, Immunity, and Illness in the Elderly.* New York: Pergamon Press; 1985: 137–142.

28. Darr D, Combs S, Dunston S, Manning T, Pinnell S. Topical vitamin C protects porcine skin from ultraviolet radiation-induced damage. *Br J Dermatol.* 1992;127(3):247–253.

29. Pathak MA, Carbonare MD. Photoaging and the role of mammalian skin superoxide dismutase and antioxidants. *Photochem Photobiol.* 1988;47:7S.

30. Pinnell SR, Murad S. Vitamin C and collagen metabolism. In: Kligman AM, Takase Y, eds. *Cutaneous Aging.* Tokyo: University of Tokyo Press; 1988: 275–292.

31. Bissett DL, Majeti S, Fu JJ, McBride JF, Wyder WE. Protective effect of topically applied conjugated hexadienes against ultraviolet radiation-induced chronic skin damage in the hairless mouse. *Photodermatol Photoimmunol Photomed.* 1990;7(2):63–67.

32. Gensler HL, Magdaleno M. Topical vitamin E inhibition of immunosuppression and tumorigenesis induced by ultraviolet irradiation. *Nutr Cancer.* 1991;15(2):97–106.

33. Jurkiewicz BA, Bissett DL, Buettner GR. Effect of topically applied tocopherol on ultraviolet radiation-mediated free radical damage in skin. *J Invest Dermatol.* 1995;104(4):484–488.

34. Slaga TJ, Bracken WM. The effects of antioxidants on skin tumor initiation and aryl hydrocarbon hydroxylase. *Cancer Res.* 1977;37(6):1631–1635.

35. Meydani SN, Barklund MP, Liu S, et al. Vitamin E supplementation enhances cell-mediated immunity in healthy elderly subjects. *Am J Clin Nutr.* 1990;52(3):557–563.

36. Trevithick JR, Xiong H, Lee S, et al. Topical tocopherol acetate reduces post-UVB, sunburn-associated erythema, edema, and skin sensitivity in hairless mice. *Arch Biochem Biophys.* 1992;296(2):575–582.

37. Bissett DL, Chatterjee R, Hannon DP. Photoprotective effect of superoxide-scavenging antioxidants against ultraviolet radiation-induced chronic skin damage in the hairless mouse. *Photodermatol Photoimmunol Photomed.* 1990;7(2):56–62.

38. Mayer P, Pittermann W, Wallat S. The effects of vitamin E on the skin. *Cosmet Toilet.* 1993;108(2):99–109.

39. Keller KL, Fenske NA. Uses of vitamins A, C, and E and related compounds in dermatology: a review. *J Am Acad Dermatol.* 1998;39(4 Pt 1):611–625.

40. Chung JH, Seo JY, Lee MK, et al. Ultraviolet modulation of human macrophage metalloelastase in human skin in vivo. *J Invest Dermatol.* 2002;119(2):507–512.

41. Werninghaus K, Meydani M, Bhawan J, Margolis R, Blumberg JB, Gilchrest BA. Evaluation of the photoprotective effect of oral vitamin E supplementation. *Arch Dermatol.* 1994;130(10):1257–1261.

42. Chan AC. Partners in defense, vitamin E and vitamin C. *Can J Physiol Pharmacol.* 1993;71(9):725–731.

43. Lin JY, Selim MA, Shea CR, et al. UV photoprotection by combination topical antioxidants vitamin C and vitamin E. *J Am Acad Dermatol.* 2003;48(6):866–874.

44. Murray JC, Burch JA, Streilein RD, Iannacchione MA, Hall RP, Pinnell SR. A topical antioxidant solution containing vitamins C and E stabilized by ferulic acid provides protection for human skin against damage caused by ultraviolet irradiation. *J Am Acad Dermatol.* 2008;59(3):418–425.

45. Thiele JJ, Hsieh SN, Ekanayake-Mudiyanselage S. Vitamin E: critical review of its current use in cosmetic and clinical dermatology. *Dermatol Surg.* 2005;31(7 Pt 2):805–813.

46. Martin A. The use of antioxidants in healing. *Dermatol Surg.* 1996;22(2):156–160.

47. Kamimura M, Matsuzawa T. Percutaneous absorption of alpha-tocopheryl acetate. *J Vitaminol (Kyoto).* 1968;14(2):150–159.

48. Pehr K, Forsey RR. Why don't we use vitamin E in dermatology? *CMAJ.* 1993;149(9):1247–1253.

49. Jenkins M, Alexander JW, MacMillan BG, Waymack JP, Kopcha R. Failure of topical steroids and vitamin E to reduce postoperative scar formation following reconstructive surgery. *J Burn Care Rehabil.* 1986 Jul;7(4):309–312.

50. Baumann LS, Spencer J. The effects of topical vitamin E on the cosmetic appearance of scars. *Dermatol Surg.* 1999;25(4):311–315.

51. Alberts DS, Goldman R, Xu MJ, et al. Disposition and metabolism of topically administered alpha-tocopherol acetate: a common ingredient of commercially available sunscreens and cosmetics. *Nutr Cancer.* 1996;26(2):193–201.

52. Gensler HL, Aickin M, Peng YM, Xu M. Importance of the form of topical vitamin E for prevention of photocarcinogenesis. *Nutr Cancer.* 1996;26(2):183–191.

53. Matsumura T, Nakada T, Iijima M. Widespread contact dermatitis from tocopherol acetate. *Contact Dermatitis.* 2004;51(4):211–212.

54. Oshima H, Tsuji K, Oh-I T, Koda M. Allergic contact dermatitis due to DL-alpha-tocopheryl nicotinate. *Contact Dermatitis.* 2003;48(3):167–168.

55. Perrenoud D, Homberger HP, Auderset PC, et al. An epidemic outbreak of papular and follicular contact dermatitis to tocopheryl linoleate in cosmetics. Swiss Contact Dermatitis Research Group. *Dermatology.* 1994;189(3):225–233.

56. Hunter D, Frumkin A. Adverse reactions to vitamin E and aloe vera preparations after dermabrasion and chemical peel. *Cutis.* 1991;47(3):193–196.

57. Bendich A, Machlin LJ. Safety of oral intake of vitamin E. *Am J Clin Nutr.* 1988;48(3):612–619.

58. Kappus H, Diplock AT. Tolerance and safety of vitamin E: a toxicological position report. *Free Radic Biol Med.* 1992;13(1):55–74.

59. Bendich A. Safety issues regarding the use of vitamin supplements. *Ann N Y Acad Sci.* 1992;669:300–310.

60. Petry JJ. Surgically significant nutritional supplements. *Plast Reconstr Surg.* 1996;97(1):233–240.

61. Dimery IW, Hong WK, Lee JJ, et al. Phase I trial of alpha-tocopherol effects on 13-cis-retinoic acid toxicity. *Ann Oncol.* 1997;8(1):85–89.

62. Strauss JS, Gottlieb AB, Jones T, et al. Concomitant administration of vitamin E does not change the side effects of isotretinoin as used in acne vulgaris: a randomized trial. *J Am Acad Dermatol.* 2000;43(5 Pt 1):777–784.

63. Ernster L, Dallner G. Biochemical, physiological and medical aspects of ubiquinone function. *Biochim Biophys Acta.* 1995;1271(1):195–204.

64. Greenberg S, Frishman WH. Co-enzyme Q10: a new drug for cardiovascular disease. *J Clin Pharmacol.* 1990;30(7):596–608.

65. Beyer R, Ernster L. The antioxidant role of Coenzyme Q10. In: Lenaz G, Barnabei O, Rabbi A, eds. *Highlights in Ubiquinone Research.* London: Taylor and Francis; 1990: 191–213.

66. Hoppe U, Bergemann J, Diembeck W, et al. Coenzyme Q10, a cutaneous antioxidant and energizer. *Biofactors.* 1999;9(2-4):371–378.

67. Ashida Y, Yamanishi H, Terada T, Oota N, Sekine K, Watabe K. CoQ10 supplementation elevates the epidermal CoQ10 level in adult hairless mice. *Biofactors.* 2005;25(1-4):175–178.

68. Tavintharan S, Ong CN, Jeyaseelan K, Sivakumar M, Lim SC, Sum CF. Reduced mitochondrial coenzyme Q10 levels in HepG2 cells treated with high-dose simvastatin: a possible role in statin-induced hepatotoxicity? *Toxicol Appl Pharmacol.* 2007;223(2):173–179.

69. Folkers K, Osterborg A, Nylander M, Morita M, Mellstedt H. Activities of vitamin Q10 in animal models and a serious deficiency in patients with cancer. *Biochem Biophys Res Commun.* 1997;234(2):296–299.

70. Rusciani L, Proietti I, Rusciani A, Paradisi A, Sbordoni G, Alfano C, et al. Low plasma coenzyme Q10 levels as an independent prognostic factor for melanoma progression. *J Am Acad Dermatol.* 2006;54(2):234–241.

71. Crane FL. Biochemical functions of coenzyme Q10. *J Am Coll Nutr.* 2001;20(6):591–598.

72. Beyer RE, Nordenbrand K, Ernster L. The role of coenzyme Q as a mitochondrial antioxidant: a short review. In: Folkers K, Yamamura Y, eds. *Biomedical and Clinical Aspects of Coenzyme Q.* Amsterdam, The Netherlands: Elsevier Science Publishers B V (Biomedical Division); 1986: 17–24.

73. Rusciani L, Proietti I, Paradisi A, et al. Recombinant interferon alpha-2b and coenzyme Q10 as a postsurgical adjuvant therapy for melanoma: a 3-year trial with recombinant interferon-alpha and 5-year follow-up. *Melanoma Res.* 2007;17(3):177–183.

74. Fuller B, Smith D, Howerton A, Kern D. Anti-inflammatory effects of CoQ10 and colorless carotenoids. *J Cosmet Dermatol.* 2006;5(1):30–38.

75. Zhang M, Dang L, Guo F, Wang X, Zhao W, Zhao R. Coenzyme Q(10) enhances dermal elastin expression, inhibits IL-1α production and melanin synthesis in vitro. *Int J Cosmet Sci.* 2012;34(3):273–279.

76. Blatt T, Mundt C, Mummert C, et al. Modulation of oxidative stresses in human aging skin. *Z Gerontol Geriatr.* 1999;32(2):83–88.

77. Lee WC, Tsai TH. Preparation and characterization of liposomal coenzyme Q10 for in vivo topical application. *Int J Pharm.* 2010;395(1-2):78–83.

78. Felippi CC, Oliveira D, Ströher A, et al. Safety and efficacy of antioxidants-loaded nanoparticles for an anti-aging application. *J Biomed Nanotechnol.* 2012;8(2):316–321.

79. Knott A, Achterberg V, Smuda C, et al. Topical treatment with coenzyme Q10-containing formulas improves skin's Q10 level and provides antioxidative effects. *Biofactors.* 2015;41(6):383–390.

80. Feigin A, Kieburtz K, Como P, et al. Assessment of coenzyme Q10 tolerability in Huntington's disease. *Mov Disord.* 1996;11(3):321–323.

81. McDaniel DH, Neudecker BA, DiNardo JC, Lewis JA2nd, Maibach HI. Idebenone: a new antioxidant - Part I. Relative assessment of oxidative stress protection capacity compared to commonly known antioxidants. *J Cosmet Dermatol.* 2005;4(1):10–17.

82. McDaniel DH, Neudecker BA, DiNardo JC, Lewis JA2nd, Maibach HI. Clinical efficacy assessment in photodamaged skin of 0.5% and 1.0% idebenone. *J Cosmet Dermatol.* 2005;4(3):167–173.

83. Montenegro L, Turnaturi R, Parenti C, Pasquinucci L. Idebenone: Novel Strategies to Improve Its Systemic and Local Efficacy. *Nanomaterials (Basel).* 2018;8(2):87.

84. Sasseville D, Moreau L, Al-Sowaidi M. Allergic contact dermatitis to idebenone used as an antioxidant in an anti-wrinkle cream. *Contact Dermatitis.* 2007;56(2):117–118.

85. Britton G. Structure and properties of carotenoids in relation to function. *FASEB J.* 1995;9(15):1551–1558.

86. Minhthy LN, Steven JS. Lycopene: chemical and biological properties. *Food Technol.* 1999;53(2):38–45.

87. Arab L, Steck S. Lycopene and cardiovascular disease. *Am J Clin Nutr.* 2000;71(6 Suppl):1691S–1695SS.

88. Chan JM, Gann PH, Giovannucci EL. Role of diet in prostate cancer development and progression. *J Clin Oncol.* 2005;23(32):8152–8160.

89. Willcox JK, Catignani GL, Lazarus S. Tomatoes and cardiovascular health. *Crit Rev Food Sci Nutr.* 2003;43(1):1–18.

90. Basu A, Imrhan V. Tomatoes versus lycopene in oxidative stress and carcinogenesis: conclusions from clinical trials. *Eur J Clin Nutr.* 2007;61(3):295–303.

91. Giovannucci E, Ascherio A, Rimm EB, Stampfer MJ, Colditz GA, Willett WC. Intake of carotenoids and retinol in relation to risk of prostate cancer. *J Natl Cancer Inst.* 1995;87(23):1767–1776.

92. Kim DJ, Takasuka N, Nishino H, Tsuda H. Chemoprevention of lung cancer by lycopene. *Biofactors.* 2000;13(1-4):95–102.

93. Narisawa T, Fukaura Y, Hasebe M, et al. Prevention of N-methylnitrosourea-induced colon carcinogenesis in F344 rats by lycopene and tomato juice rich in lycopene. *Jpn J Cancer Res.* 1998;89(10):1003–1008.

94. Nagasawa H, Mitamura T, Sakamoto S, Yamamoto K. Effects of lycopene on spontaneous mammary tumour development in SHN virgin mice. *Anticancer Res.* 1995;15(4):1173–1178.

95. Wu WB, Chiang HS, Fang JY, Hung CF. Inhibitory effect of lycopene on PDGF-BB-induced signalling and migration in human dermal fibroblasts: a possible target for cancer. *Biochem Soc Trans.* 2007;35(Pt 5):1377–1378.

96. Ahmad N, Gilliam AC, Katiyar SK, O'Brien TG, Mukhtar H. A definitive role of ornithine decarboxylase in photocarcinogenesis. *Am J Pathol.* 2001;159(3):885–892.

97. Fazekas Z, Gao D, Saladi RN, Lu Y, Lebwohl M, Wei H. Protective effects of lycopene against ultraviolet B-induced photodamage. *Nutr Cancer.* 2003;47(2):181–187.

98. Andreassi M, Stanghellini E, Ettorre A, Di Stefano A, Andreassi L. Antioxidant activity of topically applied lycopene. *J Eur Acad Dermatol Venereol.* 2004;18(1):52–55.

99. Cohly HH, Taylor A, Angel MF, Salahudeen AK. Effect of turmeric, turmerin and curcumin on H2O2-induced renal epithelial (LLC-PK1) cell injury. *Free Radic Biol Med.* 1998;24(1):49–54.

100. Ruby AJ, Kuttan G, Babu KD, Rajasekharan KN, Kuttan R. Anti-tumour and antioxidant activity of natural curcuminoids. *Cancer Lett.* 1995;94(1):79–83.

101. Maheshwari RK, Singh AK, Gaddipati J, Srimal RC. Multiple biological activities of curcumin: a short review. *Life Sci.* 2006;78(18):2081–2087.

102. Ammon HP, Wahl MA. Pharmacology of Curcuma longa. *Planta Med.* 1991;57(1):1–7.

103. Sharma OP. Antioxidant activity of curcumin and related compounds. *Biochem Pharmacol.* 1976;25(15):1811–1812.

104. Aggarwal BB, Kumar A, Bharti AC. Anticancer potential of curcumin: preclinical and clinical studies. *Anticancer Res.* 2003;23(1A):363–398.

105. Surh YJ, Han SS, Keum YS, Seo HJ, Lee SS. Inhibitory effects of curcumin and capsaicin on phorbol ester-induced activation of eukaryotic transcription factors, NF-kappaB and AP-1. *Biofactors.* 2000;12(1-4):107–112.

106. Kuttan R, Sudheeran PC, Josph CD. Turmeric and curcumin as topical agents in cancer therapy. *Tumori.* 1987;73(1):29–31.

107. Jagetia GC, Aggarwal BB. "Spicing up" of the immune system by curcumin. *J Clin Immunol.* 2007;27(1):19–35.

108. Conney AH, Lysz T, Ferraro T, et al. Inhibitory effect of curcumin and some related dietary compounds on tumor promotion and arachidonic acid metabolism in mouse skin. *Adv Enzyme Regul.* 1991;31:385–396.

109. Nakamura Y, Ohto Y, Murakami A, Osawa T, Ohigashi H. Inhibitory effects of curcumin and tetrahydrocurcuminoids on the tumor promoter-induced reactive oxygen species generation in leukocytes in vitro and in vivo. *Jpn J Cancer Res.* 1998;89(4):361–370.

110. Huang MT, Smart RC, Wong CQ, Conney AH. Inhibitory effect of curcumin, chlorogenic acid, caffeic acid, and ferulic acid on tumor promotion in mouse skin by 12-O-tetradecanoylphorbol-13-acetate. *Cancer Res.* 1988;48(21):5941–5946.

111. Cheng AL, Hsu CH, Lin JK, et al. Phase I clinical trial of curcumin, a chemopreventive agent, in patients with high-risk or pre-malignant lesions. *Anticancer Res.* 2001;21(4B):2895–2900.

112. Agrawal R, Kaur IP. Inhibitory effect of encapsulated curcumin on ultraviolet-induced photoaging in mice. *Rejuvenation Res.* 2010;13(4):397–410.

113. Heng MC. Signaling pathways targeted by curcumin in acute and chronic injury: burns and photo-damaged skin. *Int J Dermatol.* 2013;52(5):531–543.

114. Aggarwal BB, Harikumar KB. Potential therapeutic effects of curcumin, the anti-inflammatory agent, against neurodegenerative, cardiovascular, pulmonary, metabolic, autoimmune and neoplastic diseases. *Int J Biochem Cell Biol.* 2009;41(1):40–59.

115. Thongrakard V, Ruangrungsi N, Ekkapongpisit M, Isidoro C, Tencomnao T. Protection from UVB Toxicity in Human Keratinocytes by Thailand Native Herbs Extracts. *Photochem Photobiol.* 2014;90(1):214–224.

116. Sidhu GS, Singh AK, Thaloor D, et al. Enhancement of wound healing by curcumin in animals. *Wound Repair Regen.* 1998;6(2):167–177.

117. Sidhu GS, Mani H, Gaddipati JP, et al. Curcumin enhances wound healing in streptozotocin induced diabetic rats and genetically diabetic mice. *Wound Repair Regen.* 1999;7(5):362–374.

118. Thangapazham RL, Sharma A, Maheshwari RK. Beneficial role of curcumin in skin diseases. *Adv Exp Med Biol.* 2007;595:343–357.

119. Azuine MA, Bhide SV. Chemopreventive effect of turmeric against stomach and skin tumors induced by chemical carcinogens in Swiss mice. *Nutr Cancer.* 1992;17(1):77–83.

120. Huang MT, Lysz T, Ferraro T, Abidi TF, Laskin JD, Conney AH. Inhibitory effects of curcumin on in vitro lipoxygenase and cyclooxygenase activities in mouse epidermis. *Cancer Res.* 1991;51(3):813–819.

121. Limtrakul P, Lipigorngoson S, Namwong O, Apisariyakul A, Dunn FW. Inhibitory effect of dietary curcumin on skin carcinogenesis in mice. *Cancer Lett.* 1997;116(2):197–203.

122. Nagabhushan M, Bhide SV. Curcumin as an inhibitor of cancer. *J Am Coll Nutr.* 1992;11(2):192–198.

123. Bush JA, Cheung KJJr, Li G. Curcumin induces apoptosis in human melanoma cells through a Fas receptor/caspase-8 pathway independent of p53. *Exp Cell Res.* 2001;271(2):305–314.

124. Jee SH, Shen SC, Tseng CR, Chiu HC, Kuo ML. Curcumin induces a p53-dependent apoptosis in human basal cell carcinoma cells. *J Invest Dermatol.* 1998;111(4):656–661.

125. Chen J, Wanming D, Zhang D, Liu Q, Kang J. Water-soluble antioxidants improve the antioxidant and anticancer activity of low concentrations of curcumin in human leukemia cells. *Pharmazie.* 2005;60(1):57–61.

126. Hwang BM, Noh EM, Kim JS, et al. Curcumin inhibits UVB-induced matrix metalloproteinase-1/3 expression by suppressing the MAPK-p38/JNK pathways in human dermal fibroblasts. *Exp Dermatol.* 2013;22(5):371–374.

127. Vaughn AR, Branum A, Sivamani RK. Effects of Turmeric (Curcuma longa) on Skin Health: A Systematic Review of the Clinical Evidence. *Phytother Res.* 2016;30(8):1243–1264.

128. Vollono L, Falconi M, Gaziano R, et al. Potential of Curcumin in Skin Disorders. *Nutrients.* 2019;11(9):2169.

129. Hardman J, Limbird L, eds. *Goodman and Gilman's: The Pharmacological Basis of Therapeutics.* 9th ed. New York: McGraw-Hill; 1996: 1568–1672.

130. Shindo Y, Witt E, Han D, Packer L. Dose-response effects of acute ultraviolet irradiation on antioxidants and molecular markers of oxidation in murine epidermis and dermis. *J Invest Dermatol.* 1994;102(4):470–475.

131. Thiele JJ, Traber MG, Tsang K, Cross CE, Packer L. In vivo exposure to ozone depletes vitamins C and E and induces lipid peroxidation in epidermal layers of murine skin. *Free Radic Biol Med.* 1997;23(3):385–391.

132. Gey KF. Vitamins E plus C and interacting conutrients required for optimal health. A critical and constructive review of epidemiology and supplementation data regarding cardiovascular disease and cancer. *Biofactors.* 1998;7(1-2):113–174.

133. McLaren SM. Nutrition and wound healing. *J Wound Care.* 1992;1(3):45–55.

134. Kameyama K, Sakai C, Kondoh S, et al. Inhibitory effect of magnesium L-ascorbyl-2-phosphate (VC-PMG) on melanogenesis in vitro and in vivo. *J Am Acad Dermatol.* 1996;34(1):29–33.

135. Ash K, Lord J, Zukowski M, McDaniel DH. Comparison of topical therapy for striae alba (20% glycolic acid/0.05% tretinoin versus 20% glycolic acid/10% L-ascorbic acid). *Dermatol Surg.* 1998;24(8):849–856.

136. Alster TS, West TB. Effect of topical vitamin C on postoperative carbon dioxide laser resurfacing erythema. *Dermatol Surg.* 1998;24(3):331–334.

137. Scarpa M, Stevanato R, Viglino P, Rigo A. Superoxide ion as active intermediate in the autoxidation of ascorbate by molecular oxygen. Effect of superoxide dismutase. *J Biol Chem.* 1983;258(11):6695–6697.

138. Cabelli DE, Bielski BH. Kinetics and mechanism for the oxidation of ascorbic acid/ascorbate by HO_2/O_2^--(hydroperoxyl/superoxide) radicals. A pulse radiolysis and stopped-flow photolysis study. *J Phys Chem.* 1983;87(10):1809–1812.

139. Miyake N, Kim M, Kurata T. Stabilization of L-ascorbic acid by superoxide dismutase and catalase. *Biosci Biotechnol Biochem.* 1999;63(1):54–57.

140. Tu YJ, Njus D, Schlegel HB. A theoretical study of ascorbic acid oxidation and $HOO^•/O_2^{•-}$ radical scavenging. *Org Biomol Chem.* 2017;15(20):4417–4431.

141. Dunham WB, Zuckerkandl E, Reynolds R, et al. Effects of intake of L-ascorbic acid on the incidence of dermal neoplasms induced in mice by ultraviolet light. *Proc Natl Acad Sci U S A.* 1982;79(23):7532–7536.

142. Darr D, Dunston S, Faust H, Pinnell S. Effectiveness of antioxidants (vitamin C and E) with and without sunscreens as topical photoprotectants. *Acta Derm Venereol.* 1996;76(4):264–268.

143. Werninghaus K. The role of antioxidants in reducing photodamage. In: Gilchrest B, ed. *Photodamage.* London: Blackwell Science Inc.; 1995: 249–258.

144. Xu TH, Chen JZ, Li YH, et al. Split-face study of topical 23.8% L-ascorbic acid serum in treating photo-aged skin. *J Drugs Dermatol.* 2012;11(1):51–56.

145. Taniguchi M, Arai N, Kohno K, Ushio S, Fukuda S. Antioxidative and anti-aging activities of 2-O-α-glucopyranosyl-L-ascorbic acid on human dermal fibroblasts. *Eur J Pharmacol.* 2012;674(2-3):126–131.

146. Kivirikko KI, Myllylä R. Post-translational processing of procollagens. *Ann N Y Acad Sci.* 1985;460:187–201.

147. Uitto J, Hoffmann H-P, Prockop DJ. Synthesis of elastin and procallagen by cells from embryonic aorta. Differences in the role of hydroxyproline and the effects of proline analogs on the secretion of the two proteins. *Arch Biochem Biophys.* 1976;173(1):187–200.

148. Geesin JC, Darr D, Kaufman R, Murad S, Pinnell SR. Ascorbic acid specifically increases type I and type III procollagen messenger RNA levels in human skin fibroblast. *J Invest Dermatol.* 1988;90(4):420–424.

149. Davidson JM, LuValle PA, Zoia O, Quaglino DJr, Giro M. Ascorbate differentially regulates elastin and collagen biosynthesis in vascular smooth muscle cells and skin fibroblasts by pretranslational mechanisms. *J Biol Chem.* 1997;272(1):345–352.

150. Scott-Burden T, Davies PJ, Gevers W. Elastin biosynthesis by smooth muscle cells cultured under scorbutic conditions. *Biochem Biophys Res Commun.* 1979;91(3):739–746.

151. Bergethon PR, Mogayzel PJJr, Franzblau C. Effect of the reducing environment on the accumulation of elastin and collagen in cultured smooth-muscle cells. *Biochem J.* 1989;258(1):279–284.

152. Traikovich SS. Use of topical ascorbic acid and its effects on photodamaged skin topography. *Arch Otolaryngol Head Neck Surg.* 1999;125(10):1091–1098.

153. Humbert PG, Haftek M, Creidi P, et al. Topical ascorbic acid on photoaged skin. Clinical, topographical and ultrastructural evaluation: double-blind study vs. placebo. *Exp Dermatol.* 2003;12(3):237–244.

154. Colven RM, Pinnell SR. Topical vitamin C in aging. *Clin Dermatol*. 1996;14(2):227–234.

155. Perricone NV. The photoprotective and anti-inflammatory effects of topical ascorbyl palmitate. *J Geriatric Derm*. 1993;1:5.

156. Darr D, Pinnell S. U. S. Patent no. 5,140,043, 1992.

157. Pullar JM, Carr AC, Vissers MCM. The Roles of Vitamin C in Skin Health. *Nutrients*. 2017;9(8):866.

158. Al-Niaimi F, Chiang NYZ. Topical vitamin C and the skin: mechanisms of action and clinical applications. *J Clin Aesthet Dermatol*. 2017;10(7):14–17.

159. Maeda K, Fukuda M. Arbutin: mechanism of its depigmenting action in human melanocyte culture. *J Pharmacol Exp Ther*. 1996;276(2):765–769.

160. Searle T, Al-Niaimi F, Ali FR. The top 10 cosmeceuticals for facial hyperpigmentation. *Dermatol Ther*. 2020;33(6):e14095.

161. Kim J, Kim J, Lee YI, Almurayshid A, Jung JY, Lee JH. Effect of a topical antioxidant serum containing vitamin C, vitamin E, and ferulic acid after Q-switched 1064-nm Nd:YAG laser for treatment of environment-induced skin pigmentation. *J Cosmet Dermatol*. 2020;19(10):2576–2582.

162. Ud-Din S, McGeorge D, Bayat A. Topical management of striae distensae (stretch marks): prevention and therapy of striae rubrae and albae. *J Eur Acad Dermatol Venereol*. 2016;30(2):211–222.

163. Hsu S. Green tea and the skin. *J Am Acad Dermatol*. 2005;52(6):1049–1059.

164. Katiyar SK, Ahmad N, Mukhtar H. Green tea and skin. *Arch Dermatol*. 2000;136(8):989–994.

165. Katiyar SK, Elmets CA, Agarwal R, Mukhtar H. Protection against ultraviolet-B radiation-induced local and systemic suppression of contact hypersensitivity and edema responses in C3H/HeN mice by green tea polyphenols. *Photochem Photobiol*. 1995;62(5):855–861.

166. Reuter J, Merfort I, Schempp CM. Botanicals in dermatology: an evidence-based review. *Am J Clin Dermatol*. 2010;11(4):247–267.

167. Shi X, Ye J, Leonard SS, et al. Antioxidant properties of (-)-epicatechin-3-gallate and its inhibition of Cr(VI)-induced DNA damage and Cr(IV)- or TPA-stimulated NF-kappaB activation. *Mol Cell Biochem*. 2000;206(1-2):125–132.

168. Wei H, Zhang X, Zhao JF, Wang ZY, Bickers D, Lebwohl M. Scavenging of hydrogen peroxide and inhibition of ultraviolet light-induced oxidative DNA damage by aqueous extracts from green and black teas. *Free Radic Biol Med*. 1999;26(11-12):1427–1435.

169. Wang ZY, Agarwal R, Bickers DR, Mukhtar H. Protection against ultraviolet B radiation-induced photocarcinogenesis in hairless mice by green tea polyphenols. *Carcinogenesis*. 1991;12(8):1527–1530.

170. Gensler HL, Timmermann BN, Valcic S, et al. Prevention of photocarcinogenesis by topical administration of pure epigallocatechin gallate isolated from green tea. *Nutr Cancer*. 1996;26(3):325–335.

171. Khan WA, Wang ZY, Athar M, Bickers DR, Mukhtar H. Inhibition of the skin tumorigenicity of (+/-)-7 beta,8 alpha-dihydroxy-9 alpha,10 alpha-epoxy-7,8,9,10-tetrahydrobenzo[a]pyrene by tannic acid, green tea polyphenols and quercetin in Sencar mice. *Cancer Lett*. 1988;42(1-2):7–12.

172. Mittal A, Piyathilake C, Hara Y, Katiyar SK. Exceptionally high protection of photocarcinogenesis by topical application of (--)-epigallocatechin-3-gallate in hydrophilic cream in SKH-1 hairless mouse model: relationship to inhibition of UVB-induced global DNA hypomethylation. *Neoplasia*. 2003;5(6):555–565.

173. Elmets CA, Singh D, Tubesing K, Matsui M, Katiyar S, Mukhtar H. Cutaneous photoprotection from ultraviolet injury by green tea polyphenols. *J Am Acad Dermatol*. 2001;44(3):425–432.

174. Katiyar SK. Green tea prevents non-melanoma skin cancer by enhancing DNA repair. *Arch Biochem Biophys*. 2011;508(2):152–158.

175. Katiyar SK, Vaid M, van Steeg H, Meeran SM. Green tea polyphenols prevent UV-induced immunosuppression by rapid repair of DNA damage and enhancement of nucleotide excision repair genes. *Cancer Prev Res (Phila)*. 2010;3(2):179–189.

176. Stratton SP, Dorr RT, Alberts DS. The state-of-the-art in chemoprevention of skin cancer. *Eur J Cancer*. 2000;36(10):1292–1297.

177. Chung JH, Han JH, Hwang EJ, , et al. Dual mechanisms of green tea extract (EGCG)-induced cell survival in human epidermal keratinocytes. *FASEB J*. 2003;17(13):1913–1915.

178. Katiyar SK, Challa A, McCormick TS, Cooper KD, Mukhtar H. Prevention of UVB-induced immunosuppression in mice by the green tea polyphenol (-)-epigallocatechin-3-gallate may be associated with alterations in IL-10 and IL-12 production. *Carcinogenesis*. 1999;20(11):2117–2124.

179. Meeran SM, Mantena SK, Katiyar SK. Prevention of ultraviolet radiation-induced immunosuppression by (-)-epigallocatechin-3-gallate in mice is mediated through interleukin 12-dependent DNA repair. *Clin Cancer Res*. 2006;12(7 Pt 1):2272–2280.

180. Katiyar SK, Bergamo BM, Vyalil PK, Elmets CA. Green tea polyphenols: DNA photodamage and photoimmunology. *J Photochem Photobiol B*. 2001;65(2-3):109–114.

181. Vayalil PK, Mittal A, Hara Y, Elmets CA, Katiyar SK. Green tea polyphenols prevent ultraviolet light-induced oxidative damage and matrix metalloproteinases expression in mouse skin. *J Invest Dermatol*. 2004;122(6):1480–1487.

182. Pazyar N, Feily A, Kazerouni A. Green tea in dermatology. *Skinmed*. 2012;10(6):352–355.

183. Tzellos TG, Sardeli C, Lallas A, Papazisis G, Chourdakis M, Kouvelas D. Efficacy, safety and tolerability of green tea catechins in the treatment of external anogenital warts: a systematic review and meta-analysis. *J Eur Acad Dermatol Venereol*. 2011;25(3):345–353.

184. Hong YH, Jung EY, Shin KS, Yu KW, Chang UJ, Suh HJ. Tannase-converted green tea catechins and their anti-wrinkle activity in humans. *J Cosmet Dermatol*. 2013;12(2):137–143.

185. Gianeti MD, Mercurio DG, Campos PM. The use of green tea extract in cosmetic formulations: not only an antioxidant active ingredient. *Dermatol Ther*. 2013;26(3):267–271.

186. Mahmood T, Akhtar N, Khan BA, Shoaib Khan HM, Saeed T. Changes in skin mechanical properties after long-term application of cream containing green tea extract. *Aging Clin Exp Res*. 2011;23(5-6):333–336.

187. Mahmood T, Akhtar N. Combined topical application of lotus and green tea improves facial skin surface parameters. *Rejuvenation Res*. 2013;16(2):91–97.

188. Zink A, Traidl-Hoffmann C. Green tea in dermatology--myths and facts. *J Dtsch Dermatol Ges*. 2015;13(8):768–775.

189. Svobodová A, Psotová J, Walterová D. Natural phenolics in the prevention of UV-induced skin damage. A review. *Biomed Pap Med Fac Univ Palacky Olomouc Czech Repub*. 2003;147(2):137–145.

190. Krausz A, Gunn H, Friedman A. The basic science of natural ingredients. *J Drugs Dermatol*. 2014;13(8):937–943.

191. Dhanalakshmi S, Mallikarjuna GU, Singh RP, Agarwal R. Silibinin prevents ultraviolet radiation-caused skin damages in SKH-1 hairless mice via a decrease in thymine dimer positive cells and an up-regulation of p53-p21/Cip1 in epidermis. *Carcinogenesis.* 2004;25(8):1459–1465.

192. Dhanalakshmi S, Mallikarjuna GU, Singh RP, Agarwal R. Dual efficacy of silibinin in protecting or enhancing ultraviolet B radiation-caused apoptosis in HaCaT human immortalized keratinocytes. *Carcinogenesis.* 2004;25(1):99–106.

193. Gupta S, Mukhtar H. Chemoprevention of skin cancer through natural agents. *Skin Pharmacol Appl Skin Physiol.* 2001;14(6):373–385.

194. Afaq F, Adhami VM, Ahmad N, Mukhtar H. Botanical antioxidants for chemoprevention of photocarcinogenesis. *Front Biosci.* 2002;7:d784–d792.

195. Singh RP, Agarwal R. Flavonoid antioxidant silymarin and skin cancer. *Antioxid Redox Signal.* 2002;4(4):655–663.

196. Katiyar SK. Treatment of silymarin, a plant flavonoid, prevents ultraviolet light-induced immune suppression and oxidative stress in mouse skin. *Int J Oncol.* 2002;21(6):1213–1222.

197. He H, Li A, Li S, Tang J, Li L, Xiong L. Natural components in sunscreens: Topical formulations with sun protection factor (SPF). *Biomed Pharmacother.* 2021;134:111161.

198. Vostálová J, Tinková E, Biedermann D, Kosina P, Ulrichová J, Rajnochová Svobodová A. Skin Protective Activity of Silymarin and its Flavonolignans. *Molecules.* 2019;24(6):1022.

199. Netto MPharm G, Jose J. Development, characterization, and evaluation of sunscreen cream containing solid lipid nanoparticles of silymarin. *J Cosmet Dermatol.* 2018;17(6):1073–1083.

200. Berardesca E, Cameli N, Cavallotti C, Levy JL, Piérard GE, de Paoli Ambrosi G. Combined effects of silymarin and methylsulfonylmethane in the management of rosacea: clinical and instrumental evaluation. *J Cosmet Dermatol.* 2008;7(1):8–14.

201. Charurin P, Ames JM, del Castillo MD. Antioxidant activity of coffee model systems. *J Agric Food Chem.* 2002;50(13):3751–3756.

202. Farris P. Idebenone, green tea, and Coffeeberry extract: new and innovative antioxidants. *Dermatol Ther.* 2007;20(5):322–329.

203. Chen D, Milacic V, Chen MS, et al. Tea polyphenols, their biological effects and potential molecular targets. *Histol Histopathol.* 2008;23(4):487–496.

204. Halder B, Bhattacharya U, Mukhopadhyay S, Giri AK. Molecular mechanism of black tea polyphenols induced apoptosis in human skin cancer cells: involvement of Bax translocation and mitochondria mediated death cascade. *Carcinogenesis.* 2008;29(1):129–138.

205. Velazquez Pereda Mdel C, Dieamant Gde C, Eberlin S, et al. Effect of green Coffea arabica L. seed oil on extracellular matrix components and water-channel expression in in vitro and ex vivo human skin models. *J Cosmet Dermatol.* 2009;8(1):56–62.

206. Chiang HM, Lin TJ, Chiu CY, et al. Coffea arabica extract and its constituents prevent photoaging by suppressing MMPs expression and MAP kinase pathway. *Food Chem Toxicol.* 2011;49(1):309–318.

207. Draelos Z. A double-blind, randomized clinical trial evaluating the dermatologic benefits of coffee berry extract. *J Am Acad Dermatol.* 2008;58(Suppl 2):AB64.

208. Draelos ZD. Optimal skin care for aesthetic patients: topical products to restore and maintain healthy skin. *Cosmet Dermatol.* 2009;22(3):S1.

209. McDaniel DH. Clinical safety and efficacy in photoaged skin with coffeeberry extract, a natural antioxidant. *Cosmet Dermatol.* 2009;22(12):610–616.

210. Palmer DM, Kitchin JS. A double-blind, randomized, controlled clinical trial evaluating the efficacy and tolerance of a novel phenolic antioxidant skin care system containing Coffea arabica and concentrated fruit and vegetable extracts. *J Drugs Dermatol.* 2010;9(12):1480–1487.

211. Leyden JJ, Shergill B, Micali G, Downie J, Wallo W. Natural options for the management of hyperpigmentation. *J Eur Acad Dermatol Venereol.* 2011;25(10):1140–1145.

212. Hexsel D, Orlandi C, Zechmeister do Prado D. Botanical extracts used in the treatment of cellulite. *Dermatol Surg.* 2005;31(7 Pt 2):866–872.

213. Berson DS. *Natural antioxidants. J Drugs Dermatol.* 2008;7(7 Suppl):s7–s12.

214. Garcia F, Pivel JP, Guerrero A, et al. Phenolic components and antioxidant activity of Fernblock, an aqueous extract of the aerial parts of the fern Polypodium leucotomos. *Methods Find Exp Clin Pharmacol.* 2006;28(3):157–160.

215. Brieva A, Guerrero A, Pivel JP. Immunomodulatory properties of a hydrophilic extract of Polypodium leucotomos. *Inflammopharmacology.* 2001;9(4):361–371.

216. Alcaraz MV, Pathak MA, Rius F, Kollias N, González S. An extract of Polypodium leucotomos appears to minimize certain photoaging changes in a hairless albino mouse animal model. A pilot study. *Photodermatol Photoimmunol Photomed.* 1999;15(3-4):120–126.

217. González S, Pathak MA, Cuevas J, Villarrubia VG, Fitzpatrick TB. Topical or oral administration with an extract of Polypodium leucotomos prevents acute sunburn and psoralen-induced phototoxic reactions as well as depletion of Langerhans cells in human skin. *Photodermatol Photoimmunol Photomed.* 1997;13(1-2):50–60.

218. González S, Pathak MA. Inhibition of ultraviolet-induced formation of reactive oxygen species, lipid peroxidation, erythema and skin photosensitization by polypodium leucotomos. *Photodermatol Photoimmunol Photomed.* 1996;12(2):45–56.

219. Gomes AJ, Lunardi CN, Gonzalez S, Tedesco AC. The antioxidant action of Polypodium leucotomos extract and kojic acid: reactions with reactive oxygen species. *Braz J Med Biol Res.* 2001;34(11):1487–1494.

220. González S, Alonso-Lebrero JL, Del Rio R, Jaen P. Polypodium leucotomos extract: a nutraceutical with photoprotective properties. *Drugs Today (Barc).* 2007;43(7):475–485.

221. Middelkamp-Hup MA, Pathak MA, Parrado C, et al. Orally administered Polypodium leucotomos extract decreases psoralen-UVA-induced phototoxicity, pigmentation, and damage of human skin. *J Am Acad Dermatol.* 2004;50(1):41–49.

222. Middelkamp-Hup MA, Pathak MA, Parrado C, et al. Oral Polypodium leucotomos extract decreases ultraviolet-induced damage of human skin. *J Am Acad Dermatol.* 2004;51(6):910–918.

223. Caccialanza M, Percivalle S, Piccinno R, Brambilla R. Photoprotective activity of oral polypodium leucotomos extract in 25 patients with idiopathic photodermatoses. *Photodermatol Photoimmunol Photomed.* 2007;23(1):46–47.

224. Jańczyk A, Garcia-Lopez MA, Fernandez-Peñas P, et al. A Polypodium leucotomos extract inhibits solar-simulated radiation-induced TNF-alpha and iNOS expression, transcriptional activation and apoptosis. *Exp Dermatol.* 2007;16(10):823–829.

225. Alonso-Lebrero JL, Domínguez-Jiménez C, Tejedor R, Brieva A, Pivel JP. Photoprotective properties of a hydrophilic extract of the fern Polypodium leucotomos on human skin cells. *J Photochem Photobiol B*. 2003;70(1):31–37.

226. Philips N, Smith J, Keller T, Gonzalez S. Predominant effects of Polypodium leucotomos on membrane integrity, lipid peroxidation, and expression of elastin and matrixmetalloproteinase-1 in ultraviolet radiation exposed fibroblasts, and keratinocytes. *J Dermatol Sci*. 2003;32(1):1–9.

227. Capote R, Alonso-Lebrero JL, García F, Brieva A, Pivel JP, González S. Polypodium leucotomos extract inhibits trans-urocanic acid photoisomerization and photodecomposition. *J Photochem Photobiol B*. 2006;82(3):173–179.

228. Parrado C, Nicolas J, Juarranz A, Gonzalez S. The role of the aqueous extract Polypodium leucotomos in photoprotection. *Photochem Photobiol Sci*. 2020 May 20. [Online ahead of print.]

229. Parrado C, Mascaraque M, Gilaberte Y, Juarranz A, Gonzalez S. Fernblock (Polypodium leucotomos Extract): Molecular Mechanisms and Pleiotropic Effects in Light-Related Skin Conditions, Photoaging and Skin Cancers, a Review. *Int J Mol Sci*. 2016;17(7):1026.

230. Jang M, Cai L, Udeani GO, et al. Cancer chemopreventive activity of resveratrol, a natural product derived from grapes. *Science*. 1997;275(5297):218–220.

231. Ratz-Łyko A, Arct J. Resveratrol as an active ingredient for cosmetic and dermatological applications: a review. *J Cosmet Laser Ther*. 2019;21(2):84–90.

232. Afaq F, Adhami VM, Ahmad N. Prevention of short-term ultraviolet B radiation-mediated damages by resveratrol in SKH-1 hairless mice. *Toxicol Appl Pharmacol*. 2003;186(1):28–37.

233. Adhami VM, Afaq F, Ahmad N. Suppression of ultraviolet B exposure-mediated activation of NF-kappaB in normal human keratinocytes by resveratrol. *Neoplasia*. 2003;5(1):74–82.

234. Ding XZ, Adrian TE. Resveratrol inhibits proliferation and induces apoptosis in human pancreatic cancer cells. *Pancreas*. 2002;25(4):e71–e76.

235. Athar M, Back JH, Tang X, et al. Resveratrol: a review of preclinical studies for human cancer prevention. *Toxicol Appl Pharmacol*. 2007;224(3):274–283.

236. Delmas D, Rébé C, Lacour S, et al. Resveratrol-induced apoptosis is associated with Fas redistribution in the rafts and the formation of a death-inducing signaling complex in colon cancer cells. *J Biol Chem*. 2003 Oct;278(42):41482–41490.

237. Aziz MH, Afaq F, Ahmad N. Prevention of ultraviolet-B radiation damage by resveratrol in mouse skin is mediated via modulation in survivin. *Photochem Photobiol*. 2005;81(1):25–31.

238. Aziz MH, Reagan-Shaw S, Wu J, Longley BJ, Ahmad N. Chemoprevention of skin cancer by grape constituent resveratrol: relevance to human disease? *FASEB J*. 2005;19(9):1193–1195.

239. Reagan-Shaw S, Afaq F, Aziz MH, Ahmad N. Modulations of critical cell cycle regulatory events during chemoprevention of ultraviolet B-mediated responses by resveratrol in SKH-1 hairless mouse skin. *Oncogene*. 2004;23(30):5151–5160.

240. Reagan-Shaw S, Mukhtar H, Ahmad N. Resveratrol imparts photoprotection of normal cells and enhances the efficacy of radiation therapy in cancer cells. *Photochem Photobiol*. 2008;84(2):415–421.

241. Nichols JA, Katiyar SK. Skin photoprotection by natural polyphenols: anti-inflammatory, antioxidant and DNA repair mechanisms. *Arch Dermatol Res*. 2010;302(2):71–83.

242. Ferzli G, Patel M, Phrsai N, Brody N. Reduction of facial redness with resveratrol added to topical product containing green tea polyphenols and caffeine. *J Drugs Dermatol*. 2013;12(7):770–774.

243. Baxter RA. Anti-aging properties of resveratrol: review and report of a potent new antioxidant skin care formulation. *J Cosmet Dermatol*. 2008;7(1):2–7.

244. McDaniel DH, Neudecker BA, DiNardo JC, Lewis JA2nd, Maibach HI. Idebenone: a new antioxidant – Part I. Relative assessment of oxidative stress protection capacity compared to commonly known antioxidants. *J Cosmet Dermatol*. 2005;4(1):10–17.

245. Giardina S, Michelotti A, Zavattini G, Finzi S, Ghisalberti C, Marzatico F. Efficacy study in vitro: assessment of the properties of resveratrol and resveratrol + N-acetyl-cysteine on proliferation and inhibition of collagen activity. *Minerva Ginecol*. 2010;62(3):195–201.

246. Wu Y, Jia LL, Zheng YN, et al. Resveratrate protects human skin from damage due to repetitive ultraviolet irradiation. *J Eur Acad Dermatol Venereol*. 2013;27(3):345–350.

247. Waterhouse AL, Walzem RL. Nutrition of grape phenolics. In: Rice-Evans CA, Packer L, eds. *Flavonoids in Health and Disease*. New York: Marcel Dekker; 1998: 359–385.

248. Carando S, Teissedre P-L. Catechin and procyanidin levels in French wines: contribution to dietary intake. In: Gross GG, Hemingway RW, Yoshida T, eds. *Plant Polyphenols 2: Chemistry, Biology, Pharmacology, Ecology*. New York: Kluwer Academic/Plenum Publishers; 1999: 725–737.

249. Bagchi D, Garg A, Krohn RL, Bagchi M, Tran MX, Stohs SJ. Oxygen free radical scavenging abilities of vitamins C and E, and a grape seed proanthocyanidin extract in vitro. *Res Commun Mol Pathol Pharmacol*. 1997;95(2):179–189.

250. Ariga T, Hamano M. Radical scavenging action and its mode in procyanidins B-1 and B-3 from azuki beans to peroxyl radicals. *Agric Biol Chem*. 1990;54(10):2499–2504.

251. Maffei Facino R, Carini M, Aldini G, Bombardelli E, Morazzoni P, Morelli R. Free radicals scavenging action and anti-enzyme activities of procyanidines from Vitis vinifera. A mechanism for their capillary protective action. *Arzneimittelforschung*. 1994;44(5):592–601.

252. Da Silva JM, Darmon N, Fernandez Y, Mitjavila S Oxygen free radical scavenger capacity in aqueous models of different procyanidins from grape seeds. *J Agric Food Chem*. 1991;39(9):1549–1552.

253. Vinson JA, Dabbagh YA, Serry MM, Jang J. Plant flavonoids, especially tea flavonols, are powerful antioxidants using an in vitro oxidation model for heart disease. *J Agric Food Chem*. 1995;43(11):2800–2802.

254. Koga T, Moro K, Nakamori K, et al. Increase of antioxidative potential of rat plasma by oral administration of proanthocyanidin-rich extract from grape seeds. *J Agric Food Chem*. 1999;47(5):1892–1897.

255. Bagchi D, Bagchi M, Stohs SJ, et al. Free radicals and grape seed proanthocyanidin extract: importance in human health and disease prevention. *Toxicology*. 2000;148(2-3):187–197.

256. Mittal A, Elmets CA, Katiyar SK. Dietary feeding of proanthocyanidins from grape seeds prevents photocarcinogenesis in SKH-1 hairless mice: relationship to decreased fat and lipid peroxidation. *Carcinogenesis*. 2003;24(8):1379–1388.

257. Mantena SK, Katiyar SK. Grape seed proanthocyanidins inhibit UV-radiation-induced oxidative stress and activation of MAPK

and NF-kappaB signaling in human epidermal keratinocytes. *Free Radic Biol Med.* 2006;40(9):1603–1614.

258. Sharma SD, Meeran SM, Katiyar SK. Dietary grape seed proanthocyanidins inhibit UVB-induced oxidative stress and activation of mitogen-activated protein kinases and nuclear factor-kappaB signaling in in vivo SKH-1 hairless mice. *Mol Cancer Ther.* 2007;6(3):995–1005.

259. Sharma SD, Katiyar SK. Dietary grape-seed proanthocyanidin inhibition of ultraviolet B-induced immune suppression is associated with induction of IL-12. *Carcinogenesis.* 2006;27(1):95–102.

260. Yarovaya L, Waranuch N, Wisuitiprot W, Khunkitti W. Effect of grape seed extract on skin fibroblasts exposed to UVA light and its photostability in sunscreen formulation. *J Cosmet Dermatol.* 2021;20(4):1271–1282.

261. Gupta M, Dey S, Marbaniang D, Pal P, Ray S, Mazumder B. Grape seed extract: having a potential health benefits. *J Food Sci Technol.* 2020;57(4):1205–1215.

262. Devi S, Singh R. Antioxidant and anti-hypercholesterolemic potential of Vitis vinifera leaves. *Pharmacogn J.* 2017;9(4): 565–572.

263. Langley P. Why a pomegranate? *BMJ.* 2000;321(7269):1153–1154.

264. Gil MI, Tomás-Barberán FA, Hess-Pierce B, Holcroft DM, Kader AA. Antioxidant activity of pomegranate juice and its relationship with phenolic composition and processing. *J Agric Food Chem.* 2000;48(10):4581–4589.

265. Aviram M, Dornfeld L, Rosenblat M, et al. Pomegranate juice consumption reduces oxidative stress, atherogenic modifications to LDL, and platelet aggregation: studies in humans and in atherosclerotic apolipoprotein E-deficient mice. *Am J Clin Nutr.* 2000;71(5):1062–1076.

266. Wang RF, Xie WD, Zhang Z, et al. Bioactive compounds from the seeds of Punica granatum (pomegranate). *J Nat Prod.* 2004;67(12):2096–2098.

267. Afaq F, Saleem M, Krueger CG, Reed JD, Mukhtar H. Anthocyanin- and hydrolyzable tannin-rich pomegranate fruit extract modulates MAPK and NF-kappaB pathways and inhibits skin tumorigenesis in CD-1 mice. *Int J Cancer.* 2005;113(3):423–433.

268. Seeram NP, Aviram M, Zhang Y, et al. Comparison of antioxidant potency of commonly consumed polyphenol-rich beverages in the United States. *J Agric Food Chem.* 2008;56(4):1415–1422.

269. Schubert SY, Lansky EP, Neeman I. Antioxidant and eicosanoid enzyme inhibition properties of pomegranate seed oil and fermented juice flavonoids. *J Ethnopharmacol.* 1999;66(1):11–17.

270. Chidambara Murthy KN, Jayaprakasha GK, Singh RP. Studies on antioxidant activity of pomegranate (Punica granatum) peel extract using in vivo models. *J Agric Food Chem.* 2002;50(17):4791–4795.

271. Afaq F, Mukhtar H. Botanical antioxidants in the prevention of photocarcinogenesis and photoaging. *Exp Dermatol.* 2006;15(9):678–684.

272. Seeram NP, Adams LS, Henning SM, et al. In vitro antiproliferative, apoptotic and antioxidant activities of punicalagin, ellagic acid and a total pomegranate tannin extract are enhanced in combination with other polyphenols as found in pomegranate juice. *J Nutr Biochem.* 2005;16(6):360–367.

273. Syed DN, Malik A, Hadi N, Sarfaraz S, Afaq F, Mukhtar H. Photochemopreventive effect of pomegranate fruit extract on UVA-mediated activation of cellular pathways in normal human epidermal keratinocytes. *Photochem Photobiol.* 2006;82(2):398–405.

274. Hora JJ, Maydew ER, Lansky EP, Dwivedi C. Chemopreventive effects of pomegranate seed oil on skin tumor development in CD1 mice. *J Med Food.* 2003;6(3):157–161.

275. Afaq F, Malik A, Syed D, Maes D, Matsui MS, Mukhtar H. Pomegranate fruit extract modulates UV-B-mediated phosphorylation of mitogen-activated protein kinases and activation of nuclear factor kappa B in normal human epidermal keratinocytes paragraph sign. *Photochem Photobiol.* 2005;81(1):38–45.

276. Zaid MA, Afaq F, Syed DN, Dreher M, Mukhtar H. Inhibition of UVB-mediated oxidative stress and markers of photoaging in immortalized HaCaT keratinocytes by pomegranate polyphenol extract POMx. *Photochem Photobiol.* 2007;83(4):882–888.

277. Aslam MN, Lansky EP, Varani J. Pomegranate as a cosmeceutical source: pomegranate fractions promote proliferation and procollagen synthesis and inhibit matrix metalloproteinase-1 production in human skin cells. *J Ethnopharmacol.* 2006;103(3):311–318.

278. Fowler JFJr, Woolery-Lloyd H, Waldorf H, Saini R. Innovations in natural ingredients and their use in skin care. *J Drugs Dermatol.* 2010;9(6 Suppl):S72–S81.

279. Henning SM, Yang J, Lee RP, et al. Pomegranate Juice and Extract Consumption Increases the Resistance to UVB-induced Erythema and Changes the Skin Microbiome in Healthy Women: a Randomized Controlled Trial. *Sci Rep.* 2019;9(1):14528.

280. Packer L, Witt EH, Tritschler HJ. alpha-Lipoic acid as a biological antioxidant. *Free Radic Biol Med.* 1995;19(2):227–250.

281. Egan RW, Gale PH, Beveridge GC, Phillips GB, Marnett LJ. Radical scavenging as the mechanism for stimulation of prostaglandin cyclooxygenase and depression of inflammation by lipoic acid and sodium iodide. *Prostaglandins.* 1978;16(6):861–869.

282. Podda M, Tritschler HJ, Ulrich H, Packer L. Alpha-lipoic acid supplementation prevents symptoms of vitamin E deficiency. *Biochem Biophys Res Commun.* 1994;204(1):98–104.

283. Kagan VE, Shvedova A, Serbinova E, et al. Dihydrolipoic acid--a universal antioxidant both in the membrane and in the aqueous phase. Reduction of peroxyl, ascorbyl and chromanoxyl radicals. *Biochem Pharmacol.* 1992;44(8):1637–1649.

284. Podda M, Han D, Koh B, Fuchs J, Packer L. Conversion of lipoic acid to dihydrolipoic acid in human keratinocytes. *J Invest Dermatol.* 1994;102(4):598.

285. Podda M, Rallis M, Traber MG, Packer L, Maibach HI. Kinetic study of cutaneous and subcutaneous distribution following topical application of [7,8-14C]rac-alpha-lipoic acid onto hairless mice. *Biochem Pharmacol.* 1996;52(4):627–633.

286. Perricone NV. Pharmacologic cognitive enhancers: dermatologic indications. *Skin & Aging.* 1998;2:68.

287. Kubota Y, Musashi M, Nagasawa T, Shimura N, Igarashi R, Yamaguchi Y. Novel nanocapsule of α-lipoic acid reveals pigmentation improvement: α-Lipoic acid stimulates the proliferation and differentiation of keratinocyte in murine skin by topical application. *Exp Dermatol.* 2019;28(Suppl 1):55–63.

288. Zhou Z, Liu C, Wan X, Fang L. Development of a w/o emulsion using ionic liquid strategy for transdermal delivery of anti-aging component α-lipoic acid: Mechanism of different ionic liquids on skin retention and efficacy evaluation. *Eur J Pharm Sci.* 2020;141:105042.

289. Hoyer S. Abnormalities of glucose metabolism in Alzheimer's disease. *Ann N Y Acad Sci.* 1991;640:53–58.

290. Monograph: alpha-Lipoic acid. *Altern Med Rev.* 1998;3(4): 308–310.

291. Carpintero DJ. Use of thioctic acid for prevention of the adverse effects induced by benznidazole in patients with chronic Chagas' infection. *Medicina (B Aires)*. 1983;43(3):285–290.

292. Bast A, Haenen GR. Interplay between lipoic acid and glutathione in the protection against microsomal lipid peroxidation. *Biochim Biophys Acta*. 1988;963(3):558–561.

293. Rosenberg HR, Culik R. Effect of α-lipoic acid on vitamin C and vitamin E deficiencies. *Arch Biochem*. 1959;80:86–93.

294. Biewenga GP, Haenen GR, Bast A. The pharmacology of the antioxidant lipoic acid. *Gen Pharmacol*. 1997;29(3):315–331.

295. Yıldırım Baş F, Bayram D, Arslan B, et al. Effect of alpha lipoic acid on smoking-induced skin damage. *Cutan Ocul Toxicol*. 2017;36(1):67–73.

296. Bergqvist-Karlsson A, Thelin I, Bergendorff O. Contact dermatitis to alpha-lipoic acid in an anti-wrinkle cream. *Contact Dermatitis*. 2006;55(1):56–57.

297. West LG, Birac PM, Pratt DE. Separation of the isomeric isoflavones from soybeans by high-performance liquid chromatography. *J Chromatogr*. 1978 Mar;150(1):266–268.

298. Persky V, Van Horn L. Epidemiology of soy and cancer: perspectives and directions. *J Nutr*. 1995;125(3 Suppl):709S–712S.

299. Davis JN, Muqim N, Bhuiyan M, Kucuk O, Pienta KJ, Sarkar FH. Inhibition of prostate specific antigen expression by genistein in prostate cancer cells. *Int J Oncol*. 2000;16(6):1091–1097.

300. Lu LJ, Anderson KE, Grady JJ, Kohen F, Nagamani M. Decreased ovarian hormones during a soya diet: implications for breast cancer prevention. *Cancer Res*. 2000;60(15):4112–4121.

301. Lu LJ, Anderson KE, Grady JJ, Nagamani M. Effects of soya consumption for one month on steroid hormones in premenopausal women: implications for breast cancer risk reduction. *Cancer Epidemiol Biomarkers Prev*. 1996;5(1):63–70.

302. Messina MJ, Persky V, Setchell KD, Barnes S. Soy intake and cancer risk: a review of the in vitro and in vivo data. *Nutr Cancer*. 1994;21(2):113–131.

303. Wei H, Saladi R, Lu Y, et al. Isoflavone genistein: photoprotection and clinical implications in dermatology. *J Nutr*. 2003;133(11 Suppl 1):3811S–3819S.

304. Albertazzi P, Pansini F, Bottazzi M, Bonaccorsi G, De Aloysio D, Morton MS. Dietary soy supplementation and phytoestrogen levels. *Obstet Gynecol*. 1999;94(2):229–231.

305. Albertazzi P, Steel SA, Clifford E, Bottazzi M. Attitudes towards and use of dietary supplementation in a sample of postmenopausal women. *Climacteric*. 2002;5(4):374–382.

306. Wei H, Bowen R, Cai Q, Barnes S, Wang Y. Antioxidant and antipromotional effects of the soybean isoflavone genistein. *Proc Soc Exp Biol Med*. 1995;208(1):124–130.

307. Polkowski K, Mazurek AP. Biological properties of genistein. A review of in vitro and in vivo data. *Acta Pol Pharm*. 2000;57(2):135–155.

308. Widyarini S, Husband AJ, Reeve VE. Protective effect of the isoflavonoid equol against hairless mouse skin carcinogenesis induced by UV radiation alone or with a chemical cocarcinogen. *Photochem Photobiol*. 2005;81(1):32–37.

309. Wei H, Wei L, Frenkel K, Bowen R, Barnes S. Inhibition of tumor promoter-induced hydrogen peroxide formation in vitro and in vivo by genistein. *Nutr Cancer*. 1993;20(1):1–12.

310. Wei H, Barnes S, Wang Y. Inhibitory effect of genistein on a tumor promoter-induced c-fos and c-jun expression in mouse skin. *Oncol Rep*. 1996;3(1):125–128.

311. Wei H, Cai Q, Rahn RO. Inhibition of UV light- and Fenton reaction-induced oxidative DNA damage by the soybean isoflavone genistein. *Carcinogenesis*. 1996;17(1):73–77.

312. Wang Y, Zhang X, Lebwohl M, DeLeo V, Wei H. Inhibition of ultraviolet B (UVB)-induced c-fos and c-jun expression in vivo by a tyrosine kinase inhibitor genistein. *Carcinogenesis*. 1998;19(4):649–654.

313. Mazière C, Dantin F, Dubois F, Santus R, Mazière J. Biphasic effect of UVA radiation on STAT1 activity and tyrosine phosphorylation in cultured human keratinocytes. *Free Radic Biol Med*. 2000;28(9):1430–1437.

314. Silva LA, Ferraz Carbonel AA, de Moraes ARB, Simões RS, Sasso GRDS, Goes L, et al. Collagen concentration on the facial skin of postmenopausal women after topical treatment with estradiol and genistein: a randomized double-blind controlled trial. *Gynecol Endocrinol*. 2017;33(11):845–848.

315. Patriarca MT, Barbosa de Moraes AR, Nader HB, et al. Hyaluronic acid concentration in postmenopausal facial skin after topical estradiol and genistein treatment: a double-blind, randomized clinical trial of efficacy. *Menopause*. 2013;20(3):336–341.

316. Packer L, Rimbach G, Virgili F. Antioxidant activity and biologic properties of a procyanidin-rich extract from pine (Pinus maritima) bark, pycnogenol. *Free Radic Biol Med*. 1999;27(5-6):704–724.

317. Rohdewald P. Pycnogenol®, French maritime pine bark extract. In: Coates PM, Blackman MR, Cragg G, Levine M, Moss J, White J, eds. *Encyclopedia of Dietary Supplements*. New York: Marcel Dekker; 2005: 545–553.

318. Sime S, Reeve VE. Protection from inflammation, immunosuppression and carcinogenesis induced by UV radiation in mice by topical Pycnogenol. *Photochem Photobiol*. 2004;79(2):193–198.

319. Rohdewald P. A review of the French maritime pine bark extract (Pycnogenol), a herbal medication with a diverse clinical pharmacology. *Int J Clin Pharmacol Ther*. 2002;40(4):158–168.

320. Krizkova L, Chovanová Z, Duracková Z, Krajcovic J. Antimutagenic in vitro activity of plant polyphenols: Pycnogenol and Ginkgo biloba extract (EGb 761). *Phytother Res*. 2008;22(3):384–388.

321. Devaraj S, Vega-López S, Kaul N, Schönlau F, Rohdewald P, Jialal I. Supplementation with a pine bark extract rich in polyphenols increases plasma antioxidant capacity and alters the plasma lipoprotein profile. *Lipids*. 2002;37(10):931–934.

322. Saliou C, Rimbach G, Moini H, et al. Solar ultraviolet-induced erythema in human skin and nuclear factor-kappa-B-dependent gene expression in keratinocytes are modulated by a French maritime pine bark extract. *Free Radic Biol Med*. 2001;30(2):154–160.

323. Marini A, Grether-Beck S, Jaenicke T, et al. Pycnogenol® effects on skin elasticity and hydration coincide with increased gene expressions of collagen type I and hyaluronic acid synthase in women. *Skin Pharmacol Physiol*. 2012;25(2):86–92.

324. Grether-Beck S, Marini A, Jaenicke T, Krutmann J. French Maritime Pine Bark Extract (Pycnogenol®) Effects on Human Skin: Clinical and Molecular Evidence. *Skin Pharmacol Physiol*. 2016;29(1):13–17.

325. Dogan E, Yanmaz L, Gedikli S, Ersoz U, Okumus Z. The Effect of Pycnogenol on Wound Healing in Diabetic Rats. *Ostomy Wound Manage*. 2017;63(4):41–47.

326. Puizina-Ivić N, Mirić L, Carija A, Karlica D, Marasović D. Modern approach to topical treatment of aging skin. *Coll Antropol*. 2010;34(3):1145–1153.

327. Baulieu EE, Thomas G, Legrain S, et al. Dehydroepiandrosterone (DHEA), DHEA sulfate, and aging: contribution of the DHEAge Study to a sociobiomedical issue. *Proc Natl Acad Sci U S A.* 2000;97(8):4279–4284.

328. Coach C, Benghuzzi H, Tucci M. The effect of ultraviolet radiation and pre-treatment of dehydroepiandrosterone on RMK cells in culture. *Biomed Sci Instrum.* 2001;37:31–36.

329. Nestler JE, Barlascini CO, Clore JN, Blackard WG. Dehydroepiandrosterone reduces serum low density lipoprotein levels and body fat but does not alter insulin sensitivity in normal men. *J Clin Endocrinol Metab.* 1988;66(1):57–61.

330. Nouveau S, Bastien P, Baldo F, de Lacharriere O. Effects of topical DHEA on aging skin: a pilot study. *Maturitas.* 2008;59(2):174–181.

331. El-Alfy M, Deloche C, Azzi L, et al. Skin responses to topical dehydroepiandrosterone: implications in antiageing treatment? *Br J Dermatol.* 2010;163(5):968–976.

332. Dean CE. Prasterone (DHEA) and mania. *Ann Pharmacother.* 2000;34(12):1419–1422.

333. Reiter RJ, Tan DX, Osuna C, Gitto E. Actions of melatonin in the reduction of oxidative stress. A review. *J Biomed Sci.* 2000;7(6):444–458.

334. Reiter RJ, Tan DX, Cabrera J, et al. The oxidant/antioxidant network: role of melatonin. *Biol Signals Recept.* 1999;8(1-2):56–63.

335. Kumar CA, Das UN. Effect of melatonin on two stage skin carcinogenesis in Swiss mice. *Med Sci Monit.* 2000;6(3):471–475.

336. Nickel A, Wohlrab W. Melatonin protects human keratinocytes from UVB irradiation by light absorption. *Arch Dermatol Res.* 2000;292(7):366–368.

337. Bangha E, Elsner P, Kistler GS. Suppression of UV-induced erythema by topical treatment with melatonin (N-acetyl-5-methoxytryptamine). A dose response study. *Arch Dermatol Res.* 1996;288(9):522–526.

338. Dreher F, Gabard B, Schwindt DA, Maibach HI. Topical melatonin in combination with vitamins E and C protects skin from ultraviolet-induced erythema: a human study in vivo. *Br J Dermatol.* 1998;139(2):332–339.

339. Howes RA, Halliday GM, Damian DL. Effect of topical melatonin on ultraviolet radiation-induced suppression of Mantoux reactions in humans. *Photodermatol Photoimmunol Photomed.* 2006;22(5):267–269.

340. Cho JW, Kim CW, Lee KS. Modification of gene expression by melatonin in UVB-irradiated HaCaT keratinocyte cell lines using a cDNA microarray. *Oncol Rep.* 2007;17(3):573–577.

341. Fischer T, Wigger-Alberti W, Elsner P. Melatonin in dermatology. Experimental and clinical aspects. *Hautarzt.* 1999;50(1):5–11.

342. Pandi-Perumal SR, Srinivasan V, Maestroni GJ, Cardinali DP, Poeggeler B, Hardeland R. Melatonin: Nature's most versatile biological signal? *FEBS J.* 2006;273(13):2813–2838.

343. Kim TH, Jung JA, Kim GD, et al. Melatonin inhibits the development of 2,4-dinitrofluorobenzene-induced atopic dermatitis-like skin lesions in NC/Nga mice. *J Pineal Res.* 2009;47(4):324–329.

344. Kleszczyński K, Hardkop LH, Fischer TW. Differential effects of melatonin as a broad range UV-damage preventive dermato-endocrine regulator. *Dermatoendocrinol.* 2011;3(1):27–31.

345. Kleszczynski K, Fischer TW. Melatonin and human skin aging. *Dermatoendocrinol.* 2012;4(3):245–252.

346. Arendt J. Melatonin. *Clin Endocrinol (Oxf).* 1988;29(2):205–229.

347. Fischer TW, Greif C, Fluhr JW, Wigger-Alberti W, Elsner P. Percutaneous penetration of topically applied melatonin in a cream and an alcoholic solution. *Skin Pharmacol Physiol.* 2004;17(4):190–194.

348. Slominski A, Tobin DJ, Zmijewski MA, Wortsman J, Paus R. Melatonin in the skin: synthesis, metabolism and functions. *Trends Endocrinol Metabl.* 2008;19(1):17–24.

349. Fischer TW, Slominski A, Tobin DJ, Paus R. Melatonin and the hair follicle. *J Pineal Res.* 2008;44(1):1–15.

350. Murch SJ, Simmons CB, Saxena PK. Melatonin in feverfew and other medicinal plants. *Lancet.* 1997;350(9091):1598–1599.

351. Fischer TW, Trüeb RM, Hänggi G, Innocenti M, Elsner P. Topical melatonin for treatment of androgenetic alopecia. *Int J Trichology.* 2012;4(4):236–245.

352. Hatem S, Nasr M, Moftah NH, Ragai MH, Geneidi AS, Elkheshen SA. Clinical cosmeceutical repurposing of melatonin in androgenic alopecia using nanostructured lipid carriers prepared with antioxidant oils. *Expert Opin Drug Deliv.* 2018;15(10):927–935.

353. Fischer TW, Kleszczyński K, Hardkop LH, Kruse N, Zillikens D. Melatonin enhances antioxidative enzyme gene expression (CAT, GPx, SOD), prevents their UVR-induced depletion, and protects against the formation of DNA damage (8-hydroxy-2'-deoxyguanosine) in ex vivo human skin. *J Pineal Res.* 2013;54(3):303–312.

354. Fischer TW, Scholz G, Knöll B, Hipler UC, Elsner P. Melatonin suppresses reactive oxygen species in UV-irradiated leukocytes more than vitamin C and trolox. *Skin Pharmacol Appl Skin Physiol.* 2002;15(5):367–373.

355. Sierra AF, Ramírez ML, Campmany AC, Martínez AR, Naveros BC. In vivo and in vitro evaluation of the use of a newly developed melatonin loaded emulsion combined with UV filters as a protective agent against skin irradiation. *J Dermatol Sci.* 2013;69(3):202–214.

356. Bangha E, Elsner P, Kistler GS. Suppression of UV-induced erythema by topical treatment with melatonin (N-acetyl-5-methoxytryptamine). Influence of the application time point. *Dermatology.* 1997;195(3):248–252.

357. Fischer T, Bangha E, Elsner P, Kistler GS. Suppression of UV-induced erythema by topical treatment with melatonin. Influence of the application time point. *Biol Signals Recept.* 1999;8(1–2):132–135.

358. Dreher F, Denig N, Gabard B, Schwindt DA, Maibach HI. Effect of topical antioxidants on UV-induced erythema formation when administered after exposure. *Dermatology.* 1999;198(1):52–55.

359. Morganti P, Fabrizi G, Palombo P, et al. New chitin complexes and their anti-aging activity from inside out. *J Nutr Health Aging.* 2012;16(3):242–245.

360. Scheuer C, Pommergaard HC, Rosenberg J, Gögenur I. Dose dependent sun protective effect of topical melatonin: A randomized, placebo-controlled, double-blind study. *J Dermatol Sci.* 2016;84(2):178–185.

361. Milani M, Sparavigna A. Antiaging efficacy of melatonin-based day and night creams: a randomized, split-face, assessor-blinded proof-of-concept trial. *Clin Cosmet Investig Dermatol.* 2018;11:51–57.

362. Rusanova I, Martínez-Ruiz L, Florido J, et al. Protective Effects of Melatonin on the Skin: Future Perspectives. *Int J Mol Sci.* 2019;20(19):4948.

363. Day D, Burgess CM, Kircik LH. Assessing the Potential Role for Topical Melatonin in an Antiaging Skin Regimen. *J Drugs Dermatol.* 2018;17(9):966–969.

364. Slominski AT, Hardeland R, Zmijewski MA, Slominski RM, Reiter RJ, Paus R. Melatonin: A Cutaneous Perspective on its Production, Metabolism, and Functions. *J Invest Dermatol.* 2018;138(3):490–499.

365. Spallholz JE, Boylan LM, Larsen HS. Advances in understanding selenium's role in the immune system. *Ann N Y Acad Sci.* 1990;587:123–139.

366. Yoshizawa K, Willett WC, Morris SJ, et al. Study of prediagnostic selenium level in toenails and the risk of advanced prostate cancer. *J Natl Cancer Inst.* 1998;90(16):1219–1224.

367. Overvad K, Thorling EB, Bjerring P, Ebbesen P. Selenium inhibits UV-light-induced skin carcinogenesis in hairless mice. *Cancer Lett.* 1985;27(2):163–170.

368. Burke KE, Combs GFJr, Gross EG, Bhuyan KC, Abu-Libdeh H. The effects of topical and oral L-selenomethionine on pigmentation and skin cancer induced by ultraviolet irradiation. *Nutr Cancer.* 1992;17(2):123–137.

369. Rafferty TS, Beckett GJ, Walker C, Bisset YC, McKenzie RC. Selenium protects primary human keratinocytes from apoptosis induced by exposure to ultraviolet radiation. *Clin Exp Dermatol.* 2003;28(3):294–300.

370. McKenzie RC, Rafferty TS, Beckett GJ. Selenium: an essential element for immune function. *Immunol Today.* 1998;19(8):342–345.

371. Clark LC, Combs GFJr, Turnbull BW, et al. Effects of selenium supplementation for cancer prevention in patients with carcinoma of the skin. A randomized controlled trial. Nutritional Prevention of Cancer Study Group. *JAMA.* 1996;276(24):1957–1963.

372. Institute of Medicine, Food and Nutrition Board. *Dietary Reference Intakes: Vitamin C, Vitamin E, Selenium, and Carotenoids.* Washington, DC, National Academy Press; 2000.

373. Koller LD, Exon JH. The two faces of selenium-deficiency and toxicity--are similar in animals and man. *Can J Vet Res.* 1986;50(3):297–306.

374. McKenzie RC. Selenium, ultraviolet radiation and the skin. *Clin Exp Dermatol.* 2000;25(8):631–636.

375. Stewart MS, Spallholz JE, Neldner KH, Pence BC. Selenium compounds have disparate abilities to impose oxidative stress and induce apoptosis. *Free Radic Biol Med.* 1999;26(1-2):42–48.

376. Lin FH, Lin JY, Gupta RD, et al. Ferulic acid stabilizes a solution of vitamins C and E and doubles its photoprotection of skin. *J Invest Dermatol.* 2005;125(4):826–832.

377. Greul AK, Grundmann JU, Heinrich F, et al. Photoprotection of UV-irradiated human skin: an antioxidative combination of vitamins E and C, carotenoids, selenium and proanthocyanidins. *Skin Pharmacol Appl Skin Physiol.* 2002;15(5):307–315.

378. Passi S, De Pità O, Grandinetti M, Simotti C, Littarru GP. The combined use of oral and topical lipophilic antioxidants increases their levels both in sebum and stratum corneum. *Biofactors.* 2003;18(1-4):289–297.

CHAPTER 40

Cleansing Agents

Leslie S. Baumann, MD
Edmund M. Weisberg, MS, MBE

SUMMARY POINTS

What's Important?

1. Cleansers play an important role in skincare regimen efficacy.
2. Cleansers increase penetration of the products that follow in the regimen.
3. Surfactant type determines irritation potential of cleansers.

What's New?

1. Increased water temperature increases cleanser irritation.
2. Hard water causes skin irritation while ultrapure soft water does not.
3. Water filters will remove Ca^{2+} and reduce cleanser irritancy.

What's Coming?

1. Use of low-pH cleansers in the morning to increase efficacy of the products that follow.
2. Natural saponins that cleanse without irritation are being identified as demand for organic products increases.
3. More patient education about proper cleansing is needed.

INTRODUCTION

Cleansing is one of the most important steps in any skincare routine because it prepares the skin for the application of topical products. Cleansers affect the efficacy and the side-effect profile of the products that follow them in the skincare routine by influencing penetration of skincare ingredients. Cleanser choice is particularly important when treating an individual with medications that render them more susceptible to inflammation. For example, acne medications are better tolerated when the proper cleanser is used. The following discussion focuses on the various types of cleansers.

THE EFFECTS OF CLEANSERS ON SKIN

Cleansers prepare the skin for subsequently applied products. Foaming cleansers surround lipids and remove them from the skin's surface. This temporarily injures the skin barrier, increasing transepidermal water loss and penetration of applied ingredients. Creamy cleansers, referred to as nonfoaming cleansers in this chapter, deposit lipids on the skin that help nourish and strengthen the skin barrier. All cleansers, especially when applied with a cloth, loofah, or facial brush, promote exfoliation, removing desquamated skin cells from the surface of the skin. The amount of friction, type of water (hard vs. soft), and the temperature of the water all play a role in how much exfoliation the cleanser causes. Of course, the type of cleanser influences the amount of exfoliation that occurs. Low-pH cleansers, like hydroxy acid cleansers and salicylic acid cleansers, loosen the attachments between cells, promoting exfoliation. All cleansers promote exfoliation but there are two classes of cleansers that excel at enhancing desquamation through exfoliation.

Exfoliation

There are two types of cleansing products that promote desquamation and exfoliation: mechanical exfoliators and chemical exfoliators. Mechanical exfoliators use friction. These include loofas, washcloths, and facial brushes. Facial scrubs, invented by dermatologist Dr. Rose Saperstein, are also examples of mechanical exfoliators.[1] Low-pH ingredients such as glycolic, lactic, and phytic acids act as chemical exfoliators and were first described as such by dermatologist Dr. Eugene Van Scott and Ruey Yu, PhD.[2] These hydroxy acids are often used as exfoliating cleansers. A second type of acid, known as beta hydroxy acid (BHA) or salicylic acid, is also used to exfoliate skin.

Cleansers and Irritation

The surfactants in cleansers can irritate the skin. It is theorized that the surfactant absorbs into the skin, disrupts the lipids in the skin barrier, superficial keratinocytes (corneocytes), and the stratum corneum, affects epidermal hyperproliferation and differentiation through calcium effects, alters cytokine expression, and causes increased transepidermal water loss from barrier disruption.[3–13]

The irritation potential of a cleanser depends on the barrier status of the skin, class of surfactant, duration of exposure to surfactant, frequency of washing, and water used to cleanse. Surfactants with C_{10}–C_{14} chain lengths are the most aggressive because they are the most active in solution.

THE EFFECTS OF WATER ON SKIN

Types of Water

Water has different constituents that can affect cleanser function and irritancy. Tap water varies greatly depending on its source and how it is treated. "Hard water" is characterized by a high content of multivalent cations such as Ca^{2+} and Mg^{2+} while soft water (in the United States) has less than 60 mg/L of calcium carbonate. (Soft water usually contains less magnesium, but this is not in the definition of soft water.) There is no standardized definition for ultrapure soft water (UPSW) but in the dermatology literature it is usually represented as <1 mg/L of Ca^{2+} and Mg^{2+}.

Minerals in Water

Ca^{2+} and Mg^{2+} mineral salts found in hard water decrease foaming from surfactants and cause soap scum or calcium deposits in bathtubs and sinks. The decreased foaming often results in increased use of the detergent-containing cleansing product to achieve more foam and therefore an increase in exposure to detergents. Mineral salts react with the fatty acids in soaps to form a "metallic soap" that remains on the skin after rinsing unless washed off with UPSW.[14,15]

Metallic soap acts as a skin irritant and may induce an allergic response. Studies have shown that UPSW will decrease atopic dermatitis (AD) in children;[16] however, if low concentrations of metallic ions remain in the water, there is no improvement in AD. In other words, UPSW will help prevent AD while soft water with remaining metallic ions will not. Tanaka et al. showed that metallic soap induced and exacerbated AD in mice unless they were washed with UPSW

without multivalent cations.[15] The UPSW did not exacerbate AD symptoms but metallic soap did.

Metallic soap disrupts the skin barrier directly and by affecting lamellar body secretion from keratinocytes,[3] which is regulated by Ca^{2+}.[17–19] The important point is that the irritation potential of surfactants differs with the hardness (amount of Ca^{2+}) of the water.

Washing vs. Rinsing with Water

Minerals in water increase irritation from cleansers, and the timing of water exposure plays a key role. It is not the water used to wash the face with the cleanser that is the culprit; rather, it is the water used to rinse the cleanser off the skin that alters the irritation potential of the cleanser.[3] Using a UPSW to rinse the face after cleansing helps decrease irritation from cleansing. Finding UPSW may be difficult so it is generally advised to use a facial water that does not contain calcium to rinse the skin after cleansing. Different types of water have varying amounts of calcium (**Table 40-1**). Brita filters have been shown to remove about 90% of the calcium from various types of water.[20]

Water Temperature

The temperature of water used to cleanse the skin also plays a role in irritancy of skin cleansers as demonstrated in a study that applied sodium lauryl sulfate (SLS) on the volar forearm for 5 days at varying temperatures.[21] A significant correlation between high water temperature and skin irritation was found.[22,23] Anionic surfactants provoked the highest increase in irritancy with elevated water temperature.[24] Studies looking at the effect of cold water on surfactant-induced skin irritation have been conflicting. Most show that cold water reduces irritation,[25] but one revealed that cold increased barrier disruption.[26]

Water temperature can also influence the penetration of ingredients into the skin.[27] Increased skin temperature is associated with increased blood flow to the area. Barrier disruption and increased blood flow lead to increased absorption of topically applied products. Using hot water to rinse the face results in a higher risk for skin irritation.

The irritation potential of a cleanser is affected by the type and temperature of the water, frequency of washing, and the duration of surfactant exposure; however, the type of surfactant in the cleanser is the most important contributor to irritation. Facial waters with Ca^{2+} and soothing minerals such as selenium and sulfur can be used to rinse the face if a nonionic surfactant cleanser is used.

TYPES OF SURFACTANTS

Anionic (Negatively Charged) Surfactants

Anionic surfactants form generous foam and confer the highest cleansing power (**Table 40-2**). "Soap" contains the anionic surfactant alkyl carboxylate. Anionic agents are potent irritants to the skin,[28] and have been found to cause harmful swelling of cell membranes.[29,30] The anionic surfactant SLS

TABLE 40-1	Comparison of Mineral Composition of Water.[20]						
Water Type	**Brand**	**Calcium in Mg/L**	**Selenium**	**Copper**	**Magnesium**	**Notes**	
Tap water		8–130 mg				Varies by location	
Purified water	Aquafina	0 mg					
Purified water	Dasani	<10 mg			Yes		
Spring water	Fiji	17 mg					
Spring water	Volvic	9.9 mg			6 mg		
Spring water	Zepherhills	58 mg					
Mineral water	Evian	78 mg			24 mg		
Mineral water	Perrier	147 mg			4 mg		
Mineral water	San Pellegrino	204 mg			57 mg		
Mineral water	Vittel	575 mg			118 mg		
Facial water	La Roche Posay Thermal	140 mag	60 micrograms	220 micrograms		Contains other minerals	
Facial water	Vichy Volcanic	165 mg			12 mg/L	Contains other minerals	

Notes: If blank, value is unknown. Company values for LaRoche Posay provided by L'Oréal.

strips lipids from the skin, and is so irritating that it is used in the research setting to impair the skin barrier. This surfactant is one of the main reasons for the "sulfate free" trend in shampoos and conditioners. It is often confused with sodium laureth sulfate, also known as sodium lauryl ether sulfate or SLES, which is also an effective cleanser but is less likely to provoke irritation than SLS (**Table 40-2**). All anionic surfactants can cause skin irritation. They are often used in small amounts and combined with other classes of surfactants so that the final product features a vigorous foam but less irritation potential.

Cationic (Positively Charged) Surfactants

Cationic surfactants contain lower detergent properties than anionic surfactants and are very irritating. However, they are often used because of their antimicrobial properties. These surfactants often lead to the hand dermatitis seen in frequent hand washers. Cetrimide, chlorhexidine, and benzalkonium chloride are examples of cationic surfactants. Behentrimonium methosulfate and PG-dimonium chloride phosphate are cationic surfactants seen in facial cleansers.

Amphoteric Surfactants

Most facial cleansers use amphoteric, also called zwitterionic, surfactants. They have a positive and negative charge. Amphoteric surfactants exhibit changing properties depending on the pH of the solution. Amphoterics are popular in cleansers because they lather well, display effective cleansing power, are compatible with different pHs, impart moderate antimicrobial activity, and cause minimal irritation. Cocamidopropyl betaine is a commonly used amphoteric surfactant. See **Table 40-3** for more examples.

TABLE 40-2	Anionic Surfactants in Facial Cleansers
Alpha Olefin Sulfonate	
Ammonium Laureth Sulfate	
Ammonium Lauryl Sulfate	
Disodium Laureth Sulfosuccinate	
Phenoxyethanol	
Potassium Cocoate	
Sodium Cocoyl Isethionate	
Sodium Dodecyl Sulfate	
Sodium Laureth Sulfate	
Sodium Laurilsulfate	
Sodium Lauryl Sulfate	

TABLE 40-3	Amphoteric Surfactants
Behenyl Betaine	
Capryl/Capramidopropyl Betaine	
Cocamidopropyl Betaine	
Cocamidopropyl Hydroxysultaine	
Cocoaminopropionic Acid	
Coco-Betaine	
Disodium Cocoamphodiacetate	
Sodium C14-16 Olefin Sulfonate	
Sodium Cocamidopropyl	
Sodium Cocoamphoacetate	
Sodium Cocomonoglyceride Sulfate	
Sodium Lauroamphoacetate	

Nonionic Surfactants

Nonionic agents have no electric charge. They are expensive and demonstrate poor cleansing characteristics but are popular because they cause less skin irritation. Nonionic surfactants can disrupt the skin barrier by solubilizing fatty acids and cholesterol.[31] Examples of nonionic surfactants include cocoglucoside, pentaerythrityl tetraethylhexanoate, lauryl glucoside, decylglucoside, and coconut diethanolamine (cocamide DEA) (**Table 40-4**).

Other Classes of Surfactants

Newer classes of cleansers such as superfatted soaps, transparent soaps, and combination bars (combars) have been developed to diminish the irritancy of soaps through the addition of secondary components. Bars composed of synthetic surfactants are often referred to as "syndet bars." These surfactants have a neutral pH, and include ingredients such as alkyl glyceryl ether sulfonate, alpha olefin sulfonates, betaines, sulfosuccinates, sodium cocoyl monoglyceride sulfate, and sodium cocoyl isethionate.

Natural Ingredients in Cleansers

Organic plant-derived surfactants include ingredients such as saponins and sucrose laurate. Saponins are a large family of structurally related compounds derived from plants. The name is derived from the plant species *Saponaria*. Many possess foaming characteristics that render them a good option for natural or organic cleanser formulations. Saponins are composed of a steroid or triterpenoid aglycone (sapogenin) connected to one or more oligosaccharide moieties by glycosidic linkage.[32] The foaming action of saponins results from the combination of the nonpolar sapogenin and the water-soluble side chain. The *Sapindus mukorossi* (soapnut) plant has been used as a natural cleanser and shown in one study to have antimicrobial activity.[33,34] *Camellia oleifera* has been demonstrated to exhibit effective detergent abilities.[32] Several plants contain saponins, including alfalfa foliage, peas, chickpeas, horse chestnut trees, soybeans, and daisies. Desert plants, including *Yucca schidigera* and *Quillaja saponaria*, are good sources of saponins that are found in natural cleansers on the market.

CATEGORIES OF FACIAL CLEANSERS

Foaming Cleansers

Foaming cleansers are used to remove surface oil, makeup, and sunscreen. They are most appropriate for oily skin types. They contain a combination of different types of surfactants to provide the foam. Surfactants work by reducing the surface tension on the skin and emulsifying dirt.[35] These cleansers usually have a high pH of 8–10. Anionic surfactants provide the most foam but are the most irritating.[28] Anionic surfactants are often combined with other surfactants like amphoteric or nonionic surfactants to decrease irritation potential while preserving the ability to yield a vigorous foam. Patients,

TABLE 40-4	Nonionic Surfactants
C12-15 Alkyl Benzoate	
Caprylic/Capric Triglyceride	
Caprylyl/Capryl Glucoside	
Cetearyl Alcohol	
Cetyl Alcohol	
Cocamide DEA	
Coco Glucoside	
Coconut Diethanolamine	
Decyl Glucoside	
Di-PPG-2 Myreth-10 Adipate	
Glycerol Monostearate	
Glyceryl Laurate	
Glyceryl Oleate	
Glyceryl Stearate	
Glycol Distearate	
Glycol Stearate	
Isononyl Isononanoate	
Lauryl Glucoside	
Neopentyl Glycol Dicaprate	
PEG-120 Methyl Glucose Dioleate	
PEG-30 Glyceryl Cocoate	
Pentaerythrityl Tetraethylhexanoate	
Polyglyceryl-10 Distearate	
Saponins	
Sodium Lauryl Sulfate	
Stearyl Alcohol	
Sucrose Cocoate	
Sucrose Laurate	
Triethanolamine	
Triheptanoin	

especially oily skin types, like the clean feeling of the skin after using an anionic surfactant but this must be balanced with protection of the skin barrier.

Many patients will request sulfate-free cleansers. This trend emerged from publicity surrounding the irritation associated with the widely used surfactant SLS found in cleansers and shampoos. Warnings to avoid SLS resulted in the "sulfate-free" trend. (Sulfates are also unpopular due to their petroleum-based origin.) Not all sulfates are as irritating to the skin as SLS. The irritation potential of anionic surfactants like sulfates depends on the factors mentioned above.

Naturally derived surfactants like cocamidopropyl betaine and disodium cocoamphodiacetate from coconut oil or disodium laureth sulfosuccinate, which is often used in baby cleansing products, are surfactants that are gentle on the skin. Fatty acid esters of sucrose such as sucrose laurate are natural detergent options.[36]

Nonfoaming Cleansers

These agents were developed through efforts to reduce detergent irritancy. This class of cleansers includes superfatted soaps, combars, syndet bars, and lipids such as fatty acids and oils. Cream, milk, cold creams, and oil cleansers fall into this category. These products usually have a neutral pH. If these cleansers contain surfactants, they are mild and usually nonionic like caprylyl/capryl glucoside, glyceryl stearate, caprylic/capric triglyceride, and monolaurin. Saponins, as stated above, are derived from plants such as the soapnut and *Camellia oleifera*.[32,37] Nonfoaming cleansers are most appropriate for dry skin types. Individuals with oily skin types often report that they "do not feel clean" when they use these cleansers.

Hydroxy Acid Cleansers

There are several types of hydroxy acids (**Table 40-5**). These acidic cleansers lower the pH of the skin's surface below the physiological pH of the stratum corneum, which is normally 4.1–5.8 in lighter skin types and slightly lower in darker skin types. The pH of the skin influences barrier function, synthesis of lipids, as well as epidermal differentiation and desquamation. Lowering the skin pH pushes the microbiome in a healthier direction, strengthens the skin barrier, and reduces inflammation.[38] A lower pH also aids in the absorption of some cosmeceutical ingredients such as ascorbic acid. The acidity of hydroxy acids acts to loosen cell attachments, which induces exfoliation and accelerates the cell cycle. This also allows increased penetration of any skincare products that follow in the skincare routine.

The use of products with a low pH leaves some people, known as "stingers," feeling uncomfortable. This sensation is not completely understood but likely is due to activation of acid sensing ion channels (ASIC). Patients with rosacea may be stingers so hydroxy acids should be used with caution in rosacea skin types. There are three main groups of hydroxy acids found in cleansers: alpha hydroxy acids, beta hydroxy acids, and polyhydroxy acids.

The ability of a hydroxy acid cleanser to exfoliate the skin depends on the pH and the pKa, also known as the acid dissociation constant or K_a. The pKa is the pH at which the level of free acid is the same as the level of the salt form of the acid. When the pH is less than the pKa, the free acid form predominates; when the pH is greater than the pKa, the salt form predominates. A weak acid has a high pK_a, while a strong acid has a $pK_a \leq -2$. It is necessary to have the proper balance of the salt and acid forms to obtain a hydroxy acid with effective exfoliating properties but with minimal irritation.[39] Because the pKa of BHA differs from that of the AHA family, it is difficult to formulate a combination product containing both that reaches an optimal pH. For example, in a combination AHA-BHA product with a pH of 3.5, the AHA *acid* form would predominate but the BHA *salt* form would predominate. The effects of BHA would be rendered suboptimal. For this reason, hydroxy acid cleansers are often divided into three categories.

Alpha Hydroxy Acids (AHAs)

AHAs are hydrophilic and act as humectants that pull water to the skin's surface. The pKa for AHAs is 3.83.[40] The acidity increases desquamation and imparts smoothness to the skin's surface. AHAs are well suited for use by individuals with dry skin because they do not dry out the skin the way that salicylic acid cleansers can.

Beta Hydroxy Acids (BHAs)

Salicylic acid (SA) cleansers, also known as BHA, have a pKa of 2.97. They belong to the aspirin family and possess anti-inflammatory properties. Salicylic acid is lipophilic and can penetrate through the sebum-derived lipids into pores. They are the most effective cleansing ingredients to unclog pores. Therefore, SA cleansers are ideal for use by individuals with oily skin and oily skin prone to acne. Dry skin types, especially those on retinoids and benzoyl peroxide, will not tolerate SA as well as they will AHA cleansers.

Polyhydroxy Acids (PHAs)

The pKa of a popular polyhydroxy acid known as lactobionic acid is 3.8. PHAs, also known as polyhydroxy bionic acids (PHBAs), include gluconolactone and lactobionic acid. They were developed to deliver the anti-aging efficacy of alpha hydroxy acids without the irritation or increased vulnerability to ultraviolet (UV) radiation due to their antioxidant effects.[41]

Antibacterial Cleansers

Antibacterial cleansers contain ingredients that reduce *Propionibacterium acnes* and other types of bacteria on the skin. Cationic surfactants such as cetrimide, chlorhexidine, and benzalkonium chloride are antimicrobial but can be very irritating to the skin.

Other antimicrobials found in cleansers include benzoyl peroxide (BP), silver, hypochlorous acid, sodium hypochlorite, and triclosan. Triclosan has been designated by the FDA as a "contaminant of emerging concern" due to the possibility of antimicrobial resistance, endocrine dysfunction, and accumulation in wastewater that can infiltrate drinking water. Triclosan is also a known cause of contact dermatitis.

BP is the antimicrobial most often used in acne cleansers because it is among the ingredients identified in the FDA monograph for acne. (This means that when BP in a

TABLE 40-5	Hydroxy Acids
Citric acid: $C_6H_8O_7$	
Gluconolactone: $C_6H_{10}O_6$	
Glycolic acid: $C_2H_4O_3$	
Lactic acid: $C_3H_6O_3$	
Malic acid: $C_4H_6O_5$	
Mandelic acid: $C_8H_8O_3$	
Phytic acid: $C_6H_{18}O_{24}P_6$	
Salicylic acid: $C_7H_6O_3$	
Tartaric acid: $C_4H_6O_6$	

concentration of 2.5–10% is included in an acne formulation, it is regulated as an OTC product and an acne efficacy claim can be made.)[42] BP can be highly irritating and is not well tolerated by patients with dry skin.

Silver has a long history of use in medicine,[43] having been used as an antibacterial agent since the times of King Herod (74 BCE to 4 BCE). It has been shown to effectively kill viruses, fungi, and bacteria without antibiotic resistance.[44]

Hypochlorous acid is a major active component of bleach. It is used as an antimicrobial in cleansers to treat acne and prevent skin infection in eczema. It has anti-inflammatory capabilities and has been shown to decrease the activity of histamine, neutrophil-generated leukotrienes (LTB4), interleukin (IL)-6, and IL-2. Its efficacy depends upon pH and stability of the formulation.[45]

CLEANSER CHOICE BY SKIN ISSUE

Acne Cleansers

Recommending the right cleanser for acne-prone skin first depends on whether the patient has oily or dry skin. Individuals with dry skin and acne cannot tolerate drying acne medications. Choosing the correct cleanser and moisturizer can help acne patients comply with the acne treatment plan due to fewer side effects.

For Dry Skin Types

Dry skin acne types often need two different cleansers. For the morning cleanser, AHA cleansers such as glycolic acid, which act as a humectant, hydrate skin and have a relatively low pH, are recommended. *Cutibacterium acnes* are less likely to grow on skin with a lower pH. Hydroxy acids regulate desquamation and enhance exfoliation, helping prevent comedones. These hydroxy acid cleansers cause too much exfoliation to be used more than once a day in patients recently placed on retinoids. While the skin is becoming accustomed to retinoids, a creamy nonfoaming cleanser should be used once daily, preferably at night. Creamy cleansers are ideal for removing sunscreen and makeup, as well as for depositing lipids on the skin that will help the patient tolerate retinoids applied at night. Foaming cleansers should never be used on *dry* acne-prone skin. Individuals with the acne subtype of sensitive skin should also avoid using scrubs, loofahs, and other forms of mechanical exfoliation. Over exfoliation increases the number of acne lesions by disrupting desquamation in the hair follicle.

For Oily Skin Types

Salicylic acid cleansers are ideal for acne-prone patients with oily skin. Lipophilic SA penetrates into the hair follicle to unclog pores. The anti-inflammatory properties of SA help prevent the formation of papules and pustules that characterize acne.[46] Twice-daily use of SA by patients with oily skin and acne may feel too drying when combined with acne medications such as a retinoid and BP. If this is the case, a foaming cleanser can be used in the evening to remove dirt, makeup, and sunscreen. If irritation occurs, the patient should be advised to avoid foaming cleansers while continuing anionic and cationic surfactants.

Rosacea Cleansers

Rosacea patients often flush red when they wash their face, even if they only use water, because of friction. They should use soft water (calcium free) when possible to rinse the face. If they still experience redness and flushing with morning cleansing, they can omit AM cleansing and apply the morning rosacea medications followed by a sunscreen appropriate for their skin type. All rosacea patients, whether oily or dry, should be counseled to avoid mechanical exfoliation, including cleansing scrubs, chemical exfoliants, and abrasive loofahs or cloths.

For Dry Skin Types

Most rosacea patients have dry skin and may experience skin stinging. If they have dry skin, they should avoid foaming cleansers and mechanical exfoliation. If they experience stinging, they should avoid low-pH cleansers such as hydroxy acid cleansers. Creamy nonfoaming cleansers with anti-inflammatory ingredients are best for this skin type. These patients should also be counseled to avoid anion and cationic surfactants and look for products with fatty acid ester-containing surfactants such as caprylic/capric triglyceride, glyceryl stearate, or polyglyceryl fatty acids such as polyglyceryl-10 distearate.[47]

Hydroxy acid cleansers can be used in dry skin types with rosacea if they do not suffer from stinging. If the patient is beginning a retinoid, the likelihood of stinging increases, so do not begin a hydroxy acid cleanser at the same time that the patient is beginning a retinoid. Once they are accustomed to a retinoid, or if they are not on a retinoid and do not experience stinging, a hydroxy acid cleanser can be used to prevent comedones, increase exfoliation, and smooth fine lines. Hydroxy acid cleansers should be used in the morning to help increase penetration of rosacea medications, or other antioxidants.

In the evening, dry sensitive rosacea skin types should gently use a non-foaming cleanser with anti-inflammatory ingredients to remove makeup, sunscreen, and any built-up dirt or bacteria from the skin's surface. This should be followed by an anti-erythema product that targets the inflammation caused by rosacea. Anti-inflammatory ingredients that can be found in soothing cleansers and moisturizers for rosacea-prone skin include argan oil, green tea, feverfew, chamomile, licorice extract, and aloe.

For Oily Skin Types

It is less common to see patients with oily skin who have rosacea. They need to cleanse twice daily to remove excess oil to prevent comedones and acne lesions. SA cleansers are ideal for oily sensitive rosacea-prone skin types. SA cleansers should not be started at the same time as a retinoid as discussed above. Unless the patient has very oily skin, they may not be able to use the SA cleanser twice a day. If this is the case, use the SA cleanser in the morning to help increase absorption of rosacea medications and antioxidants.

Foaming cleansers can be used in rosacea patients with oily skin as long as they have a minimal amount of anionic and cationic surfactants. Amphoteric or nonionic surfactants are preferred. Soothing cleansers with anti-inflammatory ingredients such as green tea, sulfur, sulfacetamide, feverfew, licorice extract, aloe, niacinamide, green tea, and SA are a good choice for oily rosacea-prone skin types.

Eczema

Patients with eczema should choose creamy lipid-laden barrier-safe non-foaming cleansers. For patients with frequent skin infections, hypochlorous acid, hypochlorite, and silver are beneficial ingredients found in cleansers to help decrease skin bacteria and prevent infections. Foaming cleansers should never be used in eczema-prone types. Eczema-prone types should use lukewarm soft water, especially when rinsing off cleansers. They should apply any medications or treatment serums to damp skin immediately after cleansing followed by a barrier repair moisturizer. Acne medications containing retinoids or BP should be applied *after* a barrier repair moisturizer.

CONCLUSION

Cleansers play an important role in skincare because they affect the skin barrier, pH of the skin, presence of bacteria, condition of the pores, and penetration of the post-cleanser applied ingredients. Knowing which cleansing product to use based on a patient's skin type is critical to recommending the proper ingredients so that patients can achieve and maintain healthy skin. It is important to consider the types of surfactants when choosing a cleanser as well as the type of water that will be used with the cleanser.

References

1. Saperstein RB, Stiefel WK. U.S. Patent No. 3,092,111. Washington, DC: U.S. Patent and Trademark Office, 1963.

2. Baumann LS. The Interesting History of Dermatologist-Developed Skin Care. Dermatology News. August 26, 2020. https://www.mdedge.com/dermatology/article/227534/aesthetic-dermatology/interesting-history-dermatologist-developed-skin.

3. Warren R, Ertel KD, Bartolo RG, Levine MJ, Bryant PB, Wong LF. The influence of hard water (calcium) and surfactants on irritant contact dermatitis. *Contact Dermatitis.* 1996;35(6):337–343.

4. Imokawa G, Mishima Y. Cumulative effect of surfactants on cutaneous horny layers: adsorption onto human keratin layers in vivo. *Contact Dermatitis.* 1979;5(6):357–366.

5. Fulmer AW, Kramer GJ. Stratum corneum lipid abnormalities in surfactant-induced dry scaly skin. *J Invest Dermatol.* 1986;86(5):598–602.

6. Downing DT, Abraham W, Wegner BK, Willman KW, Marshall JL. Partition of sodium dodecyl sulfate into stratum corneum lipid liposomes. *Arch Dermatol Res.* 1993;285(3):151–157.

7. Denda M, Hori J, Koyama J, et al. Stratum corneum sphingolipids and free amino acids in experimentally-induced scaly skin. *Arch Dermatol Res.* 1992;284(6):363–367.

8. Rawlings AV, Watkinson A, Rogers J, Mayo AM, Hope J, Scott IR. Abnormalities in stratum corneum structure, lipid composition, and desmosome degradation in soap induced winter xerosis. *Soc Cosmet Chem.* 1994;45:203–220.

9. Wilhelm KP, Saunders JC, Maibach HI. Increased stratum corneum turnover induced by subclinical irritant dermatitis. *Br J Dermatol.* 1990;122(6):793–798.

10. White MI, Jenkinson DM, Lloyd DH. The effect of washing on the thickness of the stratum corneum in normal and atopic individuals. *Br J Dermatol.* 1987;116(4):525–530.

11. Lee SH, Elias PM, Proksch E, Menon GK, Mao-Quiang M, Feingold KR. Calcium and potassium are important regulators of barrier homeostasis in murine epidermis. *J Clin Invest.* 1992;89(2):530–538.

12. Hunziker T, Brand CU, Kapp A, Waelti ER, Braathen LR. Increased levels of inflammatory cytokines in human skin lymph derived from sodium lauryl sulphate-induced contact dermatitis. *Br J Dermatol.* 1992;127(3):254–257.

13. Denda M, Koyama J, Namba R, Horii I. Stratum corneum lipid morphology and transepidermal water loss in normal skin and surfactant-induced scaly skin. *Arch Dermatol Res.* 1994;286(1):41–46.

14. Friedman M, Wolf R. Chemistry of soaps and detergents: various types of commercial products and their ingredients. *Clin Dermatol.* 1996;14(1):7–13.

15. Tanaka A, Matsuda A, Jung K, Jang H, Ahn G, Ishizaka S, et al. Ultra-pure soft water ameliorates atopic skin disease by preventing metallic soap deposition in NC/Tnd mice and reduces skin dryness in humans. *Acta Derm Venereol.* 2015;95(7):787–791.

16. Togawa Y, Kambe N, Shimojo N, et al. Ultra-pure soft water improves skin barrier function in children with atopic dermatitis: a randomized, double-blind, placebo-controlled, crossover pilot study. *J Dermatol Sci.* 2014;76(3):269–271.

17. Menon GK, Price LF, Bommannan B, Elias PM, Feingold KR. Selective obliteration of the epidermal calcium gradient leads to enhanced lamellar body secretion. *J Invest Dermatol.* 1994;102(5):789–795.

18. Abraham W, Wertz PW, Landmann L, Downing DT. Stratum corneum lipid liposomes: calcium-induced transformation into lamellar sheets. *J Invest Dermatol.* 1987;88(2):212–214.

19. Friberg SE, Goldsmith L, Rong G. The influence of calcium ions and 2-(alkoxy)-1-((alkoyloxy)methyl)-ethyl-7-(4-heptyl-5,6)-(dicarboxy-2-cyclohexene-l-yl) heptanoate on a simplified model of stratum corneum lipids. *J Am Oil Chem Soc.* 1988; 65:1834–1837.

20. Morr S, Cuartas E, Alwattar B, Lane JM. How much calcium is in your drinking water? A survey of calcium concentrations in bottled and tap water and their significance for medical treatment and drug administration. *HSS J.* 2006;2(2):130–135.

21. Löffler H, Aramaki J, Effendy I. Response to thermal stimuli in skin pretreated with sodium lauryl sulfate. *Acta Derm Venereol.* 2001;81(6):395–397.

22. Berardesca E, Vignoli GP, Distante F, Brizzi P, Rabbiosi G. Effects of water temperature on surfactant-induced skin irritation. *Contact Dermatitis.* 1995;32(2):83–87.

23. Ohlenschlaeger J, Friberg J, Ramsing D, Agner T. Temperature dependency of skin susceptibility to water and detergents. *Acta Derm Venereol.* 1996;76(4):274–276.

24. Clarys P, Manou I, Barel AO. Influence of temperature on irritation in the hand/forearm immersion test. *Contact Dermatitis.* 1997;36(5):240–243.

25. Fluhr JW, Bornkessel A, Akengin A, et al. Sequential application of cold and sodium lauryl sulphate decreases irritation and barrier disruption in vivo in humans. *Br J Dermatol.* 2005;152(4):702–708.

26. Halkier-Sørensen L, Menon GK, Elias PM, Thestrup-Pedersen K, Feingold KR. Cutaneous barrier function after cold exposure in hairless mice: a model to demonstrate how cold interferes with barrier homeostasis among workers in the fish-processing industry. *Br J Dermatol.* 1995;132(3):391–401.

27. Clarys P, Alewaeters K, Jadoul A, Barel A, Manadas RO, Préat V. In vitro percutaneous penetration through hairless rat skin: influence of temperature, vehicle and penetration enhancers. *Eur J Pharm Biopharm.* 1998;46(3):279–283.

28. Effendy I, Maibach HI. Surfactants and experimental irritant contact dermatitis. *Contact Dermatitis.* 1995;33(4):217–225.

29. Wilhelm KP, Freitag G, Wolff HH. Surfactant-induced skin irritation and skin repair: evaluation of a cumulative human irritation model by noninvasive techniques. *J Am Acad Dermatol.* 1994;31(6):981–987.

30. Froebe CL, Simion FA, Rhein LD, Cagan RH, Kligman A. Stratum corneum lipid removal by surfactants: relation to in vivo irritation. *Dermatologica.* 1990;181(4):277–283.

31. Ananthapadmanabhan KP, Moore DJ, Subramanyan K, Misra M, Meyer F. Cleansing without compromise: the impact of cleansers on the skin barrier and the technology of mild cleansing. *Dermatol Ther.* 2004;17(Suppl 1):16–25.

32. Chen YF, Yang CH, Chang MS, Ciou YP, Huang YC. Foam properties and detergent abilities of the saponins from Camellia oleifera. *Int J Mol Sci.* 2010;11(11):4417–4425.

33. Bárány E, Lindberg M, Lodén M. Biophysical characterization of skin damage and recovery after exposure to different surfactants. *Contact Dermatitis.* 1999;40(2):98–103.

34. Corazza M, Lauriola MM, Zappaterra M, Bianchi A, Virgili A. Surfactants, skin cleansing protagonists. *J Eur Acad Dermatol Venereol.* 2010;24(1):1–6.

35. Baumann LS. Overview of Cleansing Agents. In: *Cosmeceuticals and Cosmetic Ingredients.* New York: McGraw-Hill; 2014:19–20.

36. Osipow L, Snell FD, Marra D, York WC. Surface activity of monoesters fatty acid esters of sucrose. *Ind Engineer Chem.* 1956;48(9):1462–1464.

37. Tmáková L, Sekretár S, Schmidt Š. Plant-derived surfactants as an alternative to synthetic surfactants: surface and antioxidant activities. *Chem Papers.* 2016;70(2):188–196.

38. Proksch E. pH in nature, humans and skin. *J Dermatol.* 2018;45(9):1044–1052.

39. Kligman AM. A comparative evaluation of a novel low-strength salicylic acid cream and glycolic acid products on human skin. *Cosmet Dermatol.* 1997;10(Suppl 4):11–15.

40. Davies M, Marks R. Studies on the effect of salicylic acid on normal skin. *Br J Dermatol.* 1976;95(2):187–192.

41. Green BA, Briden E. PHAs and bionic acids: next generation of hydroxy acids. In: Draelos ZD, ed. *Cosmeceuticals.* 2nd edition. Amsterdam: Elsevier; 2009: 209–215.

42. U.S. Department of Health and Human Services Food and Drug Administration Center for Drug Evaluation and Research (CDER). Guidance for Industry Topical Acne Drug Products for Overthe-Counter Human Use — Revision of Labeling and Classification of Benzoyl Peroxide as Safe and Effective. *Small Entity Compliance Guide.* June 2011 OTC. https://www.fda.gov/media/80442/download. Accessed December 6, 2020.

43. Alexander JW. History of the medical use of silver. *Surg Infect (Larchmt).* 2009;10(3):289–292.

44. Randall CP, Oyama LB, Bostock JM, Chopra I, O'Neill AJ. The silver cation (Ag+): antistaphylococcal activity, mode of action and resistance studies. *J Antimicrob Chemother.* 2013;68(1):131–138.

45. Del Rosso JQ, Bhatia N. Status Report on Topical Hypochlorous Acid: Clinical Relevance of Specific Formulations, Potential Modes of Action, and Study Outcomes. *J Clin Aesthet Dermatol.* 2018;11(11):36–39.

46. Stringer T, Nagler A, Orlow SJ, Oza VS. Clinical evidence for washing and cleansers in acne vulgaris: a systematic review. *J Dermatolog Treat.* 2018;29(7):688–693.

47. Cosmetic Ingredient Review. Safety Assessment of Polyglyceryl Fatty Acid Esters as Used in Cosmetics. *Draft Report for Panel Review.* Spring, 2016. https://www.cir-safety.org/sites/default/files/polyglyceryl%20fatty%20acid.pdf. Accessed December 6, 2020.

CHAPTER 41

Depigmenting Ingredients

Leslie S. Baumann, MD

SUMMARY POINTS

What's Important?

1. When using any type of skin lightener, it can take 12–16 weeks to see a visible decrease in skin pigmentation.
2. Fatty acids in moisturizers can affect tyrosinase activity.
3. Hydroquinone alone or in combination with a topical steroid and retinoid have the best efficacy.
4. Triple combination creams containing a tyrosinase inhibitor, a retinoid, and a corticosteroid remain the best topical skincare product to lighten skin.
5. Coenzyme Q_{10} is an antioxidant, increases ATP production, and inhibits tyrosinase activity by affecting gene transcription.

What's New?

1. Oral tranexamic acid has been shown to be safe and very effective for melasma.
2. Hydroquinone is no longer allowed in cosmetic products in the United States.

What's Coming?

1. Studies and clinical experience will evaluate the efficacy, dosing, and optimal protocols for the use of tranexamic acid intradermally or with microneedling.
2. More studies and clinical experience on oral tranexamic acid are needed to determine the most effective treatment and maintenance protocols and relapse rates.
3. More studies on the use of cysteamine in pigmentation disorders and the mechanism by which it inhibits melanin formation are needed.
4. Studies on the efficacy of oral melatonin will shed light on melatonin's role in pigment production.
5. New ingredients to replace hydroquinone and its derivatives are being developed.
6. Glutathione is not recommended until stable topical forms that can penetrate the skin have been developed; oral forms have poor bioavailability; and IV forms need far more studies evaluating safety, efficacy, and optimal dosing.

Dark spots on the skin, whether they are solar lentigos, post-inflammatory hyperpigmentation, or melasma, are a source of embarrassment and stress for many cosmetic patients. (The causes of dyschromia are discussed in Chapter 20, Skin Pigmentation Disorders.) Hyperpigmentation is difficult to treat because sun, heat, blue light, stress, hormones, and other factors that are difficult to avoid contribute to melanin development. Teaching patients the appropriate lifestyle habits for preventing pigmentation and how to use a skincare routine to erase unwanted dark spots is discussed in Chapter 14, Uneven Skin Tone. This chapter will review the ingredients in skincare products that lighten dark spots on the skin to give an even complexion. These ingredients are typically used in combination and rarely alone. A triple combination cream (TCC)

BOX 41-1	What Is an MASI Score?

The Melasma Area and Severity Index (MASI) is a reliable measure of the severity of melasma. The MASI score is calculated by subjective assessment of three factors: area (A) of involvement, darkness (D), and homogeneity (H). The areas assessed are the forehead (f), right malar region (rm), left malar region (lm), and chin (c), corresponding to 30%, 30%, 30%, and 10% of the total face, respectively.[1]

The modified MASI score (mMASI) eliminates the homogeneity measurement. The calculation of the modified MASI score is easier to use and has been shown to be scientifically valid. A higher MASI or mMASI score correlates with worse melasma.

is the most commonly used type of skincare product to lighten dark spots on the skin.

Melanin synthesis within melanosomes and their distribution to keratinocytes within the epidermal melanin unit determines skin pigmentation. Hyperpigmentation occurs when this system goes awry (see Chapter 20). Dark spots and hyperpigmented patches that lead to an uneven skin tone are unacceptable to cosmetic patients. For this reason, hundreds of products on the market are touted as "lightening creams" or "brightening creams." Although there are many product choices available, the number of effective agents to treat hyperpigmentation disorders is relatively small. Further, all of these agents require 3 to 4 months of use for improvement to be seen. Combining these formulations with retinoids (Chapter 45), sunscreens (Chapter 46), chemical peels (Chapter 24), and lights or lasers (Chapter 26) may enhance the effectiveness of these products. Currently available topical agents used to treat hyperpigmentation include tyrosinase inhibitors, melanosome-transfer inhibitors, melanocyte-cytotoxic agents, peptides, retinoids, peeling agents, and sunscreens. This chapter will discuss the ingredients commonly used for the treatment of pigmentary disorders. Several studies use a melasma area and severity index (MASI) score to assess improvement of facial pigmentation in melasma.

TRIPLE COMBINATION CREAMS

The most effective and most commonly used topical treatment for skin pigmentation, first proposed by Kligman in 1975, contains 0.1% tretinoin, 5% hydroquinone (HQ), and 0.1% dexamethasone.[2] This combination is still referred to as the "Kligman formula." Similar agents following this general formula and utilizing a steroid, a tyrosinase inhibitor, and a retinoid are known as TCCs. There is one FDA-approved TCC product on the market known as Triluma® available by prescription.[3,4] Myriad medical providers use compounding pharmacies to customize a TCC; however, stability and formulation issues must be considered because these ingredients are challenging to combine together. It is not easy to find a pharmacy that does it properly and FDA rules on compounding prescription medications have made it more difficult.

Several studies have demonstrated the efficacy of TCCs. The three ingredients facilitate each other, acting synergistically. HQ blocks tyrosinase but can cause inflammation. The steroid decreases inflammation, soothes retinoid dermatitis, and lightens skin, but can cause thinning of the dermis. The retinoid prevents skin atrophy, increases exfoliation, and lightens skin, but can cause retinoid dermatitis.[5] Using the three together eliminates many of the side effects.

When using a TCC, it can take 12–16 weeks to observe a visible decrease in skin pigmentation. Changes can be seen earlier in specialized photography as discussed in Chapter 14. Moderate to severe melasma is difficult to clear and may require multiple treatment courses. Despite these challenges, TCCs remain the most effective topical skincare treatment for melasma.[6] Several studies have demonstrated efficacy, a few of which are described below.

In a large, multicenter, randomized controlled trial of TCC (4% HQ, 0.05% tretinoin, and 0.01% fluocinolone acetonide) in 2003, the combination of the three ingredients was found to be more effective than any of the two ingredients, demonstrating the synergy of all three components.[4] In this trial, 77% of subjects achieved complete or near complete clearing. In the groups that received only two ingredients, the maximum that achieved complete or near complete clearing was 47%. Twenty-six percent of subjects using TCC achieved complete clearance by 8 weeks. A 12-month extension of the same study on 569 subjects to determine the safety and efficacy of TCC demonstrated safety with only 2.5% discontinuing treatment due to adverse events.[3]

In 2007, TCC was compared with 4% HQ alone. Both were used once daily in a controlled, open-label, 8-week trial.[7] Clearance of melasma was seen in 35% of subjects using TCC as compared to 5% clearance in those using HQ alone. In 2008, TCC was shown to be superior to 4% HQ alone in Asian patients.[8] In 2015, the efficacy of TCC in Chinese patients with melasma was demonstrated.[9]

TCCs remain the gold standard for topical treatment of skin pigmentation. They can be combined with alpha hydroxy acid or salicylic acid cleansers and defensin serums to hasten desquamation and speed clearing. Use of moisturizers with hyaluronic acid may help increase penetration of skin-lightening ingredients while moisturizers with linoleic acid or linolenic acid can aid in tyrosinase inhibition.[10] TCCs are traditionally made with HQ, but any tyrosinase inhibitor can be combined with any retinoid and a corticosteroid. Efficacy will vary depending on the type of tyrosinase inhibitor chosen and the potency of the retinoid. The important point is that skincare products for skin dyspigmentation should include combinations of retinoids, anti-inflammatories, and tyrosinase inhibitors.

TYROSINASE INHIBITORS

Tyrosinase, the enzyme that controls the synthesis of melanin, is a unique product of melanocytes. Tyrosinase converts tyrosine to dopa, resulting in melanin (**Fig. 41-1**). It is the rate-limiting enzyme for the biosynthesis of melanin in

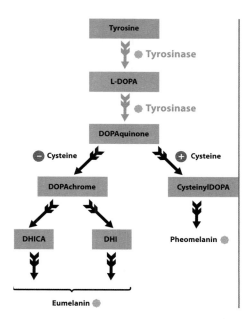

FIGURE 41-1. The synthesis of melanin from tyrosine and dopa by tyrosinase.

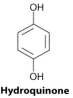

Hydroquinone

FIGURE 41-2. The chemical structure of hydroquinone.

epidermal melanocytes. Therefore, tyrosinase activity is a major regulatory step in melanogenesis and the target of the most frequently used skincare products to reduce melanin production. Tyrosinase inhibitors are the most popular type of skincare products on the market to lighten skin. Tyrosinase is a copper-containing metalloprotein and requires copper to function.[11,12] It is inhibited by copper-chelating ingredients such as flavonoids. Thiols such as glutathione and cysteine also affect tyrosinase activity.[13]

Hydroquinone

HQ (**Fig. 41-2**) was used in cosmetic products (2% concentration or less) until the U.S. CARES Act was passed in 2020. Subtitle F of this act changed the way HQ was regulated and it is now considered a drug, resulting in removal of all HQ from cosmetic products. Prescription drugs may contain HQ (4%), and custom pharmacy formulations include HQ (2% to ≥ 10%) as an ingredient. HQ is used to inhibit melanin production and yield skin lightening.

HQ occurs naturally as an ingredient in various plant-derived food and beverage products, such as vegetables, fruits, grains, coffee, tea, beer, and wine.[14] For many years, HQ has been the main treatment modality for post-inflammatory hyperpigmentation and melasma. HQ exerts its depigmenting effect by inhibiting tyrosinase and has been shown to decrease its activity by 90%.[15] HQ is cytotoxic to melanocytes.[16] It is known to cause reversible inhibition of cellular metabolism by affecting both DNA and RNA synthesis. Although useful as a sole agent, HQ is often combined with other agents such as tretinoin, glycolic acid, kojic acid, azelaic acid, and corticosteroids.[17] It is often included in TCCs as discussed above. As with all tyrosinase inhibitors, it frequently takes 6–12 weeks before any improvement becomes noticeable.

Numerous concerns about the safety of HQ have emerged in recent years and, in fact, its use was banned in Europe in 2000 for general cosmetic purposes. In Asia, its use is highly regulated. At the time that this chapter was written, HQ was banned in cosmetic formulations in the US. HQ is the most effective of the tyrosinase inhibitors, however, and has been used for several years by dermatologists to treat pigmentation disorders, with few reports of serious side effects. The reason for the scrutiny is that HQ is a metabolite of benzene and has potential mutagenic properties. Some studies have shown that large doses of HQ delivered systemically—not by topical application—resulted in some evidence of cancer in rats. However, HQ is detoxified in the liver in humans, and metabolized very differently in rats.[18,19] In humans, HQ is probably metabolized to detoxified derivatives, such as glucuronide and sulfate conjugates of HQ.[20] In the 40 years HQ has been on the market, no human cases of cancer have been attributed to its use. The most serious human health effect seen in workers exposed to HQ is pigmentation of the eye and, in a small number of cases, permanent corneal damage.[14] The main concerns of the FDA are the side effects associated with topical use of HQ, which can lead to a condition called exogenous ochronosis.[21] Ochronosis presents as asymptomatic blue-black macules in the area of HQ application, which is essentially a more permanent form of hyperpigmentation. It usually occurs after prolonged use of HQ.[22] For this reason, the FDA decided that HQ should be used only under a physician's supervision. Topical HQ products are thought to provoke exogenous ochronosis by inhibiting the enzyme homogentisic acid oxidase in the skin. This results in the local accumulation of homogentisic acid that then polymerizes to form ochronotic pigment.[23] Exogenous ochronosis seems to occur more commonly among patients with darker skin types and of Asian descent. Despite the widespread use of HQ, only 30 cases of ochronosis have been attributed to its use in North America.[19] Other side effects like skin rashes and nail discoloration may also occur, but can be resolved by simply discontinuing HQ use (**Fig. 41-3**). The incidence of side effects from HQ may also be decreased through the use of lower strengths of HQ, using a test site first to determine the presence of allergy, and taking "hydroquinone holidays" every 3 to 4 months. The debate in the FDA about the safety of HQ has increased the need for new depigmenting ingredients. Many of these share a similar chemical structure to HQ.

Aloesin

Aloesin (**Fig. 41-4**) is a *C*-glycosylated chromone naturally derived from *Aloe vera*. It competitively inhibits tyrosinase, by

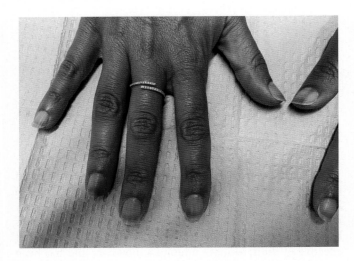

FIGURE 41-3. Pigmentation of the nails caused by hydroquinone use.

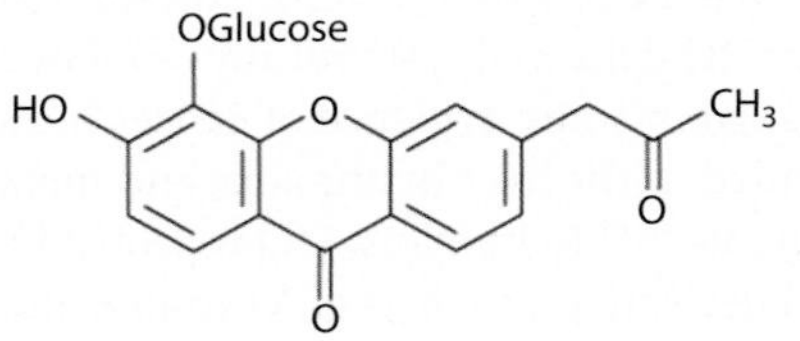

FIGURE 41-4. The chemical structure of aloesin.

TABLE 41-1	Flavonoids and Flavonoid-like Compounds[a,27]
Family	Inhibition of Melanin Formation
Hydroxystilbene derivatives	
Resveratrol	+
Oxyresveratrol	++
Piceatannol (PICE)	+++
Gnetol	++
(4-Methoxy-benzyliden)-(3-methoxy-phenyl)-amine.	+++
4,4-Dihydroxybiphenyl	+++
Rosmarinic acid, rooperol	?
Hydroxyflavanols conjugated to gallic acid	
EGCG [(–)-epigallocatechin-3-O-gallate]	
GCG [(–)-gallocatechin-3-O-gallate]	?
Proanthocyanidins	
Grape seed extract	+
Pycnogenol	+
Elaters	
Ellagic acid	+++
Flavonols	
Genistein	–
6,7,4-Trihydroxyisoflavone	+++
Apigenin	+
Quercetin (in onions)	+
Flavanones (Chalcones)	
Isoliquiritigeninchalcone	+++
Butein	+++
Aloesin	+++

[a]Flavonoids and flavonoid-like substances show varying degrees of tyrosinase inhibition. Some of these ingredients also inhibit melanin production through pathways other than tyrosinase inhibition. +, mild inhibition; ++, moderate inhibition; +++, strong inhibition; ?, not enough studies performed to rank. Flavonoids also have the ability to chelate copper, which is one way they inhibit tyrosinase activity.

suppressing both the hydroxylation of tyrosine to DOPA and oxidation of DOPA to DOPAchinone, and it blocks melanin production in cultured normal melanocytes.[24] Aloesin and a few chemically related chromones have been demonstrated to exhibit an even stronger inhibitory effect on tyrosinase than arbutin and kojic acid.[25] One study on the inhibitory effect of aloesin and/or arbutin (administered four times daily for 15 days) on pigmentation in human skin after ultraviolet (UV) radiation showed suppressed pigmentation by 34% for aloesin, 43.5% for arbutin, and 63.3% for the co-treatment with aloesin and arbutin compared with the control group.[26]

Flavonoids

More than 4,000 flavonoids have been identified in leaves, barks, and flowers. All have phenolic and pyran rings, and are therefore considered benzopyrane derivatives.[27] Many flavonoids display depigmenting effects (**Table 41-1**). They are classified into six major groups: flavanols, flavones, flavonols, flavanones, isoflavones, and anthocyanidins. These classes differ in the conjugation of rings and the position of hydroxyl, methoxy, and glycosidic groups.[28] Flavonoids exhibit antioxidant properties, but they can also directly inhibit tyrosinase and act on the distal part of the melanogenesis oxidative pathway. Flavonoids also have the ability to chelate copper. Copper is required for the function of tyrosinase, so when flavonoids form a complex with copper, this inhibits tyrosinase activity.

Resveratrol (**Fig. 41-5**) falls into the hydroxystilbene derivative group of flavonoids as do oxyresveratrol and gnetol, which are more efficient tyrosinase inhibitors than resveratrol.[29] Resveratrol induces depigmentation also by reducing microphthalmia-associated transcription factor (MITF) and tyrosinase promoter activity.[30] (See **Box 41-2.**) In a 2003 study aimed at developing a skin-whitening agent, investigators assessed the inhibitory effects on tyrosinase of 285 different herbal extracts, finding that *Ramulus mori* extracts performed

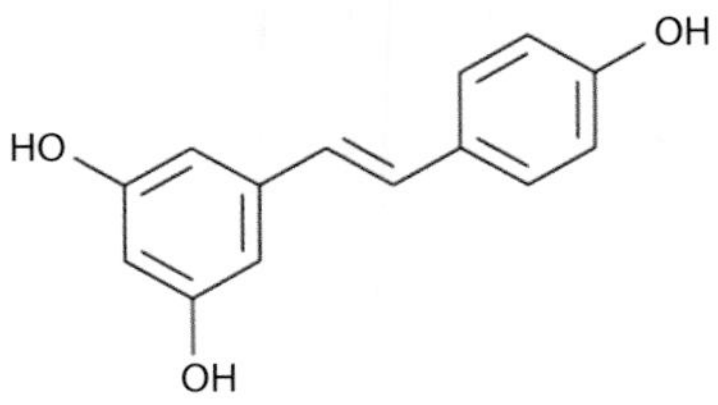

FIGURE 41-5. The chemical structure of resveratrol.

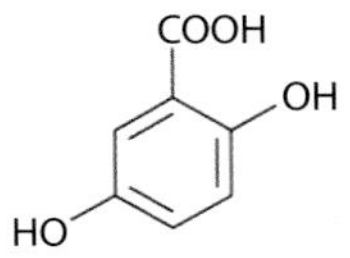

FIGURE 41-6. The chemical structure of gentisic acid.

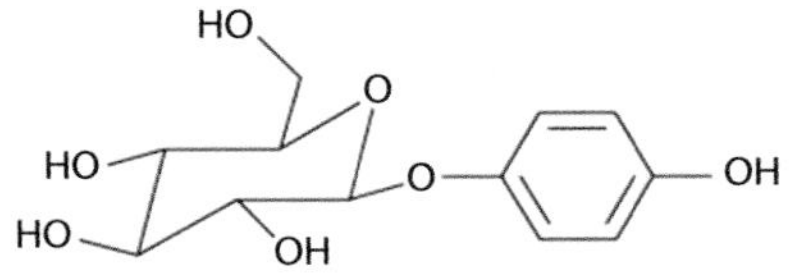

FIGURE 41-7. The chemical structure of arbutin.

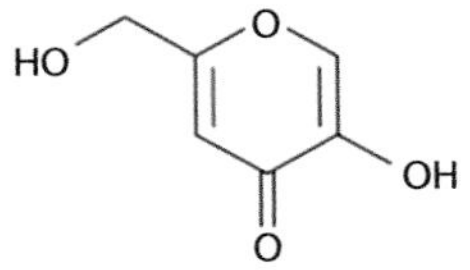

BOX 41-2   The MITF Gene

The MITF gene provides instructions for a protein called melanocyte-inducing transcription factor. The MITF protein attaches to DNA and controls the activity of particular genes involved in the development and function of melanocytes.

FIGURE 41-8. The chemical structure of kojic acid.

optimally. This extract contains 2-oxyresveratrol and showed strong inhibition of tyrosinase activity, as well as melanin synthesis in B-16 melanoma cells, and caused no toxicity or irritation in various animal tests.[31]

Ellagic Acid

A polyphenolic antioxidant, ellagic acid is isolated from various trees, nuts, and fruit, including strawberries, green tea, eucalyptus, and geraniums.[32] It is a tyrosinase inhibitor and has been shown to prevent UV-induced pigmentation. Ellagic acid seems to be more effective than kojic acid or arbutin and it is safer than HQ as it affects melanogenesis without inducing cytotoxic reactions.[33] Two small randomized controlled trials have suggested that ellagic acid in combination with other therapies was effective in treating melasma, but investigations of ellagic acid are necessary to ascertain its clinical potential.[32,34,35]

Gentisic Acid

Gentisic acid (**Fig. 41-6**) is derived from genetian roots. It has been tested *in vitro* and in cell cultures proving its inhibitory effect on tyrosinase. However, methyl gentisate seems to be more effective than the free acid. *In vitro* studies have shown HQ to be less effective and more cytotoxic to melanocytes than methyl gentisate.[36]

HYDROQUINONE-LIKE INGREDIENTS

Arbutin

Arbutin ($C_{12}H_{16}O_7$) is a naturally occurring β-D-glucopyranoside that consists of a molecule of HQ bound to glucose (**Fig. 41-7**). Traditionally used in Japan, arbutin is present in the leaves of bearberry shrubs as well as pear trees and certain herbs, such as wheat, and in small quantities in cranberry and blueberry leaves.[37–39] Its depigmenting mechanism involves a reversible inhibition of melanosomal tyrosinase activity rather than the suppression of tyrosinase expression and synthesis,[40]

without provoking melanotoxic effects.[41,42] However, the utility of arbutin as a depigmenting agent is unclear. Nakajima et al. reported that although tyrosinase activity was reduced in normal human melanocytes treated with arbutin, an increase of pigmentation occurred.[43] These results have not yet been duplicated. Arbutin serves as an ingredient in various cosmetic products available in the US.[44] Deoxyarbutin and α-arbutin, synthetic derivatives of arbutin, have shown promising *in vitro* and *in vivo* results with a greater inhibition of tyrosinase than the plant-derived compound,[37,45] with α-arbutin also found to be effective in the periorbital region.[39]

In a 2008 randomized, prospective, open-label study of 10 patients with melasma, Ertam et al. found that pigmentation was reduced by 43.5% in the five subjects topically treated with 3% arbutin gel once daily for 1 month. A decline of 7.1% was observed in the placebo group.[34] In 2015, Morag et al. conducted a randomized controlled trial of 102 women with melasma and solar lentigines. Twice daily application of a cream containing 2.51% β-arbutin (derived from *Serratulae quinquefoliae*) over 8 weeks yielded lightening and skin tone homogenization in 66% of patients.[46]

Kojic Acid

Kojic acid (5-hydroxy-2-hydroxymethyl-γ-pyrone or $C_6H_6O_4$) (**Fig. 41-8**) is a fungal metabolite commonly produced by various species of *Aspergillus, Acetobacter,* and *Penicillium*.[47,48] It is widely used as a food additive for preventing enzymatic browning and to promote reddening of unripe strawberries.[49] Kojic acid suppresses tyrosinase activity, mainly by chelating copper. This leads to a whitening effect on the skin.[50] Consequently, manufacturers, particularly in Japan, have used it extensively in cosmetic agents.[51] When used in cosmetic products, kojic acid enhances the shelf life of the formulation through its preservative and antibiotic actions.[52] This stability is one of the advantages of kojic acid when compared to HQ and other depigmenting agents.[53]

As is the case with numerous topically applied preparations, kojic acid is hydrophilic and poorly absorbed into the skin. Various formulation technologies are used to try and increase skin penetration of kojic acid.[54] Combining kojic acid with hydroxy acids that loosen attachments between corneocytes or hyaluronic acid that increases delivery of ingredients is another strategy to increase the efficacy of kojic acid-containing agents. Lee et al. reported on derivatives of kojic acid displaying greater efficiency through increased penetration into the skin.[55]

In two separate studies, kojic acid combined with glycolic acid was shown to be more effective when compared with 10% glycolic acid and 4% HQ for the treatment of hyperpigmentation.[56,57] A study by Lim compared the effect of a gel containing 10% glycolic acid and 2% HQ with and without 2% kojic acid.[58] The result was that the addition of kojic acid to the gel further improved melasma.

Products that contain kojic acid are usually used twice daily for 4 months or until the patient achieves the desired effect. Kojic acid-containing products are more effective when combined with retinoids and corticosteroids in a TCC. Unfortunately, kojic acid has been associated with contact allergy and is considered to have a high sensitizing potential,[59] with increased sunburn risk for those with sensitive skin.[48] Because preparations using 2.5% concentrations of kojic acid have resulted in facial dermatitis,[60] a concentration of 1% is usually used in topical formulations. This 1% concentration is also the recommendation of the European Union's Scientific Committee on Consumer Safety.[61] However, there have been reports of sensitization to 1% creams as well.[59]

Kojic acid has been extensively used in foods, and several reports on its oral safety are available. Toxicity resulting from an oral dose has been reported in a Japanese study recording the occurrence of hepatocellular tumors in p53-deficient mice.[62] Furthermore, convulsions may occur if kojic acid is injected.[53] It is recommended that kojic acid not be applied to broken skin.[48]

HYDROXYCOUMARINS

Coumarins are lactones of phenylpropanoid acid with an *H*-benzopyranone nucleus. They directly interact with tyrosinase. Yamamura et al. studied the antimelanogenic activity of six hydrocoumarins and α-tocopherol in normal human melanocytes. In particular, 7-allyl-6-hydroxy-4,4,5,8-tetramethylhydrocoumarin (hydrocoumarin 4) strongly inhibited melanogenesis and intracellular glutathione synthesis in normal human melanocytes. The investigators suggested that hydrocoumarin 4 may be effective in preventing hyperpigmentation and proposed a combined treatment of hydrocoumarins and α-tocopherols to enhance the hypopigmenting effect by a free radical-scavenging mechanism.[63]

OTHER TYROSINASE INHIBITORS

Difluorocyclohexyloxyphenol

TFC-1067 is a gem-difluorocompound known as 2-[2-(2,4-difluorophenyl)-2-propen-1-yl]-1,3-propanediol or difluorocyclohexyloxyphenol (**Fig. 41-9**). Difluorocyclohexyloxyphenol is a tyrosinase inhibitor without melanocyte toxicity. In a 2020 study, 48 women received either TFC-1067 or 2% HQ topically to treat facial dyschromia. TFC-1067 was found to have equivalent results to 2% HQ.[64]

Licorice Extract

Glabridin (*Glycyrrhiza glabra*) (**Fig. 41-10**) is the main ingredient of licorice extract that affects skin. *G. glabra* extract has been used to treat dermatitis, eczema, pruritus, cysts, and skin irritation.[65] In addition, *G. glabra* has demonstrated antimutagenic, anticarcinogenic, as well as tumor-suppressive capacity against skin cancer in animal models, and the National Cancer Institute has formally recognized the chemopreventive value of its primary constituent glycyrrhizin.[66–68] Glabridin is used in skin-lightening products because it inhibits tyrosinase activity

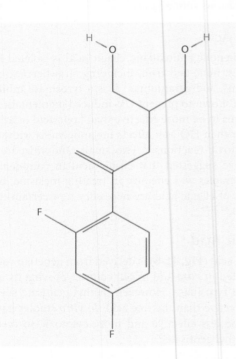

FIGURE 41-9. Structure of 2-[2-(2,4-Difluorophenyl)-2-propen-1-YL]-1,3-propanediol.

Glabridin

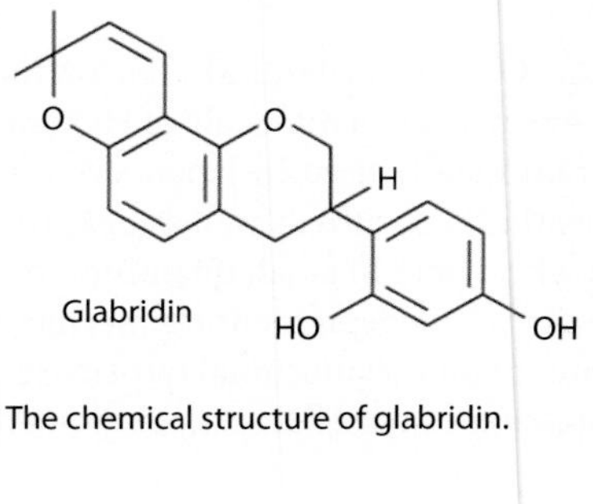

FIGURE 41-10. The chemical structure of glabridin.

in cell cultures without affecting DNA synthesis. Combined analysis of SDS-polyacrylamide gel electrophoresis and DOPA staining on the large granule fraction of these cells has shown that glabridin specifically lowered the activities of T1 and T3 tyrosinase isozymes. Topical applications of 0.5% glabridin have also been demonstrated to inhibit UVB-induced pigmentation and erythema in the skin of guinea pigs. Furthermore, the inhibition of superoxide anion production and cyclooxygenase activity revealed the anti-inflammatory effects of glabridin *in vitro*.[69] Notably, *G. glabra* has shown efficacy in the treatment of melasma.[70] One study suggested that glabridin exhibits a superior depigmenting effect compared to HQ.[71] In Europe, licorice extract is widely used as an anti-inflammatory agent.[72] However, there are no controlled clinical trials in the literature examining the efficacy of this agent to treat inflammation. Forms of licorice extract have been incorporated into skincare products to prevent inflammation. One such ingredient is licochalcone A, an oxygenated retrochalcone found in Eucerin Redness Relief™ products. Licochalone has displayed antiparasitic, antibacterial, and antitumorigenic activity as well as shown efficacy in treating rosacea.[27,73–77]

Paper Mulberry or Mulberry Extract

Paper mulberry, also known as *Broussonetia papyrifera*, is an East Asian ornamental deciduous tree. In a study in which 101 plant extracts were evaluated for inhibitory activity against tyrosinase, L-3,4-dihydroxyphenylalanine (L-DOPA) oxidation, and melanin biosynthesis in B16 mouse melanoma cells, investigators noted that the leaves and bark of *B. papyrifera*

inhibited both tyrosinase activity and L-DOPA in a concentration-dependent fashion.[78] Although it displays activity as a tyrosinase inhibitor, there are currently no peer-reviewed clinical studies evaluating its use in pigmentary disorders.

Emblicanin

Emblica is an extract from the edible *Phyllantus emblica* fruit and is thus 100% natural. The key components are the tannins emblicanin A and emblicanin B. Emblica combines all the important properties required for a skin-lightening ingredient: It acts at several different sites in the melanogenesis pathway, not only as an inhibitor of tyrosinase and/or tyrosinase-related proteins (TRP-1 and -2) and peroxidase/H_2O_2,[79] but also as a broad-spectrum cascading antioxidant. Emblica is thought to have efficacy comparable to HQ and kojic acid, but without provoking similarly harmful side effects. It is photochemically and hydrolytically stable, which facilitates its inclusion in skincare formulations.

MELANOSOME TRANSFER INHIBITORS

When melanin is synthesized (as shown in **Fig. 41-1**), it is packaged into melanosomes that store and transport it (**Fig. 41-11**). One melanocyte touches many keratinocytes with its "arms." The melanosomes accumulate in the arms of the melanocyte (**Fig. 41-12**). To enter into keratinocytes, melanosomes must traverse through a "doorway" into the keratinocytes. The doorway is protected by a receptor known as protease-activated receptor (PAR)-2. PAR-2 is a G-protein-

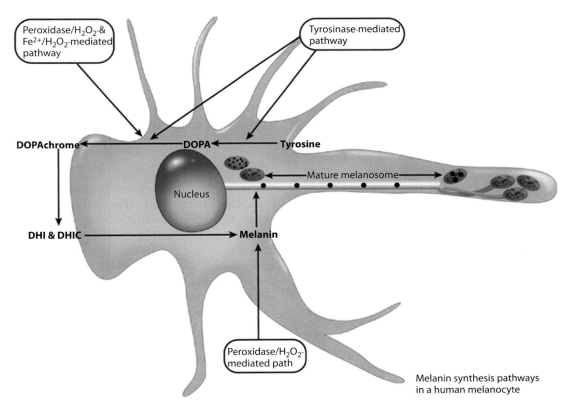

FIGURE 41-11. Melanin is synthesized in the melanocyte, packaged into melanosomes, and moves to the "arms" of the melanocyte for transport.

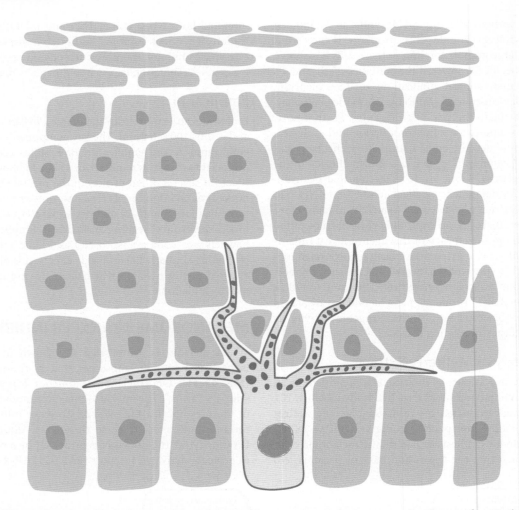

FIGURE 41-12. Melanosomes accumulate in the arms of the melanocyte. These arms traverse between many keratinocytes forming the epidermal-melanin unit.

coupled receptor (**Fig. 41-13**). When activated, PAR-2 allows melanin-carrying melanosomes to move from melanocytes into keratinocytes.[80] PAR-2 is the only PAR that is not responsive to thrombin unless it is present at high levels.[81]

PAR-2 has been found in cell cultures to regulate the ingestion of melanosomes by keratinocytes.[82] Ingredients that interfere with PAR-2 activation induce skin depigmentation by reducing melanosome transfer and distribution to the keratinocytes. These melanosome transfer-inhibiting ingredients are also called PAR-2 blockers. Soybeans, which contain the serine protease inhibitors soybean trypsin inhibitor (STI) and Bowman-Birk protease inhibitor (BBI), have been demonstrated to block melanosome transfer, resulting in an improvement of mottled facial pigmentation.[83] In addition, blocking activation of PAR-2 with trypsin and other synthetic peptides has been shown to result in visible skin darkening.[84]

PAR-2 blockers prevent transfer of melanosomes but do not break down melanin already present in keratinocytes. For this reason, skin lightening will not be seen for 8–16 weeks of using such skincare products because the melanin-containing keratinocytes must desquamate off the skin's surface before an

effect is seen. PAR-2 inhibitors work best when combined with exfoliants such as retinoids to speed desquamation and tyrosinase inhibitors to prevent the formation of new melanin.

Niacinamide

Niacinamide, also known as nicotinamide, is the biologically active amide of vitamin B_3 (**Fig. 41-14**). Niacinamide has been shown to exhibit anti-inflammatory, antioxidant, and immunomodulatory properties. In addition, it has been demonstrated to inhibit the transfer of melanosomes to epidermal keratinocytes by blocking PAR-2. Clinical trials have shown that niacinamide inhibited melanosome transfer by up to 68% in an *in vitro* model and improved unwanted facial pigmentation.[85] Significant effects on hyperpigmentation have been demonstrated by a 5% niacinamide formulation used twice daily for 8 weeks and by 3.5% niacinamide in combination with retinyl palmitate.[86] The effects on pigmentation have been shown to be reversible.[87] In a 2014 randomized, double-blind, vehicle-controlled trial with 42 Korean women (from 30 to 60 years old), a moisturizing cream combining 2% niacinamide and 2% tranexamic acid was found to be significantly more

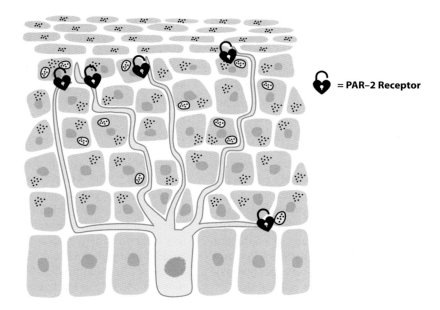

FIGURE 41-13. PAR-2 receptors function as a lock that opens a door that allows transport of melanosomes from the melanocyte to the keratinocyte. When PAR-2 is activated, the melanosomes move into the keratinocytes where they remain, providing melanin to the keratinocytes.

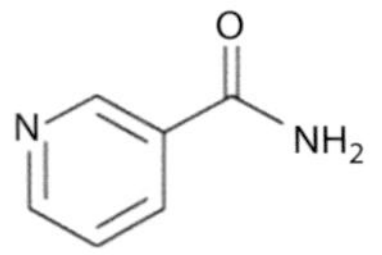

FIGURE 41-14. The chemical structure of niacinamide.

successful than control in diminishing irregular pigmentation.[88] Niacinamide is also an effective anti-inflammatory ingredient and contributes to cellular energy production in the NAD/NADH pathway (Chapter 38, Anti-Inflammatory Agents).

Soy

The soybean plant belongs to the pea family, *Leguminosae*. Soy is found in tofu products as well as in soybeans and soymilk. Chinese women who work in the tofu industry are reputed to have beautiful skin.[89] As the health benefits of soy have become known, it has been added to many skincare products.

Paine et al. demonstrated that soymilk and the soymilk-derived proteins STI and BBI are able to inhibit PAR-2 activation and thus induce skin depigmentation.[90] As the inhibition of melanosome transfer is reversible, side effects of these soy-derived proteins are negligible. This is important because the PAR-2 receptor participates in multiple cellular processes beyond regulating pigmentation.

The depigmenting activity of these melanosome transfer-inhibiting agents and their capacity to prevent UV-induced pigmentation has been demonstrated both *in vitro* and *in vivo*. In one study, dark-skinned Yucatan microswine were treated with soybean extract. Diminished skin color was observed visually and confirmed by F&M staining of histologic sections that demonstrated reduced melanin deposition in the skin biopsies of treated skin. Interestingly, the effect was seen only with fresh soymilk and not observed when pasteurized soymilk preparations were used. This suggests that a heat-labile component of the soymilk, STI, is the active depigmenting agent. Treatments with soymilk were also shown to prevent UVB-induced darkening of the swine skin. In addition, human trials have demonstrated lightening of pigmented spots after application of soybean extract.[91]

Another study examined the efficacy of a moisturizer containing non-denatured STI and BBI on skin pigmentation, skin tone, and photoaging. Sixty-five women, aged 30 to 61, with Fitzpatrick phototypes I to III and moderately severe mottled hyperpigmentation, lentigines, blotchiness, tactile roughness, and dullness were enrolled in the parallel, randomized, double-blind, and vehicle-controlled study. The moisturizer and the vehicle, respectively, were administered twice daily for a period of 12 weeks. By clinical observation, self-assessment, colorimetry, and digital photography, the researchers reported a significant improvement of mottled pigmentation, blotchiness, dullness, and fine lines, as well as overall texture, skin tone, and appearance versus the vehicle.[83] In addition to these depigmentation properties, soy contains isoflavones, which have antioxidant properties that have been found to confer cancer-preventing benefits.

MELANOCYTE-CYTOTOXIC AGENTS

HQ is cytotoxic to melanocytes when oxidized into highly reactive species such as hydroxybenzoquinone and p-benzoquinone, which are capable of disrupting fundamental cellular processes. Other tyrosinase inhibitors also form free radicals that become toxic to melanocytes.

Azelaic Acid

Azelaic acid (**Fig. 41-15**) is a naturally occurring saturated dicarboxylic acid. While topical azelaic acid is used in the management of hyperpigmentary skin disorders, the associated proposed mechanism(s) of action of azelaic acid and how azelaic acid exerts its clinical effect are not fully understood.[92,93] It is known that high amounts of azelaic acid are cytotoxic to melanocytes.[94] Azelaic acid suppresses the energy production and/or DNA synthesis of melanocytes and imparts an antiproliferative effect.[95] The clinical effectiveness of azelaic acid is thought to be due in part to its inhibitory action on neutrophil-generated reactive oxygen species, leading to a reduction of oxidative tissue injury at sites of inflammation.[96] Research has demonstrated that *in vitro* azelaic acid scavenges hydroxyl radicals and blocks oxyradical toxicity in cell cultures.[97,98] Further *in vitro* studies have demonstrated that azelaic acid is a competitive inhibitor of tyrosinase resulting in a decrease in melanin formation.[99,100] It can reversibly inhibit the activity of mitochondrial respiratory chain enzymes, such as reduced NADH-dehydrogenase, succinic acid dehydrogenase, and reduced ubiquinone cytochrome-*c* oxidoreductase.[101]

Azelaic acid has been reported to be effective for patients with melasma with fewer side effects than seen with HQ.[99,102,103] In a multicenter, randomized trial lasting 24 weeks, azelaic acid 20% cream produced significantly greater decreases in pigmentary intensity than did its vehicle both subjectively and in the chromameter analysis.[104] Another study demonstrated that the combination of azelaic acid 20% cream and glycolic acid 15% or 20% lotion was as effective as 4% HQ cream in the treatment of hyperpigmentation in darker-skinned patients, with only a slightly higher rate of mild local irritation.[105] In a subsequent study in which hyperpigmented lesions were visible only with a UVB camera, azelaic acid was found to be superior to glycolic acid in attenuating the subclinical hyperpigmentation when used over a 3-week period.[91] In the US,

topical azelaic acid is available by prescription in concentrations of a 15% gel and a 20% cream for the treatment of rosacea and acne, respectively. The use for hyperpigmentation is off-label. Topically applied azelaic acid is well tolerated, with adverse effects generally limited to mild local cutaneous irritation. Azelaic acid is an excellent alternative for patients who cannot tolerate HQ.

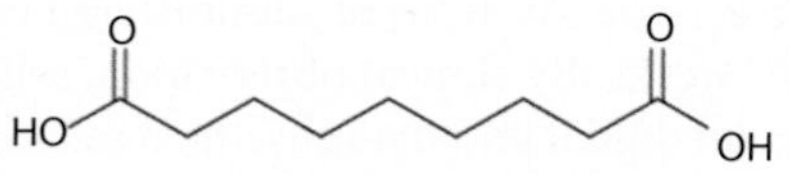

Mequinol

Chemically known as 4-hydroxyanisole, mequinol is a derivative of HQ (**Fig. 41-16**). Its exact mechanism of action is unknown; however, mequinol is a substrate to tyrosinase and acts as a competitive inhibitor of melanogenesis.[106] Notably, 2% mequinol with 0.01% tretinoin has been proven to be effective in the treatment of solar lentigines.[107,108] In a randomized, parallel-grouped, double-masked study with 216 subjects, the effects of 2% mequinol/0.01% tretinoin were compared with those of 3% HQ in the treatment of solar lentigines. With a twice-daily treatment for more than 16 weeks and a follow-up after 24 weeks, a significantly higher proportion of subjects achieved clinical success with 2% mequinol/0.01% tretinoin compared with 3% HQ.[109]

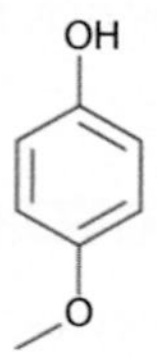

Monobenzone

The monobenzyl ether in HQ is the substance that causes permanent depigmentation of normal skin. It is often used in vitiligo patients to permanently depigment the skin surrounding depigmented areas when repigmentation is not feasible and the depigmented areas are disfiguring. Monobenzone (**Fig. 41-17**) is metabolized inside cells into quinine, which is cytotoxic to melanocytes.[110] It is usually prepared at a concentration of 20%.

Monobenzone is applied two or three times daily on pigmented skin, with depigmentation beginning around 6 to 12 months into treatment. Transfer of the agent can occur to anyone who touches the medication; therefore, contact with others should be avoided for up to 3 hours after application.[111] Potential side effects include contact dermatitis, conjunctival melanosis, skin lightening in untreated areas,[112] the possibility of an unwanted repigmentation starting from follicular melanocytes, and the need for lifelong total photoprotection. Skin treated with monobenzone may be especially sensitive to irritation. Because this agent is cytotoxic to melanocytes, it must be stressed that after depigmentation therapy with this agent, future attempts at repigmentation treatment will be completely ineffective.

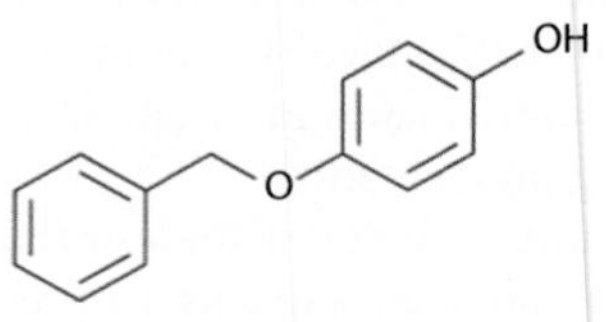

FIGURE 41-15. The chemical structure of azelaic acid.

FIGURE 41-16. The chemical structure of mequinol.

FIGURE 41-17. The chemical structure of monobenzone—a derivative of hydroquinone.

N-Acetyl-4-S-cysteaminylphenol

N-Acetyl-4-S-cysteaminylphenol is a melanocytotoxic agent consisting of phenolic and catecholic compounds with potent depigmenting properties. In addition to inhibiting tyrosinase, it interferes with the thiol system decreasing the antioxidant glutathione.[113] It favors pheomelanin synthesis, and is less irritating and more stable than HQ. A study in which 12 patients with melasma were treated with a daily application of 4% N-acetyl-4-S-cysteaminylphenol showed significant reduction in pigmentation, with results being visible as early as 2 to 4 weeks after therapy.[114]

PEPTIDES

As discussed in Chapter 37, Anti-Aging Ingredients, peptides have issues with stability, shelf life, interaction with other ingredients, and penetration into the skin. Assuming that these issues can be resolved with formulation techniques and skincare regimen design, peptides may have some utility in treating pigmentation. Oligopeptide-68 (Arg-Asp-Gly-Gln-Ile-Leu-Ser-Thr-Trp-Tyr) suppresses MITF by reducing tyrosinase activity.[115,116] Tetrapeptide PKEK has also been shown to confer skin-lightening effects through an unknown mechanism of action.[117]

ANTIOXIDANTS

Antioxidants impart anti-aging, anticarcinogenic, as well as anti-inflammatory activities, and may also decrease pigmentation that occurs after exposure to UV light and inflammation.[118] Further, antioxidants help preserve the stability of ingredients in formulations such as ascorbic acid by scavenging free radicals. Antioxidants are used orally and topically in the treatment of melasma.

Research on vitiligo has demonstrated that antioxidants affect melanin production. A comparison of normal melanocytes with melanocytes from vitiligo patients revealed lower catalase activity and higher vitamin E and ubiquinone levels in the vitiligo patients suggesting that an imbalance in the antioxidant status and increase in the intracellular peroxide levels could play a role in the disorder.[119] In addition, antioxidants, including glutathione, a naturally occurring antioxidant involved in regulating melanin synthesis,[120] have been shown to inhibit or delay hyperpigmentation.[121]

Piceatannol (PICE) is an example of an antioxidant shown to inhibit tyrosinase.[121] PICE (**Fig. 41-18**) is a phenolic compound derived from resveratrol. It has antioxidative, antitumorigenic, and apoptosis-inducing effects. In this study, investigators found that PICE inhibited melanogenesis and displayed potent antioxidant properties. The authors concluded that the antioxidant activity played a major role in the inhibition of melanin production. The flavonoid antioxidant phloretin can reduce tyrosinase activity,[122] and has been shown to hinder elastase and matrix metalloproteinase-1 activity. Phloretin is difficult to formulate because it has photoinstability and poor solubility in aqueous solutions.[123]

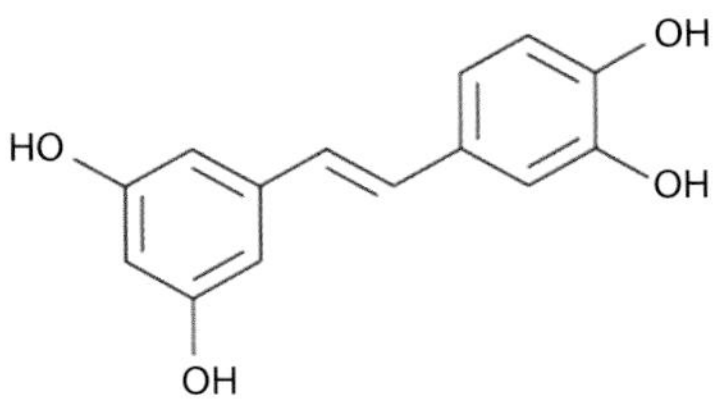

FIGURE 41-18. The chemical structure of piceatannol (PICE)—a derivative of resveratrol.

Antioxidants may prevent inflammation by directly inhibiting tyrosinase as is the case with phloretin and PICE. In addition, antioxidants decrease pigmentation by scavenging free radicals, reducing inflammation, and affecting prostaglandin and histamine levels. They likely prevent inflammation and subsequent pigmentation by several other mechanisms as well including effects on transcription factor nuclear factor-κB (NF-κB), inducible nitric oxide synthase expression, and inhibition of cyclooxygenase.[124]

Although antioxidants generally can reduce pigmentation, a few studies have shown that some antioxidants increase skin pigmentation. Consequently, the individual properties of each antioxidant should be considered before using them to decrease skin pigmentation.[125]

Antioxidants, Inflammation, and Prostaglandins

Inflammation has long been known to lead to skin pigmentation, especially in darker skin types. Prostaglandins, which are produced during inflammation, play a role in skin pigmentation and this is one of the mechanisms by which inflammation can exacerbate melasma or lead to postinflammatory pigment alteration (PIPA). Antioxidants can prevent the formation of prostaglandins,[126] thereby preventing inflammation and tyrosinase activation. The plasmin inhibitor *trans*-4-aminomethyl-cyclohexanecarboxylic acid (*trans*-AMCHA or tranexamic acid) has been proposed to decrease tyrosinase activity in the melanocytes via reduction in prostaglandin synthesis, thus preventing UV-induced pigmentation in guinea pigs. Localized intradermal microinjections of tranexamic acid were used in an Asian study with some success (see section on tranexamic acid in this chapter).[127]

The prostaglandin PGF_2 increases tyrosinase activity and stimulates melanin formation.[128] Latanoprost and Bimatoprost, analogues of prostaglandin $F_{2\alpha}$ ($PGF_{2\alpha}$), were originally used as intraocular pressure-lowering drugs and more recently have become popular for stimulating eyelash growth. Their use has been associated with hyperpigmentation of the iris and the eyelid and should be used with caution by those with darker skin types and those with a history of melasma and other pigmentation disorders.

Antioxidants, Inflammation, and Histamine

Inflammation also contributes to skin pigmentation through the effects of histamine. Histamine is released from mast cells during inflammation and increases the level of tyrosinase-mediated cAMP via actions on protein kinase A (PKA). The release of histamine stimulates melanogenesis and results in the production of eumelanin rather than pheomelanin.[129] Yoshida et al. found that blocking H2 receptors with famotidine suppressed the increase in melanogenesis, but antagonists of H1 and H3 do not have any influence.[130] The effect of histamine-related agents is difficult to predict and their use to treat hypo- and hyperpigmentation is still unreliable. However, antioxidants, especially flavonoids, have been shown to inhibit histamine release.[131]

Coenzyme Q_{10} (Ubiquinone)

Coenzyme Q_{10}, also known as ubiquinone or CoQ_{10}, is one of the most popular anti-aging ingredients because it is an antioxidant and aids in mitochondrial production of cellular energy known as ATP (**Fig. 41-19**) (see Chapter 37). As aging occurs, and when patients are placed on cholesterol-lowering statin drugs, natural levels of CoQ_{10} decline. Levels of CoQ_{10} have also been shown to decrease in aging skin. Topical CoQ_{10} has been demonstrated to improve skin wrinkles, but may have value in evening skin tone and reducing skin pigmentation.[132]

CoQ_{10} is a potent tyrosinase inhibitor. It works by down-regulating the melanogenic regulatory genes POMC, α-MSH, tyrosinase, and MITF. In addition to providing energy in the form of ATP, CoQ_{10} reduces inflammation and neutralizes free radicals. It also induces the antioxidant genes HO-1, γ-GCLC, and GSH. *In vivo* experiments on zebrafish have shown that CoQ_{10} reverses UVA-induced hyperpigmentation.[132] Oral and topical CoQ_{10} can be added to any skincare routines to treat dyschromia.

The Cosmetic Ingredient Review board evaluated CoQ_{10} in cosmetics in September 2020.[133] They stated that CoQ_{10} in cosmetics at a maximum concentration of 1% is safe. Idebenone, which is a derivative of CoQ_{10}, was deemed to be safe at concentrations up to 0.5%. Idebenone is associated with a risk of contact dermatitis; therefore, CoQ_{10} is the preferred form to use in skincare. The CIR panel noted that CoQ_{10} and idebenone, when used in large amounts, can render warfarin less effective. Therefore, these should be used with caution and on a limited amount of body surface area (e.g., only the face and neck) in patients taking warfarin anticoagulants.

Vitamin C

Vitamin C or ascorbic acid (**Fig. 41-20**) can be found in citrus fruits and green leafy vegetables. It inhibits melanin formation and reduces oxidized melanin because it is able to reduce o-DOPAquinone back to DOPA, thus avoiding melanin formation.[134] Vitamin C interacts with copper ions at

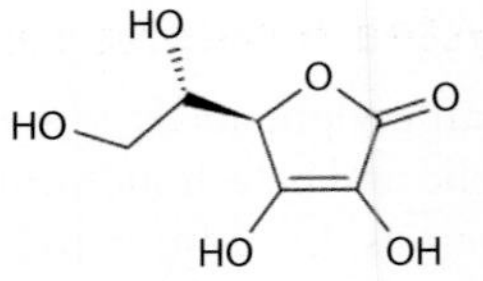

FIGURE 41-20. The chemical structure of vitamin C (L-ascorbic acid).

tyrosinase-active sites and inhibits the action of the tyrosinase.[135] A 25% vitamin C formulation was found to significantly diminish melasma pigmentation in 16 weeks.[136] Numerous forms of vitamin C demonstrate various bioactive characteristics that should be considered when choosing which vitamin C to use to lighten skin. In addition to its utility as a depigmenting agent, vitamin C displays antioxidant properties and has been shown to stimulate collagen synthesis (see Chapters 37, and 39, Antioxidants).

L-ascorbic acid is the form of ascorbic acid receiving the greatest focus in cosmeceutical research. It is mainly used for anti-aging to increase collagen synthesis (Chapter 37). It is easily broken down by air and light, requires a low pH of 2–2.5 to be absorbed into the skin, and is hydrophilic. A plethora of research supports its use as an anti-aging and antioxidant skincare product.

Ascorbyl palmitate is also used in anti-aging preparations. It is lipophilic and does not require a low pH to remain stable or to penetrate into the skin. It does not absorb into the skin as well as L-ascorbic acid does (when L-ascorbic acid is at a low pH), but is more stable with a longer shelf life, and can be formulated into creams.[137]

Magnesium-L-ascorbyl-2-phosphate (VC-PMG) is a stable derivative of ascorbic acid. This form of vitamin C seems to have the most potent ability to block tyrosinase of the vitamin C family.[138] One study examining the effects of topically applied VC-PMG on patients with melasma or senile lentigos demonstrated a significant lightening effect in 19 of 34 patients.[138] However, percutaneous absorption of magnesium ascorbyl phosphate is low because it is a charged molecule, making it difficult to traverse the stratum corneum.

Multiple topical preparations contain vitamin C; however, many of these products have problems with stability, are packaged improperly, and their utility is questionable. Proper packaging of vitamin C skincare products should limit UV, light, and air exposure to prevent rapidly oxidizing vitamin C. Once these products have been opened, they should be used within 4 weeks. Vitamin C turns dark when oxidized; therefore, once darkening occurs, the product should be discarded.

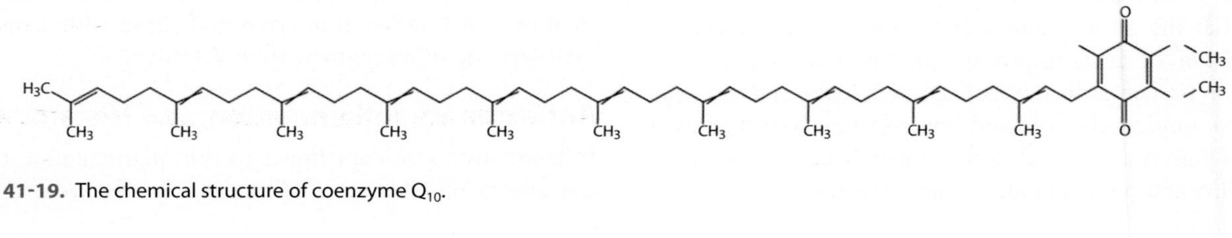

FIGURE 41-19. The chemical structure of coenzyme Q_{10}.

Various methods have been used to increase penetration of vitamin C into the skin. One easy option is to precede the use of L-ascorbic acid with a low-pH cleanser such as hydroxy acid to reduce the skin's pH and augment the absorption of vitamin C (Chapter 35, Skincare Regimen Design, and Chapter 40, Cleansing Agents). Applying vitamin C serum after a peel, microdermabrasion, facial scrubs, or dermaplaning can increase absorption, but the low pH of the L-ascorbic acid formulations causes unpleasant stinging. Another method is iontophoresis. In a randomized, double-blind, placebo-controlled study, investigators used iontophoresis to enhance the penetration of vitamin C into the skin and significantly decrease pigmentation compared to placebo.[139] Intradermal injections of vitamin C have been used in a process known as mesotherapy but delayed type hypersensitivity and granulomas have been reported, especially with the lipophilic forms of ascorbic acid.[140] Granulomas have also been reported when lipophilic forms of ascorbic acid are applied after microneedling.[141]

Vitamin E

Oral intake of vitamin E (α-tocopherol or α-T) (**Fig. 41-21**) has been reported in the Japanese literature to be effective for the treatment of facial hyperpigmentation, especially in combination with vitamin C.[142,143] Studies examining the effects of α-tocopheryl ferulate (a compound composed of α-T and ferulic acid) on melanogenesis in cultured human melanoma cells demonstrated inhibition of tyrosine hydroxylase activity in an indirect manner. The researchers found that this tocopherol derivative was a stronger inhibitor of melanin formation than arbutin and kojic acid.[144] They postulated that α-tocopheryl ferulate could be used to ameliorate and prevent facial hyperpigmentation induced by UV radiation by inhibiting tyrosinase as well as through antioxidant mechanisms.[145]

The depigmenting effect of α-T was also examined in normal human melanocytes and investigators showed that 30 μg/mL of α-T dissolved in 150 μg/mL of lecithin inhibited melanization significantly without inhibiting cell growth, and that this phenotypic change was associated with the dose-dependent inhibition of tyrosinase.[146]

Tocopherol employs four homologs (α, β, γ, and δ) with differing numbers and positions of the methyl groups in the chromatin ring. The expression of tyrosinase melanoma cells has been found to have been suppressed by γ-tocopherol (γ-T).[147] Tocopheryl-dimethyl-glycinate (TDMG) is a novel tocopherol derivative with the dimethylglycine ester linked to the sixth position of the chromanoxyl ring of tocopherol.[148] A Japanese group reported on a novel hydrophilic γ-T derivative known as γ-tocopheryl-*N,N*-di-methylglycinate

hydrochloride (γ-TDMG); this derivative converts to the antioxidant γ-T in skin and displays greater bioavailability than γ-T itself. The investigators examined whether γ-TDMG could reduce UV-induced skin pigmentation in brown guinea pigs. By topically applying 0.1% or 0.5% γ-TDMG to the skin of brown guinea pigs before and after exposure to UVB as well as UVA (three times in 1 week) and then 10 times/week for 4 weeks, they demonstrated significant skin lightening with 0.5% γ-TDMG and a dose-dependent inhibition of melanin synthesis. These data suggest that the topical application of γ-TDMG may be efficacious in preventing photo-induced skin pigmentation in humans.[149]

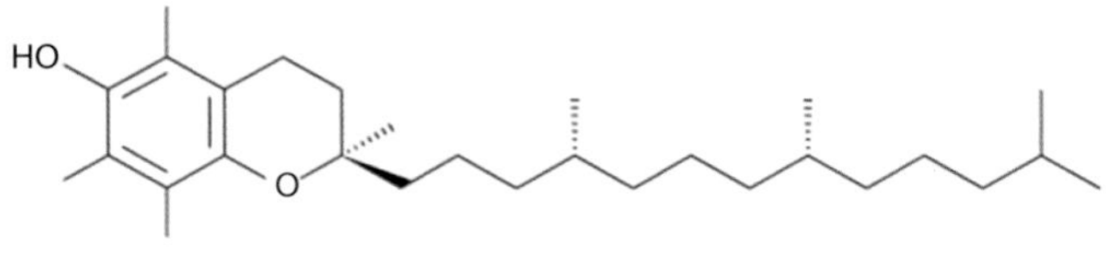

Ferulic Acid

A precursor to vanillin, ferulic acid is derived from the metabolism of phenylalanine and tyrosine and belongs to the family of polyphenolic compounds known as hydroxycinnamic acids. Ferulic acid is a potent antioxidant and a strong UV absorber.[150] A 2005 study demonstrated that the addition of 0.5% ferulic acid to a solution of 15% L-ascorbic acid (vitamin C) and 1% α-tocopherol (vitamin E) would stabilize the formulation and help prevent oxidation of ascorbic acid.[151] In addition, ferulic acid has antioxidant benefits of its own.

Alpha-tocopheryl ferulate, a vitamin E and ferulic acid compound, absorbs UV radiation and displays antioxidant properties. It was shown to inhibit melanin production in cultured human melanoma cells and normal human melanocytes *in vitro*. Further, it was found to be significantly better at blocking melanin production than arbutin, kojic acid, ascorbic acid, and tranexamic acid, suggesting potential as a whitening agent by indirectly inhibiting tyrosine hydroxylase activity.[145]

Glutathione

Glutathione is touted as a "wonder drug" to treat dark spots and melasma on the skin; however, this is due to inflated marketing claims and lack of regulatory oversight rather than scientific data.[152] Glutathione occurs naturally in leafy vegetables, walnuts, oranges, whey protein, tomatoes, and fruits, and is produced endogenously in humans.[153] It is a combination of three amino acids: glutamate, cysteine, and glycine. It functions as an electron donor and converts from the oxidized form GSSG to a reduced form (GSH) by glutathione peroxidase.[153] In addition to inhibiting tyrosinase, it promotes production of pheomelanin rather than eumelanin (**Fig. 41-1**). GSH increases production of cysteinyldopa leading to increased production of pheomelanin, a yellow-red pigment that is lighter than the dark brown eumelanin.

Glutathione is used topically, orally, sublingually, and intravenously (IV). It is difficult to formulate topically because it is highly unstable, especially with exposure to air and light. The GSSG form is more stable. Topical glutathione (the oxidized GSSG form) was studied in a concentration of 2%. This lotion formulation was applied daily by 30 women for 10 weeks. A split-face model was used with placebo on one side of the face and GSSG on the other. A significant difference in skin color and melanin index as compared to placebo was seen ($P <$

FIGURE 41-21. The chemical structure of vitamin E (α-tocopherol, α-T).

0.001) with no adverse events.[153] Oral and sublingual glutathione doses are 20–40 mg/kg in two divided doses. It is regarded as generally recognized as safe (GRAS) by the FDA when used orally. It has poor bioavailability when taken orally and, therefore, has poor efficacy.

IV doses of GSH are 600–1,200 mg one to two times weekly. IV glutathione can engender severe side effects such as potentially fatal Stevens-Johnson syndrome, kidney and/or liver dysfunction, and sepsis. IV glutathione is not recommended at this time because more studies evaluating safety, efficacy, and optimal dosing are necessary. In 2020, a study looked at animals that received injected glutathione intraperitoneally (into the abdomen) at various doses, with 40 mg/kg/day reducing skin pigmentation and the number of melanized cells.[154] No toxic effects were seen. It is expected that there will be advances in the future using this moiety.

If a stable topical form of glutathione could be developed that would penetrate into skin, this would represent a significant advance in the skin-lightening market. The effects of glutathione would likely occur much faster than current therapies because it switches melanin production from darker eumelanin to lighter pheomelanin. Most depigmenting ingredients inhibit tyrosinase and take 12–16 weeks for effects to be noticed on the skin. Glutathione effects are seen much sooner. However, at the time of publication, there were no efficacious glutathione formulations available. Topical GSSG needs more data to establish efficacy and safety.

Green Tea

Green tea is one of the most popular beverages consumed throughout the world. Of all the compounds known to exhibit antioxidant activity, green tea polyphenols (GTPs) are associated with the largest amount of scientific evidence to support their use in dermatology. Green tea has been reported to impart numerous health benefits when administered either topically or orally, due to its antioxidant, anti-inflammatory, and anticarcinogenic properties.[155-157]

Most "green tea-containing" skincare products have minimal amounts of green tea because it is expensive and products with large amounts of green tea (50%–90% polyphenols) have a tinted brown color. A special preparation process of the tea leaves, which involves short steaming and prevents any fermentation, ensures the preservation of the antioxidant polyphenols. Four major polyphenolic catechins can be isolated from the fresh leaves of the green tea plant *Camellia sinensis*: ECG [(–)-epicatechin-3-*O*-gallate], GCG [(–)-gallocatechin-3-*O*-gallate], EGCG [(–)-epigallocatechin-3-*O*-gallate], and EGC [(–)-epigallocatechin] (**Fig. 41-22**).[158] EGCG is the most studied and abundant component and comprises 30% to 40% of the dry weight of green tea leaves.[159,160]

There have been several *in vitro* and *in vivo* studies of green tea and its effects on skin. GTPs have been demonstrated to modulate biochemical pathways important in cell proliferation, inflammatory responses, and reactions of tumor promoters.[161] GTPs exert protection against UV-mediated responses such as sunburn, immunosuppression, and photoaging by

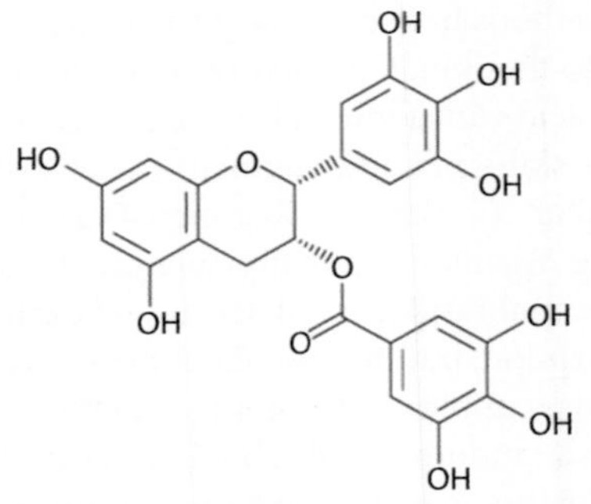

FIGURE 41-22. The chemical structure of EGCG.

inhibiting UV-induced elements of the mitogen-activated protein kinase (MAPK) pathways, Ras and activator protein AP-1 and LDH activation, as well as by the upregulation of UVA-suppressed GSH-Px and the inhibition of UVB-induced infiltration of inflammatory cells.[162] GTPs are thus thought to have the potential to protect the skin when used in combination with traditional sunscreens.[163,164] GTPs also display anticarcinogenic activity. Specifically, EGCG has been shown to exhibit antiproliferative and pro-apoptotic effects on human melanoma cells.[165]

Of the four major polyphenolic catechins, ECG, GCG, and EGCG proved to be the strongest inhibitors of tyrosinase with GCG demonstrating the greatest inhibitory effect on tyrosinase, competitively suppressing the enzyme at its active site.[166,167] Furthermore, EGCG inhibits melanin synthesis in a concentration-dependent manner. It is not cytotoxic to melanocytes; rather, it reduces MITF and tyrosinase protein levels.

Studies of GTPs in human skin have been limited in comparison to animal studies. There are three major challenges for their topical use in humans: (1) establishing a standard formulation and delivery systems that ensure the stability of these easily oxidized antioxidants, (2) increasing epidermal penetration of these hydrophilic agents into human skin, and (3) using a sufficient amount without rendering the skincare product too dark.

Pycnogenol

Pycnogenol is a standardized pine bark extract that exhibits potent antioxidant, anti-inflammatory, and anticarcinogenic activity.[168-170] A 30-day clinical trial of 30 women with melasma was performed using 25-mg pycnogenol orally at each meal, three times daily. Investigators found that the average surface area of melasma significantly decreased, revealing oral pycnogenol to be a safe treatment for this condition.[169] One study has demonstrated that pycnogenol is active when applied topically. In this study, hairless mice exposed to solar-simulated UV radiation were treated post-irradiation with lotions containing pycnogenol. Dose-dependent reductions in the inflammatory sunburn reaction and immunosuppression were observed as a result of pycnogenol treatment. Tumor formation was delayed, and tumor prevalence was also significantly reduced in mice treated with 0.2% pycnogenol.

Researchers concluded that topical pycnogenol displays potential as a photoprotective complement to sunscreens, clearly evincing biologic activity when applied after UV exposure.[168] More data are needed to determine the validity of these claims.

Silymarin

Silymarin is a naturally occurring polyphenolic flavonoid or flavonolignans compound derived from the seeds of the milk thistle plant *Silybum marianum*.[171] Milk thistle has been used for medicinal purposes for more than two millennia. Today, it is used clinically in Europe and Asia as an antihepatotoxic agent and is available as a supplement in Europe and the US. The main component of silymarin is silybin (silibinin), which is its most biologically active constituent conferring the preponderance of its antioxidant, anti-inflammatory, and anticarcinogenic properties.[172]

Topical application of silybin prior to, or immediately after, UV irradiation has been found to impart strong protection against UV-induced damage in the epidermis by a reduction in thymine dimer-positive cells and an upregulation of p53-p21/Cip1, which researchers believe may lead to the inhibition of cell proliferation and apoptosis. This study suggests that mechanisms other than sunscreen effect are integral to silybin efficacy against UV-caused skin damage.[173] Investigators have also noted that silybin enhances UVB-induced apoptosis and speculated that it acts as a UVB damage sensor to deliver its biologic action.[174]

The antioxidant activity of silymarin is well established. Chemoprotective activity against skin cancer has also been reported and continues to be the subject of much investigation.[175–177] In a study to identify the mechanism of photocarcinogenesis prevention in mouse skin by the topical treatment of silymarin, hindering UVB-induced immunosuppression and oxidative stress was found to be potentially related to the prevention of photocarcinogenesis in mice.[178] The authors concluded from this trial and related data from other studies that there are compelling arguments for the inclusion of silymarin in sunscreens or in other products in a skincare regimen. Furthermore, silymarin has been shown to inhibit UV-induced NF-κB activation in keratinocytes. Researchers have hypothesized that the inhibition of NF-κB activation and the consequent suppression of UV-induced inflammation by silymarin is a result primarily of the inhibition of UV-induced inflammation by free radical scavenging and a modulation of intracellular GSH content.[179]

Most of the milk thistle or silymarin available in the US comes in the form of oral supplements. The extant evidence on this botanical suggests potent antioxidant strength and great potential as an antiphotodamage, anticarcinogenic component in an improved medical, dermatologic armamentarium. Moreover, silymarin may favorably supplement sunscreen protection and provide additional antiphotocarcinogenic protection.[180]

Alpha-Lipoic Acid (Thioctic Acid)

Alpha-lipoic acid (also known, though less commonly, as thioctic acid) and its reduced form dihydrolipoic acid (DHLA) are antioxidants. Alpha-lipoic acid (**Fig. 41-23**) is both water and fat soluble and can thus act in the lipid cell membrane

and the aqueous compartment of the cell.[181] In addition, α-lipoic acid has been shown to inhibit the activation of NF-κB transcription factor, modulating the cellular response to UV radiation and preventing UV-induced oxidative injury. It further inhibits tyrosinase by chelating copper and suppressing DOPAquinone-derivative formation.[179] DHLA shows slightly stronger antioxidant activity than α-lipoic acid by reacting with superoxide and hydroxyl radicals.[182] Alpha-lipoic acid elevates intracellular GSH levels by increasing its *de novo* synthesis,[183] which reduces UV radiation sensitivity and promotes formation of pheomelanin rather than eumelanin.[184]

Both α-lipoic acid and DHLA have been proven to block the expression of MITF,[185] consequently inhibiting tyrosinase expression and activity.[30] There have been some reports of contact dermatitis to α-lipoic acid.[186] Alpha-lipoic acid is included in multiple topical cosmetic formulations. Further *in vivo* studies are necessary to verify the above-stated findings. In fact, one study reported that α-lipoic acid does not have antioxidant benefits, so more data are needed to assess α-lipoic acid in anti-aging skincare.[187]

Antioxidants That Stimulate Pigmentation

Rarely, some antioxidants stimulate pigmentation. Quercetin, an extract of onion, is a tyrosinase inhibitor *in vitro*;[188] however, this flavonol is a strong inductor of melanogenesis in normal and malignant human melanocytes,[189] and in reconstituted three-dimensional human epidermis models.[190] Glycyrrhizin, another popular antioxidant that is frequently used to inhibit tyrosinase, has been shown to stimulate melanogenesis in B16 melanoma cells.[191] Clinical trials of each individual antioxidant agent, combinations of ingredients, and the entire skincare regimen must be performed before one can feel confident in their ability to inhibit melanogenesis.

TRANEXAMIC ACID

Tranexamic acid (TXA) is a derivative of the amino acid lysine.[192] It is a fibrinolytic agent that prevents the conversion of plasminogen to plasmin. TXA has been shown to improve dyschromia but the mechanism is poorly understood (**Fig. 41-24**).

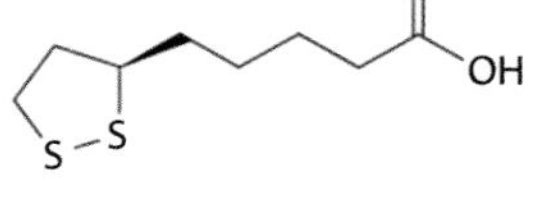

FIGURE 41-23. The chemical structure of α-lipoic acid.

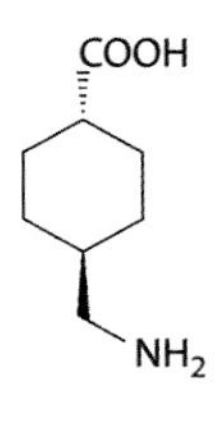

FIGURE 41-24. Structure of tranexamic acid (public domain, via Wikimedia Commons).

Oral Tranexamic Acid

Oral TXA is used off-label to treat refractory melasma.[6] Doses range from 500–1,500 mg daily. The most common dose in the medical literature is 500 mg two times daily. In the US, TXA tablets come in a 650-mg dose tablet, so most physicians recommend breaking the tablet in half and prescribe 325 mg twice daily. Patients should be carefully questioned about a medical history of thromboembolic disease such as those listed in **Table 41-2**. At the time this chapter was authored, there were no reports of blood clots in patients treated with TXA for melasma.[193] Several well-designed studies and the author's experience suggest efficacy for melasma.

In one study, 44 patients were treated with 250 mg of TXA by mouth two times daily for 3 months.[194] There was a 49% reduction of melasma as assessed by the mMASI score in subjects that received TXA. An 18% improvement in the mMASI score was noted in the placebo group. (The improvement of the placebo group was likely due to the daily use of sunscreen in the trial.) Several trials have demonstrated efficacy of oral TXA in treating melasma. What is not known is how long the beneficial effects last. In the aforementioned study, 3 months after the TXA treatment ended, 26% of patients continued to show improvement, while only 19% showed improvement in the placebo group. The most common side effects are GI complaints such as nausea and diarrhea.

Melasma tends to recur and relapse after TXA treatment as with any other melasma treatments. At this time there is no consensus on how long TXA should be used, if there should be a treatment holiday, how long it is safe to continue use, or what the likelihood or frequency is of relapse. Oral TXA is a promising medication for the treatment of melasma, but more studies and clinical experience are needed to determine the most effective treatment and maintenance protocols.

Topical Tranexamic Acid

Topical TXA is included in formulations at a dose of 2–5%.[6] The topical formulations are not as effective as oral administration or intralesional injection. In 2014, a randomized, split-face trial compared 3% topical TXA versus 3% HQ and 0.01% dexamethasone.[195] These agents were used twice daily for 12 weeks. The improvement in the TXA group was superior but the difference was not statistically significant. In 2015, a study comparing 5% TXA versus 4% HQ cream for the treatment of melasma did not find a statistically significant difference between the two groups.[196] Another study in 2017 compared 5% TXA with 2% HQ and did not show a statistical difference.[197] These studies demonstrate that TXA may work as well as 2% and 4% HQ to treat dyspigmentation.[198]

Intradermal Tranexamic Acid

TXA is used both intradermally and after microneedling in areas of increased pigmentation. It comes in a liquid form and most protocols use 4–100 mg/mL. Several studies have looked at intradermal TXA or TXA applied after microneedling;

TABLE 41-2	Contraindications and Cautions to Use of Oral Tranexamic Acid
Contraindications	
<ul><li>Acute promyelocytic leukemia patients on oral tretinoin</li><li>Breastfeeding</li><li>History of blood clots</li><li>History of deep vein thrombosis</li><li>History of pulmonary embolism</li><li>History of stroke</li><li>Kidney disease: The effects may be increased because of slower removal of the medicine from the body.</li><li>Pregnancy</li><li>Stroke</li></ul>	
Use with caution in patients on these medications because of increased risk of blood clots:	
<ul><li>Desogestrel</li><li>Dienogest</li><li>Drospirenone</li><li>Estradiol</li><li>Ethinyl estradiol</li><li>Ethynodiol</li><li>Etonogestrel</li><li>Gestodene</li><li>Levonorgestrel</li><li>Medroxyprogesterone</li><li>Mestranol</li><li>Nomegestrol</li><li>Norelgestromin</li><li>Norethindrone</li><li>Norgestimate</li><li>Norgestrel</li><li>Segesterone</li><li>Ulipristal</li></ul>	

however, different doses and protocols have been used. At this time it is too early to say if TXA is an effective treatment when used in this manner.[6]

OTHER DEPIGMENTING AGENTS

Alpha Hydroxy Acids and Beta Hydroxy Acid

Alpha hydroxy (AHA) and beta hydroxy acid (BHA) peels are prevalent in aesthetic medical practices. All AHAs have a terminal carboxyl group with one or two hydroxyl groups on the second or α carbon and a variable length carbon chain.[199] The two shortest carbon chain acids, glycolic (2-hydroxyethanoic) and lactic (2-hydroxypropanoic), are the most commonly used in dermatology (**Figs. 41-25 and 41-26**).[200] The former is a very versatile peeling agent associated with minimal complications and is used in various strengths ranging from 20% to 70%. People with virtually any skin type can be candidates for AHA and BHA peels, including Asian Americans, African Americans, LatinX, and others with deeply pigmented skin (see Chapter 24).[201]

AHAs exert different effects on the epidermis and the dermis. In the epidermis, the principal effect is diminished

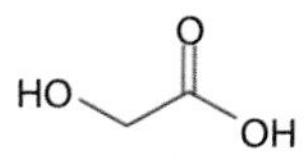

Glycolic acid
(2–Hydroxyethanoic acid)

FIGURE 41-25. The chemical structure of glycolic acid.

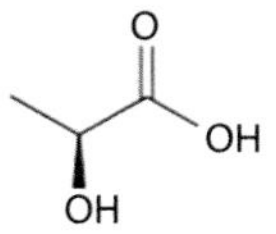

FIGURE 41-26. The chemical structure of lactic acid.

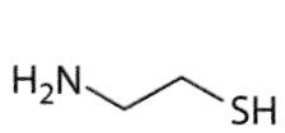

FIGURE 41-27. Chemical structure of cysteamine.

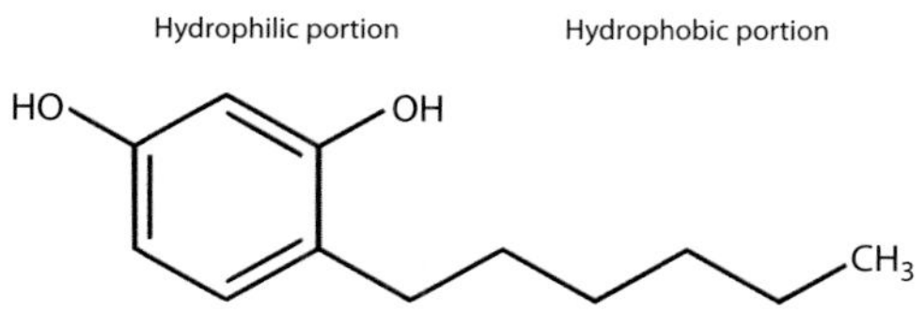

FIGURE 41-28. Hexyresorcinol (adapted from Wikimedia Commons).

corneocyte cohesion and humectant function.[202] This causes more rapid desquamation of the pigmented keratinocytes with the intention that the newly formed keratinocytes will contain less pigment. AHAs speed the keratinocyte turnover rate thereby shortening the cell cycle. In melanoma cells, AHAs directly inhibit tyrosinase activity.[203]

In 1997, Burns et al. demonstrated that serial glycolic acid peels provide benefits, with minimal adverse effects, for the treatment of post-inflammatory hyperpigmentation in individuals with dark complexions.[204] Patients who receive a chemical peel in addition to a topical treatment demonstrate a greater and more rapid improvement of pigmented lesions compared to topical treatment alone with a slight lightening of their normal facial skin tone.[205] In 2005, lactic acid in a concentration of 92% was used to treat melasma. Patients treated every 3 weeks for a maximum of six times showed significant improvement in their MASI scores.[206] Lactic acid was further shown to be as effective in decreasing pigmentation as Jessner's solution.[207] When treating PIPA with peels, it is initially important to use lower concentrations of AHA and slowly increase the strength to avoid irritating the skin, which would cause even more hyperpigmentation.[208] The use of topical HQ preparations pre- and post-peel decreases the chances of aggravating PIPA.

Cysteamine

Cysteamine is the decarboxylated derivative of the amino acid cysteine and cystamine is a disulfide that undergoes reduction into cysteamine.[209,210] Cysteamine is an aminothiol that has antioxidant characteristics (**Figure 41-27**).[211] Cystamine/cysteamine can mobilize zinc ions from metallothionein, inhibit transglutaminase, and inactivate glucose-6-phosphate dehydrogenase.[212,213] Cystamine/cysteamine activates lysosomal proteases and promotes the uptake of cysteine via a glutamate-sensitive transporter with consequent increased synthesis of glutathione.[214,215] As discussed above, glutathione nudges the melanin synthesis pathways in the direction of lighter pheomelanin and away from production of darker eumelanin. Cysteamine inhibits melanin formation without melanocyte toxicity.[13] It is unknown what the exact mechanism of action is on melanin production. It is possible that cystamine works by one of the following mechanisms[211]:

(1) Inhibition of tyrosinase
(2) Removing dopaquinone from the melanogenesis pathway
(3) Chelating iron and copper ions
(4) Increasing intracellular levels of glutathione,[216] which shifts eumelanin to pheomelanin synthesis and slows down melanin production.

Formulation of cysteamine is challenging because it is unstable and has an unpleasant odor when oxidized. New formulations have overcome these challenges resulting in topical cysteamine products for the treatment of melasma.

In 2014, a double-blind, placebo-controlled trial evaluated 53 patients that used either placebo or cysteamine 5% cream for 4 months.[217] Some subjects stated that the cream had a sulfur-like odor. There was a no statistically significant improvement of the MASI score at 2 months in the cysteamine-treated group as compared to the placebo group. However, at the 4-month visit, statistically significant improvements of the MASI scores were seen in the cysteamine group as compared to the placebo group. (No P-value was given but the publication offered some confusing statistics: t-test, 95% and a confidence interval of 0.5–8.3.)[218] Side effects included erythema, dryness, itching, and a burning sensation. Three patients had to discontinue therapy due to erythema. One patient in the study experienced an acne reaction.

In 2020, a randomized, double-blind, parallel-group study examined the safety and efficacy of a 5% cysteamine cream as compared to a TCC with 4% HQ, 0.05% retinoic acid, and 0.1% betamethasone for facial melasma.[211] The cysteamine cream showed greater improvement in the MASI score at Months 2 and 4. However, there were no statistically significant differences noted in the investigator and subject assessments at the 2- and 4-month visits. More data are needed to determine the efficacy and safety of cysteamine for dyschromia.

Octadecenedioic Acid

Octadecenedioic acid, also called dioic acid, is a monounsaturated dicarboxylic acid with a similar structure to azelaic acid.[219] The skin-lightening activity of octadecenedioic acid is mediated by the stimulation of the peroxisome proliferator-activating receptor (PPAR). The binding to PPAR leads to reduced melanin production through the reduction of the synthesis of tyrosinase mRNA.[220] PPARs are members of the nuclear receptor superfamily, which regulates important cellular functions, including cell proliferation and differentiation, as well as inflammatory responses.[221] Three subtypes of PPARs (designated α, β, and γ) are expressed in human melanocytes.[222]

Octadecenedioic acid is a PPAR-γ agonist, with a 10-fold higher affinity for this receptor than the other two PPARs.[220] This suggests a novel mechanism of skin pigmentation and consequently a new approach to treating skin pigmentation disorders. One study showed that 1% dioic acid reduced skin pigmentation the same as 2% HQ in 96 subjects. Both HQ and dioic acid groups demonstrated a 40% improvement in MASI score over 12 weeks.[223] HQ caused more itching while the dioic acid group reported some acne, which was postulated to be due to the oily vehicle.

Pyruvic Acid

Pyruvic acid is an α-keto-acid with keratolytic, antimicrobial, and sebostatic properties in addition to the ability to stimulate new collagen production. It is successfully used in the treatment of acne.[224] A treatment with 50% pyruvic acid, employed for four peeling sessions performed every 2 weeks, has been shown to effectively reduce the degree of pigmentation in melasma patients and decrease skin wrinkling. No side effects, such as persistent erythema or post-inflammatory hyperpigmentation, were observed.[225] Comparable results in terms of safety and efficacy were also seen in 20 patients treated for moderately photodamaged facial skin.[226]

Resorcinol

Resorcinol (m-dihydrobenzene) is isomeric with cathecol and HQ.[227] This bactericidal agent is soluble in water, ether, and alcohol. The primary indications for its use include PIPA as well as melasma and acne; secondary indications are sun-damaged skin and freckles. Resorcinol should not be used in pregnancy or in darker skin types (Fitzpatrick IV–VI). Some authors have mentioned the possibility of an allergic reaction to resorcinol and suggest testing the agent by applying it to a small area on the arm or behind the ear a few days before using it as a peel. One study established the skin sensitization potential of resorcinol using a local lymph node assay.[228] Shimizu et al. proved that 4-substituted resorcinols, naturally obtained or synthesized, have potent tyrosinase inhibitory ability.[229] In addition, Tasaka et al. showed a depigmenting effect for a resorcinol derivative with an isopentyl group in position 6 of resorcinol (NKO-09), with a more potent depigmenting effect than HQ by inhibiting tyrosine hydroxylation and DOPA oxidation.[230]

Hexylresorcinol

Hexylresorcinol mimics tyrosine, allowing it to inhibit tyrosinase activity. It has been shown to be a more potent inhibitor

of tyrosinase than HQ, kojic acid, or licorice extract. It poses less risk of skin sensitivity than resorcinol. It has also exhibited antioxidant, antiglycation, and anti-inflammatory activity. Its amphiphilic character (**Figure 41-28**) allows the hydrophobic portion to interact with the phospholipid layers of the cell membrane and penetrate into the cell while the hydrophilic portion allows it to share protons in aqueous media.[231]

Retinoids

The family of retinoids, which are lipophilic vitamin A derivatives that easily penetrate the epidermis, comprises several different substances (see Chapter 45). Retinoids apparently exert their depigmenting effects directly by influencing melanocytes as well as indirectly by modulating melanogenesis. Topical retinoids seem to directly affect melanogenesis via tyrosinase, TRP-1, and TRP-2 expression.[232-234] By accelerating the cell turnover of epidermal keratinocytes, topical retinoids reduce melanosome transfer to the keratinocytes and induce dispersion of keratinocyte pigment granules leading to a uniform distribution of melanin content in the epidermis. More rapid epidermal turnover also diminishes the cohesiveness of corneocytes and thus induces desquamation that consequently leads to an accelerated loss of melanin in the stratum corneum.[235] Indirectly, the changes engendered in the stratum corneum may facilitate the penetration of additional depigmenting agents into the epidermis and increase their bioavailability, thereby leading to increased depigmentation. Retinoids prevent the skin atropy seen with steroids, which are often included in depigmenting products such as TCCs.[5]

Tretinoin in concentrations of 0.05% to 0.1% is often used alone or in a TCC to treat PIPA and melasma. Studies have revealed that retinoic acid inhibits the induction of tyrosinase, and subsequently melanogenesis, in mouse melanoma cell cultures.[236] Further, clinical trials in humans have shown tretinoin to be efficacious for the treatment of melasma.[237,238] The topical retinoid tazarotene has also been demonstrated to improve irregular hyperpigmentation associated with photoaging.[239] Adapalene (0.1% and 0.3%) is a potent synthetic retinoid. In a randomized trial, adapalene 0.1% showed the same effect on reduction in MASI as 0.05% tretinoin, yet the patients treated with adapalene experienced significantly fewer side effects.[240] Oral 0.05% isotretinoin has exhibited clinically important but not statistically significant results in a randomized trial treating Thai patients with melasma.[241]

The side effects of retinoids, such as dryness, irritation, and scaling, are due to activation of EDGF as described in Chapter 45.[242] The decreased cohesiveness of corneocytes allows for other agents to more readily penetrate into the skin and enhance their efficacy, as is the case with HQ, which often is used in combination with retinoids. It is advisable to add a corticosteroid to retinoid therapy to mitigate irritation.

MOISTURIZERS

Free fatty acids have regulatory effects on melanogenesis. Unsaturated fatty acids decrease melanin synthesis and tyrosinase activity, while saturated fatty acids increase melanin synthesis and tyrosinase activity.[10,243] Table 43-3 (Chapter 43, Moisturizers) lists some popular fatty acids in skincare products and their effects on melanogenesis. Linoleic acid, linolenic acid, and oleic fatty acids have been demonstrated to decrease tyrosinase activity. Linoleic acid has been shown to inhibit tyrosinase activity in melanocytes and decrease UVB-induced pigmentation.[10,113] In a 6-week, double-blind, randomized controlled trial, the triple combination of linoleic acid, lincomycin, and betamethasone valerate yielded greater improvement than any two of the ingredients or the vehicle alone.[244]

Using moisturizers containing these fatty acids may help increase efficacy of skin-lightening products. Grape seed oil, borage seed oil, and argan oil are good sources of linoleic acid as seen in Figure 43-2 (Chapter 43). Use of hyaluronic acid moisturizers on top of skin-lightening products may help increase absorption and efficacy of the skin-lightening product.[245] As discussed in Chapter 35, moisturizers should always be placed on top (or after) skin-lightening products. The only exception is when starting a retinoid, in which case the retinoid or TCC can be placed on top of a moisturizer to help mitigate side effects. Efficacy of skin lightening will be diminished when a retinoid or TCC is placed on top of a moisturizer, but side effects will also be reduced.

SUNSCREEN

Sun and light protection play a critical role in the treatment of pigmentary disorders. UV radiation and blue light stimulate the synthesis of melanin and promote the transfer of pigments from melanocytes to keratinocytes thereby increasing pigmentation. The use of a broad-spectrum sunscreen with an SPF of 19 was shown to improve melasma. In a 2019 study, 100 melasma patients applied 3 cc of sunscreen three times daily for 12 weeks. No skin lighteners or retinoids were used. A statistically significant difference in MASI score was seen at baseline and at 12 weeks, demonstrating the utility of sun protection to treat melasma.[246]

Iron Oxide Pigments

Visible light of 400–700 nm has been shown to stimulate skin pigmentation,[247] especially in Fitzpatrick phototypes IV–VI.[248] Blue light exposure is very common because it is emitted from cell phones, computer screens, and numerous other sources. In order to improve skin pigmentation, skin must be protected from blue light as well as UV light. Iron oxide (FeO) pigments are found in makeup foundations and some tinted sunscreens. The darker the sunscreen tint or makeup foundation color, the more iron oxide is in the formulation. Tinted sunscreens help block visible light and should be included in skincare routines to lighten facial pigmentation.[249] Daily tinted sunscreen use should be a part of any skin-lightening regimen (see Chapter 46 for a discussion of the different types of sunscreens).

ORAL AGENTS TO TREAT SKIN PIGMENTATION

Polypodium Leucotomos

This antioxidant is derived from the Calaguala fern. It has been shown to have efficacy as a photoprotective agent and decreases redness from UV exposure.[250] Although it may help prevent pigmentation by reducing inflammation from sun exposure, some studies have not shown it to be very efficacious in preventing melasma.[251] Other research data suggest that its use in conjunction with topical HQ and sunscreen may be effective.[252]

Melatonin

Melatonin is an antioxidant. A small 2020 study showed that melatonin levels are lower in melasma patients as compared to patients who do not have melasma.[253] Melanin seems to have an inhibitory effect on tyrosinase activity.[254,255] In 2009, a trial using topical melatonin, oral melatonin, or HQ cream to treat melasma was performed.[256] All groups had a significant reduction in the MASI score by 90 days; however, HQ was superior to both topical and oral melatonin. It is too early to know what role melatonin, either topical or oral, plays in skin pigmentation.

CONCLUSION

The process of skin pigmentation involves many pathways and is difficult to treat clinically. Sun protection and sun avoidance are critical but exposure to light, heat, and estrogen plays a role. The most effective skin-lightening skincare routines contain combinations of ingredients. The most commonly used combination is a TCC product containing a retinoid, a tyrosinase inhibitor, and a corticosteroid. New agents are constantly being explored to treat the difficult problem of dyschromia. See Chapter 14 for suggestions on how to use these depigmenting ingredients in a skincare routine.

References

1. Pandya AG, Hynan LS, Bhore R, et al. Reliability assessment and validation of the Melasma Area and Severity Index (MASI) and a new modified MASI scoring method. *J Am Acad Dermatol.* 2011;64(1):78–83, 83.e1–2.
2. Kligman AM, Willis I. A new formula for depigmenting human skin. *Arch Dermatol.* 1975;111(1):40–48.
3. Torok H, Taylor S, Baumann L, et al. A large 12-month extension study of an 8-week trial to evaluate the safety and efficacy of triple combination (TC) cream in melasma patients previously treated with TC cream or one of its dyads. *J Drugs Dermatol.* 2005;4(5):592–597.
4. Taylor SC, Torok H, Jones T, et al. Efficacy and safety of a new triple-combination agent for the treatment of facial melasma. *Cutis.* 2003;72(1):67–72.
5. Lesnik RH, Mezick JA, Capetola R, Kligman LH. Topical all-trans-retinoic acid prevents corticosteroid-induced skin

atrophy without abrogating the anti-inflammatory effect. *J Am Acad Dermatol.* 1989;21(2 Pt 1):186–190.

6. McKesey J, Tovar-Garza A, Pandya AG. Melasma Treatment: An Evidence-Based Review. *Am J Clin Dermatol.* 2020; 21(2):173–225.

7. Ferreira Cestari T, Hassun K, Sittart A, de Lourdes Viegas M. A comparison of triple combination cream and hydroquinone 4% cream for the treatment of moderate to severe facial melasma. *J Cosmet Dermatol.* 2007;6(1):36–39.

8. Chan R, Park KC, Lee MH, et al. A randomized controlled trial of the efficacy and safety of a fixed triple combination (fluocinolone acetonide 0.01%, hydroquinone 4%, tretinoin 0.05%) compared with hydroquinone 4% cream in Asian patients with moderate to severe melasma. *Br J Dermatol.* 2008;159(3):697–703.

9. Gong Z, Lai W, Zhao G, et al. Efficacy and safety of fluocinolone acetonide, hydroquinone, and tretinoin cream in chinese patients with melasma: a randomized, double-blind, placebo-controlled, multicenter, parallel-group study. *Clin Drug Investig.* 2015;35(6):385–395.

10. Ando H, Ryu A, Hashimoto A, Oka M, Ichihashi M. Linoleic acid and alpha-linolenic acid lightens ultraviolet-induced hyperpigmentation of the skin. *Arch Dermatol Res.* 1998;290(7):375–381.

11. Noh H, Lee SJ, Jo HJ, Choi HW, Hong S, Kong KH. Histidine residues at the copper-binding site in human tyrosinase are essential for its catalytic activities. *J Enzyme Inhib Med Chem.* 2020;35(1):726–732.

12. Petris MJ, Strausak D, Mercer JF. The Menkes copper transporter is required for the activation of tyrosinase. *Hum Mol Genet.* 2000;9(19):2845–2851.

13. Qiu L, Zhang M, Sturm RA, Gardiner B, Tonks I, Kay G, et al. Inhibition of melanin synthesis by cystamine in human melanoma cells. *J Invest Dermatol.* 2000;114(1):21–27.

14. DeCaprio AP. The toxicology of hydroquinone—relevance to occupational and environmental exposure. *Crit Rev Toxicol.* 1999;29(3):283–330.

15. Nordlund JJ. Postinflammatory hyperpigmentation. *Dermatol Clin.* 1988;6(2):185–192.

16. Penney KB, Smith CJ, Allen JC. Depigmenting action of hydroquinone depends on disruption of fundamental cell processes. *J Invest Dermatol.* 1984;82(4):308–310.

17. Guevara IL, Pandya AG. Melasma treated with hydroquinone, tretinoin and a fluorinated steroid. *Int J Dermatol.* 2001;40(30):212–215.

18. Bates B. Derms react to possible FDA ban of hydroquinone: cite poor scientific reasoning, ethnic bias. *Skin and Allergy News.* 2007;38(1):1–20.

19. Nordlund JJ, Grimes PE, Ortonne JP. The safety of hydroquinone. *J Eur Acad Dermatol Venerol.* 2006;20(7):781–787.

20. Picardo M, Carrera M. New and experimental treatments of cloasma and other hypermelanoses. *Dermatol Clin.* 2007;25(3):353–362, ix.

21. Lawrence N, Bligard CA, Reed R, Perret WJ. Exogenous ochronosis in the United States. *J Am Acad Dermatol.* 1988;18(5 Pt 2):1207–1211.

22. Barrientos N, Oritz-Frutos J, Gómez E, Iglesias L. Allergic contact dermatitis from a bleaching cream. *Am J Contact Dermat.* 2001;12(1):33–34.

23. Kramer KE, Lopez A, Stefanato CM, Phillips TJ. Exogenous ochronosis. *J Am Acad Dermatol.* 2000;42(5 Pt 2):869–871.

24. Jones K, Hughes J, Hong M, Jia Q, Orndorff S. Modulation of melanogenesis by aloesin: a competitive inhibitor of tyrosinase. *Pigment Cell Res.* 2002;15(5): 335–340.

25. Piao LZ, Park HR, Park YK, Lee SK, Park JH, Park MK. Mushroom tyrosinase inhibition activity of some chromones. *Chem Pharm Bull (Tokyo).* 2002;50(3):309–311.

26. Choi S, Lee SK, Kim JE, Chung MH, Park YI. Aloesin inhibits hyperpigmentation induced by UV radiation. *Clin Exp Dermatol.* 2002;27(6):513–515.

27. Solano F, Briganti S, Picardo M, Ghanem G. Hypopigmenting agents: an updated review on biological, chemical and clinical aspects. *Pigment Cell Res.* 2006;19(6):550–571.

28. Kim YJ, Uyama H. Tyrosinase inhibitors from natural and synthetic sources: structure, inhibition mechanism and perspective for the future. *Cell Mol Life Sci.* 2005;62(15):1707–1723.

29. Ohguchi K, Tanaka T, Kido T, et al. Effects of hydroxystilbene derivatives on tyrosinase activity. *Biochem Biophys Res Commun.* 2003;307(4):861–863.

30. Lin CB, Babiarz L, Liebel F, et al. Modulation of microphthalmia-associated transcription factor gene expression alters skin pigmentation. *J Invest Dermatol.* 2002;119(6):1330–1340.

31. Lee KT, Lee KS, Jeong JH, Jo BK, Heo MY, Kim HP. Inhibitory effects of Ramulus mori extracts on melanogenesis. *J Cosmet Sci.* 2003;54(2):133–142.

32. Hollinger JC, Angra K, Halder RM. Are Natural Ingredients Effective in the Management of Hyperpigmentation? A Systematic Review. *J Clin Aesthet Dermatol.* 2018 Feb;11(2):28–37.

33. Shimogaki H, Tanaka Y, Tamai H, Masuda M. In vitro and in vivo evaluation of ellagic acid on melanogenesis inhibition. *Int J Cosmet Sci.* 2000;22(4):291–303.

34. Ertam I, Mutlu B, Unal I, Alper S, Kivçak B, Ozer O. Efficiency of ellagic acid and arbutin in melasma: a randomized, prospective, open-label study. *J Dermatol.* 2008;35(9):570–574.

35. Dahl A, Yatskayer M, Raab S, Oresajo C. Tolerance and efficacy of a product containing ellagic and salicylic acids in reducing hyperpigmentation and dark spots in comparison with 4% hydroquinone. *J Drugs Dermatol.* 2013;12(1):52–58.

36. Curto EV, Kwong C, Hermersdörfer H, et al. Inhibitors of mammalian melanocyte tyrosinase: in vitro comparisons of alkyl esters of gentisic acid with other putative inhibitors. *Biochem Pharmacol.* 1999;57(6):663–672.

37. Davis EC, Callender VD. Postinflammatory hyperpigmentation: a review of the epidemiology, clinical features, and treatment options in skin of color. *J Clin Aesthet Dermatol.* 2010;3(7):20–31.

38. Searle T, Al-Niaimi F, Ali FR. The top 10 cosmeceuticals for facial hyperpigmentation. *Dermatol Ther.* 2020;33(6):e14095.

39. Sawant O, Khan T. Management of periorbital hyperpigmentation: An overview of nature-based agents and alternative approaches. *Dermatol Ther.* 2020;33(4):e13717.

40. Maeda K, Fukuda M. Arbutin: mechanism of its depigmenting action in human melanocyte culture. *J Pharmacol Exp Ther.* 1996;276(2):765–769.

41. Draelos ZD. Skin lightening preparations and the hydroquinone controversy. *Dermatol Ther.* 2007;20(5):308–313.

42. Zhu W, Gao J. The use of botanical extracts as topical skin-lightening agents for the improvement of skin pigmentation disorders. *J Investig Dermatol Symp Proc.* 2008;13(1):20–24.

43. Nakajima M, Shinoda I, Fukuwatari Y, Hayasawa H. Arbutin increases the pigmentation of cultured human melanocytes

through mechanisms other than the induction of tyrosinase activity. *Pigment Cell Res.* 1998;11(1):12–17.

44. Grimes PE. Management of hyperpigmentation in darker racial ethnic groups. *Semin Cutan Med Surg.* 2009;28(2):77–85.

45. Boissy RE, Visscher M, DeLong MA. DeoxyArbutin: a novel reversible tyrosinase inhibitor with effective in vivo skin lightening potency. *Exp Dermatol.* 2005;14(8):601–608.

46. Morag M, Nawrot J, Siatkowski I, et al. A double-blind, placebo-controlled randomized trial of Serratulae quinquefoliae folium, a new source of β-arbutin, in selected skin hyperpigmentations. *J Cosmet Dermatol.* 2015;14(3):185–190.

47. Bhat R, Hadi SM. Photoinactivation of bacteriophage lambda by kojic acid and Fe(III): role of oxygen radical intermediates in the reaction. *Biochem Mol Biol Int.* 1994;32(4):731–735.

48. Saeedi M, Eslamifar M, Khezri K. Kojic acid applications in cosmetic and pharmaceutical preparations. *Biomed Pharmacother.* 2019;110:582–593.

49. Guttridge CG, Jarrett JM, Stinchcombe GR, Curtis PJ. Chemical induction of local reddening in strawberry fruits. *J Sci Food Agric.* 1977;28(3):243–246.

50. Higa Y, Hatae S, Inoue T, Ohyama Y. Inhibitory effects of kojic acid on melanin formation; in vitro and in vivo studies in black goldfish. *J Jpn Cosmetic Sci Soc.* 1982;6(194):3.

51. Cabanes J, Chazarra S, Garcia-Carmona F. Kojic acid, a cosmetic skin whitening agent, is a slow-binding inhibitor of catecholase activity of tyrosinase. *J Pharm Pharmacol.* 1994;46(12):982–985.

52. Uher M, Brtko J, Rajniakova O, Kovac M, Novotana E. Kojic acid and its derivatives in cosmetics and health protection. *Parfuem Kosmet.* 1993;74:554–556.

53. Burdock GA, Soni MG, Carabin IG. Evaluation of health aspects of kojic acid in food. *Regul Toxicol Pharmacol.* 2001;33(1):80–101.

54. Khezri K, Saeedi M, Morteza-Semnani K, Akbari J, Rostamkalaei SS. An emerging technology in lipid research for targeting hydrophilic drugs to the skin in the treatment of hyperpigmentation disorders: kojic acid-solid lipid nanoparticles. *Artif Cells Nanomed Biotechnol.* 2020;48(1):841–853.

55. Lee YS, Park JH, Kim MH, Seo SH, Kim HJ. Synthesis of tyrosinase inhibitory kojic acid derivative. *Arch Pharm (Weinheim).* 2006;339(3):111–114.

56. Ellis DA, Tan AK, Ellis CS. Superficial micropeels: glycolic acid and alpha-hydroxy acid with kojic acid. *Facial Plast Surg.* 1995;11(1):15–21.

57. Garcia A, Fulton JE Jr. The combination of glycolic acid and hydroquinone or kojic acid for the treatment of melasma and related conditions. *Dermatol Surg.* 1996;22(5):443–447.

58. Lim JT. Treatment of melasma using kojic acid in a gel containing hydroquinone and glycolic acid. *Dermatol Surg.* 1999;25(4):282–284.

59. Nakagawa M, Kawai K, Kawai K. Contact allergy to kojic acid in skin care products. *Contact Dermatitis.* 1995;32(1):9–13.

60. Nakayama H, Watanabe H, Nishioka K, Hayakawa R, Higa Y. Treatment of chloasma with kojic acid cream. *Rinsho Hifuka.* 1982;36:715–722.

61. Scientific Committee on Consumer Safety. European Commission. Opinion on kojic acid (updated 26–27 June 2012). https://ec.europa.eu/health/sites/health/files/scientific_committees/consumer_safety/docs/sccs_o_098.pdf. Accessed April 8, 2021.

62. Takizawa T, Mitsumori K, Tamura T, et al. Hepatocellular tumor induction in heterozygous p53-deficient CBA mice by a 26-week dietary administration of kojic acid. *Toxicol Sci.* 2003;73(2):287–293.

63. Yamamura T, Onishi J, Nishiyama T. Antimelanogenic activity of hydrocoumarins in cultured normal human melanocytes by stimulating intracellular glutathione synthesis. *Arch Dermatol Res.* 2002;294(8):349–354.

64. Draelos ZD, Deliencourt-Godefroy G, Lopes L. An effective hydroquinone alternative for topical skin lightening. *J Cosmet Dermatol.* 2020;19(12):3258–3261.

65. Saeedi M, Morteza-Semnani K, Ghoreishi MR. The treatment of atopic dermatitis with licorice gel. *J Dermatolog Treat.* 2003;14(3):153–157.

66. Wang ZY, Nixon DW. Licorice and cancer. *Nutr Cancer.* 2001;39(1):1–11.

67. Agarwal R, Wang ZY, Mukhtar H. Inhibition of mouse skin tumor-initiating activity of DMBA by chronic oral feeding of glycyrrhizin in drinking water. *Nutr Cancer.* 1991;15(3-4):187–193.

68. Craig WJ. Health-promoting properties of common herbs. *Am J Clin Nutr.* 1999;70(3 Suppl):491S–499S.

69. Yokota T, Nishio H, Kubota Y, Mizoguchi M. The inhibitory effect of glabridin from licorice extracts on melanogenesis and inflammation. *Pigment Cell Res.* 1998;11(6):355–361.

70. Amer M, Metwalli M. Topical liquiritin improves melasma. *Int J Dermatol.* 2000;39(4):299–301.

71. Holloway VL. Ethnic cosmetic products. *Dermatol Clin.* 2003;21(4):743–749.

72. Rico MJ. Rising drug costs: the impact on dermatology. *Skin Therapy Lett.* 2000;5(4):1–2,5.

73. Friis-Møller A, Chen M, Fuursted K, Christensen SB, Kharazmi A. In vitro antimycobacterial and antilegionella activity of licochalcone A from Chinese licorice roots. *Planta Med.* 2002;68(5):416–419.

74. Barfod L, Kemp K, Hansen M, Kharazmi A. Chalcones from Chinese liquorice inhibit proliferation of T cells and production of cytokines. *Int Immunopharmacol.* 2002;2(4):545–555.

75. Rafi MM, Rosen RT, Vassil A, et al. Modulation of bcl-2 and cytotoxicity by licochalcone-A, a novel estrogenic flavonoid. *Anticancer Res.* 2000;20(4):2653–2658.

76. Tsukiyama R, Katsura H, Tokuriki N, Kobayashi M. Antibacterial activity of licochalcone A against spore-forming bacteria. *Antimicrob Agents Chemother.* 2002;46(5):1226–1230.

77. Shibata S, Inoue H, Iwata S, et al. Inhibitory effects of licochalcone A isolated from Glycyrrhiza inflata root on inflammatory ear edema and tumour promotion in mice. *Planta Med.* 1991;57(3):221–224.

78. Hwang JH, Lee BM. Inhibitory effects of plant extracts on tyrosinase, L-DOPA oxidation, and melanin synthesis. *J Toxicol Environ Health A.* 2007;70(5):393–407.

79. Chaudhuri RK. Emblica cascading antioxidant: a novel natural skin care ingredient. *Skin Pharmacol Appl Skin Physiol.* 2002;15(5):374–380.

80. Baumann LS. Cosmeceutical marketing claims. *Cosmeceuticals and Cosmetic Ingredients.* New York: McGraw-Hill, 2014, p. 125.

81. Heuberger DM, Schuepbach RA. Protease-activated receptors (PARs): mechanisms of action and potential therapeutic modulators in PAR-driven inflammatory diseases. *Thromb J.* 2019;17:4.

82. Seiberg M, Paine C, Sharlow E, et al. Inhibition of melanosome transfer results in skin lightening. *J Invest Dermatol.* 2000;115(2):162–167.

83. Wallo W, Nebus J, Leyden JJ. Efficacy of a soy moisturizer in photoaging: a double-blind, vehicle-controlled, 12-week study. *J Drugs Dermatol.* 2007;6(9):917–922.

84. Seiberg M, Paine C, Sharlow E, et al. The protease-activated receptor 2 regulates pigmentation via keratinocyte-melanocyte interactions. *Exp Cell Res.* 2000;254(1):25–32.

85. Hakozaki T, Minwalla L, Zhuang J, et al. The effect of niacinamide on reducing cutaneous pigmentation and suppression of melanosome transfer. *Br J Dermatol.* 2002;147(1):20–31.

86. Otte N, Borelli C, Korting HC. Nicotinamide—biologic actions of an emerging cosmetic ingredient. *Int J Cosmet Sci.* 2005;27(5):255–261.

87. Greatens A, Hakozaki T, Koshoffer A, et al. Effective inhibition of melanosome transfer to keratinocytes by lectins and niacinamide is reversible. *Exp Dermatol.* 2005;14(7):498–508.

88. Lee DH, Oh IY, Koo KT, et al. Reduction in facial hyperpigmentation after treatment with a combination of topical niacinamide and tranexamic acid: a randomized, double-blind, vehicle-controlled trial. *Skin Res Technol.* 2014;20(2):208–212.

89. Liu J-C, Seiberg M. Applications of total soy in skin care. In: Baran R, Maibach H, eds. *Textbook of Cosmetic Dermatology.* 3rd ed. New York, NY: Taylor & Francis Informa Healthcare; 2004: 115.

90. Paine C, Sharlow E, Liebel F, Eisinger M, Shapiro S, Seiberg M. An alternative approach to depigmentation by soybean extracts via inhibition of the PAR-2 pathway. *J Invest Dermatol.* 2001;116(4):587–595.

91. Hermanns JF, Petit L, Martalo O, Piérard-Franchimont C, Cauwenbergh G, Piérard GE. Unraveling the patterns of subclinical pheomelanin-enriched facial hyperpigmentation: effect of depigmenting agents. *Dermatology.* 2000;201(2):118–122.

92. Nazzaro-Porro M. The use of azelaic acid in hyperpigmentation. *Rev Contemp Pharmacother.* 1993;4(415):223.

93. Nguyen QH, Bui TP. Azelaic acid: pharmacokinetic and pharmacodynamic properties and its therapeutic role in hyperpigmentary disorders and acne. *Int J Dermatol.* 1995;34(2):75–84.

94. Pathak MA, Ciganek ER, Wick M, Sober AJ, Farinelli WA, Fitzpatrick TB. An evaluation of the effectiveness of azelaic acid as a depigmenting and chemotherapeutic agent. *J Invest Dermatol.* 1985;85(3):222–228.

95. Leibl H, Stingl G, Pehamberger H, Korschan H, Konrad K, Wolff K. Inhibition of DNA synthesis of melanoma cells by azelaic acid. *J Invest Dermatol.* 1985;85(5):417–422.

96. Akamatsu H, Komura J, Asada Y, Miyachi Y, Niwa Y. Inhibitory effect of azelaic acid on neutrophil functions: a possible cause for its efficacy in treating pathogenetically unrelated diseases. *Arch Dermatol Res.* 1991;283(3):162–166.

97. Passi S, Picardo M, Zompetta C, De Luca C, Breathnach AS, Nazzaro-Porro M. The oxyradical-scavenging activity of azelaic acid in biological systems. *Free Radic Res Commun.* 1991;15(1):17–28.

98. Passi S, Picardo M, De Luca C, Breathnach AS, Nazzaro-Porro M. Scavenging activity of azelaic acid on hydroxyl radicals "in vitro". *Free Radic Res Commun.* 1991;11(6):329–338.

99. Fitton A, Goa KL. Azelaic acid. A review of its pharmacological properties and therapeutic efficacy in acne and hyperpigmentary skin disorders. *Drugs.* 1991;41(5):780–798.

100. Nazzaro-Porro M, Passi S. Identification of tyrosinase inhibitors in cultures of Pityrosporum. *J Invest Dermatol.* 1978;71(3):205–208.

101. Passi S, Picardo M, Nazzaro-Porro M, Breathnach A, Confaloni AM, Serlupi-Crescenzi G. Antimitochondrial effect of saturated medium chain length (C8-C13) dicarboxylic acids. *Biochem Pharmacol.* 1984;33(1):103–108.

102. Verallo-Rowell VM, Verallo V, Graupe K, Lopez-Villafuerte L, Garcia-Lopez M. Double-blind comparison of azelaic acid and hydroquinone in the treatment of melasma. *Acta Derm Venereol Suppl (Stockh).* 1989;143:58–61.

103. Baliña LM, Graupe K. The treatment of melasma. 20% azelaic acid versus 4% hydroquinone cream. *Int J Dermatol.* 1991;30(12):893–895.

104. Lowe NJ, Rizk D, Grimes P, Billips M, Pincus S. Azelaic acid 20% cream in the treatment of facial hyperpigmentation in darker-skinned patients. *Clin Ther.* 1998;20(5):945–959.

105. Kakita LS, Lowe NJ. Azelaic acid and glycolic acid combination therapy for facial hyperpigmentation in darker-skinned patients: a clinical comparison with hydroquinone. *Clin Ther.* 1998;20(5):960–970.

106. Riley PA. Mechanism of pigment cell toxicity produced by hydroxyanisole. *J Pathol.* 1970;101(2):163–169.

107. Fleischer AB Jr, Schwartzel EH, Colby SI, Altman DJ. The combination of 2% 4-hydroxyanisole (mequinol) and 0.01% tretinoin is effective in improving the appearance of solar lentigines and related hyperpigmented lesions in two double-blind multicenter clinical studies. *J Am Acad Dermatol.* 2000;42(3):459–467.

108. Draelos ZD. The combination of 2% 4-hydroxyanisole (mequinol) and 0.01% tretinoin effectively improves the appearance of solar lentigines in ethnic groups. *J Cosmet Dermatol.* 2006;5(3):239–244.

109. Jarratt M. Mequinol 2%/tretinoin 0.01% solution: an effective and safe alternative to hydroquinone 3% in the treatment of solar lentigines. *Cutis.* 2004;74(5):319–322.

110. Huang CL, Nordlund JJ, Boissy R. Vitiligo: a manifestation of apoptosis? *Am J Clin Dermatol.* 2002;3(5):301–308.

111. Halder RM, Richards GM. Management of dyschromias in ethnic skin. *Dermatol Ther.* 2004;17(2):151–157.

112. Canizares O, Uribe Jaramillo F, Kerdel Vegas F. Leukomelanoderma subsequent to the application of monobenzylether of hydroquinone. *AMA Arch Derm.* 1958;77(2):220–223.

113. Sarkar R, Bansal A, Ailawadi P. Future therapies in melasma: What lies ahead? *Indian J Dermatol Venereol Leprol.* 2020;86(1):8–17.

114. Jimbow K. N-acetyl-4-S-cysteaminylphenol as a new type of depigmenting agent for the melanoderma of patients with melasma. *Arch Dermatol.* 1991;127(10):1528–1534.

115. Pratchyapurit WO. Combined use of two formulations containing diacetyl boldine, TGF-β1 biomimetic oligopeptide-68 with other hypopigmenting/exfoliating agents and sunscreen provides effective and convenient treatment for facial melasma. Either is equal to or is better than 4% hydroquinone on normal skin. *J Cosmet Dermatol.* 2016;15(2):131–144.

116. Lima TN, Pedriali Moraes CA. Bioactive peptides: applications and relevance for cosmeceuticals. *Cosmetics.* 2018;5(1):21.

117. Marini A, Farwick M, Grether-Beck S, et al. Modulation of skin pigmentation by the tetrapeptide PKEK: in vitro and in vivo evidence for skin whitening effects. *Exp Dermatol.* 2012;21(2):140–146.

118. Yamakoshii J, Otsuka F, Sano A, et al. Lightening effect on ultraviolet-induced pigmentation of guinea pig skin by oral administration of a proanthocyanidin-rich extract from grape seeds. *Pigment Cell Res.* 2003;16(6):629–638.

119. Maresca V, Roccella M, Roccella F, et al. Increased sensitivity to peroxidative agents as a possible pathogenic factor of melanocyte damage in vitiligo. *J Invest Dermatol.* 1997;109(3):310–313.

120. Benathan M, Alvero-Jackson H, Mooy AM, Scaletta C, Frenk E. Relationship between melanogenesis, glutathione levels and melphalan toxicity in human melanoma cells. *Melanoma Res.* 1992;2(5-6):305–314.

121. Yokozawa T, Kim YJ. Piceatannol inhibits melanogenesis by its antioxidative actions. *Biol Pharm Bull.* 2007;30(11):2007–2011.

122. Chen J, Li Q, Ye Y, Huang Z, Ruan Z, Jin N. Phloretin as both a substrate and inhibitor of tyrosinase: Inhibitory activity and mechanism. *Spectrochim Acta A Mol Biomol Spectrosc.* 2020;226:117642.

123. Anunciato Casarini TP, Frank LA, Pohlmann AR, Guterres SS. Dermatological applications of the flavonoid phloretin. *Eur J Pharmacol.* 2020;889:173593.

124. Biesalski HK. Polyphenols and inflammation: basic interactions. *Curr Opin Clin Nutr Metab Care.* 2007;10(6):724–728.

125. Postaire E, Jungmann H, Bejot M, Heinrich U, Tronnier H. Evidence for antioxidant nutrients-induced pigmentation in skin: results of a clinical trial. *Biochem Mol Biol Int.* 1997;42(5):1023–1033.

126. Staniforth V, Chiu LT, Yang NS. Caffeic acid suppresses UVB radiation-induced expression of interleukin-10 and activation of mitogen-activated protein kinases in mouse. *Carcinogenesis.* 2006;27(9):1803–1811.

127. Lee JH, Park JG, Lim SH, et al. Localized intradermal microinjection of tranexamic acid for treatment of melasma in Asian patients: a preliminary clinical trial. *Dermatol Surg.* 2006;32(5):626–631.

128. Dutkiewicz R, Albert DM, Levin LA. Effects of latanoprost on tyrosinase activity and mitotic index of cultured melanoma lines. *Exp Eye Res.* 2000;70(5):563–569.

129. Lassalle MW, Igarashi S, Sasaki M, Wakamatsu K, Ito S, Horikoshi T. Effects of melanogenesis-inducing nitric oxide and histamine on the production of eumelanin and pheomelanin in cultured human melanocytes. *Pigment Cell Res.* 2003;16(1):81–84.

130. Yoshida M, Takahashi Y, Inoue S. Histamine induces melanogenesis and morphologic changes by protein kinase A activation via H2 receptors in human normal melanocytes. *J Invest Dermatol.* 2000;114(2):334–342.

131. Kawai M, Hirano T, Higa S, et al. Flavonoids and related compounds as anti-allergic substances. *Allergol Int.* 2007;56(2):113–123.

132. Hseu YC, Ho YG, Mathew DC, Yen HR, Chen XZ, Yang HL. The in vitro and in vivo depigmenting activity of Coenzyme Q10 through the down-regulation of α-MSH signaling pathways and induction of Nrf2/ARE-mediated antioxidant genes in UVA-irradiated skin keratinocytes. *Biochem Pharmacol.* 2019;164:299–310.

133. Consumer Ingredient Review. Safety Assessment of Ubiquinone Ingredients as Used in Cosmetics. September 14–15, 2020. https://www.cir-safety.org/sites/default/files/Ubiquinone.pdf. Accessed April 11, 2021.

134. Ros JR, Rodríguez-López JN, García-Cánovas F. Effect of L-ascorbic acid on the monophenolase activity of tyrosinase. *Biochem J.* 1993;295(Pt 1):309–312.

135. Ando H, Kondoh H, Ichihashi M, Hearing VJ. Approaches to identify inhibitors of melanin biosynthesis via the quality control of tyrosinase. *J Invest Dermatol.* 2007;127(4):751–761.

136. Hwang SW, Oh DJ, Lee D, Kim JW, Park SW. Clinical efficacy of 25% L-ascorbic acid (C'ensil) in the treatment of melasma. *J Cutan Med Surg.* 2009;13(2):74–81.

137. Pinnell SR, Yang H, Omar M, et al. Topical L-ascorbic acid: percutaneous absorption studies. *Dermatol Surg.* 2001;27(2):137–142.

138. Kameyama K, Sakai C, Kondoh S, et al. Inhibitory effect of magnesium L-ascorbyl-2-phosphate (VC-PMG) on melanogenesis in vitro and in vivo. *J Am Acad Dermatol.* 1996;34(1):29–33.

139. Huh CH, Seo KI, Park JY, Lim JG, Eun HC, Park KC. A randomized, double-blind, placebo-controlled trial of vitamin C iontophoresis in melasma. *Dermatology.* 2003;206(4):316–320.

140. Soltani-Arabshahi R, Wong JW, Duffy KL, Powell DL. Facial allergic granulomatous reaction and systemic hypersensitivity associated with microneedle therapy for skin rejuvenation. *JAMA Dermatol.* 2014;150(1):68–72.

141. Cervantes J, Hafeez F, Badiavas EV. Erythematous Papules After Microneedle Therapy for Facial Rejuvenation. *Dermatol Surg.* 2019;45(10):1337–1339.

142. Hayakawa R. Clinical research group on a combination preparation of vitamins E and C. Effects of combination preparation of vitamin E and C in comparison with single preparation to the patients of facial hyperpigmentation: a double-blind controlled clinical trial. *Nishinihon J Dermatol.* 1980;42:1024–1034.

143. Takigawa M. YEC-1 clinical research group. Clinical evaluation of YEC-1 (UNKER EC) to female patients with facial hyperpigmentation. *Kiso Rinsho.* 1991;25:312–322.

144. Funasaka Y, Chakraborty AK, Komoto M, Ohashi A, Ichihashi M. The depigmenting effect of alpha-tocopheryl ferulate on human melanoma cells. *Br J Dermatol.* 1999;141(1):20–29.

145. Ichihashi M, Funasaka Y, Ohashi A, et al. The inhibitory effect of DL-alpha-tocopheryl ferulate in lecithin on melanogenesis. *Anticancer Res.* 1999;19(5A):3769–3774.

146. Funasaka Y, Komoto M, Ichihashi M. Depigmenting effect of alpha-tocopheryl ferulate on normal human melanocytes. *Pigment Cell Res.* 2000;13(Suppl 8):170–174.

147. Kamei Y, Ohtsuka Y. *Fragrance J.* 2003;56–63.

148. Takata J, Hidaka R, Yamasaki A, et al. Novel d-gamma-tocopherol derivative as a prodrug for d-gamma-tocopherol and a two-step prodrug for S-gamma-CEHC. *J Lipid Res.* 2002;43(12):2196–2204.

149. Kuwabara Y, Watanabe T, Yasuoka S, et al. Topical application of gamma-tocopherol derivative prevents UV-induced skin pigmentation. *Biol Pharm Bull.* 2006;29(6):1175–1179.

150. Baumann LS. Cosmeceutical marketing claims. *Cosmeceuticals and Cosmetic Ingredients.* New York: McGraw-Hill; 2014: 171–175.

151. Lin FH, Lin JY, Gupta RD, et al. Ferulic acid stabilizes a solution of vitamins C and E and doubles its photoprotection of skin. *J Invest Dermatol.* 2005;125(4):826–832.

152. Sonthalia S, Jha AK, Lallas A, Jain G, Jakhar D. Glutathione for skin lightening: a regnant myth or evidence-based verity? *Dermatol Pract Concept.* 2018;8(1):15–21.

153. Watanabe F, Hashizume E, Chan GP, Kamimura A. Skin-whitening and skin-condition-improving effects of topical oxidized glutathione: a double-blind and placebo-controlled

clinical trial in healthy women. *Clin Cosmet Investig Dermatol.* 2014;7:267–274.

154. AlGhamdi KM, Kumar A, Al-Rikabi AC, Mubarak M. Safety and efficacy of parenteral glutathione as a promising skin lightening agent: A controlled assessor blinded pharmacohistologic and ultrastructural study in an animal model. *Dermatol Ther.* 2020;33(2):e13211.

155. Khan N, Mukhtar H. Tea Polyphenols in Promotion of Human Health. *Nutrients.* 2018;11(1):39.

156. Tipoe GL, Leung TM, Hung MW, Fung ML. Green tea polyphenols as an anti-oxidant and anti-inflammatory agent for cardiovascular protection. *Cardiovasc Hematol Disord Drug Targets.* 2007;7(2):135–144.

157. Cabrera C, Artacho R, Giménez R. Beneficial effects of green tea—a review. *J Am Coll Nutr.* 2006;25(2):79–99.

158. Yang CS, Wang ZY. Tea and cancer. *J Natl Cancer Inst.* 1993;85(13):1038–1049.

159. Wright TI, Spencer JM, Flowers FP. Chemoprevention of non-melanoma skin cancer. *J Am Acad Dermatol.* 2006;54(6):933–946.

160. Katiyar SK, Elmets CA. Green tea polyphenolic antioxidants and skin photoprotection (Review). *Int J Oncol.* 2001;18(6):1307–1313.

161. Katiyar SK, Ahmad N, Mukhtar H. Green tea and skin. *Arch Dermatol.* 2000;136(8):989–994.

162. Hsu S. Green tea and the skin. *J Am Acad Dermatol.* 2005;52(6):1049–1059.

163. Yusuf N, Irby C, Katiyar SK, Elmets CA. Photoprotective effects of green tea polyphenols. *Photodermatol Photoimmunol Photomed.* 2007;23(1):48–56.

164. Wang ZY, Agarwal R, Bickers DR, Mukhtar H. Protection against ultraviolet B radiation-induced photocarcinogenesis in hairless mice by green tea polyphenols. *Carcinogenesis.* 1991;12(8):1527–1530.

165. Nihal M, Ahmad N, Mukhtar H, Wood GS. Anti-proliferative and proapoptotic effects of (-)-epigallocatechin-3-gallate on human melanoma: possible implications for the chemoprevention of melanoma. *Int J Cancer.* 2005;114(4):513–521.

166. No JK, Soung DY, Kim YJ, et al. Inhibition of tyrosinase by green tea components. *Life Sci.* 1999;65(21):PL241–L246.

167. Kim DS, Park SH, Kwon SB, Li K, Youn SW, Park KC. (-)-Epigallocatechin-3-gallate and hinokitiol reduce melanin synthesis via decreased MITF production. *Arch Pharm Res.* 2004;27(3):334–339.

168. Sime S, Reeve VE. Protection from inflammation, immunosuppression and carcinogenesis induced by UV radiation in mice by topical Pycnogenol. *Photochem Photobiol.* 2004;79(2):193–198.

169. Ni Z, Mu Y, Gulati O. Treatment of melasma with Pycnogenol. *Phytother Res.* 2002;16(6):567–571.

170. Bito T, Roy S, Sen CK, Packer L. Pine bark extract pycnogenol downregulates IFN-gamma-induced adhesion of T cells to human keratinocytes by inhibiting inducible ICAM-1 expression. *Free Radic Biol Med.* 2000;28(2):219–227.

171. Svobodová A, Psotová J, Walterová D. Natural phenolics in the prevention of UV-induced skin damage. A review. *Biomed Pap Med Fac Univ Palacky Olomouc Czech Repub.* 2003;147(2):137–145.

172. Soleimani V, Delghandi PS, Moallem SA, Karimi G. Safety and toxicity of silymarin, the major constituent of milk thistle extract: An updated review. *Phytother Res.* 2019;33(6):1627–1638.

173. Dhanalakshmi S, Mallikarjuna GU, Singh RP, Agarwal R. Silibinin prevents ultraviolet radiation-caused skin damages in SKH-1 hairless mice via a decrease in thymine dimer positive cells and an up-regulation of p53-p21/Cip1 in epidermis. *Carcinogenesis.* 2004;25(8):1459–1465.

174. Dhanalakshmi S, Mallikarjuna GU, Singh RP, Agarwal R. Dual efficacy of silibinin in protecting or enhancing ultraviolet B radiation-caused apoptosis in HaCaT human immortalized keratinocytes. *Carcinogenesis.* 2004;25(1):99–106.

175. Singh RP, Agarwal R. Flavonoid antioxidant silymarin and skin cancer. *Antioxid Redox Signal.* 2002;4(4):655–663.

176. Gupta S, Mukhtar H. Chemoprevention of skin cancer through natural agents. *Skin Pharmacol Appl Skin Physiol.* 2001;14(6):373–385.

177. Prasad RR, Paudel S, Raina K, Agarwal R. Silibinin and non-melanoma skin cancers. *J Tradit Complement Med.* 2020;10(3):236–244.

178. Katiyar SK. Treatment of silymarin, a plant flavonoid, prevents ultraviolet light-induced immune suppression and oxidative stress in mouse skin. *Int J Oncol.* 2002;21(6):1213–1222.

179. Saliou C, Kitazawa M, McLaughlin L, et al. Antioxidants modulate acute solar ultraviolet radiation-induced NF-kappa-B activation in a human keratinocyte cell line. *Free Radic Biol Med.* 1999;26(1-2):174–183.

180. Katiyar SK. Silymarin and skin cancer prevention: anti-inflammatory, antioxidant and immunomodulatory effects (Review). *Int J Oncol.* 2005;26(1):169–176.

181. Kagan VE, Shvedova A, Serbinova E, et al. Dihydrolipoic acid—a universal antioxidant both in the membrane and in the aqueous phase: reduction of peroxyl, ascorbyl and chromanoxyl radicals. *Biochem Pharmacol.* 1992;44(8):1637–1649.

182. Packer L, Witt EH, Tritschler HJ. alpha-Lipoic acid as a biological antioxidant. *Free Radic Biol Med.* 1995;19(2):227–250.

183. Han D, Handelman G, Marcocci L, et al. Lipoic acid increases de novo synthesis of cellular glutathione by improving cystine utilization. *Biofactors.* 1997;6(3):321–338.

184. Tyrrell RM, Pidoux M. Correlation between endogenous glutathione content and sensitivity of cultured human skin cells to radiation at defined wavelengths in the solar ultraviolet range. *Photochem Photobiol.* 1988;47(3):405–412.

185. Fisher DE. Microphthalmia: a signal responsive transcriptional regulator in development. *Pigment Cell Res.* 2000;13(Suppl 8):145–149.

186. Bergqvist-Karlsson A, Thelin I, Bergendorff O. Contact dermatitis to alpha-lipoic acid in an anti-wrinkle cream. *Contact Dermatitis.* 2006;55(1):56–57.

187. Lin JY, Lin FH, Burch JA, et al. Alpha-lipoic acid is ineffective as a topical antioxidant for photoprotection of skin. *J Invest Dermatol.* 2004;123(5):996–998.

188. Kubo I, Kinst-Hori I. Flavonols from saffron flower: tyrosinase inhibitory activity and inhibition mechanism. *J Agric Food Chem.* 1999;47(10):4121–4125.

189. Nagata H, Takekoshi S, Takeyama R, Homma T, Yoshiyuki Osamura R. Quercetin enhances melanogenesis by increasing the activity and synthesis of tyrosinase in human melanoma cells and in normal human melanocytes. *Pigment Cell Res.* 2004;17(1):66–73.

190. Takeyama R, Takekoshi S, Nagata H, Osamura RY, Kawana S. Quercetin-induced melanogenesis in a reconstituted

three-dimensional human epidermal model. *J Mol Histol.* 2004;35(2):157–165.

191. Jung GD, Yang JY, Song ES, Par JW. Stimulation of melanogenesis by glycyrrhizin in B16 melanoma cells. *Exp Mol Med.* 2001;33(3):131–135.

192. Kaur A, Bhalla M, Sarkar R. Tranexamic acid in melasma: a review. *Pigment Int.* 2020;7(1):12.

193. Kim HJ, Moon SH, Cho SH, Lee JD, Kim HS. Efficacy and Safety of Tranexamic Acid in Melasma: A Meta-analysis and Systematic Review. *Acta Derm Venereol.* 2017;97(7):776–781.

194. Del Rosario E, Florez-Pollack S, Zapata L Jr., et al. Randomized, placebo-controlled, double-blind study of oral tranexamic acid in the treatment of moderate-to-severe melasma. *J Am Acad Dermatol.* 2018;78(2):363–369.

195. Ebrahimi B, Naeini FF. Topical tranexamic acid as a promising treatment for melasma. *J Res Med Sci.* 2014;19(8):753–757.

196. Banihashemi M, Zabolinejad N, Jaafari MR, Salehi M, Jabari A. Comparison of therapeutic efects of liposomal Tranexamic Acid and conventional Hydroquinone on melasma. *J Cosmet Dermatol.* 2015;14(3):174–177.

197. Atef N, Dalvand B, Ghassemi M, Mehran G, Heydarian A. Therapeutic efects of topical tranexamic acid in comparison with hydroquinone in treatment of women with Melasma. *Dermatol Ther (Heidelb).* 2017;7(3):417–424.

198. Wang JV, Jhawar N, Saedi N. Tranexamic Acid for Melasma: Evaluating the Various Formulations. *J Clin Aesthet Dermatol.* 2019;12(8):E73–E74.

199. Clark CP3rd. Alpha hydroxy acids in skin care. *Clin Plast Surg.* 1996;23(1):49–56.

200. Brody HJ. *Chemical Peeling and Resurfacing.* St. Louis, MO: Mosby-Year Book; 1997: 90–100.

201. Murad H, Shamban AT, Premo PS. The use of glycolic acid as a peeling agent. *Dermatol Clin.* 1995;13(2):285–307.

202. Slavin JW. Considerations in alpha hydroxy acid peels. *Clin Plast Surg.* 1998;25(1):45–52.

203. Usuki A, Ohashi A, Sato H, Ochiai Y, Ichihashi M, Funasaka Y. The inhibitory effect of glycolic acid and lactic acid on melanin synthesis in melanoma cells. *Exp Dermatol.* 2003;12(Suppl 2):43–50.

204. Burns RL, Prevost-Blank PL, Lawry MA, Lawry TB, Faria DT, Fivenson DP. Glycolic acid peels for postinflammatory hyperpigmentation in black patients. A comparative study. *Dermatol Surg.* 1997;23(3):171–174.

205. Lim JT, Tham SN. Glycolic acid peels in the treatment of melasma among Asian women. *Dermatol Surg.* 1997;23(3):177–179.

206. Sharquie KE, Al-Tikreety MM, Al-Mashhadani SA. Lactic acid as a new therapeutic peeling agent in melasma. *Dermatol Surg.* 2005;31(2):149–154.

207. Sharquie KE, Al-Tikreety MM, Al-Mashhadani SA. Lactic acid chemical peels as a therapeutic modality in melasma in comparison to Jessner's solution chemical peels. *Dermatol Surg.* 2006;32(12):1429–1436.

208. Rubin MG. The clinical use of alpha hydroxy acids. *Australas J Dermatol.* 1994;35(1):29–33.

209. Jeitner TM, Pinto JT, Cooper AJL. Cystamine and cysteamine as inhibitors of transglutaminase activity in vivo. *Biosci Rep.* 2018;38(5):BSR20180691.

210. Paul BD, Snyder SH. Therapeutic Applications of Cysteamine and Cystamine in Neurodegenerative and Neuropsychiatric Diseases. *Front Neurol.* 2019;10:1315.

211. Karrabi M, David J, Sahebkar M. Clinical evaluation of efficacy, safety and tolerability of cysteamine 5% cream in comparison with modified Kligman's formula in subjects with epidermal melasma: A randomized, double-blind clinical trial study. *Skin Res Technol.* 2021;27(1):24–31.

212. Birckbichler PJ, Orr GR, Patterson MKJr, Conway E, Carter HA. Increase in proliferative markers after inhibition of transglutaminase. *Proc Natl Acad Sci U S A.* 1981;78(8):5005–5008.

213. Terada T. Thioltransferase can utilize cysteamine as same as glutathione as a reductant during the restoration of cystamine-treated glucose 6-phosphate dehydrogenase activity. *Biochem Mol Biol Int.* 1994;34(4):723–727.

214. Pisoni RL, Acker TL, Lisowski KM, Lemons RM, Thoene JG. A cysteine-specific lysosomal transport system provides a major route for the delivery of thiol to human fibroblast lysosomes: possible role in supporting lysosomal proteolysis. *J Cell Biol.* 1990;110(2):327–335.

215. Issels RD, Nagele A, Eckert KG, Wilmanns W. Promotion of cystine uptake and its utilization for glutathione biosynthesis induced by cysteamine and N-acetylcysteine. *Biochem Pharmacol.* 1988;37(5):881–888.

216. de Matos DG, Furnus CC. The importance of having high glutathione (GSH) level after bovine in vitro maturation on embryo development effect of beta-mercaptoethanol, cysteine and cystine. *Theriogenology.* 2000;53(3):761–771.

217. Mansouri P, Farshi S, Hashemi Z, Kasraee B. Evaluation of the efficacy of cysteamine 5% cream in the treatment of epidermal melasma: a randomized double-blind placebo-controlled trial. *Br J Dermatol.* 2015;173(1):209–217.

218. du Prel JB, Hommel G, Röhrig B, Blettner M. Confidence interval or p-value?: part 4 of a series on evaluation of scientific publications. *Dtsch Arztebl Int.* 2009;106(19):335–339.

219. Wiechers JW, Groenhof FJ, Wortel VA, Miller RM, Hindle NA. Octadecenedioic acid for a more even skin tone. *Cosmetics and Toiletries.* 2002;117(7):55–68.

220. Wiechers JW, Rawlings AV, Garcia C, et al. A new mechanism of action for skin whitening agents: binding to peroxisome proliferator activated receptor. *Int J Cosmet Sci.* 2005;27(2):123–132.

221. Berger J, Moller DE. The mechanisms of action of PPARs. *Annu Rev Med.* 2002;53:409–435.

222. Michalik L, Wahli W. Peroxisome proliferator-activated receptors (PPARs) in skin health, repair and disease. *Biochim Biophys Acta.* 2007;1771(8):991–998.

223. Tirado-Sánchez A, Santamaría-Román A, Ponce-Olivera RM. Efficacy of dioic acid compared with hydroquinone in the treatment of melasma. *Int J Dermatol.* 2009;48(8):893–895.

224. Cotellessa C, Manunta T, Ghersetich I, Brazzini B, Peris K. The use of pyruvic acid in the treatment of acne. *J Eur Acad Dermatol Venereol.* 2004;18(3):275–278.

225. Berardesca E, Cameli N, Primavera G, Carrera M. Clinical and instrumental evaluation of skin improvement after treatment with a new 50% pyruvic acid peel. *Dermatol Surg.* 2006;32(4):526–531.

226. Ghersetich I, Brazzini B, Peris K, Cotellessa C, Manunta T, Lotti T. Pyruvic acid peels for the treatment of photoaging. *Dermatol Surg.* 2004;30(1):32–36.

227. Karam PG. 50% resorcinol peel. *Int J Dermatol.* 1993; 32(8):569–574.

228. Basketter DA, Sanders D, Jowsey IR. The skin sensitization potential of resorcinol: experience with the local lymph node assay. *Contact Dermatitis.* 2007;56(4):196–200.

229. Shimizu K, Kondo R, Sakai K. Inhibition of tyrosinase by flavonoids, stilbenes and related 4-substituted resorcinols: structure-activity investigations. *Planta Med.* 2000;66(1):11–15.

230. Tasaka K, Kamei C, Nakano S, Takeuchi Y, Yamato M. Effects of certain resorcinol derivatives on the tyrosinase activity and the growth of melanoma cells. *Methods Find Exp Clin Pharmacol.* 1998;20(2):99–109.

231. Fidalgo J, Deglesne PA, Arroya R, Ranneva E, Deprez P. 4-Hexylresorcinol a New Molecule for Cosmetic Application. *J Biomol Res Ther.* 2018;8(170):2.

232. Ortonne JP. Retinoid therapy of pigmentary disorders. *Dermatol Ther.* 2006;19(5):280–288.

233. Nair X, Parah P, Suhr L, Tramposch KM. Combination of 4-hydroxyanisole and all trans retinoic acid produces synergistic skin depigmentation in swine. *J Invest Dermatol.* 1993;101(2):145–149.

234. Orlow SJ, Chakraborty AK, Boissy RE, Pawelek JM. Inhibition of induced melanogenesis in Cloudman melanoma cells by four phenotypic modifiers. *Exp Cell Res.* 1990;191(2):209–218.

235. Kasraee B, Handjani F, Aslani FS. Enhancement of the depigmenting effect of hydroquinone and 4-hydroxyanisole by all-trans-retinoic acid (tretinoin): the impairment of glutathione-dependent cytoprotection? *Dermatology.* 2003;206(4):289–291.

236. Orlow SJ, Chakraborty AK, Pawelek JM. Retinoic acid is a potent inhibitor of inducible pigmentation in murine and hamster melanoma cell lines. *J Invest Dermatol.* 1990;94(4):461–464.

237. Kimbrough-Green CK, Griffiths CE, Finkel LJ, et al. Topical retinoic acid (tretinoin) for melasma in black patients. A vehicle-controlled clinical trial. *Arch Dermatol.* 1994;130(6):727–733.

238. Griffiths CE, Finkel LJ, Ditre CM, Hamilton TA, Ellis CN, Voorhees JJ. Topical tretinoin (retinoic acid) improves melasma. A vehicle-controlled, clinical trial. *Br J Dermatol.* 1993;129(4):415–421.

239. Phillips TJ, Gottlieb AB, Leyden JJ, et al. Efficacy of 0.1% tazarotene cream for the treatment of photodamage: a 12-month multicenter, randomized trial. *Arch Dermatol.* 2002;138(11):1486–1493.

240. Dogra S, Kanwar AJ, Parasad D. Adapalene in the treatment of melasma: a preliminary report. *J Dermatol.* 2002;29(8):539–540.

241. Leenutaphong V, Nettakul A, Rattanasuwon P. Topical isotretinoin for melasma in Thai patients: a vehicle-controlled clinical trial. *J Med Assoc Thai.* 1999;82(9):868–875.

242. Weinstein GD, Nigra TP, Pochi PE, et al. Topical tretinoin for treatment of photodamaged skin. *Arch Dermatol.* 1991;127(5):659–665.

243. Ando H, Watabe H, Valencia JC, et al. Fatty acids regulate pigmentation via proteasomal degradation of tyrosinase: a new aspect of ubiquitin-proteasome function. *J Biol Chem.* 2004;279(15):15427–15433.

244. Lee MH, Kim HJ, Ha DJ, Paik JH, Kim HY. Therapeutic effect of topical application of linoleic acid and lincomycin in combination with betamethasone valerate in melasma patients. *J Korean Med Sci.* 2002;17(4):518–523.

245. Brown MB, Jones SA. Hyaluronic acid: a unique topical vehicle for the localized delivery of drugs to the skin. *J Eur Acad Dermatol Venereol.* 2005;19(3):308–318.

246. Sarkar R, Ghunawat S, Narang I, Verma S, Garg VK, Dua R. Role of broad-spectrum sunscreen alone in the improvement of melasma area severity index (MASI) and Melasma Quality of Life Index in melasma. *J Cosmet Dermatol.* 2019;18(4):1066–1073.

247. Ramasubramaniam R, Roy A, Sharma B, Nagalakshmi S. Are there mechanistic differences between ultraviolet and visible radiation induced skin pigmentation? *Photochem Photobiol Sci.* 2011;10(12):1887–1893.

248. Mahmoud BH, Ruvolo E, Hexsel CL, et al. Impact of long-wavelength UVA and visible light on melanocompetent skin. *J Invest Dermatol.* 2010;130(8):2092–2097.

249. Lyons AB, Trullas C, Kohli I, Hamzavi IH, Lim HW. Photoprotection beyond ultraviolet radiation: A review of tinted sunscreens. *J Am Acad Dermatol.* 2020:S0190–9622(20)30694-0.

250. Parrado C, Nicolas J, Juarranz A, Gonzalez S. The role of the aqueous extract Polypodium leucotomos in photoprotection. *Photochem Photobiol Sci.* 2020 May 20.

251. Ahmed AM, Lopez I, Perese F, et al. A randomized, double-blinded, placebo-controlled trial of oral Polypodium leucotomos extract as an adjunct to sunscreen in the treatment of melasma. *JAMA Dermatol.* 2013;149(8):981–983.

252. Goh CL, Chuah SY, Tien S, Thng G, Vitale MA, Delgado-Rubin A. Double-blind, Placebo-controlled Trial to Evaluate the Effectiveness of *Polypodium Leucotomos* Extract in the Treatment of Melasma in Asian Skin: A Pilot Study. *J Clin Aesthet Dermatol.* 2018;11(3):14–19.

253. Sarkar R, Devadasan S, Choubey V, Goswami B. Melatonin and oxidative stress in melasma - an unexplored territory; a prospective study. *Int J Dermatol.* 2020;59(5):572–575.

254. Valverde P, Benedito E, Solano F, Oaknin S, Lozano JA, García-Borrón JC. Melatonin antagonizes alpha-melanocyte-stimulating hormone enhancement of melanogenesis in mouse melanoma cells by blocking the hormone-induced accumulation of the c locus tyrosinase. *Eur J Biochem.* 1995;232(1):257–263.

255. Kim TK, Lin Z, Tidwell WJ, Li W, Slominski AT. Melatonin and its metabolites accumulate in the human epidermis in vivo and inhibit proliferation and tyrosinase activity in epidermal melanocytes in vitro. *Mol Cell Endocrinol.* 2015;404:1–8.

256. Hamadi SA, Mohammed MM, Aljaf AN, Abdulrazak A. The role of topical and oral melatonin in management of melasma patients. *J Arab Univ Basic Appl Sci.* 2009;8:30–42.

CHAPTER 42

Fragrance

Edmund M. Weisberg, MS, MBE
Leslie S. Baumann, MD

SUMMARY POINTS

What's Important?

1. Contact allergy to fragrance is a common problem often seen throughout the world, with fragrances consistently placed among the top 10 contact dermatitis allergens.
2. Fragrance is the second most common allergen family associated with allergic contact dermatitis (after nickel), as well as the most often cited cause of such reactions to cosmetic products.

What's New?

1. The use of the synthetic fragrance hydroxyisohexyl 3-cyclohexene carboxaldehyde (HICC) was banned by the European Union in August 2019.
2. The most common fragrance screeners in most baseline series include FM I, FM II, and balsam of Peru.
3. Although banned in the EU, HICC may be deemed by some to be useful for screening, along with hydroperoxides of limonene and linalool, to diagnose fragrance allergy.

What's Coming?

1. Continual retrospective studies will help to calibrate evolving patch test standards, helping to identify up-to-date allergens that are most appropriate to include in screening.

Innovative products and procedures inundate medicine and the specialty of dermatology at a dizzying pace. At the same time, the billion-dollar beauty industry continues to expand, with few if any signs of a decline. The global fragrance and flavor market represents a significant and lucrative subdivision of the beauty market. Players in this subdivision are constantly testing various fragrance ingredients to stay ahead of encroaching regulation and increased rates of sensitization. Indeed, while contact allergy to fragrance is not a presentation seen in the dermatologist's office as frequently as acne, for example, it is a common problem seen often throughout the world. This is not surprising since fragrances are virtually omnipresent in products that are placed on the skin, such as soaps, body lotions and moisturizers, shampoos, deodorants, shaving products, cosmetics, perfumes, sunscreens, and dental products, as well as food products, detergents, and even air fresheners. Furthermore, as stated in Chapter 19, Contact Dermatitis to Cosmetic Ingredients, fragrances consistently place among the top 10 contact dermatitis allergens. Fragrances are also the second most common allergen family associated with allergic contact dermatitis, following only nickel, as well as the most often cited cause of such reactions to cosmetic products.[1] Indeed, most fragrance ingredients can elicit allergic reactions and thereby act as allergens or raise the risk of sensitization, noted Kumar et al.[2] This looms as an especially important realization given the general rise in the incidence of contact allergy to various fragrances and the fact that epidemiologic and human allergen sensitization studies have shown that individuals who are found to be sensitive to one allergen through patch testing are at significantly greater risk of having a second allergen identified.[3–5] Given the greater expertise expected of cosmetic dermatologists regarding agents intended to beautify the skin, it is incumbent upon such specialists to have a strong working knowledge of the primary fragrances identified as provoking allergic reactions. This chapter will focus briefly on selected problematic fragrances, primarily on the worst offenders found within Fragrance Mix (FM) I and FM II.

DEMOGRAPHICS, REACTIONS, AND SIGNIFICANCE

An epidemiologic survey in the United Kingdom published in 2004 reported that 23% of women and 13.8% of men displayed adverse reactions to a personal care product (e.g., deodorants and perfumes, skincare products, hair care products, and nail cosmetics) over the course of a year.[6] More recently, in a 1999 to 2006 Brazilian study of 176 patients (154 women and 22 men) seen in a private office who complained of dermatoses resulting from cosmetics, 45% exhibited dermatoses linked to cosmetics and 14% had skin lesions that were found to be caused by inappropriate use of cosmetics.[7] Further, several studies indicate that approximately 10% of dermatologic patients who are patch tested for 20 to 100 ingredients exhibit allergic sensitivity to at least one ingredient common in cosmetic products.[6]

Fragrances and preservatives are the most common allergens and women aged 20 to 60 years old represent the demographic group that experiences the majority of these reactions.[8] Individuals who are overexposed to skincare products and patients with an impaired stratum corneum, as manifested by dry skin, reportedly have increased susceptibility to allergic reactions.[9] Contact allergy caused by fragrances is typically seen as axillary dermatitis, dermatitis of the face (including the eyelids) and neck, hand dermatitis, and eruptions in locations where perfume may be dabbed on or sprayed such as the wrists and behind the ears.[10] It is important to note that while the overall risk of allergic reaction to fragrances is low, the absolute numbers of individuals affected by fragrance allergy are significant. The prevalence of fragrance allergy in the general population is believed to range from 0.7% to 2.6%, with the positive reaction rate to fragrances spanning 5% to 11% in patch-test populations, according to Reeder.[11]

In 2016, Diepgen et al. performed a cross-sectional study of a random sample from the general populations (from 18 to 74 years old) in Germany, Italy, the Netherlands, Portugal, and Sweden to estimate the prevalence of contact allergy in Europe. A random sample of 3,119 were patch tested (after 12,377 subjects were interviewed) and more than one-quarter of the population was found to have a contact allergy to at least one allergen in the European baseline series. Greater prevalence was identified in women than in men, with the highest prevalences found, in descending order, for nickel, thiomersal, cobalt, FM II, FM I, hydroxyisohexyl 3-cyclohexene carboxaldehyde (HICC), p-tert-butylphenol formaldehyde resin, and para-phenylenediamine.[12] The same team previously gleaned from these data, in trying to ascertain the prevalence of fragrance contact allergy in the European general population, that the highest prevalence for contact allergy was for FM I in

petrolatum, with a high content of atranol and chloratranol, followed by FM II in petrolatum.[13]

FRAGRANCE MIX I

FM I is composed of eight different substances: α-amyl cinnamic aldehyde, cinnamic alcohol, cinnamic aldehyde, eugenol, geraniol, hydroxycitronellal, isoeugenol, oak moss.[14] FM I (**Table 42-1**), known simply as the FM for several years, was introduced in 1977 by Larsen and widely adopted.[15] This was a full 20 years after the first report of an allergic reaction to fragrance-based chemicals in 1957.[16]

In a review of patch test data for 25,545 patients from 1980 to 1996, Buckley et al. found that oak moss was the most common allergen. Oak moss contains the potent allergens chloroatranol and atranol.[17,18] Sensitivity to isoeugenol and α-amyl cinnamic aldehyde increased during the 16-year period under review; sensitivity to eugenol and geraniol remained stable; reaction to hydroxycitronellal declined slowly; and precipitous drop-offs in sensitivity frequency were associated with cinnamic aldehyde and cinnamic alcohol. Consequently, the authors identified the latter two FM I ingredients as rare fragrance allergens at that juncture.[19] Bruze et al. have subsequently shown, however, that cinnamic aldehyde in the concentration range of 0.01% to 0.32% when applied twice daily on healthy skin induces axillary dermatitis within a few weeks.[20]

Significantly, a 2006 study of related pairs found in the FM (i.e., cinnamal/cinnamic alcohol and isoeugenol/eugenol) as assessed through records of 23,660 patients patch tested to the FM from 1984 to 1998, indicated that there were substantial isolated reactions to the individual fragrance chemicals, justifying their continued usage as individual constituents in FM I.[21]

In a study intended to evaluate the changing frequencies of sensitization to the FM as well as single compounds *Myroxylon pereirae* (balsam of Peru), and oil of turpentine, investigators analyzed the data amassed by the Information Network of Departments of Dermatology multicenter project that ran from 1996 to 2002. They found significant increases between 1996 and 1998 in the proportions of patients exhibiting sensitivity to both single compounds and the FM. However, a significant decline was observed after 1999 in sensitization to the FM, which the researchers attributed to reduced exposure due to the use of less potent allergens in fine fragrances, and

TABLE 42-1	Fragrance Mix (FM) I	
α-Amyl cinnamic aldehyde		
Cinnamic alcohol		
Cinnamic aldehyde		
Eugenol		
Geraniol		
Hydroxycitronellal		
Isoeugenol		
Oak moss		

the potential lower use of natural ingredient-based cosmetics. Investigators also found the relative share of sensitivity to individual ingredients of the FM to be increased for compounds such as isoeugenol and oak moss. This increase could not be ascribed to their use, which for the top allergen oak moss was reported to be 0.4% as compared to the lower-potency geraniol, thought to be represented in 50% of the product market.[14] In fact, researchers noted that the International Fragrance Association (IFRA) and the Research Institute for Fragrance Materials (RIFM) had recommended the use of lower concentrations of isoeugenol and oak moss (**Table 42-2**). Such findings helped to illuminate the emerging belief that some ingredients within the FM were much more significant allergens than others and that re-evaluation might be warranted, including omission from the FM of some of the less troublesome components. In addition, one of the primary complaints regarding FM I had been the emergence of false positives and false negatives, and the detection of only approximately 70% of the patients allergic to fragrances.[10]

FRAGRANCE MIX II

In addition to the perceived imbalance in potency of the FM I compounds and the debate over whether certain chemicals continue to merit inclusion, a report in 1993 estimated that FM I failed to identify at least 15% of perfume allergies.[22] Five years later, Larsen found that as much as 33% of fragrance sensitivity may go undetected if it is tested in isolation as the only test compound.[23,24]

The incomplete detection of fragrance allergens through use of FM I and the identification of additional sensitizing allergens through clinical experience, and subsequent reporting and confirmation of such findings, eventually led to the development of FM II (**Table 42-3**). For instance, a multicenter trial in Europe completed in 2002 that evaluated 14 frequently used chemicals laid the groundwork as it identified the six most sensitizing chemicals, all of which were ultimately included as FM II.[25,26] These chemicals—HICC (also known as Lyral®), citral, farnesol, citronellol, α-hexyl-cinnamic aldehyde, and coumarin—were evaluated in 1,701 consecutive patients who were patch tested in six European centers. In all six centers, the team of investigators found the numbers of patients who reacted to the three different concentrations of FM II, which would have gone undetected by FM I, to be significant enough to warrant the codification of this new FM. Overall, FM II (14%) elicited a reaction in 2.9% of patients; of these, 33% were negative to FM I. In a more recent study in Germany of 6,968 patients, 7.7% reacted to FM I and 4.6% reacted to FM II.[27]

In 2008, investigators writing on behalf of the European Society of Contact Dermatitis (ESCD) and the European Environmental Contact Dermatitis Research Group (EECDRG), after conducting a literature review, recommended that FM II at a concentration of 14% w/w (5.6 mg/cm²) and Lyral, specifically, at 5% w/w (2.0 mg/cm²), be included in the European baseline patch test series. (The ESCD has delegated the major responsibility for the European patch test series to the EECDRG.) Lyral is the most common sensitizer among the FM II fragrances, followed by farnesol,[24] and is the most important sensitizer of the six fragrance substances included in FM II.[28]

HICC/Lyral

The synthetic fragrance hydroxyisohexyl 3-cyclohexene carboxaldehyde (HICC, or Lyral®), an aldehyde sufficiently lipophilic to penetrate the skin, is a common allergen that also happens to be used in numerous cosmetic and household products, including more than 50% of marketed deodorants,[29] and often provokes contact sensitization.[30]

Frosch et al. tested Lyral (5% in petrolatum) along with FM I and 11 other fragrances on consecutive patients in six European dermatology departments in 1999. Lyral elicited a positive reaction in 2.7% of 1,855 patients (range 1.2%–17%) and ranked next to 11.3% with FM allergy, leading the investigators to call for testing of Lyral in patients thought to be suffering from contact dermatitis.[31] Geier et al. reported on a subsequent test of Lyral 5% in petrolatum in 3,245 consecutive patch test patients in 20 dermatology departments, with 1.9% reacting to the fragrance. As part of this study, Lyral and FM I were tested in parallel in 3,185 patients, with 9.4% reacting to FM I and 1.9% to Lyral. A reaction to both occurred in 40 patients, corresponding to 13.3% of those reacting to FM I

TABLE 42-2	Member Nations of the International Fragrance Association (IFRA)
Australia	
Brazil	
France	
Germany	
Indonesia	
Italy	
Japan	
Mexico	
Netherlands	
Singapore	
Spain	
Switzerland	
Turkey	
United Kingdom	
United States	

TABLE 42-3	Fragrance Mix (FM) II
α-Hexyl cinnamal	
Citral	
Citronellol	
Coumarin	
Farnesol	
Hydroxyisohexyl 3-cyclohexene carboxaldehyde (Lyral®)	

and 67.8% of those reacting to Lyral. As a result of this study, the German Contact Dermatitis Research Group (DKG) opted to include Lyral as part of its standard patch test series.[32] In 2002, Frosch et al. supervised the evaluation of 1,855 patients patch tested in six European dermatology centers to determine the frequency of responses to 8% FM and 14 other often used fragrances. The six chemicals displaying the greatest reactivity after FM were, in descending order, Lyral, citral, farnesol, citronellol, hexyl cinnamic aldehyde, and coumarin. As a precursor to the codification of FM II, they found these six substances worthy of using in patch testing of contact dermatitis patients, with Lyral as the most notable of these chemicals.[26]

In 2006, the North American Contact Dermatitis Group (NACDG) conducted a multicenter study comparing three concentrations of Lyral (5%, 1.5%, and 0.5% in petrolatum) to the NACDG screening tray, which includes FM I, balsam of Peru, cinnamic aldehyde, ylang ylang oil, jasmine absolute, and tea tree oil. Data collected from 1,603 patients at six sites identified balsam of Peru (6.6%) and FM I (5.9%) to be the most common patch-test-positive fragrance allergens, followed by cinnamic aldehyde (1.7%), ylang ylang oil (0.6%), jasmine absolute (0.4%), Lyral (0.4% for 5% Lyral, 0.3% for 1.5% Lyral, and 0.2% for 0.5% Lyral), and tea tree oil (0.3%). The investigators concluded that Lyral is an uncommon allergen in North America, and that the 5% concentration should be used in patch tests for patients suspected of having a fragrance allergy.[33]

In a small 2007 study, researchers demonstrated that Lyral causes allergic contact dermatitis in a high percentage of sensitized individuals at usage concentrations typically found in deodorants.[29] Previously, Lyral had been found to provoke contact allergic reactions in 2% to 3% of eczema patients undergoing patch testing. In a small study of 18 eczema patients and seven control subjects, Johansen et al. examined a dose-response relationship of Lyral contact allergy. A serial dilution of Lyral in ethanol 6% to 6 ppm was administered to the volar forearm in a 2-week, repeated open application test. Upon no reaction to this dosage, cases were tested for 2 additional weeks at a higher dose. Eleven cases reacted to the low dose, five to the high, and two to neither. There was no reaction to the ethanol vehicle-control. Control subjects failed to react to either Lyral concentration or the ethanol vehicle. With a statistically significant difference between the groups, the investigators concluded that Lyral was causing skin sensitivity. They recommended reductions in usage concentrations to prevent allergic contact dermatitis in response to this fragrance.[34]

The ensuing year, Bruze et al. determined, based on a survey of the literature, that the European baseline patch test series (baseline series) should include FM II and Lyral. They added that a positive response to FM II should prompt additional patch testing with the six FM II ingredients, or five if there are simultaneous positive reactions to Lyral and FM II.[24]

In 2011, Carvalho et al. reported on a retrospective study including all patients submitted to patch test from January 2007 to December 2009 in a contact dermatitis unit to characterize the frequency of contact allergy to HICC. They found the frequency of positive reactions was 2.7% (17 of 629), with

a significant history of eczema among those who had tested positive. The investigators concluded that their data supported the inclusion of HICC in the baseline patch test series.[30]

In 2017, Engfeldt et al. followed up on the 2014 decision to exclude HICC from the Swedish baseline series and studied whether FM II with 5% HICC could detect more positive reactions than the normal FM II with 2.5% HICC. Evaluating the findings from 2,118 dermatitis patients at five Swedish dermatology departments, the investigators concluded that FM II with 5% HICC did not detect more positive reactions than FM II with 2.5% HICC. Further, HICC did not detect an adequate proportion of patients reacting only to HICC, justifying its exclusion from the Swedish baseline series.[35]

FM I/II AND THE 26 FRAGRANCES REQUIRED TO BE LABELED IN EUROPE

The creation of FM II was quickly followed by additional regulation of the fragrance market in Europe. As of March 2005, as mandated by the seventh amendment of the European Union (EU) Cosmetics Directive (and further clarified in EU regulation No. 1223/2009), all cosmetic products were required to indicate on their labels the presence of 26 individual fragrances if present at > 10 ppm in leave-on products and > 100 ppm in rinse-off products (**Table 42-4**).[1] Similar regulations were instituted regarding detergents as of October 2005, with labeling mandated for any of the 26 fragrances present at > 100 ppm.[36]

During the four 6-month periods between January 2003 and January 2005, Schnuch et al. patch tested 21,325 individuals for the 26 fragrances in addition to the standard series of fragrances. Frequencies of sensitization were noted as follows: tree moss (2.4%), Lyral (2.3%), oak moss (2.0%), hydroxycitronellal (1.3%), isoeugenol (1.1%), cinnamic aldehyde (1.0%), farnesol (0.9%), cinnamic alcohol (0.6%), citral (0.6%), citronellol (0.5%), geraniol (0.4%), eugenol (0.4%), coumarin (0.4%), lilial (0.3%), amyl-cinnamic alcohol (0.3%), benzyl cinnamate (0.3%), benzyl alcohol (0.3%), linalool (0.2%), methylheptin carbonate (0.2%), amyl-cinnamic aldehyde (0.1%), hexyl-cinnamic aldehyde (0.1%), limonene (0.1%), benzyl salicylate (0.1%), γ-methylionon (0.1%), benzyl benzoate (0.0%), and anisyl alcohol (0.0%). Given such percentages, the investigators concluded that clearly the 26 fragrances range in importance as risks to eliciting contact sensitivity, with some of great concern and others of no significance at all.[37]

In 2007, Buckley evaluated the exposure patterns to fragrances on the UK product market by surveying 300 products including the words "parfum" or "aroma" for any of the 26 listed fragrances. The fragrances that were most frequently identified were linalool (63%), limonene (63%), citronellol (48%), geraniol (42%), butylphenyl methylpropional (Lilial™) (42%), and hexyl cinnamal (42%). Besides geraniol, all the other FM I ingredients were represented: eugenol (27%), hydroxycitronellal (17%), isoeugenol (9%), cinnamic alcohol (8%), amyl cinnamal (7%), cinnamal (6%), and oak moss absolute (4%). FM II ingredients, in addition to citronellol and hexyl cinnamal, were also found in the product survey

	The 26 Individual Fragrances Required by the EU Cosmetics Directive (as of March 11, 2005) to be Labeled on Cosmetic Products If Present at > 10 ppm in Leave-On Products and > 100 ppm in Rinse-Off Products
TABLE 42-4	
A-isomethyl ionone	
Amyl cinnamal	
Amyl cinnamic alcohol	
Anisyl alcohol	
Benzyl alcohol	
Benzyl benzoate	
Benzyl cinnamate	
Benzyl salicylate	
Butylphenyl methylpropional (BPMP, Lilial™)	
Cinnamal	
Cinnamic alcohol	
Citral	
Citronellol	
Coumarin	
Eugenol	
Farnesol	
Geraniol	
Hexyl cinnamal	
Hydroxycitronellal	
Isoeugenol	
Limonene	
Linalool	
Lyral	
Methyl heptine carbonate	
Oak moss (*Evernia prunastri*)	
Tree moss (*Evernia fufuracea*)	

in significant numbers: coumarin (30%), Lyral (29%), citral (25%), and farnesol (8%). Buckley concluded that exposure levels to key allergens in FM I and II continue for the British population. Given the frequent use of the fragrances linalool and limonene, Buckley also suggested that these two chemicals be included in the test series for patients suspected of fragrance allergy.[36]

During the same year, Rastogi et al. conducted a survey of four primary fragrance allergens—isoeugenol, Lyral, atranol, and chloroatranol—included in 22 popular Danish as well as international brands purchased on the Danish retail market. Isoeugenol was identified in 56% of the products, Lyral in 72%, atranol in 59%, and chloroatranol in 36%. While isoeugenol was found to be included in concentrations below the recommended maximum level of 0.02% in each case, Lyral concentration attained a maximum of 0.2%, which is 10-fold higher than the EU Scientific Committee's identification of the safest maximum tolerable concentration. The concentration levels

for atranol and chloroatranol were similar to those found in 2003 and the frequency of use of the latter represented a significant reduction.[38]

Noting that the prestige perfumes intended for women have been the products demonstrated to contain the highest concentrations of allergens, Rastogi et al. evaluated 10 fine fragrances, five introduced between 1921 and 1990 and five launched since then by the same companies. They found that the five older perfumes included a mean of 5 allergens in FM I, whereas the five newer products contained a mean of 2.8 of the FM I allergens. In addition, the mean concentrations of the FM allergens in the old perfumes were 2.6 times higher than the mean for the new products. The investigators concluded that a concerted effort by the fragrance industry to curtail the use of offending ingredients or, perhaps, changes in fashion may have contributed to this decrease in the use of FM I allergens in prestige perfumes.[39]

It is important to note that even in products touted as containing only natural ingredients, fragrance substances represented in FM I and II, including hydroxycitronellal, coumarin, cinnamic alcohol, and α-amyl cinnamic aldehyde, have been identified. In a study of natural products, Rastogi et al. noted that the presence of hydroxycitronellal and α-hexylcinnamic aldehyde showed that artificial fragrances can be found in products marketed for their natural ingredients.[40]

In 2017, Bennike et al. conducted a cross-sectional study on consecutive dermatitis patients patch tested using the 26 fragrances and European baseline series from 2010 to 2015, finding that 15.7% of 6,004 patients were sensitized to fragrance. Further, they observed that non-mix fragrances were the most important single fragrance allergens, including Lin-OOH, *Evernia furfuracea*, Lim-OOH, and HICC.[41]

The next year, Ung et al. conducted a retrospective review of patch test records of all patients with eczema evaluated using the European baseline series FM I, FM II, *Myroxylon pereirae*, HICC, as well as individual fragrance substances from 2015 to 2016. They found that patch testing with these baseline series is no longer adequate for screening for fragrance allergy, with oxidized linalool, oxidized limonene, and *Evernia furfuracea* revealed as frequent allergens.[42]

In 2020, a retrospective study by the International Contact Dermatitis Research Group (ICDRG) set out to identify the prevalence of contact allergy to FM II and HICC from 2012 to 2016, particularly looking at simultaneous responses and undetected contact allergy to HICC when only FM II was tested (noting that HICC is included in FM II and also tested separately per the ICDRG baseline series). Contact allergy to FM II and HICC was identified in 3.9% and 1.6%, respectively, of the 25,019 consecutive dermatitis patients patch tested with FM II and HICC in 13 dermatology clinics in 12 countries across five continents. The ICDRG reported that the frequency of missed contact allergy to HICC when testing only with FM II was less than 0.5%, casting doubt on the need for separate testing.[28]

A retrospective study by Geier and Brans determined in 2020 that fewer positive test reactions to the fragrance mixes could be ascribed to decreasing use of oak moss containing atranol and chloroatranol, as well as HICC, the use of which was banned in the EU as of August 2019. They added that further reductions in the sensitization frequencies should be expected based on this prohibition.[1] Currently, the most common fragrance screeners in the majority of baseline series include FM I, FM II, and balsam of Peru, with HICC, hydroperoxides of limonene, and hydroperoxides of linalool also useful for inclusion to screening for diagnosis of fragrance allergy.[11]

CONCLUSION

Fragrances are ubiquitous chemical constituents in a significant proportion of the products that people use every day. A substantial minority of individuals develop allergic contact dermatitis to at least one of the many hundreds of fragrances used in the wide variety of products that come into contact with the skin. In addition, with the advent of aromatherapy, an increasing number of patients have come to enjoy the olfactory sensation that they experience from using such products. Ironically, the very ingredients that may bring some therapeutic relief by dint of their scents may cause some irritation to the skin. The roster of fragrances in products, as well as the range of products with fragrances added, has expanded as has the list of fragrances included in patch testing for sensitivity since the first allergy to fragrance-based chemicals was identified in 1957. It is important that cosmetic dermatologists and aestheticians be aware of the plethora of chemicals that have been recognized for provoking cutaneous reactions in a distinct but sizable minority of patients as well as the range of substances used in baseline patch test series.

References

1. Geier J, Brans R. How common is fragrance allergy really? *Hautarzt*. 2020;71(3):197–204.
2. Kumar M, Devi A, Sharma M, Kaur P, Mandal UK. Review on perfume and present status of its associated allergens. *J Cosmet Dermatol*. 2021;20(2):391–399.
3. Heydorn S, Johansen JD, Andersen KE, et al. Fragrance allergy in patients with hand eczema – a clinical study. *Contact Dermatitis*. 2003;48(6):317–323.
4. Nielsen NH, Linneberg A, Menné T, et al. Allergic contact sensitization in an adult Danish population: two cross-sectional surveys eight years apart (the Copenhagen Allergy Study). *Acta Derm Venereol*. 2001;81(1):31–34.
5. Friedman PS. The immunology of allergic contact dermatitis: the DNCB story. *Adv Dermatol*. 1990;5:175–195.
6. Orton DI, Wilkinson, JD. Cosmetic allergy: incidence, diagnosis, and management. *Am J Clin. Dermatol*. 2004;5(5):327–337.
7. Duarte I, Campos Lage AC. Frequency of dermatoses associated with cosmetics. *Contact Dermatitis*. 2007;56(4):211–213.
8. Mehta SS, Reddy BS. Cosmetic dermatitis—current perspectives. *Int J Dermatol*. 2003;42(7):533–542.
9. Jovanović M, Poljacki M, Duran V, Vujanović L, Sente R, Stojanović S. Contact allergy to Compositae plants in patients with atopic dermatitis. *Med Pregl*. 2004;57(5-6):209–218.
10. de Groot AC, Frosch PJ. Adverse reactions to fragrances. A clinical review. *Contact Dermatitis*. 1997;36(2):57–86.
11. Reeder MJ. Allergic Contact Dermatitis to Fragrances. *Dermatol Clin*. 2020;38(3):371–377.
12. Diepgen TL, Ofenloch RF, Bruze M, et al. Prevalence of contact allergy in the general population in different European regions. *Br J Dermatol*. 2016;174(2):319–329.
13. Diepgen TL, Ofenloch R, Bruze M, et al. Prevalence of fragrance contact allergy in the general population of five European countries: a cross-sectional study. *Br J Dermatol*. 2015;173(6):1411–1419.
14. Schnuch A, Lessmann H, Geier J, Frosch PJ, Uter W; IVDK. Contact allergy to fragrances: frequencies of sensitization from 1996 to 2002. Results of the IVDK. *Contact Dermatitis*. 2004;50(2):65–76.
15. Larsen WG. Perfume dermatitis. A study of 20 patients. *Arch Dermatol*. 1977;113(5):623–626.
16. Chatard H. Case of sensitization to perfumes with cutaneous and general reactions. *Bull Soc Fr Dermatol Syphiligr*. 1957;64(3):323.
17. Johansen JD, Andersen KE, Svedman C, et al. Chloroatranol, an extremely potent allergen hidden in perfumes: a dose-response elicitation study. *Contact Dermatitis*. 2003;49(4):180–184.
18. Rastogi SC, Bossi R, Johansen JD, et al. Content of oak moss allergens atranol and chloroatranol in perfumes and similar products. *Contact Dermatitis*. 2004;50(6):367–370.
19. Buckley DA, Wakelin SH, Seed PT, et al. The frequency of fragrance allergy in a patch-test population over a 17-year period. *Br J Dermatol*. 2000;142(2):279–283.
20. Bruze M, Johansen JD, Andersen KE, et al. Deodorants: an experimental provocation study with cinnamic aldehyde. *J Am Acad Dermatol*. 2003;48(2):194–200.
21. Buckley DA, Basketter DA, Smith Pease CK, Rycroft RJ, White IR, McFadden JP. Simultaneous sensitivity to fragrances. *Br J Dermatol*. 2006;154(5):885–888.
22. de Groot AC, van der Kley AM, Bruynzeel DP, et al. Frequency of false-negative reactions to the fragrance mix. *Contact Dermatitis*. 1993;28(3):139–140.
23. Larsen W, Nakayama H, Fischer T, et al. A study of new fragrance mixtures. *Am J Contact Dermat*. 1998;9(4):202–206.
24. Bruze M, Andersen KE, Goossens A; ESCD; EECDRG. Recommendation to include fragrance mix 2 and hydroxyisohexyl 3-cyclohexene carboxaldehyde (Lyral) in the European baseline patch test series. *Contact Dermatitis*. 2008;58(3):129–133.
25. Frosch PJ, Pirker C, Rastogi SC, et al. Patch testing with a new fragrance mix detects additional patients sensitive to perfumes and missed by the current fragrance mix. *Contact Dermatitis*. 2005;52(4):207–215.
26. Frosch PJ, Johansen JD, Menné T, et al. Further important sensitizers in patients sensitive to fragrances. I. Reactivity to 14 frequently used chemicals. *Contact Dermatitis*. 2002;47(2):78–85.
27. Nardelli A, Carbonez A, Ottoy W, Drieghe J, Goossens A. Frequency of and trends in fragrance allergy over a 15-year period. *Contact Dermatitis*. 2008;58(3):134–141.
28. Bruze M, Ale I, Andersen KE, et al; International Contact Dermatitis Research Group. Contact Allergy to Fragrance Mix II and Hydroxyisohexyl 3-Cyclohexene Carboxaldehyde: A Retrospective Study by International Contact Dermatitis Research Group. *Dermatitis*. 2020;31(4):268–271.
29. Jørgensen PH, Jensen CD, Rastogi S, Andersen KE, Johansen JD. Experimental elicitation with hydroxyisohexyl-3-cyclohexene

carboxaldehyde-containing deodorants. *Contact Dermatitis.* 2007;56(3):146–150.

30. Carvalho R, Maio P, Amaro C, Santos R, Cardoso J. Hydroxyisohexyl 3-cyclohexene carboxaldehyde (Lyral®) as allergen: experience from a contact dermatitis unit. *Cutan Ocul Toxicol.* 2011;30(3):249–250.

31. Frosch PJ, Johansen JD, Menné T, et al. Lyral is an important sensitizer in patients sensitive to fragrances. *Br J Dermatol.* 1999;141(6):1076–1083.

32. Geier J, Brasch J, Schnuch A, et al. Lyral has been included in the patch test standard series in Germany. *Contact Dermatitis.* 2002;46(5):295–297.

33. Belsito DV, Fowler JF Jr, Sasseville D, Marks JG Jr, De Leo VA, Storrs FJ. Delayed-type hypersensitivity to fragrance materials in a select North American population. *Dermatitis.* 2006;17(1):23–28.

34. Johansen JD, Frosch PJ, Svedman C, et al. Hydroxyisohexyl 3-cyclohexene carboxaldehyde—known as Lyral: quantitative aspects and risk assessment of an important fragrance allergen. *Contact Dermatitis.* 2003;48(6):310–316.

35. Engfeldt M, Hagvall L, Isaksson M, et al. Patch testing with hydroxyisohexyl 3-cyclohexene carboxaldehyde (HICC) – a multicentre study of the Swedish Contact Dermatitis Research Group. *Contact Dermatitis.* 2017;76(1):34–39.

36. Buckley DA. Fragrance ingredient labeling in products on sale in the U.K. *Br J Dermatol.* 2007;157(2):295–300.

37. Schnuch A, Uter W, Geier J, Lessmann H, Frosch PJ. Sensitization to 26 fragrances to be labeled according to current European regulation. Results of the IVDK and review of the literature. *Contact Dermatitis.* 2007;57(1):1–10.

38. Rastogi SC, Johansen JD, Bossi R. Selected important fragrance sensitizers in perfumes—current exposures. *Contact Dermatitis.* 2007;56(4):201–204.

39. Rastogi SC, Menné T, Johansen JD. The composition of fine fragrances is changing. *Contact Dermatitis.* 2003;48(3):130–132.

40. Rastogi SC, Johansen JD, Menné T. Natural ingredients based cosmetics. Content of selected fragrance sensitizers. *Contact Dermatitis.* 1996;34(6):423–426.

41. Bennike NH, Zachariae C, Johansen JD. Non-mix fragrances are top sensitizers in consecutive dermatitis patients – a cross-sectional study of the 26 EU-labelled fragrance allergens. *Contact Dermatitis.* 2017;77(5):270–279.

42. Ung CY, White JML, White IR, Banerjee P, McFadden JP. Patch testing with the European baseline series fragrance markers: a 2016 update. *Br J Dermatol.* 2018;178(3):776–780.

CHAPTER 43

Moisturizers

Leslie S. Baumann, MD

SUMMARY POINTS

What's Important?

1. Occlusives, humectants, and emollients treat the symptoms of dry skin, while barrier repair ingredients treat the causes of dry skin.
2. Hyaluronic and oleic acids increase penetration of other ingredients.
3. The type of water used in a moisturizer can affect its efficacy.
4. Using the wrong ratio of ceramides, fatty acids, and cholesterol will injure the skin barrier and worsen dehydration.

What's New?

1. Unsaturated fatty acids decrease melanin synthesis and tyrosinase activity, while saturated fatty acids increase melanin synthesis and tyrosinase activity.
2. Barrier repair moisturizers can diminish inflammation and reduce inflammatory cytokine levels in serum.

What's Coming?

1. New technologies to increase penetration using nanotechnology and other methods will increase the ability to add ingredients to moisturizers.

Moisturization research was spearheaded in the 1950s when Blank demonstrated that low moisture content of the skin is a prime factor in dry skin conditions.[1] In the last 50 years, scores of scientists have devoted their lives to researching moisturization and have begun to unravel the mysteries of skin hydration (see Chapter 12, Dry Skin). It is now known that the symptoms of dry skin can be treated by increasing the hydration state of the stratum corneum (SC) with occlusive or humectant ingredients and by smoothing the rough surface with an emollient. Moisturizers represent a multibillion-dollar market in the United States. Commonly used moisturizers are oil-in-water emulsions and water-in-oil emulsions. In some cases, oils are used as a moisturizer. This chapter will identify and discuss the mechanisms of action of the main components found in popular moisturizers.

MECHANISM OF ACTION OF MOISTURIZERS

There are numerous moisturizers on the market but they all have the same goal: to increase water content in the SC. This can be accomplished by preventing water evaporation from the skin through the use of occlusive ingredients or by augmenting the integrity of the skin barrier (see Chapter 12). The mainstay of enhancing the skin barrier's integrity involves providing fatty acids, ceramides, and cholesterol in moisturizers. Ensuring a healthy skin barrier is the best way to combat skin dehydration.

Improving the skin's ability to hold on to water is another strategy for moisturizing skin. Increasing levels of natural moisturizing factor (NMF), glycerin (glycerol), and other humectants such as hyaluronic acid (HA) and heparan sulfate

(HS) will help skin retain water. Lastly, increasing the ability of the epidermis to absorb important components for the circulation, such as glycerol and water through aquaporin (AQP) channels, will also aid in increasing skin hydration.

Moisturizers play a larger role than just hydrating the skin. They can affect the calcium gradient, pH, and fatty acid distribution of the skin. Moisturizers can also influence mRNA expression of genes such as involucrin, transglutaminase, and kallikrein. In addition, they can modify keratinocyte differentiation and desquamation.[2]

Moisturizers also affect skin penetration. If they are placed on the skin before a second product, they can either increase or decrease the penetration of that product depending on the ingredients in the moisturizer. This should be considered when designing a skincare routine (see Chapter 35, Skincare Regimen Design).

MOISTURIZERS AND INFLAMMATION

Moisturizers help prevent and treat inflammation. Dry skin is more likely to become inflamed because water is necessary for many cell functions. However, the reduction of inflammation seen with moisturizer use transcends helping the skin hold on to water. The components in moisturizers can combat inflammation directly. Also, barrier repair moisturizers can decrease inflammation by helping the skin maintain barrier homeostasis. One study looked at 33 human subjects who used a moisturizer containing myristoyl/palmitoyl oxostearamide/arachamide mea (a multi-lamellar emulsion, or MLE, technology) twice daily for 30 days.[3] This study showed that use of the barrier repair moisturizer normalized levels of cytokines that cause inflammation (IL-1β, IL-6) and decreased levels of TNF-α. They postulated that the use of MLE technology-containing moisturizers may help prevent systemic inflammatory diseases such as heart disease, diabetes, and Alzheimer's. Several studies have shown that moisturizing newborns will help prevent food allergies and asthma and stop the "atopic march" that begins with an impaired skin barrier.[4] Fatty acids function as signal molecules and can activate the body's immune response.[5] Moisturizers often contain various types of fatty acids that can help reduce inflammation. Microbes on the skin can break down lipids in moisturizers (and sebum) into short chain fatty acids. Short chain fatty acids affect inflammatory reactions and help maintain a balanced microbiome.

INGREDIENTS IN MOISTURIZERS

Occlusives

Occlusives coat the SC to slow transepidermal water loss (TEWL). They are usually oily, full of lipids, or contain silicone. Sebum is an occlusive moisturizer. An occlusive moisturizer alone does not improve the skin barrier but can contribute fatty acids to the barrier. For the barrier to be repaired, fatty acids must be combined with ceramides and cholesterol. In other words, occlusive moisturizers can treat the symptoms of dry skin, but they do not treat the underlying cause—an impaired skin barrier. Adding to the level of fatty acids already on the skin without ceramides and cholesterol can actually injure the skin barrier. For this reason, it is best to use barrier repair technology to treat dry skin. Nevertheless, there are myriad moisturizers on the market that contain only occlusive ingredients.

Occlusive ingredients provide an emollient (smoothing) effect and reduce TEWL. Two of the best occlusive ingredients currently available are petrolatum and mineral oil. Petrolatum, for example, exhibits a water vapor loss resistance 170 times that of olive oil.[6] However, petrolatum has a greasy feeling that may render agents containing it cosmetically unacceptable. Other commonly used occlusive ingredients include paraffin, squalene, dimethicone, soybean oil, grapeseed oil, propylene glycol, lanolin, and beeswax.[7] In addition, "natural" oils such as sunflower oil have been increasing in popularity. Occlusive agents are only effective while present on the skin; once removed, TEWL returns to the previous level. It is not desirable to lower TEWL by more than 40% because excess hydration with maceration leading to alteration of the microbiome can result.[8] In moisturizers, occlusives are usually combined with humectant ingredients or included in barrier repair moisturizers. Oils are an example of occlusive ingredients.

Petrolatum

Petrolatum was considered by many, including Kligman, to be one of the best moisturizers.[9] It has been used as a skincare product since 1872. However, now the trend is towards more natural ingredients, particularly ones that do not have a carbon footprint on the environment or appear obviously to the consumer as chemically based. Consequently, petrolatum has declined in popularity.

Petrolatum is a purified mixture of hydrocarbons derived from petroleum (crude oil). The hydrocarbon molecules present in petrolatum prevent oxidation, giving petrolatum a long shelf life. Because petrolatum is one of the most occlusive moisturizing ingredients known, it is often the gold standard to which other occlusive ingredients are compared.[10] Petrolatum is also well known for being noncomedogenic.[11] The possibility of an individual being allergic to petrolatum is so unlikely that some authors believe it to be a non-sensitizing agent, but allergic contact dermatitis to petrolatum has been reported in the literature.[12–14] The greasy, oily texture makes this ingredient cosmetically inelegant (and is yet another reason for its reduced popularity). Therefore, petrolatum is often combined with other ingredients to minimize the greasy feeling.

Lanolin

Lanolin is a complex animal-derived natural product that cannot be synthesized. The method of refinement used determines the composition and quality of the resulting product, so not all lanolin products display the same properties.[15] Lanolin is derived from the sebaceous secretions of sheep; however, its composition is significantly different from human skin.[16] Lanolin shares two important characteristics with SC lipids: (a) lanolin contains cholesterol, an essential component of SC lipids, and (b) lanolin and SC lipids can coexist as solids and liquids at physiologic temperatures. Unfortunately, there is a subset of individuals who develop contact sensitization to lanolin.[17] Many moisturizing products are now labeled as "lanolin free."

Oils

With the surge in popularity of natural and organic ingredients, oils are now commonly used in moisturizing products or as moisturizing agents themselves. In addition, moisturizing "cleansing oils" are also commercially available. Oil is a substance that is liquid at room temperature and insoluble in water. Oils contain copious lipids, which the skin requires for the proper formation and function of cell membranes to prevent TEWL. Vegetable oils are pressed out of seeds and essential oils are steamed from several plant parts, including stems, leaves, and roots. Not all oils are of botanical origin. Mineral oil, or liquid petrolatum, is derived from the distillation of petroleum in the production of gasoline.

Essential oils are extracts of oils that include the essence of the fragrance and none of the lipids. For this reason, essential oils are not good moisturizers and have no hydrating effects but pose a risk of allergenicity. Essential oils have significantly increased in popularity in recent years. However, it is crucial to realize that these ingredients are common allergens.[18] Massage therapists and others who are routinely exposed to essential oils should try to limit their exposure to lower their risk for developing an allergy to a topically applied oil that can translate to an allergy to the related oil in food products.[19]

Mineral oil

With a history of cosmetic uses spanning two millennia and inclusion in modern cosmetic agents for more than 100 years, mineral oil is one of the most frequently used oils in skincare products.[20] In 1989, investigators found that an emulsion containing mineral oil was more effective than several linoleic acid emulsions in diminishing skin vapor loss induced in volunteers by the topical application of the surfactant sodium lauryl sulfate.[21] A randomized, double-blind, controlled trial in 2004 showed that mineral oil and extra virgin coconut oil were equally efficacious and safe as moisturizers in treating mild-to-moderate xerosis in 34 patients, with surface lipid level and skin hydration significantly enhanced in both groups.[22] Because of its source, though, several criticisms, and some myths, have emerged regarding mineral oil. In fact, in 1997, an epidemiologic review of the relationship between mineral oil exposure and cancer revealed several associations.[23] Importantly, however, any such evidence linking mineral oil exposure (via dermal contact or inhalation) and specific forms of cancer has been derived from cases of protracted exposure to industrial grade mineral oil. Cosmetic grade mineral oil has never been associated with cancer etiology. Furthermore, a 2005 study suggested that even though industrial grade mineral oil may be comedogenic, cosmetic grade mineral oil patently is not, and, consequently, should not be excluded from appropriate cosmetic formulations because of lingering myths or extrapolations from industrial grade mineral oil regarding comedogenicity.[20] While mineral oil is fragrance-free, inexpensive, colorless, and effective, it is cosmetically inelegant and more popular when used in combination with other ingredients. For an increasing segment of the population concerned about the carbon footprint associated with mineral oil and its impact on the environment, this ingredient is not very popular. Nevertheless, mineral oil remains an exceedingly effective emollient and occlusive agent.[24]

Natural oils

Natural oils contain fatty acids that are important in maintaining the skin barrier. Linoleic acid, an ω-6 fatty acid present in sunflower, safflower, and other oils, is an example of an essential fatty acid that must be obtained from the diet or through topical application. In addition to providing structural lipids needed for barrier integrity, linoleic acid is used by the body to produce γ-linolenic acid (GLA). GLA is a polyunsaturated essential *cis*-fatty acid important in the production of prostaglandins; therefore, it plays a role in the inflammatory process. Many oils and foods contain linoleic acid (**Table 43-1**). Several of these oils are found in skincare products that supply fatty acids while functioning as occlusive agents. Oils are a common source of fatty acids used in skincare products. Each oil contains different levels of fatty acids that affect the activity of the oil. See **Table 43-2** for fatty acid composition of oils commonly found in moisturizers.

Argan Oil (*Argania spinosa* kernel oil)

Approximately 37% of argan oil is composed of linoleic acid, rendering it a great oil to treat inflammation. Argan oil comes from the nut of an argan tree. When the nuts are roasted the oil is suffused with a nutty flavor that is used in cooking. Unprocessed oil is used in cosmeceutical products due to the high amounts of antioxidants and linoleic acid. Argan oil is noncomedogenic and has a very low risk of allergy. It can be used as an oil alone or combined in moisturizing products. In

TABLE 43-1	Oils and Foods That Contain Linoleic Acid
Oils	**Foods**
Coconut	Egg yolks
Grape seed	Grass-fed cow milk
Hemp	Lard
Macadamia	Okra
Olive	Soybean
Palm	Spirulina
Peanut	
Pistachio	
Poppy seed	
Rice bran	
Safflower	
Sesame	
Sunflower	
Walnut	
Wheat germ	

TABLE 43-2	Fatty Acid Content of Various Oils Used in Moisturizers				
Oil	Oleic	Linoleic	Linolenic	Palmitic	Stearic
Argan	42.8%	36.8%	<0.5%	12%	6%
Almond	32%	13%	0%	10%	
Borage seed	18.5%	36.6%	21.1%	10.7%	6.4%
Coconut	6.5%	2%		9.5%	2%
Grape seed	15.8%	69.6%	0.1%	7%	4%
Macadamia	60%	1–3%	1–2%		
Olive	70%	15%	0.5%	13%	1.5%
Safflower	13.75%	76.22%		6.02%	2.37%

a 2013 study in 30 postmenopausal women, the topical application of argan oil displayed a statistically significant improvement in skin hydration after 2 months of treatment.[25]

Sunflower Seed Oil (*Helianthus annus*)

The primary constituents of sunflower oil are oleic and linoleic acids. In a study by Darmstadt et al. intended to identify safe and inexpensive vegetable oils effective in enhancing epidermal barrier function and available in developing countries, researchers testing various oils on mouse epidermal barrier function found that mustard, olive, and soybean oils significantly delayed recovery compared to controls or skin treated with Aquaphor, which is used to ameliorate skin barrier function. However, one application of sunflower seed oil significantly accelerated skin barrier function recovery within an hour and sustained this result 5 hours after application.[26] Some of the same investigators subsequently compared the effects of the topically applied emollients sunflower seed oil and Aquaphor in the prevention of nosocomial infections in very low birthweight premature infants in Bangladesh. Infants born before week 33 of gestation after hospital admission were randomly assigned to daily massage with either agent (159 subjects in each group) and results were compared with 181 untreated controls by intention-to-treat analysis. Infants treated with sunflower seed oil were 41% less likely to develop nosocomial infections as compared to controls. (Aquaphor performed slightly better than no treatment but did not significantly reduce infection risk.) This study also fulfilled one of the aims of the earlier study by Darmstadt et al., finding sunflower seed oil an effective, affordable, and available emollient option for patients in developing countries.[27]

Evening Primrose Oil (*Oenothera biennis*)

Evening primrose oil (EPO) is rich in ω-6 fatty acids, containing both linoleic and γ-linolenic acids. Indeed, EPO is thought to be the best source of GLA. Linoleic acid, which helps to maintain SC cohesion and contributes to TEWL reduction, is also used by the body to synthesize GLA.[28] EPO is usually taken as an oral supplement but is also included in topical skincare products. Some studies of EPO have revealed significant effects in the treatment of atopic dermatitis; however, studies have been largely inconsistent regarding such an application.[29] Nevertheless, the presence of linoleic and γ-linolenic

acids may justify the use of EPO in patients with dry skin or poor nutrition.

Olive Oil (*Olea europaea*)

Used by the ancient Greeks, Egyptians, and Romans for bathing as well as medicinal purposes, olive oil is used in contemporary times as a healthy component, and the primary source of fat, in the Mediterranean diet, considered one of the healthiest in the world. The leaves and fruits of the olive plant have also been used as external emollients to treat skin ulcers and inflammatory wounds.[30] Olive oil contains various potent compounds, many with antioxidant properties, such as polyphenols, squalene, fatty acids (especially oleic acid), triglycerides, tocopherols, carotenoids, sterols, and chlorophylls.[31] In particular, the phenols in virgin olive oil are known to scavenge reactive oxygen and nitrogen species active in human disease; however, it is unknown whether the influence of these compounds extends beyond the extracellular environment.[31,32] Adverse side effects associated with olive oil are very rare, as this natural oil is generally regarded as safe and very weakly irritant.[33] However, oleic acid in olive oil helps increase penetration. If a patient suffers from allergic contact dermatitis, use of olive oil can increase their susceptibility to contact dermatitis by impairing the skin barrier. Therefore, olive oil is not a good choice for skin hydration.[34,35]

Jojoba (*Buxus chinensis* or *Simmondsia chinensis*)

Jojoba (pronounced ho-ho-ba) oil is derived from the cold-pressed peanut- or small olive-sized seeds of the jojoba plant and contains triglycerides as well as several fatty acids including oleic, linoleic, linolenic, and arachidonic acids.[31] Jojoba oil is similar in consistency to human sebum and is cosmetically elegant, making it popular in skincare products. Both a humectant and an occlusive, jojoba oil has been found to exhibit significant beneficial properties as an analgesic, antibacterial, anti-inflammatory, antioxidant, antiparasitic, and antipyretic agent.[31]

Humectants

Humectants are water-soluble substances with high water absorption capabilities. They can attract water from the atmosphere and hold it on the skin's surface making it feel dewy and moist. Although humectants may draw water from the environment to help hydrate the skin, in low-humidity conditions they may take water from the deeper epidermis and dermis resulting in increased skin dryness.[36] For this reason, they work better when combined with occlusives. Humectants are also popular additives to cosmetic moisturizers because they prevent product evaporation and thickening, thereby extending the shelf life of various moisturizers. Some humectants display bacteriostatic activity as well.[37] Humectants draw water into the skin, causing a slight swelling of the SC that gives the perception of smoother skin with fewer wrinkles. Accordingly, several manufacturers tout moisturizers as "anti-wrinkle creams" even though they impart no long-term anti-wrinkling effect. Examples of commonly used humectants include HA, HS, glycerin, sorbitol, sodium hyaluronate, urea, propylene glycol, alpha hydroxy acids, and sugars.

Glycerin

Glycerin (glycerol) is a robust humectant and has a hygroscopic ability that closely resembles that of NMF (see Chapter 12).[38] This also allows the SC to retain a high water content even in a dry environment. Research by Choi et al. has shown that glycerol plays an important role in skin hydration because glycerol levels correlate with SC hydration levels.[39]

Orth et al. compared two high-glycerin moisturizers to 16 other popular moisturizers in 394 patients with severely dry skin.[40] The high-glycerin products were superior to all other products tested over this 5-year period because they rapidly restored dry skin to normal hydration. They also helped prevent the return to dryness for a longer period than the other formulations, even those containing petrolatum. Ultrastructural analysis of skin treated with "high glycerin" formulations shows that glycerin causes an expansion of the SC because of increased thickness of the corneocytes and larger spaces between layers of corneocytes.[41] These findings suggest that glycerin appears to create a reservoir of moisture-holding ability that renders the skin more resistant to drying as seen in Orth's study. Glycerin also functions by stabilizing and fluidizing cell membranes and by hydrating enzymes needed for desmosome degradation.[40]

Glycerin can be obtained from topical preparations but can also be transported from the circulation into the epidermis through AQP channels (see Chapter 11, Oily Skin). Recent studies have shown that normal SC hydration requires endogenous glycerol.[42] Two unrelated inbred mouse models demonstrated the potential importance of endogenous glycerol for normal SC hydration. Knockout mice, which lack the AQP-3 water channel, are unable to transport glycerol from the circulation into the epidermis and they exhibit abnormal SC hydration and reduced SC glycerol levels.[43] This defect in mice is corrected when glycerol is applied topically.[44] Glycerin has been available for several years but the discovery that it can modulate AQP-3 channels in the skin suggests that it is here to stay.[45]

Urea

Urea is a component of the NMF. It has been used in hand creams since the 1940s.[46] In addition to acting as a humectant,

urea displays a mild antipruritic effect.[47] Although there is some disagreement in the literature, several studies have shown that the combination of urea with hydrocortisone, retinoic acid, and other agents increases penetration of these agents.[48,49] In a double-blind experiment, 3% and 10% urea creams were shown to be more effective in dry skin than the vehicle-control. Interestingly, TEWL was unchanged after treatment with the 3% urea cream, while the 10% urea cream caused a decrease in TEWL although the creams were reported clinically to be equally effective.[50] At concentrations below 10%, urea has consistently been found to function as a moisturizer.[51]

Hydroxy Acids

Alpha hydroxy acids (AHAs) are a family of naturally occurring organic acids that function as humectants; they also exhibit exfoliating properties. Glycolic (derived from sugar cane) and lactic (derived from sour milk) acids are the most commonly used AHAs in moisturizing products and were the first to be marketed. Other AHAs include malic acid, derived from apples, citric acid, derived from acidic fruits, and tartaric acid, derived from grapes.[52] Topical preparations that contain AHAs have long been known to exert significant influence on epidermal keratinization.[53] Salicylic acid, a chemical exfoliant and the lone beta hydroxy acid (BHA), is derived from willow bark, wintergreen leaves, and sweet birch, but is also available in synthetic form.[54]

The cosmetic effects of hydroxy acids include normalization of SC exfoliation resulting in increased plasticization and decreased formation of dry scales on the surface of the skin. AHAs and BHA function by degrading the desmosomes and allowing desquamation to proceed. They also influence corneocyte cohesiveness at the basement levels of the SC,[55] where they affect its pH and improve desquamation.[56] The application of AHAs and BHA in high concentrations leads to detachment of keratinocytes and epidermolysis; application at lower concentrations degrades intercorneocyte cohesion directly above the granular layer, which furthers desquamation and thinning of the SC. A thinner SC is more flexible and compact, giving the skin a more youthful appearance. This increased flexibility obtained from the use of AHAs has been shown to persist even in low-humidity situations.[57] A thinner, more compact SC is also desirable because it better reflects light, making the skin appear more luminous.[56]

A thinner SC, however, does have some purported disadvantages. For instance, exfoliants have been demonstrated to lower the minimal erythema dose (MED) of the skin.[58] Although one study showed that glycolic acid imparted a photoprotective effect,[59] all subsequent studies have revealed increased photosensitivity following the application of AHAs.[60,61] The FDA has reviewed the research on AHAs and now requires that these products include a label warning that they be used in conjunction with sun protection.

Lactic Acid

Lactic acid is unique because it is an AHA as well as a component of the NMF. This means that it confers the same benefit as other AHAs by promoting desquamation but offers other beneficial effects as well. The benefits of lactic acid on photoaged skin are well understood, as demonstrated by a double-blind vehicle-controlled study that found that an 8% L-lactic acid formula was superior to vehicle for the treatment of photoaged skin. Statistically significant improvements were seen in skin roughness and signs of photodamage (mottled hyperpigmentation and sallowness).[62] However, the benefits of lactic acid in dry skin are just being elucidated. This AHA was first used in 1943 for the treatment of ichthyosis.[63] Lactic acid (especially the L-isomer) has been found *in vitro* and *in vivo* to increase the production of ceramides by keratinocytes.[46,64] In addition, application of the L-isomer of lactic acid to keratinocytes not only increased the ceramide content but appeared to increase the ratio of ceramide 1 linoleate to ceramide 1 oleate. This is likely an important finding because a reduced ratio of ceramide 1 linoleate to ceramide 1 oleate is seen in diseases such as atopic dermatitis and acne.[65,66] The increased levels of ceramides, particularly ceramide 1 linoleate, may partly explain why patients treated with the L-isomer of lactic acid exhibited an improved water barrier with less TEWL after a surfactant patch test than did patients treated with vehicle alone. The effect of lactic acid on epidermal turnover is dependent on both pH and concentration. It has been shown that at a fixed lactic acid concentration the pH is the influential factor in epidermal turnover, while at fixed pH the desquamation of the skin is dependent on lactic acid concentration.[67] Currently, lactic acid is thought of as a reliable moisturizing substance that helps to maintain epidermal barrier integrity.[68]

Propylene Glycol

Propylene glycol (PG) is an odorless liquid that functions as both a humectant and an occlusive. It displays antimicrobial and keratolytic activity. PG has been shown to enhance the penetration of drugs such as minoxidil and steroids. Although PG is known to be a weak sensitizer itself, it may contribute to contact dermatitis by enhancing penetration of other allergens.[69] Propylene glycol is added to moisturizers as a penetration enhancer.

Emollients

Emollients are compounds added to cosmetics to soften and smooth the skin. They function by filling the spaces between desquamating corneocytes to yield a smooth surface.[70] These products provide increased cohesion causing a flattening of the curled edges of the individual corneocytes.[38] This leads to a smoother surface with less friction and greater light refraction. Several emollients function as humectants and occlusive moisturizers as well. Lanolin, mineral oil, and petrolatum are examples of occlusive ingredients that also impart an emollient effect.

Barrier Repair Ingredients

It is well known that the application of the primary skin barrier lipid components—ceramides, cholesterol, and fatty acids—strengthens the skin barrier function and improves skin hydration. Using a barrier repair moisturizer in dry skin

types is preferred because humectants, emollients, and occlusives treat the symptoms but not the cause. Barrier repair moisturizers help the skin hold on to water and protect itself from allergens, irritants, and microbes. Barrier repair moisturizers should be the frontline therapy for dry skin.

Using the wrong ratio of ceramides, fatty acids, and cholesterol will injure the skin barrier and worsen dehydration. In 1993, Man et al. showed that ceramide and fatty acid together, when applied without cholesterol, *delayed* barrier recovery.[71] In addition, two other mixtures of cholesterol plus fatty acid or cholesterol plus ceramide delayed barrier repair. These incomplete mixtures produced abnormal lamellar bodies, leading to abnormal SC intercellular membrane bilayers.

Complete mixtures of ceramide, fatty acid, and cholesterol in a 1:1:1 ratio results in normal barrier recovery.[71] Studies in young mice (< 10 weeks) and humans (20–30 years of age) have demonstrated that applying a mixture of cholesterol, ceramides, and essential/nonessential free fatty acids (FFAs) in an equimolar ratio allows normal barrier recovery, but any 3:1:1:1 ratio of these four ingredients hastens barrier recovery.[72] Currently, the goal of the best barrier repair moisturizers is to supply these vital components in a 3:1:1:1 ratio. The other way to determine if a moisturizer mimics the skin's natural barrier is to look at the moisturizer under a cross-polarized microscope and see if optical anisotropy occurs in the shape of a Maltese cross pattern. Lipids that form a multilamellar pattern that mimics physiologic lipids demonstrate this Maltese cross pattern.

Pseudoceramides

Pseudoceramides are now commonly used in skincare products instead of ceramides because it is expensive and difficult to use naturally derived ceramides typically extracted from microorganisms. Pseudoceramides can replace natural ceramides to form the lipid bilayer in the SC.[73] The length of the chains can be customized to affect ceramide function, making pseudoceramides a popular skincare ingredient to treat dry skin and eczema. MLE-PC is an example of a pseudoceramide formulation shown to mimic natural ceramides.[74] Pseudoceramides can be combined with fatty acids and cholesterol in a 1:1:1 ratio to repair the skin barrier.

Myristoyl/Palmitoyl Oxostearamide/Arachamide Mea

This barrier repair ingredient is manufactured in South Korea and is known as MLE technology. It contains pseudoceramides, cholesterol, and fatty acids and mimics the skin's natural skin barrier. When viewed under a cross-polarized microscope, anisotropy is evident.[74] (See Chapter 12.) Optical anisotropy is a pattern of light that resembles a Maltese cross pattern and demonstrates an intact skin barrier (see Figure 1–7 in Chapter 1, Basic Science of the Epidermis, for the Maltese cross image). Myristoyl/palmitoyl oxostearamide/arachamide mea can be thought of as fatty acids, cholesterol, and ceramides in the proper ratio and 3D shape to strengthen the skin barrier.

Physiologic Lipid Emulsion

Another South Korean innovation includes pseudoceramides, fatty acids, as well as cholesterol and is known as PSL technology. This combination of lipids demonstrates anisotropy under the cross-polarized microscope as seen in **Fig. 43-1**. There are so many new barrier repair emulsions designed to mimic the skin barrier that the visualization of the Maltese cross pattern is considered a primary way to determine the more effective barrier repair moisturizers.

Fatty Acids

Fatty acids are chain compounds composed of carbon, oxygen, and hydrogen with a hydrocarbon on one end and a carboxyl group on the other. FFAs on the skin's surface are derived from sebum and extruded lamellar granule content from keratinocytes. FFAs on the skin's surface may also be by-products from skin microbes or components in cleansers or moisturizers.

Fatty acids have a hydrophilic head and hydrophobic tails. They can be saturated or unsaturated. Fatty acids make up one-third of the skin barrier along with ceramides and cholesterol. The shape of the fatty acid affects the integrity of the skin barrier. For example, the hydrophobic tails of stearic acid are closer together, so this fatty acid is one of the best to help the skin barrier prevent water evaporation (**Fig. 43-2**). Conversely, oleic acid has tails that do not pack together as well and can result in holes in the skin barrier (**Figs. 43-3, 43-4A** and **43-4B**). In fact, oleic acid has been shown to facilitate the penetration of skincare ingredients.[75,76] Fatty acids are found in oils. (**Table 43-2** lists the percentage of various fatty acids found in oils frequently used in moisturizers.) Fatty acids have different characteristics. Protein kinase C (PKC) is a critical signaling pathway for cells. PKC is activated by *cis*-unsaturated fatty acids like oleic, linoleic, linolenic, arachidonic, and docosahexaenoic acids. Saturated fatty acids do not have the same effect on PKC.

Fatty acids and inflammation

Fatty acids act as signal molecules and can activate or turn off immune cells. In the skin, fatty acids of different lengths play various regulatory roles. Polyunsaturated acids are precursors to molecules that affect inflammation such as eicosanoids.

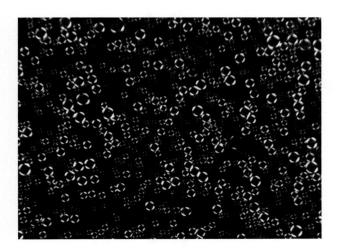

FIGURE 43-1. When a moisturizer mimics the natural multilamellar membranes of the skin's lipid bilayer, a Maltese cross pattern is visualized under the polarized microscope. (This image of PSL technology appears courtesy of Dr. Jong-Kyung Youm.)

Linoleic acid is a fatty acid that has anti-inflammatory capabilities in addition to providing structural support for the cell membrane. The linoleic acid derivatives eicosapentaenoic and docosahexaenoic acids reduce the capacity of immune cells to synthesize inflammatory factors.[5] Linoleic acid is found in a wide range of foods, which can be recommended to patients to reduce skin inflammation (**Table 43-1**). Numerous studies examine the effects of fatty acids on inflammatory pathways.

Fatty acids and pigmentation

FFAs have regulatory effects on melanogenesis. Unsaturated fatty acids decrease melanin synthesis and tyrosinase activity, while saturated fatty acids increase melanin synthesis and tyrosinase activity.[77,78] **Table 43-3** lists some popular fatty acids in skincare products and their effects on melanogenesis.

Extracellular Matrix Components

Collagen

Many expensive moisturizers contain collagen, and some manufacturers claim that the collagen in such formulations can replace the collagen lost during the aging process. This claim is unfounded, however, because most of the collagen "extracts" have a molecular weight of 15000 to 50000 daltons. Only substances with a molecular weight of 5000 daltons or less can penetrate the SC.[8] The popularity of these products may stem from their emollient properties: they leave a film on the skin that fills in surface irregularities and smooths skin temporarily. This is very similar to the way that hair conditioners work. Once the product dries, the protein films shrink slightly causing a subtle stretching out of fine skin wrinkles. Of course, this effect is *temporary* but can be enhanced with the addition of humectants to further *temporarily* plump out the tiny wrinkles. These products are usually labeled as firming creams as well as moisturizers, although they have little to no effect on TEWL.

Hyaluronic Acid

HA is a hygroscopic sugar that can bind over 1,000 times its weight in water. It is the most abundant glycosaminoglycan found in the human dermis. The recent popularity of HA fillers for injection into the dermis to correct wrinkles has led to a plethora of HA-containing moisturizers on the market. HA functions as a humectant on the skin's surface. The size of HA determines whether it can penetrate the epidermis and enter the dermis when applied topically.[79] Crosslinking HA affects the ability of HA to enter the dermis.[80] Smaller low molecular weight HA can more easily enter the dermis. HA has special properties that are not completely understood that render it a favorite adjunct to increase penetration of other ingredients.[81] Use of HA can amplify the side effects of benzoyl peroxide and retinoids by increasing penetration of these ingredients. HA can be used on top of peptide, growth factor, and ascorbic acid serums to augment penetration (see Chapter 35).

Heparan Sulfate

HS is a glycosaminoglycan component of the ECM that avidly binds water. It increases cellular response to growth factors

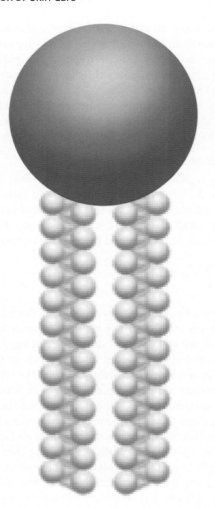

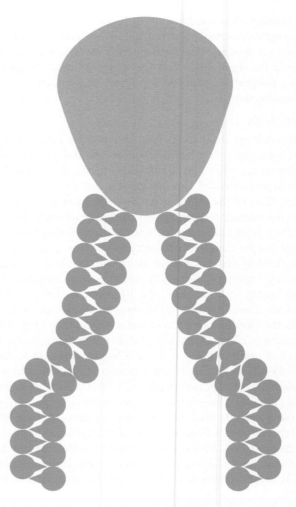

FIGURE 43-2. Stearic acid is a fatty acid that has straight hydrophobic tails that allow for close packing together of molecules and a strong skin barrier.

FIGURE 43-3. The hydrophobic tails of oleic acid are not straight and therefore cannot pack as tightly into the bilayer membranes.

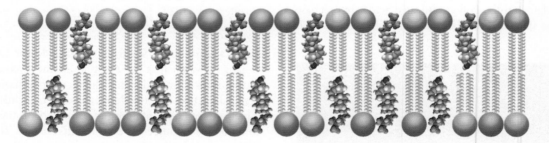

FIGURE 43-4A. When stearic acid is used as the fatty acid in bilayer membranes, the lipids are able to pack in tightly and strengthen the skin barrier (green is stearic acid, purple is cholesterol, and orange is ceramides).

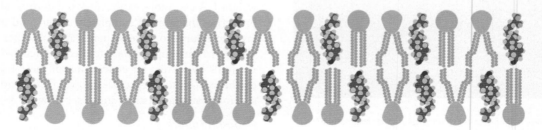

FIGURE 43-4B. When oleic acid is used as the fatty acid in bilayer membranes, there are spaces between oleic acid and the other lipids due to the tail shape of oleic acid. This impairs the skin barrier (pink is oleic acid, purple is cholesterol, and orange is ceramides).

TABLE 43-3	Fatty Acids in Skincare and Their Effects on Melanogenesis		
Fatty Acid	**Saturation State**	**Activity**	**Notes**
Linoleic	Unsaturated	Anti-inflammatory	Decreases melanogenesis
Linolenic	Unsaturated	Anti-inflammatory	Decreases melanogenesis
Oleic	Unsaturated	Increases skin penetration	Decreases melanogenesis
Palmitic	Saturated	Anti-inflammatory	Increases melanogenesis
Stearic	Saturated	Decreases skin penetration	Increases melanogenesis

and plays a significant role in intercellular communications. HS also binds and stores growth factors and protects them until they arrive at their target receptors. Once at the receptor, they present the growth factor or cytokine to the appropriate binding site.[82] HS chaperones the cell signals until they get to their destination. HS, in the form of a proprietary HS analogue, has been found to rejuvenate photodamaged skin by improving skin hydration, firmness, elasticity, and barrier function.[83]

Natural Ingredients

Oatmeal

Wild oats (*Avena sativa*) have been used for over 2000 years in traditional folk medicine, particularly as a poultice or soak. Whole oat flour is thought to be protective in nature and to exhibit antioxidant activity, inhibit prostaglandin synthesis, and display a cleansing capacity. Another oat compound, oat β-glucan, is believed to be immunomodulatory. Oat proteins exert various beneficial effects, including emulsifying activity, fat-binding activity, water-hydration capacity, low foaming potential, and antioxidant activity (courtesy of superoxide dismutase). It is thought that oat lipids influence viscosity and pasting properties and decrease TEWL. For decades, colloidal oat grain suspensions have been used as adjuncts in the treatment of atopic dermatitis.[84] Better benefits are generally seen with the use of oat fractions than whole oatmeal,[31] and colloidal oatmeal has replaced rolled oats and oatmeals in skincare products. Significantly, oatmeal has been shown to have moisturizing and anti-inflammatory properties. In a study on 12 healthy individuals, researchers assessing the anti-inflammatory activity of two topically applied oatmeal extracts (*Avena sativa* and *Avena rhealba*), using the sodium lauryl sulfate irritation model, found that both extracts displayed preventive effects on skin irritation.[85] Notably, oatmeal is one of the few botanically derived or natural products labeled by the FDA as an effective skin protectant.

Shea Butter

Used widely in cosmetic products as a moisturizer, particularly as an emollient, shea butter (*Butyrospermum parkii*)

is a natural fat derived from the shea or karite tree, which grows naturally across 19 African countries. A study in 2002 revealed that shea butter manifests anti-inflammatory activity.[86] Composed mainly of oleic and stearic acids, shea butter is also notable for containing a higher percentage of unsaponifiables than other vegetable oils.[87] Shea butter is included and touted in various skin and hair care products, especially high-end skincare products, for conferring rich emollient benefits, and is thought to maintain moisture and to provide benefits as an adjuvant moisturizer in the treatment of skin conditions such as atopic dermatitis, dry skin, acne, scars, and striae alba.

Other Ingredients

Several moisturizers contain antioxidants such as vitamins C and E, coffeeberry, green tea, and coenzyme Q_{10}. These are popular ingredients because antioxidants are thought to reduce the levels of free radicals attacking the skin and related organs, a process believed to contribute to cutaneous aging (see Chapter 39, Antioxidants). Niacinamide and soy are also popular additives in cosmetic moisturizers (see Chapter 41, Depigmenting Ingredients). Anti-aging ingredients are often added to moisturizers (see Chapter 37, Anti-Aging Ingredients).

Manufacturers are adding to moisturizers ingredients that affect calcium and potassium levels. However, water plays a more important role in exposing skin to calcium as discussed in Chapter 40, Cleansing Agents. Such formulations may play a role in maintaining skin barrier function as fluctuations in Ca^{2+} and potassium levels have been shown to influence skin barrier function.[88]

PREBIOTICS IN MOISTURIZERS

Prebiotics provide nutrients for some bacteria. Probiotics are live organisms that provide a health benefit. Both prebiotics and probiotics may have a role in skin products to support maintenance of the normal skin microbiome.[89] However, it remains unknown which bacteria are most beneficial to preserve skin health. Many studies suggest that the key is diversity. Using pre- and probiotics incorrectly could decrease diversity and end up being detrimental. Currently, it is too early to make suggestions about which pre- and probiotics to use in skincare products (see Chapter 4, Skin Microbiome).

WATER IN MOISTURIZERS

The type of water that is used in a moisturizer can greatly affect the properties of the moisturizer. Water can contain various minerals that act on the skin or affect cleansers used on the skin (see Table 40–1 in Chapter 40 for a table on different types of water). Thermal water is a type of water used in some moisturizers. It contains various minerals such as Ca^{2+}, bicarbonate (HCO^-_3), silicates, iron compounds, sodium and magnesium salts, selenium, sulfur compounds, strontium, and metals.[89] Selenium has antioxidant and anti-inflammatory properties and provides protection against toxic heavy metals.

MOISTURIZER EFFECT ON SKINCARE ROUTINE

Where the moisturizer is placed in the skincare regimen significantly influences the efficacy of the regimen because moisturizers affect penetration. If a moisturizer with numerous occlusive ingredients is placed over a treatment skincare product, the occlusion can enhance absorption of that treatment product. If the moisturizer is placed before the treatment product, then less of the treatment product will be absorbed (Chapter 35). This fact can be used to help patients begin a retinoid. Applying a retinoid over the moisturizer will reduce side effects of retinoids. Once the patient acclimates, the moisturizer can be placed on top of the retinoid to increase penetration (see Chapter 45, Retinoids).

Dry skin types should be treated with a barrier repair moisturizer while oily skin types can be treated with a humectant moisturizer. Occlusive ingredients should be used either as a skin protectant to prevent what follows from getting into the skin or as a penetration enhancer when placed on top of a skincare product. HA moisturizers have no barrier repair abilities but can be used to increase penetration of other skincare products. **Table 43-4** lists ingredients in moisturizers that increase penetration of other skincare products.

SIDE EFFECTS OF MOISTURIZERS

Moisturizers are generally very safe, with few reports of side effects. Allergic contact dermatitis can result from the use of preservatives, perfumes, solubilizers, sunscreens, and other skincare product constituents. Ingredients that may lead to contact dermatitis include fragrances, preservatives, propylene glycol,[90] vitamin E,[91] and Kathon CG (see Chapter 19, Contact Dermatitis to Cosmetic Ingredients, for more information).

CONCLUSION

While the ultimate purpose of all moisturizers is to enhance the hydration state of the SC, moisturizing ingredients operate in distinctly specific ways. Occlusives coat the SC and reduce TEWL; humectants attract water from the atmosphere and hold it on the skin's surface; and emollients soften and smooth the skin. In order to recommend the best moisturizers for patients' skin, the medical provider should understand that occlusives, humectants, and emollients treat the symptoms of dry skin, while barrier repair ingredients treat the causes of dry skin.

References

1. Blank IH. Factors which influence the water content of the stratum corneum. *J Invest Dermatol*. 1952;18(6):433–440.
2. Buraczewska I, Berne B, Lindberg M, Lodén M, Törmä H. Moisturizers change the mRNA expression of enzymes synthesizing skin barrier lipids. *Arch Dermatol Res*. 2009;301(8):587–594.
3. Ye L, Mauro TM, Dang E, et al. Topical applications of an emollient reduce circulating pro-inflammatory cytokine levels in chronically aged humans: a pilot clinical study. *J Eur Acad Dermatol Venereol*. 2019;33(11):2197–2201.
4. Lowe AJ, Leung DYM, Tang MLK, Su JC, Allen KJ. The skin as a target for prevention of the atopic march. *Ann Allergy Asthma Immunol*. 2018;120(2):145–151.
5. Yang M, Zhou M, Song L. A review of fatty acids influencing skin condition. *J Cosmet Dermatol*. 2020;19(12):3199–3204.
6. Spruit D. The interference of some substances with the water vapour loss of human skin. *Dermatologica*. 1971;142(2):89–92.
7. Draelos Z. Moisturizers. In: Draelos Z, ed. *Atlas of Cosmetic Dermatology*. New York, NY: Churchill Livingstone; 2000:83.
8. Wehr RF, Krochmal L. Considerations in selecting a moisturizer. *Cutis*. 1987;39(6):512–515.
9. Kligman AM. Regression method for assessing the efficacy of moisturizers. *Cosmet Toilet*. 1978;93:27–35.
10. Morrison D. Petrolatum. In: Loden M, Maibach H, eds. *Dry Skin and Moisturizers*. Boca Raton, FL: CRC Press; 2000: 251.
11. American Academy of Dermatology Invitational Symposium on Comedogenicity. *J Am Acad Dermatol*. 1989;20(2 Pt 1):272–277.
12. Schnuch A, Lessmann H, Geier J, Uter W. White petrolatum (Ph. Eur.) is virtually non-sensitizing. Analysis of IVDK data on 80 000 patients tested between 1992 and 2004 and short discussion of identification and designation of allergens. *Contact Dermatitis*. 2006;54(6):338–343.
13. Tam CC, Elston DM. Allergic contact dermatitis caused by white petrolatum on damaged skin. *Dermatitis*. 2006;17(4): 201–203.
14. Ulrich G, Schmutz JL, Trechot P, Commun N, Barbaud A. Sensitization to petrolatum: an unusual cause of false-positive drug patch-tests. *Allergy*. 2004;59(9):1006–1009.
15. Harris I, Hoppe U. Lanolins. In: Loden M, Maibach H, eds. *Dry Skin and Moisturizers*. Boca Raton, FL: CRC Press; 2000: 259.
16. Proserpio G. Lanolides: emollients or moisturizers? *Cosmet Toilet*. 1978; 93:45–48.
17. Kligman AM. The myth of lanolin allergy. *Contact Dermatitis*. 1998;39(3):103–107.
18. Boonchai W, Iamtharachai P, Sunthonpalin P. Occupational allergic contact dermatitis from essential oils in aromatherapists. *Contact Dermatitis*. 2007;56(3):181–182.
19. Bleasel N, Tate B, Rademaker M. Allergic contact dermatitis following exposure to essential oils. *Australas J Dermatol*. 2002;43(3):211–213.
20. DiNardo JC. Is mineral oil comedogenic? *J Cosmet Dermatol*. 2005;4(1):2–3.
21. Blanken R, van Vilsteren MJ, Tupker RA, Coenraads PJ. Effect of mineral oil and linoleic-acid-containing emulsions on the skin

TABLE 43-4	Ingredients That Penetrate Other Skincare Products
Glycerin	
Glycerol	
Hyaluronic acid	
Isopropyl myristate	
Oleic acid	
Propylene glycol	

vapour loss of sodium-lauryl-sulphate-induced irritant skin reactions. *Contact Dermatitis.* 1989;20(2):93–97.

22. Agero AL, Verallo-Rowell VM. A randomized double-blind controlled trial comparing extra virgin coconut oil with mineral oil as a moisturizer for mild to moderate xerosis. *Dermatitis.* 2004;15(3):109–116.

23. Tolbert PE. Oils and cancer. *Cancer Causes Control.* 1997; 8(3):386–405.

24. Rawlings AV, Lombard KJ. A review on the extensive skin benefits of mineral oil. *Int J Cosmet Sci.* 2012;34(6):511–518.

25. Boucetta KQ, Charrouf Z, Aguenaou H, Derouiche A, Bensouda Y. Does Argan oil have a moisturizing effect on the skin of postmenopausal women? *Skin Res Technol.* 2013;19(3):356–357.

26. Darmstadt GL, Mao-Qiang M, Chi E, et al. Impact of topical oils on the skin barrier: possible implications for neonatal health in developing countries. *Acta Paediatr.* 2002;91(5):546–554.

27. Darmstadt GL, Saha SK, Ahmed AS, et al. Effect of topical treatment with skin barrier-enhancing emollients on nosocomial infections in preterm infants in Bangladesh: a randomised controlled trial. *Lancet.* 2005;365(9464):1039–1045.

28. Berbis P, Hesse S, Privat Y. Essential fatty acids and the skin. *Allerg Immunol (Paris).* 1990;22(6):225–231.

29. Williams HC. Evening primrose oil for atopic dermatitis. *BMJ.* 2003;327(7428):1358–1359.

30. Koca U, Süntar I, Akkol EK, Yilmazer D, Alper M. Wound repair potential of Olea europaea L. leaf extracts revealed by in vivo experimental models and comparative evaluation of the extracts' antioxidant activity. *J Med Food.* 2011;14(1-2): 140–146.

31. Aburjai T, Natsheh FM. Plants used in cosmetics. *Phytother Res.* 2003;17(9):987–1000.

32. de la Puerta R, Martínez Domínguez ME, Ruíz-Gutiérrez V, Flavill JA, Hoult JR. Effects of virgin olive oil phenolics on scavenging of reactive nitrogen species and upon nitrergic neurotransmission. *Life Sci.* 2001;69(10):1213–1222.

33. Kränke B, Komericki P, Aberer W. Olive oil—contact sensitizer or irritant? *Contact Dermatitis.* 1997;36(1):5–10.

34. Danby SG, AlEnezi T, Sultan A, et al. Effect of olive and sunflower seed oil on the adult skin barrier: implications for neonatal skin care. *Pediatr Dermatol.* 2013;30(1):42–50.

35. Weisberg EM, Baumann LS. The foundation for the use of olive oil in skin care and botanical cosmeceuticals. In: *Olives and Olive Oil in Health and Disease Prevention.* Cambridge, MA: Academic Press; 2021: 425–434.

36. Idson B. Dry skin: moisturizing and emolliency. *Cosmet Toilet.* 1992;107(7):69–78.

37. Mitsui T. Humectants. Mitsui T, ed. *New Cosmetic Science.* New York, NY: Elsevier; 1997: 134.

38. Chernosky ME. Clinical aspects of dry skin. *J Soc Cosmet Chem.* 1976;27:365–376.

39. Choi EH, Man MQ, Wang F, et al. Is endogenous glycerol a determinant of stratum corneum hydration in humans? *J Invest Dermatol.* 2005;125(2):288–293.

40. Orth D, Appa Y. Glycerine. a natural ingredient for moisturizing skin. In: Loden M, Maibach H, eds. *Dry Skin and Moisturizers.* Boca Raton, FL: CRC Press; 2000: 217.

41. Orth D, Appa Y, Contard E, et al. Effect of High Glycerin Therapeutic Moisturizers on the Ultrastructure of the Stratum Corneum. Poster presentation at the 53rd Annual Meeting of the American Academy of Dermatology. New Orleans, LA. February, 1995:3–8.

42. Fluhr JW, Mao-Qiang M, Brown BE, et al. Glycerol regulates stratum corneum hydration in sebaceous gland deficient (asebia) mice. *J Invest Dermatol.* 2003;120(5):728–737.

43. Hara M, Ma T, Verkman AS. Selectively reduced glycerol in skin of aquaporin-3-deficient mice may account for impaired skin hydration, elasticity, and barrier recovery. *J Biol Chem.* 2002;277(48):46616–46621.

44. Hara M, Verkman AS. Glycerol replacement corrects defective skin hydration, elasticity, and barrier function in aquaporin-3-deficient mice. *Proc Natl Acad Sci U S A.* 2003;100(12): 7360–7365.

45. Draelos ZD. Active agents in common skin care products. *Plast Reconstr Surg.* 2010;125(2):719–724.

46. Harding C, Bartolone J, Rawlings A. Effects of natural moisturizing factor and lactic acid isomers on skin function. In: Loden M, Maibach H, eds. *Dry Skin and Moisturizers.* Boca Raton, FL: CRC Press; 2000: 236.

47. Kligman AM. Dermatologic uses of urea. *Acta Derm Venereol.* 1957;37(2):155–159.

48. Wohlrab W. The influence of urea on the penetration kinetics of topically applied corticosteroids. *Acta Derm Venereol.* 1984;64(3):233–238.

49. Wohlrab W. Effect of urea on the penetration kinetics of vitamin A acid into human skin. *Z Hautkr.* 1990;65(9):803–805.

50. Serup J. A double-blind comparison of two creams containing urea as the active ingredient. Assessment of efficacy and side-effects by non-invasive techniques and a clinical scoring scheme. *Acta Derm Venereol Suppl (Stockh).* 1992;177:34–43.

51. Celleno L. Topical urea in skincare: A review. *Dermatol Ther.* 2018;31(6):e12690.

52. Lawrence N, Brody HJ, Alt TH. Chemical peeling. In: Coleman W, Hanke W, eds. *Cosmetic Surgery of the Skin.* 2nd ed. St. Louis, MO: CV Mosby; 1997: 85–111.

53. Van Scott EJ, Yu RJ. Control of keratinization with alpha-hydroxy acids and related compounds. I. Topical treatment of ichthyotic disorders. *Arch Dermatol.* 1974;110(4): 586–590.

54. Draelos ZD. Rediscovering the cutaneous benefits of salicylic acid. *Cosm Derm.* 1997;10(Suppl 4):4.

55. Van Scott EJ, Yu R. Hyperkeratinization, corneocyte cohesion, and alpha hydroxy acids. *J Am Acad Dermatol.* 1984;11(5 Pt 1): 867–879.

56. Berardesca E, Distante F, Vignoli GP, Oresajo C, Green B. Alpha hydroxyacids modulate stratum corneum barrier function. *Br J Dermatol.* 1997;137(6):934–938.

57. Takahashi M, Machida Y, Tsuda Y. The influence of hydroxy acids on the rheological properties of the stratum corneum. *J Soc Cosmet Chem.* 1985;36(2):177–187.

58. Draelos ZD. Therapeutic moisturizers. *Dermatol Clin.* 2000;18(4):597–607.

59. Perricone NV, DiNardo JC. Photoprotective and antiinflammatory effects of topical glycolic acid. *Dermatol Surg.* 1996;22(5): 435–437.

60. Kaidbey K, Sutherland B, Bennett P, et al. Topical glycolic acid enhances photodamage by ultraviolet light. *Photodermatol Photoimmunol Photomed.* 2003;19(1):21–27.

61. Tsai TF, Bowman PH, Jee SH, Maibach HI. Effects of glycolic acid on light-induced skin pigmentation in Asian and Caucasian subjects. *J Am Acad Dermatol.* 2000;43(2 Pt 1):238–243.

62. Stiller MJ, Bartolone J, Stern R, et al. Topical 8% glycolic acid and 8% L-lactic acid creams for the treatment of photodamaged skin. A double-blind vehicle-controlled clinical trial. *Arch Dermatol.* 1996;132(6):631–636.

63. Stern EC. Topical application of lactic acid in the treatment and prevention of certain disorders of the skin. *Urol Cutaneous Rev.* 1943;50:106.

64. Rawlings AV, Davies A, Carlomusto M, et al. Effect of lactic acid isomers on keratinocyte ceramide synthesis, stratum corneum lipid levels and stratum corneum barrier function. *Arch Dermatol Res.* 1996;288(7):383–390.

65. Yamamoto A, Serizawa S, Ito M, Sato Y. Stratum corneum lipid abnormalities in atopic dermatitis. *Arch Dermatol Res.* 1991;283(4):219–223.

66. Wertz PW, Miethke MC, Long SA, Strauss JS, Downing DT. The composition of the ceramides from human stratum corneum and from comedones. *J Invest Dermatol.* 1985;84(5):410–412.

67. Thueson DO, Chan EK, Oechsli LM, Hahn GS. The roles of pH and concentration in lactic acid-induced stimulation of epidermal turnover. *Dermatol Surg.* 1998;24(6):641–645.

68. Algiert-Zielińska B, Mucha P, Rotsztejn H. Lactic and lactobionic acids as typically moisturizing compounds. *Int J Dermatol.* 2019;58(3):374–379.

69. Hannuksela M. Glycols. In: Loden M, Maibach H, eds. *Dry Skin and Moisturizers.* Boca Raton, FL: CRC Press; 2000: 413–415.

70. Draelos Z. Moisturizers. In: Draelos Z, ed. *Atlas of Cosmetic Dermatology.* New York, NY: Churchill Livingstone; 2000:85.

71. Man MQ, Feingold KR, Elias PM. Exogenous lipids influence permeability barrier recovery in acetone-treated murine skin. *Arch Dermatol.* 1993;129(6):728–738.

72. Zettersten EM, Ghadially R, Feingold KR, Crumrine D, Elias PM. Optimal ratios of topical stratum corneum lipids improve barrier recovery in chronologically aged skin. *J Am Acad Dermatol.* 1997;37(3 Pt 1):403–408.

73. Ishida K, Takahashi A, Bito K, Draelos Z, Imokawa G. Treatment with Synthetic Pseudoceramide Improves Atopic Skin, Switching the Ceramide Profile to a Healthy Skin Phenotype. *J Invest Dermatol.* 2020;140(9):1762–1770.e8.

74. Park BD, Youm JK, Jeong SK, Choi EH, Ahn SK, Lee SH. The characterization of molecular organization of multilamellar emulsions containing pseudoceramide and type III synthetic ceramide. *J Invest Dermatol.* 2003;121(4):794–801.

75. Naik A, Pechtold LA, Potts RO, Guy RH. Mechanism of oleic acid-induced skin penetration enhancement in vivo in humans. *J Control Release.* 1995;37(3):299–306.

76. Jiang SJ, Zhou XJ. Examination of the mechanism of oleic acid-induced percutaneous penetration enhancement: an ultrastructural study. *Biol Pharm Bull.* 2003;26(1):66–68.

77. Ando H, Watabe H, Valencia JC, et al. Fatty acids regulate pigmentation via proteasomal degradation of tyrosinase: a new aspect of ubiquitin-proteasome function. *J Biol Chem.* 2004;279(15):15427–15433.

78. Ando H, Ryu A, Hashimoto A, Oka M, Ichihashi M. Linoleic acid and alpha-linolenic acid lightens ultraviolet-induced hyperpigmentation of the skin. *Arch Dermatol Res.* 1998;290(7):375–381.

79. Rieger MM. Hyaluronic acid in cosmetics. A review of its chemistry and biochemistry. *Cosmet Toilet.* 1998;113(3):35–42.

80. Berkó S, Maroda M, Bodnár M, et al. Advantages of cross-linked versus linear hyaluronic acid for semisolid skin delivery systems. *Eur Polymer J.* 2013;49(9):2511–2517.

81. Brown MB, Jones SA. Hyaluronic acid: a unique topical vehicle for the localized delivery of drugs to the skin. *J Eur Acad Dermatol Venereol.* 2005;19(3):308–318.

82. Simon Davis DA, Parish CR. Heparan sulfate: a ubiquitous glycosaminoglycan with multiple roles in immunity. *Front Immunol.* 2013;4:470.

83. Gallo RL, Bucay VW, Shamban AT, et al. The potential role of topically applied heparan sulfate in the treatment of photodamage. *J Drugs Dermatol.* 2015;14(7):669–674.

84. Pigatto P, Bigardi A, Caputo R, et al. An evaluation of the allergic contact dermatitis potential of colloidal grain suspensions. *Am J Contact Dermat.* 1997;8(4):207–209.

85. Vié K, Cours-Darne S, Vienne MP, Boyer F, Fabre B, Dupuy P. Modulating effects of oatmeal extracts in the sodium lauryl sulfate skin irritancy model. *Skin Pharmacol Appl Skin Physiol.* 2002;15(2):120–124.

86. Thioune O, Ahodikpe D, Dieng M, Diop AB, Ngom S, Lo I. Inflammatory ointment from shea butter and hydro-alcoholic extract of Khaya senegalensis barks (Cailcederat). *Dakar Med.* 2002;45(2):113–116.

87. Lodén M, Andersson AC. Effect of topically applied lipids on surfactant-irritated skin. *Br J Dermatol.* 1996;134(2):215–220.

88. Denda M, Tsutsumi M, Inoue K, Crumrine D, Feingold KR, Elias PM. Potassium channel openers accelerate epidermal barrier recovery. *Br J Dermatol.* 2007;157(5):888–893.

89. Baldwin HE, Bhatia ND, Friedman A, Eng RM, Seite S. The Role of Cutaneous Microbiota Harmony in Maintaining a Functional Skin Barrier. *J Drugs Dermatol.* 2017;16(1):12–18.

90. Gonzalo MA, de Argila D, García JM, Alvarado MI. Allergic contact dermatitis to propylene glycol. *Allergy.* 1999 Jan;54(1):82–83.

91. Baumann LS, Spencer J. The effects of topical vitamin E on the cosmetic appearance of scars. *Dermatol Surg.* 1999;25(4):311–315.

CHAPTER 44

Preservatives

Edmund M. Weisberg, MS, MBE
Leslie S. Baumann, MD

SUMMARY POINTS

What's Important?

1. Parabens are more likely to cause contact dermatitis on skin with a compromised barrier such as tape-stripped skin.
2. Preservatives in paraben-free products currently on the market are more likely to cause an allergic rection than parabens.
3. Only intact skin should come in touch with products containing parabens to prevent irritant reactions.

What's New?

1. Experts have concluded that current scientific knowledge is insufficient to demonstrate a clear cancer risk due to the topical application of cosmetics that contain parabens on *normal intact skin*.

What's Coming?

1. New preservatives will be developed that have no estrogenic activity and decreased allergic potential.
2. Organic skincare product choices without preservatives are becoming more efficacious.

Preservatives are integral ingredients in various food, pharmaceutical, cosmetic, and skincare formulations. As water is included in most such products, preservatives are added to prevent the growth of microorganisms and the resultant rapid deterioration or decomposition of the formulation. Indeed, without preservatives, which are biocidal chemicals, these items important to daily life would exhibit little to no shelf life and become quickly invaded and permeated by numerous bacteria, fungi, and molds. As such, preservatives are intended to maintain the integrity of the product and protect the user from infection.[1] While antimicrobial preservatives are essential components in the majority of cosmetics and skincare products, these ingredients have been cited frequently as causes of allergic contact dermatitis.[1-3] Such occurrences are most often associated with topical application on damaged or broken skin. Of greater concern in recent years has been the reports linking the use of some skincare products with cancer incidence. This chapter will focus on the most frequently used class of preservatives, recent data regarding the estrogenic potential of these compounds, and the controversy regarding possible associations between the chronic use of chemical preservatives that make contact with the skin and cancer.

PARABENS

Parabens, alkyl esters of *p*-hydroxybenzoic acid (PHBA), were commonly found in skin, hair, and body care products until the last 15 years when consumers became afraid of them. Parabens are found naturally in raspberries, blackberries, carrots, and cucumbers and are common ingredients in food and pharmaceuticals. Parabens were the most widely used preservatives in cosmetics and included in the vast majority of skincare formulations.[4,5] In fact, in the early to mid-1980s, it was estimated that at least 90% of personal care products, including deodorants, toothpastes, shampoos, body creams, shower gels, moisturizers, etc., contained one or more parabens as a preservative.[6] For decades, parabens had a strong record of efficacy, safety, and stability and were well tolerated except for occasional allergic reactions.[7] Now paraben-free products prevail.

Allergic Reactions to Parabens

For years parabens had been thought to cause allergic reactions in susceptible individuals. The penetration ability of parabens is influenced by the inclusion in cosmetic preparations of penetration enhancers, which facilitate the rapid absorption of parabens through intact skin.[8,9] It is now known that parabens do not absorb well into the skin without high-tech penetration enhancers and are not likely to cause allergy unless the skin barrier is compromised. In fact, the incidence of contact dermatitis to parabens is the lowest of all the preservatives. In 2019, the American Contact Dermatitis Society declared parabens the "(non)-allergen of the year" because of a low incidence of reactions in patch tests.[10] Products containing parabens should be avoided by people who know they are allergic to parabens, which can be determined by patch testing.

Safety of Parabens

The fear of parabens is based on findings that *in vitro* some parabens have been shown to display weak estrogenic effects. This has led to concern about parabens contributing to breast cancer in women or reproductive system effects in men such as reduced sperm counts. The Cosmetic Ingredient Review (CIR) panel evaluated all of the paraben safety data in 2018 and determined that parabens were safe.[11] The CIR amended the report in March 2019 to make the following points:

1. Parabens can accumulate in human tissue, but do not remain there for long.[12]
2. The available evidence does not show a significant association between parabens and any systemic disease.
3. The major exposure humans have to parabens is in cosmetic products.

There are several reasons experts have concluded that parabens are safe. Parabens have minimal penetration through intact skin.[13] If they do penetrate into skin, they are rapidly metabolized to *p*-hydroxybenzoic acid and quickly excreted in the urine.[14] Although *in vitro* some parabens have been shown to have estrogenic effects, these are extremely weak.[14] The four most commonly used parabens in cosmetic products are 10,000-fold or *less potent* than 17ß-estradiol. Another reason cited to exonerate parabens is that geographic differences in paraben exposures internationally do not correlate with the frequency or incidence of breast cancer in developed nations. Experts have concluded that current scientific knowledge is insufficient to demonstrate a clear cancer risk due to the topical application of cosmetics that contain parabens on *normal intact skin*.

Types of Parabens

The family of parabens includes methyl paraben, ethyl paraben, butyl paraben, isobutyl paraben, propyl paraben, isopropyl paraben, and benzyl paraben.[15] Methyl, ethyl, propyl, and butyl paraben are the most frequently used parabens in cosmetic formulations (**Table 44-1**).[12] Notably, these chemicals

TABLE 44-1	The Most Commonly Used Parabens and Their Chemical Structures and Molecular Formulas	
Paraben	Chemical Structure	Molecular Formula
Methyl paraben	CH_3	$C_8H_8O_3$
Ethyl paraben	CH_2CH_3	$C_9H_{10}O_3$
Propyl paraben	$(CH_2)_2CH_3$	$C_{10}H_{12}O_3$
Butyl paraben	$(CH_2)_3CH_3$	$C_{11}H_{14}O_3$

can be absorbed through the skin and migrate into the bloodstream and bodily tissues.

Methyl Paraben

Methyl paraben is the most common of the various forms of parabens. The methyl ester of *p*-hydroxybenzoic acid is found in many skincare products. It is readily absorbed through the skin and GI tract. It is quickly hydrolyzed and excreted in the urine and does not accumulate in the body. Studies have shown that methyl paraben is nontoxic, non-irritating, and non-sensitizing. It is not teratogenic, embryotoxic, nor carcinogenic. Methyl paraben, because of its shorter side chain groups and greater lipophilicity, has been demonstrated to be more readily absorbed by the skin than other paraben chemicals.[12,16] It is also on the low order of ingredients provoking acute and chronic toxicity.[3] Studies have concluded that methyl paraben is safe.[17,18]

Propyl Paraben

Propyl paraben is the ester form of *p*-hydroxybenzoic acid that has been esterified with *n*-propanol. It is the most commonly used antimicrobial preservative in foods, cosmetics, and drugs. Propyl paraben is readily absorbed through the skin and GI tract. It is rapidly hydrolyzed and excreted in the urine and does not accumulate in the body. Studies have shown that this commonly used paraben is safe.[19]

GENERAL STUDIES ON PRESERVATIVES

El Hussein et al. set out to ascertain the permeation of methyl, ethyl, propyl, and butyl parabens through the epidermal and dermal layers as well as accumulation in the skin layers and/or passage to other bodily tissues. They found that the capacity of the various parabens to penetrate the skin was based on their relative lipophilicity—with the more lipophilic, the less they were likely to penetrate or cross skin layers.[12] Butyl paraben is the most lipophilic of the four, followed by propyl, ethyl, and methyl parabens. Butyl paraben displayed comparatively weak passage through the skin, and has been shown elsewhere to have the potential for accumulating in the skin, particularly after multiple or frequent applications.[20]

Nicotinamide, the biologically active amide of vitamin B_3, is a hydrophilic molecule used as an active ingredient in cosmetic formulations for its moisturizing and depigmenting activity (see Chapter 41, Depigmenting Ingredients).[21] In 2008, nicotinamide, also known as niacinamide, was shown to have the capacity to influence the transdermal permeation of methyl, ethyl, propyl, and butyl parabens. Specifically, nicotinamide was found to promote the dissolution of parabens in solutions and gels as well as lower paraben partitioning in the oily phase thus ensuring an effective water-phase concentration in emulsion. Investigators concluded that nicotinamide interacts with parabens by ultimately decreasing transdermal penetration, thereby diminishing the risk or potential for toxicity.[22]

Hyaluronic and oleic acids have been demonstrated to increase penetration of skincare ingredients.[23,24] Liposomes and other vehicles are also used. The presence of these ingredients in the skincare regimen should be considered when deciding whether to avoid parabens.

Lee et al. set out to evaluate the side effects of cosmetic preservatives alone or in combination as product ingredients and to assess objective and subjective sensory skin irritation (representing symptoms such as burning, stinging, and itching absent visual inflammation). The researchers found no significant differences among methyl paraben, ethyl paraben, propyl paraben, butyl paraben, phenoxyethanol, and chlorphenesin in objective skin irritation potential at the minimal inhibitory concentration. However, chlorphenesin was found to exhibit greater potential in subjective irritation. They also found that formulation type influenced sensory irritation and that the combination of phenoxyethanol and chlorphenesin significantly increased irritation.[25]

It is worth recalling that in a 2004 review of the major classes of preservatives as well as agents such as Euxyl K 400 and isopropynyl butylcarbamate, Sasseville concluded that the parabens, which had been used for three-quarters of a century at that time, were still the most frequently used preservatives while inducing sensitivity less often than newer biocides.[1]

There are several preservatives used in paraben-free products. The most gentle is phenoxyethanol; however, it does not kill yeast and fungus, which is problematic in a hot, humid environment. Many preservatives release formaldehyde, which has its own safety issues in addition to being a strong allergen in numerous people (see Chapter 19, Contact Dermatitis to Cosmetic Ingredients, and **Table 44-2**). In some cases, such as organic products, preservatives are not used. This dramatically lowers the shelf life of these skincare products.

WHAT IS THE DAILY AVERAGE EXPOSURE TO PARABENS?

It is estimated that parabens are found in 10% of personal care products.[10] In most cases, these products contain 1% or less of parabens. If the average patient uses 50 g of personal care products a day, then the average daily exposure to parabens topically is 0.05 g. Parabens are also found in food and drugs, so the total paraben exposure per day is assumed to be about 1 mg/day.[19] When food, personal care product, and drug exposure rates are added, the average person is exposed to 1.29 mg/kg/day or 77.5 mg/day for a 60 kg individual. Clearly, personal care products account for a fraction of exposure as most paraben exposure comes from food.

TABLE 44-2	Paraben Alternatives	
Preservative	Allergenicity	Downside
2-bromo-2-nitropropane-1,3-diol	Formaldehyde releasing	
Benzyl alcohol		Incompatible with non-ionic surfactants
Diazolidinyl urea	Formaldehyde releasing	
DMDM hydantoin	Formaldehyde releasing	
Hydroxymethylglycinate	Formaldehyde releasing	
Imidazolidinyl urea	Formaldehyde releasing	
Phenoxyethanol		Weak against yeast and mold
Quaternium-15	Formaldehyde releasing	
Sodium benzoate		Weak against bacteria; forms benzene when combined with ascorbic acid
Trishydroxymethylnitromethane	Formaldehyde releasing	

CONCLUSION

Parabens have not been linked to carcinogenicity, cytotoxicity, or mutagenicity.[10,16] Some estrogenic effects or activity that mimic estrogen have been associated with parabens *in vitro*, but this activity has been noted as very weak and there are no established reports of human cases in which parabens have elicited an estrogen-mediated adverse event. Concerns about a possible link between parabens and breast cancer have diminished. Present knowledge provides no established link between the topical application of paraben-containing skincare formulations on healthy skin and cancer risk.[16] **There are no data to support discouraging patients from using paraben-containing products, which are often safer than other preservative alternatives.** Only intact skin should come in touch with products containing parabens to prevent irritant reactions.

References

1. Sasseville D. Hypersensitivity to preservatives. *Dermatol Ther.* 2004;17(3):251–263.
2. Wilkinson JD, Shaw S, Andersen KE, et al. Monitoring levels of preservative sensitivity in Europe: a 10-year overview (1991–2000). *Contact Dermatitis.* 2002;46(4):207–210.
3. Ishiwatari S, Suzuki T, Hitomi T, Yoshino T, Matsukuma S, Tsuji T. Effects of methyl paraben on skin keratinocytes. *J Appl Toxicol.* 2007;27(1):1–9.
4. Cashman AL, Warshaw EM. Parabens: a review of epidemiology, structure, allergenicity, and hormonal properties. *Dermatitis.* 2005;16(2):57–66.

5. Rastogi SC, Schouten A, De Kruijf N, Weijland JW. Contents of methyl-, ethyl-, propyl-, butyl- and benzylparaben in cosmetic products. *Contact Dermatitis*. 1995;32(1):28–30.

6. Elder RL. Final report on the safety assessment of methylparaben, ethylparaben, propylparaben and butylparaben. *J Am Coll Toxicol*. 1984;3(5):147–209.

7. Gilman AG, Goodman LS, Gilman A, eds. *Goodman and Gilman's The Pharmacological Basis of Therapeutics*, 6th ed. New York, NY: Macmillan; 1980: 969.

8. Pozzo AD, Pastori N. Percutaneous absorption of parabens from cosmetic formulations. *Int J Cosm Sci*. 1996;18(2):57–66.

9. Kitagawa S, Li H, Sato S. Skin permeation of parabens in excised guinea pig dorsal skin, its modification by penetration enhancers and their relationship with n-octanol/water partition coefficients. *Chem Pharm Bull (Tokyo)*. 1997;45(8):1354–1357.

10. Fransway AF, Fransway PJ, Belsito DV, et al. Parabens. *Dermatitis*. 2019;30(1):3–31.

11. Heldreth B. CIR Conclusion: Parabens Are Safe. *Cosmet Toilet*. November 16, 2018. https://www.cosmeticsandtoiletries.com/regulatory/region/northamerica/CIR-Conclusion-Parabens-Are-Safe-500174801.html. Accessed April 26, 2021.

12. El Hussein S, Muret P, Berard M, Makki S, Humbert P. Assessment of principal parabens used in cosmetics after their passage through human epidermis-dermis layers (ex-vivo study). *Exp Dermatol*. 2007;16(10):830–836.

13. Loretz LJ, Api AM, Barraj LM, et al. Exposure data for cosmetic products: lipstick, body lotion, and face cream. *Food Chem Toxicol*. 2005;43(2):279–291.

14. Fransway AF, Fransway PJ, Belsito DV, Yiannias JA. Paraben Toxicology. *Dermatitis*. 2019;30(1):32–45.

15. Golden R, Gandy J, Vollmer G. A review of the endocrine activity of parabens and implications for potential risks to human health. *Crit Rev Toxicol*. 2005;35(5):435–458.

16. Soni MG, Carabin IG, Burdock GA. Safety assessment of esters of p-hydroxybenzoic acid (parabens). *Food Chem Toxicol*. 2005; 43(7):985–1015.

17. Soni MG, Taylor SL, Greenberg NA, Burdock GA. Evaluation of the health aspects of methyl paraben: a review of the published literature. *Food Chem Toxicol*. 2002;40(10):1335–1373.

18. European Commission Directorate-General for Health and Consumers. Scientific Committee on Consumer Safety Opinion on Parabens. Revised March 22, 2011. https://ec.europa.eu/health/scientific_committees/consumer_safety/docs/sccs_o_041.pdf. Accessed April 26, 2021.

19. Soni MG, Burdock GA, Taylor SL, Greenberg NA. Safety assessment of propyl paraben: a review of the published literature. *Food Chem Toxicol*. 2001;39(6):513–532.

20. Darbre P. Underarm cosmetics and breast cancer. *Eur J Cancer Prev*. 2004;13:153.

21. Baumann LS. Niacinamide. In: *Cosmeceuticals and Cosmetic Ingredients*. New York: McGraw-Hill; 2014: 126–128.

22. Nicoli S, Zani F, Bilzi S, Bettini R, Santi P. Association of nicotinamide with parabens: effect on solubility, partition and transdermal permeation. *Eur J Pharm Biopharm*. 2008;69(2): 613–621.

23. Brown MB, Jones SA. Hyaluronic acid: a unique topical vehicle for the localized delivery of drugs to the skin. *J Eur Acad Dermatol Venereol*. 2005;19(3):308–318.

24. Naik A, Pechtold LA, Potts RO, Guy RH. Mechanism of oleic acid-induced skin penetration enhancement in vivo in humans. *J Control Release*. 1995;37(3):299–306.

25. Lee E, An S, Choi D, Moon S, Chang I. Comparison of objective and sensory skin irritations of several cosmetic preservatives. *Contact Dermatitis*. 2007;56(3):131–136.

CHAPTER 45

Retinoids

Leslie S. Baumann, MD

SUMMARY POINTS

What's Important?

1. UVB exposure and free radicals cause a decrease in collagen production by blocking the TGF-β/SMAD pathway and an increase in breakdown of collagen by increasing matrix metalloproteinases (MMPs). Retinoids block both of these pathways, leading to increased collagen in the skin.
2. Retinoids are the most proven of any anti-aging ingredients and are FDA approved for photoaging.
3. Retinoids improve extrinsically and intrinsically aged skin.
4. Retinol turns into all-*trans* retinoic acid inside the cell cytoplasm.
5. Scaling and peeling occur within 2 to 4 days of beginning topical treatment.
6. Pretreating skin with retinoids 2 weeks prior to a cosmetic procedure speeds wound healing.
7. Retinoids can, and should, be used in patients who have excessive sun exposure along with antioxidants to protect skin from UV damage and MMPs.
8. Retinoids are unstable when exposed to air, light, oxidizing agents, high temperature, and low pH.

What's New?

1. Retinol has been proven in many studies to reduce fine lines and wrinkles.
2. Retinoid dermatitis is mediated in part by epidermal derived growth factor.
3. Genistein can be used to block epidermal-derived growth factor and reduce peeling.

What's Coming?

1. Combining retinoids with anti-aging ingredients as discussed in Chapter 37, Anti-Aging Ingredients.
2. More stable formulations of retinols are in the pipeline.
3. Retinoid/genistein products are being developed with technologies that promote penetration of genistein.
4. Trifarotene has not yet been studied for the treatment of photoaged skin, but it is likely that it will demonstrate efficacy.

A family of compounds derived from vitamin A, retinoids include β-carotene, carotenoids, retinol, tretinoin, tazarotene, trifarotene, and adapalene. For decades retinoids have been used topically and systemically for the treatment of dermatologic disorders, particularly acne, psoriasis, and photoaging. The efficacy of retinoids for the treatment and prevention of photoaging has been proven unequivocally over the last two decades. Understanding the mechanism of action of retinoids on photoaged skin has led to a greater understanding of the etiology of skin aging (see Chapters 5, Intrinsic Aging, and 6, Extrinsic Aging).

HISTORY OF RETINOIDS IN DERMATOLOGY

The history of the discovery of retinoids is interesting, lengthy, and very much worth reviewing.[1] Retinol is said to have been discovered in 1909, isolated in 1931, and first synthesized in 1947, becoming commercially available soon thereafter.[2] Since that time, the retinoid field has proliferated with compounds, now numbering more than 2,500 products.[3] In fact, many generic forms of tretinoin are currently available in the United States (U.S.) and retinoids are even combined with medications such as antibiotics and hydroquinone. Topical retinoids were first used in dermatology to treat acne. The first anecdotal evidence that retinoids could improve aged skin was seen in female patients being treated for acne. These patients reported that their skin felt smoother and less wrinkled after treatment.[4] This observation was followed by a clinical trial by Albert Kligman, MD, and Jim Leyden, MD, at the University of Pennsylvania. They showed that patients treated with tretinoin demonstrated improvement of sunlight-induced epidermal atrophy, dysplasia, keratosis, and dyspigmentation.[5]

In a *Dermatology News* podcast from October 15, 2020, Dr. Jim Leyden recounted that when the research retinoid arrived for the first acne research trials, it came in amber bottles and worked to clear acne.[6] However, the second batch of study drug came in clear glass bottles and efficacy was not seen. This is when they discovered that retinoids were light sensitive. If they had not realized this fact, retinoids might not have been developed to treat acne and photoaging.

Myriad clinical trials have confirmed such early observations that retinoids improve photoaged skin. The data were submitted to the U.S. Food and Drug Administration (FDA), which later approved tretinoin (brand name Renova™) for use against photodamage. Although there are numerous topical retinoids on the market today that are also useful against photodamage, tretinoin and tazarotene are the only topical drugs approved by the FDA to treat photodamaged skin. Retinol, the metabolic precursor of tretinoin, is often added to cosmetic formulations and has been shown to improve wrinkles. This chapter will focus on the anti-aging activity of retinoids.

MECHANISM OF ACTION

Chemical Structure

Retinoids are in the vitamin A family. Initially, a retinoid was defined as a compound the structure and action of which resembled the parent compound retinol. (The Latin suffix -*oid* means "resemble" so retinoid means "resembles retinol.") Through the last several decades, chemists have made extensive modifications to the naturally occurring molecule. These have resulted in the development of three generations of retinoids (**Fig. 45-1**). The latest retinoids bear little structural resemblance to retinol but still qualify as retinoids because they can exert their biologic action through the same retinoic acid nuclear receptors modulated by the active natural metabolite of vitamin A, retinoic acid.

Retinoids can act directly by inducing transcription from genes with promoter regions that contain retinoid response elements or indirectly by inhibiting the transcription of certain genes.[7] Three domains within the retinoic acid molecule govern its biologic activity: an acidic function at one extreme and a lipophilic domain at the other, linked by a group that determines their relative spatial orientation.[8] Synthetic retinoids also require an acidic function pointing away from a lipophilic portion for receptor affinity and transcription. The successive generations of retinoids are the result of modification to the retinoic acid skeleton with structural rigidification, through addition of aromatic rings in place of the vulnerable

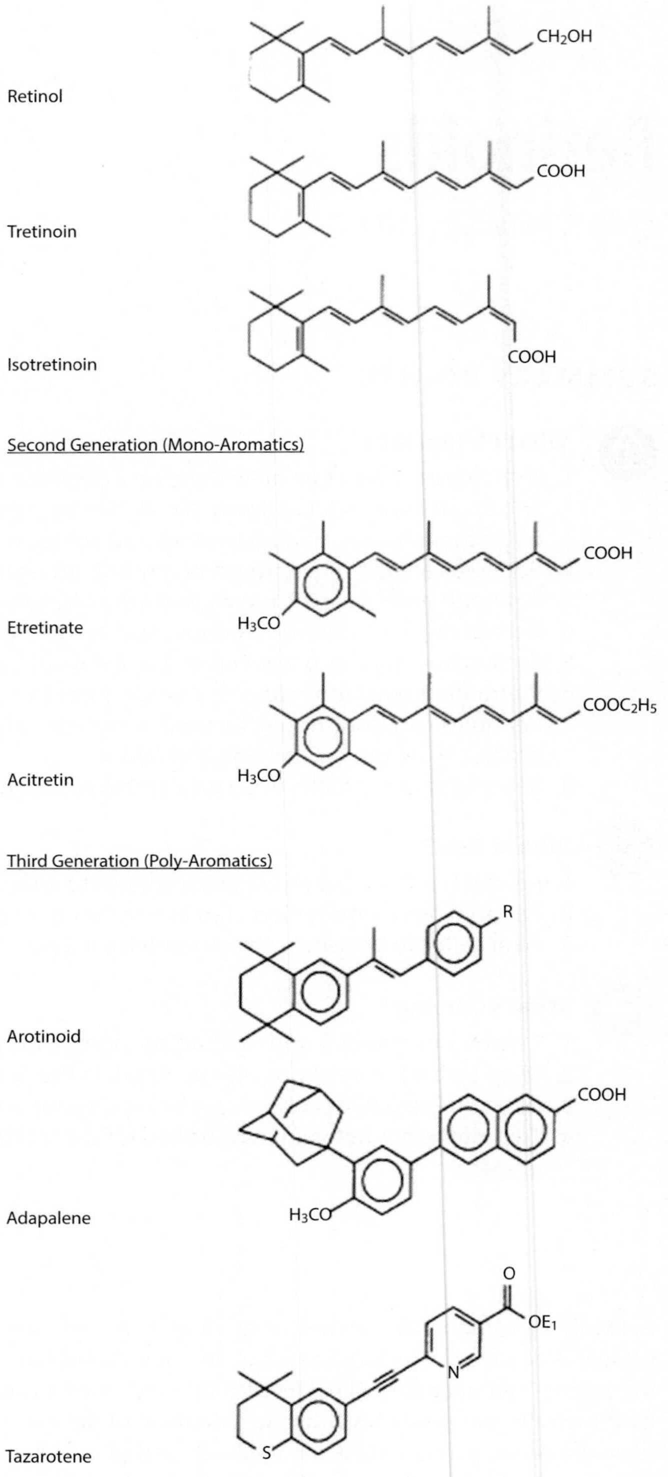

FIGURE 45-1. Chemical structures of the three generations of retinoids. Addition of aromatic rings has made third-generation retinoids more stable and more specific for certain receptors.

double bonds found in retinoic acid. This has rendered the third-generation retinoids more photostable when compared to the first- and second-generation molecules; some compounds within this family have displayed significantly reduced irritation potential.[9]

Retinoic acid is a lipid-soluble molecule known to affect cell growth, differentiation, homeostasis, apoptosis, and embryonic development. In fact, retinoids elicit their effects at the molecular level by regulating gene transcription and affecting functions such as cellular differentiation and proliferation, matrix metalloproteinase (MMP) production, T-cell differentiation, Toll-like receptor 2 (TLR-2) activity, as well as collagen, hyaluronic acid, and elastin synthesis (**Fig. 45-2**). When retinol is applied to the skin, it passes into the cytoplasm and turns into retinaldehyde and then all-*trans* retinoic acid (ATRA). ATRA moves into the nucleus and confers numerous effects such as activating heterodimerization (working together) of retinoic acid receptors (RARs) and retinoid X receptors (RXRs), upregulating the TGF-β/SMAD pathway, and downregulating c-Jun. The ultimate effects of retinoids lead to decreased breakdown of collagen and increased synthesis of collagen. Inhibition of TLR-2 activity leads to reduced inflammation and diminished acne.

ATRA has activity on over 3,000 genes in keratinocytes that play a role in many important pathways such as DNA synthesis and repair, cell cycle, RNA metabolism, apoptosis, and protein kinase activity. Retinoic acid strongly influences keratinocyte differentiation and proliferation and regulates keratin production.[10]

Retinoid Receptors

Retinoid-binding proteins were first discovered in the 1970s.[11] In 1987, the discovery of retinoic acid receptors led to the realization that tretinoin is a hormone.[12,13] Since that time, much research has been performed to determine the exact roles of the retinoid binding proteins and receptors. The biologic effects of retinoic acid are now known to be mediated by several biologic systems: binding proteins such as cellular retinoic acid-binding proteins I and II (CRABP-I and -II); cellular retinol-binding protein (CRBP);[4] and nuclear receptors that are divided into two categories, the RARs and the RXRs.[14] All of these nuclear receptors are members of a large superfamily called nuclear hormone superfamily receptors, which includes the receptors for vitamin D, estradiol, glucocorticoids, and thyroid hormone.[15]

The retinoic acid receptor family is composed of two types of receptors, the RARs and the RXRs. RARs and RXRs are divided into α, β, and γ subtypes. The RARα, RARβ, and RARγ genes have been localized to chromosomes 17q21, 3p24, and 12q13, respectively, and the RXRα, RXRβ, and RXRγ genes have been mapped to chromosomes 9q34.3, 6p21.3, and 1q22–23, respectively.[16] These receptors are able to regulate gene expression in two ways: (1) they induce gene expression by binding to specific DNA sequences known as retinoic acid responsive elements (RAREs), or (2) they inhibit gene expression by downregulating the actions of other transcription factors, such as activator protein (AP)-1 and NF-IL6. All the α, β, and γ subtypes exhibit distinct affinities for retinoic acid and manifest a characteristic tissue distribution. For example,

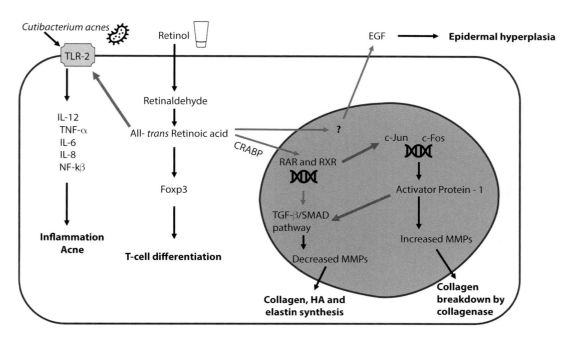

FIGURE 45-2. Retinol penetrates into skin and turns into retinaldehyde and then all-*trans* retinoic acid (ATRA). ATRA inhibits TLR-2 activation by *Cutibacterium acnes*. ATRA causes heterodimerization of RAR/RXR leading to increased collagen, elastin, and hyaluronic acid synthesis and a decrease of MMPs. ATRA inhibits c-Jun heterodimerization, blocking the production of MMPs. ATRA increases expression of epidermal growth factor through an unknown mechanism involving heparin-binding-EGF and amphiregulin. ATRA increases T-cell differentiation through Foxp3. Green arrows = activation. Red arrows = inhibition.

epidermis is a privileged tissue for the expression of RARγ and RXRα, the major isoforms of their respective families in this tissue, whereas RARα is ubiquitous. In the skin, RARβ is primarily found in the dermis, and it is also found in other body tissues.[8] Ninety percent of the RARs in the epidermis and cultured keratinocytes are RARγ, which is the receptor associated with terminal differentiation; therefore, this receptor is the target of the retinoids used in dermatology.[17]

The interactions of the retinoid receptors among themselves and other receptors of the nuclear hormone superfamily are complex. RARs are known to heterodimerize with RXR in order to interact with their RAREs and mediate classic retinoid activity and toxicity. RXRs, however, are more promiscuous, heterodimerizing with several other members of the steroid receptor superfamily including peroxisome proliferator-activated receptors (PPARs), vitamin D receptors, thyroid hormone receptors, and various orphan receptors, such as LXR, PXR, and FXR.[18] The interactions of these receptors are complex and beyond the scope of this chapter.

RARα, RARγ, and RXR are highly expressed in keratinocytes and fibroblasts. RARα is more abundant in the fibroblasts. At baseline, RARβ is either not present or expressed at a low level; however, once RARβ is exposed to retinoic acid, it is rapidly expressed. The RARα/RXRα complex is dominant in the basal layer whereas the RARγ/RXRα complex is most common in the layers above the basal layer.[10]

Retinoids and Stem Cells

Retinoids modulate stem cell pluripotency and promote stem cell differentiation through the expression of mRNA and microRNA and by altering expression of genes involved in DNA methylation. DNA methylation is increased by retinoic acid. Short-term treatment with retinoic acid promotes pluripotency of induced pluripotent stem cells by inhibiting the Wnt pathway and positively modulating AKT/mTOR signaling.[19] A complete discussion of retinoids and stem cells is beyond the scope of this chapter.

Retinoids and Aquaporin

Ultraviolet (UV) light downregulates aquaporin (AQP)-3 in keratinocytes. AQP-3 is important in skin hydration and helps water move between cells (see Chapter 12, Dry Skin). ATRA, when applied to keratinocyte cultures, blocks the downregulation of AQP-3 by activating epidermal-derived growth factor.[20] This means that retinoids can improve transport of solutes between cells through AQP channels.

RETINOIDS AS ANTI-AGING AGENTS

Photodamage and Wrinkles

Retinoids improve wrinkles caused by both intrinsic and extrinsic aging. Copious research demonstrates the efficacy of retinoids to treat and improve photoaged skin and wrinkles and the FDA has approved tazarotene and tretinoin for this purpose. Retinoids are FDA approved for the *treatment* of photoaging, but there is much evidence to show that they also play a role in the *prevention* of aging (**Box 45-1**). Retinoids can "prejuvenate" the skin by rendering it less vulnerable to free radicals and extrinsic factors known to engender aging by blocking pathways induced by free radicals and UV light.

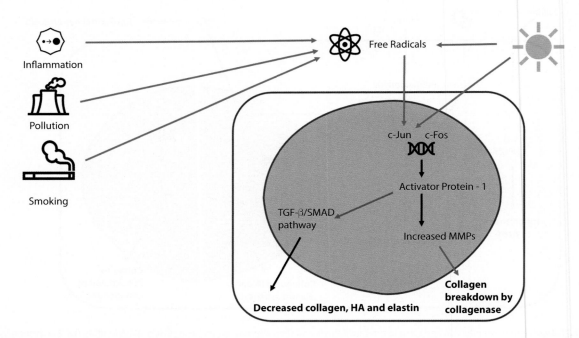

FIGURE 45-3. Pollution, smoking, inflammation, and UV exposure result in increased free radicals. Free radicals and UV light increase expression of the gene c-Jun. c-Jun heterodimerizes with the gene c-Fos and makes activator protein (AP)-1 and inhibits the TGF-β/SMAD pathway. This results in decreased collagen, hyaluronic acid, and elastin production and an increase in MMP enzymes that break down collagen and hyaluronic acid. Green arrows = stimulation. Red arrows = inhibition.

As discussed in Chapter 6, Extrinsic Aging, UV light, pollution, smoking, stress, inflammation, and normal metabolism lead to an increase in free radicals. Both free radicals and UV light activate pathways that lead to an increase in MMPs and a decrease in collagen production (**Fig. 45-3**). UVB exposure and free radicals diminish skin collagen in two major ways: 1) decrease collagen production by blocking the TGF-β/SMAD pathway, and 2) increase breakdown of collagen by MMPs.

Fisher et al. demonstrated that expression of collagen Types I and III is substantially reduced within 24 hours after a single UV exposure.[21] Pretreatment of the skin with ATRA (tretinoin) was shown to inhibit this loss of procollagen synthesis. Therefore, pretreatment of the skin with topical retinoids, when used consistently, is beneficial in preventing as well as treating photodamage.[22] UV light also causes activation of MMP genes resulting in production of collagenase, gelatinase, and stromelysin, which degrade skin collagen and components of the extracellular matrix.[23,24] Fisher et al. showed that application of tretinoin inhibits the induction of all three of these harmful MMPs.[25]

Retinoids and Matrix Metalloproteinases

Two transcription factors, c-Jun and c-Fos, must heterodimerize to produce AP-1. AP-1 blocks the TGF-β/SMAD pathway and

| BOX 45-1 | How Retinoids Prevent Skin Aging |

- Increase production of collagen
- Decrease production of MMPs

activates MMP genes resulting in production of collagenase, gelatinase, and stromelysin. ATRA hinders the UV-induced increase in c-Jun protein. Although high levels of c-Jun mRNA are still present, signifying that the c-Jun gene has been activated, the levels of c-Jun protein are decreased when exposed to retinoids (**Fig. 45-4**). When c-Jun is inhibited by retinoids, AP-1 activity decreases, leading to reduced production of MMPs.

Retinoids and Stress

Psychological stress is known to hasten extrinsic aging. Stress-induced epinephrine heightens oxidative damage and increases inflammation. In a 2019 study, researchers found that epinephrine reduced keratinocyte proliferation.[26] When retinol was added to the cell cultures, increased keratinocyte proliferation was seen even in the presence of epinephrine. This suggests that retinoids may be able to overcome some of the skin stress responses. Retinoids also increased expression of epidermal-derived growth factor in stressed and non-stressed cells. Researchers postulated that retinoids may help decrease aging risk from stress.

HISTOLOGIC CHANGES SEEN WITH RETINOIDS

Retinoid treatment reverses the flattening of the dermal-epidermal junction seen in aged skin and induces the development of rete ridges. Other histologically observed changes with the use of retinoids include abolition of cellular atypia, increased compaction of the stratum corneum

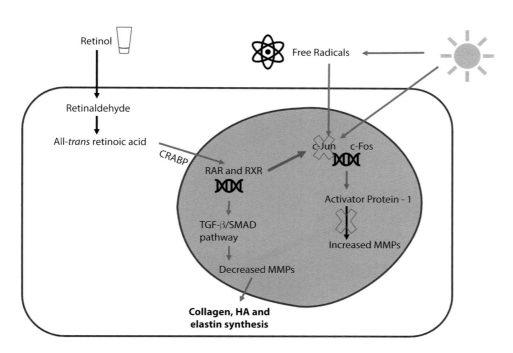

FIGURE 45-4. Retinoids protect skin from extrinsic aging by blocking activation of c-Jun. This prevents activation of AP-1 and allows the TGF-β/SMAD pathway to lead to decreased MMPs and increased collagen, hyaluronic acid, and elastin synthesis.

(SC), less clumping of melanin in basal cells, and a correction of polarity of keratinocytes, with more orderly differentiation as cells move upward. The ultrastructural changes seen with retinoid use include evidence of hyperproliferation of keratinocytes (e.g., larger nuclei, increased ribosomes, etc.) and a reduction in the size of melanosomes.

As described in Chapter 6, changes in collagen and the ratio of collagen I to collagen III have been found to be important in the photoaging process. Retinoids have been shown to increase collagen synthesis in photoaged individuals.[27] In addition to preventing the breakdown of collagen as described above, topical application of tretinoin 0.1% to photodamaged skin increases collagen production and restores levels of collagen I. An increase in anchoring fibrils (collagen VII) is also seen after application of tretinoin 0.1%, leading to stronger and more resilient skin.[27]

Retinol in cosmetic skincare products is effective to treat cutaneous aging as shown in several studies.[28] In an investigation of topical retinol and retinoic acid used for 4 weeks, increases were seen in epidermal thickness, expression of collagen I and III genes, and increased levels of procollagens I and III.[29] These findings seen under the microscope preceded improvement of facial wrinkles that was evident at 12 weeks. This is important because it reveals that skin improves with retinoids even before the improvement is noticeable to the naked eye. It also shows that retinol has efficacy in treating photoaged skin. This is not surprising because retinol is converted into retinoic acid in the skin (**Fig. 45-5**).

VISIBLE CHANGES IN SKIN WITH RETINOIDS

Several studies demonstrate the efficacy of retinol as well as prescription retinoids for the treatment of photoaging.[22,30,31] The first of these clinical trials using tretinoin to demonstrate clinical improvement of photoaged skin were published in 1986 and 1988.[5,32] Since then, many other studies and much clinical experience have shown similar results. Only tretinoin and tazarotene are FDA approved for the treatment of photoaging. However, any retinoid that can penetrate the skin and enter the cell's nucleus to bind the RAR should yield improvement in photodamage. Adapalene, for example, has not been FDA approved for photoaging, but some studies have demonstrated efficacy.[33] Trifarotene has not yet been studied as a treatment for photoaging; however, it is expected to show similar improvement on fine wrinkles and mottled pigmentation.

Although histologic changes after retinoid use are visible under the microscope after a few weeks and changes on gene expression are seen almost immediately, it takes much longer for the skin to synthesize enough collagen to make noticeable changes on the skin. In one study, improvements of facial wrinkles were seen in 12 weeks.[29] This study illustrates that the visible findings of the effects of retinoids on wrinkles are not instantaneous and can take 12 weeks or longer. In two 52-week, double-blind, placebo-controlled studies of topical retinol, 44% of subjects had a significant improvement of crow's feet lines and 84% of subjects experienced improvement of mottled pigmentation.[34] Many studies have clearly demonstrated the efficacy of retinoids and their ability to improve

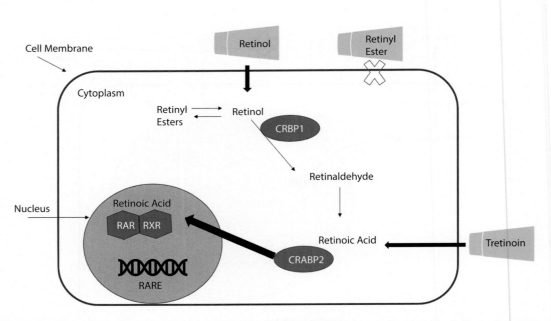

FIGURE 45-5. Retinyl esters do not penetrate very well into the cytoplasm of skin cells. Retinol, tretinoin, adapalene, trifarotene, and tazarotene penetrate easily into the skin. Retinol is converted into retinoic acid inside the cell. Retinol, adapalene, tazarotene, and trifarotene directly bind the retinoic acid receptors. When RAR and RXR heterodimerize and bind to retinoic acid response elements (RAREs), gene transcription occurs.

fine lines and even skin tone, but patients are often not compliant because they want to see changes sooner.[35] Educating patients that retinoids improve both extrinsically and intrinsically aged skin is helpful in promoting compliance.[28]

How Long Does It Take to See Improvement in Wrinkles with Retinoids?

A 1997 study showed that most subjects are improved by 24 weeks, but those that do not respond in the first 24 weeks often see improvement in the second 24 weeks.[36] This same study showed that higher doses of tretinoin (0.1%) result in faster improvement as compared to 0.05%.

Another study in 1997 demonstrated that lower doses of retinoids take longer to see results.[37] In the 48-week study, divided into two 24-week time frames, 126 subjects were treated with tretinoin emollient cream 0.05% and 133 subjects with tretinoin emollient cream 0.01%. In the first 24 weeks, a higher percentage improvement was seen in the 0.05% group. The 0.05% group continued to improve during the second 24 weeks but at a slower rate. The 0.01% group showed less improvement at 24 weeks but demonstrated a higher rate of improvement than the 0.05% group in the second 24 weeks. Subjects receiving the 0.01% formulation improved more during the second 24 weeks of therapy than in the first but still did not achieve the levels of response observed with the 0.05% formulation over 48 weeks of treatment. These results demonstrate that higher doses yield a faster response, but most subjects improved.

These findings contradicted a 1995 study that compared the effects of placebo with tretinoin 0.1% and 0.025% creams.[30] This study found that at 48 weeks both groups that received tretinoin improved as compared to placebo and there was not a statistically significant difference in improvement between the 0.025% and 0.1% creams. However, the 0.025% cream was associated with fewer side effects.

In 2001, an investigator-masked, vehicle-controlled, parallel comparison study considered 0.01%, 0.025%, 0.05%, and 0.1% tazarotene creams as compared to tretinoin 0.05% cream.[38] These were applied once daily for 24 weeks. All study creams improved mottled hyperpigmentation and fine wrinkles. Overall, 0.1% tazarotene had the best efficacy at 8, 12, and 20 weeks. There was a higher rate of adverse events in the 0.1% tazarotene group. By the end of the 24 weeks, tretinoin 0.05% and tazarotene 0.1% had similar efficacy. This demonstrates that improvement can be achieved faster with tazarotene 0.1% as compared to tretinoin 0.05% and lower doses of tazarotene.

Myriad medical providers start patients, especially sensitive skin types, on a low-dose retinoid. In the author's experience, it can take 6–12 months to see results when retinoids are begun at a low dose and slowly increased to higher doses. Titrating retinoids this way helps decrease side effects and improve compliance. Adding in other products to the regimen that will give patients a quicker result such as a facial scrub, defensin, or hyaluronic acid product will show rapid results to keep the patient on track with their retinoid. These "quick result" products deliver instant changes that are temporary while retinoid results take longer but yield enduring changes to the skin.

How Long Does Skin Improvement Remain After Stopping Retinoids?

Long-lasting improvement of skin treated with retinoids was demonstrated in a 22-month trial of retinoic acid.[39] This investigation, which was a continuation of a previous tretinoin study, showed that patients treated with 0.1% tretinoin experienced improvement of wrinkles after 6 to 10 months of treatment. When a patient's retinoid regimen was changed to 0.1% every other day or a lowered dose of 0.05% every day, the benefits that had been achieved with the tretinoin 0.1% remained. Although this study was not designed to determine the best maintenance dose of retinoids, it demonstrated that changes seen with retinoids are sustained. When the retinoids were completely stopped, the changes lasted for at least 2 months and were followed by a partial regression to baseline.

In 1997, the same 126 subjects who had completed the 48-week study of tretinoin 0.05% emollient cream mentioned above were then entered into one of three groups to examine how long the skin improvement remained. Tretinoin 0.05% emollient cream was the retinoid used in this study. Group 1 used no retinoid, group 2 used the retinoid one day a week, and group 3 used the retinoid three times a week.[37] Data showed that improvement was maintained on the 3 doses/week regimen and to a lesser extent on the once/week regimen. The no-retinoid treatment group experienced a reversal of some of the benefits at 6 months.

Topical Retinoids

Retinoids have shown benefits in the treatment of acne (Chapter 16, Acne), psoriasis, photoaging, stretch marks, dyspigmentation, and keratosis pilaris in addition to various other conditions. In fact, there are more than 125 distinct dermatologic disorders for which there is credible evidence of retinoid efficacy.[3]

The higher the retinoid dose is, the faster changes will be seen in the skin. However, side effects from stronger retinoids amplify adverse events and lower compliance. There is a plethora of retinoids from which to choose. Retinol is found in cosmetic products and is the least expensive and most accessible for patients. Adapalene 0.1% is now available as an OTC without a prescription. (Adapalene 0.3% still requires a prescription.) Tretinoin and tazarotene are FDA approved for photoaging but are expensive and not covered by insurance in most cases. Adapalene and trifarotene are approved for acne but can be used off-label for photoaging.

Selection of Topical Retinol

Prescription retinoids are manufactured and packaged in a regulated manner that is overseen by the FDA. For this reason, prescription retinoids have good quality control. Cosmetic retinol products have no oversight or regulations to ensure their efficacy. In fact, retinol is often listed as an inactive ingredient in order to prevent any biologic claims that would subject the product to regulation as a drug rather than a cosmetic (see Chapter 32, Cosmetics and Drug Regulations). Cosmetic retinol products have varying degrees of efficacy depending on several factors (**Table 45-1**). In many cases, cosmetic products that claim to contain retinol actually have retinyl esters or retinaldehyde. In some cases, there is a small amount of retinol and a larger amount of retinyl esters. Retinyl esters do not penetrate well into the skin and are therefore not very potent.[40] They are often the type of retinoids used in brands that claim to be "nonirritating." If scaling, redness, and peeling do not occur, the ability of the retinoid to bind RAR should be doubted. So, if the retinoid is nonirritating, it is likely ineffective. To be clear, irritation is *not* necessary for efficacy and does not signal efficacy in any way; rather, it is a sign that the retinoid is active and binding the RAR.

All retinoids that bind the RAR receptors will increase epidermal-derived growth factor activity, which leads to scaling.[41] Studies have shown that genistein included in a retinoid formula can decrease scaling, but penetration of genistein is difficult and there are very few formulations that contain retinol and genistein together. Currently, the presence of peeling is the best way to ascertain the potency of a retinoid product.

Retinoids that are FDA approved have standards and guidelines to follow, so one can be certain that these are packaged and manufactured properly. Retinol, as mentioned earlier, is not regulated because it is a cosmetic. Consequently, there is a wide range of potency in retinol products. If two 0.1% retinols are compared, they may not have the same potency. One researcher in Slovenia developed a way to quantify active retinol in 21 commercially available retinol-containing skincare products.[42] His quantitative methodology revealed that over half of the products tested had discrepancies between the retinoid amount reported to be contained in the product and what was actually in the product. Many cosmetic retinol products did not have the amount of retinol that they claimed on the label and the ingredient labeling was incorrect. The most common abnormality was the presence of a retinoid not declared on the label. For example, one label read "retinol" but retinyl esters were actually in the formula. The lack of regulations on retinol-containing cosmetic products in the US means that the medical provider must take special care to choose an efficacious retinol product from a reputable company. There are multiple reasons that a retinoid cosmetic product has limited efficacy as listed in **Table 45-1**. In many cases, when retinol products are produced, they are stirred in huge vats that look like a Kitchen Aid mixer—open to the air. The air and light inactivate the retinol before it is even packaged. To be properly made, a vacuum or inert gas should be used instead of air.[43] In other instances, when the formula is fed into the tubes and bottles, it is exposed to light and air. It is uncommon to find a retinol manufacturer who uses a closed system free of air and light to manufacture and package retinol. This accounts for why there are so many ineffective versions of retinols on the market. The best example is retinol in a jar. In these jars, when they are opened, the retinol loses efficacy almost immediately. Retinol is sensitive to air, high temperature, oxidizing agents, UV light, and a low pH.[44] Addition of antioxidants can help preserve the efficacy of retinol.

TABLE 45-1	Factors That Affect Retinoid Efficacy

- Form of retinoid used
- Purity of retinoid used
- Percent of retinoid in formulation
- Air or light exposure during mixing of the formula
- Air or light exposure during transfer into the pump or tube packaging
- Air or light exposure once opened

USE OF RETINOIDS IN A SKINCARE ROUTINE

Retinoids are lipophilic and easily cross the skin barrier into the epidermis and dermis to reach the retinoid receptors. Drug delivery to the dermis is not problematic with retinoids as they penetrate rapidly into skin. In fact, some skincare regimens prescribe a short contact time of 15 minutes before the retinoid is washed off to facilitate the patient adapting to the retinoid. This short contact time is not necessary when the proper dose, amount, and frequency of retinoid use are combined with the proper cleanser and moisturizer.

Retinoids should be included in every skincare routine for acne, anti-aging, dyspigmentation, and, when possible, rosacea. Retinoids impart profound beneficial effects on pigmentation, collagen content, and skin texture. Although the short-term side effects as well as the need to wait over 16 weeks to see results reduce compliance, encouraging patients to use their retinoids is worth the effort. The medical provider should ask the patient at every visit if they are using their retinoids. In the author's experience, the answer is no in at least 25% of patients. Consistent encouragement and education can increase compliance with retinoids.

Using Retinoids in Rosacea Patients

Rosacea patients are known to have very sensitive skin that turns red, stings, and burns, sometimes even in contact with water. For this reason, it is difficult to start a rosacea patient on a retinoid. Rosacea is partially caused by dilation of blood vessels (Chapter 17, Rosacea). Loss of collagen around blood vessels due to sun exposure can predispose patients with significant sun damage to rosacea. Use of a retinoid can improve symptoms; however, rosacea patients are very prone to inflammation so retinoids should be started slowly. In these patients, it is recommended to hydrate the skin and reduce inflammation for the first 4 weeks. If the skin is hydrated and the barrier seems to be intact, begin a low-dose retinoid every 3 days on top of a moisturizer. Use moisturizers with anti-inflammatory ingredients (Chapter 38, Anti-Inflammatory Ingredients). Most rosacea patients can tolerate retinoids when they are used in this manner.

Cleanser and water choice will greatly affect the side-effect profile of rosacea patients on retinoids (Chapter 40, Cleansing Agents). Dry skin types should always use nonfoaming cleansers such as creamy lipid-filled cleansers when starting a retinoid. The retinoids are tolerated much better when the skin barrier is intact. Use of hard water and foaming cleaners can injure the skin barrier allowing greater penetration of retinoids and an increased side-effect profile. Oily skin types can use foaming cleansers because their skin barrier is protected by the occlusive lipids found in sebum.

Moisturizer choice also greatly affects the ability to tolerate retinoids. Use of hyaluronic acid-containing moisturizers increases penetration of retinoids and can lead to significant side effects in dry skin types beginning retinoids as indicated for acne, melasma, or cutaneous aging. It is best to avoid hyaluronic acid moisturizers when beginning a retinoid. Instead, choose a moisturizer with barrier repair ingredients such as myristoyl/palmitoyl oxostearamide/arachamide mea or a 1:1:1 ratio of ceramides, fatty acids, and cholesterol (Chapter 43, Moisturizers). Applying the retinoid on top of a barrier repair moisturizer will decrease delivery of the retinoid into the skin and allow the skin to slowly acclimate to the retinoid.

Side Effects

Adverse effects of retinoids include redness, peeling, stinging, and sensitivity (**Fig. 45-6**). These side effects are extremely common and greatly reduce patient compliance. They are not allergic reactions although many patients believe they are allergic to retinoids if they have experienced the side effects in the past. Educating patients on how to prevent and manage these side effects is a major factor in compliance. Side effects can be managed by limiting dose, frequency of use, and employing the proper cleansers and moisturizers.

Side effects from retinoid use occur from activation of epidermal growth factor, which causes the scaling. Side effects can also occur when the retinoid binds undesired receptor subtypes. The more specific the binding pattern a retinoid exhibits, the fewer side effects it will elicit. The newer generation of retinoids destined for dermatologic use have been designed to reduce side effects by creating compounds that bind more selectively to the RARγ receptor subtype. However, with these improved molecules, the side effects from topically applied retinoids still persist due to intrinsic RARγ activation and epidermal-derived growth factor.

Scaling and Peeling

When beginning a retinoid in a new patient, the medical provider should be suspicious if peeling is not seen in the first few weeks of use. If a patient does not peel or experience flaking when they begin retinoids, this means:

1. The product has lost efficacy. It may be an inferior form of retinoid such as a retinaldehyde or retinyl ester. In many cases, the retinol product is not made correctly and may have lost activity during manufacturing, packaging, or a long life on the shelf due to exposure to light or air.
2. The patient is not using the product as directed.
3. The patient is an oily skin type and the sebum on the skin is preventing entry of the retinoid into the skin. Addition

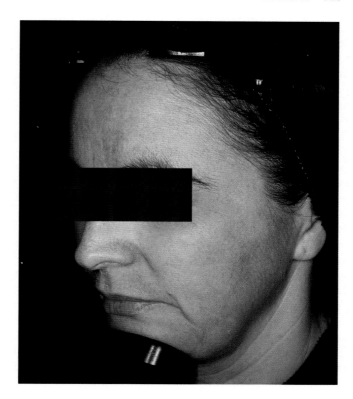

FIGURE 45-6. Redness, flaking, and stinging tender skin are common symptoms after beginning a retinoid. These symptoms usually improve with time. Using a low dose less often over a moisturizer can decrease the risk of retinoid dermatitis. This is not an allergic reaction.

of a foaming cleanser or a hydroxy acid cleanser can help improve penetration.
4. The patient is applying the retinoid over a moisturizer that contains an occlusive ingredient that prevents penetration of the retinoid. Switch the retinoid to be applied before the moisturizer.
5. The patient is a resistant skin type who is not very susceptible to inflammation. Review how they are using the retinoid product. If they are using it properly, it is likely that they are a resistant skin type and the retinoid strength, application frequency, as well as amount can be increased faster than in other skin types.
6. The other products in the regimen have genistein or other agents that block epidermal-derived growth factor.
7. The patient is following directions and titrating the retinoid as prescribed.

Peeling and scaling from retinoids is *not required* to see efficacy. However, these signs can be used to determine the strength and quality of a retinoid product. The increased desquamation and resultant flaking of the skin correspond with increased proliferation of keratinocytes, as indicated by a greater number of mitotic figures and enhanced expression of differentiation markers.[45] These findings are related to the type and dose of the retinoid with stronger doses showing increased amounts of peeling. Scaling and peeling usually occur within 2 to 4 days of beginning topical treatment.[46]

Studies demonstrate that patients may achieve maximum clinical improvement of photoaged skin without developing retinoid dermatitis. In other words, the irritation produced by retinoids is separate from the photoaging benefits of retinoids. This was revealed in the study that compared two different strengths of tretinoin (0.1% and 0.025%). Although both strengths were equally efficacious in the treatment of photoaging, the degree of irritation differed markedly between the two treatment groups, with the 0.1% tretinoin-treated group exhibiting approximately a three-fold greater incidence of irritation than the 0.025% tretinoin-treated group.[30] This irritation is now known to be caused by RAR activation of epidermal growth factor.[41] Before the role of epidermal growth factor was elucidated, evidence that the topical application of tretinoin to the skin of transgenic mice deficient in RARs did not result in any apparent epidermal hyperplasia or desquamation showed that RAR activation played a role in scaling and peeling.[47] The scaling seen with retinoids can be reduced by epidermal growth factor receptor inhibitors such as genistein. Use of anti-inflammatory and antioxidant ingredients and the proper cleanser and moisturizer can help reduce retinoid dermatitis.

Erythema is another side effect of topical retinoids that elicits noncompliance from patients. This symptom is caused by a different mechanism that appears not to be receptor mediated.[48] Patients with rosacea and naturally pink skin tend to be particularly disturbed by this side effect. Using the techniques described in **Table 45-2** may decrease the incidence of all types of skin irritation.

Dry skin is also a common complaint of patients treated with retinoids. The flaking that patients experience when using retinoids often leads them to believe that their skin is dry, although the observed flaking is caused by epidermal growth factor and not by reduced skin hydration. In fact, retinoids increase AQP levels in the skin. Retinoids can even be used to treat dry skin disorders like keratosis pilaris and ichthyosis.[49] The dry skin noted by retinoid users is likely due in part to an increase in transepidermal water loss, which accompanies topical retinoid use. The increase in transepidermal water loss is an effect typical of topically applied retinoids and is thought to be associated with a perturbation of the SC water barrier function.[50,51] Although retinoids increase cell proliferation, this leads to a decrease in ceramide biosynthesis (at least in the short term). This decline in ceramides, a vital component of the water barrier of the SC, may partly explain the xerosis seen with retinoid use.[52]

It is important not to begin other irritating agents, such as facial scrubs, facial brushes, chemical peels, or microdermabrasion, when retinoid therapy is begun. These can be added later once the retinoid is sufficiently tolerated. However, many dermatologists have observed that patients who have been on hydroxy acids for extended periods before beginning retinoids may exhibit less irritation from the retinoids. The reason for this is currently unclear. However, it is believed that the hydroxy acids enhance the function of the skin barrier,

TABLE 45-2	Instructions for Patients Using Retinoids for the First Time
AM: Use cleanser, moisturizer, and sunscreen as directed by your skincare specialist.	
PM:	

PM:
1. Cleanse face.
2. Apply eye cream to protect the delicate eye area.
3. Apply treatment product for anti-aging, acne, dyspigmentation, or rosacea.
4. Apply moisturizer.
5. Apply ¼ teaspoon of retinoid product to face. Apply another ¼ teaspoon to neck and chest.

Notes:
1. Use retinoid every third night for the first 2 weeks.
2. If you have no redness, increase to every other night for 2 weeks.
3. If you have no redness, increase to every night.
4. Once you have used it every night for 3 months, ask your medical provider to recommend the next strongest formulation.
5. You may only be able to use the product on your neck twice a week. The neck is more sensitive than the face.
6. Use the retinoid on top of a moisturizer.
7. Do not use facial scrubs, facial brushes, loofas, microdermabrasion, or at-home chemical peels when beginning a retinoid.
8. Stop retinoid products 1 week before facial waxing to avoid skin burning from the wax or tell the aesthetician to use cool wax or threading.

leading to less absorption of the retinoids. Using barrier repair moisturizers in addition to the retinoids can be very helpful to increase tolerability.

Teratogenicity

It is well established that teratogenicity is a significant risk associated with the use of retinoids, especially via oral administration. The advisability of topical retinoid use by women of childbearing age has been the subject of debate because of the potential risk of systemic absorption. As a general rule, great care should be taken when prescribing these drugs to women of childbearing age, and prescriptions should be restricted to those drugs for which a high safety margin has been clinically demonstrated (e.g., in the courses of treatment for psoriasis or acne). It is recommended to have pregnant and breastfeeding patients cease using topical retinoids, although there are multiple studies that show some topical retinoids have no adverse effect when used during pregnancy. For example, in one controlled study in which 0.025% tretinoin gel was applied daily to the face, neck, and upper part of the chest for 14 days, fluctuations in plasma levels of endogenous retinoids were lower than those of diurnal and nutritional factors.[53] Another study demonstrated no significant increase in the rate of fetal malformation in a large group of patients treated with topical tretinoin during the first trimester of pregnancy, as compared with those who were not exposed to the drug.[54] Even cosmetic retinols should be used carefully in pregnancy because studies show that there is inconsistency in the amount of retinol found in products. In fact, the retinoids found in these products may not match what is on the label. Researchers fear that use of a high-dose retinol on a large surface area of the body during pregnancy could result in high serum levels of vitamin A, although this has not been proven.[42]

Retinoids and Sun Exposure

Many patients and physicians have worried that use of topical tretinoin may lead to increased photosensitivity because the nightly use of retinoids causes the SC to become thinner and more compact. This concern has been due, at least in part, to the fact that early tretinoin users were warned to apply the product only at night. The precaution stemmed from the product's poor stability when exposed to UV light, though, not to any reported photosensitivity provocation. In fact, it has now been established that there is no decrease of the minimal erythema dose for human skin that has been pretreated with topical tretinoin and irradiated with UV light of a defined energy. This shows that retinoids possess neither phototoxic nor photosensitizing activity.[25] However, retinoids do make the SC more compact, reducing natural sun protection factor (SPF). When used in conjunction with hydroxy acids or exfoliants, care should be taken to wear SPF daily because combinations of exfoliants can slightly reduce the skin's natural SPF. The benefits that retinoids provide in blocking MMPs outweigh the slight loss of SPF; therefore, retinoids can, and should, be used in patients who have excessive sun exposure along with antioxidants.

RETINOIDS PRE- AND POST-PROCEDURE

Retinoids should be used prior to wounding to increase collagen production and expedite healing. Multiple studies support the use of pretreatment with tretinoin to accelerate wound healing (Chapter 36, Pre- and Post-Procedure Skincare).[55–57] Punch biopsies on arms pretreated with tretinoin cream 0.05% to 0.1% were shown to heal faster.[58] Using retinoids for 2 to 4 weeks prior to cosmetic procedures or intentional wounding such as microneedling is supported by a preponderance of studies,[59] as peak epidermal hypertrophy emerges after 7 days of tretinoin application and normalizes after 14 days of continued treatment.[60] Such an approach gives the skin time to recover from any retinoid dermatitis before the scheduled surgery. Pretreatment with adapalene should be introduced 5 to 6 weeks before any procedure because it exhibits a longer half-life and requires an earlier initiation period.[61]

Topical retinoids should not be used after procedures until epithelialization is complete. A study by Hung et al. in a porcine model demonstrated that while 0.05% tretinoin cream daily for 10 days prior to partial-thickness skin wounding accelerated re-epithelialization, use of tretinoin after wounding slowed healing.[62]

AVAILABLE TYPES OF TOPICAL RETINOIDS

All retinoids affect RAR receptors, but which RAR receptor subtype they affect may vary (**Table 45-3**). RARγ and RXRα are located in the epidermis while RARβ is found in the dermis. Although topically applied retinoids seem similar upon cursory inspection, they actually exhibit important differences, which fall beyond the scope of this chapter. Addressing the second-generation oral retinoids acitretin and etretinate also lies outside the range of this discussion.

First Generation

Tretinoin

Tretinoin, the natural retinoid ATRA, is a first-generation retinoid and was the first available topical retinoid, initially marketed as Retin-A˚. Once the photoaging benefits of tretinoin were described, a new formulation, Renova˚, was approved by the FDA and marketed for the treatment of photodamage. Although the other retinoids are also beneficial in treating photodamage, Renova is currently the only tretinoin approved specifically for this purpose. Tretinoin is a nonselective retinoid that activates all RAR pathways (α, β, and γ) directly and RXR pathways indirectly through conversion of ATRA to 9-*cis*-retinoic acid (the natural ligand for RXRs).[63] Other brands of tretinoin are FDA approved to treat acne. Tretinoin is available as a generic.

Given its availability as a generic drug, tretinoin is currently found in several products. Notably, two combination products have been introduced to the market. Ziana is a medication that contains tretinoin 0.025% and clindamycin 1.2%. It is used at night in patients with acne. This product is ideal for use in adult acne sufferers who can also benefit from an anti-aging component in their skin regimen. Tri-Luma combines tretinoin, hydroquinone, and a mild steroid. It has shown utility in pigmentary disorders such as melasma and as a first-line therapy for photoaging (Chapter 33, Choosing Skincare Products).

Retinol

Retinol, also known as vitamin A, is a first-generation retinoid as well. It is converted to retinaldehyde and then to ATRA by a dedicated metabolic machinery within the keratinocytes to become active in the epidermis. Although it is a precursor to retinoic acid, retinol is classified as a cosmetic rather than a

TABLE 45-3	Receptor Selectivity (for Both Receptor Binding and Gene Transactivation)	
	RARs	**RXRs**
Tretinoin	α, β, γ	(α, β, γ)[a]
Isotretinoin	α, β, γ	(α, β, γ)[a]
Adapalene	β, γ	—
Tazarotene	β, γ	—
Trifarotene	γ	

[a]Weak binding because of isomerization to *9-cis*-retinoic acid.

drug; therefore, it is found in a plethora of cosmetic formulations. It is interesting to note that because cosmetic companies cannot claim that their retinol products exert a biologic action, retinol is listed on scores of cosmetic products as an "inactive ingredient." This regulatory quirk, in addition to the fact that early forms of retinol were very unstable and exhibited a brief shelf life, has led many to believe that retinol exerts minimal, if any, biologic activity. Moreover, homeopathic doses of retinol and its esters are often listed on cosmetic labels, adding to the poor reputation of retinol, although retinol has been shown to have significant biologic action and efficacy at the proper doses.

Even though retinol is approximately 20 times less potent than retinoic acid, retinol exhibits greater penetration into the skin when compared to retinoic acid. Once inside the cell it is converted to retinoic acid. There is great variability in doses of retinol, usually 0.025%, 0.05%, or 0.1% (these percentages cannot be compared to the tretinoin percentages because they are different molecules). The wide variety in strengths of retinol products allows the medical provider to choose from many doses. Sensitive skin patients, even rosacea patients, can usually tolerate the lower doses of retinol such as 0.025% if combined in the proper skincare regimen for the patient's skin type. Unfortunately, some manufacturers do not list the concentration of retinol on product packages. Another obstacle in this area is the inclusion of ineffective esters such as retinyl palmitate.[3] In some cases the label says "retinol" when it contains a retinyl ester.[42] Retinol products should be packaged in airless pumps or in small mouth aluminum tubes to limit exposure to light and air. Jars of retinol are not acceptable.

Third Generation
Adapalene
Adapalene is a third-generation retinoid approved for the treatment of acne. It has selective affinity only for RARγ receptors and does not interact with any of the RXR subtypes.[64] The drug was intentionally designed for increased receptor specificity in order to maximize the beneficial effects, and for mitigation of the unwanted effects usually seen with the topical application of retinoids. In fact, adapalene has been demonstrated to be less irritating than tretinoin in several studies.[8] Moreover, it has been shown to possess a comfortable safety margin with regard to teratogenicity, and is the only synthetic retinoid without the X-classification (signifying a teratogenic compound). Pharmacologic and preclinical studies of adapalene have revealed the drug to exhibit excellent follicular penetration, comedolytic activity, and anti-inflammatory properties.[65-67] In addition, adapalene is more chemically stable than tretinoin and does not break down in the presence of light, as does tretinoin.[68] Differin is the only available formulation of adapalene and is now available without a prescription as an OTC drug. It is available in a 0.1% OTC and a 0.3% form by prescription.

Tazarotene
In 1997, the FDA approved tazarotene for the treatment of both facial acne vulgaris and plaque psoriasis. It is currently

available in 0.1% and 0.05% gels and in 0.1% and 0.05% creams. Tazarotene activates the gene expression of RARβ and RARγ, but does not interact with any of the RXR subtypes.[7] Tazarotene, like other retinoids, has been shown to be effective against photoaging. One small double-blind, placebo-controlled trial compared the effects of tazarotene 0.1% gel on the forearm to the effects of vehicle alone for a 12-week period.[69] Not surprisingly, tazarotene was associated with improvement in some of the signs of photodamage, such as reduced skin roughness and fine wrinkling, at the end of the study period. Beneficial histologic changes characteristic of retinoid treatment occurred in the epidermis and SC. There is clinical evidence that tazarotene is well tolerated by acne patients, but there are conflicting data on this subject in the literature. Specifically, a split-face study demonstrated that the tolerability of tazarotene 0.1% gel is clinically comparable to that of tretinoin 0.1% gel microsphere, tretinoin 0.025% gel, and adapalene 0.1% gel,[70] while tazarotene has otherwise been shown to display significantly higher irritation than other retinoids, justifying every-other-day regimens to improve patient compliance. The efficacy of every-other-day tazarotene 0.1% gel was examined in acne patients and was found to offer comparable efficacy to once-daily adapalene 0.1% gel.[71] Tazarotene 0.1% is FDA approved for the treatment of photoaging.

Fourth Generation
Trifarotene (Aklief)
In October 2019, the FDA approved trifarotene for the treatment of acne on the face and trunk.[72] Trifarotene is the only retinoid on the market that exclusively targets the RARγ receptor. The RARγ receptor is the most common RAR found in the skin. Two pivotal clinical trials of 2,420 patients showed that trifarotene 0.005% cream demonstrated significant improvement in acne as compared to placebo.[73] This agent is new and there are no published studies of its effects on photoaging at this time.

AGENTS THAT BIND RXR

RXRs are important in controlling apoptosis. Alitretinoin, or 9-cis-retinoic acid (Pan-Retin), which is currently approved by the FDA for the treatment of Kaposi's sarcoma, binds the RXRα, β, and γ receptors. Its use in acne and photoaging has not yet been studied. Targretin gel is another RXR-selective retinoid. Targretin selectively binds all three RXRs, α, β, and γ, and is now being reviewed in trials for psoriasis. It can repress AP-1 function, though not as well as retinoids such as ATRA or 9-cis-retinoic acid.[1] The use of RXR ligands in cancer treatments implies that these drugs may have utility in preventing some of the benign neoplasms seen in aging skin; however, this has not yet been studied.

---

1 Personal communication with Reid Bissonnette, PhD, Nuclear Receptor Discovery Department of Ligand Pharmaceuticals.

CONCLUSION

Retinoids are the most effective treatment for wrinkles. The use of retinoids and sunscreen remain the best way to prevent skin aging besides sun avoidance, exercise, eating fruits and vegetables, and limiting stress. Patients need to be educated about the benefits of retinoids to help them persevere through the troublesome first 2 to 4 weeks of redness and peeling that can occur. Education, encouragement, and frequent reminders to use the product are critical for retinoid success. Fortunately, studies have suggested that once skin appearance has been improved with retinoids, taking the prescribed retinoid three times per week will maintain the beneficial effects.

References

1. Wolf G. A history of vitamin A and retinoids. *FASEB J.* 1996; 10(9):1102–1107.

2. Machlin LJ. Beyond deficiency. New views on the function and health effects of vitamins. Introduction. *Ann N Y Acad Sci.* 1992;669:1–6.

3. Kligman AM. The growing importance of topical retinoids in clinical dermatology: a retrospective and prospective analysis. *J Am Acad Dermatol.* 1998;39(2 Pt 3):S2–S7.

4. Kligman L, Kligman AM. Photoaging—Retinoids, alpha hydroxy acids, and antioxidants. In: Gabard B, Elsner P, Surber C, Treffel P, eds. *Dermatopharmacology of Topical Preparations.* New York, NY: Springer; 2000: 383.

5. Kligman AM, Grove GL, Hirose R, Leyden JJ. Topical tretinoin for photoaged skin.*J Am Acad Dermatol.* 1986;15(4 Pt 2):836–859.

6. Dermatology News Podcast. Looking back on retinoid discovery and development with Dr. James Leyden. October 15, 2020. https://www.mdedge.com/podcasts/dermatology-weekly/looking-back-retinoid-discovery-and-development-dr-james-leyden?sso=true. Accessed April 27, 2021.

7. Chandraratna RA. Tazarotene—first of a new generation of receptor-selective retinoids. *Br J Dermatol.* 1996;135(Suppl 49):18–25.

8. Millikan LE. Adapalene: an update on newer comparative studies between the various retinoids. *Int J Dermatol.* 2000;39(10):784–788.

9. Weiss JS. Current options for topical treatment of acne vulgaris. *Pediatr Dermatol.* 1997;14(6):480–488.

10. Szymański Ł, Skopek R, Palusińska M, Schenk T, Stengel S, Lewicki S, et al. Retinoic Acid and Its Derivatives in Skin. *Cells.* 2020;9(12):2660.

11. Chytil F, Ong D. Cellular retinoid-binding proteins. In: Sporn MB, Roberts A, Goodman D, eds. *The Retinoids*, Vol. 2. Orlando, FL: Academic Press; 1984: 89–123.

12. Giguere V, Ong ES, Segui P, Evans RM. Identification of a receptor for the morphogen retinoic acid. *Nature.* 1987; 330(6149):624–629.

13. Petkovich M, Brand NJ, Krust A, Chambon P. A human retinoic acid receptor which belongs to the family of nuclear receptors. *Nature.* 1987;330(6147):444–450.

14. Pfahl M. The molecular mechanism of retinoid action–retinoids today and tomorrow. *Retinoid Dermatol.* 1996;44:2–6.

15. Petkovich M. Regulation of gene expression by vitamin A: the role of nuclear retinoic acid receptors. *Annu Rev Nutr.* 1992;12:443–471.

16. Chambon P. A decade of molecular biology of retinoic acid receptors. *FASEB J.* 1996;10(9):940–954.

17. Nagpal S, Chandraratna RA. Recent developments in receptor-selective retinoids. *Curr Pharm Des.* 2000;6(9):919–931.

18. Lippman SM, Lotan R. Advances in the development of retinoids as chemopreventive agents. *J Nutr.* 2000;130(2S Suppl): 479S–482S.

19. Godoy-Parejo C, Deng C, Zhang Y, Liu W, Chen G. Roles of vitamins in stem cells. *Cell Mol Life Sci.* 2020;77(9):1771–1791.

20. Cao C, Wan S, Jiang Q, Amaral A, Lu S, Hu G, et al. All-trans retinoic acid attenuates ultraviolet radiation-induced down-regulation of aquaporin-3 and water permeability in human keratinocytes. *J Cell Physiol.* 2008;215(2):506–516.

21. Fisher GJ, Datta S, Wang Z, Li XY, Quan T, Chung JH, et al. c-Jun-dependent inhibition of cutaneous procollagen transcription following ultraviolet irradiation is reversed by all-trans retinoic acid. *J Clin Invest.* 2000;106(5):663–670.

22. Fisher GJ, Talwar HS, Lin J, Voorhees JJ. Molecular mechanisms of photoaging in human skin in vivo and their prevention by all-trans retinoic acid. *Photochem Photobiol.* 1999;69(2):154–157.

23. Fisher GJ, Wang ZQ, Datta SC, Varani J, Kang S, Voorhees JJ. Pathophysiology of premature skin aging induced by ultraviolet light. *N Engl J Med.* 1997;337(20):1419–1428.

24. Shapiro SD. Matrix metalloproteinase degradation of extracellular matrix: biological consequences. *Curr Opin Cell Biol.* 1998;10(5):602–608.

25. Fisher GJ, Datta SC, Talwar HS, et al. Molecular basis of sun-induced premature skin ageing and retinoid antagonism. *Nature.* 1996;379(6563):335–339.

26. Romana-Souza B, Silva-Xavier W, Monte-Alto-Costa A. Topical retinol attenuates stress-induced ageing signs in human skin ex vivo, through EGFR activation via EGF, but not ERK and AP-1 activation. *Exp Dermatol.* 2019;28(8):906–913.

27. Woodley DT, Zelickson AS, Briggaman RA, et al. Treatment of photoaged skin with topical tretinoin increases epidermal-dermal anchoring fibrils. A preliminary report. *JAMA.* 1990;263:3057.

28. Kafi R, Kwak HS, Schumacher WE, et al. Improvement of naturally aged skin with vitamin A (retinol). *Arch Dermatol.* 2007;143(5):606–612.

29. Kong R, Cui Y, Fisher GJ, et al. A comparative study of the effects of retinol and retinoic acid on histological, molecular, and clinical properties of human skin. *J Cosmet Dermatol.* 2016;15(1):49–57.

30. Griffiths CE, Kang S, Ellis CN, et al. Two concentrations of topical tretinoin (retinoic acid) cause similar improvement of photoaging but different degrees of irritation. A double-blind, vehicle-controlled comparison of 0.1% and 0.025% tretinoin creams. *Arch Dermatol.* 1995;131(9):1037–1044.

31. Fisher GJ, Voorhees JJ. Molecular mechanisms of photoaging and its prevention by retinoic acid: ultraviolet irradiation induces MAP kinase signal transduction cascades that induce Ap-1-regulated matrix metalloproteinases that degrade human skin in vivo. *J Investig Dermatol Symp Proc.* 1998;3(1):61–68.

32. Weiss JS, Ellis CN, Headington JT, Tincoff T, Hamilton TA, Voorhees JJ. Topical tretinoin improves photoaged skin: a double-blind vehicle-controlled study. *JAMA.* 1988;259(4):527–532.

33. Rusu A, Tanase C, Pascu GA, Todoran N. Recent Advances Regarding the Therapeutic Potential of Adapalene. *Pharmaceuticals (Basel).* 2020;13(9):217.

34. Randhawa M, Rossetti D, Leyden JJ, et al. One-year topical stabilized retinol treatment improves photodamaged skin in a double-blind, vehicle-controlled trial. *J Drugs Dermatol.* 2015;14(3):271–280.

35. Pedersen ES, Voorhees JJ, Sachs DL. Topical Retinoids for the Treatment of Photoaged Skin. *Cutaneous Photoaging.* 2019;19:341.

36. Olsen EA, Katz HI, Levine N, et al. Sustained improvement in photodamaged skin with reduced tretinoin emollient cream treatment regimen: effect of once-weekly and three-times-weekly applications. *J Am Acad Dermatol.* 1997;37(2 Pt 1):227–230.

37. Olsen EA, Katz HI, Levine N, et al. Tretinoin emollient cream for photodamaged skin: results of 48-week, multicenter, double-blind studies. *J Am Acad Dermatol.* 1997;37(2 Pt 1):217–226.

38. Kang S, Leyden JJ, Lowe NJ, et al. Tazarotene cream for the treatment of facial photodamage: a multicenter, investigator-masked, randomized, vehicle-controlled, parallel comparison of 0.01%, 0.025%, 0.05%, and 0.1% tazarotene creams with 0.05% tretinoin emollient cream applied once daily for 24 weeks. *Arch Dermatol.* 2001;137(12):1597–1604.

39. Ellis CN, Weiss JS, Hamilton TA, Headington JT, Zelickson AS, Voorhees JJ. Sustained improvement with prolonged topical tretinoin (retinoic acid) for photoaged skin. *J Am Acad Dermatol.* 1990;23(4 Pt 1):629–637.

40. Duell EA, Kang S, Voorhees JJ. Unoccluded retinol penetrates human skin in vivo more effectively than unoccluded retinyl palmitate or retinoic acid. *J Invest Dermatol.* 1997;109(3):301–305.

41. Rittié L, Varani J, Kang S, Voorhees JJ, Fisher GJ. Retinoid-induced epidermal hyperplasia is mediated by epidermal growth factor receptor activation via specific induction of its ligands heparin-binding EGF and amphiregulin in human skin in vivo. *J Invest Dermatol.* 2006;126(4):732–739.

42. Temova Rakuša Ž, Škufca P, Kristl A, Roškar R. Quality control of retinoids in commercial cosmetic products. *J Cosmet Dermatol.* 2021;20(4):1166–1175.

43. Eitenmiller RR, Lee J. *vitamin E: food chemistry, composition, and analysis.* Boca Raton, FL: CRC Press; 2004: 16.

44. Lee SC, Lee KE, Kim JJ, Lim SH. The effect of cholesterol in the liposome bilayer on the stabilization of incorporated Retinol. *J Liposome Res.* 2005;15(3-4):157–166.

45. Rosenthal DS, Griffiths CE, Yuspa SH, Roop DR, Voorhees JJ. Acute or chronic topical retinoic acid treatment of human skin in vivo alters the expression of epidermal transglutaminase, loricrin, involucrin, filaggrin, and keratins 6 and 13 but not keratins 1, 10, and 14. *J Invest Dermatol.* 1992;98(3):343–350.

46. Griffiths CE, Finkel LJ, Tranfaglia MG, Hamilton TA, Voorhees JJ. An in vivo experimental model for effects of topical retinoic acid in human skin. *Br J Dermatol.* 1993;129(4):389–394.

47. Feng X, Peng ZH, Di W, et al. Suprabasal expression of a dominant-negative RXR alpha mutant in transgenic mouse epidermis impairs regulation of gene transcription and basal keratinocyte proliferation by RAR-selective retinoids. *Genes Dev.* 1997;11(1):59–71.

48. Kang S, Voorhees JJ. Photoaging therapy with topical tretinoin: an evidence-based analysis. *J Am Acad Dermatol.* 1998;39(2 Pt 3):S55–S61.

49. Digiovanna JJ, Mauro T, Milstone LM, Schmuth M, Toro JR. Systemic retinoids in the management of ichthyoses and related skin types. *Dermatol Ther.* 2013;26(1):26–38.

50. Tagami H, Tadaki T, Obata M, Koyama J. Functional assessment of the stratum corneum under the influence of oral aromatic retinoid (etretinate) in guinea-pigs and humans. Comparison with topical retinoic acid treatment. *Br J Dermatol.* 1992;127(5):470–475.

51. Effendy I, Kwangsukstith C, Lee LY, Maibach HI. Functional changes in human stratum corneum induced by topical glycolic acid: comparison with all-trans retinoic acid. *Acta Derm Venereol.* 1995;75(6):455–458.

52. Griffiths CE, Voorhees JJ. Human in vivo pharmacology of topical retinoids. *Arch Dermatol Res.* 1994;287(1):53–60.

53. Buchan P, Eckhoff C, Caron D, Nau H, Shroot B, Schaefer H. Repeated topical administration of all-trans-retinoic acid and plasma levels of retinoic acids in humans. *J Am Acad Dermatol.* 1994;30(3):428–434.

54. Jick SS, Terris BZ, Jick H. First trimester topical tretinoin and congenital disorders. *Lancet.* 1993;341(8854):1181–1182.

55. Vagotis FL, Brundage SR. Histologic study of dermabrasion and chemical peel in an animal model after pretreatment with Retin-A. *Aesthetic Plast Surg.* 1995;19(3):243–246.

56. Stuzin JM. Discussion. A randomized controlled trial of skin care protocols for facial resurfacing: lessons learned from the Plastic Surgery Educational Foundation's Skin Products Assessment Research study. *Plast Reconstr Surg.* 2011;127(3):1343–1345.

57. Elson ML. The role of retinoids in wound healing. *J Am Acad Dermatol.* 1998;39(2 Pt 3):S79–S81.

58. Popp C, Kligman AM, Stoudemayer TJ. Pretreatment of photoaged forearm skin with topical tretinoin accelerates healing of full-thickness wounds. *Br J Dermatol.* 1995;132(1):46–53.

59. Orringer JS, Kang S, Johnson TM, et al. Tretinoin treatment before carbon-dioxide laser resurfacing: a clinical and biochemical analysis. *J Am Acad Dermatol.* 2004;51(6):940–946.

60. Kim IH, Kim HK, Kye YC. Effects of tretinoin pretreatment on TCA chemical peel in guinea pig skin. *J Korean Med Sci.* 1996;11(4):335–341.

61. Basak PY, Eroglu E, Altuntas I, Agalar F, Basak K, Sutcu R. Comparison of the effects of tretinoin, adapalene and collagenase in an experimental model of wound healing. *Eur J Dermatol.* 2002;12(2):145–148.

62. Hung VC, Lee JY, Zitelli JA, Hebda PA. Topical tretinoin and epithelial wound healing. *Arch Dermatol.* 1989;125(1):65–69.

63. Levin AA, Sturzenbecker LJ, Kazmer S, et al. 9-cis retinoic acid stereoisomer binds and activates the nuclear receptor RXR alpha. *Nature.* 1992;355(6358):359–361.

64. Shalita A, Weiss JS, Chalker DK, Ellis CN, Greenspan A, Katz HI, et al. A comparison of the efficacy and safety of adapalene gel 0.1% and tretinoin gel 0.025% in the treatment of acne vulgaris: a multicenter trial. In: *J Am Acad Dermatol.* 1996;34(3):482–485.

65. Chandraratna RA. Tazarotene: the first receptor-selective topical retinoid for the treatment of psoriasis. *J Am Acad Dermatol.* 1997;37(2 Pt 3):S12–S17.

66. Burke BM, Cunliffe WJ. The assessment of acne vulgaris—the Leeds technique. *Br J Dermatol.* 1984;111(1):83–92.

67. Verschoore M, Bouclier M, Czernielewski J, Hensby C. Topical retinoids. Their uses in dermatology. *Dermatol Clin.* 1993;11(1):107–115.

68. Verschoore M, Poncet M, Czernielewski J, Sorba V, Clucas A. Adapalene 0.1% gel has low skin-irritation potential. *J Am Acad Dermatol.* 1997;36(6 Pt 2):S104–S109.

69. Sefton J, Kligman AM, Kopper SC, Lue JC, Gibson JR. Photodamage pilot study: a double-blind, vehicle-controlled study to assess the efficacy and safety of tazarotene 0.1% gel. *J Am Acad Dermatol*. 2000;43(4):656–663.

70. Leyden J. Split-face evaluation of the facial tolerability of tazarotene gel compared with tretinoin gels and adapalene gel. Poster presented at the 58th Annual Meeting of the American Academy of Dermatology. San Francisco, CA, March 10–15, 2000.

71. Kakita L. Tazarotene versus tretinoin or adapalene in the treatment of acne vulgaris. *J Am Acad Dermatol*. 2000;43(2 Pt 3): S51–S54.

72. Petronelli M. *Trifarotene cream proves safe, effective for acne vulgaris. Dermatology Times*. May 11, 2020. https://www.dermatologytimes.com/view/trifarotene-cream-proves-safe-effective-acne-vulgaris. Accessed April 30, 2021.

73. Tan J, Thiboutot D, Popp G, et al. Randomized phase 3 evaluation of trifarotene 50 μg/g cream treatment of moderate facial and truncal acne. *J Am Acad Dermatol*. 2019;80(6):1691–1699.

CHAPTER 46

Sunscreens

Leslie S. Baumann, MD
Edmund M. Weisberg, MS, MBE

SUMMARY POINTS

What's Important?

1. Over the last 30 years in the United States, the incidence of melanoma has increased by 270% despite dermatologists' consistent warnings to engage in skin-protective behaviors.
2. Physical sunscreens are often preferred over chemical sunscreens, but physical sunscreens may not block all wavelengths of UV light and are less aesthetically appealing, as they appear white or violet on the skin.
3. The daily use of sunscreen is not the first-line defense against the ravages of the sun and does not indemnify a person from photodamage or give one license to stay out longer because of one application. It must be used in conjunction with other skin-protective behaviors.
4. Sunscreen is the most effective anti-aging skincare product.

What's New?

1. After many years of debate, the US Food and Drug Administration has not yet released a final monograph for nonprescription OTC sunscreen formulations.

What's Coming?

1. Hopefully new effective and environmentally safe SPF ingredients will be developed soon.
2. More educational campaigns on the importance of daily SPF use are needed.

For several years, dermatologists have exhorted their patients to avoid or, at the very least, severely limit exposure to the sun since ultraviolet (UV) radiation is the primary cause of skin cancer, exogenous skin aging, wrinkles, and blotchy pigmentation.[1] In spite of these attempts to educate the public, the incidence of skin cancer is climbing at a disturbing rate. Over the last 30 years in the United States US, the incidence of melanoma has increased by 270%, with rises in UV exposure as well as surveillance cited among several factors for the higher incidence.[2,3] Alarmingly, there were 82,054 new cases of melanoma in the US in 2019, with 11,906 deaths due to this most potent and fatal of the skin cancers.[4] Cosmetic patients offer a captive and interested audience that can be educated about the hazards of the sun and the need for corresponding protective behavior. Of all the skincare advice doled out to patients, this is likely the most important, because proper protection from the sun will make a great difference in the patient's future appearance. Patients should be advised that if they do not avoid the sun and practice protective measures, they are wasting their money on cosmetic products and procedures.

With the ever-present potential for year-round solar exposure, it is always that time of year for dermatologists. That is, every patient interaction is an appropriate time for dermatologists to suggest the use of a daily broad-spectrum sunscreen and other skin-protective behavior (e.g., wearing SPF clothing, hats, as well as sunglasses, and sun avoidance between 10 AM and 4 PM) that shields the skin from the deleterious effects of solar exposure. One strategy is to remind patients that a daily SPF is the most effective anti-aging skincare product.

There are significant differences between physical (inorganic) and chemical (organic) sunscreen ingredients, though, with much greater confidence expressed by scientists in the safety of physical sunscreens. Many patients also present with questions related to reports on the relative safety of sunscreen ingredients issued by the Environmental Working Group (EWG), which claimed that 260 products among more than 750 sunscreen formulations met their criteria in 2021.[5,6] The focus here will be on some recent studies related to salient sunscreen issues, with an emphasis on the preferred physical sunscreens, attitudes about sunscreen use, and what patients need to know. This chapter also discusses the practical aspects of sunscreen formulations and selection, which should enhance the practitioner's ability to help patients find the best sunscreen protection for their skin type and lifestyle as well as answer patients' numerous product questions.

ULTRAVIOLET A AND B

On a typical summer day, UVA comprises approximately 96.5% of the UV radiation reaching earth, leaving UVB only with the remaining 3.5%.[7] When compared with all kinds of light reaching the earth's surface, UVA makes up 9.5% (**Fig. 46-1**). While UVA is the predominant UV light reaching the earth's surface, UVB exposure is more likely to cause squamous cell carcinoma in an experimental setting.[8] This supports the usage of sunscreens intended to block UVB. The first sunscreens developed were designed to prevent erythema (skin reddening) and sunburns by blocking UVB, and did little to block UVA. UVA exposure leads to immunosuppression and is thought to play a role in the development of melanoma.[9] Therefore, both UVA and UVB sunscreens should be used. UV light exerts its carcinogenic effect on the skin by inducing mutations in DNA. DNA is considered a chromophore for UV light. Although maximum UV absorption by DNA occurs at 260 nm, UVB is considered a major source of DNA damage.[10] UV irradiation results in DNA damage by formation of two dimers between adjacent pyrimidines, cyclobutane pyrimidine dimers (CPDs), and pyrimidine 6 to 4 photoproducts. Nucleotide excision repair (NER) enzymes are responsible for removal of these carcinogenic products. If not repaired, mutations in the DNA sequence—also known as UV "signature mutations"—may occur.

UVB is blocked by glass and the amount of UVB that reaches the earth's surface varies by the time of day, with maximal rays reaching the earth from 10 AM to 4 PM. UVA radiation, on the other hand, can pass through glass (**Fig. 46-2**). Its ability to reach the earth's surface remains more constant regardless of the time of day or the amount of cloud cover (**Fig. 46-3**). UVA penetrates deeper into the skin, contributing to cutaneous wrinkling and aging. UVA radiation is also known to cause damage to the dermal layer of the skin (**Fig. 46-4**). In a study performed by Lavker et al., repeated exposures to suberythemic doses of UVA resulted in greater epidermal thickness, in addition to deposition of lysosomes on elastin fibers, as well as decreased Langerhans cells and dermal inflammatory infiltrates.[11] Unfortunately, the sun protection factor (SPF) primarily assesses the protective effects against UVB light, leaving UVA out of the picture. In other words, if SPF 45 is on a label, this applies to UVB protection only and provides no information about protection against UVA radiation.

SUN PROTECTION FACTOR

The SPF represents the ability of a sunscreen to delay sun-induced skin erythema, which is a visible sign of damage mainly caused by UVB radiation. SPF is defined technically as the

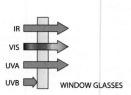

FIGURE 46-2. UVB is blocked by glass while infrared (IR), visible (VIS), and UVA light can penetrate glass. New plastic coatings are available to coat glass to prevent UVA penetration.

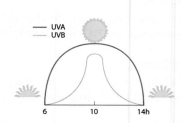

FIGURE 46-3. UVA rays reach the earth's surface throughout the day, as opposed to UVB, which reaches the earth maximally between 10 AM and 4 PM.

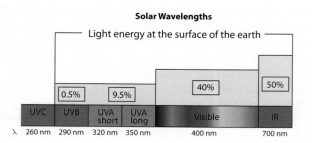

FIGURE 46-1. Solar wavelengths. On a normal day, UVA is the predominant UV type at the surface of the earth.

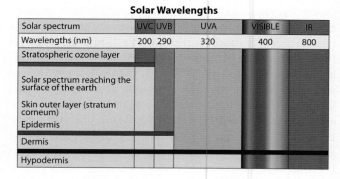

FIGURE 46-4. UVA, visible light, and infrared radiation can penetrate into the dermis, while UVB cannot.

level of sun exposure needed to produce a minimal erythema dose divided by the amount of energy required to produce the same erythema on unprotected skin. In theory, a subject that applies an SPF 10 sunscreen on uncovered skin could stay in the sun 10 times longer without incurring a visible skin erythemal reaction. The SPF is determined through testing on the untanned skin of human volunteers (generally the back or the upper part of the buttocks).

The internationally agreed upon standard quantity of sunscreen per unit of skin surface (i.e., the sunscreen thickness) required to measure the SPF in humans is 2 mg/cm^2 of skin.[12] For an adult to apply this amount of sunscreen to the entire body, 30 mL of sunscreen would be required to obtain that thickness.[13] In most cases people do not apply enough sunscreen.[14] Facial powders, for example, are exceedingly difficult to apply in an amount sufficient to equal the 2 mg/cm^2 of skin that is used in testing to determine the SPF. The average face is about 600 cm^2; therefore, a person would need to apply about 1.2 g of facial powder to get the SPF stated on the product's label. The primary author has found in her practice that most women apply only about 0.085 g of powder at a time. In other words, one would have to apply 14 times the amount of powder normally used to be sufficiently protected against the sun (**Fig. 46-5A and B**). Facial SPF lotion applications tend to amount to about 0.8 g per average application, as measured in the primary author's practice. Therefore, individuals would need to use about 1.5 times the amount of facial lotion they are accustomed to using in order to achieve the SPF on the label. In fact, a recent study demonstrated that most users probably achieve a mean SPF of between 20% and 50% of that expected from the product label because they do not apply the sunscreen as thickly as is performed in laboratory conditions.[15] The key is to apply a sufficient amount of sunscreen evenly across a given area to achieve the intended solar protection.

The notion of inadequate sunscreen application was also suggested by a study of European students that found that the students used approximately one-fifth of the recommended sunscreen quantity.[13] A useful rule-of-thumb is that the protection most people ultimately obtain from a sunscreen is equal to about one-third of the SPF. So applying an SPF-15 sunscreen at a typical application thickness to the face provides about five-fold protection, not 15-fold.[16] While still counseling patients on the proper amount of sunscreen to apply, it is advisable to recommend the highest SPF sunscreen that the patient can tolerate to compensate for this discrepancy.

In the past, the SPF system was based mainly on UVB (280–315 nm) exposure, which is responsible for the immediate reddening seen on the skin. It is important to remember that UVA-associated reddening is seen much later and, therefore, UVA exposure and dose would not be accounted for in the current methods of measuring SPF. UVA light is also responsible for darkening pigment seen after sun exposure. Because of the damaging effects of UVA, there is new research regarding the incorporation of UVA (320–400 nm) into the sun protection index. Globally, there are several UVA rating systems and the FDA is currently trying to decide which rating system to make the standard in the US. Because there is no consensus standard for UVA testing, products in the US do not provide any UVA coverage information on the product label. This is obviously a significant problem.

THE FDA AND SUNSCREEN

More than a decade ago, the FDA was considering the problem of UVA and sunscreen labeling. In August 2007, the FDA proposed the creation of a new rating system for UVA sunscreen products.[17] This system would be based on a scale of one to four stars, with one star representing low UVA protection, two stars, medium protection, three stars, high protection, and four stars, the highest UVA protection available in an over-the-counter (OTC) sunscreen product. Under this proposal, a sunscreen product that fails to provide at least a low level (one star) of protection would bear a "no UVA protection" marking on the front label near the SPF value. In addition, a warning would be

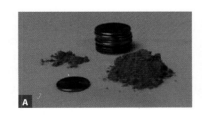
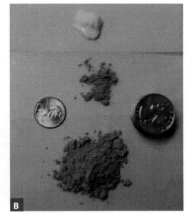

FIGURE 46-5. A. The powder on the left is the amount of powder the average woman uses, while the powder pile on the right is the amount of powder necessary to use to meet the SPF on the sunscreen label. The white lotion is the amount of facial lotion required to use on the face to meet the SPF on the label. **B.** The same image viewed from above. In the upper portion of this photo is the amount of facial lotion required to use on the face to meet the SPF on the product label, while the large pile of powder is the amount needed to cover the face with powder to achieve the SPF on the label.

required on labels stating: "UV exposure from the sun increases the risk of skin cancer, premature skin aging, and other skin damage. It is important to decrease UV exposure by limiting time in the sun, wearing protective clothing, and using a sunscreen." It was hoped that this warning would increase awareness that sun avoidance and limiting sun exposure are also necessary. This proposal has not yet been accepted and the star rating system, or any comparable system, is not yet in place.

Dermatologists have long recommended sunscreen use for all ages beyond 6 months, with infants to be completely shielded from the sun; in more recent times, these suggestions have included daily sunscreen use to protect against photoaging, nonmelanoma skin cancers, and melanoma. Notably, a meta-analysis reviewing over 1,300 article titles and covering 270 articles in detail revealed in 2008 that melanoma risk rises with an increasing number of sunburns during all periods of life, not just childhood.[18] For several years, the FDA has discussed issuing a final monograph for nonprescription OTC sunscreen formulations. Such guidelines would be helpful to disseminate to patients. As of publication, the final monograph had not yet been produced. Nevertheless, there remains a copious amount of information and advice to filter for patients. However, in issuing proposed rules in advance of a final monograph for nonprescription OTC sunscreens, the FDA has described the conditions under which such products are generally recognized as safe and effective (GRASE) and not misleadingly labeled, with the physical sunblocks identified as sufficiently safe.[19] Search www.fda.gov to find out the current sunscreen rulings.

TESTING TO DETERMINE UVA PROTECTION

As suggested above, ascertaining the optimal UVA rating method is difficult and even contentious. Each manufacturer believes that the method they use is the best. L'Oréal developed the persistent pigment darkening (PPD) method,[20] while Johnson & Johnson created the protection factor UVA (PFA) method.[21] The PPD and PFA are very similar approaches in that they both measure end-result tanning.[22] The FDA has not yet determined which UVA measurement method is best because all methods lack an endpoint measure that is a true surrogate marker for long wavelength (i.e., > 340 nm) UVA-induced skin damage (i.e., skin cancer or photoaging).[22] The FDA seems to be most seriously considering two methods of UVA testing: the critical wavelength method and the PFA (PA) method. The critical wavelength was developed in 1994 and is an *in vitro* testing method.[23] It involves placing a certain amount of sunscreen on a slide and exposing the slide to progressively higher wavelengths of light starting at 290 nm, the beginning of the UVB range. When 10% of the incident light passes through the slide, or the protection provided by the sunscreen has dropped to 90%, the corresponding wavelength of light is recorded. For sunscreens with SPF 15 or above, this is a good measure of UVA protection. If one is testing a low-SPF product, below SPF 15, this is thought to be a suboptimal method.

The PFA (PA) method is similar to the UVB SPF rating insofar as it is an *in vivo* test that measures what is in essence the tanning effect of short wavelength UVA rays (320–350 nm).[24] This is widely used in Europe. However, the PFA (PA) system measures an observed effect (tanning), not the biologic endpoint. It is possible that the FDA will recommend a combination of the critical wavelength and PFA (PA) methods (see **Tables 46-1 and 46-2** for a brief summary of the three types of tests to ascertain sunscreen efficacy and for related non-US standards).

Another approach to measuring UVA involves the quantitative measurement of free radicals in human skin induced

TABLE 46-1	Three Types of Tests to Determine Sunscreen Efficacy		
	Sun Protection Factor (SPF)	**UVA Protection Factor (UVAPF)**	**Broad-Spectrum Protection and Photostability**
Goal	To protect skin against UVB (and some UVA) wavelengths	To protect skin from developing persistent pigment darkening (PPD) induced by UVA exposure	To provide broad-spectrum protection against UVB and UVA; to prevent rapid degradation from UV exposure
Method(s)	Testing on humans to compare time of exposure necessary to induce mild skin reddening, or minimum erythema dose (MED), in absence of the product with time needed to induce the same MED in the presence of the product.	Testing on humans to compare the time of exposure necessary to induce mild skin darkening in the absence of the product with the time required to induce the same level of darkening in the presence of the product.	Laboratory testing to measure the absorbance of light at each wavelength, arriving at a relative ratio of absorbance in the UVB and UVA ranges as well as photostability. The most common measure of broad-spectrum efficacy is critical wavelength (CW).[a] Photostability is measured as the ratio of the absorbance of the formula before irradiation to the absorbance of the formula after irradiation with a particular UV amount.
Result	This ratio = SPF	This ratio = UVAPF	Broad spectrum, if CW ≥ 370 nm[b]; the photostability value = Beta-value

[a]The FDA may use the same test with a slightly different measurement, considering the ratio of longer wavelength UVA1 (340–400 nm) compared to the total UV (UVA+UVB absorbance).
[b]This is the standard in the European Union (EU) and will be soon adopted in the Association of Southeast Asian Nations (ASEAN).

TABLE 46-2	EU and ASEAN Standards for Sunscreens		
SPF	PPD	CW	Label
≥ 6	≥ one-third of the SPF value (e.g., the PPD ≥ 5 for an SPF 15 product; PPD ≥ 10 for SPF 30)	≥ 370 nm	Products that meet all 3 criteria = labeled as broad spectrum; products that do not = labeled as NOT providing UVA protection

by UV radiation.[25] Reactive free radicals have been correlated with the occurrence of skin damage such as cancer and skin aging. The method of measuring free radicals is known as electron spin resonance (ESR) spectroscopy. This technique incorporates the radical trapping properties of nitroxides. Nitroxides are antioxidant and anticancer substances. In a 2003 study, the nitroxides TEMPO, PCM, and PCA were used because of their known capacity to trap reactive free radicals in skin exposed to UV irradiation. The effects of UV radiation on the nitroxides can be measured because they reduce to hydroxylamines. The nitroxide PCA is found universally in skin and is solely reduced by UV-generated free radicals and reactive oxygen species (ROS), thus making it possible to estimate the penetration of UVA and UVB irradiation. UV irradiation decreases the PCA intensity, and this reduction has been shown to be engendered mainly by UVA radiation. Therefore, using ESR, the *in vivo* detection of UV-generated free radicals/ROS via the reduction of the nitroxide PCA in human skin should be possible.[26]

An additional method used to assess UVA radiation damage is comparing the accumulation levels of p53, which is known to be an important tumor suppressor gene. Mutations in p53 have been noted in more than 90% of squamous cell carcinomas, 50% of basal cell carcinomas (BCCs), and 60% of actinic keratoses.[27] Expression of p53 is used to quantify harm associated with UV-related skin damage and can be used to evaluate the effectiveness of sunscreens.

In a 2000 study, two sunscreens with identical SPF but varying UVA protection factors were evaluated using the PPD method.[28] The PPD is a measure of the amount of darkening pigment present a day or so after sun exposure. The SPF of the sunscreens was 7, while the UVA protection factor (UVA-PF) determined *in vivo* using the PPD method was 7 for one product and 3 for the other. The amount of p53 was also measured in skin exposed to UV radiation. The results showed that only partial protection was afforded by the two sunscreens with identical SPF, but there was a lower level of p53 in the areas of skin treated with the sunscreen of higher UVA protection factor. The results portrayed a marked increase in the amount of p53 in the skin with increasing exposure to higher levels of UVA radiation. These results confirmed that SPF based on erythemal reaction caused by UVB does not accurately predict the level of protection conferred against UVA damage from sun exposure.[28]

Other Sunscreen Terminology

A sunscreen is considered **water resistant** if the SPF level is determined effective after 40 minutes of water immersion. The testing procedure for these sunscreens is as follows: the subjects must swim in an indoor pool for 20 minutes followed by air drying (not towel drying) the skin. The subjects are then asked to swim for another 20 minutes followed by an air-drying period. The water-resistant sunscreen SPF is then measured after the total 40 minutes of water contact.[29] The FDA requires that the SPF listed on the label reflect the SPF that is achieved after this water-resistant testing rather than the SPF value present before testing.

Sunscreens that are labeled **very water resistant** have been shown to exhibit an effective SPF after undergoing the following testing: the subjects swim in an indoor pool for 20 minutes then air dry for 20 minutes. The procedure is repeated for a total of 80 minutes of water immersion. If a sunscreen retains its protective integrity after four 20-minute water immersions, it is considered **very water resistant.** It is important to note that the word "waterproof" is no longer allowed in labeling because it is misleading. No sunscreen is completely waterproof.

The lipophilic base of the vehicle used in these "water-resistant" formulations allows the products to adhere well to the skin, though their typically greasy feel is not often welcome by users. Depending on the ingredients used, the higher SPF formulations tend to be oilier or more opaque.

SUNSCREEN CLASSIFICATION

The two generally recognized major types of sunscreen products are chemical and physical. Chemical sunscreens absorb UV energy but also can generate free radicals, engender skin allergies, and pose the risk of systemic absorption. Some chemical sunscreen ingredients have been demonstrated to display estrogenic activity. Physical sunscreens provide a protective coating to the skin while reflecting harmful UV rays. While strongly preferred by dermatologists, physical sunscreens may not block all wavelengths of UV light and are less aesthetically appealing, as they appear white or violet on the skin.

Physical Sunscreens

Barrier sunscreens, known more commonly as physical sunscreens, scatter or reflect UV radiation and are rarely associated with allergic reactions. These sunscreens block the widest range of light including UV, visible, and infrared spectra, and are recommended for use especially when intense sun exposure, such as at the beach or at high altitudes, is expected. Patients with sensitive skin are more likely to tolerate this type of sunscreen, as opposed to the chemical variety. Titanium dioxide (TiO_2), magnesium oxide, iron oxide, and zinc oxide (ZnO) are the primary ingredients in physical sunscreens. The older formulations require a thick layer of application, melt in the sun, stain clothing, and can be comedogenic. Some of these agents are so opaque that they are visible and, consequently, often cosmetically unacceptable to most people. Some manufacturers have marketed opaque products in bright colors specifically designed for use by children.

Zinc Oxide and Titanium Dioxide

Discovered in the 1960s as essential for human health and development, zinc is a trace element not synthesized by the human body. However, it acts as a cofactor in over 300 enzymes necessary for cell function. Zinc deficiency has been linked to skin alterations, delayed wound healing, and hair loss. Zinc oxide (ZO), a metal oxide best known as a physical sunblock ingredient, has a significant profile in the dermatologic armamentarium. It is the main active ingredient in calamine lotion, an antipruritic compound used to treat various mild conditions, such as bites and stings from insects, eczema, poison ivy, rashes, and sunburn. ZnO is also found in OTC ointments or suppository form for healing hemorrhoids and fissures, and is used widely in baby powders, barrier creams, moisturizers, antiseptic ointments, anti-dandruff shampoos, athletic bandage tape, and, of course, sunscreens.[30,31] In addition, it has been shown to exhibit antibacterial properties (particularly in nanoparticle form as opposed to bulk),[32] and found to be effective in compression dressings for surgical wounds,[33,34] as well as in combination with 4% hydroquinone and 10% L-ascorbic acid to alleviate early signs of photodamage in normal to oily skin.[35]

Cosmetically acceptable translucent or colloidal suspensions consisting of micronized preparations of ZnO and TiO_2 have been recently developed. These formulations are popular because they remain on the skin's surface and are not systemically absorbed, which minimizes irritation and sensitization, and maximizes their safety profile.[36] In fact, reports of contact allergy to either of these components are exceedingly rare.[36,37] In the early 1990s, microfine ZnO became available.[38] Microfine ZnO absorbs appreciably more UV light in the long-wave UVA spectrum (340–380 nm). The only other sunscreen ingredient approved for use in the US that protects against this UVA spectrum is the organic chemical avobenzone (butylmethoxydibenzoylmethane). Because avobenzone is photolabile in UV light, its protective ability is uncertain.[39] Notably, ZnO and TiO_2 are not photolabile. However, newer photostable formulations of avobenzone have been developed. Formulations containing micronized ZnO or TiO_2 are the most often recommended products for sensitive skin types; however, ZnO or TiO_2 products are not interchangeable. Microfine TiO_2 effectively attenuates UVB (290–320 nm) and UVA2 (320–340 nm); however, it is less effective than ZnO in the UVA1 range (> 340 nm).[38,40] Microfine ZnO has a particle size of less than 0.2 μm. At this size, visible light scattering is minimized, and the particles appear transparent in thin films.[41] TiO_2 has a higher refractive index in visible light than ZnO (2.6 for TiO_2 and 1.9 for ZnO)[38]; therefore, TiO_2 is whiter and more difficult to incorporate into transparent products than is ZnO.

One problem with metal oxides that contain physical sunscreens, though, is that they may produce oxygen free radicals at their surface when irradiated. The photoreactivity of metal oxides has been extensively studied,[42] and it even has been suggested that photoactive metal oxides may initiate deleterious events in the skin. Generally, TiO_2 is much more photoactive than ZnO as shown in a report by Mitchnick et al.[38] TiO_2 has even been shown to damage DNA in *in vitro* studies.[43] However, to affect skin, the particles would have to traverse the stratum corneum (SC). Since particles of microfine ZnO and TiO_2 are too large to enter the skin, they would not be expected to be biologically active. Most companies minimize the photoreactivity of these agents by coating the surface with dimethicone or silicone.[44]

In large particle form, TiO_2 and ZnO are non-chemical sunscreens favored by physicians for their very nature. These compounds have been shown in nanoparticle form to be effective barriers against UV-induced damage, rendering more robust protection against UV insult, while leaving less white residue, than previous generations of the physical sunblocks. They absorb UV radiation, leading to photocatalysis and the release of ROS.[45]

Safety Studies

In 2009, Filipe et al. assessed the localization and potential skin penetration of TiO_2 and ZnO nanoparticles, dispersed in three sunscreen formulations, under realistic *in vivo* conditions in normal and altered skin. They considered a test hydrophobic formulation containing coated 20-nm TiO_2 nanoparticles and two commercially available sunscreen products containing TiO_2 alone or combined with ZnO, with respect to how consumers actually use sunscreens as compared to the recommended standard condition for the SPF test. The researchers observed that traces of the physical blockers could be detected only at the skin surface and uppermost area of the SC in normal human skin after 2 hours of exposure. After 48 hours, layers deeper than the SC contained no detectable TiO_2 or ZnO nanoparticles. The investigators also found preferential deposition of the nanoparticles in the openings of pilosebaceous follicles but no penetration into viable skin tissue. They concluded that significant penetration of TiO_2 or ZnO nanoparticles to keratinocytes is unlikely.[46]

The following year, Gulson et al. determined, in a small study with 20 individuals, that trace amounts of zinc from ZnO in sunscreens applied for 5 consecutive days outdoors were absorbed in the skin. Levels of the stable isotope tracer (68)Zn in blood and urine from females who received the nano-sunscreen were higher than in males receiving the same sunscreen and higher than all participants who received the bulk sunscreen.[47] As Wang and Tooley have cautioned, the concerns regarding the safety of nanoparticles in sunscreens relates to potential toxicity and the capacity to penetrate the skin.[48] However, as zinc is a safe and essential mineral, there is no concern with zinc-containing sunscreens.

In 2011, Kang et al. demonstrated that TiO_2 nanoparticles, but not normal-sized TiO_2, and UVA synergistically promote rapid ROS production and breakdown of mitochondrial membrane potential, leading to apoptosis, and that TiO_2 nanoparticles are more phototoxic than larger ones.[49] Also that year, though, Tyner et al. found that barrier function was not diminished by nanoscale TiO_2 use and that optimal UV attenuation resulted when TiO_2 particles are stabilized with a coating and evenly dispersed (i.e., as with non-agglomerated coated nanoscale materials). They concluded that nanoscale TiO_2 is nontoxic and may impart greater efficacy.[50]

According to Schilling et al., evidence suggests minimal risks to human health from the use of TiO_2 or ZnO nanoparticles at concentrations of up to 25% in cosmetic preparations or sunscreens, regardless of coatings or crystalline structure. In their safety review of these ingredients, the researchers explained that the TiO_2 and ZnO nanoparticles featured in sunscreen formulations occur as aggregates of primary particles 30–150 nm in size that bond in a manner that renders them impervious to the force of product application. With structure of the nanoparticles unaffected, no primary particles are released. The nanoparticles also display equivalence with larger particles in terms of distribution and duration and, therefore, recognition and elimination from the body, the authors concluded.[51] Safety studies conducted between 2009 and 2011 indicated that TiO_2 and ZnO nanoparticles are safe when applied to intact human skin, with no data suggesting significant penetration of the particles beyond the SC.[48,52–54] Currently, most authorities concur that TiO_2 and ZnO nanoparticles do not penetrate into viable skin layers and that evidence suggests the benefits of using such products far outweigh the risks.[55] A 2017 risk assessment of ZnO by Kim et al. showed that all forms (cream, lotion, spray, and propellant) were within safe ranges for human use in up to 25% concentrations.[56] Dréno et al. reported in 2019 that TiO_2 nanoparticles do appear to be safe at the cutaneous level (not penetrating beyond the outer SC to the general circulation in healthy or impaired skin) in concentrations of up to 25% but note that sprayable products or powders may present some risk to the lungs based on some animal studies, adding that the EU Cosmetic Regulation authorizing nano-TiO_2 as a UV filter excludes formulations that can reach the lungs.[57]

Summary

TiO_2 and ZnO have long been used safely and effectively as the two primary inorganic physical sunscreens. ZnO is a particularly versatile substance with multiple indications in dermatology, warranting its inclusion in various sunscreens, moisturizers, and shampoos. The use of both of these metal oxides in nanoparticle form represents one of the many subjects debated within the larger sunscreen context. Their use in nanoparticle form appears to be most effective but the different physicochemical qualities of the metal oxide in nanosize form have prompted questions regarding safety. Most such questions have been answered, as current data suggest minimal risk to intact skin but ongoing studies in real-world conditions (i.e., UV exposure, sunburn) continue.

Chemical Sunscreens

Chemical sunscreens are usually combined with physical sunscreens or with each other to form high-SPF products that can be used during times of significant sun exposure. However, there are several disadvantages to these products. Chemical sunscreens absorb UV radiation. The absorbed radiation must then be dissipated as either heat or light, or else be used in some chemical reaction. This may result in the creation of ROS or photoproducts that can attack other chemicals in a formulation; if absorbed, such by-products can attack the skin itself (see Chapter 39, Antioxidants, for a discussion of free radicals and antioxidants). However, in most cases, the radiation simply is emitted again at a longer wavelength and does not lead to free radical formation.[38]

Chemical sunscreens are composed of synthetically prepared organic chemicals that can be broadly labeled as UVB- or UVA-absorbing substances. These colorless, often-odorless agents prevent UV radiation from penetrating the epidermis by acting as filters as they absorb and reflect UV radiation. Many chemical sunscreens have been reported to cause allergic or photoallergic reactions in susceptible patients. Another drawback of chemical sunscreens is that some of them are unstable when exposed to UV radiation. For example, a 15-minute exposure to solar-simulated light has been reported to destroy 36% of avobenzone.[39] Moreover, as avobenzone degrades, other organic sunscreen agents in the formula may be destroyed as well.[58] Some chemical sunscreens are systemically absorbed and levels have been demonstrated in the urine of humans using the product.[59] For this reason, chemical sunscreens should not be used in children younger than 2 years of age. Several popular chemical sunscreen additives will be discussed below.

STABILITY OF SUNSCREENS

A viable sunscreen product must be photostable or maintain its intended protection for a limited time before inevitable breakdown caused by UV exposure. Photostability is characterized by the effect of light on the degradation of certain substances. The photostability of a sunscreen depends on varying factors such as which filters were used, as well as the types of UV filters, solvents, and vehicles. A common means of measuring and quantifying photostability is through the comet assay test, which assesses DNA damage in cells. It is categorized as a gel-electrophoresis-based test.[60] Recent studies have attempted to evaluate the stability of sunscreens. Avobenzone, a common filter in sunscreens and potent absorber of UV radiation, has been shown to be increasingly photolabile. For this reason, photostable forms of avobenzone (such as Helioplex™) have been developed. Subsequent findings have suggested adding Tinosorb, a UVA filter, in conjunction with avobenzone to improve the photostability of avobenzone. When Tinosorb is combined with avobenzone, it prevents avobenzone's degradation caused by UV irradiation.[61] In one study, four different UV filters commonly used in SPF-15 sunscreens were compared using HPLC analysis and spectrophotometry.

The following were the UV filter combinations tested: octyl methoxycinnamate (OMC), benzophenone (BP)-3, and octyl salicylate (OS) (formulation 1); OMC, avobenzone (AVB), and 4-methylbenzilidene camphor (MBC) (formulation 2); OMC, BP-3, and octocrylene (OC) (formulation 3); and OMC, AVB, and OC (formulation 4). The results showed that all four of the UV filter combinations presented varying photostability. The best results were demonstrated by formulation 3 (OMC, BP-3, and OC), followed by, in descending order, formulations 4, 1, and 2. In addition, OC improved the photostability of OMC, AVB, and BP-3.[62] For this reason, many sunscreens on the market contain combinations of sunscreen ingredients.

A formulation called UV Pearls utilizes microencapsulation technology to entrap organic sunscreen chemicals in a sol-gel silica glass. This enables the incorporation of hydrophobic UV filters into the aqueous phase of sunscreen formulations. The "encapsulation of sunscreens" allows physical separation between organic and inorganic ingredients. This results in an increased overall photostability in sunscreen products. In addition, it is believed that encapsulating UV filters will significantly decrease the dermal uptake of these UV filters, and reduce the amount of free radicals generated by keeping the organic filters on the top layers of the skin. This diminishes penetration into the deeper layers and decreases the risk of contact dermatitis.[63]

UVB-ABSORBING SUNSCREEN FORMULATIONS

Para-aminobenzoic Acid

Poorly soluble in water, thus only suitable for alcohol-containing vehicles, para-aminobenzoic acid (PABA) was one of the first commonly used sunscreen ingredients. PABA established a reputation for inducing a stinging sensation in the skin and staining both cotton and synthetic fabrics. Subsequent formulations were labeled as "PABA-free" because of the widespread negative publicity associated with such characteristics. To skirt this problem, manufacturers developed PABA derivatives, which are water soluble and unable to penetrate the SC. Octyl diethyl PABA or padimate O, a potent absorber of UVB, is the main derivative used. Photoallergic reactions have been reported in association with the use of PABA and its derivatives.

Cinnamates

This category of compounds has largely replaced PABA derivatives. OMC, with a UV absorption maximum of 310 nm, is the most commonly used. Several cosmetic products, including makeup foundations, lipsticks, and leave-in hair conditioners, contain this compound. The Freeze 24/7 Iceshield uses the UV Pearl technology in which OMC is encapsulated in sol-gel silica glass and formulated into a wash-on sunscreen. In other words, it is a cleanser that deposits sunscreen on the skin with cleansing. This is a great option for people who do not like the greasy feel of sunscreen (men, in particular, are reputed to complain about greasy formulations).

Because cinnamates are poorly soluble in water, they do not wash off with cleansing and are often included in water-resistant and very water-resistant sunscreens. Although allergy to these agents is unusual, photoallergic reactions have been reported in association with the use of formulations containing cinnamates. It is believed that coating the particles with the sol-gel silica glass may decrease the incidence of allergy. Patients allergic to this compound may also be allergic to fragrances and flavorings that contain cinnamic aldehyde and cinnamon oil.[64]

Salicylates

With a UV absorption maximum at 310 nm, salicylates are used to augment the UVB protection in sunscreens. OS (2-ethyl hexyl salicylate) and homosalate (homomethyl salicylate) are the most popular salicylates in sunscreens. These compounds are stable, nonsensitizing, and water insoluble, yielding high substantivity. The chemical properties of salicylates render them highly suitable for combination with other chemical sunscreen agents, such as benzophenones, in cosmetic formulations. In fact, salicylates are used only in combination with other UV filters because they are too weak to be the sole active filtering ingredients. Contact allergy to salicylates is quite rare.

Phenylbenzimidazole Sulfonic Acid

In contrast to other UV filters that are soluble in the oil phase, phenylbenzimidazole sulfonic acid (PSA) is water soluble. As a result, this ingredient imparts a less oily feel to sunscreen formulations. Unfortunately, PSA, like salicylates, is a selective UVB filter and allows almost full UVA transmission. This compound may be more suitable in combination with other filters.

UVA-ABSORBING SUNSCREEN FORMULATIONS

Benzophenones

The absorption range for benzophenones is predominantly in the UVA portion of the light spectrum between 320–350 nm. Oxybenzone, which is frequently used to augment UVB protection, has an absorption maximum at 326 nm. This compound is also one of the best blockers of UVA2 (shorter UVA wavelengths) available in the US. Oxybenzone is a very common sunscreen ingredient, and it is estimated that 20% to 30% of sunscreens contain this chemical.[65] Unfortunately, oxybenzone is one of the common sunscreen agents to cause photoallergic contact dermatitis.[64,66] One case report described a 22-year-old female that developed anaphylaxis after widespread application of a sunscreen containing oxybenzone.[65] The allergy to oxybenzone was later confirmed by skin testing. Further, it has been well established that systemic absorption of oxybenzone occurs. A study in the *Lancet* demonstrated in humans that application of substantial amounts of a sunscreen containing oxybenzone resulted in the oxybenzone being absorbed and subsequently excreted in urine.[59] Oxybenzone has low acute toxicity as reported from animal studies yet little is known about its chronic toxicity and disposition after topical application in humans, though it is emerging as a potential contaminant.[67,68] For this reason, sunscreens containing this agent are not recommended for use in children.

Menthyl Anthranilate

The absorption peak for this compound is at 340 nm. Consequently, it is a weak UVB filter, but offers effective UVA2 protection. Menthyl anthranilate is less widely used than benzophenone because it is less effective.

Parsol 1789

Parsol 1789 (AVB or butyl methoxydibenzoylmethane) has an absorption maximum at 355 nm and provides superior UVA protection. This ingredient was approved by the FDA in the late 1990s. Parsol 1789 has also been frequently reported to cause photoallergic dermatitis.[64] AVB is one of the most commonly used UVA-blocking ingredients. The initial formulations had significant issues with stability. However, since 2007 several stabilized forms of AVB have become commercially available, including Helioplex by Neutrogena and Active Photobarrier Complex by Aveeno. Sunscreens manufactured before 2007 should be discarded.

Mexoryl®

After years of negotiations, the FDA approved the UVA filter Mexoryl. It is found in many L'Oréal brands including La Roche-Posay, Vichy, and Lancôme. Mexoryl SX is the formulation approved in the US. It does not block UV light quite as effectively as Mexoryl XL, which is not yet available in the US. However, Mexoryl SX is a water-soluble formulation and therefore feels less greasy on the skin and more suitable for everyday use. In contrast, Mexoryl XL is oil soluble, making it more suitable as a water-resistant sunscreen. Mexoryl SX is an organic filter found to be very effective against shorter UVA wavelengths. These short UVA waves (320–340 nm) constitute 95% of UV radiation that reaches the earth. Mexoryl can be added in combination with other UV filters. In contrast to AVB, Mexoryl is photostable and does not degrade when exposed to UV radiation.[69]

Sunscreen Combinations

Many sunscreen formulations contain combinations of active sunscreen ingredients to enhance protection and alter the aesthetics of the product. The FDA regulates which sunscreens can be combined with others, recognizing that certain sunscreen ingredients are incompatible and can actually lower the SPF rating of a product when combined.[29] Combinations are employed to achieve a higher SPF using a lower concentration of sunscreen ingredients.

ROLE OF ANTIOXIDANTS IN SUNSCREENS

Just as the body has its own immune defense system, the skin has its own antioxidant defense system. This system protects the skin from UV-induced oxidative damage. Excess UV radiation can prevent free radicals in the skin from being absorbed by this natural defense mechanism, thus leading to cancer, wrinkling, and aging. This excess of UV exposure calls for the induction and use of antioxidant enzymes.[27] Such enzymes act as UV filters and capture the free radicals before they cause damage. Retinyl esters, a storage form of vitamin A, have been found to absorb UV radiation with a maximum at 325 nm.[70] Along with enzymatic antioxidants, nonenzymatic forms exist as well. GSH, α-tocopherol, and β-carotene are among a few of the nonenzymatic antioxidants administered. Some examples of enzymatic forms include catalase, superoxide dismutase, and GSH peroxidase.[27] Antioxidants can be administered in oral or topical forms (see Chapter 39). Oral forms tend to be more beneficial because they do not wear away from skin by daily rubbing and washing. In addition, topical antioxidants may not have the capacity to be properly absorbed into the skin. Consequently, topical antioxidants do not protect well against UV radiation alone and have a low SPF. Thus, antioxidants should be used in conjunction with a sunscreen to increase their efficiency.

One antioxidant of note is *Polypodium leucotomos*, a botanically derived compound that belongs to the genus of ferns. It has been used in the treatment of various inflammatory disorders as well as vitiligo. In a study by González et al., the *in vivo* properties of polypodium were identified. In the study, 21 volunteers were divided into two groups. One group was treated with orally ingested psoralens (8-MOP or 5-MOP) and the other group was not treated. These volunteers were then exposed to solar radiation. The following clinical parameters were evaluated: immediate pigment darkening (IPD), minimal erythema dose (MED), minimal melanogenic dose (MMD), and minimal phototoxic dose (MPD) before and after topical or oral administration of polypodium leucotomos.[71] The results showed that polypodium was photoprotective after topical application as well as oral administration.

ADVERSE EFFECTS OF SUNSCREENS

Current data suggest that adverse effects induced by chemical sunscreens have included no systemic problems but have entailed local cutaneous manifestations such as contact dermatitis, irritant and allergic, as well as phototoxic and photoallergic reactions. In fact, sunscreens are one of the most common causative agents of photoallergic contact dermatitis in the US.[72] These agents can also cause contact dermatitis in the absence of sun exposure. PABA, benzophenones, cinnamates, and methoxydibenzoylmethane are the most common ingredients in chemical sunscreens implicated in provoking allergic contact dermatitis (see Chapter 19, Contact Dermatitis).[73–75] Physical sunscreens containing TiO_2 and ZnO have never been reported to cause contact allergy and, therefore, are suitable for patients with a history of sunscreen hypersensitivity.[76]

It is important to remember that additives to sunscreen preparations such as fragrances and preservatives are also likely to cause allergic reactions in susceptible patients (see Chapters

42, Fragrance, and 44, Preservatives). One study of 603 patients found that although 19% of the subjects complained of some sort of reaction to the sunscreen, none of the subjects were allergic to the sunscreen active ingredients, as revealed by patch testing. In fact, only 10% of the reactions were found to have an allergic component. Most adverse responses were consistent with an irritant reaction.[77] Sunscreen vehicles, particularly the oily preparations, can also exacerbate acne, as can acute UV exposure. Research suggests that it is not the individual sunscreen oil but the vehicle that can cause the development of comedones.[78,79]

The misconception that sunscreen offers total protection is insidious insofar as it leads some consumers to increase the length or frequency of their sun exposure. No sunscreen completely blocks the sun. In fact, the FDA no longer allows the term "sunblock" to be used on product labeling. Because the protection offered by many sunscreens is limited to UVB (280–315 nm) and short-wavelength UVA2 (320–340 nm), the use of such products may paradoxically increase exposure to long-wavelength UVA1 (340–400 nm).[80] UVA (320–400 nm) comprises the major portion of UV radiation reaching the surface of the earth and has been shown to play a role in skin carcinogenesis, photodermatosis induction, and other skin diseases provoked by the sun. UVA has been recognized as a component in the genesis of solar elastosis,[81] and studies by Lavker[11] and Lowe[82] provide evidence that repeated exposure to an artificial source of long-wavelength UVA produces morphologic changes in human skin indicative of photodamage.

In a study by Bissonnette et al., the pigmentation darkening method was used to compare UVA protection afforded by six commercially available sunscreens with an SPF of 20 or more.[83] These products claimed on their labels to offer UVA and UVB protection. Researchers found that the sunscreens that allowed the lowest amount of pigment darkening, and therefore the best UVA coverage, contained Parsol 1789. Interestingly, the sunscreens that protected the least against UVA-induced pigmentation were the sunscreens with the second and third highest SPF (45 and 50), revealing that selection of a high SPF sunscreen cannot be used as the only guide to compare UVA protection afforded by sunscreens. Fortunately, many stabilized avobenzone formulations and Mexoryl have increased the UVA protection of easily available sunscreens.

VITAMIN D AND SUNSCREEN

Another current controversy that is far from being resolved pertains to vitamin D and sun exposure. Vitamin D is important for the prevention of several types of cancers. Studies have shown that vitamin D may prevent or reduce the risk of lung, breast, and prostate cancers.[84,85] Unfortunately, the best method for obtaining a healthy and proper dose of vitamin D is through the sun (**Fig. 46-6**). Supplements, pills, and fortified milk do not contain the proper recommended dose of daily vitamin D. Lying on a sunny beach for 20 minutes can generate 10,000 IU of vitamin D while a glass of milk produces only 100 IU.[86] Thus emerges the controversy, as the best way of obtaining vitamin D is through sun exposure, yet too much sun exposure is known to cause skin cancer. In addition, sunscreens block most UVB light. It is UVB that promotes the synthesis of vitamin D. UVB is the source of sunburns and suntans as well. Research on this topic is ongoing and a final conclusion has not yet been reached. One study showed that there is no correlation between skin cancer prevention and vitamin D. In this study, 165 melanoma patients and 209 controls were questioned using a food-frequency questionnaire. Investigators controlled for age, hair color, and family history,

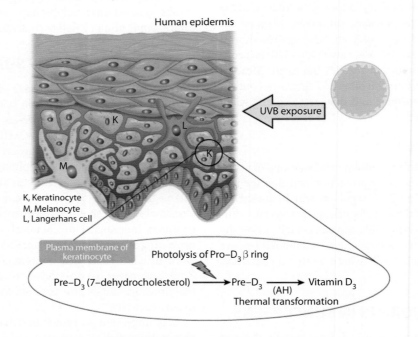

FIGURE 46-6. Vitamin D conversion in the skin.

and the results showed no evidence of vitamin D conferring protection against melanoma or reducing its risk.[87] A parallel study implied that sunscreen application does not decrease vitamin D levels.[88] On the other hand, some evidence has emerged indicating that sunscreen application does in fact decrease vitamin D levels. In one particular study, 20 long-term users of sunscreen with PABA were tested and found to have significantly lower vitamin D serum levels as compared to normal controls.[89] Although this controversy is far from being settled, the damaging effects of UV radiation are thought to outweigh the benefits of limited solar exposure, particularly since diet and supplementation may be safer ways of achieving sufficient vitamin D levels.[90]

INTERMITTENT USE OF SUNSCREEN

Many sunscreen users may have the misconception that intermittent use of a high-SPF product is as effective as daily use of a lower-SPF product. For instance, dermatologists are in a position to hear anecdotally that a distinct subset of sunscreen users consider themselves regular users of sunscreen, every time they go to the beach. One study demonstrated that sunscreens must be applied properly, regularly, and in appropriate amounts to be optimally effective in preventing UV-induced skin damage. The findings suggest that missing an application of sunscreen, even a potent one, can have negative consequences for the skin, with regular use of an SPF-15 sunscreen revealed to be more effective than intermittent use of a higher-SPF product in protecting the skin.[91] Therefore, patients should be advised to use sunscreen on a daily basis, even when not planning to go into the sun. This will help protect them from the UVA rays transmitted indoors through glass, and from unanticipated sun exposures.

There are so many different product formulations on the market that an appropriate sunscreen should be available for every patient, though in some cases, identifying one may take some effort. At this point, given the amassed body of research, the benefits of wearing daily sunscreen, at least on exposed areas such as the face, appear to outweigh any risks.

VEHICLES FOR DELIVERY OF ACTIVE INGREDIENTS

Sunscreen product efficacy and aesthetic results are influenced by the manufacturer's choice of vehicle to deliver active ingredients. Emulsions, known as lotions and creams, are the most common sunscreen vehicles. Of course, several kinds of formulations are commercially available and are typically selected according to individual preferences.

Cleansers

One cleanser on the market called IceShield by Freeze 24/7 claims to deposit sunscreen on the skin. This is a great option to use for those who do not like the feel of greasy sunscreens. However, there is a dearth of data as to how effective these wash-on sunscreens are. While more evidence is needed, it is presently recommended that this product be combined with a more reliable sunscreen when prolonged sun exposure is anticipated.

Lotions and Creams

For people with normal to oily skin, lotions tend to be preferred because lotions have lower viscosity, spread more easily, and are less greasy. Combination skin is also amenable to lotions, but patients with dry skin typically prefer creams. These products make ideal sunscreens because the most effective active ingredients can be introduced into the lipid phase of an emulsion. Products with a higher SPF contain more sunscreen oil and impart a heavy and greasy feel.[92,93]

Oils

The only advantage to oils is that they spread easily. Unfortunately, they also spread thinly on the skin rendering less sun protection. Consumers tend not to like oils because of the greasy, messy feel on the skin.

Gels

Male patients and those with oily skin tend to prefer gels. For people that are preparing to exercise while wearing sunscreen, water-based gels are appropriate because alcohol-based gels can cause burning and stinging of the eyes.

Sprays

Sprays have become popular in the last few years, especially for use in children. These products are a good option for tending to large areas of the body. One must take care to ensure that all exposed body surfaces are covered and that a sufficient amount of spray is used.

Sticks

Lipid-soluble sunscreen ingredients are contained in sticks. Waxes and petrolatum are added to thicken the formulations. Sticks are effective in protecting narrow and prominent areas such as the lips, ears, nose, and around the eyes. For use during exercise and water activities, sticks are superior to other formulations because they last longer and do not have the tendency to melt, which can irritate the eyes.

PROTECTIVE EFFECTS OF MAKEUP AND OTHER SKINCARE PRODUCTS

Sunscreen ingredients are now commonly found in many makeup foundations. Most facial foundations provide some sun protection due to the inclusion of ingredients such as TiO_2 and the pigments used to color the product. TiO_2 is added specifically to augment the SPF of some of these products, but it does result in a foundation that is more opaque. Consequently, chemical sunscreens are more often added to impart protection. Not every sunscreen ingredient is suitable for inclusion in makeup foundations, however. For example, Parsol effectively blocks UVA, but is inactivated upon exposure to iron oxide and other pigments used in makeup foundations. In addition, as stated above, the SPF on the label of a sunscreen powder and facial foundation is not an accurate reflection of how much sun protection these products offer. This is because the average person applies much less sunscreen product than is used in FDA testing.[14]

Within the last few years, manufacturers have produced hair care products, notably shampoos and conditioners, that contain sunscreen ingredients. Such ingredients are probably rinsed away and rendered ineffective because several sunscreen ingredients are water soluble and many of the hair care products are intended to be rinsed out. Although there are no data establishing their effectiveness, leave-in hair care products are more likely to provide some protection to the hair shaft. The FDA has not recognized any of these products as having protective effects against the sun. Until proper studies have been completed and data made available, including SPF-labeling, one should not rely on these products. The best recommendation is to wear a hat to prevent sun damage to the hair.

Insect Repellent and Sunscreen Combinations

A study by Montemarano et al. found that insect repellent interferes with sunscreen efficacy.[94] However, a subsequent study by Murphy and Montemarano disputed this finding, showing that insect repellent has the same efficacy even when sunscreen is applied with it.[95] At this time, it is advisable to apply these products separately until further information is available.

Sun Protection with Clothing

The UV Protection Factor (UPF) is a useful measurement guideline for clothing similar to the SPF that is used for sunscreens.[96] The most common, in vitro, method of ascertaining the UPF of clothing involves the use of a UV radiation source and a photodetector to record the intensity of the UV before and after passing through the fabric. The UPF is simply the ratio of the two measurements. The clothing industry has largely accepted, and embraced in some cases, the concepts of sun protection provided by clothing and the UPF. There is even a British standard for the measurement of UPF.[97] Because clothing is not subject to the wide variation or inconsistency of sunscreen application, a fabric really does provide the level of sun protection that its UPF suggests.[16] Further, it is believed that approximately 90% of summer clothes have a UPF higher than 10 and offer protection equal to that of sunscreens of SPF 30 or higher; the UPF of approximately 80% of such clothing exceeds a reading of 15, and offers nearly complete protection under normal sun exposure patterns.[98,99]

Washing clothes appears to strengthen the UPF. It is well known that cotton clothes shrink from the washing process. Therefore, it is reasonable to infer that the spaces, also known as "pores," between a fabric's threads shrink from washing. In fact, Welsh and Diffey demonstrated such a capacity in their study on the effects of fabric shrinkage (from laundry with water alone and detergent alone) on UPF measurement.[100] The relative size of these pores plays a significant role in limiting UV radiation transmission through clothing.[101] Wang et al. compiled fabric porosity data that demonstrated a reduction in the total area of pores between threads or yarns in fabrics laundered by various methods.[102] They concluded that the reduction of pore size after washing was responsible for the observed increase in UPF measurements and the ensuing decrease in UV transmission through the fabric.

UPF can be further increased by washing fabrics with detergents that contain UV-absorbing agents. Tinosorb, the UV-absorber used in the study by Wang et al., has a stilbene disulfonic acid triazine backbone that, when added to laundry, enables the chemical to vigorously bind to cotton fabric.[102] The result is a reduction in UV transmission through absorption of UV energy onto the ring structures of the compound. The study results showed that the UPF increased significantly after multiple washings with detergent and UV absorber, though there was no noticeable change in the whiteness or texture of the fabric. More UVA was transmitted through the fabrics than UVB, according to the authors.

While clothing obviously plays an integral role in protecting skin exposed to the sun, hats are also useful apparel adjuncts. Wearing a broad-brimmed hat can provide an SPF of about 5.[103] Hats can also add additional protection to the coverage that sunglasses provide by cutting down on the angles of sun exposure (**Fig. 46-7**).

Window Shields

UVA rays can penetrate glass, while UVB rays cannot. Because UVB rays are the ones that cause initial reddening, a significant amount of UVA exposure can go unnoticed. For patients with photosensitive skin disorders and those who want to take a step further to prevent UVA exposure, window shields are available that block UVA rays. The Llumar UV Shield is recommended by the Skin Cancer Foundation because it has been shown to block 99.9% of the UVA radiation in the range of 320–380 nm. These shields can be placed on car, boat, and house windows to decrease UVA exposure.

Chemoprevention of Photodamage

Chemoprevention is another potential option for protection against sunlight-related skin disorders.[104] Chemoprevention refers to the prevention of disease through dietary manipulation or pharmacologic intervention. Among the agents that have been identified as having potential chemopreventive activities in humans are retinoids and low-fat diets.[105,106] In addition, a polyphenolic fraction isolated from green tea has been shown to exhibit multiple chemopreventive activities in animal models and in in vitro systems (see Chapter 9, Nutrition and the Skin).[107–109] Investigations are ongoing regarding the potential chemopreventive properties of several other botanicals and nutritional components.

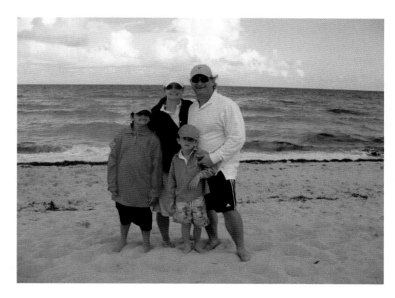

FIGURE 46-7. In addition to sunscreen, sunglasses, broad-brimmed hats, and sun-protective clothing should be worn when exposed to sunlight for any significant length of time.

ATTITUDES ON SUNSCREEN USE AND EFFECTS OF ITS OMISSION

When recommending particular sunscreens to patients, the most important consideration is which product they will most likely accept using daily. The best choice should be based on the patient's skin type and lifestyle factors, with a higher SPF formulation suggested for intended prolonged sun exposure. Patients should be reminded that facial foundation makeup and powders should not be relied upon for daily sun protection as these are used in insufficient quantities to actually deliver the SPF listed on the label.

Obviously, the daily use of sunscreen is an important adjunct to skin-protective behavior. However, because no sunscreen can effectively block all parts of the UV spectrum, sun avoidance, protective clothing and hats, and window shields can all be utilized to lessen acute and cumulative sun exposure. Patients should be instructed about the proper use of sunscreen and asked about sunscreen use at every visit. This constant nagging will help them realize how important it is to protect their skin from the sun. Even if patients claim to use sunscreen and know about the hazards of the sun, studies have shown that they still do not get enough sun protection. In fact, it is known that mothers provide more sun protection to their children than to themselves,[110] and that while sun protection awareness increases with age, sun protection attitudes and behaviors tend to wane from childhood to adolescence.[111] Even well-intentioned sunscreen users can forget the rules. For example, one study found that 98% of 352 family groups applied their sunscreen after arrival at the beach, instead of 30 minutes before as is suggested for optimal sun protection.[112]

In 2013, Hughes et al. conducted a randomized, controlled, community-based intervention with 903 adults under 55 years old (out of 1,621 randomly selected adults) in Nambour, Australia to ascertain how regular sunscreen use compared with discretionary use or the use of β-carotene supplements compared with placebo in preventing or slowing skin aging. They found that regular sunscreen use mitigated skin aging in healthy, middle-aged individuals and there was no effect of β-carotene supplements on cutaneous aging.[113]

Of course, skin cancer is known to be the most deleterious consequence of sun exposure. Sunscreen remains a key element in protecting against it. In 2012, Chesnut et al. highlighted the one randomized controlled study on the role of sunscreen in preventing BCC, the most common human malignancy. They noted that while the study found no significant protective effects from sunscreens, epidemiologic and direct evidence have shown UV exposure to be the paramount risk factor for engendering BCC. Further, they observed that the lone randomized controlled study on the influence of sunscreen on BCC neglected to account for sunscreen abuse, sunscreen misuse, sunscreen formulation, and cumulative UV exposure, thus lacking an authentic perspective on how sunscreen is actually used.[114]

An interesting 2015 mediation analysis of decision-making regarding sun avoidance and sunscreen use suggested the usefulness of evaluating the status of underlying risk ideas among patients to help physicians increase the likelihood of compliance with sun protection behavior advice.[115]

Two years later, Pratt et al. called for some form of public health announcement or other intervention to address their finding that UV imaging shows that facial areas susceptible to skin cancer are disproportionately omitted in the application of sunscreens. They also suggested that UV blocking sunglasses should be touted as an additional protective measure against UV-induced harm.[116]

What Patients Should Know

The American Academy of Dermatology (AAD) touts several randomized controlled trials as evidence that sunscreens play a key role in preventing the development of actinic keratoses, squamous cell carcinomas, nevi, melanomas, photoaging, and photoimmunosuppression. In addition, the AAD has called for global standardization of ways to measure the efficacy of sunscreens and continued public education so as to better inform sunscreen users of proper application and optimal photoprotection approaches.[117]

Sunless Tanning

Discouraging patients from sunbathing and tanning remains a challenge despite the much greater awareness of the potential harm from UV rays. Sunless tanning agents have been available for more than half a century. They have long been known to protect against visible light and longwave UVA, and in 2004 Faurschou et al. demonstrated that DHA also yields a small but significant SPF.[118,119] The sunless tan results from the interaction between DHA and SC amino acids.[120] Researchers have found that the addition of antioxidants to DHA formulations could render sunless tanners more natural looking.[121] However, physicians should advise consumers not to consider sunless tanners a substitute for adequate skin-protective behavior. In 2008, Jung et al. found, in an analysis of three self-tanning agents, that sun exposure engendered 180% additional free radicals in DHA-treated skin as compared to untreated skin.[122]

Acne

Another disadvantage of sun exposure that warrants mentioning to patients is that, for several decades, prolonged sun exposure or "sunbathing" has been thought to exacerbate acne by enhancing the comedogenicity of sebum.[92]

Sunscreen Bans

The fourth national report by the US Centers for Disease Control and Prevention on human exposure to environmental chemicals revealed early in 2018 that approximately 97% of the individuals tested had oxybenzone in their urine.[123] Notably, various concentrations of oxybenzone (BP-3) have also been found in waterways and fish around the world, with the chemical noted for engendering toxic reactions in coral (bleaching) and fish (mortality).[123] In July 2018, the State of Hawai'i announced that it would ban the use of two key sunscreen ingredients with an eye toward preservation of the surrounding marine life, particularly coral reefs. The bill took effect on January 1, 2021, and prohibits the sale of OTC sunscreens containing oxybenzone and octinoxate, the two most popular chemical sunscreen ingredients.[124]

Raffa et al. recently considered whether this new regulation aimed at environmental preservation will pose the risk of a concomitant rise in human skin cancers. It is known that multiple factors have contributed to the declining health, bleaching, and death of coral reefs, including alterations in ocean temperature and chemistry, pathogens, entrance of non-native, invasive species, harmful fishing practices, and pollution. Studies have shown that sunscreens, via direct or indirect influence such as virus promotion, represent a significant portion of the pollution responsible for coral reef bleaching. Raffa and colleagues noted that while advocates push for additional such bans around the world and opponents decry the possible spike in skin cancers, researchers are busy trying to develop sunscreens that will protect skin and at least do no harm to the environment.[125] The South Pacific archipelago nation of Palau, the Caribbean island nation of Bonaire, and Key West, FL have also signed laws intended to ban sunscreens containing oxybenzone and octinoxate that took effect on January 1, 2021.[126–128]

CONCLUSION

There are numerous sunscreen choices on the market. It is important to help patients find the sunscreen that is most suitable for their needs and skin type to increase the likelihood of compliance to a daily sunscreen regimen. It is even more important to emphasize that the daily use of sunscreen is not the first-line defense against the ravages of the sun and that sunscreen use does not indemnify a person from photodamage or give one license to stay out longer because of a coating of sunscreen. The daily use of sunscreens is a key component, though, in the continuing effort to keep the skin looking young and healthy.

The importance of using sunscreen on a daily basis cannot be overstated. Sun exposure affects almost every skin condition. Trying to appeal to patients' vanity by broaching the prospect of wrinkle formation remains an effective strategy to achieve better adherence to skin-protective behaviors. The primary author suggests considering an individual's skin type in determining an optimal skin-protection regimen, as a general guideline, and urges patients to first layer their exposed skin with an antioxidant formulation followed by an antioxidant-containing sunscreen or two different types of sunscreens, intended to block both UVA and UVB (particularly one of the physical sunscreens ZnO or TiO_2, to block UVA). Finally, for individuals who opt to get their vitamin D through sun exposure rather than supplementation and diet (given the few dietary sources), exposing only their legs and arms to the sun for about 15 minutes each day is recommended.

References

1. Taylor CR, Stern RS, Leyden JJ, Gilchrest BA. Photoaging/photodamage and photoprotection. *J Am Acad Dermatol.* 1990;22(1):1–15.
2. Carr S, Smith C, Wernberg J. Epidemiology and Risk Factors of Melanoma. *Surg Clin North Am.* 2020;100(1):1–12.
3. Rastrelli M, Tropea S, Rossi CR, Alaibac M. Melanoma: epidemiology, risk factors, pathogenesis, diagnosis and classification. *In Vivo.* 2014;28(6):1005–1011.
4. Aggarwal P, Knabel P, Fleischer AB Jr. United States burden of melanoma and non-melanoma skin cancer from 1990 to 2019. *J Am Acad Dermatol.* 2021:S0190-9622(21)00755-6.
5. EWG's Guide to Sunscreens. https://www.ewg.org/sunscreen/report/executive-summary/. Accessed July 1, 2021.

6. EWG's Best Beach and Sport Sunscreens. https://www.ewg.org/sunscreen/best-sunscreens/best-beach-sport-sunscreens/. Accessed July 1, 2021.

7. Diffey BL. What is light? *Photodermatol Photoimmunol Photomed*. 2002;18(2):68–74.

8. de Gruijl FR. Photocarcinogenesis: UVA vs. UVB radiation. *Skin Pharmacol Appl Skin Physiol*. 2002;15(5):316–320.

9. Poon TS, Barnetson RS, Halliday GM. Prevention of immunosuppression by sunscreens in humans is unrelated to protection from erythema and dependent on protection from ultraviolet a in the face of constant ultraviolet B protection. *J Invest Dermatol*. 2003;121(1):184–190.

10. Vink AA, Roza L. Biological consequences of cyclobutane pyrimidine dimers. *J Photochem Photobiol B*. 2001;65(2-3):101–104.

11. Lavker RM, Gerberick GF, Veres D, Irwin CJ, Kaidbey KH. Cumulative effects from repeated exposures to suberythemal doses of UVB and UVA in human skin. *J Am Acad Dermatol*. 1995;32(1):53–62.

12. Diffey BL. Sunscreens, suntans and skin cancer. People do not apply enough sunscreen for protection. *BMJ*. 1996;313(7062):942.

13. Autier P, Boniol M, Severi G, Doré JF; European Organizatin for Research and Treatment of Cancer Melanoma Co-operative Group. Quantity of sunscreen used by European students. *Br J Dermatol*. 2001;144(2):288–291.

14. Azurdia RM, Pagliaro JA, Rhodes LE. Sunscreen application technique in photosensitive patients: a quantitative assessment of the effect of education. *Photodermatol Photoimmunol Photomed*. 2000;16(2):53–56.

15. Stokes R, Diffey B. How well are sunscreen users protected? *Photodermatol Photoimmunol Photomed*. 1997;13(5-6):186–188.

16. Diffey BL. Sun protection with clothing. *Br J Dermatol*. 2001;144(3):449–450.

17. Skin Inc. FDA Proposes New Rule for Sunscreen Products. June 6, 2008. https://www.skininc.com/spabusiness/regulations/9874517.html. Accessed July 1, 2021.

18. Dennis LK, Vanbeek MJ, Beane Freeman LE, Smith BJ, Dawson DV, Coughlin JA. Sunburns and risk of cutaneous melanoma: does age matter? A comprehensive meta-analysis. *Ann Epidemiol*. 2008;18(8):614–627.

19. Federal Register. The Daily Journal of the United States Government. Sunscreen drug products for over-the-counter human use. A proposed rule by the Food and Drug Administration. https://www.federalregister.gov/documents/2019/02/26/2019-03019/sunscreen-drug-products-for-the-over-the-counter-human-use. Accessed July 1, 2021.

20. Chardon A, Moyal D, Hourseau C. Persistent pigment darkening response as a method for evaluation of ultraviolet A protection assays. In: Lowe NJ, Shaath MA, Pathak MA, eds. *Sunscreens Development, Evaluation and Regulatory Assays*. 2nd ed. New York, NY: Marcel Dekker; 1997: 559–582.

21. Cole C, Van Fossen R. Measurement of sunscreen UVA protection: an unsensitized human model. *J Am Acad Dermatol*. 1992;26(2 Pt 1):178–184.

22. Nash JF, Tanner PR, Matts PJ. Ultraviolet A radiation: testing and labeling for sunscreen products. *Dermatol Clin*. 2006;24(1):63–74.

23. Cole C. Sunscreen protection in the ultraviolet A region: how to measure the effectiveness. *Photodermatol Photoimmunol Photomed*. 2001;17(1):2–10.

24. Moyal D, Chardon A, Kollias N. UVA protection efficacy of sunscreens can be determined by the persistent pigment darkening (PPD) method. (Part 2). *Photodermatol Photoimmunol Photomed*. 2000;16(6):250–255.

25. Haywood R, Wardman P, Sanders R, Linge C. Sunscreens inadequately protect against ultraviolet-A-induced free radicals in skin: implications for skin aging and melanoma? *J Invest Dermatol*. 2003;121(4):862–868.

26. Herrling T, Fuchs J, Rehberg J, Groth N. UV-induced free radicals in the skin detected by ESR spectroscopy and imaging using nitroxides. *Free Radic Biol Med*. 2003;35(1):59–67.

27. Kullavanijaya P, Lim HW. Photoprotection. *J Am Acad Dermatol*. 2005;52(6):937–958.

28. Seité S, Moyal D, Verdier MP, Hourseau C, Fourtanier A. Accumulated p53 protein and UVA protection level of sunscreens. *Photodermatol Photoimmunol Photomed*. 2000;16(1):3–9.

29. Draelos ZD. A dermatologist's perspective on the final sunscreen monograph. *J Am Acad Dermatol*. 2001;44(1):109–110.

30. Schauber J. Topical therapy of perianal eczema. *Hautarzt*. 2010;61(1):33–38.

31. Xhauflaire-Uhoda E, Henry F, Piérard-Franchimont C, Piérard GE. Electrometric assessment of the effect of a zinc oxide paste in diaper dermatitis. *Int J Cosmet Sci*. 2009;31(5):369–374.

32. Padmavathy N, Vijayaraghavan R. Enhanced bioactivity of ZnO nanoparticles – an antimicrobial study. *Sci Technol Adv Mater*. 2008;9(3):1–7.

33. Parboteeah S, Brown A. Managing chronic venous leg ulcers with zinc oxide paste bandages. *Br J Nurs*. 2008;17(6):S30, S32, S34–6.

34. Treadwell T. Commentary: Enhanced healing of surgical wounds of the lower leg using weekly zinc oxide compression dressings. *Dermatol Surg*. 2011;37(2):166–167.

35. Bruce S, Watson J. Evaluation of a prescription strength 4% hydroquinone/10% L-ascorbic Acid treatment system for normal to oily skin. *J Drugs Dermatol*. 2011;10(12):1455–1461.

36. de Graaf NPJ, Feilzer AJ, Kleverlaan CJ, Bontkes H, Gibbs S, Rustemeyer T. A retrospective study on titanium sensitivity: Patch test materials and manifestations. *Contact Dermatitis*. 2018;79(2):85–90.

37. Shaw T, Simpson B, Wilson B, Oostman H, Rainey D, Storrs F. True photoallergy to sunscreens is rare despite popular belief. *Dermatitis*. 2010;21(4):185–198.

38. Mitchnick MA, Fairhurst D, Pinnell SR. Microfine zinc oxide (Z-cote) as a photostable UVA/UVB sunblock agent. *J Am Acad Dermatol*. 1999;40(1):85–90.

39. Deflandre A, Lang G. Photostability assessment of sunscreens. Benzylidene camphor and dibenzoylmethane derivatives. *Int J Cosmet Sci*. 1988;10(2):53–62.

40. Beasley DG, Meyer TA. Characterization of the UVA protection provided by avobenzone, zinc oxide, and titanium dioxide in broad-spectrum sunscreen products. *Am J Clin Dermatol*. 2010;11(6):413–421.

41. Fairhurst D, Mitchnik MA. Particulate sun blocks: general principles. In: Lowe NJ, Shaath NA, Pathak MA, eds. *Sunscreens—Development, Evaluation, and Regulatory Aspects*. New York, NY: Marcel Dekker; 1997: 313–352.

42. Wamer WG, Yin JJ, Wei RR. Oxidative damage to nucleic acids photosensitized by titanium dioxide. *Free Radic Biol Med*. 1997;23(6):851–858.

43. Hidaka H, Horikoshi S, Serpone N, Knowland J. In vitro photochemical damage to DNA, RNA and their bases by an inorganic sunscreen agent on exposure to UVA and UVB radiation. *J Photochem Photobiol A: Chemistry.* 1997;111(1-3):205–213.

44. Gillies R, Kollias N. Noninvasive in vivo determination of sunscreen ultraviolet A protection factors using diffuse reflectance spectroscopy. In: Lowe NJ, Shaath NA, Pathak MA, eds. *Sunscreens—Development, Evaluation, and Regulatory Aspects.* New York, NY: Marcel Dekker; 1997: 601–610.

45. Tran DT, Salmon R. Potential photocarcinogenic effects of nanoparticle sunscreens. *Australas J Dermatol.* 2011;52(1):1–6.

46. Filipe P, Silva NJ, Silva R, et al. Stratum corneum is an effective barrier to TiO2 and ZnO nanoparticle percutaneous absorption. *Skin Pharmacol Physiol.* 2009;22(5):266–275.

47. Gulson B, McCall M, Korsch M, et al. Small amounts of zinc from zinc oxide particles in sunscreens applied outdoors are absorbed through human skin. *Toxicol Sci.* 2010;118(1):140–149.

48. Wang SQ, Tooley IR. Photoprotection in the era of nanotechnology. *Semin Cutan Med Surg.* 2011 Dec;30(4):210–213.

49. Kang SJ, Lee YJ, Kim BM, Choi YJ, Chung HW. Cytotoxicity and genotoxicity of titanium dioxide nanoparticles in UVA-irradiated normal peripheral blood lymphocytes. *Drug Chem Toxicol.* 2011;34(3):277–284.

50. Tyner KM, Wokovich AM, Godar DE, Doub WH, Sadrieh N. The state of nano-sized titanium dioxide (TiO2) may affect sunscreen performance. *Int J Cosmet Sci.* 2011;33(3):234–244.

51. Schilling K, Bradford B, Castelli D, et al. Human safety review of "nano" titanium dioxide and zinc oxide. *Photochem Photobiol Sci.* 2010;9(4):495–509.

52. Newman MD, Stotland M, Ellis JI. The safety of nanosized particles in titanium dioxide- and zinc oxide-based sunscreens. *J Am Acad Dermatol.* 2009;61(4):685–692.

53. Burnett ME, Wang SQ. Current sunscreen controversies: a critical review. *Photodermatol Photoimmunol Photomed.* 2011;27(2):58–67.

54. Wiesenthal A, Hunter L, Wang S, Wickliffe J, Wilkerson M. Nanoparticles: small and mighty. *Int J Dermatol.* 2011;50(3):247–254.

55. Vujovic M, Kostic E. Titanium dioxide and zinc oxide nanoparticles in sunscreens: a review of toxicological data. *J Cosmet Sci.* 2019;70(5):223–234.

56. Kim KB, Kim YW, Lim SK, et al. Risk assessment of zinc oxide, a cosmetic ingredient used as a UV filter of sunscreens. *J Toxicol Environ Health B Crit Rev.* 2017;20(3):155–182.

57. Dréno B, Alexis A, Chuberre B, Marinovich M. Safety of titanium dioxide nanoparticles in cosmetics. *J Eur Acad Dermatol Venereol.* 2019;33(Suppl 7):34–46.

58. Sayre RM, Dowdy JC, Gerwig AJ, Shields WJ, Lloyd RV. Unexpected photolysis of the sunscreen octinoxate in the presence of the sunscreen avobenzone. *Photochem Photobiol.* 2005;81(2):452–456.

59. Hayden CG, Roberts MS, Benson HA. Systemic absorption of sunscreen after topical application. *Lancet.* 1997;350(9081):863–864.

60. Olive PL, Banáth JP. The comet assay: a method to measure DNA damage in individual cells. *Nat Protoc.* 2006;1(1):23–29.

61. Chatelain E, Gabard B. Photostabilization of butyl methoxydibenzoylmethane (Avobenzone) and ethylhexyl methoxycinnamate by bis-ethylhexyloxyphenol methoxyphenyl triazine (Tinosorb S), a new UV broadband filter. *Photochem Photobiol.* 2001;74(3):401–406.

62. Gaspar LR, Maia Campos PM. Evaluation of the photostability of different UV filter combinations in a sunscreen. *Int J Pharm.* 2006;307(2):123–128.

63. Lapidot N, Gans O, Biagini F, Sosonkin L, Rottman C. Advanced sunscreens: UV absorbers encapsulated in Sol-Gel glass microcapsules. *J Sol-Gel Sci Tech.* 2003;26(1):67–72.

64. Rietschel R, Fowler J, eds. *Fisher's Contact Dermatitis.* 5th ed. Philadelphia, PA: Lippincott Williams & Wilkins; 2001: 403.

65. Emonet S, Pasche-Koo F, Perin-Minisini MJ, Hauser C. Anaphylaxis to oxybenzone, a frequent constituent of sunscreens. *J Allergy Clin Immunol.* 2001;107(3):556–557.

66. Heurung AR, Raju SI, Warshaw EM. Adverse reactions to sunscreen agents: epidemiology, responsible irritants and allergens, clinical characteristics, and management. *Dermatitis.* 2014;25(6):289–326.

67. Cosmetic Ingredient Review. Final report on the safety of benzophenone-1, -3, -4, -5, -9, and -11. *J Am Coll Toxicol.* 1983;2:3577.

68. DiNardo JC, Downs CA. Dermatological and environmental toxicological impact of the sunscreen ingredient oxybenzone/benzophenone-3. *J Cosmet Dermatol.* 2018;17(1):15–19.

69. Moyal D. Prevention of ultraviolet-induced skin pigmentation. *Photodermatol Photoimmunol Photomed.* 2004;20(5):243–247.

70. Antille C, Tran C, Sorg O, Carraux P, Didierjean L, Saurat JH. vitamin A exerts a photoprotective action in skin by absorbing ultraviolet B radiation. *J Invest Dermatol.* 2003;121(5):1163–1167.

71. González S, Pathak MA, Cuevas J, Villarrubia VG, Fitzpatrick TB. Topical or oral administration with an extract of Polypodium leucotomos prevents acute sunburn and psoralen-induced phototoxic reactions as well as depletion of Langerhans cells in human skin. *Photodermatol Photoimmunol Photomed.* 1997;13(1-2):50–60.

72. Rietschel R, Fowler J, eds. *Fisher's Contact Dermatitis.* 5th ed. Philadelphia, PA: Lippincott Williams & Wilkins; 2001: 402.

73. DeBuys HV, Levy SB, Murray JC, Madey DL, Pinnell SR. Modern approaches to photoprotection. *Dermatol Clin.* 2000;18(4):577–590.

74. Davis S, Capjack L, Kerr N, Fedosejevs R. Clothing as protection from ultraviolet radiation: which fabric is most effective? *Int J Dermatol.* 1997;36(5):374–379.

75. González E, González S. Drug photosensitivity, idiopathic photodermatoses, and sunscreens. *J Am Acad Dermatol.* 1996;35(6):871–885.

76. Rietschel R, Fowler J, eds. *Fisher's Contact Dermatitis.* 5th ed. Philadelphia, PA: Lippincott Williams & Wilkins; 2001: 404.

77. Foley P, Nixon R, Marks R, Frowen K, Thompson S. The frequency of reactions to sunscreens: results of a longitudinal population-based study on the regular use of sunscreens in Australia. *Br J Dermatol.* 1993;128(5):512–518.

78. Collins P, Ferguson J. Photoallergic contact dermatitis to oxybenzone. *Br J Dermatol.* 1994;131(1):124–129.

79. Funk JO, Dromgoole SH, Maibach HI. Sunscreen intolerance. Contact sensitization, photocontact sensitization, and irritancy of sunscreen agents. *Dermatol Clin.* 1995;13(2):473–481.

80. Autier P, Doré JF, Négrier S, et al. Sunscreen use and duration of sun exposure: a double-blind, randomized trial. *J Natl Cancer Inst.* 1999;91(15):1304–1309.

81. Fourtanier A, Labat-Robert J, Kern P, Berrebi C, Gracia AM, Boyer B. In vivo evaluation of photoprotection against chronic ultraviolet-A irradiation by a new sunscreen Mexoryl SX. *Photochem Photobiol.* 1992;55(4):549–560.

82. Lowe NJ, Meyers DP, Wieder JM, et al. Low doses of repetitive ultraviolet A induce morphologic changes in human skin. *J Invest Dermatol.* 1995;105(6):739–743.

83. Bissonnette R, Allas S, Moyal D, Provost N. Comparison of UVA protection afforded by high sun protection factor sunscreens. *J Am Acad Dermatol.* 2000;43(6):1036–1038.

84. The Associated Press. Vitamin D research may have doctors prescribing sunshine. USA Today. April 20, 2005. http://www.usatoday.com/news/nation/2005-05-21-doctors-sunshine-good_x.htm. Accessed July 2, 2021.

85. Nair R, Maseeh A. Vitamin D: The "sunshine" vitamin. *J Pharmacol Pharmacother.* 2012;3(2):118–126.

86. Lambert C. Too much sunscreen? *Harvard Magazine.* 2005;108(1):11–13.

87. Weinstock MA, Stampfer MJ, Lew RA, Willett WC, Sober AJ. Case-control study of melanoma and dietary vitamin D: implications for advocacy of sun protection and sunscreen use. *J Invest Dermatol.* 1992;98(5):809–811.

88. Marks R, Foley PA, Jolley D, Knight KR, Harrison J, Thompson SC. The effect of regular sunscreen use on vitamin D levels in an Australian population. Results of a randomized controlled trial. *Arch Dermatol.* 1995;131(4):415–421.

89. Matsuoka LY, Wortsman J, Hanifan N, Holick MF. Chronic sunscreen use decreases circulating concentrations of 25-hydroxyvitamin D. A preliminary study. *Arch Dermatol.* 1988;124(12):1802–1804.

90. Jou PC, Tomecki KJ. Sunscreens in the United States: current status and future outlook. *Adv Exp Med Biol.* 2014;810:464–484.

91. Phillips TJ, Bhawan J, Yaar M, Bello Y, Lopiccolo D, Nash JF. Effect of daily versus intermittent sunscreen application on solar simulated UV radiation-induced skin response in humans. *J Am Acad Dermatol.* 2000;43(4):610–618.

92. Mills OH, Porte M, Kligman AM. Enhancement of comedogenic substances by ultraviolet radiation. *Br J Dermatol.* 1978;98(2):145–150.

93. Mills OHJr, Kligman AM. Acne aestivalis. *Arch Dermatol.* 1975;111(7):891–892.

94. Montemarano AD, Gupta RK, Burge JR, Klein K. Insect repellents and the efficacy of sunscreens. *Lancet.* 1997;349(9066):1670–1671.

95. Murphy ME, Montemarano AD, Debboun M, Gupta R. The effect of sunscreen on the efficacy of insect repellent: a clinical trial. *J Am Acad Dermatol.* 2000;43(2 Pt 1):219–222.

96. Gies HP, Roy CR, Elliott G, Zongli W. Ultraviolet radiation protection factors for clothing. *Health Phys.* 1994;67(2):131–139.

97. British Standards Institution. *Method of Test for Penetration of Erythemally Weighted Solar Ultraviolet Radiation Through Clothing Fabrics BS 7914.* London, UK: British Standards Institution; 1998.

98. Gies HP, Roy CR, McLennan A. Textiles and sun protection. In: Volkmer B, Heller H, eds. *Environmental UV-Radiation, Risk of Skin Cancer and Primary Prevention.* Stuttgart, Germany: Gustav Fischer; 1996: 213–234.

99. Driscoll C. *Clothing Protection Factors.* Radiological Protection Bulletin. Oxfordshire, England: Chilton National Radiological Protection Board, 2000, p. 222.

100. Welsh C, Diffey B. The protection against solar actinic radiation afforded by common clothing fabrics. *Clin Exp Dermatol.* 1981;6(6):577–582.

101. Menzies SW, Lukins PB, Greenoak GE, et al. A comparative study of fabric protection against ultraviolet-induced erythema determined by spectrophotometric and human skin measurements. *Photodermatol Photoimmunol Photomed.* 1991;8(4):157–163.

102. Wang SQ, Kopf AW, Marx J, Bogdan A, Polsky D, Bart RS. Reduction of ultraviolet transmission through cotton T-shirt fabrics with low ultraviolet protection by various laundering methods and dyeing: clinical implications. *J Am Acad Dermatol.* 2001;44(5):767–774.

103. Diffey BL, Cheeseman J. Sun protection with hats. *Br J Dermatol.* 1992;127(1):10–12.

104. Greenwald P. Chemoprevention of cancer. *Sci Am.* 1996;275 (3):96–99.

105. DiGiovanna JJ. Retinoid chemoprevention in the high-risk patient. *J Am Acad Dermatol.* 1998;39(2 Pt 3):S82–S85.

106. Black HS, Herd JA, Goldberg LH, et al. Effect of a low-fat diet on the incidence of actinic keratosis. *N Engl J Med.* 1994;330(18):1272–1275.

107. Katiyar SK, Mukhtar H. Tea in chemoprevention of cancer epidemiologic and experimental studies. *Int J Oncol.* 1996;8:221–238.

108. Yang CS, Wang ZY. Tea and cancer. *J Natl Cancer Inst.* 1993;85(13):1038–1049.

109. Elmets CA, Singh D, Tubesing K, Matsui M, Katiyar S, Mukhtar H. Cutaneous photoprotection from ultraviolet injury by green tea polyphenols. *J Am Acad Dermatol.* 2001;44(3):425–432.

110. Autier P, Doré JF, Cattaruzza MS, et al. Sunscreen use, wearing clothes, and number of nevi in 6- to 7-year-old European children. European Organization for Research and Treatment of Cancer Melanoma Cooperative Group. *J Natl Cancer Inst.* 1998;90(24):1873–1880.

111. Dixon H, Borland R, Hill D. Sun protection and sunburn in primary school children: the influence of age, gender, and coloring. *Prev Med.* 1999;28(2):119–130.

112. Robinson JK, Rademaker AW. Sun protection by families at the beach. *Arch Pediatr Adolesc Med.* 1998;152(5):466–470.

113. Hughes MC, Williams GM, Baker P, Green AC. Sunscreen and prevention of skin aging: a randomized trial. *Ann Intern Med.* 2013;158(11):781–790.

114. Chesnut C, Kim J. Is there truly no benefit with sunscreen use and Basal cell carcinoma? A critical review of the literature and the application of new sunscreen labeling rules to real-world sunscreen practices. *J Skin Cancer.* 2012;2012:480985.

115. Santiago-Rivas M, Velicer WF, Redding C. Mediation analysis of decisional balance, sun avoidance and sunscreen use in the precontemplation and preparation stages for sun protection. *Psychol Health.* 2015;30(12):1433–1449.

116. Pratt H, Hassanin K, Troughton LD, et al. UV imaging reveals facial areas that are prone to skin cancer are disproportionately missed during sunscreen application. *PLoS One.* 2017;12(10):e0185297.

117. Young AR, Claveau J, Rossi AB. Ultraviolet radiation and the skin: Photobiology and sunscreen photoprotectioni. *J Am Acad Dermatol.* 2017;76(3S1):S100–S109.

118. Faurschou A, Wulf HC. Durability of the sun protection factor provided by dihydroxyacetone. *Photodermatol Photoimmunol Photomed.* 2004;20(5):239–242.

119. Faurschou A, Janjua NR, Wulf HC. Sun protection effect of dihydroxyacetone. *Arch Dermatol*. 2004;140(7):886–887.

120. Nguyen BC, Kochevar IE. Factors influencing sunless tanning with dihydroxyacetone. *Br J Dermatol*. 2003;149(2):332–340.

121. Muizzuddin N, Marenus KD, Maes DH. Tonality of suntan vs sunless tanning with dihydroxyacetone. *Skin Res Technol*. 2000;6(4):199–204.

122. Jung K, Seifert M, Herrling T, Fuchs J. UV-generated free radicals (FR) in skin: their prevention by sunscreens and their induction by self-tanning agents. *Spectrochim Acta A Mol Biomol Spectrosc*. 2008;69(5):1423–1428.

123. DiNardo JC, Downs CA. Dermatological and environmental toxicological impact of the sunscreen ingredient oxybenzone/benzophenone-3. *J Cosmet Dermatol*. 2018;17(1):15–19.

124. HNN Staff. Hawaii's ban on coral-harming sunscreens goes into effect New Year's Day. Hawaii News Now. December 31, 2020. https://www.hawaiinewsnow.com/2020/12/31/hawaiis-ban-coral-harming-sunscreens-goes-into-effect-new-years-day/. Accessed July 7, 2021.

125. Raffa RB, Pergolizzi JVJr, Taylor RJr, Kitzen JM, NEMA Research Group. Sunscreen bans: Coral reefs and skin cancer. *J Clin Pharm Ther*. 2019;44(1):134–139.

126. Sullivan E. Palau, in Western Pacific, is first nation to ban 'reef-toxic' sunscreens. NPR, November 2, 2018. https://www.npr.org/2018/11/02/663308800/palau-in-western-pacific-is-first-nation-to-ban-reef-toxic-sunscreens. Accessed July 2, 2021.

127. Pappas S. Another tropical paradise enacts a sunscreen ban. Live Science, May 17, 2018. https://www.livescience.com/62598-bonaire-island-bans-sunscreen.html. Accessed July 2, 2021.

128. Kaur H. Key West bans certain sunscreens to protect coral reef. CNN, February 6, 2019. https://www.cnn.com/2019/02/06/us/key-west-bans-sunscreens-to-protect-reef/index.html. Accessed July 2, 2021.

Index

FOREWORD BY **PAT SUMMERALL**   AFTERWORD BY **ROGER STAUBACH**

GREATEST

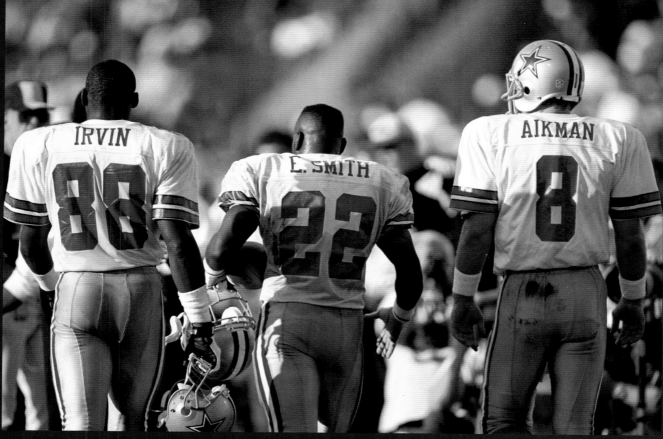

TEAM EVER

 THE **DALLAS COWBOYS** DYNASTY OF THE 1990s

RON ST. ANGELO • NORM HITZGES

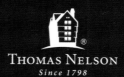

THOMAS NELSON
Since 1798

NASHVILLE   DALLAS   MEXICO CITY   RIO DE JANEIRO   BEIJING

© 2008 by Norm Hitzges

Cover & Interior Photography by Ron St. Angelo

Cover & Interior Design by Bill Chiaravalle, DeAnna Pierce , Mark Mickel • Brand Navigation, LLC

Published in Nashville, Tennessee. Thomas Nelson is a trademark of Thomas Nelson, Inc.

Thomas Nelson, Inc., titles may be purchased in bulk for educational, business, fundraising, or sales promotional use. For information, please email SpecialMarkets@ThomasNelson.com.

Previously published in 2007, ISBN 1-4016-0340-8. This edition has been updated with a special section for the commemoration of Texas Stadium.

ISBN : 978-1-4016-0437-0

Printed in China
08 09 10 11 RRD 5 4 3 2 1

To Rodney,
Enjoy these wonderful Cowboy
memories.

Norm Hitzges

FOREWORD BY PAT SUMMERALL   AFTERWORD BY ROGER STAUBACH

GREATEST TEAM EVER

THE **DALLAS COWBOYS** DYNASTY OF THE 1990s

RON ST. ANGELO • NORM HITZGES

Ron St. Ayb
Stay Focused!

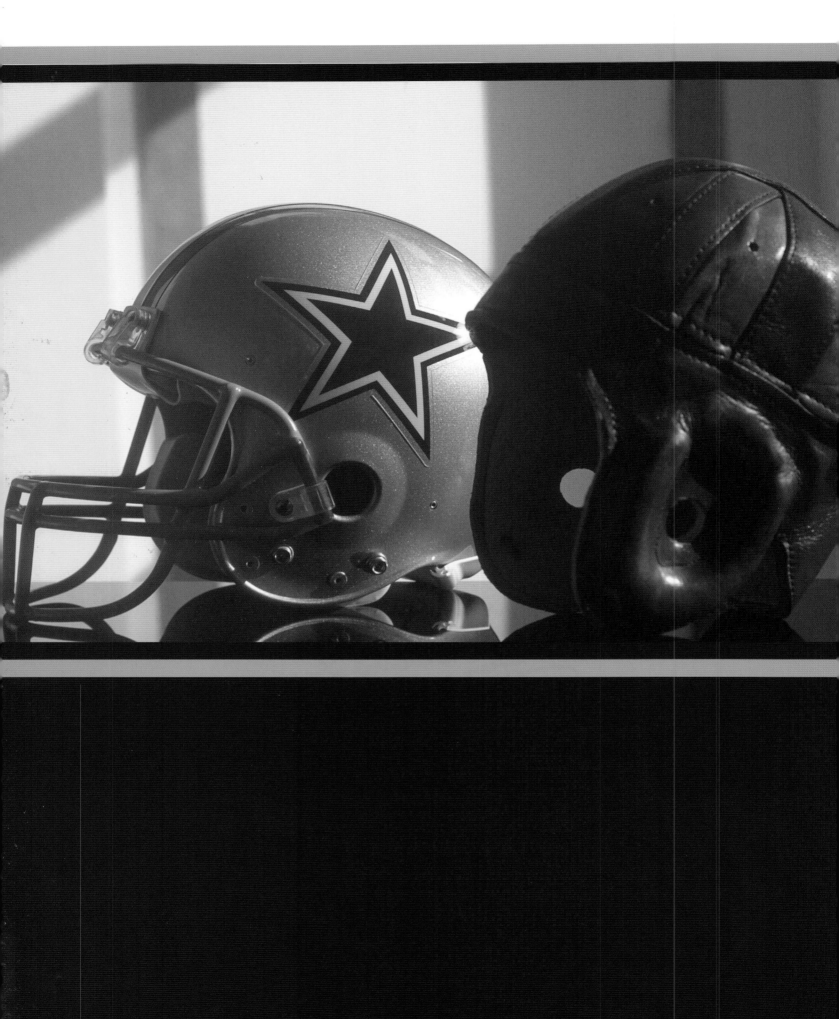

TABLE OF CONTENTS

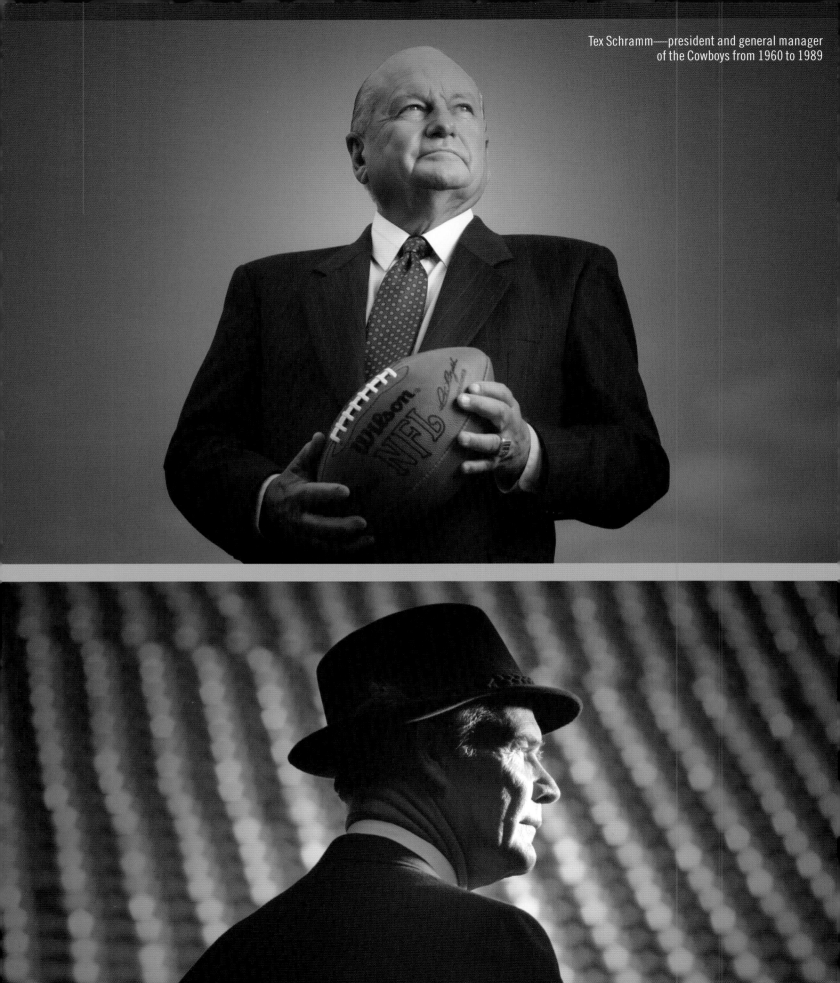

Coach Tom Landry, Dallas Cowboys, Super Bowl Champions 1972, 1978

A UNIQUE PERSPECTIVE

by PAT SUMMERALL

By sheer luck or the grace of God, or both, I've had a front-row seat for National Football League games for more than half a century—first as a player for more than a decade and then for forty-plus years as a television play-by-play announcer. Over that time, I have either played against or seen in person all of the great pro teams, permitting me to witness the handful of dynasties, and mini-dynasties that have made their mark in the NFL. These are the great teams that have pretty much dominated the league for years at a time, proving themselves much more than just one- or even two-year wonders.

I lined up against the legendary Vince Lombardi's Green Bay Packers in the sixties and then called hundreds of games involving those Packers, the Pittsburgh Steelers and Miami Dolphins of the seventies, the San Francisco Forty-niners in the late eighties, the Dallas Cowboys of the early nineties, and the New England Patriots of the early 2000s. So, while I still have my memory intact, it's time I decided which of those dominating champions is indeed the best of the best.

Forget that "Packers" nickname. The NFL should have called them the Green Bay Bruisers. Lombardi taught toughness, and his players learned their lessons well. Very little finesse was involved. They perfected the small number of plays in their offensive playbook and ran them over and over with precision. They played basic, disciplined defense. Forget substitutions—Lombardi pretty much played the same eleven on offense and the same eleven on defense. You *knew* what they'd do and they dared you to stop them. Very few opponents could. Green Bay was good—*very* good—with every ingredient of a champion.

Watching Don Shula's Dolphins was like watching major surgery being performed. Everything was so well planned out, so beautifully executed. They were so singular-minded and oftentimes matter-of-fact and almost cold in their approach. Yet, they had such skill and unity of purpose. There truly wasn't what you'd call a superstar on the entire team. In fact, the nickname of their defensive unit said it all—the No Name Defense. Their goal appeared to be the same as any other group of employees. There was a job to do . . . and they did it every day as well as possible. In fact, they did it perfectly for that magical 1972 season.

The Steelers of the seventies decimated almost everyone, particularly with their Steel Curtain defense. Led by Joe Greene and Jack Lambert, they became famous for being mean, but they were as gifted as any stop unit ever assembled. Many of their victories were born simply out of the fear opponents had of them. On offense Pittsburgh had dangerous receivers such as Lynn Swann who went deep exceptionally well. Terry Bradshaw, a big, physical quarterback, perfectly fit the Steelers mold. The record of this Chuck Noll-coached machine speaks for itself.

In the eighties the Forty-niners sort of appeared out of nowhere, with quarterback Joe Montana, a third-round draft pick, becoming an overnight superstar. Coach Bill Walsh became a genius and was dubbed a guru. The man hailed as the greatest receiver of all time, Jerry Rice, came to San Francisco from the most unlikely of places—tiny Mississippi Valley State. Running backs Roger Craig, Ricky Watters, Wendell Tyler, and Tim Rathman all fit and filled roles remarkably well. The defense became the unheralded critical part of the Niners' success. Other than Hall of Fame safety Ronnie Lott, that "D" was virtually faceless but very consistent. When the Forty-niners were right, they were nearly unbeatable.

By 2000 the New England Patriots had become a good team. Solid. Respected. But they had never truly been taken seriously until they stunned the two-touchdown favorite St. Louis Rams in Super Bowl XXXVI. No one thought of Bill Belichick as a great coach until that day—February 3, 2002. Now he's considered one of the finest of all time. Quarterback Tom Brady emerged that season as a Super Bowl MVP, and the scrappy Patriots eventually inspired talk of a dynasty, winning three Super Bowls in a span of four years. The organization became the model for others to emulate, especially with their uncanny knack for retooling at a few positions every year by finding just the right new players to replace those whose production had begun to drop off. Despite all their success, New England has never been dominating or intimidating. Just incredibly efficient, the consummate team, with everyone committed to winning instead of polishing individual resumes.

All those franchises approached and attained greatness at times. All managed to stay at or near the top for several seasons—the modern definition of "dynasty." The most brutal and successful team of them all, however, was the Dallas Cowboys of the early to mid nineties. And in their case, you could *see* greatness coming.

Jimmy Johnson quickly molded his 'Boys into a ruthless machine, forging ahead in whatever fashion was called for in any particular situation. Throw it if need be. Power blast on the ground. Shake it loose defensively. Then, once ahead, grind down the other guys with a thundering running game featuring all-time leading rusher Emmitt Smith, punishing blocker Daryl Johnston, and a massive offensive line. When it was time to throw the ball, Aikman did so with uncanny accuracy to wide receiver Michael Irvin, tight end Jay Novacek, and others.

The Dallas defense looked nothing like their powerful offense. It featured speed and quickness (and, yes, there is a real difference between the two) like the NFL had never seen before. The Cowboys attacked in an almost-collegiate style. No opponent passer felt safe from oppressive pressure, especially after Dallas added star defensive end Charles Haley to the roster early in the Johnson regime. With all the Cowboys' glittering names on offense, few noticed the defensive "clinics" they put on Sunday after Sunday. It's impossible to gauge, but I've often wondered how many rings Dallas might have won had free agency not started siphoning off their remarkable depth of talent just as that group began to achieve greatness.

The chore of labeling any one of these incredible clubs as *the best* approaches impossibility. But of those dynasties over the last fifty years, I have to go with those Dallas Cowboys as the best of them all. They had it all . . . and then some.

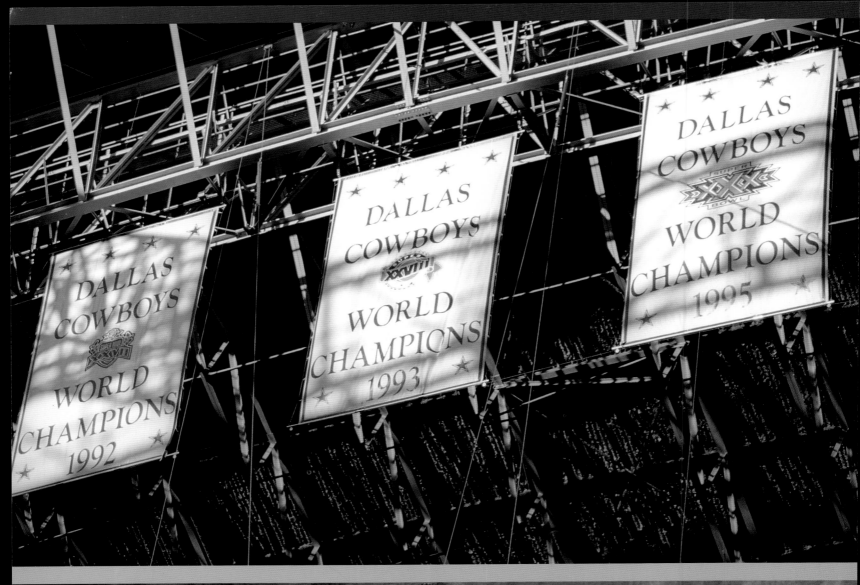

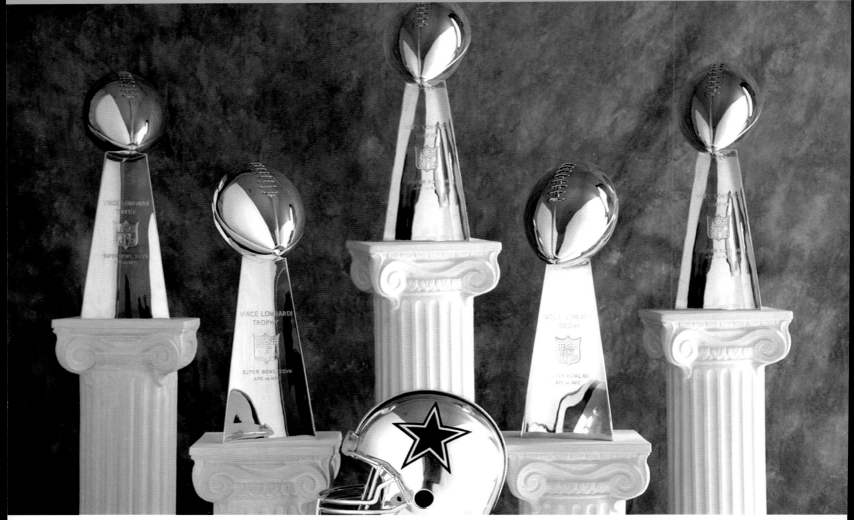

A CASE FOR GREATNESS

by NORM HITZGES

Over the more than a half century of the NFL, legions of players and thousands of teams could see the mountain. Each season one group reaches the peak. But in the league's history only a precious handful of franchises have gotten to spend any significant time perched on the summit.

To determine who might be the best *player* involves weighing the importance of the position, considering the player's ability to raise the level of play among his teammates, and measuring the impact of varying rules and styles of play on stars from very different eras. Determining the best *team* of all-time, however, might, quite oddly, be a far less daunting task than picking the finest player if only for one reason—there are so few possibilities.

For the sake of our analysis we've chosen to begin by setting a pair of absolutely fixed parameters for judging the Greatest Team Ever.

1. The nominees are graded over a five-year period exactly. Any length of dominance shorter really cannot be considered a dynasty. Some teams may have remained near the peak longer. But there also may have been factors at work in certain eras making such superiority significantly easier.

2. Every club must have won at least two championships during its five-year window and had to have remained extremely competitive for that entire half decade. (This last qualifier eliminates, for example, the late '90s Denver Broncos who did capture back-to-back Super Bowls in '97 and '98 but posted sub-par seasons on either side of those titles.)

We are left with six contenders:

1.	1963–67	Green Bay Packers
2.	1970–74	Miami Dolphins
3.	1975–79	Pittsburgh Steelers
4.	1988–92	San Francisco 49ers
5.	1991–95	Dallas Cowboys
6.	2001–05	New England Patriots

Those are your finalists for title of The Greatest Ever. We'll compare each side by side in a handful of categories together.

1. Number of Victories

A logical place to start. In our table we've totaled the number of triumphs—regular season plus playoffs—followed by the Super Bowls won for each of our six best.

	Team	Wins	Super Bowls
#1	'91–'95 Cowboys	71	'92, '93, '95
#2	'88–'92 Niners	70	'88, '89
#3	'01–'05 Patriots	68	'01, '03, '04
#4	'75–'79 Steelers	67	'75, '78, '79
#5	'70–'74 Dolphins	65	'72, '73
#6	'63–'67 Packers	57	'66, '67*

*The Super Bowl did not come into being until the last two seasons of the Packer reign ('66 and '67). Green Bay also won the NFL title in 1965, the year before the merged NFL and AFL began meeting in what quickly became known as the Super Bowl.

The top three on our wins list all did so under the present sixteen-game regular season format. Green Bay and Miami played fourteen-game schedules throughout their stretches. The sixteen-game slate became reality three years into the Steelers run. All teams after the Packers had an opportunity to win as many as three playoff games in any single season. Actually, since 1990, wild card teams could win four playoff games in one year, but none of our "dynasties" did so. Only the 1997 Broncos, 2000 Ravens, and 2005 Steelers have won four post-season games en route to their Super Bowl triumphs.

Green Bay, Miami, and Pittsburgh would all have certainly won more total games had there simply been more regular season games to play. But at what cost? More games would have meant more wear and tear and, quite possibly, more injuries. Might this have had a long-term negative effect? There certainly would have been more year-after-year fatigue. For example: during their five-year reign, the Pack played 77 games. Dallas played 93! That's the equivalent of one full season of games more for those Cowboys and their bodies.

A look at the winning percentages of each franchise might offer more insight:

1.	'70–'74	Dolphins	81.1%
2.	'63–'65	Packers	76.6%
3.	'75–'79	Steelers	76.5%
4.	'88–'92	Niners	76.4%
5.	'91–'95	Cowboys	76.3%
6.	'01–'05	Patriots	74.7%

Although the '70–'74 Dolphins have a phenomenal winning percentage, they didn't win any playoff game in the first and last year of their dominance and captured just two total championships, as did the Niners. Dallas, Pitt, New England, and the Packers can all claim three rings. Also note the razor-thin differences between numbers 2, 3, 4 and 5—three-tenths of 1 percent!

However, we *must* address one other enormous factor—free agency. The Packers, Dolphins, Steelers, and Niners faced absolutely no threat of other teams outbidding them for the services of key players. Only Dallas and New England had that challenge. And, during the infancy of free agency ('93 and '94), the "Rooney Rule" dramatically limited Dallas' ability to sign other players in the marketplace. During those two years the rule mandated that Dallas and the other three teams who reached the conference championship the previous season could only spend on free agents the amounts in salary given to the players lured away from them and no more. The rule worked as intended. In those initial two seasons of free agency, the Pokes lost ten players and signed two.

How would those earlier dynasties have fared had free agency existed during their supremacy? Who knows? Outstanding organizations usually adjust very well to change. But, the reality of the situation is that they never had to.

Finally, let's tackle another dicey question. How do we measure the varying levels of competition each faced? For example, in the '70s Miami and Pittsburgh had to outplay each other to win the AFC. Once there, they often encountered those excellent Tom Landry Cowboys in title games.

Consider for a moment, though, the NFC of the early '90s that Dallas ruled. Just to win the NFC East they had to conquer the New York Giants, who'd won the 1990 Super Bowl; Washington, who'd taken home the '91 trophy; and a Philadelphia team that had *three* ten-win seasons during that same period of Cowboy dominance. Once past their division, those wonderful Niners stood in Dallas' way. San Francisco won the '88, '89, and '93 Super Bowls. In addition to all those fine teams, five other NFC franchises (Detroit, Chicago, Minnesota, Atlanta, and New Orleans) all had at last one ten-win campaign of their own between '91 and '95. Talk about a *loaded* NFC! At one point that conference swept the Super Bowl a whopping 16 straight years (1981–1996)!

2. Play-off Victories

During their dominant half decades who totaled the most playoff wins? Here's the list of NFL all-time leaders in this category:

Rank	Years	Team	# Wins
#1	'91–'95	Cowboys	11
#2	'01–'05	Patriots	10
#3	'75–'79	Steelers	10
#4	'88–'92	Niners	8
#5	'70–'74	Dolphins	8
#6	'63–'67	Packers	7

Again, the Packers suffer from the lack of extra layers in the playoff structure. But Green Bay, the Niners, and the Patriots all had at least one year during their streaks in which they did not even make the playoffs.

Miami, Pittsburgh, and Dallas each reached the post-season in all five of their campaigns. But one, and only one, posted at least one playoff victory in each of their dynasty seasons—the Cowboys. In fact, by doing so Dallas became the first NFL team to ever record at least one playoff victory five consecutive years. The Pokes extended that mark to six in a row in '96, a record that still stands.

One final, fascinating and remarkable note: From '92 through '95, Dallas posted a gaudy 10–1 playoff record. But inside that sparkling won-loss total lies one incredible fact. All ten of those post-season triumphs came by double figures—a stretch unparalleled in pro football history! Their margins of victory in those ten wins were by, in order: 24, 10, 35, 10, 17, 17, 26, 19, 11, and 10. That's an average of an extraordinary *eighteen points per game*! Imagine a stretch in which you won three Super Bowls in four seasons and never had to sweat out the last two minutes in any playoff victory. Should you have difficulty recalling the names of Cowboy placekickers during those glory seasons, there's an excellent reason. They were simply never called on to attempt any crucial playoff-winning field goals.

3. The "Dozen-A-Year" Club

Ask any coach the quality he most values in his team, and at or near the top of all of their checklists would be consistency. Simply by their presence on our "greatest ever" roll call, and by the parameters we've put in place, each of the candidates should be considered models of consistency. But again, who's the best of the best?

To separate the contenders we'll use twelve-win-seasons as a yardstick, including regular season and post-season victories. No matter how you add them together (eleven regular season wins plus one post-season, ten regular season and two playoffs, etc.) that total of twelve represents a grand accomplishment.

Before going any further, we must address the burden this number puts on the Packers and Dolphins who played those fourteen-game rather than sixteen-game schedules. Extra games would not have helped the 8-5-1 '64 Packers get anywhere close to twelve that season. Miami missed getting to that number twice—ten wins in '70 and eleven in '74. So, conceivably, an extra pair of regular season contests in each of these years could have enabled Miami to reach that magic "twelve" in those campaigns.

Three of the other clubs (San Francisco, Pittsburgh, and New England) all missed reaching twelve at least once during their incredible half decades.

Only one franchise, only one NFL team ever, has piled up at least twelve wins for five straight years—the '91–'95 Dallas Cowboys.

4. Player Honors

To gauge the level of respect across the league for a team's talent, we've researched Pro Bowl rosters. Though the selection process has often created controversy and caused disagreement, it remains our only real measuring stick for the league's opinion on the skill level of its players.

In this particular category, schedule lengths mean nothing. And, while Pro Bowl rosters have expanded some over the years, so have the number of teams in the league. For example: in, say 1965, for a Packer to make the Pro Bowl he'd have competition only from players on the other six teams in the NFL Western Conference. The '70s Dolphins competed in a thirteen-team AFC. Ditto for those '70s Steelers. In the late '80s, the Niners were part of a fourteen-team NFC as were the Cowboys. The Patriots were one of sixteen AFC franchises.

Here's the list of the most total Pro Bowl selections ever over a three-year period:

Rank	Years	Team	# of Pro Bowlers
#1	'93–'95	Cowboys	32
#2	'72–'74	Dolphins	30
#3	'90–'92	Bills	28
#4	'71–'73	Dolphins	27
#5	'74–'76	Steelers	25
#6	'61–'63	Packers	25
#7	'77–'79	Steelers	24

Only one of the above seven teams faced the possibility of the loss of some excellent players through the process of free agency—the Cowboys. Following the '93, '94, and '95 seasons, three Cowboys who'd been named to one or more Pro Bowls left for "greener pastures."

5. The Impact of Free Agency

Only one of these "Superb Six" had to bridge a major change in the NFL economic policy during its tenure. Full free agency and the accompanying salary cap arrived after the '92 season in which Dallas had taken the first of its three Super Bowls.

Nearly a decade later the Patriots also encountered such a potential talent drain. But they'd had time to prepare for it, to study how others had approached the task, and to develop strategies for dealing with the cap.

So, how much damage did free agency do to that very young and very deep Cowboys roster? The Dallas organization, headed by owner/general manager Jerry Jones and coach Jimmy Johnson, decided that to stay as competitive as possible for as long as possible they would opt to use available cap dollars to lock up core players like quarterback Troy Aikman, running back Emmitt Smith, wide receiver Michael Irvin, tight end Eric Williams, guard Nate Newton, and others. They badly wanted to keep all the talent they had assembled. The cap rules simply wouldn't allow it.

What transpired was a slow, steady siphoning off of some significant ability. From the inception of free agency after that '92 season through the off-season immediately, following the '95 campaign that saw the last of the Cowboys three Super Bowls, Dallas lost twenty-five players and signed just seven.

Here's a partial list of the big names and big talents who got away:

LB	Ken Norton	G	Kevin Gogan
WR	Alvin Harper	LB	Dixon Edwards
C	Mark Stepnoski	DT	Tony Casillas
DT	Russell Maryland	S	James Washington
CB	Larry Brown	MLB	Robert Jones

Some random facts about what the Cowboys lost:

★ Thirteen could be considered "regulars," three had been Pro Bowlers, and another a Super Bowl MVP.

★ Combined, the "departed" made 582 starts during that '91–'95 period and ninety more in the playoffs.

★ Eleven had been in the opening lineup of one or more of Dallas' Super Bowls.

★ In total, those twenty-five lost to free agency in that four-year period started 842 games in their combined Cowboy careers.

What might that team have accomplished had free agency not come along? The mind boggles with possibilities:

Butch Davis, former Cowboy Defensive Coordinator:
"We weren't losing declining veterans. We lost marquee players. Young veterans. Players in their prime. Leaders. Had nothing changed there's no telling the possible accomplishment levels."

Charles Haley, defensive end who'd also starred with another of our "Greatest Ever" nominees, the '88–'92 49ers:
"I used to think the 49ers had the best talent until I came to the Cowboys. When one player left, another would step in and then another. It was just talent out the ying-yang. We'd lose three, four, five starters every year and still come back and fight. Without free agency I think we'd probably have gone on and won five or six Super Bowls."

Regardless of what might have happened, so many around the NFL look back and admire what did happen.

Jim Nantz, CBS NFL announcer and childhood Dallas fan complete with Cowboys bed sheets, lunch box, rain poncho, etc.:
"They had such swagger, such speed, aggression, confidence that bordered on and became arrogance. I don't think people realize what it takes to go from the very worst team in the league to the very best in just four years. If it were that easy why are there so, so many teams who NEVER figure out how to do it? Only now when I look back and examine some of these numbers do I understand how remarkable those teams were."

Bart Starr, Hall of Fame quarterback of those legendary '60s Green Bay Packers:
"It was thrilling to watch Dallas play because I remember exactly what it took to get us to the top and remain there. Every player on a team that's won multiple championships appreciates the level of unselfish commitment required to achieve that goal."

Chris Berman, high profile ESPN announcer and studio host of "NFL Live":
"I look at who they had to beat to win those championships: the Giants, Redskins, Niners, Bills. All of 'em terrific teams. And the J J's did it their way. It took courage to believe they had the right approach and to stick with it."

Which team was "The Greatest Ever?" When you review all the numbers, all the records and evidence, are there any questions?

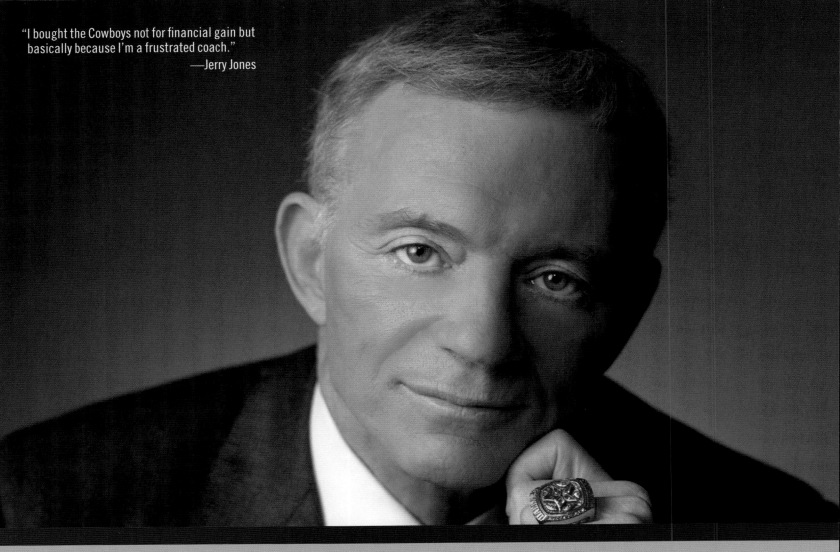

"I bought the Cowboys not for financial gain but basically because I'm a frustrated coach."
—Jerry Jones

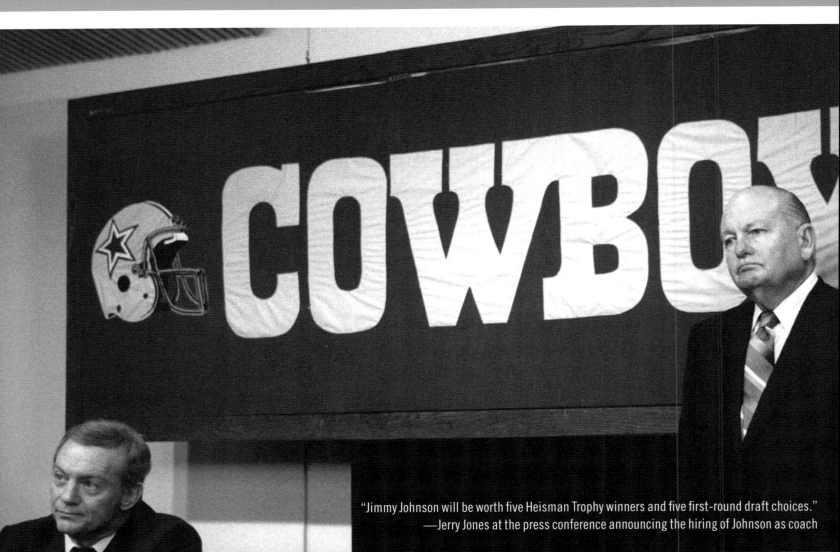

"Jimmy Johnson will be worth five Heisman Trophy winners and five first-round draft choices."
—Jerry Jones at the press conference announcing the hiring of Johnson as coach

FEBRUARY 25, 1989

"JETHRO" BUYS THE 'BOYS

Shock waves ripped through the Cowboys nation.

The Dallas Cowboys had been sold to someone named Jerral Wayne Jones from (Oh, my God) *Arkansas*. In the club's twenty-nine-year history only two men had owned the Pokes—Clint Murchison and Bum Bright. Both Texans. Both had made big bucks doing "big bidness" the way "real men" made money! Oil. Trucking. There's an old joke about some folks from the state being "fake Texans who are all hat and no cattle." These two had cattle.

They also shared the same philosophy while owning the club. *Keep your hands off. Get out of the way. Find a seat far, far in the background and stay there.*

Then along came Jones.

Jerry Jones was raised in a not-so-nice section of North Little Rock known as "Dogtown." He grew up in the rooms above his father Pat's grocery store, where stocking shelves was Jerry's first job. Pat Jones hustled all his life selling everything from those groceries to insurance to billboard space. The day Jerry called him to tell him he'd just bought the Dallas Cowboys, his dad gave a response that wasn't exactly what Jerry had anticipated. Pat had also had a good day. "I sold three boards today. Made good deals on 'em, too."

Now the Dallas Cowboys belonged to a former co-captain and guard on the University of Arkansas Hogs football team. *Sooooeee Pig!* He'd later struck it rich by borrowing money and finding Oklahoma crude. He was also vice president of a poultry company. Now Jerry Jones owned all the Cowboys' wings, breasts, and thighs.

The press conference announcing the sale served immediate notice that the football world in Texas had tilted on its axis. Murchison and Bright had been invisible as owners, staying out of the limelight. Not Jerry Jones. Energy and exuberance bubbled out of him like Oklahoma crude. He wasn't shy of cameras, microphones, or notepads and spoke with an exaggerated twang. He could at times sound like a naïve country boy—which he wasn't.

Few liked the sounds coming from Jones that first day.

"I want to be part of every decision," he proclaimed. "I won't leave anything to the football people. I'm not saying I'm coming in to be the football coach, but I intend to have an understanding of the complete situation, an understating of the player situation, of the socks and jocks."

Any chance that Jones had of a honeymoon period in Dallas had disappeared long before that first press conference. The previous Friday night, bursting with anticipation, Jones and his coach-to-be Jimmy Johnson, who'd flown into town and registered at the Mansion under a phony name, decided to chow down on some Mexican food at Mia's, a seventy-five-seat restaurant a mile from the hotel.

Room service would have been a *much* better idea.

Dallas Morning News sports reporter Ivan Maisel just happened to also be waiting for a table. The cat had escaped the bag. The next morning the world woke up to the news of Dallas' new owner-coach combo.

That Saturday afternoon, hours before the purchase and new coach announcement, Jones and Cowboys General Manager Tex Schramm had flown to Austin to tell coach Tom Landry of his fate. They delivered the news at Hidden Hills Country Club, where Landry and some family members had completed fifteen holes of golf before being summoned to the clubhouse. The reaction of the only coach the Cowboys had ever had? "You've taken my team away from me."

"American's Team" had fired "America's Tom."

Between the clumsy leaking of the news and the awkward firing of Landry, early indications were that this guy from Arkansas, this vice president of poultry, wouldn't be just a hands-on owner, he'd be a "hands-all-over" one. The reaction was fast, furious, and frighteningly negative.

★ Callers to the team's flagship radio station KRLD ranged from one describing this as a "dark day" to another announcing the canceling of his season tickets to a third saying it was Dallas' worst moment since the assassination of President John F. Kennedy.

★ *Dallas Morning News* columnist Randy Galloway: "First impression? No clue. Lost. A disaster."

★ Even NFL Commissioner Pete Rozelle, who'd always chosen his words carefully, chimed in: "This is like Lombardi's death."

★ One columnist dubbed Jones "Jethro" referring to the dimwitted Jethro Bodine of TV's suddenly oil-rich family on *The Beverly Hillbillies*.

got some bad advice and took it."

As many as seventy-five prospective buyers had kicked the tires to see if they wanted to purchase Bum Bright's Cowboys. Folks like L.A. Lakers boss Jerry Buss, New York-based Loews Corporation, and Donald Carter, the owner of the National Basketball Association's Dallas

"This is like Lombardi's death."

The nasty reaction both surprised and puzzled Jones, who would later admit that the level of venom in the comments directed at him had stung him badly. "I was going to be involved in every detail," he said. "I thought that's what they'd want to hear—that I'd be a committed owner. That's being on the floor of the manufacturing company. That's being in the store when a customer comes in."

Within days of taking control, Jones gave himself an "F" for the way everything was handled. Now, more than a decade and a half removed from that historic day, what grade would he give? "Still an F," he said. "I

Mavericks. There'd also been a serious Japanese bidder, but Bright simply couldn't stomach selling America's Team to Japan. Jones eventually got the team for $150 million. No partners. Just Jerry.

In truth, at that Saturday night introduction of Jones as the new owner, he actually hadn't closed the deal. That wouldn't happen until *weeks* later.

Jones: "The agreement we had was very informal. Handwritten. Almost a handshake deal with twenty-one, twenty-two aspects of the agreement still to be worked out involving several million dollars . . . *several million!* It was enough of a difference that either one of

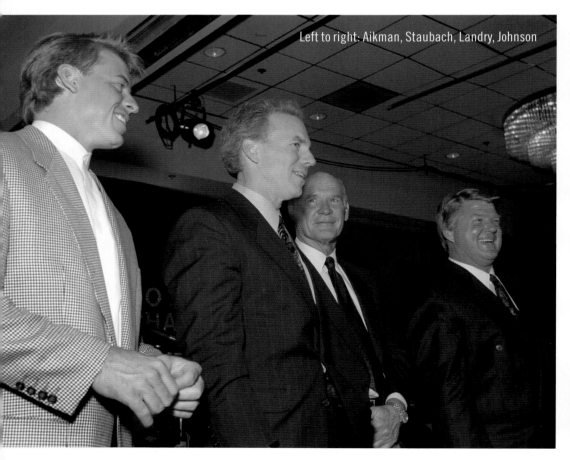

Left to right: Aikman, Staubach, Landry, Johnson

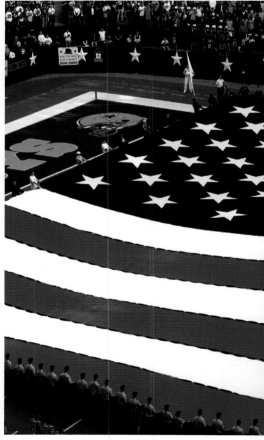

us could have voided the deal. That's how tenuous it was. At one point (weeks after the already announced sale) we're at a real log jam, and I asked Bum what happens if we can't settle things and he says, 'Well, then, I've got me a new football coach.'"

The final contractual item involved $300,000. To settle this one last agreement obstacle, they flipped a coin for that final $300 grand.

Said Jones, "After Bum won the coin flip, he put that quarter in a block where I could only see one side and attached a note that said something like, 'You'll never know if it was a two-headed coin.' I thought he was such a straight shooter I've never torn that coin out of the block to see the other side."

For his $150 million Jones had purchased a team leaking oil, not the kind you sell by the barrel. The Cowboys were coming off three consecutive losing seasons, and they had not won a playoff game in six years. And it was a franchise losing a million bucks a month. Factor in what Jones could have been earning on the millions of dollars of cash he'd put into the purchase as well as what it was costing him in terms of the interest on the millions and millions he'd borrowed using his gas and oil properties as collateral, and you've got a bottom line as ugly as those previous Cowboys win-loss records.

"At the start it was costing me $100,000 a day to own the Dallas Cowboys," Jones said.

But Jones had found himself in debt and in Dallas long before then. Years earlier, just out of school and new to the business world, Jones had flown to Love Field and proceeded to the car rental counter. "The woman at the counter took my credit card and looked down this long list. Then she took out scissors and cut it in two right in front of me and some other customers and told me, 'Young man, you need to learn how to pay your bills.' I was dead broke and didn't know it."

Once that 9:00 PM start press conference ended, Jones still had two items left on his long day's agenda. He and Bright picked up Jerry's wife Gene, a former Miss Arkansas USA, and headed for Bum's house and a celebratory visit. Then "I went out to Texas Stadium and had them turn on all the lights and walked out to the 50-yard line and laid down on my back in the middle of the blue star."

Who could have ever imagined that this son of an Arkansas grocer, the fellow who'd made money in Oklahoma crude and chickens, the man they mockingly called "Jethro," could, within four years, go back to midfield at Texas Stadium and lay down on that star wearing his very own Super Bowl ring.

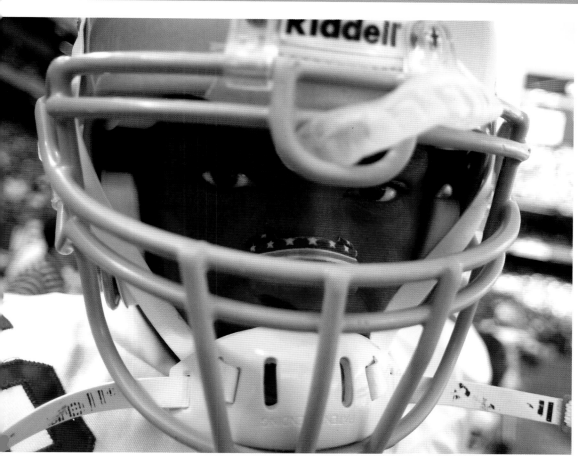

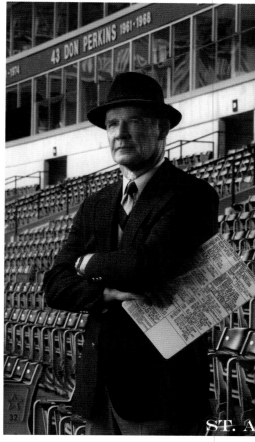

15

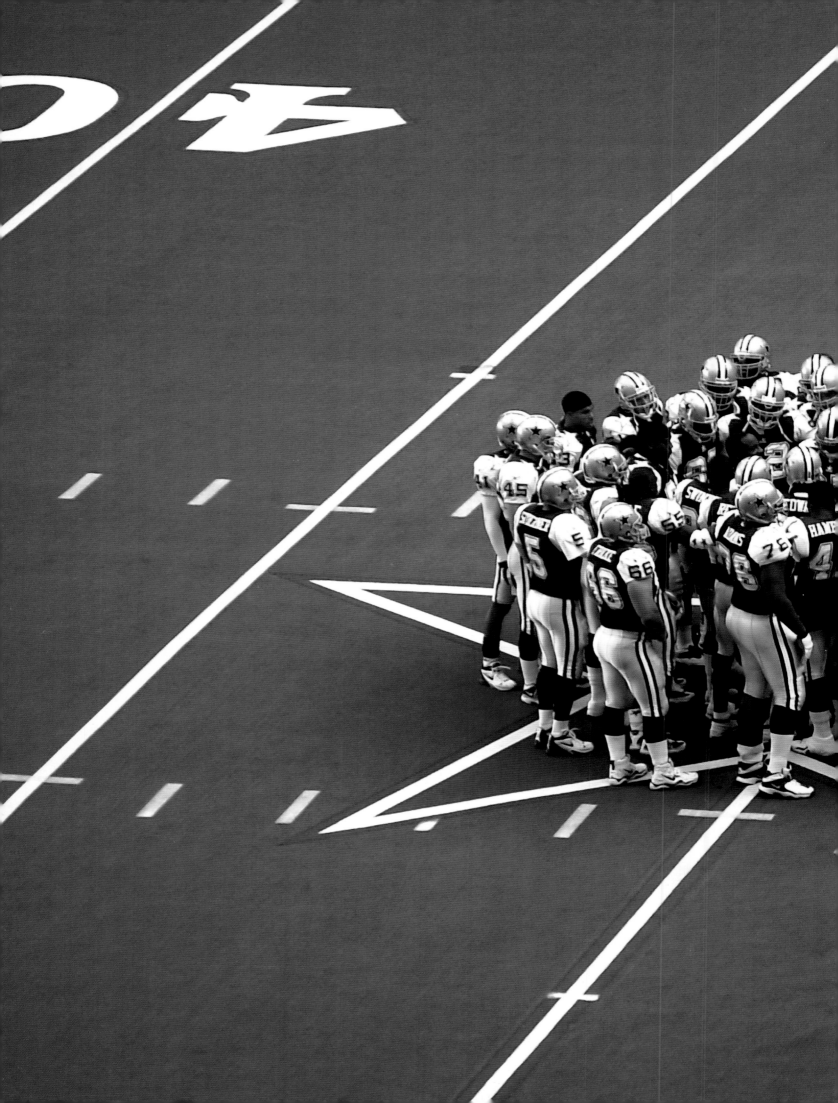

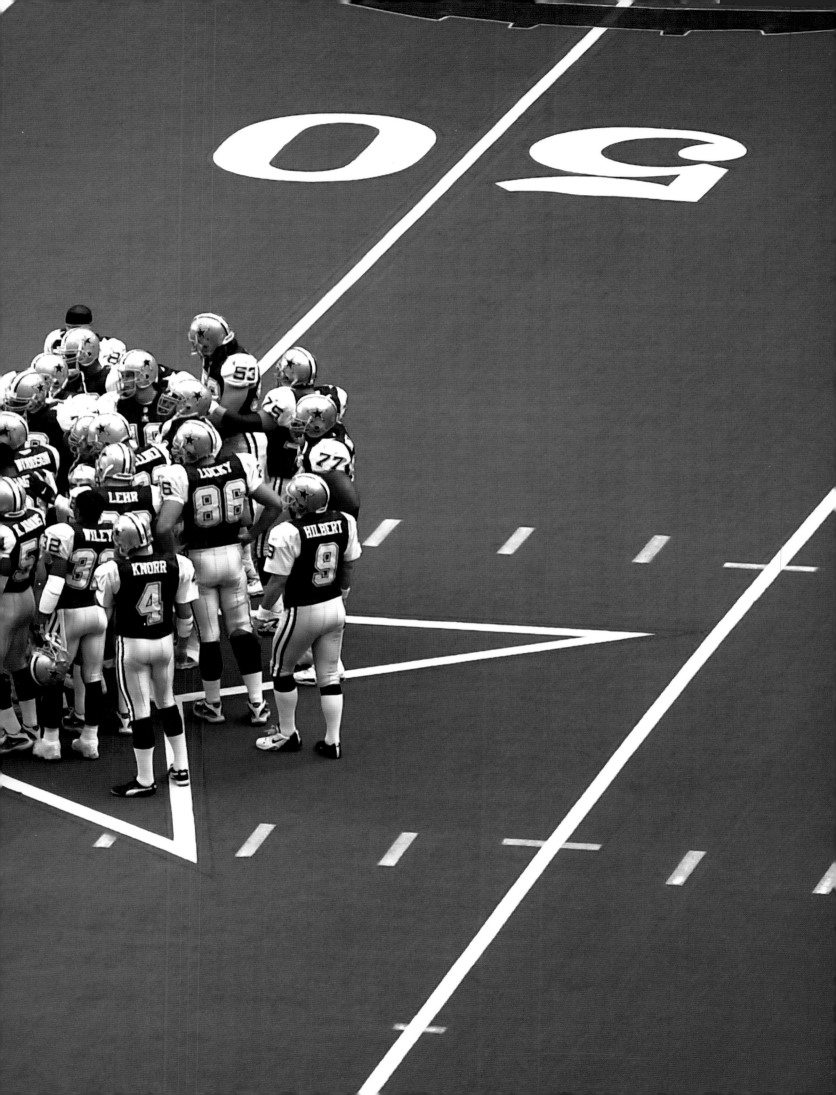

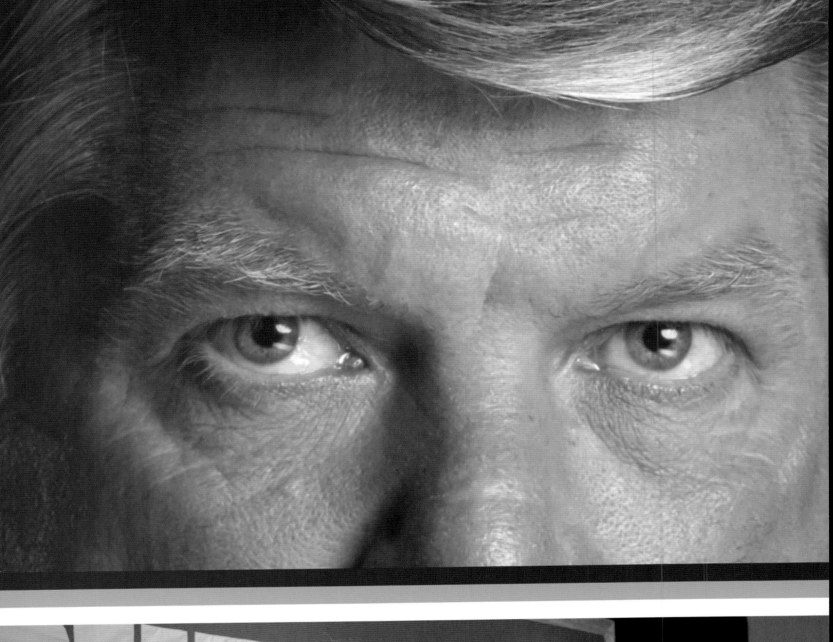
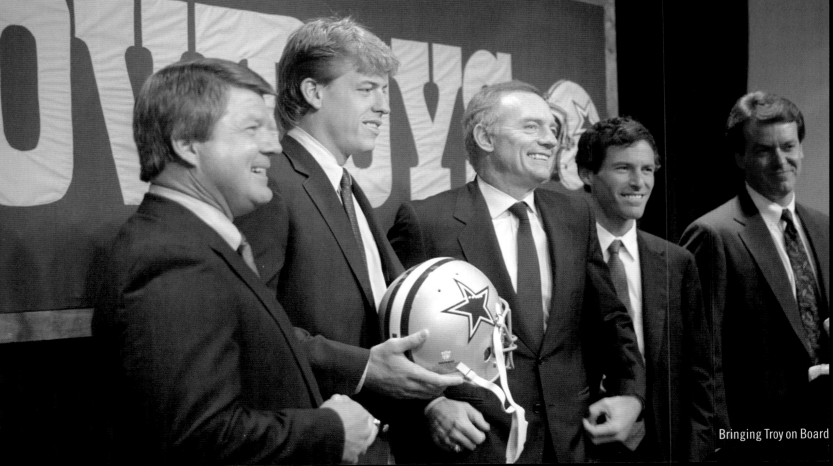

Bringing Troy on Board

HIT THE GROUND RUNNING

Fifty-six days.

That's how long Jimmy Johnson had between the day Jerry Jones named him head coach and his first NFL draft.

Fifty-six days to hire an entire staff, six of whom, like Jimmy, had never coached a day of pro football and nearly a dozen of whom he'd never even worked with.

Fifty-six days to familiarize himself with all the talent on his roster. "Not all that hard to do," remembers Jimmy. "We didn't have that much."

Fifty-six days to organize his team's off-season workout program and training camp regimen and to get up to speed on players around the league.

Fifty-six days to learn the names of executive assistants, secretaries, and key organizational people. To get to know other pro coaches and, in particular, personnel directors with whom he'd be dealing. To give himself a crash course of NFL rules, guidelines, and union matters.

Fifty-six days to move into his Valley Ranch office and to find and buy a new home in between everything else.

Fifty-six days to hammer out the parameters of his working relationship with Jerry Jones.

"We decided we'd try to never, ever let anyone or anything come between us," Jerry recalled.

Fifty-six days without a day off for Johnson or anyone on his staff. "Day off? A day off? I didn't have a day off until after that first season ended," Johnson said.

Fifty-six days to pull together all the pre-draft scouting reports on hundreds of players. During those eight weeks assistant coaches and scouts scoured the country evaluating draftable players. They were all starting from scratch.

"I had my assistant coaches, all of whom once worked the college game, phone their friends," Johnson said. "Their buddies were all college coaches, and we could get some inside information. I had my strength coaches call their peers in college. One thing you'll discover is that those guys will fudge the truth if *you're* talking to them, but they'll be straight with their friends one-on-one. Through the years I rarely found a strength coach embellishing a kid to my strength coach.

"We even talked to beat writers around the country. You look at some of these writers' mock drafts, and a lot of them were pretty accurate because they had a good idea of who their coaches really liked."

Imagine that! A team milking reporters for information. J. J. left no stone unturned.

On the Friday preceding the start of the Saturday draft, more than fifty thousand Dallasites swarmed into downtown for a parade honoring Tom Landry. By virtue of Landry's last team being the worst team in the league in 1988, Dallas had the first selection of the entire draft, and they had already decided to pick UCLA quarterback Troy Aikman, a no-brainer of a choice.

Small world: the new Cowboys coach and his first No. 1 pick had a history. It went like this: In 1984 Johnson had gotten Aikman to make an oral commitment to accept a scholarship to Oklahoma State, then coached by Johnson (and they, too, were called the Cowboys, no less). But Aikman changed his mind, decommitted, and switched to Oklahoma, which was then coached by one Barry Switzer, giving Aikman, sort of, a succession of coaches that, as fate would have it, would later repeat itself in Dallas. In another irony, in 1985, Aikman would break his leg playing for the Sooners in a game against the Miami Hurricanes, by then coached by none other than one Jimmy Johnson.

After that 1985 season, Aikman opted to transfer to UCLA despite Johnson's overtures to come join him in Miami. But finally, five years later, Jimmy got his man. Three days prior to the draft Jones had already locked up the quarterback with a six-year, $11.037 million contract. Before finalizing that deal, however, Johnson had turned down a New England trade offer of their top three picks in the 1989 draft plus a 1990 first-rounder for the rights to Aikman.

With Aikman signed, Johnson crossed his fingers that either Florida defensive end Trace Armstrong or Miami defensive end Bill Hawkins would slip to the second round, where Dallas had the top pick, number twenty-nine overall. No such luck. Chicago took Armstrong at No. 12, and the Rams grabbed Hawkins at No. 21.

On to Plan B. Johnson knew who he wanted next—Daryl Johnston, a punishing blocker at fullback for Syracuse and a player Johnson coached in the East-West college all-star Shrine game. But Dallas believed Johnston would slide well down in the second round, meaning the Cowboys could probably afford to trade down, still pick Johnston, and get something extra in return for that No. 29 pick. So, Jimmy went looking for a trading partner and found one in, of all places, Oakland. Raiders owner Al Davis and the Cowboys' general manager Tex Schramm had once been friends. But many years earlier Davis and Schramm had a major falling out over NFL Commissioner Pete Rozelle, who had been a Schramm crony and a Davis adversary.

It's no wonder the Cowboys and Raiders hadn't made a draft-day deal in fifteen years, whereas Dallas had traded with seventeen other teams during that same period. So, would the Pokes have even considered such a swap were Schramm still in charge? "Probably not," offered Gil Brandt, the personnel guru who had run Cowboys drafts for three decades. Let's just say Davis' phone number wasn't on Schramm's speed dial. But here was Johnson, basically, sleeping with the enemy.

Davis offered Oakland's later second-rounder (No. 39) and a third-round selection for that Cowboys' No. 29 and a sixth-rounder. That wasn't good enough: Jimmy wanted more. He asked for the best of Davis' three fifth-rounders instead of the sixth-rounder offered. The Raider boss balked. A few minutes later they talked again, but Davis wouldn't budge.

As the time to make the twenty-ninth pick approached for the Cowboys, the phone rang again. It was Davis, and this time he agreed to the swap. In his first-ever NFL trade, Johnson had played "sweat" with one of the league's heavyweights, and he'd won. As pre-arranged with Davis, Dallas selected Penn State guard Steve Wisniewski with that No. 29 pick and shipped him on to the Raiders. Johnston slipped as predicted and was available at No. 39.

The next two rounds produced two more players Johnson had circled on the shrinking list of available players. In the third round the Cowboys grabbed highly accomplished though smallish Pittsburgh center Mark Stepnoski. Then in Round Four they took Texas-El Paso defensive end Tony Tolbert.

"Tolbert was just a tall, skinny kid," Johnson recalled. "We thought if we could get him from 233 pounds to about 245, we might have something because he could really rush the passer."

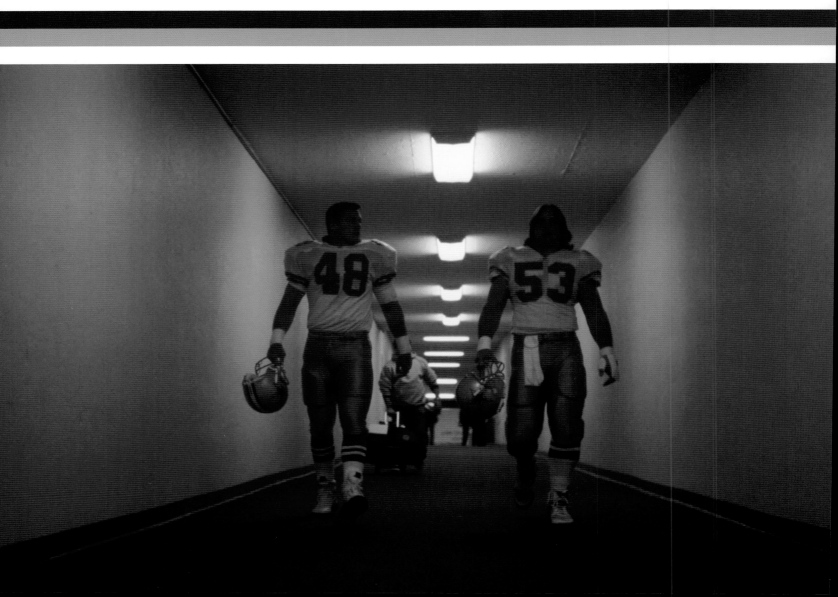

Draft analysts regarded all four as excellent prospects. All were "Johnson types."

"We got three academic all-Americans and a guy (Tolbert) who captained his team in both his junior and senior years."

Time would prove how shrewd Johnson had been with his first NFL crop. Aikman would play twelve seasons, Johnston eleven, and Stepnoski and Tolbert (eventually at *265 pounds*) nine each. They combined to start an astounding 529 games in the silver and blue.

All were selected to Pro Bowls. Among them they own eleven Super Bowl rings.

The rebuilding had begun, as had Johnson's reputation as the NFL's version of Monty Hall from *Let's Make a Deal*. That Raider swap would be the first of many. "I believe I made more trades in my five-year period than the rest of the league put together," Johnson later boasted of his Cowboys years, during which he completed an astounding fifty-one draft-related deals.

Fifty-one!

"I believe I made more trades in my five-year period than the rest of the league put together."

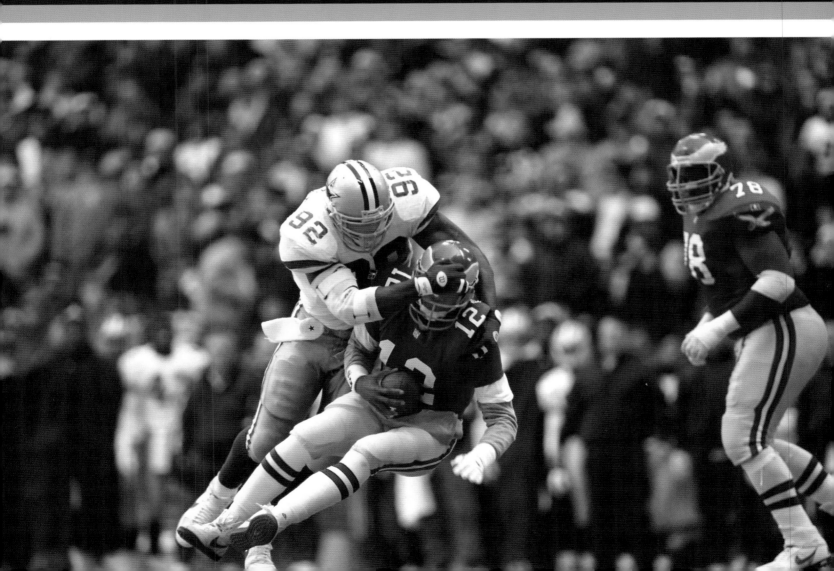

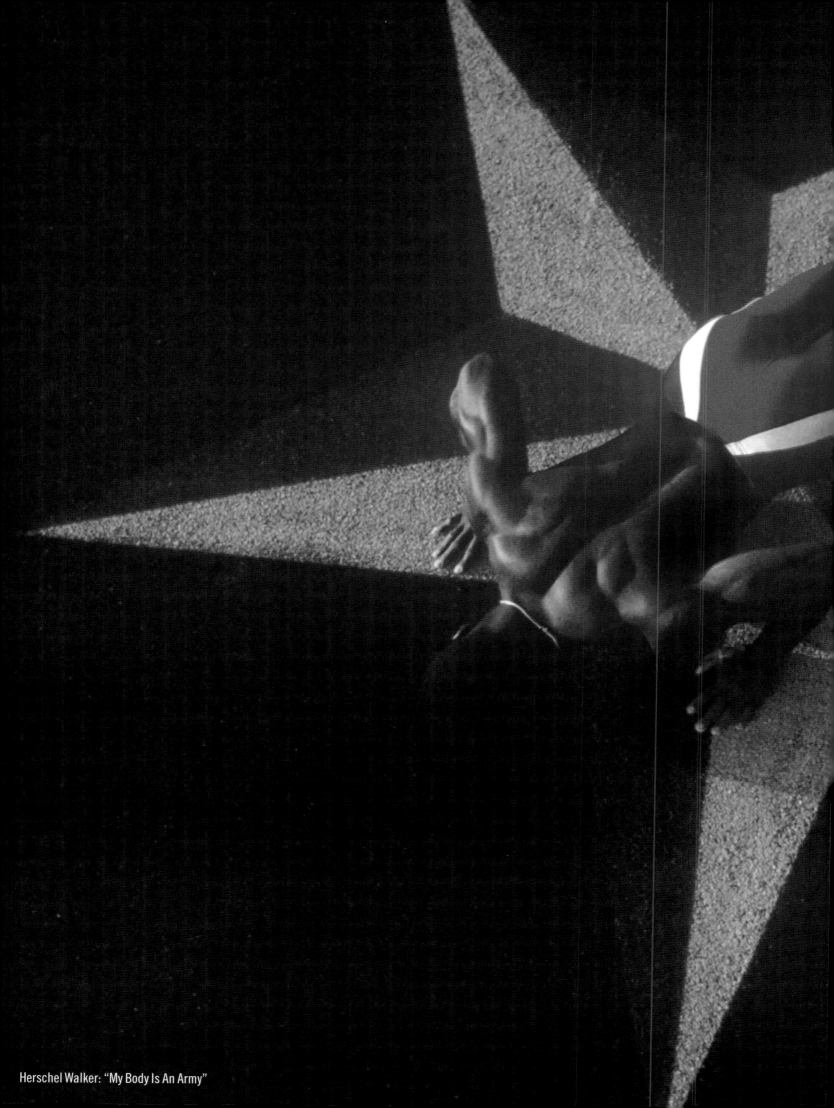
Herschel Walker: "My Body Is An Army"

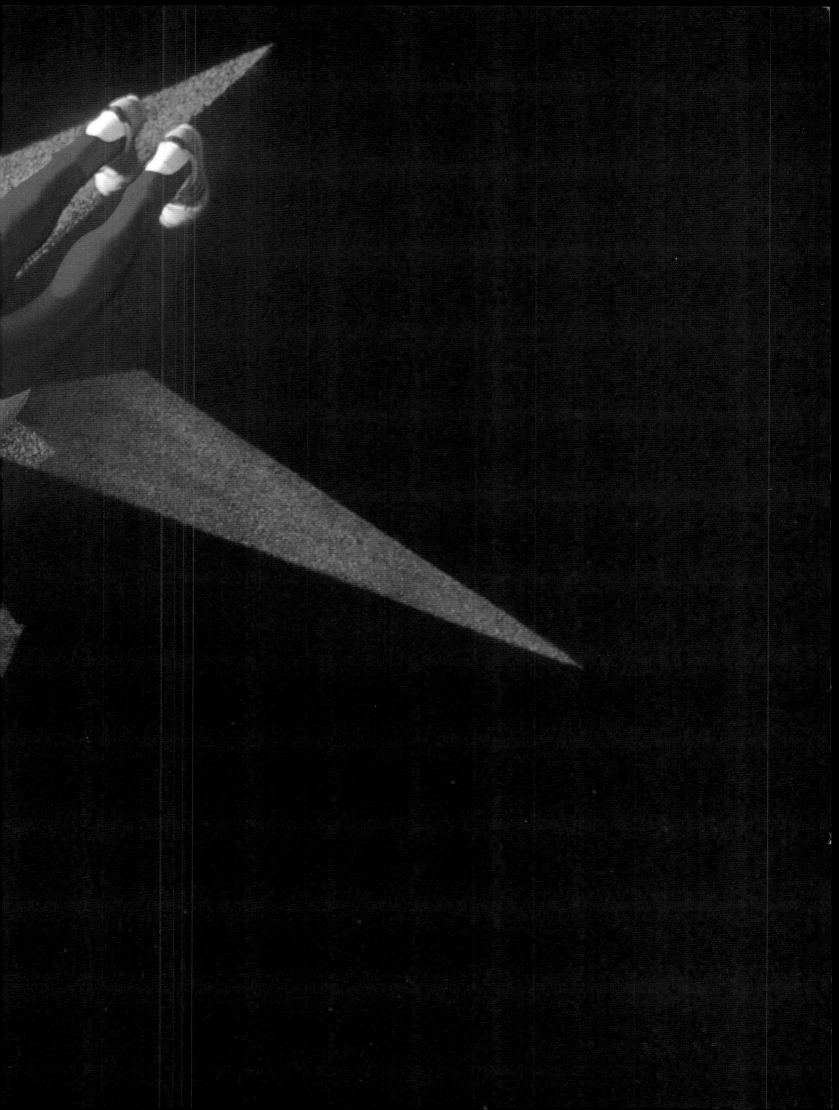

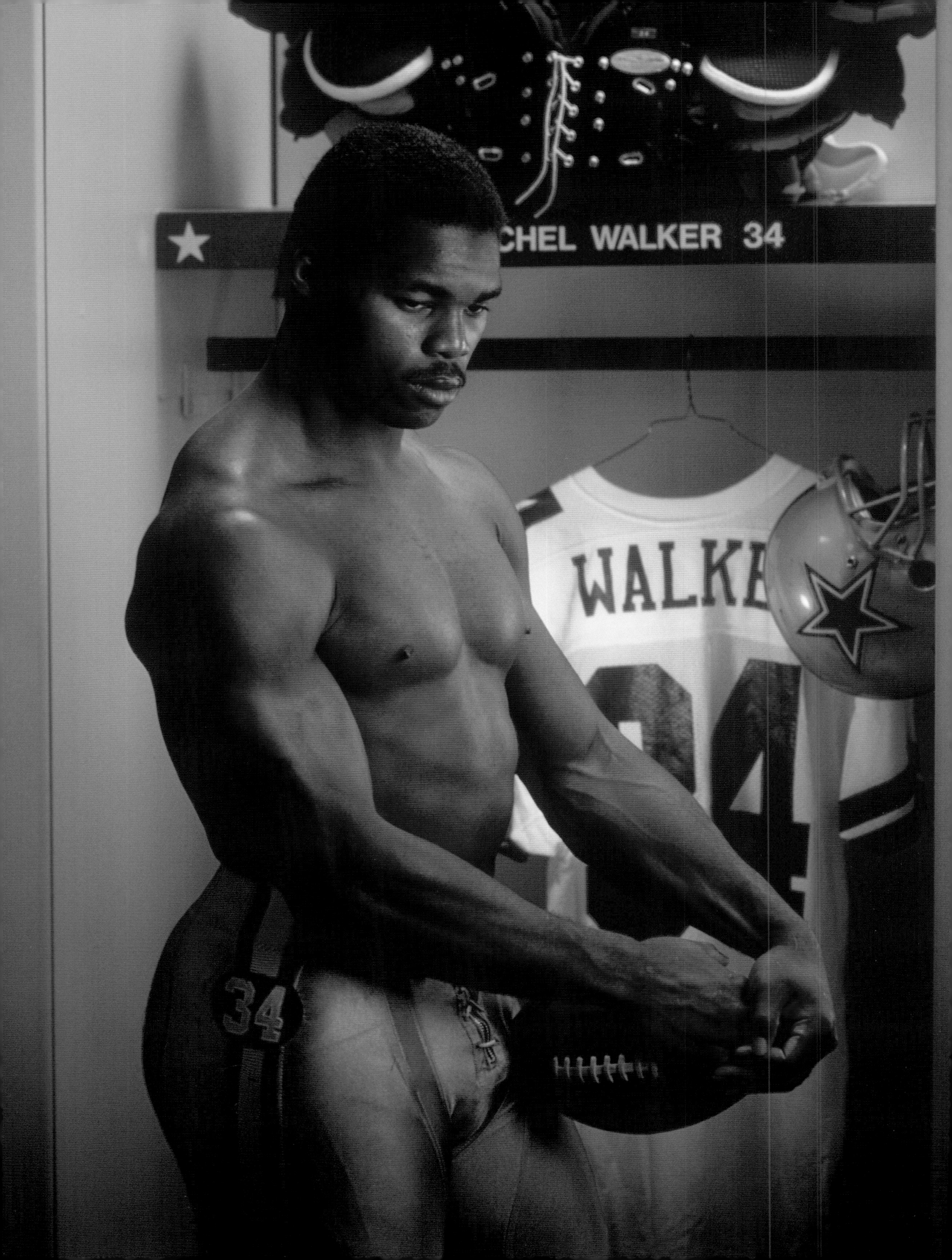
CHEL WALKER 34
WALKE
34

BLOCKBUSTER

New Orleans	28	Dallas	0
Atlanta	27	Dallas	21
Washington	30	Dallas	7
New York Giants	30	Dallas	13

After just one month of games in the new Jones-Johnson era, losing was quickly becoming a Cowboys habit.

Another routine had developed as well, off the field—Johnson and his coaching staff taking regular group jogs through the neighborhood surrounding the club's Valley Ranch complex in Irving. The runs often turned into brainstorming sessions. But one early October run, just weeks into their first season, an irked Johnson had already seen way more than enough.

"We were terrible," Johnson said (referring to his team, not his running mates) "Slowest team I'd ever seen. We had to do something way out of the ordinary, because otherwise rebuilding would have taken forever."

As all those pairs of Nikes shuffled along residential streets with names such as Staubach Drive, Howley Court, and White Lane, an idea crystallized inside Johnson's ever-working brain. *Let's make a whopper of a trade*, he reasoned in yet another of his "A-ha!" moments.

Parting with Aikman was out of the question. Ditto for second-year wide receiver Michael "the Playmaker" Irvin, although Johnson briefly flirted with that notion in discussions with his newfound pal Al Davis. "He asked me, 'You sure you wanna do that? Who's gonna catch passes for you?'" Jimmy said.

It became crystal clear to Johnson that they had but one true bargaining chip. It was the one player they had who already had substantial value in the league—star running back Herschel Walker.

Walker had won the Heisman Trophy while at Georgia, before leaving school early and getting millions to sign with the United States Football League's New Jersey Generals, where he ran absolutely wild. The Cowboys' draft manager, Brandt, had used a fifth-round pick in the 1985 draft to get Walker's rights just in case that financially wobbly league went under.

Genius move! A year later, in 1986, Walker was wearing the helmet with the big silver star on it. That first season, while sharing tailback duties with future Hall of Famer Tony Dorsett, Walker rushed for 737 yards and led the Cowboys in pass receptions and touchdowns. A year later he would lead Dallas in all three categories. In 1988 Walker was the only bright spot in an otherwise dreadful 3-13 season, piling up 1,541 yards on the ground and 505 more receiving. He was the diamond in the Cowboys coal bin.

One person who didn't "ooh" and "ahh" over Walker was Johnson, who saw Walker as unfit for the kind of team he was quickly rebuilding, and therefore expendable.

"Everyone thought he was a tremendous talent. But he wasn't necessarily a natural player," Johnson said. "I knew he could help our team. But I didn't think he was nearly as good as what we could get for him."

Not everyone agreed with "The World According to Jimmy." "Jerry Rhome and David Shula (assistant coaches) said we wouldn't win a game that year if we traded Herschel. Johnson told them "Hell, we might not win a game even if we keep 'im."

The Cowboys didn't even have to float Walker's name around the league. Several teams came calling, although one thing Dallas wasn't about to do was send Walker to another team in the NFC East, their own division, so that crossed the mildly interested New York Giants off the list. In Georgia, where the legend of Herschel lived on, the Atlanta Falcons worried that he'd drive too hard a salary bargain when his contract ran out. Remove the Falcons from the bidding.

One team with a strong level of interest was the Cleveland Browns.

"They offered us a player, a couple of future number ones and three number twos," Johnson said. "Good offer." Good enough, in fact, that the Cowboys were ready to bite.

The Cowboys and Browns planned to finalize the swap later that night. But Johnson thought they might squeeze even more out of the deal if they could just get another franchise interested, someone to give the Cowboys some leverage with the Browns. "Really, we were just looking to get the Browns to sweeten the pot," said Jimmy.

Johnson and owner/general manager Jerry Jones huddled. Each would contact other clubs to drum up interest. Johnson called Minnesota General Manager Mike Lynn.

Hello leverage!

Now Dallas had two teams interested for the very same reason. Each regarded Walker as the missing piece needed to make a run for the Super Bowl.

"The Great Train Robbery"

Johnson told Lynn: "Hey, I'm about to deal Herschel Walker this afternoon (to Cleveland). If you're interested, here's what it's going to take." He laid out a complicated request that consisted of players, draft picks, conditional picks, and provisions. "You need to get back to me by 6:30 or else the deal will already be done," Johnson told Lynn.

When Johnson returned to his office following practice, there was a fax from Lynn waiting for him. Further negotiations ate up the next few hours. Dallas kept holding out for more. Lynn, visions of Super Bowl rings dancing in his head and afraid the Cowboys might at any moment take the Browns' offer, finally caved.

Before this, the largest swap in the history of the NFL, could be finalized, it needed third-party approval: Walker's. He had to be convinced, massaged, stroked, compensated. Call it what you want. Although Herschel's contract didn't contain a no-trade clause, he could still blow up the deal by simply refusing to report to the Vikings. So it was now time for Jones to go to work with Walker's agent, Peter Johnson.

"Herschel had various commitments in Dallas—relationships, endorsements, radio shows. I sat there with just the two of them (Walker and Peter Johnson) till two or three in the morning," Jones recalls. At one point Jones hadn't slept in forty-eight hours.

The sides settled on an "exit bonus" of $1.25 million. Jones even had the nerve to try to get Minnesota to pay that, but the Vikings had to draw the line somewhere. The Vikes did, however, toss in free use of a house comparable to Walker's home in Dallas and the Mercedes Benz of his choice. By 6:15 AM Walker had arrived at Valley Ranch to clean out his locker.

All that remained was announcing the details of the blockbuster. That would include trying to explain one of the most complicated NFL deals ever consummated. Said New York Giants General Manager George Young: "The trade agreement may be longer than the Magna Carta."

The bombshell dropped on the same day league owners were meeting in the Dallas suburb of Grapevine to choose Paul Tagliabue as their new commissioner. Here's how the deal ultimately worked: Dallas sent Walker to the Vikings, along with the Cowboys' third- and tenth-round picks in 1990 and their third-rounder in 1991. In return, the Cowboys would get from Minnesota linebackers Jesse Solomon and David Howard, defensive end Alex Stewart, running back

Darrin Nelson, and cornerback Isaac Holt, along with the Vikings' first-, second-, and sixth-rounders in 1990.

But there was more, and here's where things started to get fuzzy. Minnesota *also* included, as conditional picks, their first- and second-rounders in 1991 and their first-, second-, and third-round picks of the 1992 draft.

Whew!

The conditions keyed this mammoth deal. The trade stipulated if any of the players sent to Big D were not on the Dallas roster on February 1, 1990, the Cowboys would receive the conditional pick or picks attached to that player. For example: Dallas cut Stewart almost immediately. "He turned out to be lazy," Johnson remembers vividly. "I cut him and took the second-rounder instead."

When the deal came down, the Vikings faithful celebrated. Despite Johnson proclaiming the swap as "The Great Train Robbery," Dallas fans, players, and media disagreed. In giving up what arguably was a franchise player in Walker, skeptics looked at the deal and figured that the Cowboys had gotten nothing in return but a bunch of retreads and questionable future picks.

"Love that steal for Minnesota."

"They've thrown in the towel. It's a punt offense."

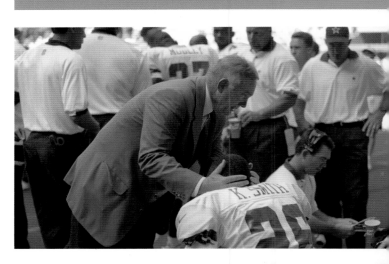

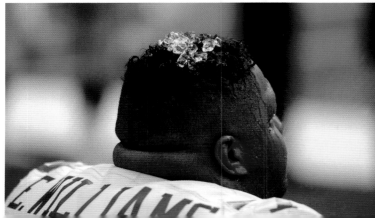

"The Cowboys got nothing more than a handful of Minnesota smoke."

"They've just shown us they're panicking."

Au contraire! What the JJs knew and almost no one else could fathom (including the Vikings) was that Dallas never intended to keep *any* of the Viking players. In fact, Johnson had decided to not even let anyone be tempted to keep them. "I told my assistant coaches not to start any of them," Johnson said. "I didn't want everyone falling in love with them and thus make the decision (to eventually cut them) harder.

"Mike Lynn thought he'd gotten a great deal. And virtually everybody else thought he'd pulled off a masterstroke on an idiot named Jimmy Johnson."

The early returns gave the edge to Lynn. Just three days later, and with only two and a half hours of practice with his new team, Walker raced fifty-one yards with a kickoff return the first time he touched the ball in a Vikings uniform. He chewed up forty-seven yards on his first carry from scrimmage. By game's end he'd piled up 148 on eighteen carries, the best rushing day by a Viking back in six years. Minnesota whipped archrival Green Bay 26–14. "Herschelmania" lived. Tampa and Super Bowl XXV would surely follow.

Well, maybe not. That 148-yard performance would be the high point of Walker's Twin Cities career. The Vikings lost in round one of the playoffs. In 1990, they slipped to 6–10 and Walker never rushed for as many as eighty yards in any one game. By mid-1991 he'd become a part-timer. The Vikes went 8–8. Walker left for Philadelphia. By '96, ironically, he'd re-signed with Dallas for the last two years of his career.

And Dallas?

The Cowboys eventually got every one of those conditional picks, winding up with three first-rounders, three seconds, a third, and a sixth. They even finagled a way to keep cornerback Isaac Holt for a few years—long enough for him to win a ring as a Cowboy. Then "Trader Jimmy" began flipping and swapping and picking. By the end of that '92 draft, the Cowboys, by using and/or dealing the choices acquired in the massive transaction, had acquired:

★ RB Emmitt Smith ★
★ DT Russell Maryland ★
★ CB Kevin Smith ★
★ S Darren Woodson ★
★ CB Clayton Holmes ★

That list includes the NFL's future all-time leading rusher (Emmitt Smith) plus three other Pro Bowlers (Maryland, Kevin Smith, and Woodson). Four of them started multiple Super Bowls. All earned multiple Super Bowl rings.

In those early turnaround years, Dallas would pull off some memorable upsets. They'd look back at certain games where team growth became wonderfully evident. But, as he reflected back over his seasons in Dallas, Johnson zeroed in on his personal turning point.

"It came on that early October jog with my crew."

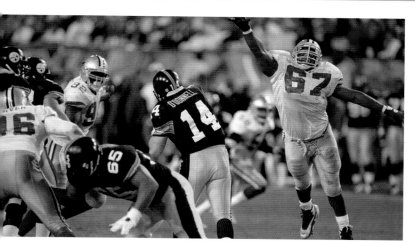

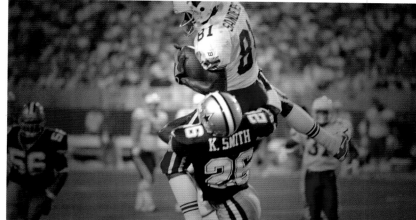

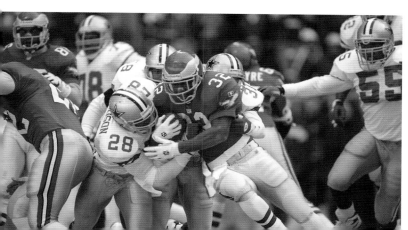

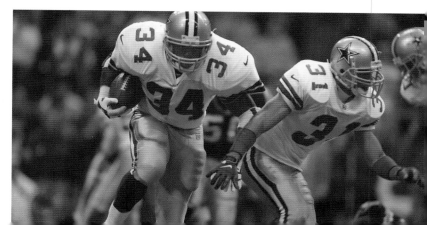

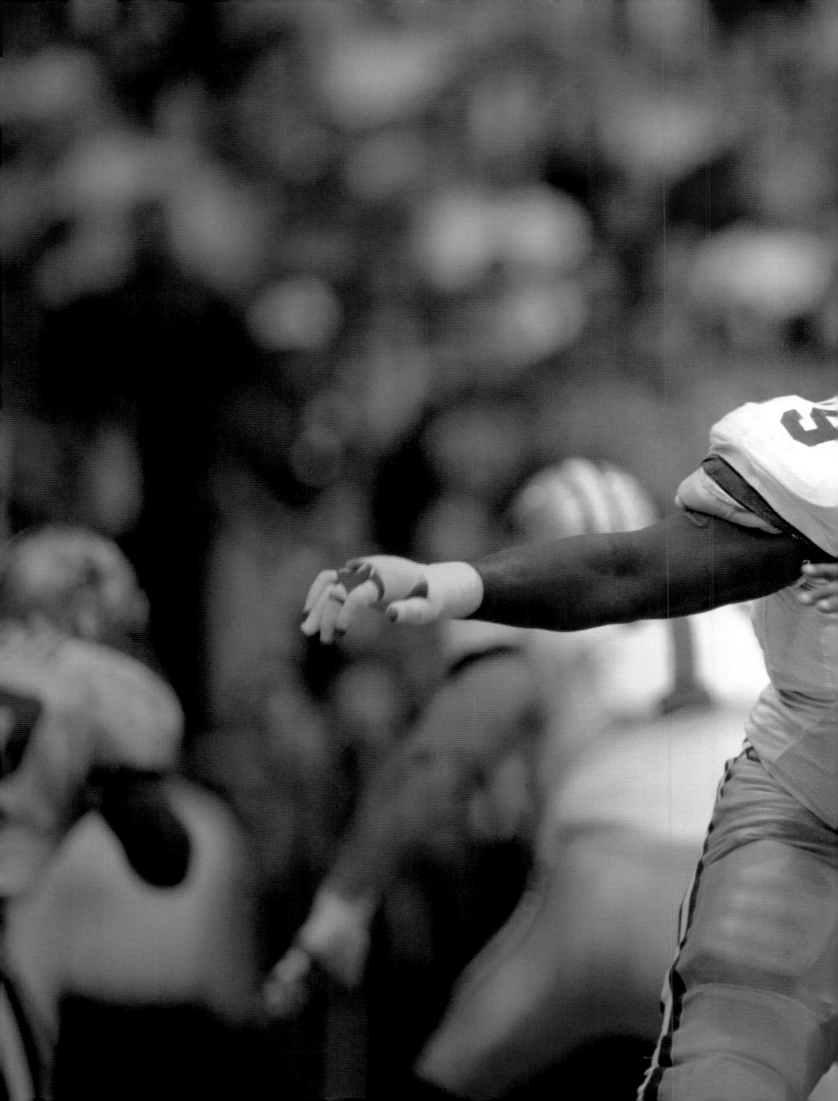

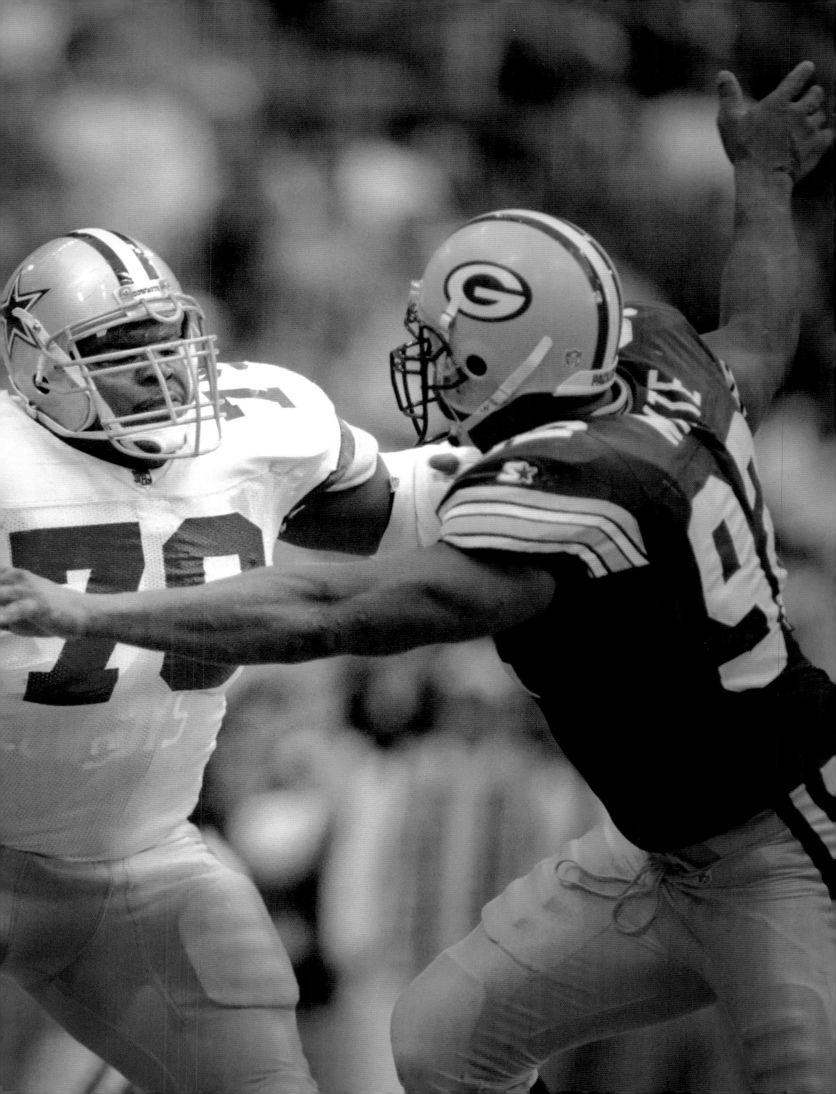

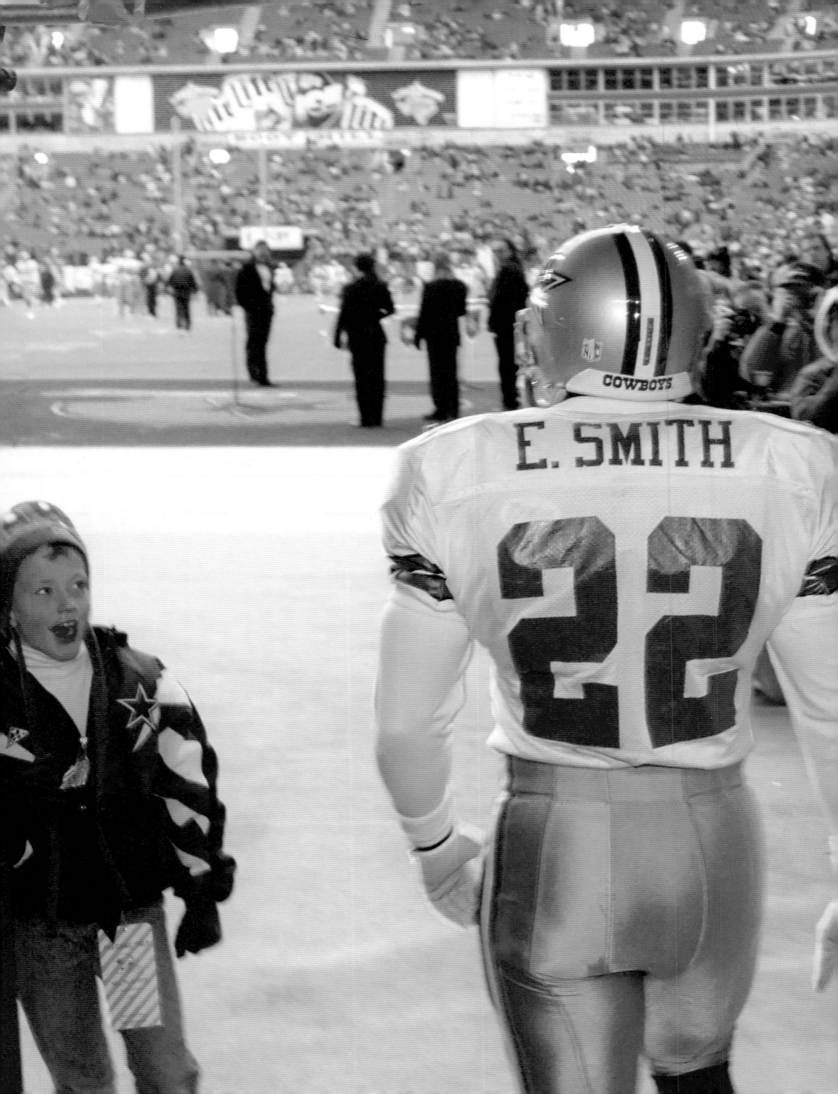

APRIL 22, 1990

SO WHAT'S PLAN C?

Another NFL Draft day arrived.

Jimmy Johnson, his staff of assistant coaches and scouts and owner Jerry Jones filled every corner of the "war room" inside the Cowboys Valley Ranch compound. Phone banks sat waiting. Everything was ready.

Dallas knew what they needed:

DEFENSE!

Dallas knew who they wanted:

Baylor Linebacker James Francis!

For weeks the entire crew had studied the dossiers of hundreds of draftable college players from No. 1 to numbers 300, 400, 500, and beyond. At the same time the organization had, with brutal honesty, evaluated the talent level of its current players. They concluded that much of their roster was flotsam and jetsam—players who had NFL jobs only because they had played on the pitiful 1–15 Cowboys.

After just that one season the Pokes did, however, feel pretty good about their offense. In the '89 draft Dallas had shored up that side of the ball with its first three selections—Aikman, Johnston, and Stepnoski. The cupboard inherited from Tom Landry was pretty bare, for the most part, but it did contain emerging wide receiver Michael Irvin and two solid offensive linemen in tackle Mark Tuinei and guard Nate Newton.

This draft, rich in defensive talent, would fit the Cowboys' needs beautifully. Dallas had the twenty-first and twenty-sixth picks overall, plus a slew of later-round choices from the Herschel Walker trade and the thirteen other deals the Johnson-Jones combo had made in one year.

The draft is the NFL's version of Christmas. Each team makes up a wish list, and one by one the gifts get opened. Dallas had been making a list and checkin' it twice. With their top pick they wanted a defensive player. This is how they had the top available defensive players ranked:

1. Southern Cal linebacker Junior Seau
2. Miami defensive tackle Cortez Kennedy
3. Baylor linebacker James Francis
4. Houston linebacker Lamar Lathon
5. N.C. State defensive tackle Ray Agnew

Dallas assumed Seau and Kennedy would go quickly, and they did. Both went off the board in the first five selections. The Cowboys could have put together a package attractive enough to jump up to get either. Such a swap, though, would have been cost prohibitive and counter productive. The braintrust concluded that packaging several high picks to move far up for one player didn't, with all their holes to fill, make much sense.

Francis became *the* target. Some scouts had compared him to New York Giants superstar linebacker Lawrence Taylor. Some thought he'd wind up as a superb pass rushing defensive end. Almost everyone agreed with Cowboys chief scout Dick Mansperger: " . . . a dominating player . . . He is a can't-miss, if that's a possibility. I would like to have him not miss here."

Dallas' "Get Francis" machine started humming. The Cowboys called Chicago asking the Bears what they wanted for their overall No. 6 pick. But the Bears liked Francis, too. Chicago spent the fifteen minutes allotted between picks trying to convince Francis to accept a $1.5 million bonus as part of a five-year, $4-million-dollar contract. The Bears insisted that their choice agree to terms before being drafted, thus avoiding ugly public negotiations and/or a prolonged holdout. When Francis balked, the Bears selected Southern Cal safety Mark Carrier, who happily accepted that cash.

Joy broke out in Cowboyville.

Their strategy crystallized.

Plan A: Believing Detroit at No. 7 and New England at No. 8 almost certainly wouldn't choose Francis, Dallas focused on trading for the No. 9, No. 10, or No. 11 pick to move up high enough to secure rights to what they thought would be the next star NFL linebacker.

Plan B: If those attempts failed, they would hone in on acquiring the University of Houston linebacker Lamar Lathon. *Finally*: Agnew represented their fallback position. All their pre-draft intelligence indicated that he'd almost certainly still be available at their No. 21 pick.

Johnson and his lieutenants started burning up the phone lines. They called Miami, which had the ninth pick and New England, which owned the tenth. Neither team bit on the deal offered, although the Dolphins subsequently passed on Francis anyway.

"It was a case of those teams asking way too much for us to trade up," said Johnson. And Trader Jimmy refused to overpay.

New England then announced a shocker at No. 10. They grabbed Agnew! The choice stunned Dallas, and it was a mixed bag: Francis was still available, but their fallback option of Agnew was off the board, and ten picks still remained before Dallas' turn came up at No. 21. The good news was that with each step down the first-round ladder, Dallas would have to pay less to move up.

Al Davis's Raiders owned pick No. 11, to be followed by Cincinnati at No. 12 and Kansas City at No. 13. Dallas dialed Davis . . . and Cincy and Kansas City just in case Francis passed the Raiders, well, maybe?

Dallas offered L.A. its first and a third to move up ten spots. But remember that '85 draft when Johnson held Davis' feet to the fire in his first trade? Now that lit match was on the other foot. Davis pushed for more. The sides got very close before time ran out. But it turned out the Raiders didn't want Francis either, taking instead Arizona defensive end Anthony Smith.

The player Dallas rated fourth-best overall in the entire draft (behind Seau, Kennedy and Francis), still hadn't been taken—Florida running back Emmitt Smith. But if Smith was that good, why had everyone else passed on him?

Some scouts believed Smith represented the worst possible combination for an NFL runner—small and slow. At five-foot-nine and around two hundred pounds, he would need to break stopwatches to be successful as a pro. He become a Florida legend gaining an incredible 8,000 yards plus at Escambia High and another 4,232 in three years at Florida. But clocks don't lie. Dallas scouts timed him at 4.48 in the forty-yard dash. The New York Giants' watches stopped at a dismal 4.70.

Smith did have one huge fan in Cowboys running backs coach Joe Brodsky, who had tried to recruit him to the University of Miami while Brodsky coached there as part of Johnson's staff: "He was a tough, hardnosed runner and every time he moved to a higher level there wasn't any drop in his production," Brodsky said. "From the time he was an eighty-pound tailback, he was prolific."

"From the time he was an eighty-pound tailback, he was prolific."

Suddenly the Cowboys *did* have a trade partner. The Chiefs at No. 13, believed the linebacker they craved, Michigan State's Percy Snow, would fall (so to speak) all the way to No. 21. If Francis slipped past Cincy at No. 12, the Chiefs would make the swap, and Dallas would have its man.

Dallas had also tried to work a trade with Cincy but to no avail. The clock ticked down toward the deadline for the Bengals to choose. No trade made sense to them.

The Bengals selected Francis.

Dallas' hopes melted.

Kansas City then took Snow.

The Cowboys called the Bengals back with a sweetened offer for Francis, but Cincy gave them the cold shoulder.

Dallas had to regroup, and the Cowboys cranked up Plan B, which called for acquiring the rights to Lathon, who they were confident wouldn't slide all the way to No. 21. They tried New Orleans. Then Houston. The Oilers passed on the swap and grabbed Lathon, the college hometown hero.

There sat the Cowboys looking and feeling like a line from a popular James Taylor ballad: "Sweet dreams and flying machines in pieces on the ground."

The defensive help Dallas so desperately craved had disappeared. So, what would Plan C be?

Meanwhile, down in Florida, Smith was becoming a nervous wreck. He'd opted to turn pro after his junior year with the Gators. But, just like Dallas, Smith's draft-day dreams had just about vanished. A couple of teams had told him they'd take him in the first five picks. But Smith found out what Johnson already knew about the NFL draft: "It's a liar convention." Somewhere in the top ten seemed more realistic to Smith. The draft had now passed No. 15. Smith remained unclaimed as he waited out the process at a buddy's home in Pensacola.

"I walked out of my friend's house," Smith said. "I couldn't watch one more minute. I was so anxious. Staring out at the Gulf, I let all these negative thoughts invade my head . . . Maybe I should have stayed in college . . . Maybe I just made the biggest mistake of my life."

Back at Valley Ranch, the Cowboys had refocused on Smith. That still, however, left two bothersome situations.

First, everyone knew that both Green Bay, which had picks 18 and 19, and Atlanta at 20, wanted runners. Surely Smith wouldn't get past both. So a deal had to happen with either Buffalo at 16 or Pittsburgh at 17.

Second, Dallas had *already* traded for a halfback. Just days before they'd sent a second-rounder to the Forty-niners for Terrence Flagler. He'd been a first-

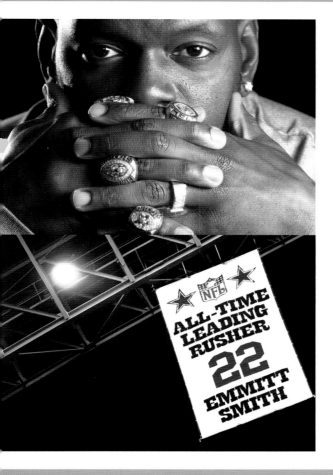

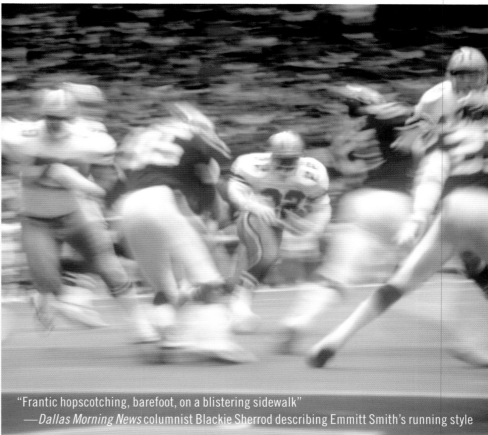

"Frantic hopscotching, barefoot, on a blistering sidewalk"
—*Dallas Morning News* columnist Blackie Sherrod describing Emmitt Smith's running style

round choice for San Francisco in '87 but had since spent three years gathering dust on the Niners bench behind star running back Roger Craig.

Johnson wanted one more evaluation from his running backs coach Brodsky, who put it as succinctly as possible: "Emmitt Smith will take your breath away. Terrence Flagler will take your breath away—but you'll get it back."

Pittsburgh at No. 17 accepted a late-third-rounder to swap first-round positions with the Cowboys. The phone rang in Pensacola. Delirium broke out in the Smith camp, and over the years for Cowboy fans the feeling would be mutual.

Emmitt eventually had a fabulous 15-year career that *would* take your breath away.

★ 18,355 rushing yards—best in NFL history

★ 164 rushing touchdowns—best in NFL history

★ Eight Pro Bowls

★ League MVP

★ Sportsman of the Year in America

★ Three Super Bowl rings

★ Two Super Bowl MVP's

★ Hall of Fame induction

But what of all those other plans that had come and gone that day?

★ James Francis: Nine solid seasons with the Bengals interrupted by a broken leg in '95. Finished his career as a backup in Washington for one season. Never a star but a consistent contributor.

★ Lamar Lathon: Five seasons as an Oiler. Four more at Carolina. Three excellent years in mid-career piling up thirty sacks. Injuries shortened his career. Out of the NFL by age thirty.

★ Ray Agnew: Eleven good years for New England, the New York Giants, and St. Louis as a run-stuffing defensive tackle. Never flashy. A blue-collar worker.

★ Terrence Flagler: Never played a single game in the silver and blue. Shuffled off to Phoenix in a trade before the '90 season began. In two seasons as a Cardinal he carried the ball only fourteen times for ninety-two yards. Had "personal issues." Out of the NFL at age twenty-seven.

Looking back on that day—the close calls, the disappointments, the incredible various possibilities—you are left with one single gigantic question:

What if?

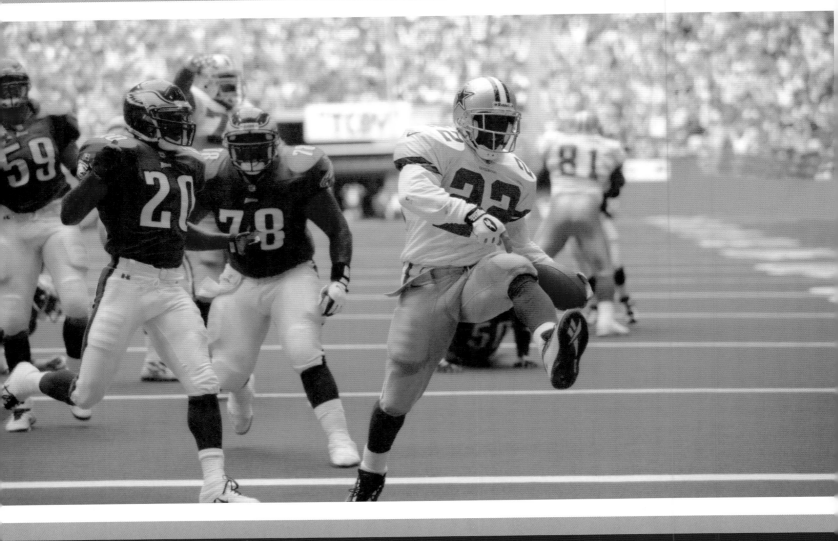

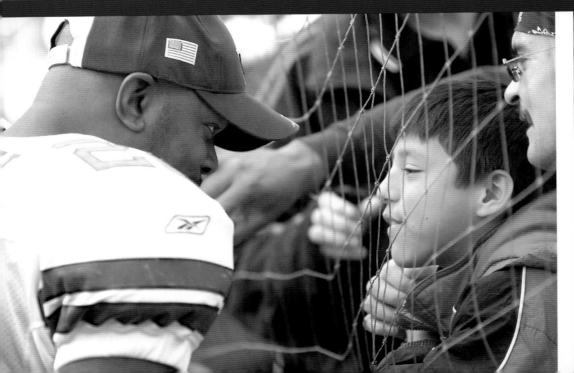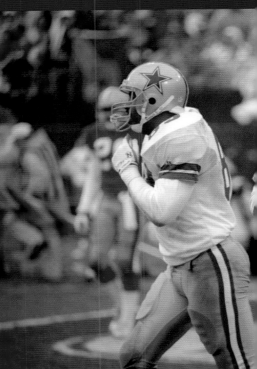

EMMITT SMITH

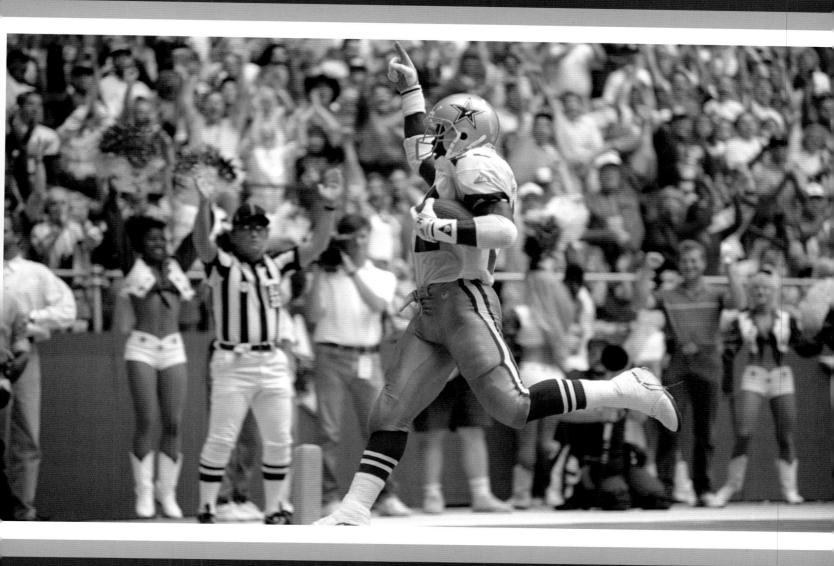

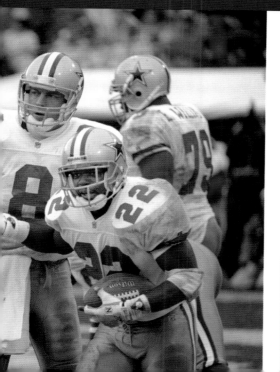

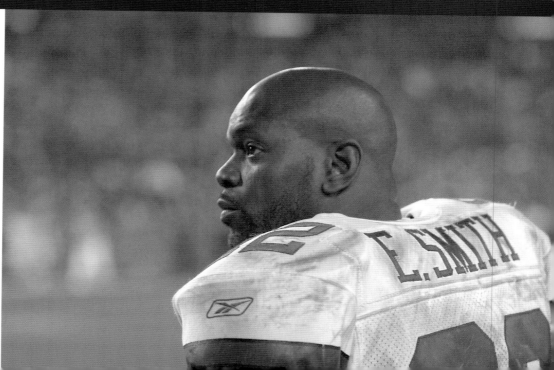

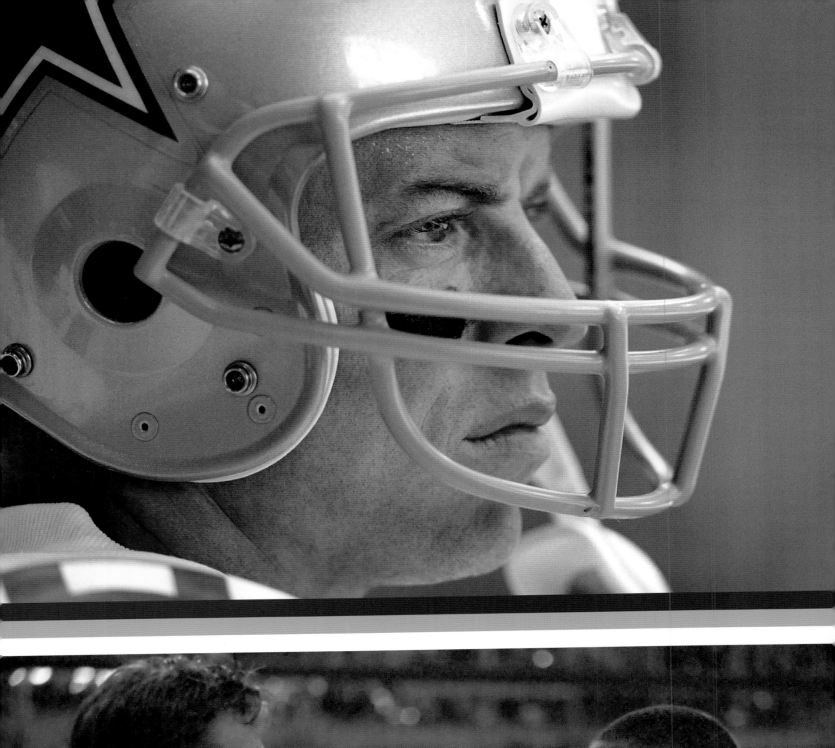
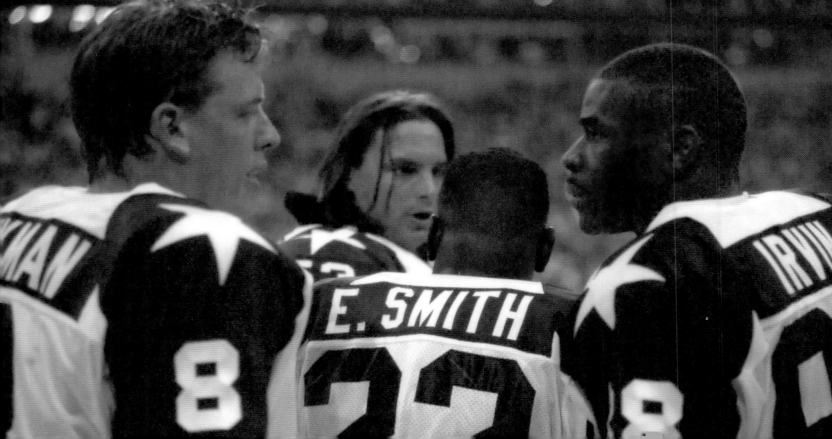

SEPTEMBER 29, 1991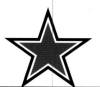

EVIDENCE OF PROGRESS

Five minutes forty-one seconds remained on the Texas Stadium clock. The defending Super Bowl champion New York Giants had just taken a 16–14 lead on a nineteen-yard pitch and catch from Jeff Hostetler to Stephen Baker "the Touchdown Maker."

Five minutes forty-one seconds to either record a signature Cowboys victory or let an opportunity to earn respect slip through their fingers.

Four games into this third year of the Johnson-Jones Dallas revival plan, a ripple of uneasiness drifted through the Cowboys nation. The Pokes had followed a dismal 1–15 first season with an encouraging 7–9 mark in '90. Dallas fans had reasons aplenty for enthusiasm. Drafts had swelled the talent base considerably. The trio of Aikman, Smith, and Irvin looked like the core of a future offensive buzzsaw. Several young faces dotted a defensive lineup that had allowed eighty-five fewer points in '90 than they had in '89.

Across the league the opinion seemed nearly unanimous—here come the Cowboys.

But '91 hadn't started like most envisioned. A pair of narrow road wins at Cleveland and Phoenix bracketed home losses to hated division rivals Washington (33–31) and Philadelphia (24–0). That brought Jimmy Johnson's record for two-and-a-quarter seasons to a somewhat disturbing 10–26.

But this wasn't Phoenix or Tampa Bay the Cowboys were hoping to chase down. New York, the defending Super Bowl champs, had taken over as kings of the NFL hill. Plus, Dallas couldn't use the memories of recent successes versus these Giants to ignite thoughts of a comeback—they didn't have any. New York had beaten up on Dallas six straight times over the last three years winning by a composite score of 145–68! In fact, when Emmitt Smith plunged in from three yards out late in the second quarter to put Dallas up 7–3, it marked the first time the Pokes had led at any point of a Giants game since 1987—a span of nearly twenty-six quarters.

Game stats of this rivalry gave Smith even more reason for apprehension. No Cowboys runner had reached one hundred yards rushing against New York's tough-as-nails defense since Tony Dorsett in November of 1980—more than a decade earlier!

With 5:41 left, the scoreboard read New York 16-Dallas 14, but the stat sheet showed the Giants' superiority. For the entire game Dallas had neither been able to force one Giants punt nor produce a single sack. The Giants' offense had averaged a staggering 8.1 yards a play. The Dallas defense had bent all day but had seldom broken. They'd forced a pair of fumbles, and New York missed a long field goal try. Seven times New York drove into Dallas territory, and yet the favored Giants had but sixteen points to show for what at game's end would be 487 yards of total offense.

The Cowboys attack, virtually stalled for the second half (45 total yards), went to work backed up to their own 16-yard line. The play-by-play of the next three and a half minutes tells the story:

★ Irvin dropped a pass.

★ Aikman hit Alexander Wright for thirteen yards.

★ Aikman's arrow down the left sideline found Irvin for 30 more.

★ Smith straight ahead for two.

★ Aikman dumped a pass to tight end Jay Novacek for five.

★ Third and three at the Giants 39. An Aikman bullet to Novacek gained thirteen. The play moved Dallas well within field goal range for kicker Kevin Willis. New York expected three Cowboys runs to exhaust the Giants time-outs and then a field goal try to take the 17–16 lead. On first down they guessed correctly.

★ A blitz swallowed up Smith two yards behind the line of scrimmage at the twenty-three. But on second down the Giants again sold out to stop the run. Dallas, meanwhile, gambled on going for all of it.

★ Aikman hit Irvin in stride on a slant at the three, and "the Playmaker" wrestled cornerback Roger Brown into the end zone.

Dallas 21–16. But 2:13 still remained. That's an eternity of time in the NFL. Again Dallas "D" bent. The Giants hurried forty-five yards forward to the Cowboys 30. But again the New York offense broke. Cornerback Isaac Holt, who'd taken heavy heat for his poor play in previous weeks, intercepted Hostetler in the end zone.

Dallas had gone toe-to-toe with the champs and won. "We all know what we did," owner Jones proclaimed. "We beat Mike Tyson."

"We took a big step as a team, as a franchise today," Johnson beamed. "A very big step."

"That's the game we started believing in what he (Johnson) was telling us," remembers enormous offensive lineman Nate Newton. "Up until that point I just kind of looked at him more out of fear than respect . . . it started to sink in that maybe we do, maybe there is something to what this cat's talking about."

A turning point for the team? That's too strong.

It was more like a coming-out party for one of its young building blocks.

"I think there are various moments for a quarterback that elevate your status within the locker room with your teammates," Akiman recalled while looking back on that still-vivid victory. "Throughout college and even here, I get in stride and there are times I feel I can't miss."

Aikman's stat line was impressive: 20 of 27 passing to ten different receivers for 277 yards and a touchdown, and without an interception.

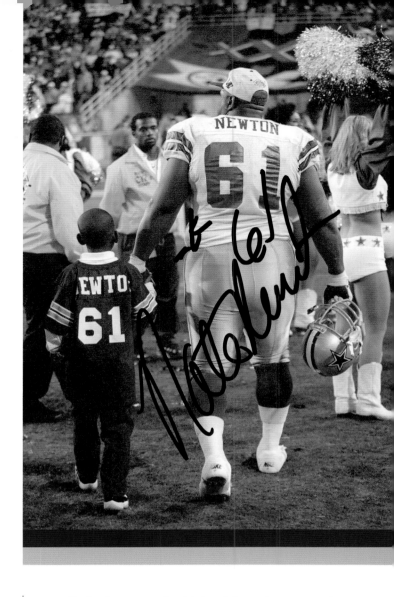

"I don't necessarily think of that win as a turning point for the team, but it was definitely for me," Aikman said in retrospect.

That triumph, that drive over the last 5:41, signaled the emergence of the new Cowboys. Again, recall that Dallas had entered the Giants contest 10–26 under Johnson. Beginning with this comeback victory, the Cowboys would go an outrageous 69–20 over the next four-plus seasons!

"I don't necessarily think of that win as a turning point for the team, but it was definitely for me."

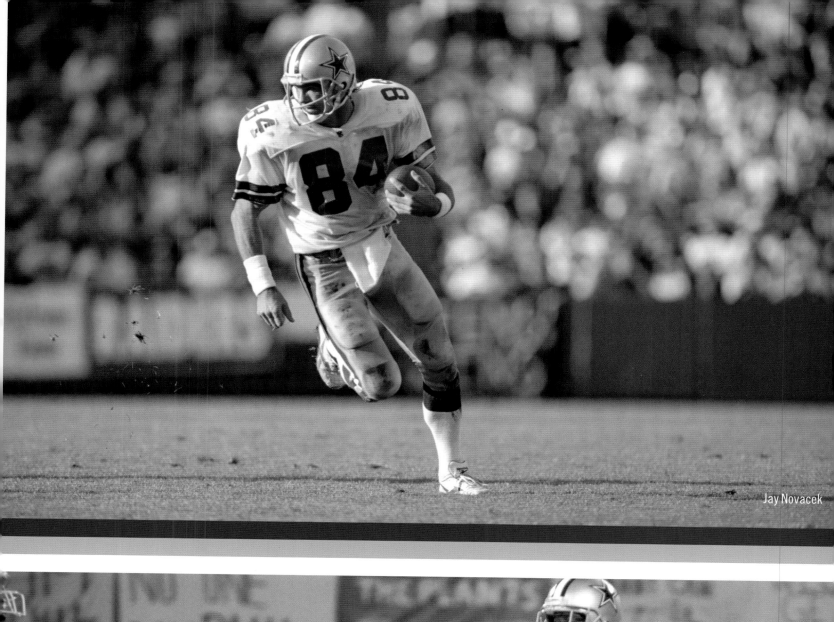

Jay Novacek

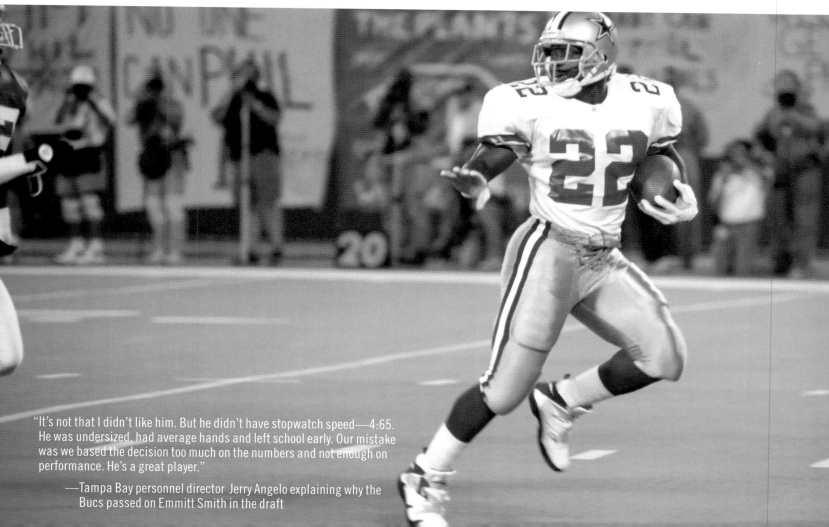

"It's not that I didn't like him. But he didn't have stopwatch speed—4:65. He was undersized, had average hands and left school early. Our mistake was we based the decision too much on the numbers and not enough on performance. He's a great player."

—Tampa Bay personnel director Jerry Angelo explaining why the Bucs passed on Emmitt Smith in the draft

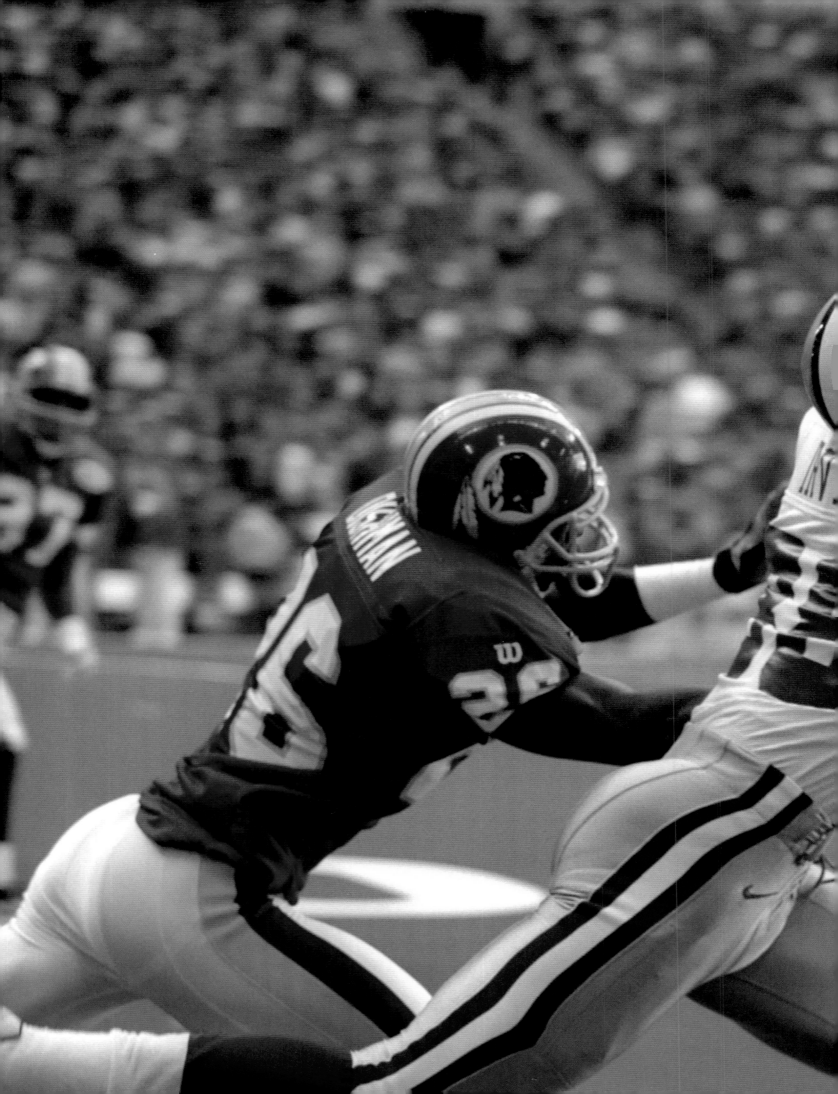

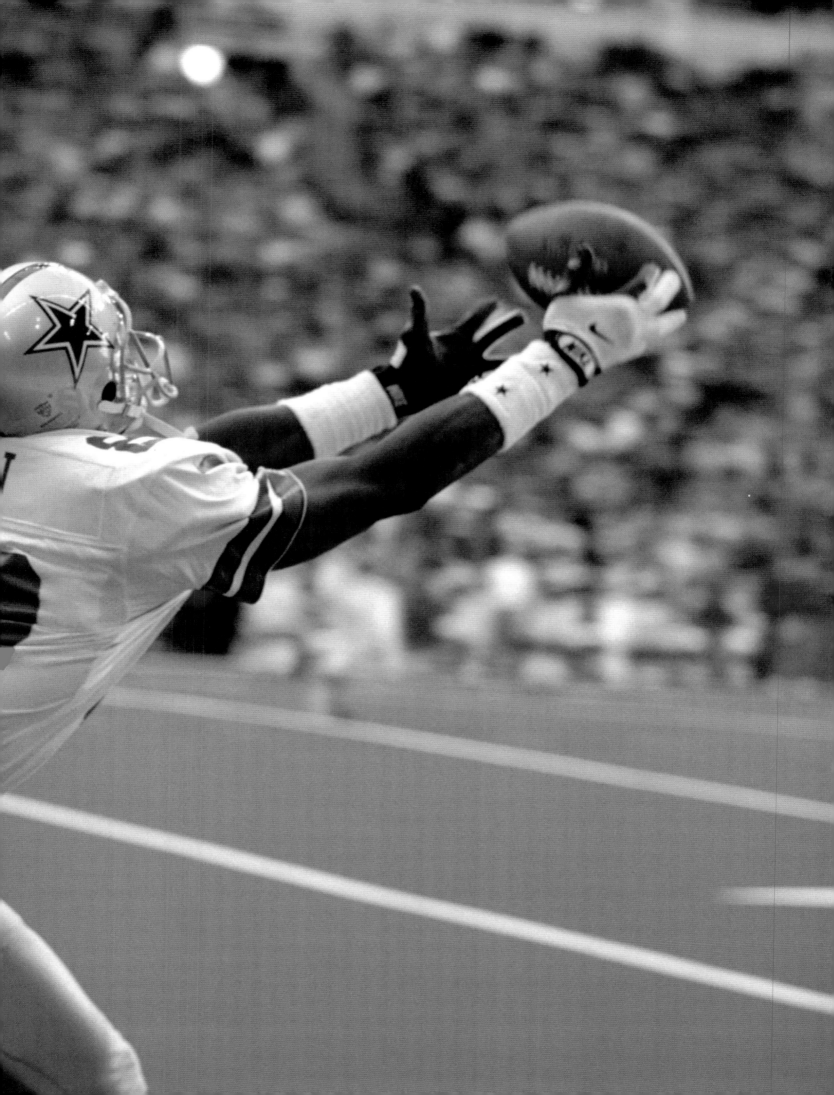

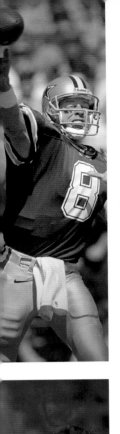
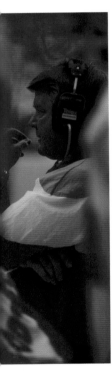
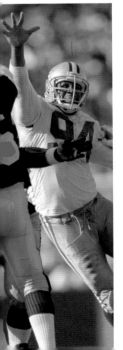
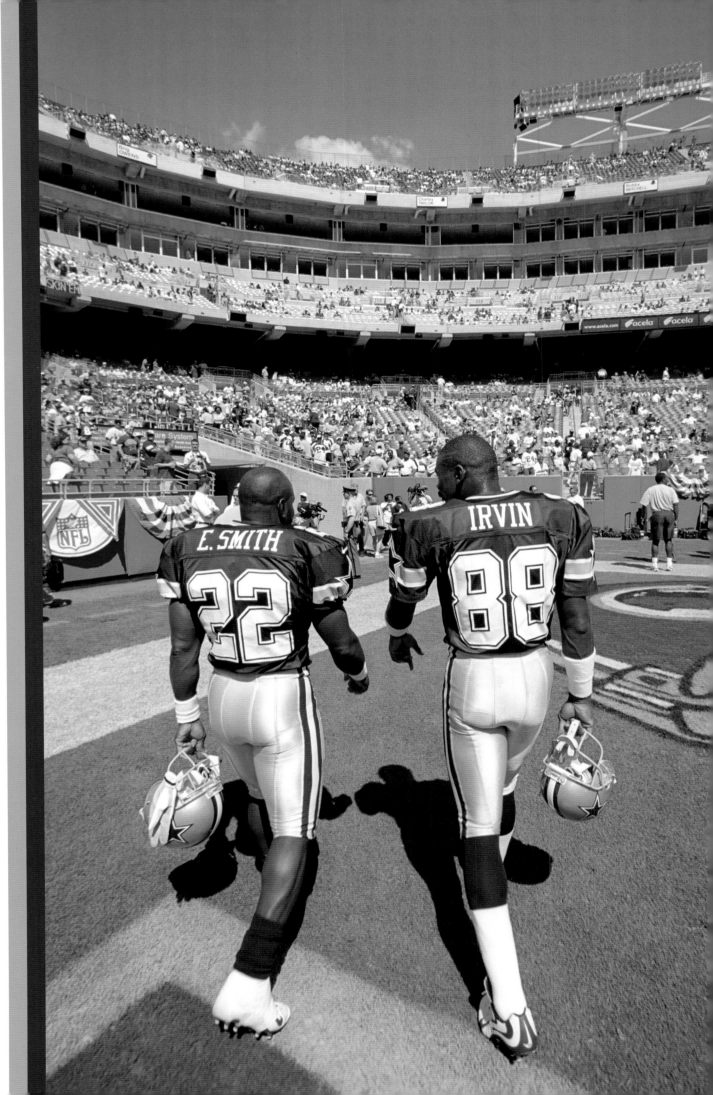

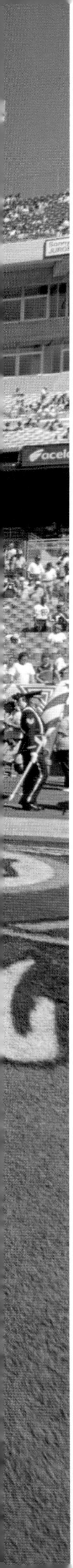

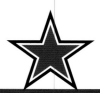

"THINGS ARE TURNING"

"If you got a big gorilla and you're gonna try to beat 'em, don't go tiptoeing around. You sneak up behind him with a big ole stick, and you swing as hard as you can and hit 'em in the head."

Jimmy Johnson's advice had nothing to do with actually hurting gorillas. Rather, it outlined his approach to knocking off the Washington Redskins, who had emerged as the two thousand-pound gorilla of the NFL.

"You've gotta take chances, onside kicks, go for it on fourth down," Johnson said. "If you're not the best team, normally you're not gonna win. Your strategy must involve 'upset thinking.' Get 'em off balance. Get 'em wondering what you'll try next. Get 'em reeling."

So far during the '91 season no team had inflicted so much as a flesh wound on the Washington Gorillas. Through eleven games they had eaten the league alive. Eleven consecutive wins by an *average* of 20.2 points per game. The last franchise to devour opponents at such a remarkable rate was another big old animal from the NFL woods—the 1942 Chicago Bears. Washington just didn't defeat teams. They *humiliated* them.

Check the 'Skins rankings in critical statistical areas after eleven weeks:

- Scoring—first
- Scoring defense—second
- Scoring offense—third
- Passing offense—fourth
- Rushing defense—fifth
- Passing defense—fifth
- Turnover margin—first

Dallas faced this pro football version of a killing machine in Week Twelve. Experts gave them about as much chance of stunning the thirteen-point favorite Redskins as David would have had against Goliath *without* his sling shot.

★ TV analyst Dan Fouts: "How big is your mortgage? I'll bet your mortgage. I don't think there's any such thing as a "lock." But if there is, this (Washington) team is one."

★ Redskins radio color man Sonny Jurgensen: "Washington would have to lay an egg for somebody to beat them."

★ Star TV analyst John Madden had already looked past this Cowboys battle and several others predicting that Washington would be the first team to ever go 16–0 in a regular season. (The unbeaten '72 Dolphins played a fourteen-game slate.)

The reasons for thinking an upset unthinkable kept piling up:

★ Washington had whipped Dallas eleven consecutive times at home by an average score of 30–12.

★ In their storied history the Skins had won 68 percent of all home games dating back thirty years.

★ This would be Dallas' third consecutive road game. The previous sixty teams assigned such a gauntlet by the NFL schedule maker had gone 20–40 in the final game of the three pack.

★ Perhaps the league's best tight end, Jay Novacek, and Pro Bowl level guard Nate Newton had been left in Dallas nursing injuries.

★ 55,677 out-of-their-gourds 'Skins faithful—many painted burgundy and gold and many more wearing rubber pig snouts to celebrate Washington's terrific offensive line "the Hogs"—shoe-horned into RFK Stadium for a 196th consecutive home sellout.

NFL games are not, however, won because of sportscasters' predictions, gaudy stats, rivalry history, unfavorable scheduling, or even injuries.

Games are won or lost on the field. Jimmy Johnson and his 6–5 Cowboys, armed with a "big ole stick," set off on safari, hoping to bag a gorilla. A great big one.

It wouldn't be easy. On Dallas' second possession of the game, 'Skins cornerback Martin Mayhew stole an Aikman pass and sped thirty-one yards for a touchdown. Redskin fans settled comfortably back in their seats and ordered a couple more cold ones preparing to witness yet another gorging. What they would end up seeing, however, was a Washington team shut out for the next forty-one minutes.

Johnson, defensive coordinator Butch Davis, and offensive coordinator Norv Turner began throwing the entire Dallas playbook (and a few other things as well) at the 'Skins. Early in the second quarter Dallas had already gone for it and converted on a fourth and five at the Washington 33. Remember, "no tiptoeing around." Later in that drive, with Dallas facing third and fifteen at the 32, the 'Skins braced for a long pass. Remember "you've gotta keep 'em off balance." The Cowboys ran a draw play. Thirty-two yards later Emmitt Smith had scored and Dallas had drawn even with the stunned 'Skins at 7–7.

Then—"you gotta swing as hard as you can"—Dallas tried an onside kick and recovered it. On the ensuing possession, Dallas reached the Redskins' 31 and had a fourth and nine. Again Dallas would forsake a field-goal try. The Cowboys would fail to get the first down, but Johnson had made his statement in going for it: "You gotta take chances."

Later, with thirteen seconds remaining in the first half, the Cowboys had the ball at the Washington 34, fourth and seven. Dallas had used its final time-out. Johnson and Aikman stood on the sideline plotting strategy. Try a long field goal? Not a chance.

"I looked at Troy, and he was thinking the same thing I was thinking," Jimmy said. "I said, 'Heck, let's take a shot at it.'"

Aikman rejoined the huddle and called "Rocket"—Dallas' terminology for the "Hail Mary pass." The play sent six-foot-three wide receiver Alvin Harper, a former collegiate high-jump champion, to the deep right corner of the end zone to try to catch what amounted to a jump ball.

Said Harper: "I looked at their roster (earlier in the week) and thought 'They're nothin' but five-foot-eight guys. Just throw it up to me.'"

Aikman let it fly, and Harper outleaped a squadron of Smurfs for the first touchdown of his NFL career and his only score of the year. Dallas led 14–7 at the half. The gorilla had suffered a significant flesh wound.

Gruesome slow-motion replays showed a right shin bent at a severe angle and a knee ominously twisted.

Aikman: "The pain was excruciating. As soon as it happened, my leg went numb. I couldn't feel my toes. I thought I'd totally blown my knee out. I was thinking my season was over, maybe more."

Aikman would not play again that day or that season. Fortunately only the video tape and not the injury would prove to be horrific.

Out came backup quarterback Steve Beuerlein, who in August had been acquired from the Raiders for a fourth-round draft choice. New signal caller but with the same game plan—go for it. Michael Irvin's spectacular juggling touchdown catch early in the fourth quarter extended Dallas' lead to 21–7. At that point the vaunted Redskin offense had not driven the ball past midfield *all day*.

Midway through the fourth quarter, the Redskins scored a touchdown to pull within 21–14.

Johnson knew it was time to swing that stick and "hit 'em in the head." Dallas would have to confront Washington mano a mano.

After a pair of passes to begin Dallas' next drive, the game boiled down to trench warfare. Emmitt Smith would slam the ball at the 'Skins the next five plays. Then a pass to Irvin. Then five more Smith blasts. A Kevin Willis field goal with 1:14 left clinched the 24–14 shocker. That final grinding drive had covered only forty-eight yards, but it lasted fifteen plays and ate 7:07 off the clock. In the end a Cowboys team that had snuck up on the gorilla most of the day wound up arm wrestling him into submission.

Jerry Jones called the result "a watershed moment."

Fullback Daryl "Moose" Johnston recalls: "We'd been watching the puzzle be put together . . . then that week we saw what we could really do when we were really focused and executed very well."

"Heck, let's take a shot at it."

Seconds later, while leaving the field at halftime, Johnson said to Aikman, "I think things are turning."

Not so fast. Five plays into the second half things turned for the worse, much worse for Dallas and Aikman. As Aikman released a pass to Kelvin Martin that resulted in a gain of twenty-seven yards, and deep into Washington territory, Redskins defensive tackle Jumpy Geathers grabbed the Dallas quarterback around the waist. With Aikman's right leg extended and planted for the delivery, defensive end Charles Mann drilled him in the back.

Aikman screamed.

"All my weight fell on his leg while it was all bent up," Geathers recollected. "I heard him holler. I knew it was bad. I was praying and hoping that it wasn't too bad."

Center Mark Stepnoski: "That's how it really got kickin'. We were playing an undefeated team . . . we lost our quarterback . . . but somehow we just kind of clicked and got going."

Aikman: "That was probably as good as the team had ever felt since I'd been there. As I look back on my career that was the turning point for our organization."

The final summation would be left for Madden who, along with Pat Summerall, had broadcast the stunner nationally and witnessed his predictions of a 16–0 Redskins season go down the drain.

"Of all the games I've ever done, Jimmy Johnson's done more with less," Madden said. "It's the best coaching job I've ever seen."

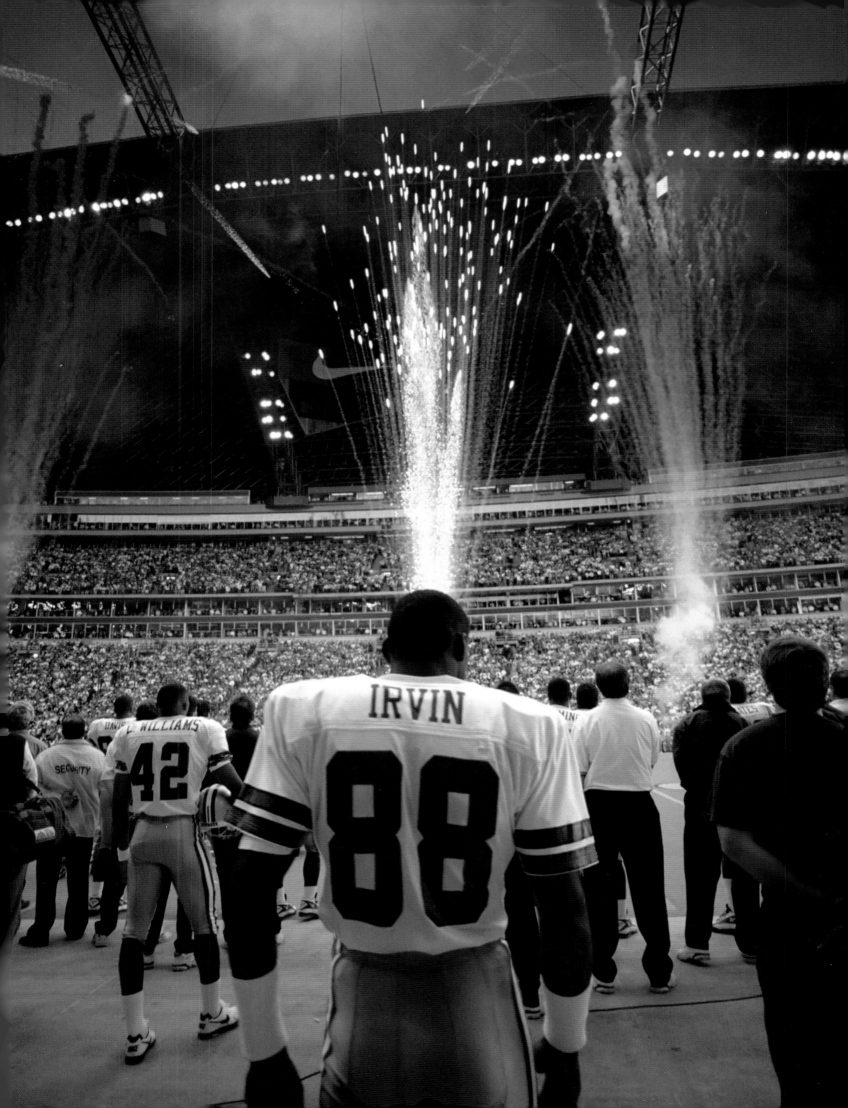

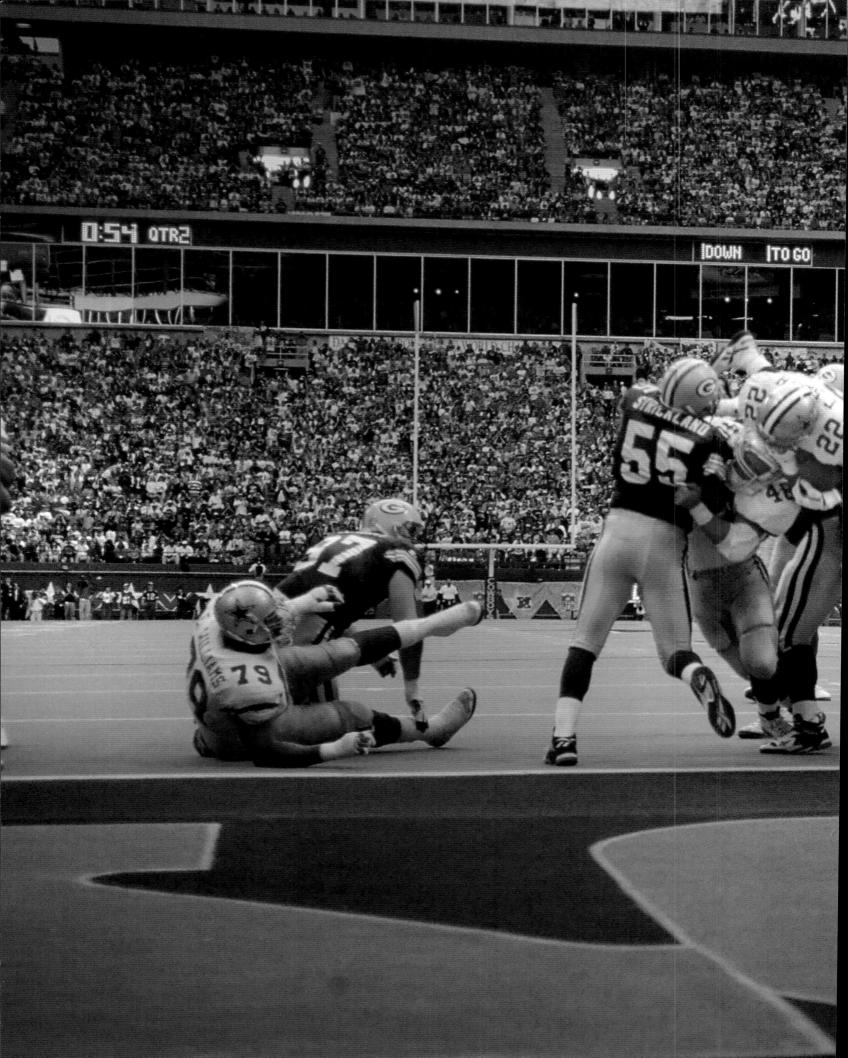

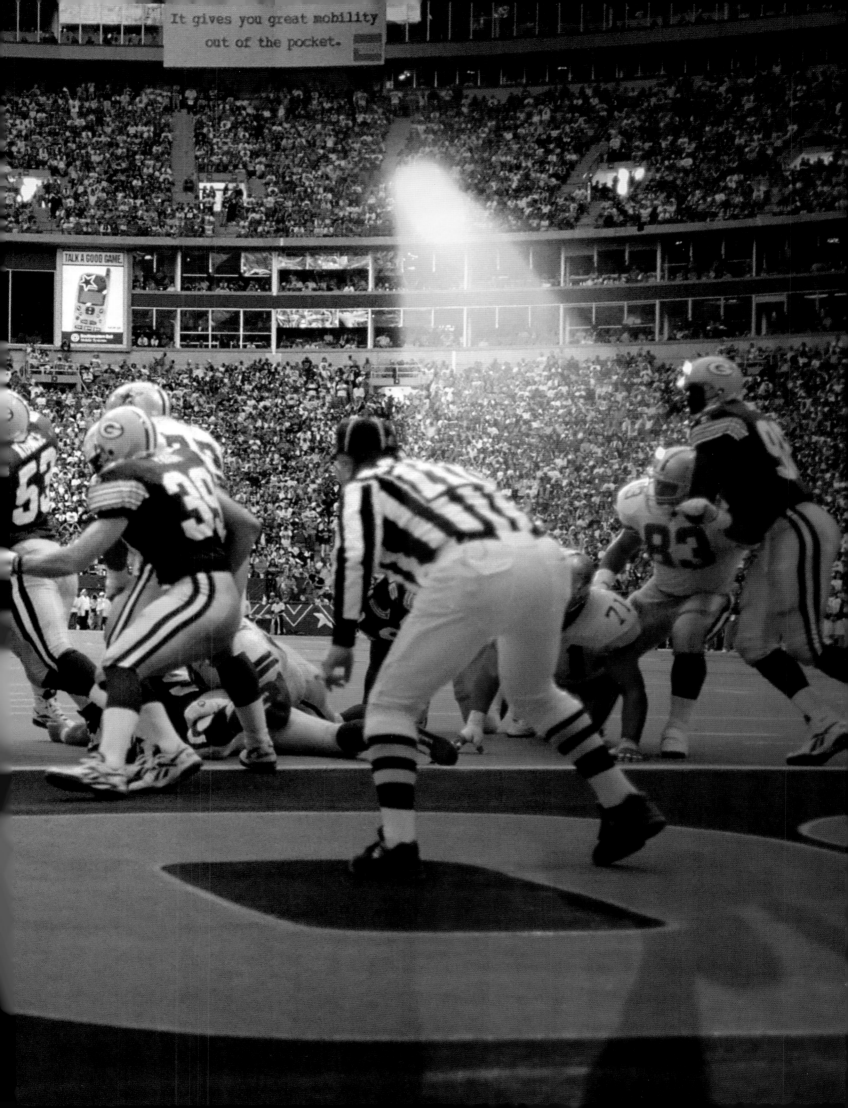

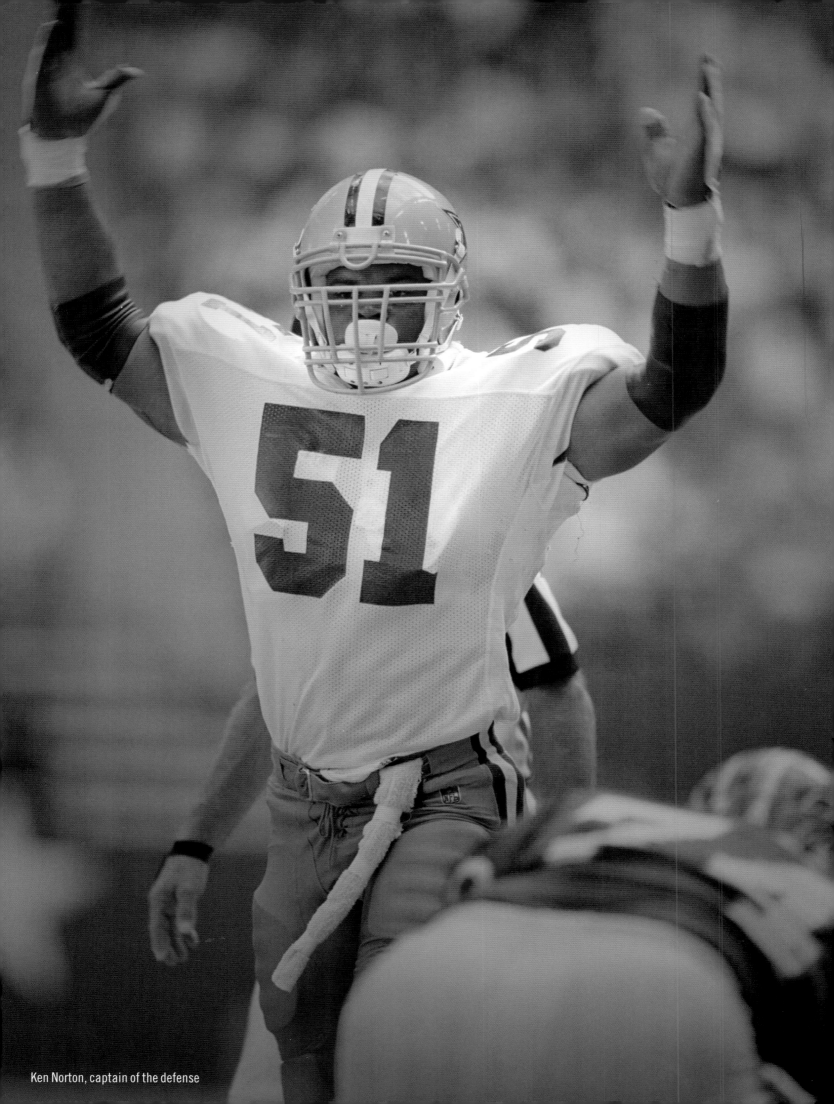

Ken Norton, captain of the defense

DECEMBER 29, 1991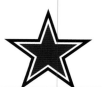

BIG "D"

A disappointed, frustrated, angry, soul-searching Chicago Bears team lingered in their Soldier Field locker room trying to make sense of what had just happened.

There's a noticeable difference in reaction between teams right after they've ended losing regular seasons and those who've just lost a playoff. In November and/or December, the regular season's end approaches steadily measured in days and weeks. Those teams with losing records and dwindling shots at the playoffs can see the end coming from a distance, whereas playoff defeats happen abruptly. Just three hours earlier these Bears, playing at home, felt confident their off-season was at least another week away. Perhaps more.

But suddenly it was over, courtesy of the Cowboys.

Some playoff losses are digested more easily than others. A team leaves the field knowing they'd fallen to a superior opponent. There's little second guessing or finger pointing.

Other defeats, however, are downright cruel—as this one was. Bears players and coaches sifting through the final numbers in their 17–13 loss to Dallas were eventually left with one question: "How did we lose this game?"

For the afternoon Chicago had:

- Run 82 plays to Dallas' 48
- Outgained the Cowboys by 84 yards
- Won time of possession by the whopping margin of 37½ to 22½ minutes.

Chicago had driven into Dallas territory on seven of their nine possessions. Twice they had the ball inside the Cowboys' 10-yard line but would get *no points*, either time. The stat sheet trumpeted Chicago's domination, but the scoreboard proclaimed a Dallas victory.

In the joyful Dallas locker room everybody understood exactly how the Cowboys had accomplished their first post-season victory in nearly nine years. With D E E E–F E N S E !

That delighted Coach Johnson. "The way we won had such significance," he said. "Everyone talked about our talent on offense, and the Triplets. Nobody noticed we'd gotten so good on defense."

Indeed!

Even though Emmitt Smith had become the first running back to ever gain more than one hundred yards rushing against the Bears in a playoff game—a span of twenty-six games dating back to *1920*—the underappreciated and underpublicized defense had carried this day.

- ★ On the game's first possession, veteran Dallas safety Bill Bates forced a fumble by quarterback Jim Harbaugh at the Dallas 49. Defensive end Tony Hill recovered, helping to set up a Dallas field goal.
- ★ Darrick Brownlow blocked a punt, giving the offense the ball at the Bears 10. Smith punched it in. Dallas led 10–0 after twelve minutes.
- ★ The Cowboys "D" drilled runner Neal Anderson on a fourth and one at the Dallas two. Chicago turned it over on downs.
- ★ Cornerback Larry Brown intercepted Harbaugh in the end zone, ending another Bears journey deep into Dallas territory.
- ★ Just before halftime the Cowboys again stuffed three Chicago runs, halting a Bears drive just three feet from the Dallas goal line. Da frustrated Bears settled for a chip shot field goal.

Second half—same script.

- ★ The Bears turned it over on downs when the Pokes defended three passes at their seven-yard line.
- ★ Finally, Bates snuffed out Chicago's last hope with an interception at the Bears 25 with 1:12 remaining.

The manner of victory satisfied Johnson: "I've always taught, all the way back to Oklahoma State (his first head coaching job): defense, special teams, and no turnovers."

During Tom Landry's last few years as coach, the Cowboys' talent base had eroded steadily. His defense over his last three years had scored just four touchdowns on fumble and interception returns, while the less-than-special teams hadn't scored at all in that time. In Johnson's first three seasons, though, the Cowboys' "D" scored seven times and the special teams added five more. Lost turnovers shrunk from forty-two in '89 to thirty-three in '90 and then to only

49

twenty-four in '91. This Dallas turnover-free victory over the Bears extended the Cowboys' winning streak to six in a row. During that run Dallas gave the ball away just three times.

Offensive players had long ago spotted the emphasis being put on the other side of the ball.

"I'm gonna tell you a little secret," guard Nate Newton divulged. "Jimmy had come into the offensive meeting and said, 'You know, fellas, we're going to do this or that,' but he really wouldn't say much. But the key was, Jimmy believed in that defense. He'd tell

. . . and we just had a sense of what we had here going forward," Jones said. "I felt like I was just in heaven."

Well, maybe not *heaven*. But they'd crept closer. Detroit rudely booted Dallas out of title contention the next weekend 38–6.

Dallas, however, would not suffer another playoff loss for three years, and they would rumble to ten victories in their next eleven playoff games. And Jones, Johnson, that glorious offense, and that unheralded defense would make three different trips to "NFL heaven."

"...and we just had a sense of what we had here going forward. I felt like I was just in heaven."

'em, 'Ya'll got to come up big!' A lotta people don't know Jimmy designed that attack defense way back at Oklahoma State."

That attack defense returned to anonymity almost immediately after this triumph in the Windy City while accolades for offensive players kept piling up. Voting by NFL players put four Cowboys in that season's Pro Bowl—all from the offense.

That number grew to six in '92—all from the offense. In '93 a remarkable eleven Cowboys journeyed to Hawaii for the all-star game—eight from the offense. Safety Thomas Everett, DT Russell Maryland, and LB Ken Norton Jr. became the first Cowboys defenders so honored in eight years. By the 1992 season Dallas would boast of having the league's No. 1-rated defense. But, again, very few noticed.

Owner Jerry Jones remembers making his way through that jubilant Cowboys locker room at Soldier Field.

"I was just so appreciative of just getting to be part of everything . . . every time I walked on the practice field or the sideline

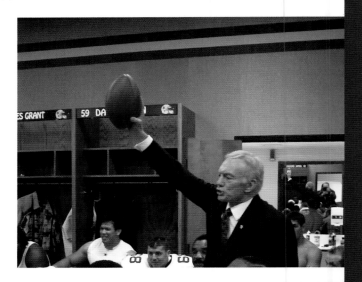

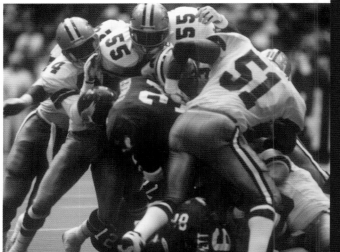

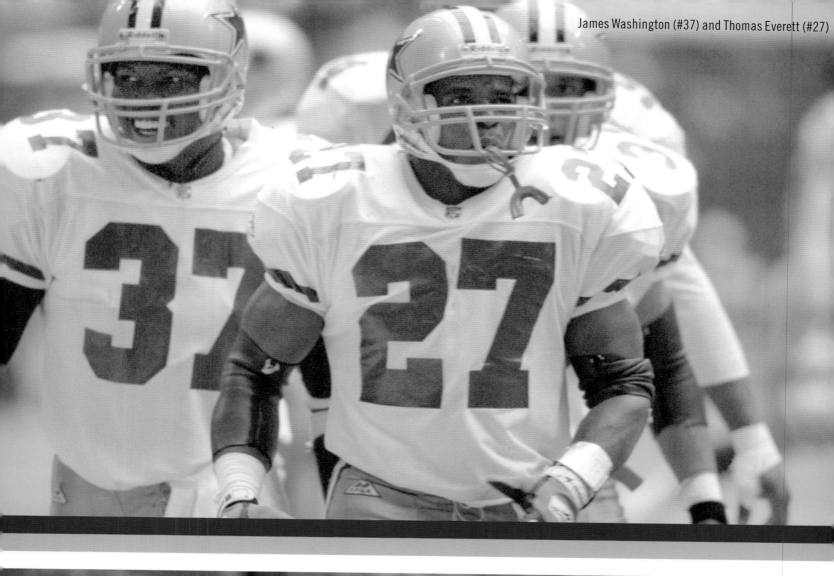

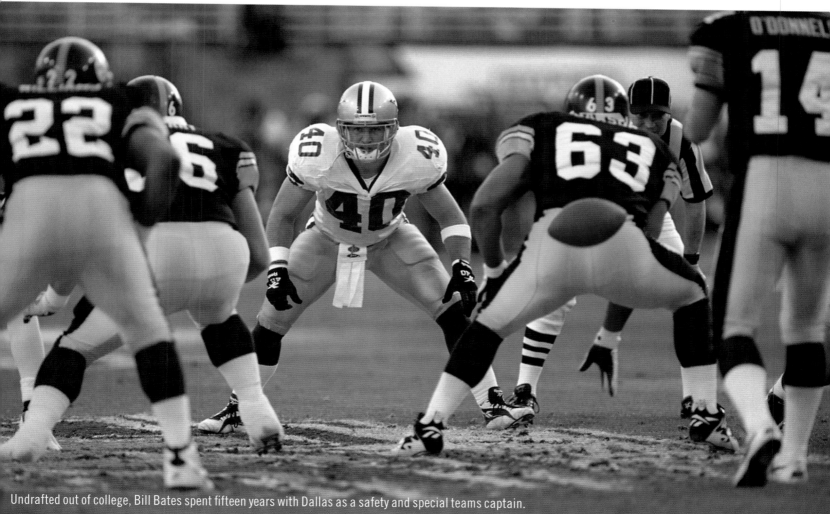

Undrafted out of college, Bill Bates spent fifteen years with Dallas as a safety and special teams captain.

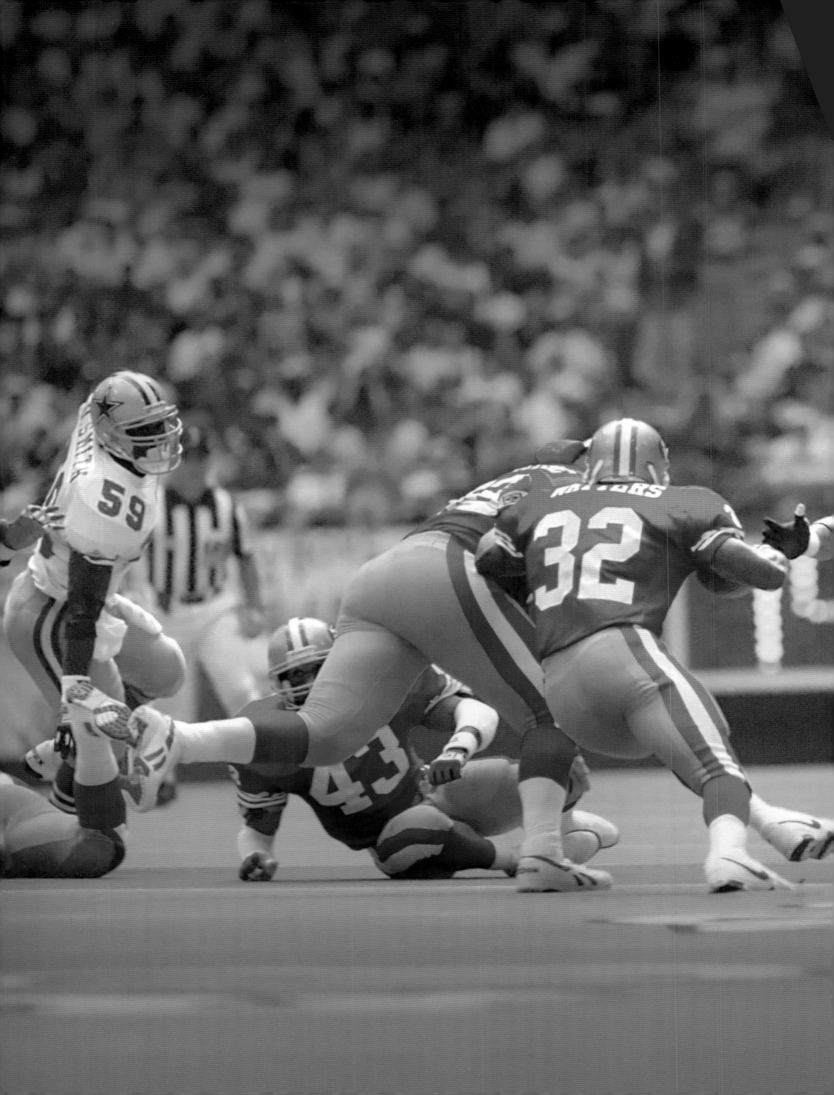

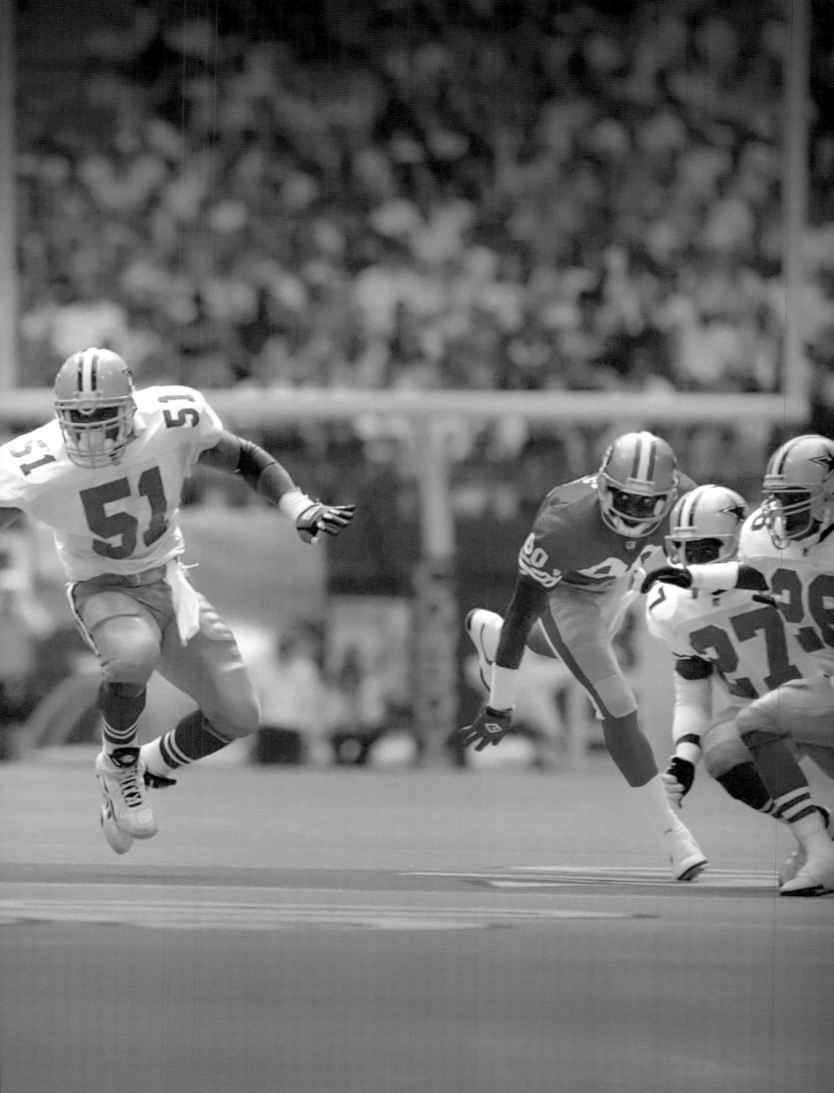

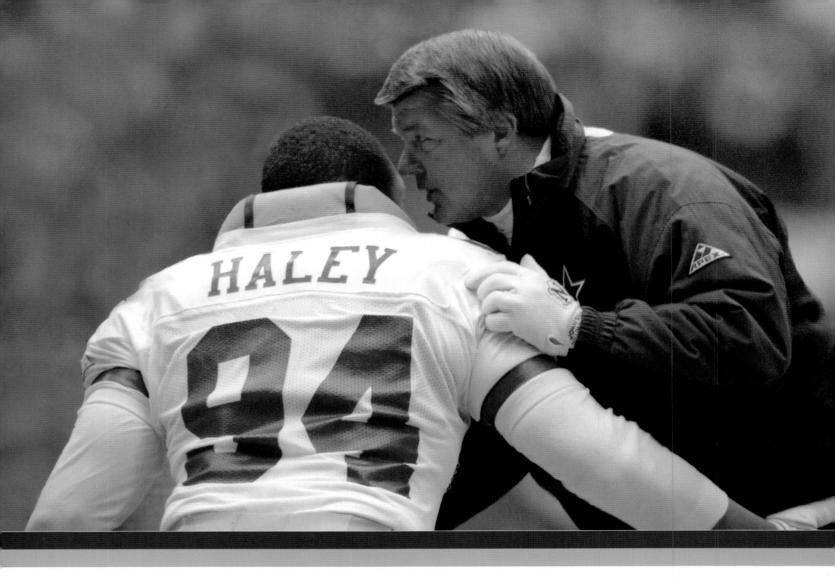

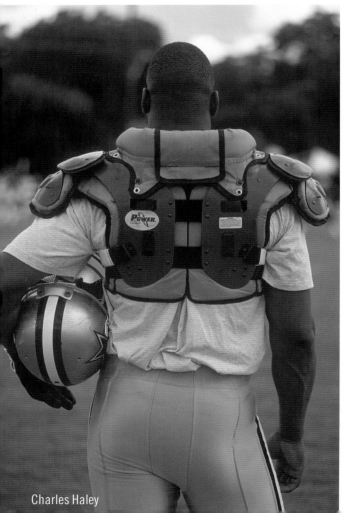

Charles Haley

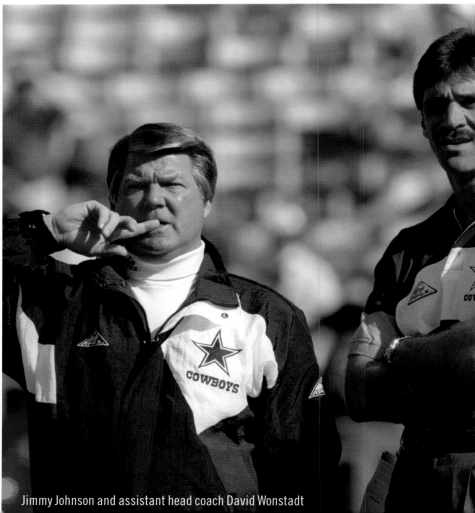

Jimmy Johnson and assistant head coach David Wonstadt

LET'S GET READY TO RUMMMBLLE

In this corner, wearing the slacks and golf shirt outfit of the Dallas coaching staff and unbeaten in countless career confrontations with players— Jimmeeee JOHNson.

And in the far corner, wearing the blue Cowboys road uniform with silver number 94 and a silver helmet with blue star, the volatile and some believe uncontrollable Charrrrles HAAAley.

Johnson vs. Haley in a Denver locker room. The NFL heavyweight division couldn't dream of a bigger bout.

The 10–2 Cowboys squared off against 7–5 Denver in nineteen-degree weather at Mile High Stadium. Coach Dan Reeves' club had won nine in a row at home and sixteen of their last seventeen. The Broncos had posted a sensational 93–29 all-time mark at home, making Mile High *the* toughest place in NFL history for a visitor to get a win.

The wounded Broncos that Dallas faced this day, however, appeared far less formidable. They'd lost future Hall of Fame quarterback John Elway to injury. Without him Denver had suffered back-to-back road losses while scoring only thirteen points. And on this frigid Sunday afternoon Coach Reeves had settled on a pretty bizarre plan to replace Elway. He would alternate twenty-year-old rookie Tommy Maddox with twenty-three-year-old Shawn Moore, whose NFL career to date consisted of one passing attempt. The Maddox-Moore tandem wouldn't just flip-flop by series, either. Sometimes the Broncos would shuffle them in and out after each play.

For Dallas, who'd brutalized the proud Giants 30–3 the week before (giving them eight victories in nine outings), this looked like a piece of cake.

And it started out that way. Cornerback Kevin Smith intercepted Maddox on the game's first play. Aikman-to-Irvin made it 7–0. Safety James Washington added another interception of a Maddox pass. Aikman-to-Irvin made it 14–0 with less than seven minutes gone.

Game over? No, sir. Game on!

Denver bounced back, driving eighty yards in nine plays. After Dallas went three and out, the Broncos traveled sixty-seven yards in just six plays to score again. Only a botched snap on the extra point kept the Broncos from a 14–14 tie. Except for a booming fifty-three-yard-line Elliott field goal for the Cowboys, the rest of the half turned into a punting exhibition. Dallas trudged toward their locker room clinging to an uneasy 17–13 lead.

Over the first thirty minutes Denver had out-gained Dallas by sixty yards. The Cowboys had averaged less than 2.7 yards per carry and committed six penalties. Despite getting three gift turnovers from Denver's still-wet-behind-the-ears quarter-backs, the Pokes led by a measly four points.

Mount Johnson was about to erupt. All he needed was something or someone to set him off. Enter Charles Haley.

In August Johnson had given NFC rival San Francisco second- and third-round picks for the talented but sometimes troubled defensive end. Even Haley concedes the Niners thought of him as "a lunatic." Uncoachable. That he'd reached the point of causing more trouble inside the club than in opposing backfields.

Johnson saw something else.

"He'd had his own way throughout his career," Johnson observed. "People became afraid to deal with him. But Charles was a competitor. Worked hard in practice. Players would follow him. He was smart. That's why I dealt for him. You can't reason with dumb players."

Despite what Johnson said, Haley was not some kind of pussycat curled up at his master's feet. Haley took medication to control his manic depression. Even Haley knew Haley could be a handful: "My mood swings are rapid and, I don't know, it depended on the day or the time whether I just took stuff or would explode at other stuff . . . I'd be excited one day and down in the dumps the next."

Haley could cuss out a reporter for a simple question and then quietly go into the community to help kids. He'd play wonderfully while battling pain from a ruptured disc in his back but occasionally seemed to disappear from games when perfectly fit. He'd matter-of-factly say things like: "A man might have saved somebody's life yesterday and go out and kill somebody the next day."

Everyone seemed to have their own personal picture of Charles Haley.

Fellow defensive lineman Jimmie Jones described him as "very humorous . . . always causing comical havoc in meetings."

The Forty-niners labeled him a "cancer."

Dallas defensive tackle Chad Hennings knew yet one more Haley. "He dictated a lot of tone in the locker room: Very verbal. Would ride players, also boost players up. A great catalyst."

Whoever or whatever the identity of Haley might be, he was about to go toe to toe with the calculating, mind-games-playing control freak and master psychologist coach of the Cowboys. For the first time since taking over as Cowboys coach, Johnson would get to put his psychology degree to work with a clinical case all his own.

Everyone paid close attention—everyone, that is, except Haley, who'd played poorly that first half, making just one tackle. If anyone needed to be paying attention, it was him. But he stood thirty feet away, completely across the room from the squeaking chalk, almost immune to the situation and tucked inside another of his funks.

Jimmy . . . went . . . ballistic!

"I told him, 'pick your BLEEP up or I'll cut your BLEEP. I've got nothing to BLEEPin' lose. You'll be gone in a heartbeat.'"

Usually, Johnson chastised Haley only in private. "He's a proud man and usually didn't respond to public humiliation in front of the team," Johnson said. "But occasionally others needed to see. Charles was such a free spirit, if you didn't (chew him out in front of others), he'd run over you."

But in this case Johnson's cork had just begun to blow.

"He dictated a lot of tone in the locker room: Very verbal. Would ride players, also boost players up. A great catalyst."

Jimmy Johnson was fried. He detested complacency anywhere or anytime. In his soul he believed he'd assembled the makings of a Super Bowl champion. Maybe not this year, with thirteen of the twenty-two starters being twenty-six or younger. But then again, why *not* this year? In the first half his Cowboy team appeared smug, unfocused, overconfident, on cruise control. Call it whatever you might, Jimmy hated every one of those descriptions.

As Johnson entered the one large main area of the visitor's locker room, assistant coaches Butch Davis and Dave Wannstedt stood at the chalkboard diagramming adjustments to stop a Broncos running play that had bugged Dallas all during the first half. The Broncos tight ends or wing men kept cutting back to "wham" block Dallas' middle linebacker, effectively blindsiding him and opening holes for runs that kept Bronco drives alive.

"I told him 'you'll be on the BLEEPin' street tomorrow. If you think I give a damn what Jerry Jones thinks then go ahead and keep playing like this because when we get back to Dallas, if things don't change, I'm gonna cut you."

"My language could get pretty spicy back then," Johnson admitted.

Haley takes the high road in recalling the butt chewing. "I think Jimmy and me had something, some chemistry," he said. "I don't think there was an attitude thing. I was in my own little world in a way. I stretched the imagination to the limit, and the coaches had a lot dealing with me because of my antics and stuff."

Others had seen or experienced Johnson's rage before.

Troy Aikman: "Some of those guys he was yelling at were scared to death. They would almost pee in their pants."

James Washington: "Most of the times he went after me it was in front of everybody. He only went after guys that could understand it and bear it. (Like Haley?) He never went after guys who would break and fold."

For others, memories of Johnson's tantrums actually elicited laughter.

Larry Brown: "His facial expression would be like, I have so much I want to tell you . . . how do I get all this out, you know, like he's ready to explode . . . he was red and his little lips would be like, not licking his lips, but like chopping his lips."

Daryl Johnston: "Arms folded, lips pursed, brow furrowed. It's the only time I ever saw his hair move. He'd furrow and unfurrow his brow and all his hair would go straight up and down."

Others like guard Nate Newton and assistant coach Joe Avezzano understood that every Johnson move, barb, or cuss word, had a motive behind it.

Newton: "He played mind games, man. Jimmy always sent messages through his studs. Troy, Emmitt, Mike, Haley, Woodson, Norton—he'd get their attention, then he knew all us grunts would fall in place."

Coach Joe: "Jimmy never did *anything* off the wall."

Once Johnson had blistered that paint off that Denver wall, Haley and all the other studs and grunts got the message. A Haley sack inside the two-minute warning helped preserve a narrow victory.

The next day behind closed doors the two talked out their differences. Each would live to fight again another day . . . literally.

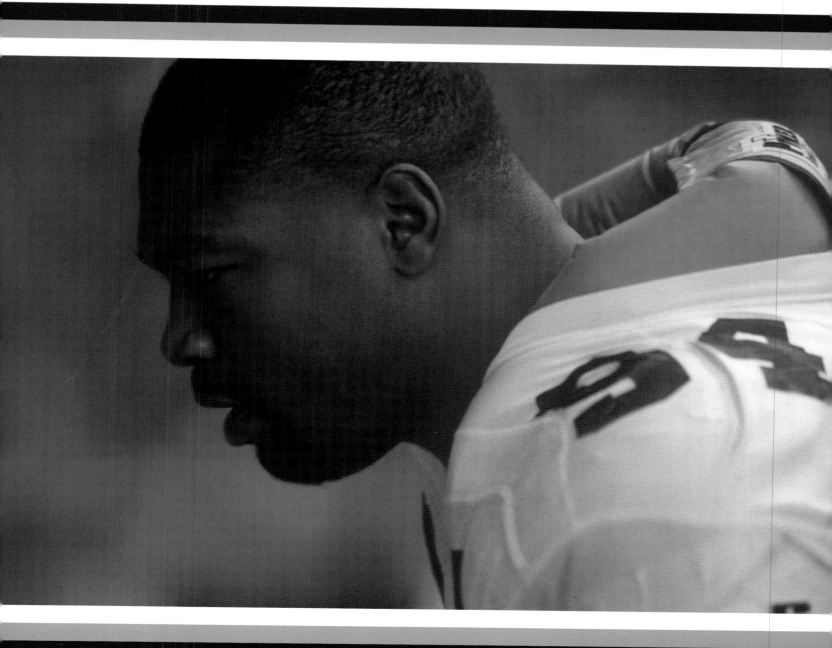

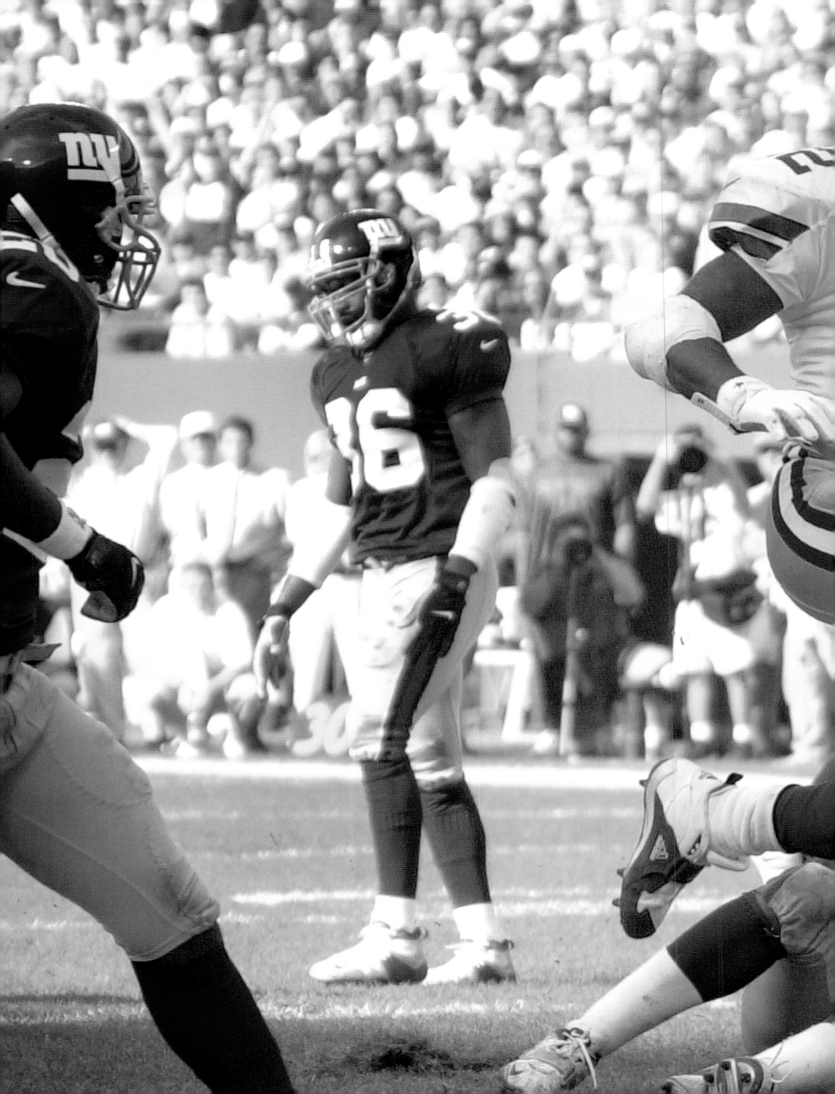

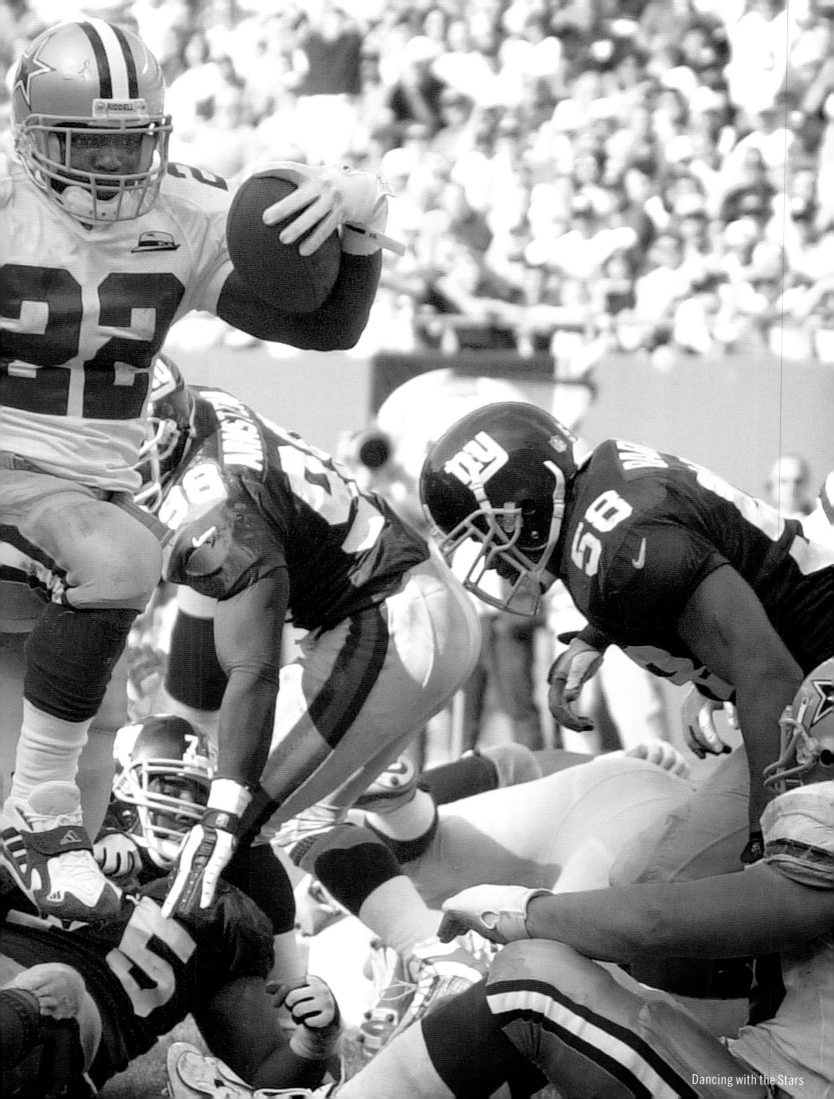

Dancing with the Stars

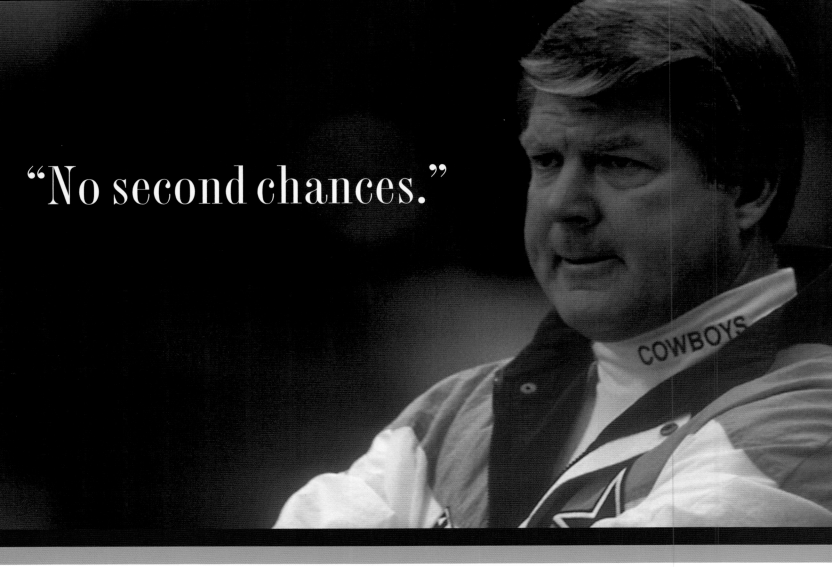

"No second chances."

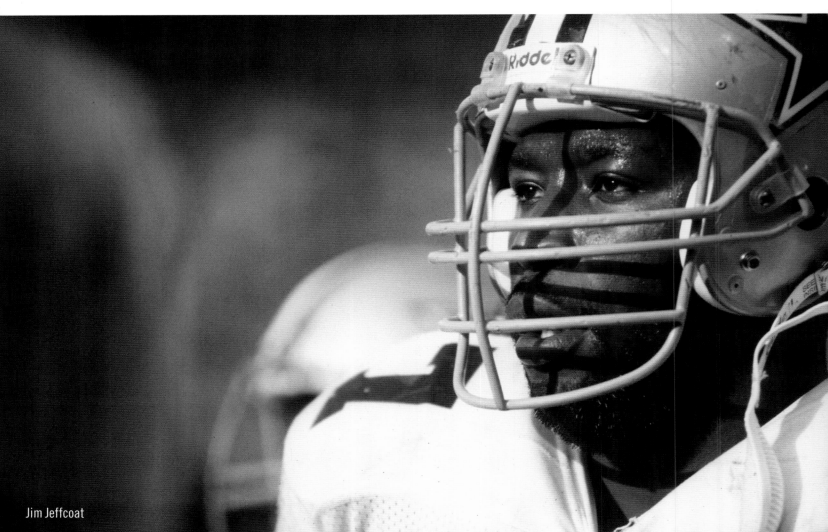

Jim Jeffcoat

BAH HUMBUG

By all appearances this second day after Christmas couldn't have gone better for the Cowboys and their fans.

They'd drilled Chicago 27–14 for their thirteenth win, becoming the first Dallas team to ever reach that victory total in a regular season.

Emmitt Smith began the day needing 109 yards to pass Pittsburgh's Barry Foster for his second consecutive NFL rushing title. A thirty-one-yard touchdown scamper early in the third quarter carried him well past the number needed. With the game safely in hand, Smith spent the rest of his afternoon watching his backup Curvin Richards score his first NFL touchdown.

Dallas put the game out of reach a minute after Smith's run. Chicago halfback Darren Lewis coughed up a fumble. Cowboys defensive tackle Russell Maryland snatched it out of the air and set sail for the Bears end zone thirty yards away for his first ever touchdown as well. At the goal line the fun started. To celebrate, Maryland launched his 275-pound body toward the heavens. That, apparently, was also where Maryland's party planning ended.

"I didn't know what to do," Maryland said. "I saw the crossbar and thought about trying to spike the ball over it."

Gravity would not permit that. So Maryland improvised in midair with a reverse spike complete with a full flat-on-his-face landing that would be the first, and almost certainly the last, NFL touchdown celebration ever called "the beached whale."

The victory brought Jimmy Johnson to .500 in his NFL coaching career. His Cowboys tenure began with a dismal 10–26 mark. But Dallas had now surged to 23–7 over their last thirty games.

So, with so many reasons for holiday cheer, why did a visibly grumpy Johnson barge into the locker room and sputter out this abbreviated post-game speech: "Sick call is at 10 AM Make sure you get your two weightlifting sessions in this week. See you tomorrow." He spun around and barged out.

To understand Johnson's lack of ho, ho, hoing, one must time travel back to that moment in the third quarter where the coach decided to take the Cowboys' foot off the Bears' throat. Dallas had clinched the NFC East crown the week before by torching Atlanta. With the victory over Chicago adding more frosting to the cake, Jimmy had opted to send in the reserves and rest several key players for the upcoming playoffs.

After all, the Bears had offered little resistance to that point. For the game, Dallas outgained them, 354 yards to 92. In none of their thirteen possessions did Chicago keep the ball for more than six snaps. Their longest drive? Twenty-five yards. Their biggest play? A sixteen-yard pass completion. Not a single yard rushing in the third quarter and absolutely none passing in the fourth.

So what turned Jimmy from Santa into the Grinch who stole Christmas?

"I don't like sloppy play," said Johnson, who wasn't about to accept the flimsy excuse that putting the bench guys in meant a letdown. "I will *never* accept sloppy play. It doesn't matter what the situation is, what the score is, or who the opponent is. I don't want us to go out there and flop around."

After three solid quarters, Dallas had stunk it up over the final fifteen minutes. Richards, who'd wanted a Johnson high-five but settled for a hearty handshake after his first career touchdown earlier, fumbled on the quarter's second play. Upon returning to the bench, Richards this time got an encouraging pat on the back from the coach.

Backup quarterback Steve Beuerlein threw an interception, and Chicago quickly converted that turnover into seven points.

Richards (him again?) scuffled with Bears defensive tackle Chris Zorich, which got Richards one of Johnson's colorful tongue lashings. Then, Richards fumbled *again*! Zorich returned it for a touchdown. Moments later wide receiver Alvin Harper lost another fumble. In the first 15 3/4 games of the season the Cowboys had committed only twenty turnovers. Now they had *four* in less than nine minutes!

Veteran Tommy Agee came in to get the final eight carries in place of Smith. Richards got the bench. His afternoon and his Cowboys career were over.

"I was fuming . . . I knew as soon as he (Richards) had that second fumble, I was cutting him as soon as the game was over," Johnson wrote in his book. *Turning the Thing Around*. "I had had enough of it, and I emphasized to the rest of the players (the next day)—I don't care who you are—we're not going to put up with turnovers."

after the last game of the year when they had the playoffs sewn up."

Did Jimmy really want to release Richards, or scream at Charles Haley in Denver, or throw that still legendary tantrum on the plane coming back to Dallas after a gut-wrenching loss to Washington (when he ordered the *flight attendants* to sit down and stop service to the players)?

"At times I have to be the bad guy just to keep things in check."

Dallas released Richards on Monday. The move totally puzzled the league. Why would anyone cut their No. 1 backup at halfback *after* the regular season had ended and with post-season play dead ahead? A league official phoned Johnson Tuesday to confirm what seemed like a wacky move.

"Coach, why'd you cut Curvin Richards yesterday? You know that you're going to have to pay him total playoff money; it's not like you're saving any money," the league official said

Johnson: "I know all of that."

Official: "So why?"

Johnson: "Because I couldn't depend on him. Why are you asking me?"

Official: "Well, it's just something that's never been done. I don't think anybody has ever cut somebody

"At times I have to be the bad guy just to keep things in check."

Years down the road Johnson would admit he often disliked having to be Scrooge. Being contrary. Often downright nasty. That the burnout created by so often playing "bad Jimmy" was one of the factors in a career that saw him never stay anywhere more than five years.

In that Monday meeting with the players to explain the waiving of Richards, Johnson delivered a passionate and succinct keep-your-eyes-on-the-prize message:

"I didn't want to go into the playoffs with a guy I couldn't depend on. If it's in the regular season and a guy fumbles, even if we lose the game, we've got other games to play to situate ourselves. . . . In the playoffs, you get *No Second Chances!*

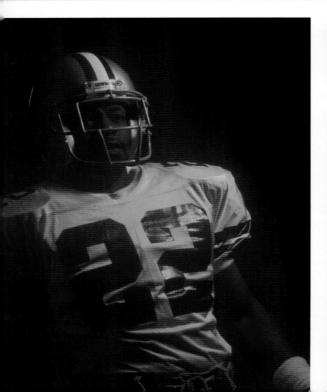
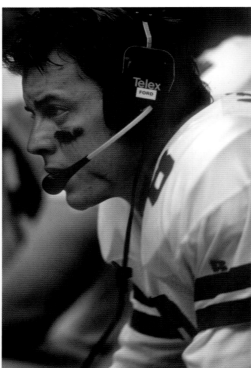
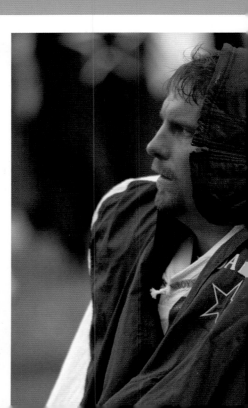

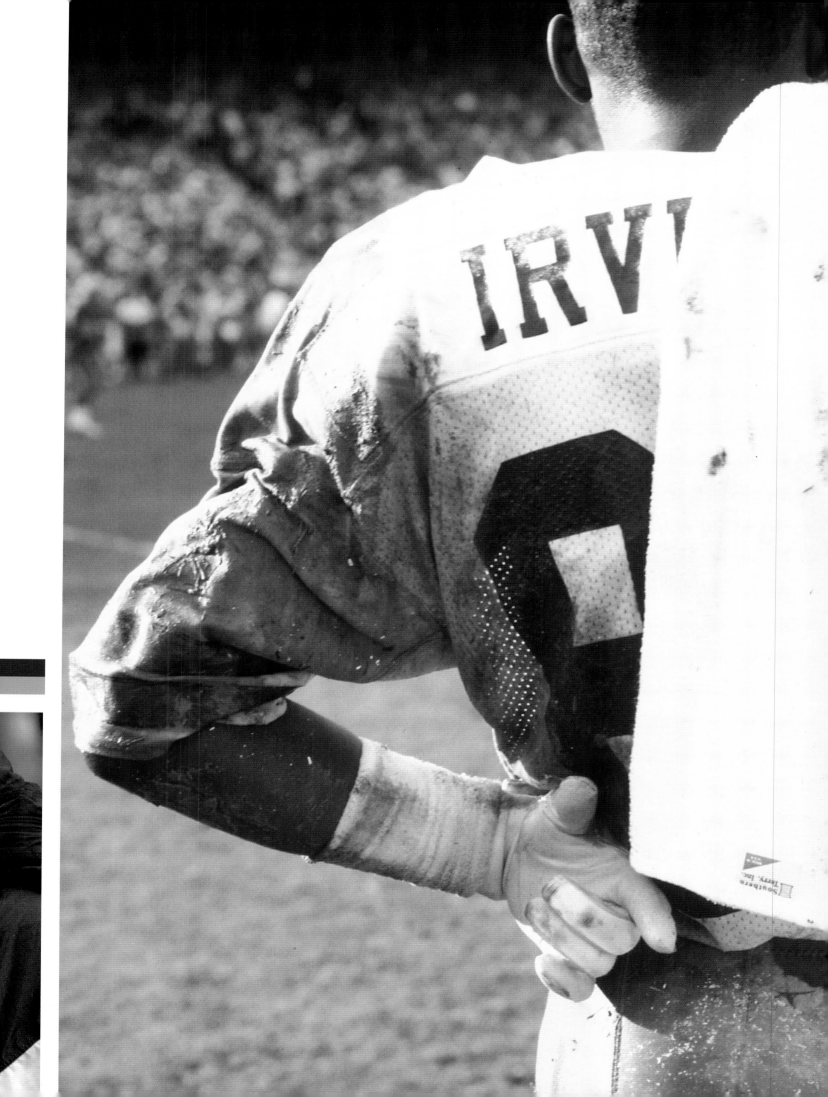

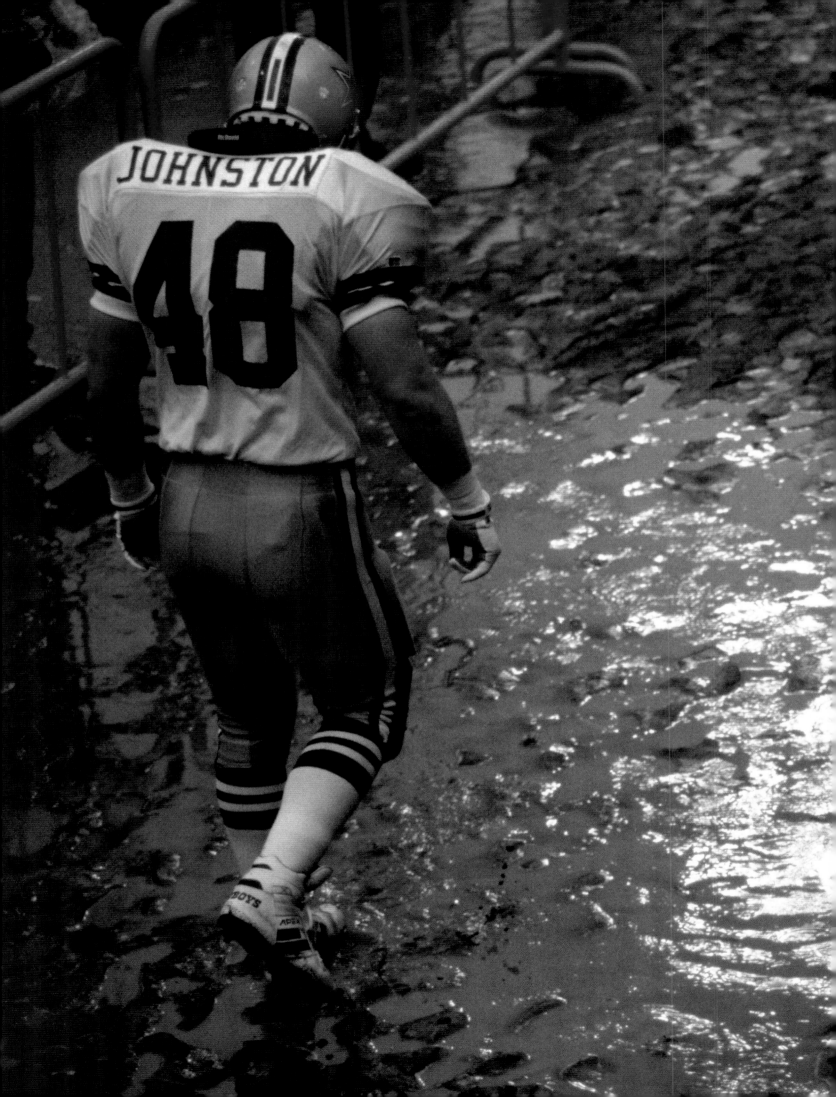

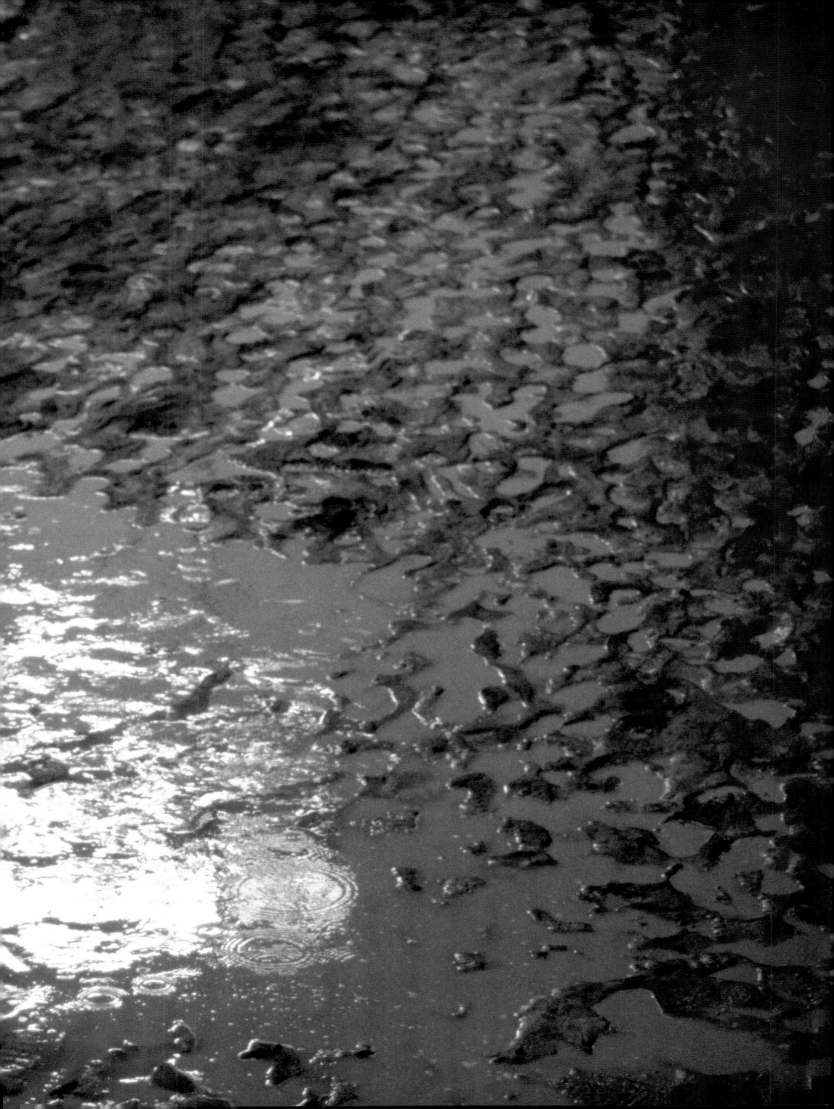

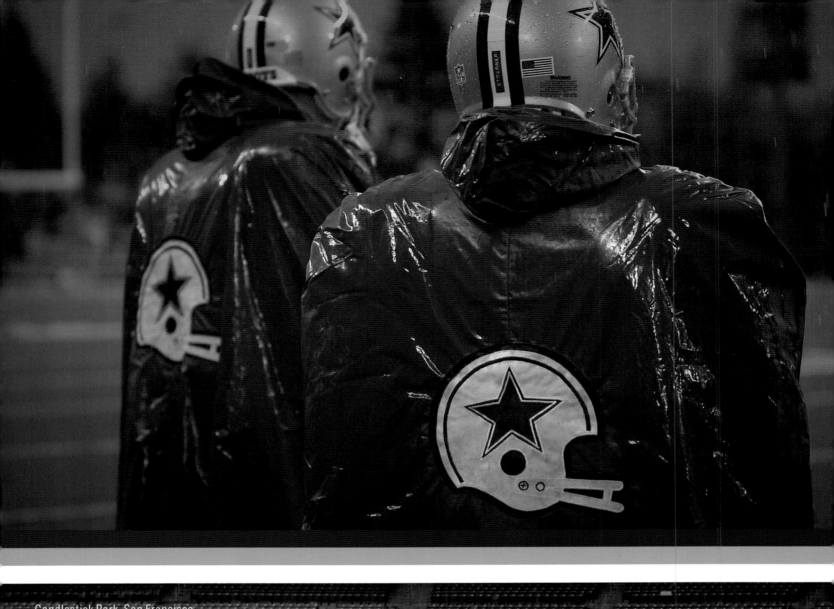

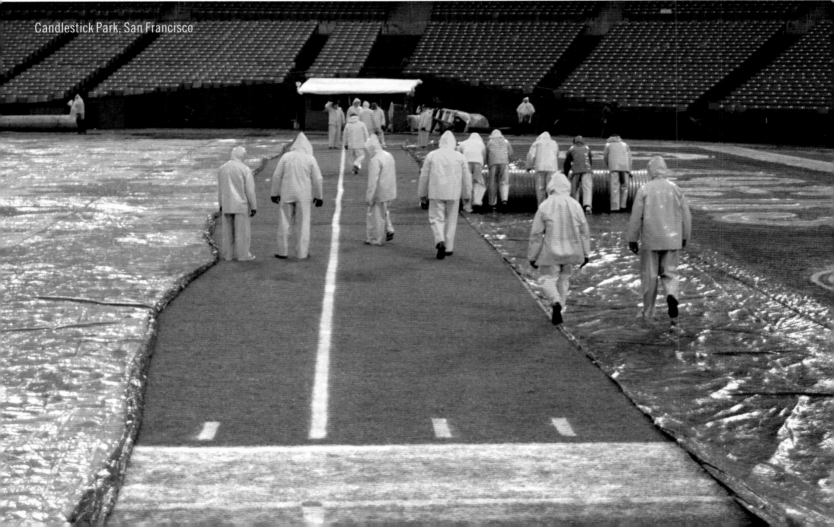

Candlestick Park, San Francisco

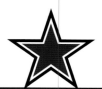
A TRULY CALCULATED GAMBLE

It's four o'clock Sunday morning in San Francisco. Nine hours until the two best teams in the NFL, the 14–3 Cowboys and the 15–2 Forty-niners, clash in the NFC championship game. Jimmy Johnson's already awake and worried. But not necessarily about the Forty-niners. He's more concerned about the sorry state of the Candlestick Park turf.

Monsoon rains had struck the Bay area that week, saturating a playing field already regarded as one of the worst in the league. The 'Stick sat right on the edge of San Francisco Bay and its playing surface actually rested a few inches *below* sea level. Even a moderate amount of rain meant drainage problems, and this had been an extended downpour.

The horrible conditions so concerned the league that they brought in the country's finest groundskeeper, George "the Sod God" Toma, to perform some kind of miracle. He'd been rehabbing playing surfaces for nearly half a century.

"This is hands down the worst field I've ever seen," Toma observed.

That's tantamount to a veteran plumber coming to your home and exclaiming: "This is absolutely the worst mess I've ever had to clean up!"

Toma's army of twenty-six joined with the park's regular crew and replaced all the grass in the middle of the field—ninety feet across and goal line to goal line. At one end they extended the repairs all the way from sideline to sideline.

In San Francisco, the epicenter during the sixties and seventies for phenomena such as flower children and hippies, along with the make-love-not-war and legalize-marijuana movements, grass had again become topic No. 1, only this time it wasn't about the kind of grass you smoked. There were even whispers of switching the contest to Stanford Stadium, a few miles south in Palo Alto. All week the water as well as the questions about the field's readiness rained down. It got to the point that the subject started annoying some Cowboys players.

Emmitt Smith: "The field is the one that ought to be worried. It has to deal with us, and we're gonna tear it up."

Mark Stepnoski: "What are we going to do, practice slipping?"

On Saturday, Johnson and other staffers toured the saturated 'Stick with Toma, who gave them a map showing the exact locations of the old and newly installed turf.

Now it's 4 AM and Johnson's studying that map, looking for any edge it might provide. By 7 o'clock Johnson, armed with a blizzard of notes, had assembled his staff.

"We went through our entire game plan—offensively, defensively, special teams, every phase," Jimmy remembers. "We got out all our call sheets and went over what parts of the field we could or couldn't blitz on, what end we had to return kickoffs up the middle as opposed to cutting outside. We made asterisks regarding the footing for Emmitt specifically. If it was a critical down, we were going to run the ball inside rather than using the toss play to the outside where Emmitt might slip."

With six hours to kickoff, Johnson had just doubled or even tripled the complexity of the game plan for offensive coordinator Norv Turner, special teams boss Joe Avezzano, and defensive coordinator Dave Wannstedt.

For some, Johnson's field-condition obsession might amount to fixation on minutia. Hours later, however, that attention to detail would pay enormous dividends.

Through nearly fifty-six minutes the two NFC heavyweights battled on even terms. Each side had scored once in each quarter. Underdog Dallas led 24–20 because they had converted their opportunities into three touchdowns and a field goal while the Niners had a pair of touchdowns and two field goals. For the game, first downs and yards gained would be nearly identical.

With 4:14 left, the NFC championship, and accompanying role of favorite in Super Bowl XXVII had come down to one critical possession. The Niners had just scored to narrow Dallas' lead to four points, and now the Cowboys had the ball. Nearly sixty-five thousand screaming Niners fans begged for a

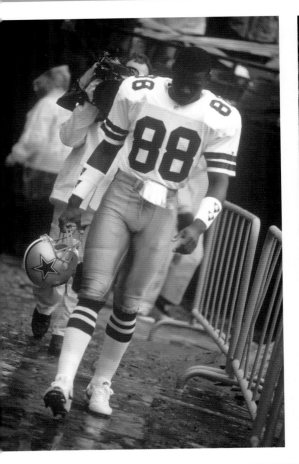

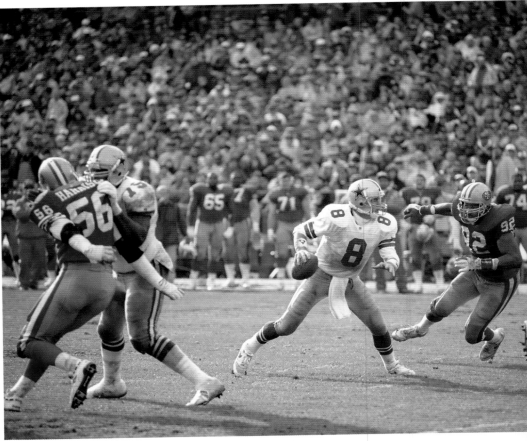

defensive stop. Dallas knew it needed at least one first down or there would be a lot of time for San Francisco to come back, especially for a potent offense that featured Steve Young, Jerry Rice, John Taylor, Ricky Watters, and others.

"The Niners expected we'd try to sit on it, run the ball, force them to use their timeouts, milk the clock," Johnson recalls. In other words, to not take any chances. Play it safe. But, along with hated things like turnovers, sloppiness, and complacency, Johnson seemed to detest playing "safe football."

During the television time-out following San Francisco's kickoff, the head coach talked it over on the headset with Turner, his offensive play caller stationed up in the coaches booth.

"The only way to make a first down is to throw it," Johnson directed. "Let's go ahead and open it up. What do we have?"

Turner: "The slant to Michael (Irvin)."

Johnson: "Okay, let's throw the slant."

Turner sent in a play called "Ace Right 896 F Flat" to Aikman. Here's how that play shaped up:

★ "Ace Right" indicates the offensive line's blocking scheme.
★ The first option dictates zipping the ball to Irvin, who splits left and, on the snap, immediately angles across the middle—the 8 route or "skinny post" in Cowboys lingo.

★ The receiver in the slot to the right sprints deep down the middle—the 9 route.
★ Alvin Harper sets up far right and runs a 12-yard curl—the 6 route.
★ Emmitt Smith, unless he must stay in to block a blitzing defensive player, slides out into the flat on a check-down route, giving Aikman a safety valve in case his downfield receivers are covered.

That's how it's *supposed* to work. And it had worked. Dallas had already executed "Ace Right 896 F Flat" a handful of times with excellent results, but never by hitting option No. 1, which was Irvin on the skinny post. The Niners, worried about the damage Irvin could do, constantly rolled their defense toward him by using a safety to help cornerback Don Griffin in coverage. Aikman had read the schemes correctly, going away from the primary receiver and consistently finding Harper or Smith for significant gains on the play.

First down at their 21 . . . up four points . . . 4:14 to go. As Dallas headed for the line of scrimmage, Irvin wanted the glory.

Aikman: "Michael got greedy. He was tired of running the 8 route and not getting the ball. He knew the ball had been going to Harper on the 6 route or to Emmitt. So, as we're breaking the huddle, Michael says to Alvin, 'You take the 8, I'm taking the 6' (swapping sides of the field)."

Remember, though, Frisco believed Dallas would play conservatively. Run the ball. Work the clock. The Niners jumped into an eight-man front. At all costs they *would* stop Smith, who'd already gashed their defense for more than a hundred yards rushing. That left Niners cornerbacks one-on-one, covering Dallas wideouts.

might or might not work depending on exactly where they lined up on the Candlestick slop.

Turner's play selection, Ace Right 896 F Flat, did not require Harper to cut on the treacherous footing, but only to sprint diagonally. Cornerback Griffin, all alone in coverage, had to instantly read Harper and cut inside (left) or outside to track him.

Roll the picture in your mind.

. . . Harper slanted.

"How 'bout them Cowboys!"

Aikman's pre-snap reads instantly told him San Francisco intended to blitz. That meant the first option—that 8 route—should be open. That's good. Very good. Or, that also might be bad.

Johnson: "We rarely threw the ball to Alvin on the slant because, sometimes, he'd get those short arms, "alligator arms" (he wouldn't stretch out to make the catch). He was great on takeoffs and sideline patterns, but he was never the primary receiver on slants."

Aikman shared Johnson's concern: "So, I'm wondering, Gosh, is Alvin gonna run this route the way he's supposed to? So, this is going through my mind and the ball is snapped and I said, 'You know, you just gotta trust the guy.' "

Center Mark Stepnoski's snap slammed into Aikman's palms. Very large men collided. In the stands, breaths were held. Harper . . .

For a moment freeze that picture in your mind. Track back hours to those early morning frenzied alterations Dallas had made to its game plan, based on that field condition chart. They'd rethought what calls

Aikman threw.

Griffin slipped on an area where the old turf had not been replaced.

The pass, the catch, the decision to gamble worked perfectly. Harper raced seventy yards to the Niners' nine. Three plays later, still not playing it safe, Dallas scored on a six-yard pass from Aikman to Kelvin Martin.

Dallas 30, San Francisco 20.

Moments later, with CBS cameras live inside the pandemonium that was the Dallas locker room, Johnson bellowed out what would be the single most famous line of his entire career.

"How 'bout them Cowboys!!!"

For one final time, however, return to those few seconds as Harper dashed along the sidelines past an exploding Dallas bench. Amongst many others, Harper sped by Dallas public relations director Rich Dalrymple who recalls that play as though it happened yesterday: "I remember standing there and thinking, We're going to the *Super Bowl* . . . and that our lives would never be the same."

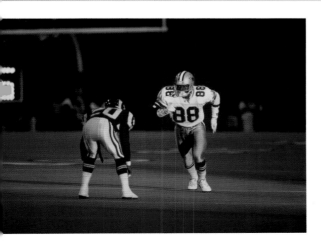
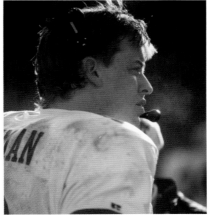
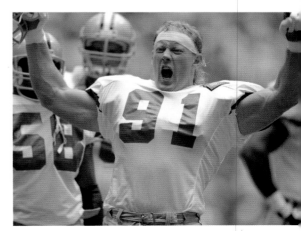

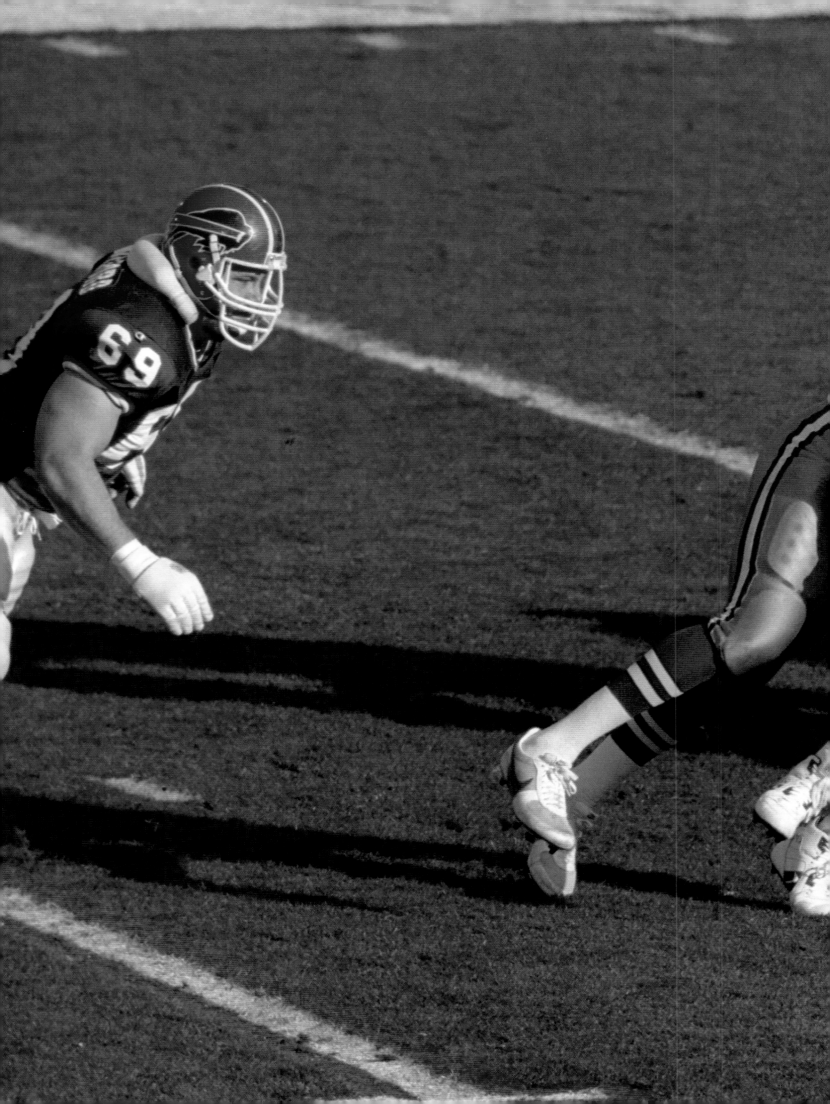

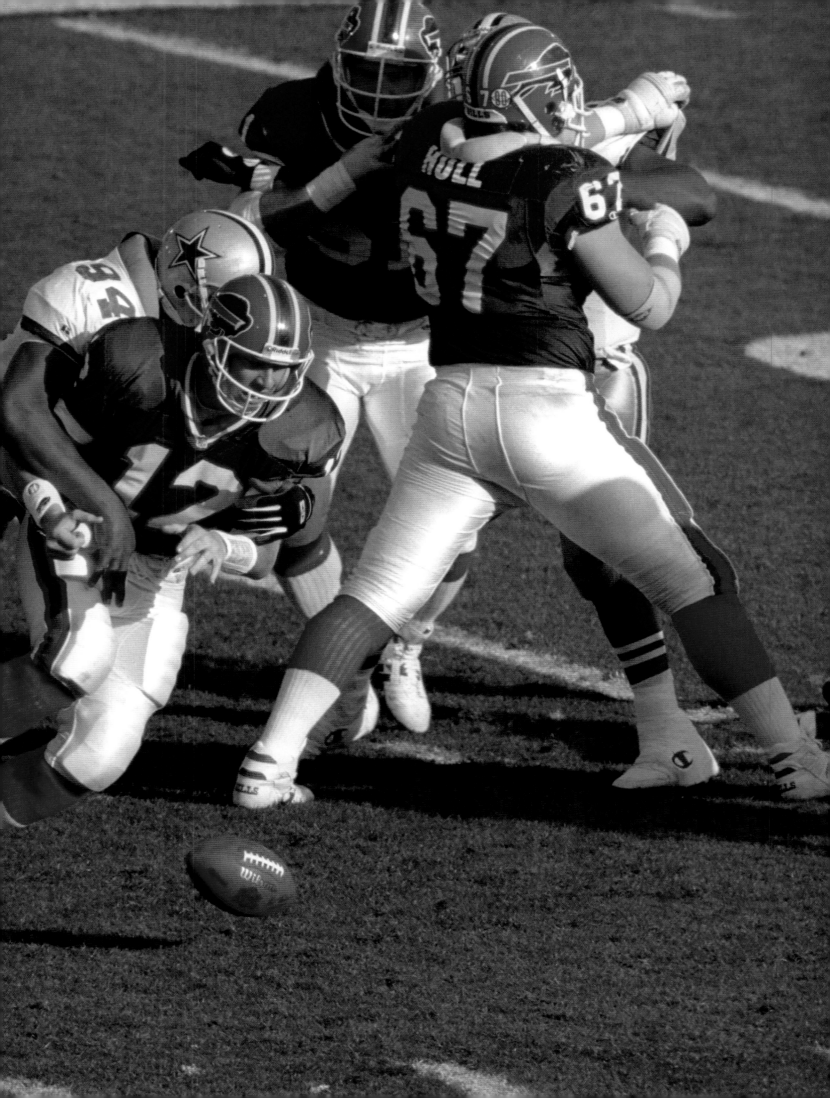

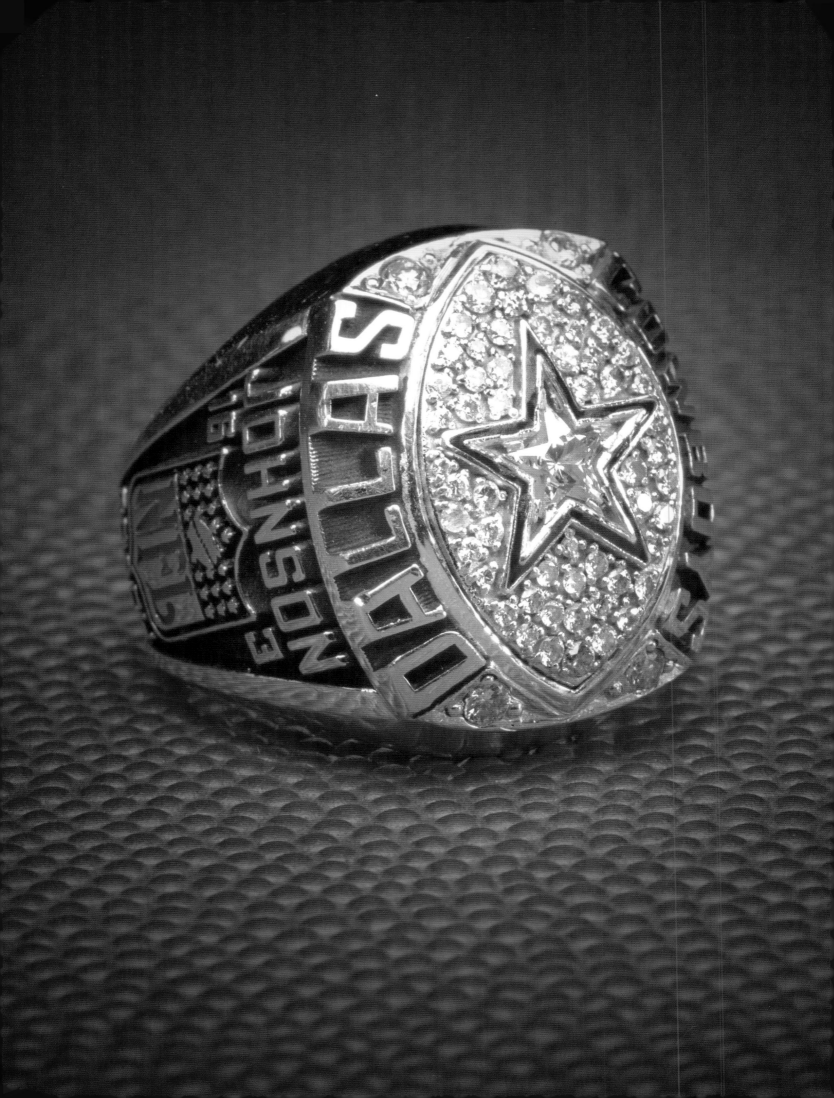

JOY RIDE

The jet helicopter lifted off the pad outside the Rose Bowl and began what would be a surreal journey through the night sky across Los Angeles. An unusual foursome sat cramped inside—Dallas owner Jerry Jones, his wife Gene, starting center Mark Stepnoski, and a radio sports talk show host who would anchor the live telecast of the Dallas Super Bowl victory party.

Earlier that day the largest crowd to ever see a Cowboys game (98,374) and the largest audience to ever watch a live event in TV history (133.4 million) had witnessed a destruction. Dallas had annihilated Buffalo, 52–17, in Super Bowl XXVII. After a drought of fifteen years, Dallas again ruled the NFL.

Only an hour and a half before, late in the fourth quarter, Jones had hurried along the sideline toward coach Jimmy Johnson repeating the same phrase: "Dallas Cowboys, World Champions."

In the euphoria of the post-game locker room Jones, getting ready for the trophy presentation, had pulled a comb from his pocket to straighten Johnson's never-before-seen-out-of-place hair that had been soaked by the traditional Gatorade shower and mussed gleefully by Emmitt Smith.

Then in the post-game celebration Jones's emotional dam began to break:

"When Commissioner (Paul) Tagliabue handed me that trophy, I got chills and a rush like none I'd had in a long time," Jones said. "None of them knows what it's like to be 1–15. That'll burn a hole in your brain and make you appreciate what it feels like to be standing here today."

As the copter floated along just above the ocean of light that is L.A. at night, Jones turned to Gene and said, "Here I am back where I started life. I was born right down there in (L.A. suburb) El Segundo."

One could only wonder the memories racing through the mind of a man who'd owned the Cowboys for 1,436 days, twenty-five short of four years.

Memories of:

★ The sharp-edged criticism he'd taken for the clumsy way he'd handled the purchase of the team.

★ Cars that still traveled Dallas streets with aging bumper stickers that read "You Can't Buy Class, Mr. Jones."

★ The 28–0 drilling New Orleans put on Dallas in the first game of his ownership and the post-game comments from Saints coach Jim Mora calling the Cowboys' game plan "simple and elementary."

★ Getting a 4:00 AM wake-up call on Christmas Eve that first season telling him all the pipes at Texas Stadium had frozen and there would be absolutely no restroom facilities for fans at that afternoon's Green Bay game. It would have to be considered oddly fortunate that only forty-one thousand tickets sold, leaving more than twenty-three thousand seats empty.

★ San Diego General Manager Bobby Beathard telling him at the midpoint of that '89 season that he'd never seen an NFL team with a lower talent level.

Through those early years, the failures, the setbacks, and all that personal criticism never seemed to bog Jones down. It never wiped that almost constant smile-grin off his face. None of the barbs appeared to even draw blood. But his wife Gene knew differently: "He's far more sensitive than he ever lets on. He has a way of taking those negatives and turning them into positives."

And during that flight Gene perceived a noticeable difference. "It was like a weight had been lifted off of him," she said. "After all the second guessing, he'd never altered course. Now, suddenly, we were living this fairy tale. I don't know if, other than our children being born, I'd ever seen him so happy."

As the roll call of suburbs slipped beneath the steady racket of the chopper blades, fragments of thoughts poured out of Jones. He'd start talking of one game memory, then switch to another, then another, on and on.

The victory had been much simpler than

expected. *Sports Illustrated* had predicted a Buffalo upset, reasoning the twice-beaten-in-the-Super-Bowl Bills were "due." And Buffalo did jump to an early 7–0 lead.

Then, the roof caved in on the Bills. In a span of precisely fifteen minutes—from 13:24 gone in the first quarter to that exact point of quarter number two—Buffalo's dreams imploded. Troy Aikman, the eventual Super Bowl Most Valuable Player, threw three touchdown passes. A Charles Haley sack forced a fumble by Bills quarterback Jim Kelly at the Bills' two-yard line. Defensive tackle Jimmie Jones picked up the ball and stepped into the end zone for another score. An injured Kelly would not return. Neither would the Bills, as far as that goes.

"As we flew, the scene out the window was very serene and beautiful," Stepnoski said. "You could see how happy Jerry was. People said he didn't know what he was doing. I'd come on the team only a couple months after Jerry bought it so I felt a tremendous sense of satisfaction both for myself and for him. We'd gone from the worst team to the best in so short a period."

It had been quite a week for Jones, one in which he and Gene had celebrated their thirtieth wedding anniversary, along with the fact he had become the first NFL owner to ever have his own microphone, placard, and designated interview area at Super Bowl media day. Waiting just ahead at the Santa Monica Civic Center were four planeloads

"We'd gone from the worst team to the best in so short a period."

Jimmy Johnson skipped jubilantly on to the Rose Bowl turf and thrust his fists in the air to celebrate. And that was at the end of the *first half*, with the Cowboys ahead 28–10.

By early in the fourth quarter, the Bills had crept back to within fourteen points. But that was as close as they would get. In a stretch of less than three minutes, Aikman threw for his fourth touchdown, Dallas intercepted a Frank Reich pass, Emmitt Smith sliced in from ten yards out, and linebacker Ken Norton Jr. scooped up a Reich fumble and returned it for a score. All that in *2:33!* For the game, Buffalo had sixteen possessions and turned it over *nine* times.

That helicopter flight, only the second of Stepnoski's life, still brings back vivid impressions for him. Stepnoski had been grabbed and put aboard at the last minute so that the party would immediately have a star player in attendance.

of friends he'd flown to LA during the week for what he believed would be a raucous post-victory party.

Jones recalls: "I remember walking out there on that parking lot with that copter sitting there. I can remember that better than what happened to me last week. . . . How could you write a better story than to have reached this point after first being perceived as having taken a team to the depths of degradation?"

Even with all the accomplishments still ahead, Jones always refers to this triumph, this ring, this improbable story line, as his sweetest triumph.

"When the helicopter took off, it was like our spirit being lifted to the heavens."

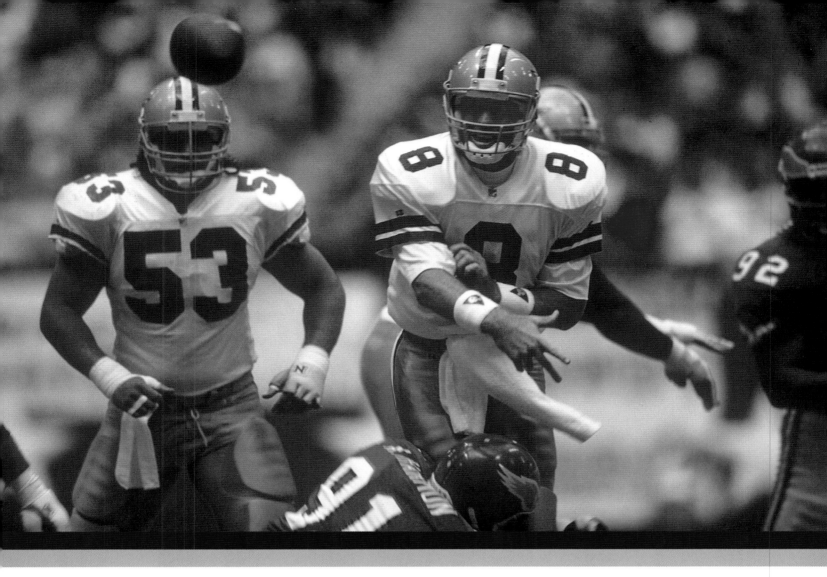

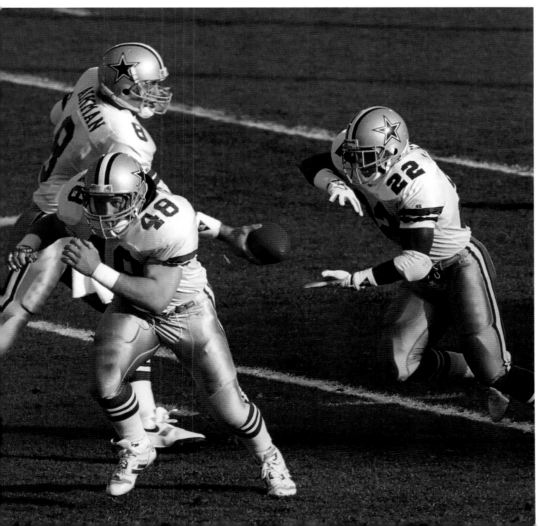

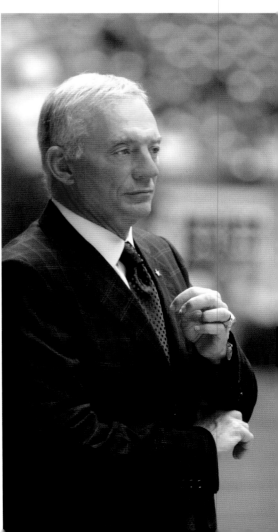

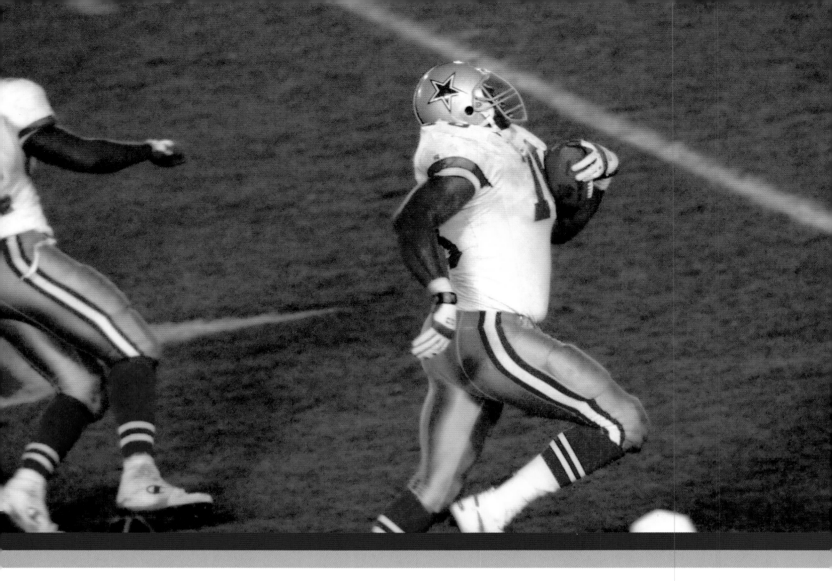
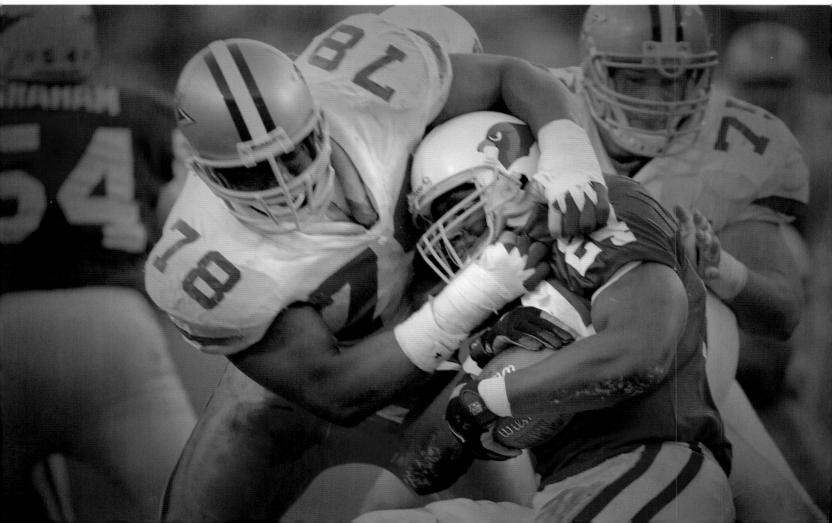

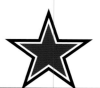

LETT IT BE

Six-foot-six, 300-plus-pound Cowboys defensive tackle Leon Lett, wearing only his thermal underwear, sat on the training room table sobbing.

His incredible blunder in the waning seconds of their Thanksgiving Day game against Miami had cost Dallas a victory they dearly needed. No amount of consolation from teammates could stem the flow of tears down the cheeks of the man they called "Big Cat." The entire nation watching on TV and 60,198 frozen-to-the-bone Texas Stadium fans had seen the Big Cat become the "Big Goat."

The game had begun with the temperature at the freezing point. Wind chill of nineteen. The worst weather conditions ever for a Cowboys home game. By the late fourth quarter, the artificial turf field had become pure white but not from snow. Worse than snow. Freezing rain, then sleet, then ice pellets. Thermometers descended to twenty degrees.

With fifteen seconds left in the game and Dallas ahead 14–13, Miami lined up for what amounted to a desperation 41-yard Pete Stoyanovich field-goal attempt. He'd tried a 44-yarder in the first quarter, only for the kicked ball to flutter just 25 yards before Dallas safety Thomas Everett caught it and ran it back to the 39.

This time holder Doug Pederson scraped away some ice to create a clean spot to place the ball. Greg Baty snapped it, Pederson got it down, and Stoyanovich skated forward. From the second his foot struck the ball, the kick had no chance. It was far too low to have a shot at clearing the crossbar. But the play was far from over.

Cowboys special teams coach Joe Avezzano had sent in a special-teams play called "block one." That put defensive tackle Jimmie Jones squarely over the nose of the deep snapper. The play call worked perfectly.

Jones: "I just did a quick swim move with him and was able to get penetration and get my hands up."

The kick ricocheted off Jones paw, landed a few yards beyond the line of scrimmage, and skittered down the right hash mark as the seconds ticked away. Safety Darren Woodson performed a brief victory dance and then sprinted toward the warmth of the locker room. Ecstatic, shivering Cowboys fans began streaming for the exits and on to their turkey day gatherings. The Cowboys had this game on ice. Literally! So many of them—players, coaches, fans—never actually saw Leon Lett turn himself into another kind of turkey.

As the ball skidded inside the 10-yard line, members of the Cowboys kick-block special team did something they had practiced countless times, yelling out the code word for such a situation—"Peter."

"Peter! Peter! Peter!" hollered Elvis Patterson, Darrin Smith, Thomas Everett, and others.

"That term 'Peter' originated years before," Avezzano said later, "because it means, uh, don't play with it."

Did Leon Lett hear the shouts of "Peter?" Or did he instead picture Everett catching that missed first quarter field goal and running with the ball? Did he know the rule simply states that, if the ball rolls to a stop, it belongs to the defense (Cowboys)? What was he thinking as he went slip-sliding toward a pigskin that the rest of his teammates hurried away from? Three Dolphin players encircled a ball still barely moving. One, maybe two more revolutions and it would wiggle to a "dead ball" stop. The videotape later would show a hesitant Lett slowing down and then going into the kind of slide quarterbacks use to avoid open field hits.

Lett's left foot nudged the ball toward the goal line. Miami lineman Jeff Dellenbach alertly flopped onto it and slid into the end zone. Suddenly, those celebrating Cowboys knew *something* had gone wrong; they just didn't know what. Neither did national TV viewers. NBC had cut away from the wobbling ball to a reaction shot of a joyful Jerry Jones.

"We didn't know what had actually happened," Avezzano remembers, "until they showed it on the big screen."

The officials huddled. The clock had stopped at :03. They ruled—Miami ball at the Dallas one-yard line with time for one final play. This time a Stoyanovich 19-yarder iced it.

"He thought I was going to cut him," Jimmy Johnson remembers. "He believed his career as a Cowboy had ended."

Dallas had lost for the second time in five days. At 7–4 they dropped behind the 8–3 Giants and into a messy wild-card race. Miami improved to 9–2, the best record in the NFL.

Inside the locker room Lett's friends tried to console him, teammates such as Tony Tolbert, Larry Brown, and at the time Lett's best friend on the team Charles Haley.

"We came to Leon's aid. We just wanted him to know everybody makes mistakes and that he'd get a second chance," said Haley.

But back in the locker room, not far from the entrance to the training room where Lett had gone for refuge, a helmet-sized hole in the wall next to the locker of defensive end Jim Jeffcoat spoke volumes of the team's level of frustration.

Outside, Avezzano was telling NBC, "There were eleven guys on the field, and ten of them knew what to do." That interview would eventually become far more prominent nationally than Lett's gaffe because the interviewer was none other than NBC analyst O. J. Simpson wearing a pair of Bruno Magli shoes. Pictures of that moment would later become evidence in Simpson's double murder mega-trial.

No amount of teammate reasoning could uplift the crestfallen Lett even though his botch job had simply been the last one in a game filled with Dallas errors.

★ Fourth-quarter drives reaching the Miami 34, 29, 44, and 14 yard lines produced no points.

★ Eddie Murray missed a 32-yard field goal.

★ Alvin Harper committed two offensive-interference penalties during one wasted third-quarter drive.

★ The defense had somehow allowed 255-pound Dolphin back Keith Byars to rumble 77 yards across the ice for a touchdown.

★ Aikman threw an interception at the Dolphin 32.

★ Two failed fourth-down attempts.

★ An outrageous 287 passing yards allowed (on a day like that?!).

Somehow fate chose the Cowboy least able to handle such a screwup. So large a man with so little certainty of who he was. This was Leon Lett, shy to the point of being introverted. So nervous on Super Bowl media day about the prospect of being interviewed that sweat poured out of him *before* the cream puff questions began. A man so tight that he suffered nose bleeds when distressed. A person so self-conscious that, at times, he had not gone to class at Emporia State simply out of embarrassment. A gentle giant who once had to be coaxed to leave his hotel room to attend the team's pre-game meal.

But the enormity of Lett's guilt didn't compare with the fear he felt closing in on him.

"He thought I was going to cut him," Jimmy Johnson remembers. "He believed his career as a Cowboy had ended."

Lett had some reason to think that. After all, earlier that year Johnson had cut linebacker John Roper for falling asleep in a meeting. And only ten months earlier an angry Johnson had released backup running back Curvin Richards because of two fourth quarter fumbles in a game Dallas *won* by two touchdowns.

The enraged coach Lett feared he would face and the one he actually encountered couldn't have been more different.

Johnson: "He was devastated. I had to be understanding with him . . . of what he was like. I didn't want to lose him mentally."

The gentle Johnson surprised those who'd grown accustomed to his outbursts.

Haley: "For the first time he didn't even go crazy . . . he was sympathetic to him."

Avezzano: "Jimmy was very soft, kind to Leon. He handled that in a way he thought best so as not to destroy a young man."

No one's ever truly determined why Lett did what he did. Several days later the club's PR department issued a simple statement on his behalf: "I'm deeply hurt for my teammates because of the judgment error I made at the end of last week's game. In my efforts to try to help my team win, I made a poor decision. Hopefully, my performance in the future will in some small way make up for my mistake."

Someone else had undoubtedly written those words, not that it mattered. Throughout the rest of the season, Lett came and went virtually ignored by a press corps that seemed to accept his fragility and need of privacy. As for Lett, he wasn't volunteering anything. Even two months later at the Super Bowl, he politely refused to answer any inquiries into what had happened during that incredulous play.

After that bizarre moment in time, however, yet one more twisted ending awaited both the Cowboys and the Dolphins.

Miami never won again in '93. Five consecutive defeats dropped them to 9–7. That giddy Dolphin team that left Dallas with the best record in the NFL did not even make the playoffs.

That depressed Dallas team would not lose again that season. Five straight regular season wins. Then three double-digit playoff triumphs on the road to repeating as Super Bowl champions.

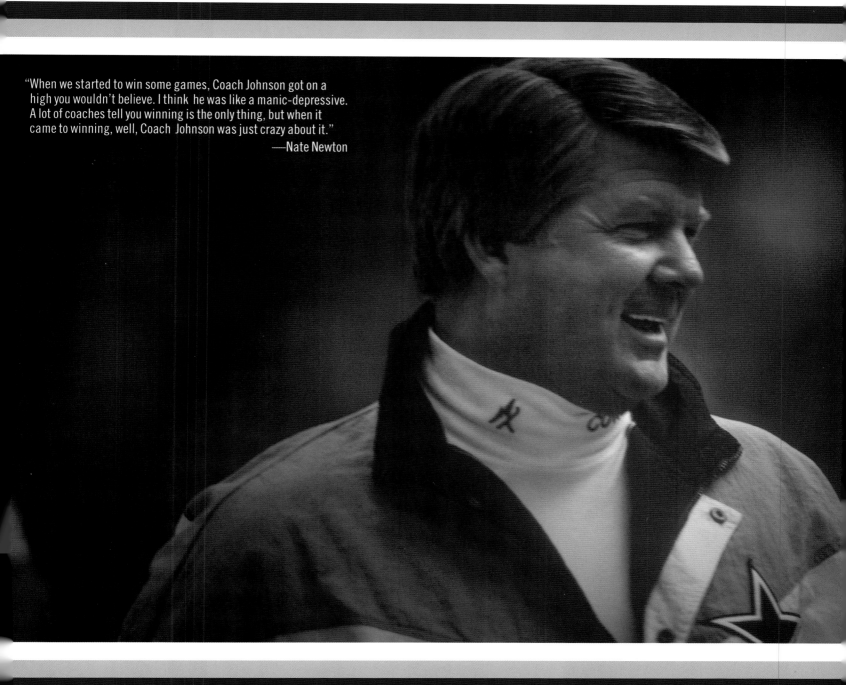

"When we started to win some games, Coach Johnson got on a high you wouldn't believe. I think he was like a manic-depressive. A lot of coaches tell you winning is the only thing, but when it came to winning, well, Coach Johnson was just crazy about it."
—Nate Newton

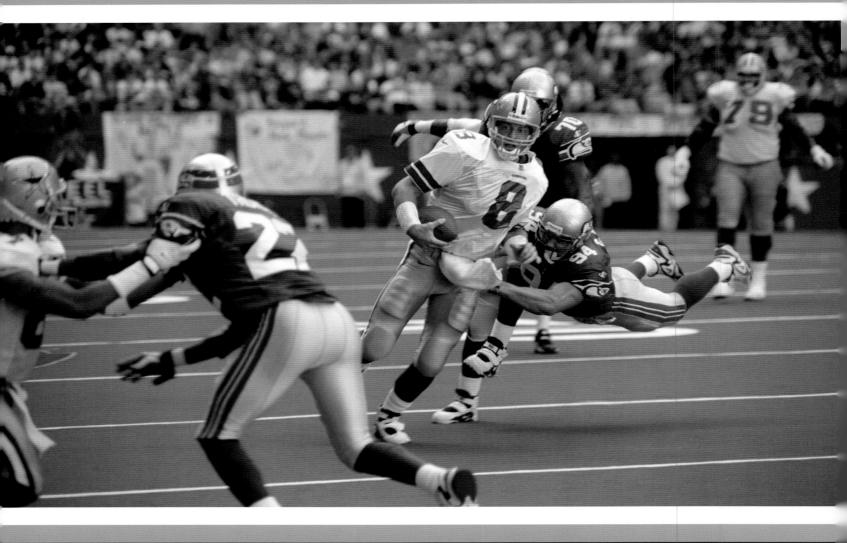
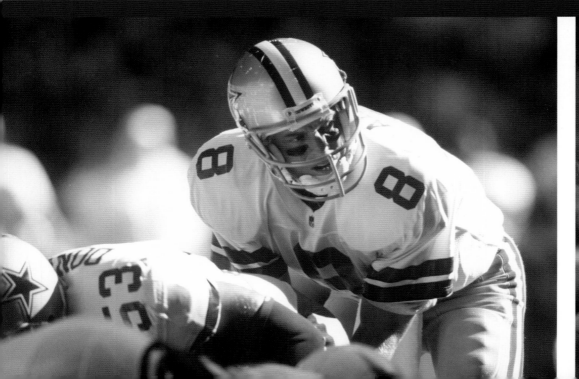
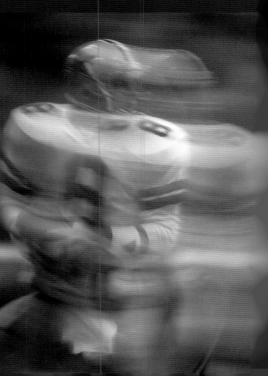

TROY AIKMAN

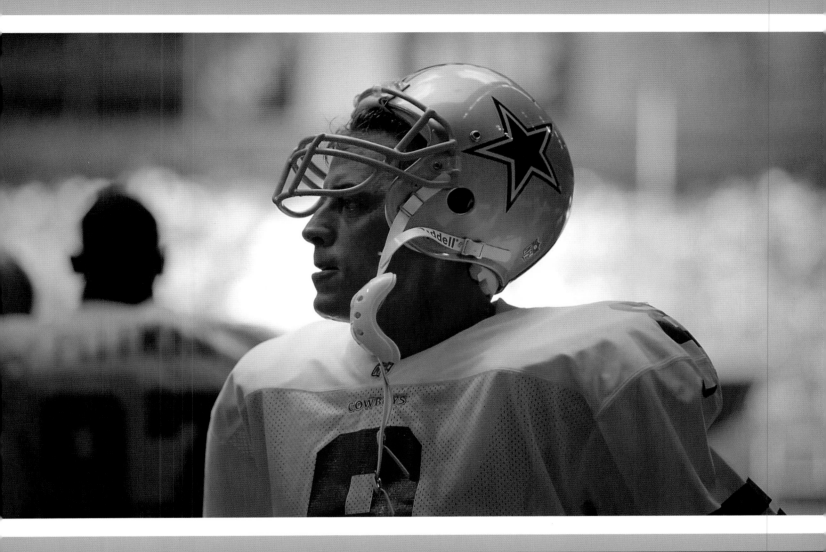

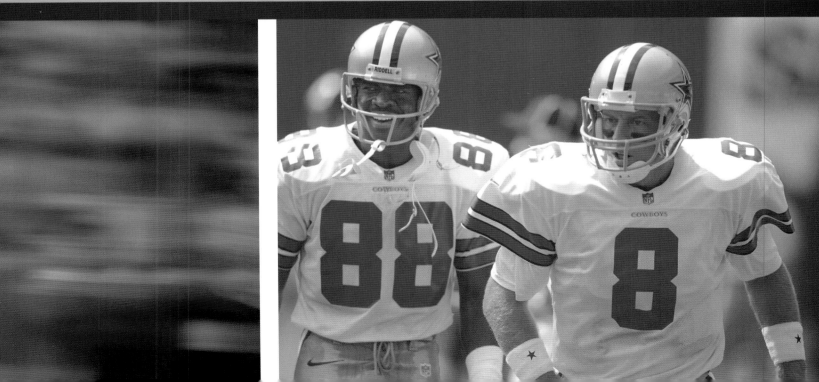

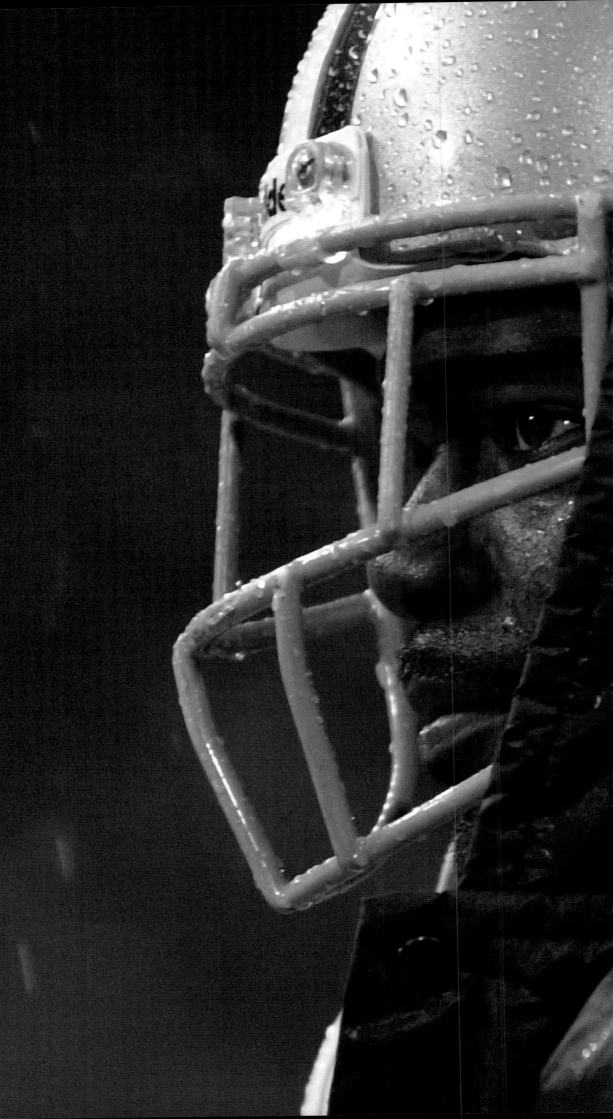

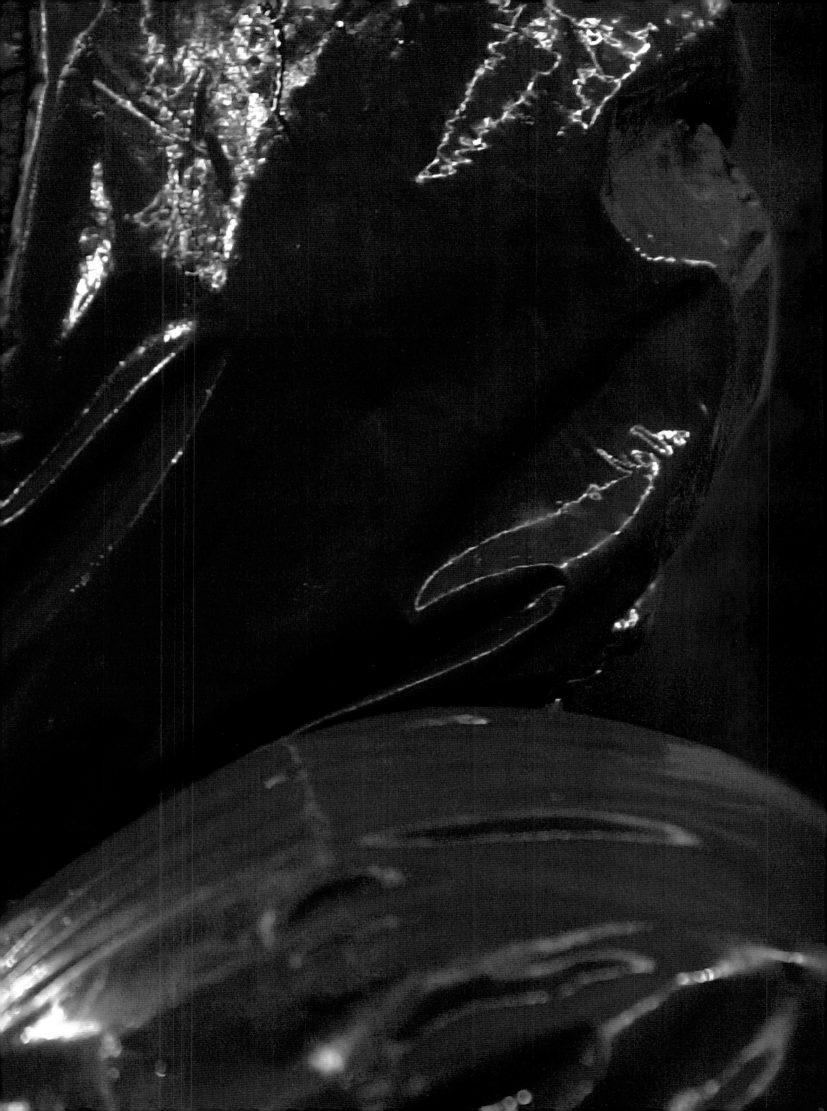

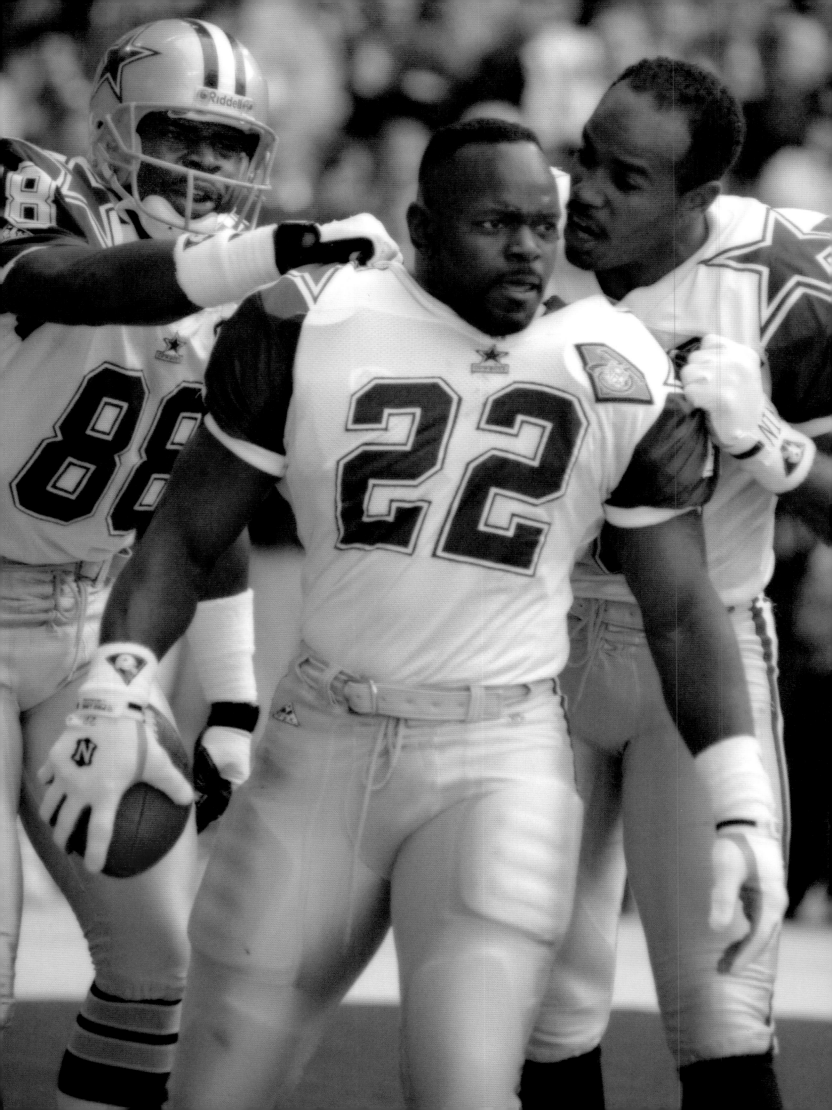

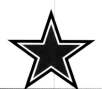
THE WARRIOR

Late in the second quarter, with the Cowboys at their own 18, running back Emmitt Smith burst through a gigantic hole off right tackle. It was one of those gaping openings runners almost never see. There were no defenders around. Lots of green artificial turf and white lines ahead. Forty-six yards downfield, New York Giants safety Greg Jackson collared Smith and the two, running at full tilt, tumbled forward. Smith landed on his right shoulder.

"Right away I knew my shoulder wasn't right. I didn't know if I could come back," Smith said. "All I knew is that my shoulder was jacked up."

Smith didn't want to go to the locker room. The Cowboys' medical staff left him no choice.

X-rays showed no break. The diagnosis? A sprain and severe separation. Trainers taped a knee pad over the shoulder and gave Smith Vicodin to mask the pain.

"I could barely move my arm," Smith recalled. "I had no range of motion."

Trainer Kevin O'Neill told him he'd feel some pain. Smith already knew that very well.

Were this Giants-Cowboys meeting just another regular season game, allowing Smith to return would have been absurd. But this wasn't just any other game. So much rode on its outcome.

The two teams, both 11-4, shared first place in the NFC East. The winner would get the division crown, a bye week to prepare for the post-season, and home-field advantage throughout the playoffs. The loser would have to suck it up and go head-banging again the next week as a playoff wild-card team.

"I wouldn't say this is a winner-take-all game," Jerry Jones said during the week. "I'd say this is a winner take a bunch. The loser still gets a scrap. It's a small crumb but it is a scrap."

The defending Super Bowl champion Cowboys had found themselves in this standings deadlock almost certainly because Smith had sat out the season's first two games while entangled in a salary dispute with Jones. Without their star runner, Dallas got drilled 35–16 by Washington and then upset 13–10 at home by Buffalo. Following the defeat to the Bills, volatile defensive end Charles Haley, with

Jones standing *very* nearby, signaled the depth of his and his teammates' frustration by slamming his helmet into a locker room wall, leaving a huge hole.

Jones got the point. The next week Smith got his money. Lots of it. Four years at $13.5 million per year.

With "Deuce Deuce" (No. 22) back in uniform, Dallas ripped off eleven victories in thirteen weeks, drawing even with the Giants and creating this Game 16 showdown.

New York had the league's stingiest defense. Only two of their fifteen opponents had managed to scratch out as many as twenty points against them this season. Dallas, however, had been one of those two higher-scoring opponents, drubbing New York 31–10 in early November.

As though the enormity of the Cowboys-Giants rematch wasn't enough, during the week of the game there was buzz around the league about Jimmy Johnson's being "intrigued" with the possibility of becoming the first coach and general manager of the expansion Jacksonville Jaguars. Just to ratchet things up one more notch, the Redskins made public their infatuation for Cowboys offensive coordinator Norv Turner, conceding that his was the lone name on their head coaching "wish list."

Never a dull moment in Dallas.

By halftime the Cowboys had carved out a 13–0 lead in what had amounted to brutal hand-to-hand combat. At the point the injured Smith left, the Pokes had run thirty-six plays. Smith runs or pass receptions accounted for twenty-five of them. Dallas had gained 228 yards—151 by Smith and 77 by everyone else.

Should Smith risk more serious injury by playing the second half? Would the pain and strapped-down shoulder even permit it?

"He said, 'Let me play until I can't play,'" Coach Johnson recalled.

The man who blocked for Smith preferred he not try it. Fullback Daryl "Moose" Johnston had memories of his own when it came to shoulder injuries.

"It's excruciating," Moose said. "You can't cough. You can't sneeze. You can't take a deep breath . . . One of the things that hurts more than anything is to raise

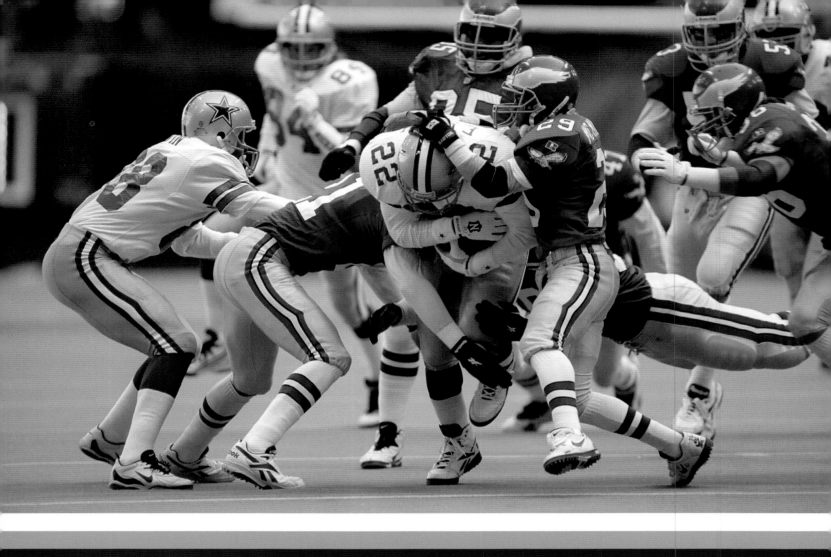

your hands above your head . . . to be out there running pass routes and put a hand up . . . you know you'll feel a shooting pain down the entire side of your body."

Johnston tried to reason with Emmitt: "What good is it going to do if we pull this game out and you can't play two weeks from now? So just let us handle this one. Go out. We can do this."

Smith would have none of it. He and Johnston addressed the question just that once. Smith told him: "I'm not going out. I'm not going out of the lineup."

All chance of further dialogue ended when Cowboys punt returner Kevin Williams fumbled two minutes into the second half. New York recovered and drove for a score, thus narrowing the Dallas advantage to 13–7.

Emmitt did have one request. So that the Giants might not know the severity of the injury, he asked his offensive linemen to help him up after plays.

Guard Nate Newton: "I was tired as hell after that game 'cause I'm like man, he's making all the money and I gotta run behind and pick him up. But damn, whatever it took to win. And man, he went to runnin' the rock. I felt like I was outside the box, watchin' the game. It was so sweet, man, so physical, so super."

The Giants rock-ribbed No. 1 defense, meanwhile, had shut Dallas down. The Phil Simms-led New York offense wedged

out enough yardage for a late third quarter David Treadwell field goal and another with ten seconds left in regulation to pull even at 13–13 and force overtime.

The pain in Smith's shoulder had worn him down. During one huddle, tears streamed down his face, "Michael (Irvin) was leaning over whispering in my ear 'Hang in there. Hang in there . . .' Troy asked me if I was alright. Nobody else said anything."

Dallas stopped New York's first OT possession with help from a 15-yard illegal block penalty against Giants center Brian Williams. Dallas got the ball at their 25. Same game plan.

★ Smith off right tackle for two yards.

★ Aikman to Smith for six more.

★ Aikman to Smith again for 11 and a first down.

★ Smith at left end for one.

★ A Giants' holding call gave Dallas another set of downs.

★ Lincoln Coleman replaced Smith and pounded for a yard. "Jimmy told me to go in but then Emmitt told me to get out," Coleman recalled.

★ Aikman to Smith for seven yards. "Every time he would get hit, he was sort of squinching his face a little bit," Giants' middle linebacker Michael Brooks would say during post-game interviews. "Squinching."

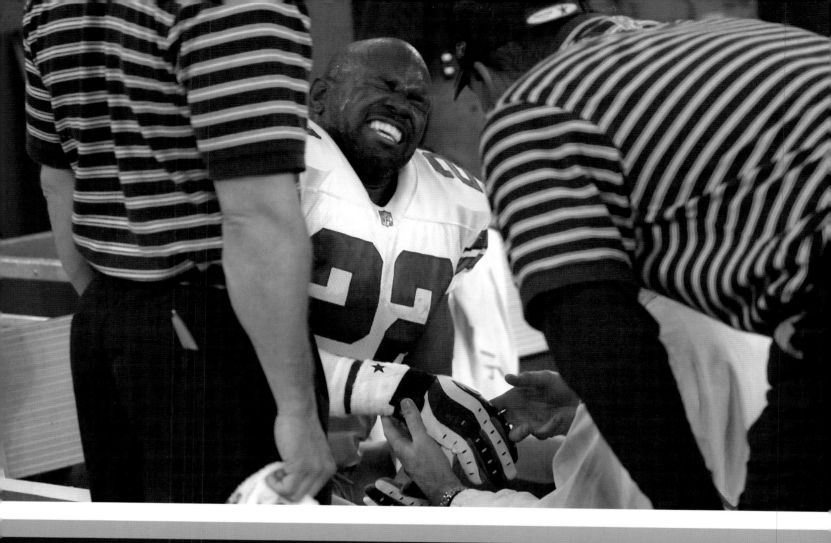

- ★ Smith off right tackle for three.

- ★ Smith up the middle for 10.

- ★ Smith over left tackle for one.

- ★ Hall of Fame linebacker Lawrence Taylor totaled eight tackles that day—seven brought Smith down.

- ★ Newton: "It got to a point, man, even a couple Giants said, 'You alright?' They were trying to punish him, but later in the game they was like, 'Emmitt, you alright?'"

- ★ Smith rammed the middle one more time.

But he had traded pain for admiration.

Johnston: "This was the first time we saw him hurt . . . the way he responded . . . the way he played through it. I think he gained everybody's respect including announcer John Madden, who, I hear, had never before walked into a locker room to congratulate a player on his performance."

Smith's 168 yards rushing pushed him past Jerome Bettis for his third consecutive rushing title—only Jim Brown, Earl Campbell, and Steve Van Buren had ever won three in a row before Emmitt.

"Let me play until I can't play."

In ten plays, nine of them featuring Smith, Dallas had driven close enough for Eddie "Money" Murray's 41-yard field goal, and the Cowboys won the war, 16–13. Smith, after what he called "the worst plane ride of my life," would spend the night in the Baylor Medical Center with an IV for the pain.

The Dallas offense gained 339 total yards—229 on Smith runs or catches.

In four-and-a-half quarters the Cowboys ran seventy total plays—42 of them were Smith rushes or receptions.

That last number—42—still remains the all-time Dallas single-game record.

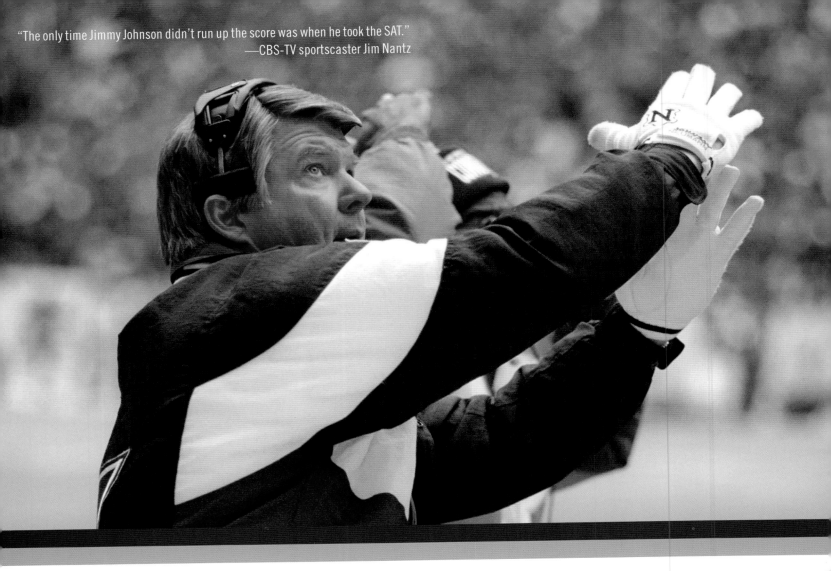

"The only time Jimmy Johnson didn't run up the score was when he took the SAT."
—CBS-TV sportscaster Jim Nantz

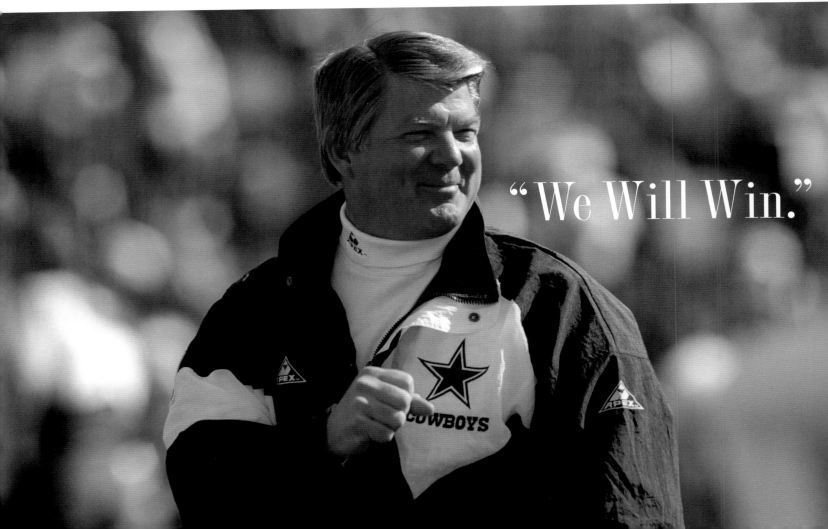

"We Will Win."

JIMMY'S BIG BRASSY BOAST

For popular *Fort Worth Star-Telegram* columnist and radio sports talk host Randy Galloway, the format for that evening's "Sports at Six" show was strictly a no-brainer. Talk Cowboys. Talk more Cowboys. Then, when you're done talking about that, talk some more Cowboys.

In three days, defending Super Bowl champion Dallas would tangle with the formidable Forty-niners, who the Cowboys had upset in the previous season's NFC title game. Galloway had just finished analyzing the contest with his guest, Denver Broncos coach and former Dallas player and assistant Dan Reeves, when the station's hotline rang! It was Jimmy Johnson calling, and not just to chat but to offer an eyebrow-raising prediction.

"We will win the ballgame," Jimmy promised, "and you can put it in three-inch headlines. We will win the ballgame. We're going to beat their rear ends, and then we're going to the Super Bowl."

Producer David Hatchett had been the one to answer the blinking hotline for Jimmy's call. "I was stunned," Hatchett said. "Shocked. The guy's preparing for one of the biggest games of his life and he's calling a talk show."

Why'd Jimmy's fingers start dialing?

"My girlfriend Rhonda and I were headed to Campisi's restaurant and I heard Randy and Dan debating who would win the game," Johnson remembered. "I was *so* cocky back then. I thought, *I'll solve this debate!*"

So, what did Troy Aikman think when he heard Jimmy?

"I thought he may have had a few too many Heinekens."

So had he?

"No, I might have had one . . . or maybe two . . . then a few more after," Johnson admitted.

Within minutes Hatchett had called the Associated Press. Everyone wanted to hear the tape—ESPN, CNN, you name it. Galloway made it home by about a half an hour after the show. "I bet I had twenty calls from all over the country, from everybody."

Sure enough, by the next morning Johnson had gotten precisely what he'd asked for—"WE WILL WIN" in exactly three-inch-high newspaper headlines. And everyone could read them, including Cowboys players. None of them disagreed.

"It's true. He took the words right out of my mouth."—linebacker Ken Norton, Jr.

"Jimmy has always told us don't play with scared money. Our butt's in the frying pan. Now bring on some heat."—guard Nate Newton.

"The man is just speaking the gospel."—safety James Washington.

Emmitt Smith even managed to mix in a reference to a high-profile pop star with his reaction. "There are no guarantees, except you stay the same color, you pay taxes, and you die. Michael Jackson just got lost somewhere along the way there."

But perhaps Johnson's comments were meant more for Cowboys ticketholders than Dallas players. In the midst of his five minutes with Galloway, Johnson also offered this: "I believe our (fans) are going to come out there and give us the homefield advantage that I want."

It's important to remember Johnson's widespread reputation, the one about his never shooting off his mouth without knowing exactly where he's aiming his bullet-like words.

That following morning a San Francisco radio station played the tape of Johnson' opinions during a live interview with Forty-niners Coach George Seifert. His take? "Well, the man's got balls, I'll say that. I don't know if they're brass or papier-mâché. We'll find out here pretty soon."

And find out we did. On Sunday, in front of an out-of-their minds, standing-room-only crowd of bonkers Cowboys fans, Dallas immediately leaped to a 7–0 advantage, led by twenty-one at the half and never looked back on the way to a seventeen-point blowout (38–21).

Even now, years and years after that "Are you kidding me?" phone call, Johnson's reminded of the moment every time he walks into the office of his Florida Keys home. A gift from a friend sits on his bookshelf. It's a cedar box with the top propped open and inside are two actual large brass balls. The bottom of the box bears this inscription: "It takes a pair of these to be a winner."

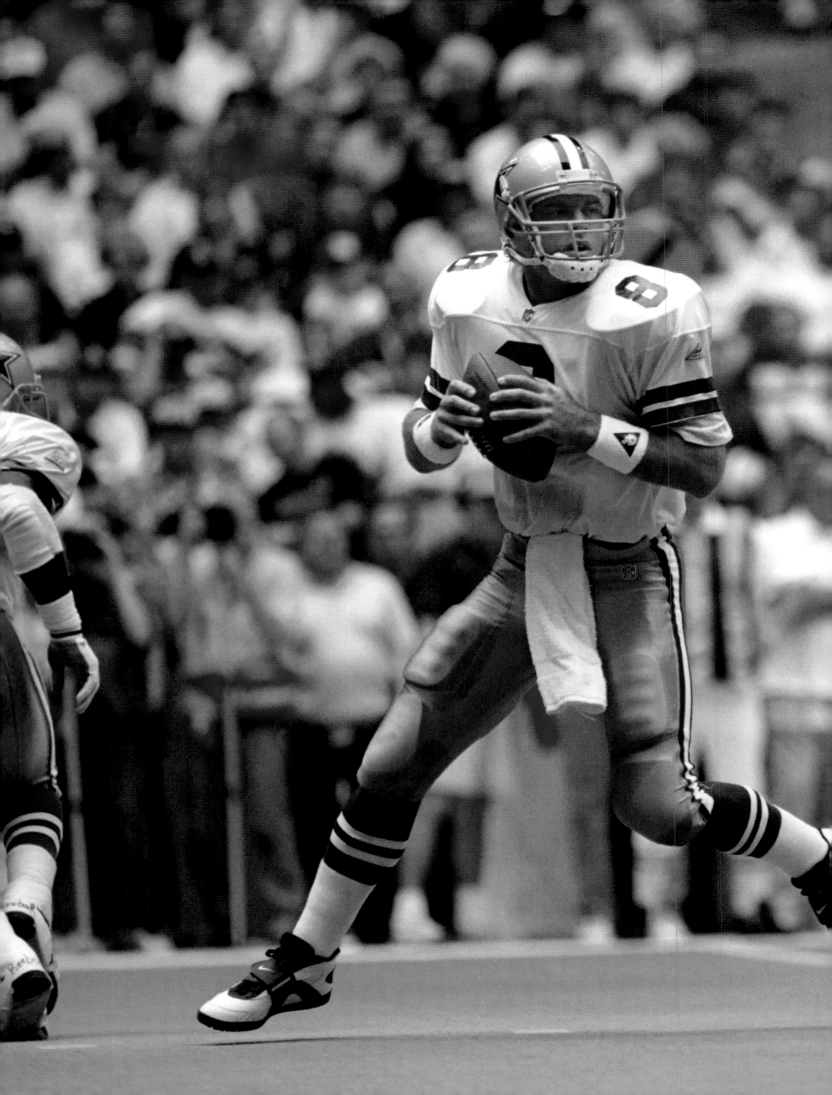

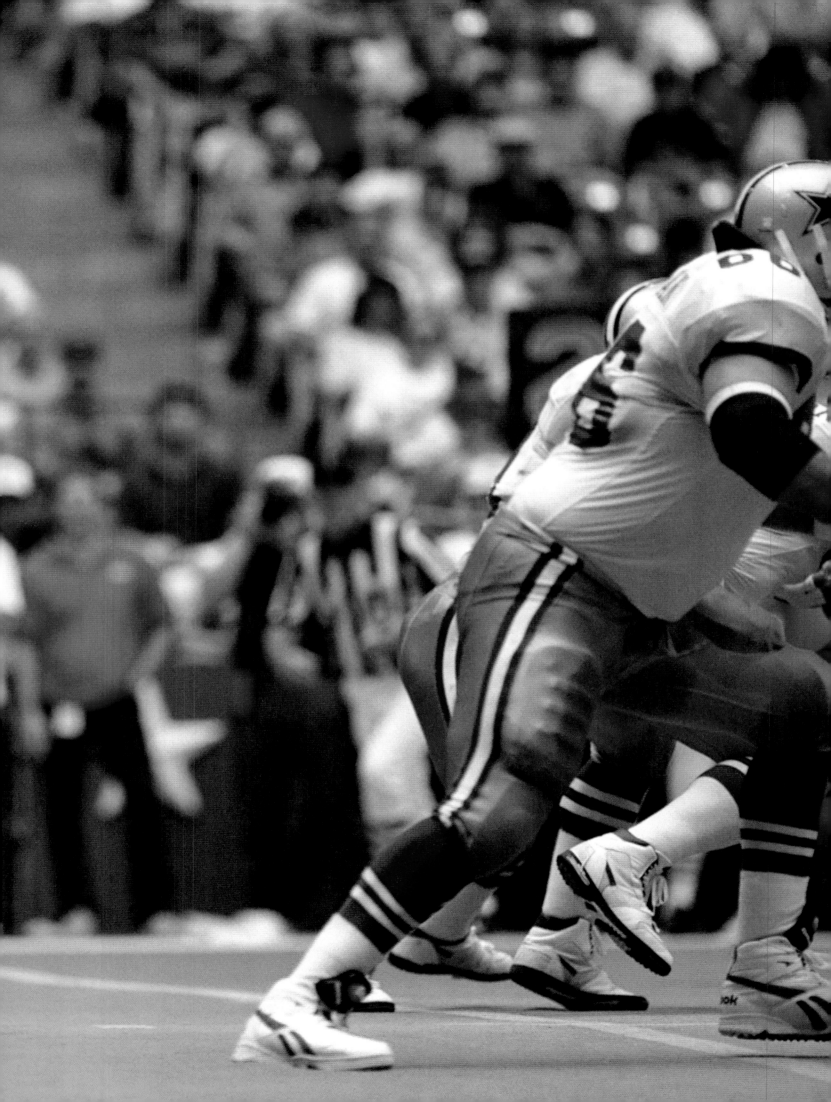

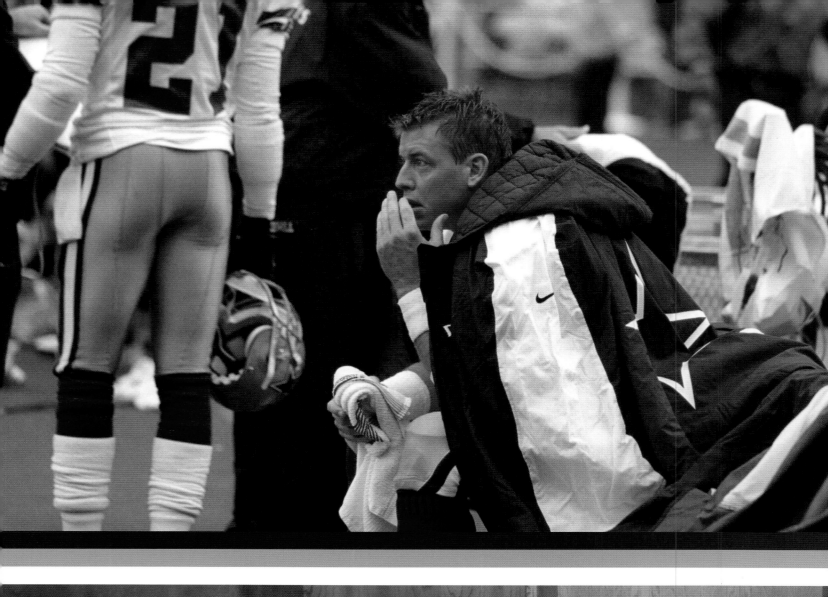
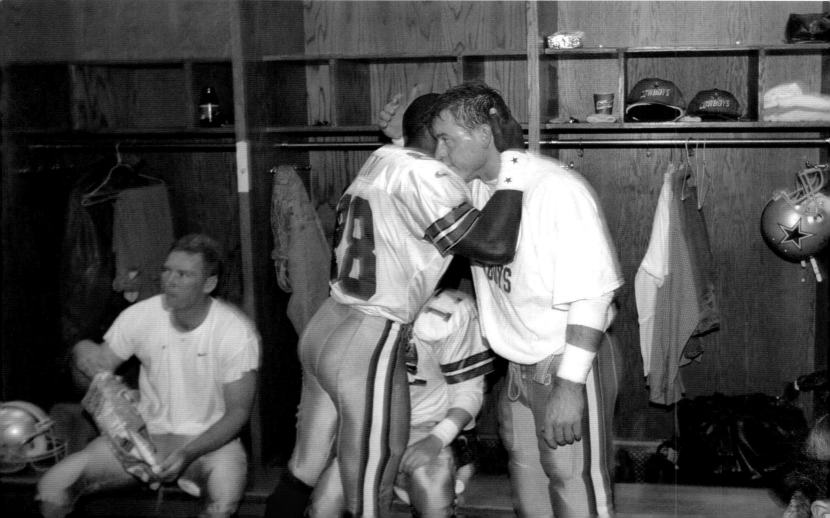

A VICTORY WORTH REMEMBERING

Two minutes into the third quarter, the outcome of the NFC Championship game had pretty much been decided. Dallas had quickly put the Forty-niners in their rearview mirror and led, 28–7.

The *star* of the game? No doubt—Troy Aikman. The *stars* of the game? They were all inside Aikman's head. He couldn't remember anything that had happened. More than a decade later, that afternoon remains a blank sheet of paper.

"Nothing. I don't remember anything," Aikman said. "I shouldn't say that; the only thing I do remember is a scuffle in pre-game warm-ups right around the goal posts, but that's it."

Too bad. Aikman missed a heckuva Cowboys victory.

Driven into a frenzy by Jimmy Johnson's impromptu prediction of a Cowboys win on a Thursday radio sports talk show, perhaps the most raucous crowd in Dallas history greeted the 49ers. The eclectic foursome of ultra-liberal Texas governor Ann Richards, actor Mickey Rooney, eccentric Texas billionaire investor T. Boone Pickens, and right-wing talk host Rush Limbaugh were among the many high profile guests of Jerry Jones at the game.

The normally well-behaved but now obviously ticked-off Niners had turned surly. (Another effect of that Johnson prediction?) When cornerback Kevin Smith approached the usually gentlemanly superstar receiver Jerry Rice for a pre-game "good luck" handshake, Rice flipped him the bird. That started the scuffle—the lone shred of memory Aikman retains of the contest.

At the coin toss, the San Francisco captains shook hands with honorary Dallas captain Roger Staubach but refused sharing any such niceties with any Cowboys players. On San Francisco's third offensive play, Rice took a swing at Smith, drawing a fifteen-yard personal-foul penalty.

"How can you be a team that wants to fight when you ain't never fought nobody," safety James Washington wondered. "All the renegades are on *this* team. I don't know what they were thinking. All that did was piss us off."

Trying to use tailback and NFL MVP Emmitt Smith sparingly because of the lingering effects of the shoulder injury he'd suffered three weeks earlier against the Giants, the Pokes' offense relied on Aikman's ultra-accurate arm.

Dallas drove 75 yards on its first possession for a score. They traveled 80 more for another touchdown on their third possession. Following a Thomas Everett interception of a Steve Young pass, the Cowboys tacked on seven more. The Dallas "D" forced a punt, and 72 yards later the offense again found the Niners' end zone.

Four drives . . . four touchdowns . . . 251 yards . . . 34 plays without a sack, fumble, interception, or penalty. Ten plays of 10 yards or more. Fourteen first downs. During those marches Dallas used three different ball carriers and five different pass receivers. Aikman's stat line: 16 attempts—13 completions—166 yards—2 touchdowns.

He remembers none of it.

On the Cowboys' second snap of that third quarter, Aikman dropped back to pass. His pocket of protection collapsed, and 292-pound Niners defensive end Dennis Brown sacked him and inadvertently kneed him in the head. Aikman's lights went out.

Somehow, functioning on a kind of human cruise control, he stayed in to call and execute one more play.

"At that time there were no headset communications with the sidelines," he said. "Not only did I call the play but I actually got the play from the sidelines via signals. I don't know what the play was. I don't know how it happened."

A groggy Aikman wandered back to the bench and spotted center Mark Stepnoski, who'd blown out a knee six weeks earlier, standing on the sidelines on crutches dressed in street clothes. Stepnoski, sensing something amiss, tried to find out how badly Aikman's bell had been rung.

"So I just went over to say, 'How ya doing'"Stepnoski said. "He goes, 'I'm alright. I'm fine. What happened to you?'"

At that point Stepnoski realized his quarterback had left for la-la-land.

"I didn't want to say anything to alarm him, because when you have a concussion you're already a little disoriented. Things have a surreal quality to them and you don't want to throw any more elements into that bizarre dream," Stepnoski said.

Next on Aikman's list of bench visits? Fullback Daryl Johnston.

Said Johnston, "He walked up with an ammonia cap in his hand, waving it in front of his face, and he said, 'I'm doing good . . . I got a question though.' And I said, 'What's that?' and he looks at the scoreboard and he goes, 'It's 28–7. How'd we get up on them so

he stopped me and would say, 'Just read the legal pad. Just read the legal pad.'"

Over the next few hours Aikman would have two telephone conversations with his mother Charlene. He saw a message pad with a phone number on it. At 12:30 AM he dialed the number, whosoever it was. But Nancy, the wife of offensive coordinator Norv Turner, said Norv was sound asleep. Somewhere in the middle of the night he wanted to put his clothes on and leave only to be stopped by Steinberg. Still, Aikman, who by then had suffered several concussions in his career, recalls none of it.

"How'd we get up on them so far?"

far?' I immediately waved my hand for the trainer and said, 'You gotta come over here. He's not with us right now.'"

Dr. J. R. Zambrano and trainer Kevin O'Neill tried to determine just how mentally far away Aikman might have traveled.

Question: "Where is next week's Super Bowl being played?"

Aikman (guessing): "Henryetta?"

No. The correct answer was Atlanta. Henryetta's the tiny town in Oklahoma Aikman grew up in.

Question: "Who won last year's Super Bowl?"

Aikman: "Uhhh . . . " That would be Dallas.

Question: "Who was last year's Super Bowl MVP?"

Aikman: Blank look. The MVP of Super Bowl XXVII had been—Troy Aikman!

The medical staff escorted Aikman to the locker room and then to Baylor Medical Center. He doesn't remember either trip. Some gaps have been filled in by those around him. His agent, Leigh Steinberg, spent the night at the hospital with him.

Said Aikman, "I kept asking him (Steinberg) over and over and over again, 'Did we win?' 'Yes.' By how much (38–21)? Did I play well? What did I do?' About five minutes would go by and I'd ask again. He finally wrote down all the answers on a legal pad and every time I'd start asking,

The amnesia brought on by such head trauma can be a frightening experience. For weeks after his concussion, Steelers linebacker Merrill Hoge had to carry around in his wallet a slip of paper with his phone number on it. He simply couldn't remember it. Atlanta QB Chris Miller appeared to be recovering well when, one afternoon, he called his own home and asked for directions on how to get there. He simply couldn't remember.

During the Super Bowl prep week that followed Aikman's concussion, he sat down and watched Dallas' dismantling of the Forty-niners.

"I thought maybe I'd get some of it back, but I couldn't," he said. "It was a very strange experience watching a game and watching myself perform but yet not remembering having done any of it."

Aikman played pretty well in that next Sunday's 30–13 Super Bowl triumph over Atlanta—a contest in which the Cowboys offense relied more on their running game with the now-healthier-than-Aikman— Emmitt Smith. The now Hall-of-Fame quarterback admits he's still a bit foggy about the events of that week and game also.

"I was absolutely amazed to learn I played well," Aikman said, "and that we were going to the Super Bowl, and that the Super Bowl wasn't in Henryetta."

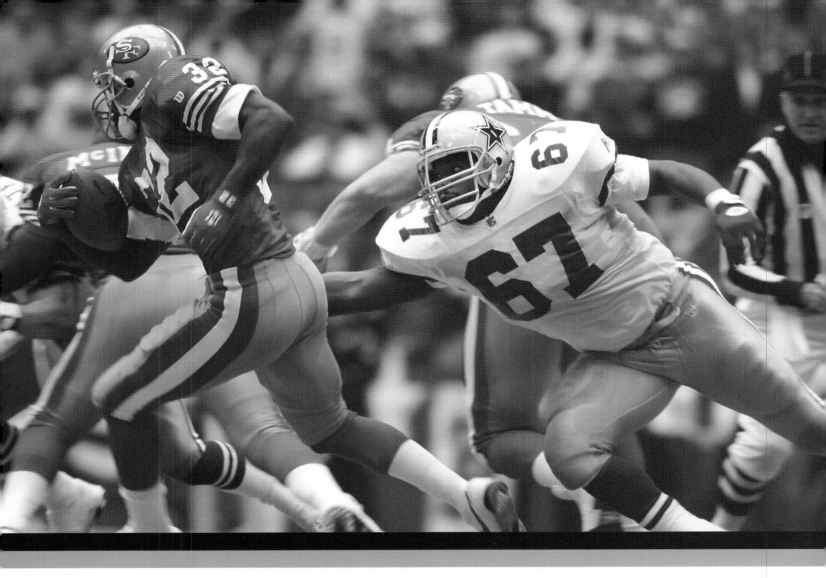
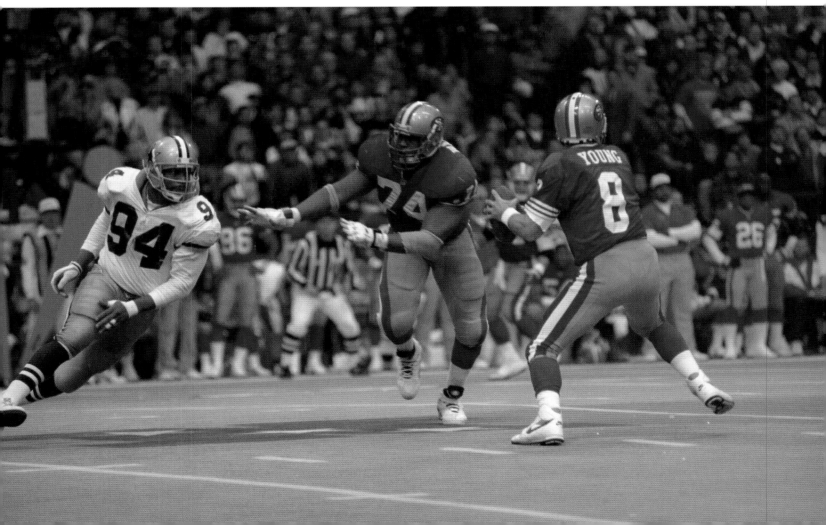

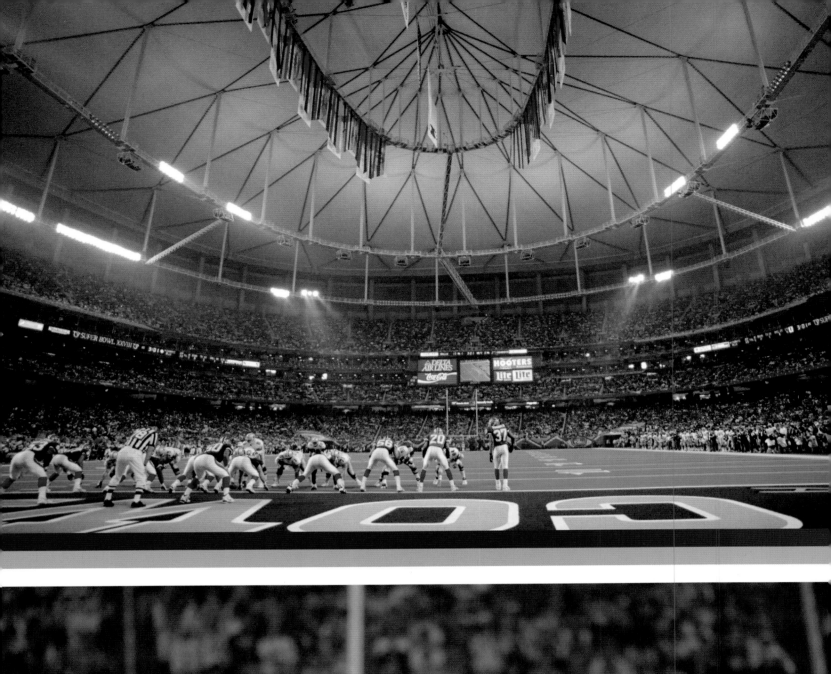
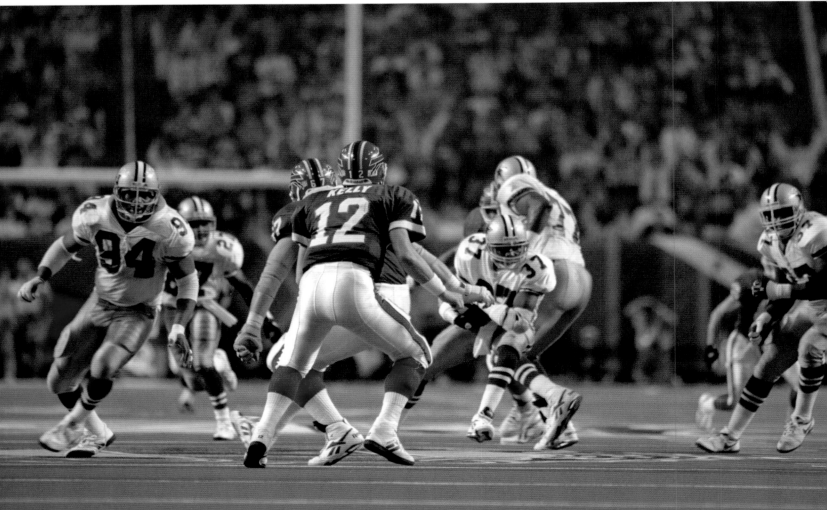

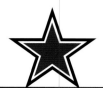

I KNOW IT'S TRUE 'CAUSE I SAW IT ON TV

Thirty minutes.

That's all that separated the Buffalo Bills from ending their frustrating three-year Super Bowl losing streak. They'd outplayed Dallas for a half and would get the kickoff to open the third quarter of Super Bowl XXVIII.

Disaster, however, would strike on the third play of the second half.

Bills quarterback Jim Kelly, with star halfback Thurman Thomas lined up on his left, set up about six yards behind center in a formation Buffalo called their K-Gun (instead of shotgun). At the snap, though, Thomas darted in front of his quarterback, grabbed the ball and sped right, hoping that a surprised Dallas defense would be confused just long enough for him to swing outside and down the right sideline for a sizable gain.

That's how the Bills playbook diagrammed the play. But that's not how it turned out. Not-fooled-for-a-second Cowboys defensive tackle Leon Lett burst through the hole left by the pulling guard and smashed Thomas. The ball squirted free. Safety James Washington, hurrying forward to help on the tackle, saw the loose ball bounce perfectly into his hands. Washington bobbed, weaved, juked, got a critical block from Lett, and sprinted 46 yards for the tying score.

Buffalo's gadget play had exploded in their face. It's almost like Lett *knew* what play the Bills called.

He did!

On the Saturday before the title game, Dallas had completed all its preparations. All that remained was killing time until kickoff. Defensive coordinator Butch Davis and several others perched in front of a hotel TV. ESPN cut to a live interview with Bills Coach Marv Levy. The Dallas group noticed, in the background behind Levy, a few Buffalo players walking through a play obviously ironing out some last details.

"Thomas would line up predominantly on Kelly's right in the shotgun, maybe 75 to 80 percent of the time," Davis recalled. "Well, ironically, as we're watching, he's lined up on his left and they ran a direct snap to him.

"We'd never seen them do that . . . *ever* . . . and here they are practicing the play *live on television*. So, we actually met with the defense and said 'Be alert' if Thomas is misplaced."

On that early third-quarter play that changed the momentum of Super Bowl XXVIII so dramatically, Lett recognized the odd formation. So did the Dallas linebackers who screamed warnings. The play never had a chance, all because Dallas happened to be watching TV as Buffalo happened to be polishing up its trick play.

James Washington's starring role had a lot to do with self-motivation. In the season-opening loss to the Redskins, Washington had performed so poorly that the defensive coaches decided to give his starting spot to second-year safety Darren Woodson. Washington still saw plenty of action in nickel and dime defenses and on special teams, but the lost starting job still irked him. He saw this game as a shot at redemption. A big performance might convince some other NFL team to trade for him and make him a starter again. That would also mean bigger paychecks.

Washington: "I was talking to Michael Irvin and Ken Norton in the training room . . . I told them, 'You know, this is *my* game, *my* opportunity. I was definitely walking around with attitude."

That Washington had the possibility of starring on this huge national stage resulted only from a decision made by the very people who'd demoted him in the first place.

Dallas—the defending NFL champions, winners of thirty-six of their last forty-four games and clear favorites in this Super Bowl—opted to shuffle its defensive lineup. Top dogs simply don't do things like that.

By now these opponents had become pretty familiar with each other. Dallas had plastered Buffalo in the previous Super Bowl. The Bills had upset the Cowboys early in this regular season using a punishing, two-back running attack instead of their usual three-receiver, hurry-up offense. The Dallas defensive coaches believed, however, Buffalo would have their K-Gun cranked up again this time.

Davis: "We felt they would try to go up-tempo and spread us out, like a fastbreak in basketball. You don't huddle. You call everything at the line of scrimmage. We felt like the 4–2–5 scheme gave us the best opportunity to execute our defensive game plan, whether it be blitzes, different kinds of zones, disguising coverages or coming after them with pressure."

Dallas normally ran a 4–3–4; that is, four defensive linemen, three linebackers, and four defensive backs. The 4–2–5 necessitated removing a linebacker (Dixon Edwards) and inserting another defensive back (Washington).

The new alignment and that fortuitous TV-watching party simply added two more unusual elements to what had been a bizarre and tumultuous Super Bowl week.

★ Michael Irvin demanded a contract renegotiation or he'd sit out the start of the next season.

★ The NFL fined star tackle Eric Williams for skipping media day and then docked five more Dallas players for failure to attend the next day's mandatory press conference.

★ Leon Lett, still embarrassed by his last-minute Thanksgiving Day gaffe that cost the Cowboys a victory over Miami, remained mum as he had for nine weeks.

★ Rumors of Jimmy Johnson's interest in the Coach/GM job of the expansion Jacksonville franchise echoed through Atlanta.

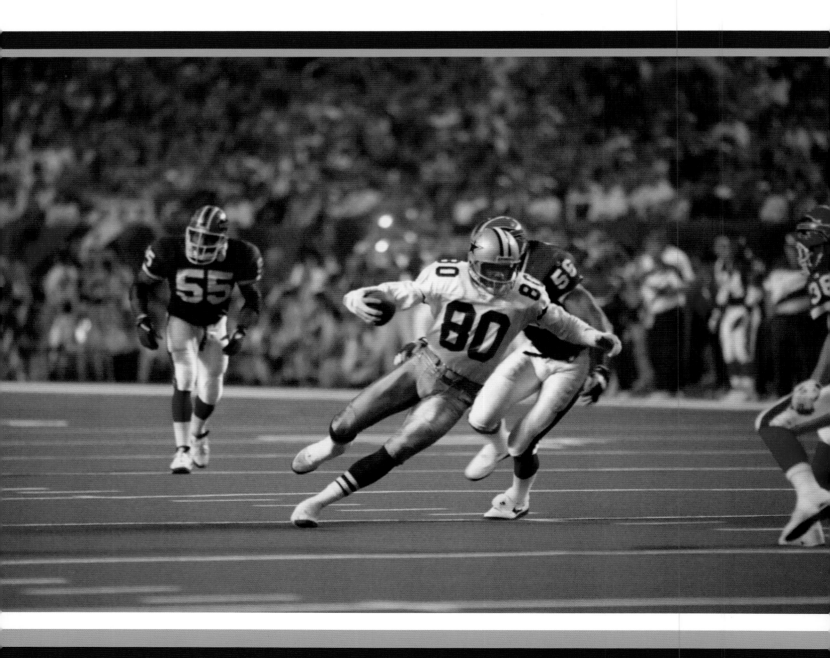

★ Aikman's brain still seemed a tad foggy at times from the effects of the concussion and slight amnesia suffered the week before against San Francisco. When asked what memory he had of that San Francisco game, Aikman said: "I remember driving to the stadium (pause) . . . What did you say?"

★ A guy stood outside the Georgia Dome on game day holding a sign that read "Six months to live. Need two tickets. Last wish."

★ And, speaking of tickets. On Monday, Dallas passed out the league-allotted thirteen per player at their training facility before departing for Atlanta. Defensive tackle Chad Hennings put his down, turned away for a few moments, turned back and they were gone. Coach Johnson found out about the ticket snatching on the plane ride. Upon arrival he called a meeting at the hotel.

On the Bills second possession "J Dub," as teammates called him, forced a Thomas fumble that Woodson recovered leading to a Cowboys field goal. By halftime he'd racked up four other tackles and deflected a pass. He made the first tackle of the second half. And the next one also. Then came Lett's wipeout of Thomas and the fumble Washington "took to the house" to tie the Super Bowl at 13-13. The air went out of Buffalo's balloon.

On the Pokes' next possession, an Aikman pass and seven Emmitt Smith runs covered 64 yards. Dallas seized a lead they would never relinquish.

The fourth quarter began with a Washington interception of a Kelly pass intended for Don Beebe on a crossing route. Beebe had replaced star Bills receiver Andre Reed, who'd been knocked out of the game on a big hit by who else but James Washington. Nine plays later, seven of them runs or catches by Smith, the Cowboys scored the title-clinching touchdown in an eventual 30–13 triumph.

"Dad, why weren't you the MVP?"

With NFL security chief Ben Nix at his side, Johnson unveiled his method of dealing with the crime and the criminal. "We've got a little bit of a problem. Evidently, someone *accidentally* picked up Chad Henning's tickets. Let me just say this: If those tickets end up back in Chad's hands in the next twelve hours, it will be a dead issue. I don't want to know who *accidentally* took them and there will be no repercussions—as long as he gets the tickets back. But if Chad doesn't get those tickets back, Ben Nix, our league security officer will take over . . . And let me say to the individual responsible right here and now: When I find out I will fine you to the maximum. In all probability I will cut you from the team. On top of that I will make sure the word gets around and you will never play in this league again . . . if he doesn't get those tickets back, come hell or high water, believe me, we'll find out who took them. And I don't think you're going to like what I'll do."

At breakfast the next morning Nix handed Hennings' tickets to Johnson. They'd been left with the bellman along with instructions that they be delivered to Nix.

At last, the actual game arrived. And Washington, the annoyed, psyched-up, and reinstated starter, played the hero's role from virtually the opening kickoff.

The Super Bowl numbers for Washington, who started only because Dallas had the nerve to switch defenses, leaped off the stat sheet. A game-high eleven tackles. One interception. One pass broken up. One forced fumble. One fumble recovery. One touchdown. One helluva performance.

"Michael Irvin came up to me near the end of the game and said, 'J Dub, congratulations on the MVP,'" Washington said. "I said, 'Man, you know they're not gonna give it to me no matter what I did today, because the politically best thing to do is to give it to Emmitt.'"

Washington, as he'd been all day, was right on. Smith, who'd rushed for 132 yards and two scores, won the MVP vote, 7½-5½.

Added Washington, "I was kinda sad. I was kinda hopin' they might split it. But they were voting with their heart, knowing the kindness of Emmitt and what he brought to the Cowboys. But I had such a good game, some big hits that changed the tempo early, and I wasn't even a guy that started."

Ten years passed. During that period, Washington, who grew up on the nasty streets of south central LA, never knew his father and was given to his grandparents to be raised when he was four, had never watched the replay of that Super Bowl. When he finally did sit down in front of the TV, he did so with his seven-year-old son at his side. "And he asked me, 'Dad, why weren't you the MVP?'"

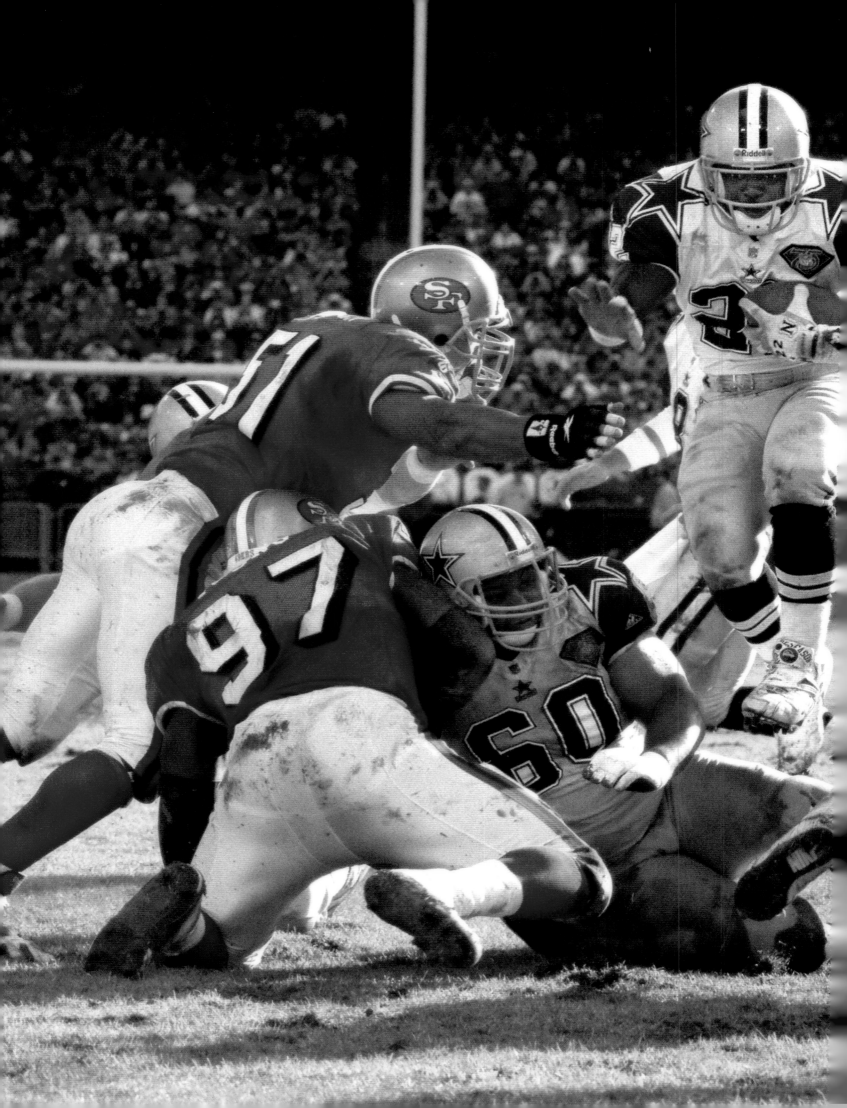

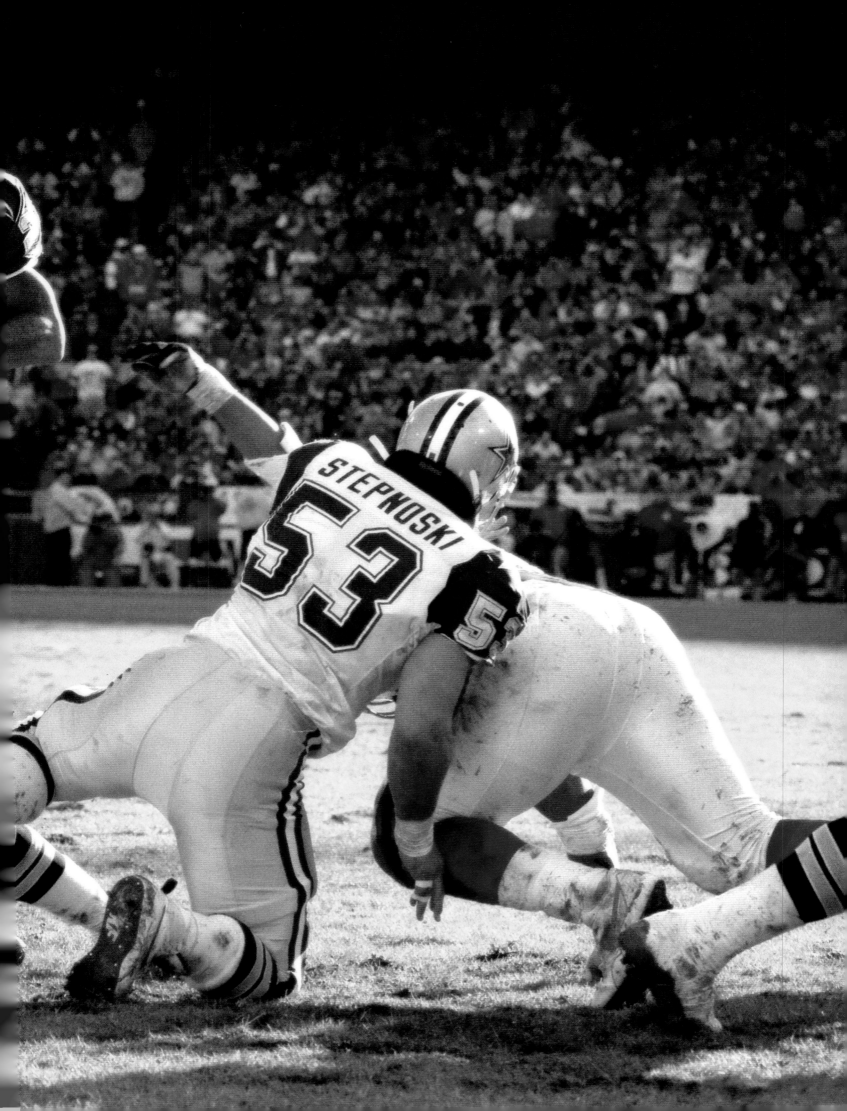

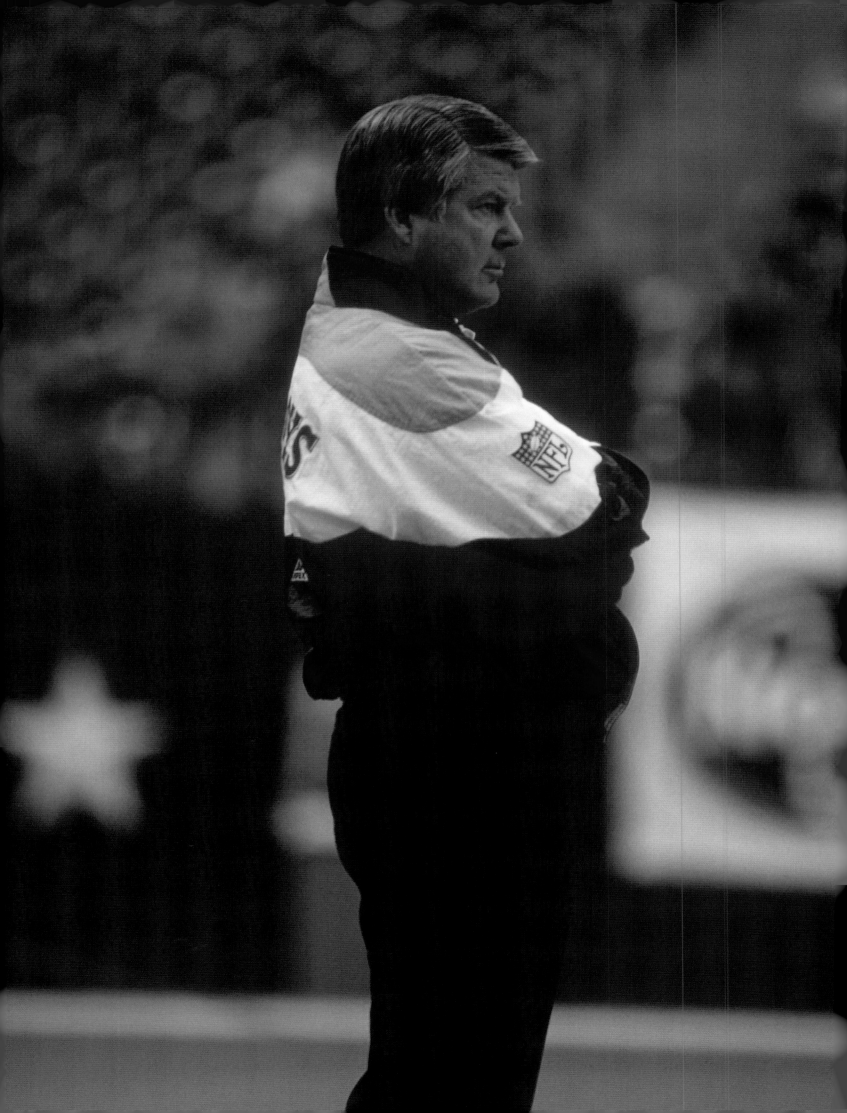

A MESSY DIVORCE

The announcement both stunned and puzzled the world of pro football. It shocked and angered Cowboys fans and players. What happened that could possibly explain why owner Jerry Jones fired head coach Jimmy Johnson? Or, did Jimmy quit? Or, had it been a mutual parting of the ways?

Regardless of what had occurred, the owner of the two-time defending Super Bowl champions and their volatile, highly successful and much-honored coach had reached a fork in the road and decided to go their separate ways. Many twists and turns in that road had brought them to this point.

As Dallas rose from the abyss of their '89 (3–13) and '90 (1–15) seasons and shot to the top of the NFL mountain in just four years, applause and acclamation rolled in for the Jones-Johnson tandem. They'd resurrected "America's Team," taking it from the outhouse to the penthouse. There appeared to be far more than enough credit to go around.

There apparently wasn't. And it's at this juncture the "he said, he said" dispute emerges.

An intense, driven, often fanatical Johnson took rightful pride in the talent accumulation and coaching job done under his watch.

The consumed, hard-charging, entrepreneurial Jones basked in the glory of the about-face he'd engineered. He'd purchased a pig's ear and turned it into a silk purse.

In truth, both Johnson and Jones had pictured their roles and resulting accomplishments perfectly.

Jerry almost certainly wouldn't have overseen Dallas' rise from the ashes without Johnson's all-consuming fire. And, without Jones' tireless efforts to overhaul and make profitable again a moribund Cowboys organization, Jimmy would not have had the freedom and financial resources so vital to his and his team's success.

Jimmy needed Jerry.

Jerry needed Jimmy.

Did they ever truly fathom that?

Small cracks, little things, in the relationship began showing up well before the divorce made headlines. Whispers that Johnson didn't appreciate Jones showing up on the sidelines during games with guests such as Prince Bandar of Saudia Arabia. That Jones, on the other hand, chaffed at Johnson's somewhat consistent refusal to publicly include the owner's contributions at or near the top of the list of factors behind the Dallas revival. Suggestions were made that Johnson leaked information to reporters contradicting the public impression of Jones being integrally involved in every aspect of the football team.

Little things, you say? Yes!

But also little wounds? Without question!

Ironically, as the Cowboys' star rose higher and higher, the gap between the two inched farther apart. During the week before the critical regular-season finale against the Giants, Johnson, whose Cowboys contract ran through 1998, had admitted being "intrigued" by the prospect of next season becoming the first head coach and general manager of the expansion Jacksonville Jaguars. Even years later, Jones still bristles at the memory of Jimmy's flirtation with another job.

"First of all, it was illegal . . . it was against all NFL rules," Jones answered a bit abruptly. Then his tone softens. "But, in answer to your question, yes it bothered me, it certainly did."

During Super Bowl week Jones stated that he and Johnson talked two or three times a day. The coach later contradicted that by saying they spoke an average of maybe once a week. Once again, Jones' persona of being "a football man" had taken a hit.

Two nights after the Cowboys victory in Super Bowl XXVIII Johnson appeared on the *Late Show with David Letterman*. The coach joked that the NFL had provided $60,000 for a Cowboys post-game party but that Jerry had pocketed $20,000 of it. (Cue the laughter.) Jones didn't laugh. And he certainly never would have chuckled at any punchline that intimated he might be "cheap" or a penny pincher. The Cowboys owner might be a variety of things, but cheap surely wasn't one of them.

Who was right? Who was wrong? That seemed to matter far less than who had *been wronged*.

"There are 500 coaches who would love to coach the Dallas Cowboys."

The final blowup in the Jones-Johnson, or, if you prefer Johnson-Jones, relationship came at the league meetings in late March in Orlando. At an NFL-sponsored party at Pleasure Island, a Disney resort in Orlando, Jones approached a table surrounded by familiar faces—Johnson and his girlfriend Rhonda, Chicago coach and former Dallas defensive coordinator Dave Wannstedt, Norv Turner (who'd just left the Dallas offensive coordinator's post to take the Redskins head-coaching job), former Dallas front office assistant Bob Ackles and his wife and former Cowboys TV coordinator Brenda Bushell. Jones had fired both Ackles and Bushell. As it turns out the group was reliving old stories about Jones, when the Cowboys owner arrived and proposed a toast to recent Cowboys glories.

Nobody toasted. Jones offered a second and a bit restructured but still positive toast. The group offered a lukewarm response at best. Jones whirled around and left more than a bit miffed. But was being ignored at the heart of Jones's displeasure at Pleasure Island?

"No, ignore is right. I've never been ignored. I'm 'in-ignorable,'" Jones chuckled as he looked far back in time. "I'm gonna have to see if that's in Merriam's—'in-ignorable.' It was more a feeling that they just didn't sense how we got to be here . . . of their perspectives of how the Cowboys were sitting here celebrating another Super Bowl."

An unhappy Jones and his personnel man and personal friend, Larry Lacewell, returned to the Hyatt Grand Cypress for a drink in the hotel bar "Trellises."

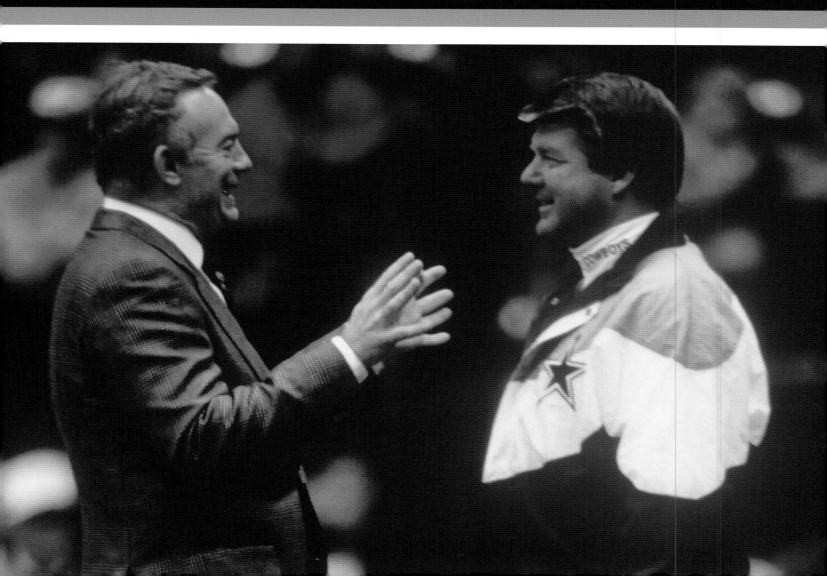

Dallas Morning News pro-football writers Rick Gosselin and Ed Werder were sharing a few "pops" with a couple other NFL beat writers in the same bar. Jones stopped by to exchange pleasantries. A bit later the writers began to depart, thinking their evening had reached "closing time." Oh, how wrong that would be.

"Jerry grabbed me by my left pants leg as I walked by, " Werder recalled, "and he says to me 'Don't leave now or you're going to miss the story of the year.'"

Not wishing to share this "story of the year," Werder and Gosselin faked going to their rooms to shake off their reporter friends and returned to "Trellises" for what would be, in media circles, a nuclear bomb of a story.

Jones, Werder, and Gosselin began an "off the record" conversation.

"But Jerry knew who he was talking to," Gosselin remembers. "He was clearly agitated, had selected his audience and knew exactly what he wanted to say."

Jones dropped the bombshell—he was thinking about firing Johnson and hiring former Oklahoma University head coach Barry Switzer. Both writers remember Jones's anger at Johnson for his "betrayal." Of calling Johnson a "disloyal SOB."

Jones then fired the shot soon to be heard 'round the NFL world. "There are five hundred coaches who would love to coach the Dallas Cowboys."

Five hundred who would love to or five hundred who *could?*

"I think there are five hundred who could have coached this team to the Super Bowl. I really believe that," Jones replied.

Five hours later those same reporters had a second, planned meeting with Jones for breakfast. During that discussion the Cowboys owner agreed that his statements be put "on the record."

Within minutes, a livid Johnson, who'd already been tipped about the crux of Jones's comments, loaded stuff into his car and bolted for his Florida home.

From the perspective of a dozen years later, Jones now both explains and regrets his "five hundred coaches" remarks.

"If you've spent any time around me, you know I express myself in hyperbole. 'He threw the ball a thousand yards,' saying things that way . . . I really to this day am amazed that anybody would look at that and say, 'Well, did Jerry actually think there were five hundred people that could coach that team? . . . But I think it (the statement) did offend him. That was a mistake. I shouldn't have said that. But I felt that strongly about the personnel of the team we had put together."

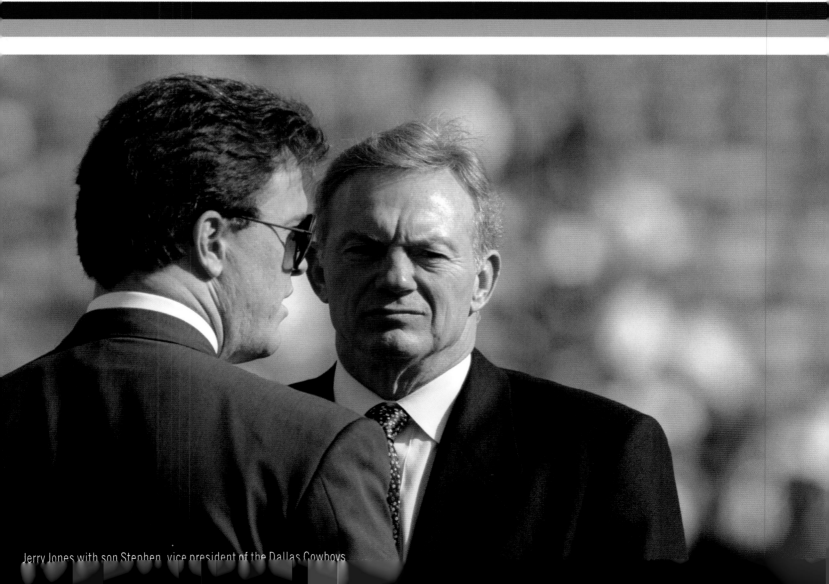

Jerry Jones with son Stephen, vice president of the Dallas Cowboys

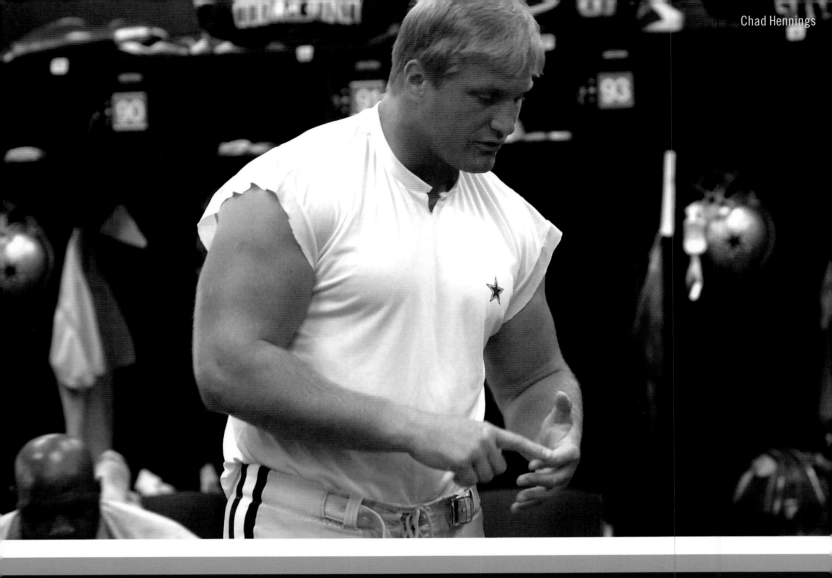

The following week would be a blur of:

★ Johnson reacting: "I'm not the greatest in the world to get along with. I know I'm arrogant. I know I'm self-serving. But somebody please tell me what I've done wrong . . . What have I done so wrong to be ripped the way I have? To my mind, I just got to the pinnacle of my profession. What did I do wrong?"

★ Stinging player rebukes like those of Emmitt Smith: "The team would be in turmoil to lose the head coach over some bull after he won two Super Bowls. I don't understand popping off like that. I think Jerry is trying to stir up controversy because the man can't live straight unless there is controversy in his life."

★ Noncommittal reaction like that of Troy Aikman: "I met with Jimmy once and got called in to meet with Jerry. I told both of them what I felt, and I left it at that. I really have no gut feeling about what's going to happen."

★ Jones clarifying why he'd even be thinking about who might coach Dallas should Jimmy leave: "My job is to stay ahead of the game. The future always begins tomorrow. If I'm not considering it, no one is. My *job* is the future of the Dallas Cowboys."

For a week the decision hung in the balance. Jones and Johnson had multiple meetings. They agreed their long-term relationship had probably run its course. The question then became Would Jimmy stay one more season to shoot for the unprecedented achievement of three consecutive Super Bowls or exit in as civil a manner as possible.

"We had pretty much decided 'Let's make it work' for one more year," Jones remembers. "We agreed neither of us would talk to any reporters. Then, the next morning's *Fort Worth Star-Telegram* had a headline saying 'Jones Tells Johnson My Way or the Highway.' At that point we looked at each other and said, 'This just isn't gonna work, is it?'"

On this Tuesday afternoon, Dallas witnessed live on TV perhaps the most bizarre press conference ever held in this city or any other. Jones and Johnson sat side by side patiently, introspectively discussing why they'd decided to divorce. No harshness. No vitriol. In fact, at times, they did and said the things that old friends of more than thirty years would be expected to say.

Johnson: "We've had hours of candid discussions the last two days, and I can sincerely tell you I feel better today about Jerry Jones as a friend than I have our entire relationship."

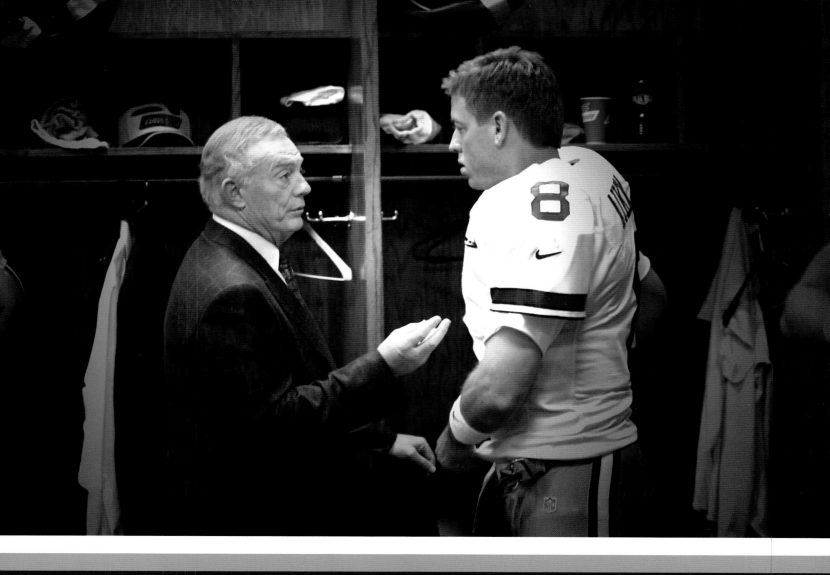

Jones: "Jimmy, did I ever try to call a play? The facts are that we never had a disagreement when it came to football."

Johnson: "It's fantastic what we were able to do. And when I say 'we' I mean 'we.' I appreciate what he's done for me."

At times Jones even patted Johnson on the knee as he spoke. Smiles all around. Like it was just another day home on the Texas range.

And never was heard a discouraging word and the skies were not cloudy all day.

Jones handed Johnson a $2 million severance check. This remarkable press conference example of "synchronized swimming" was complete.

The tale, however, does not end there. Twelve years later, speaking from the office of his Florida home, now TV football analyst Johnson drops his own bombshell:

"I was leaving anyway," he said. "I had already written down the actual date I was going to resign in my personal itinerary. It was just a few weeks away, before the draft. I was just going to say 'I'm gone.'"

All those scuffles with Jones, the behind the scenes sniping, that "five hundred coaches" comment, none of those had been the straw that broke the coach's back.

"I wanted to leave," Johnson said. "I had accomplished what I wanted to. I think even Jerry sensed that. I'd grown tired of being the bad guy, the drill sergeant, demanding that your stars give more and more. Cutting guys because they fumble. If I'd stayed, I would have had to be an even bigger SOB at the next Super Bowl than I'd been at the last one. That voice inside simply said it was time!"

In retrospect, how should we evaluate this pair who'd transformed a wallowing franchise into one now on the verge of being a dynasty? Did working too closely in the pressurized world of the NFL ruin a friendship that tracked back to their days at the University of Arkansas where they'd been starters and road roommates on a Hogs national championship club?

Were they both guilty of ignoring the danger signs of an approaching implosion? Why hadn't anyone in the organization intervened hoping to prevent the split? Or, had someone actually tried to help but failed? Were they too different or too much alike? How had the efforts of two people, apparently "poles apart," resulted in back-to-back titles?

In the end, we are left with one simple conclusion regarding this football divorce. All along this might have been a bad marriage, but it was one that on the field had produced great children.

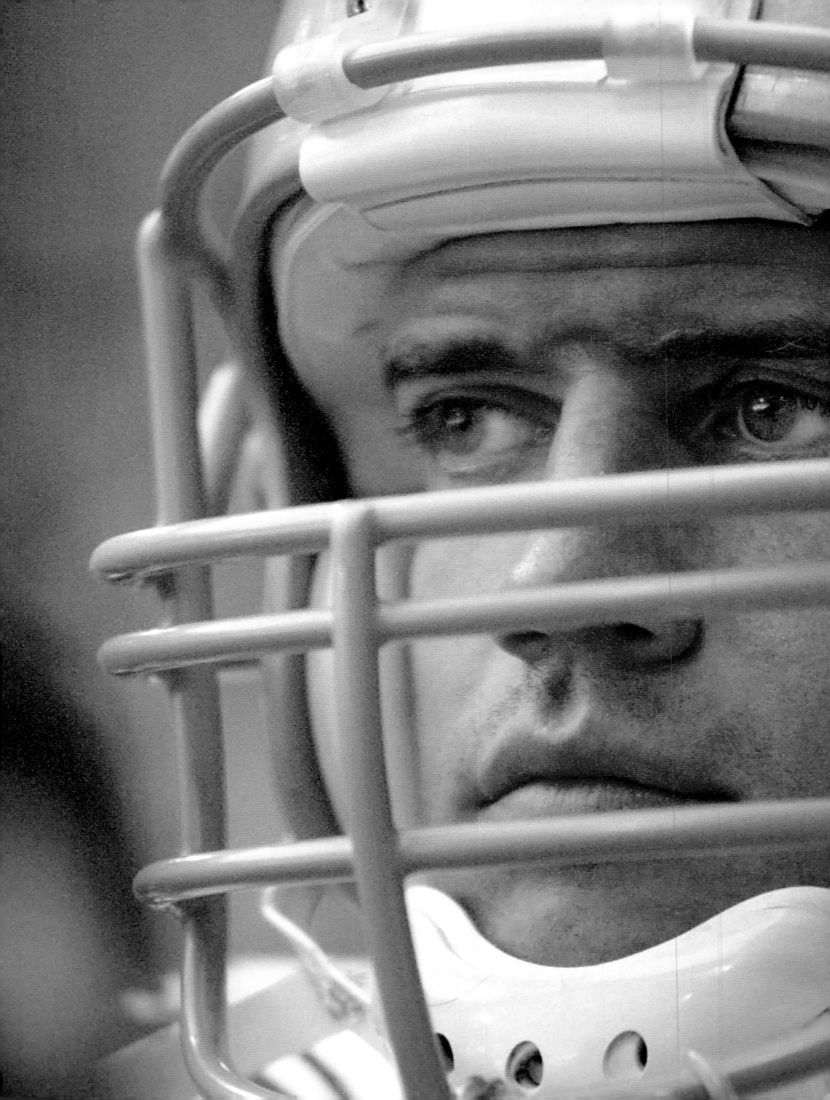

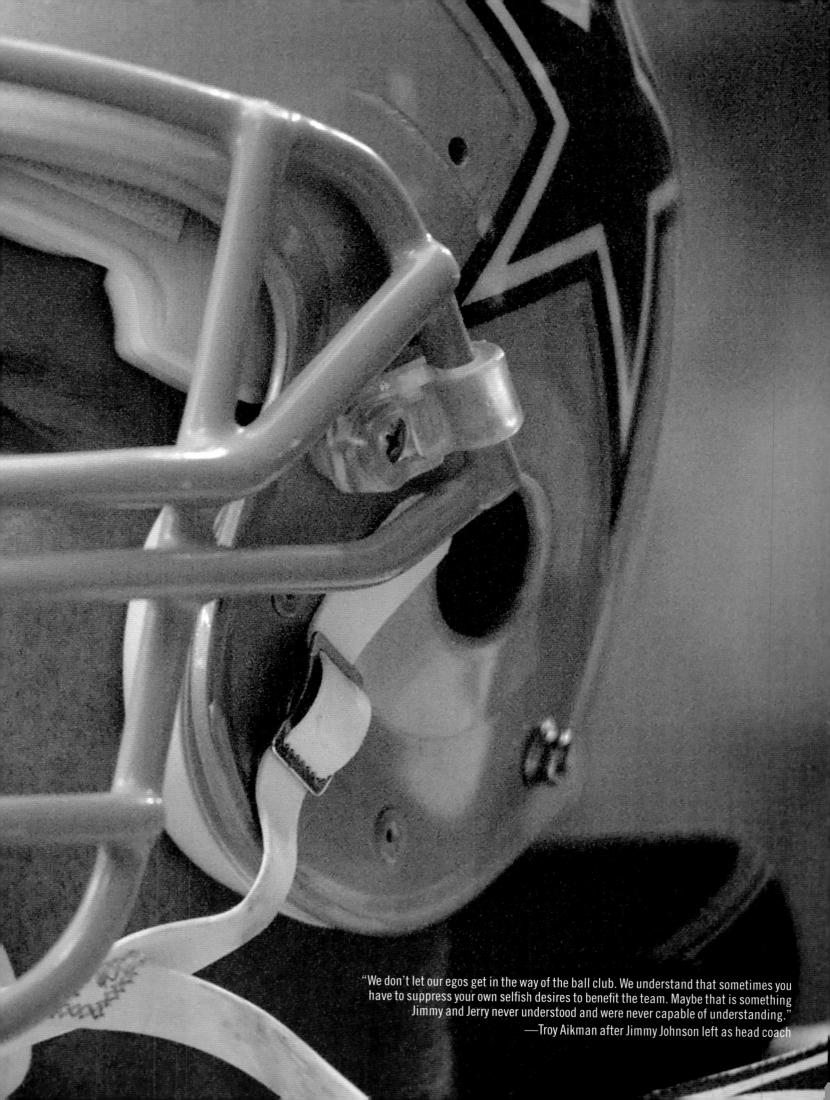

"We don't let our egos get in the way of the ball club. We understand that sometimes you have to suppress your own selfish desires to benefit the team. Maybe that is something Jimmy and Jerry never understood and were never capable of understanding."
—Troy Aikman after Jimmy Johnson left as head coach

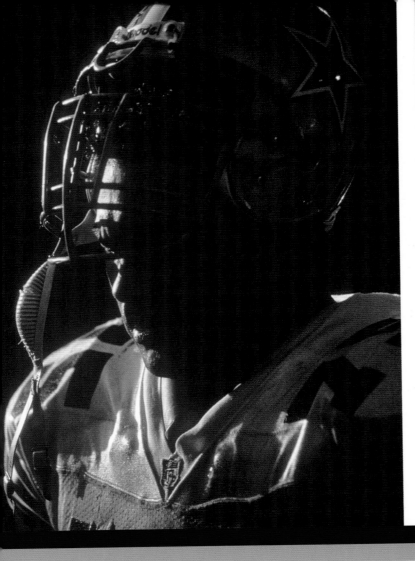
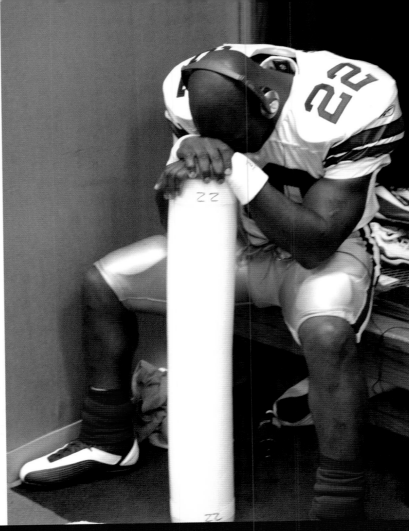
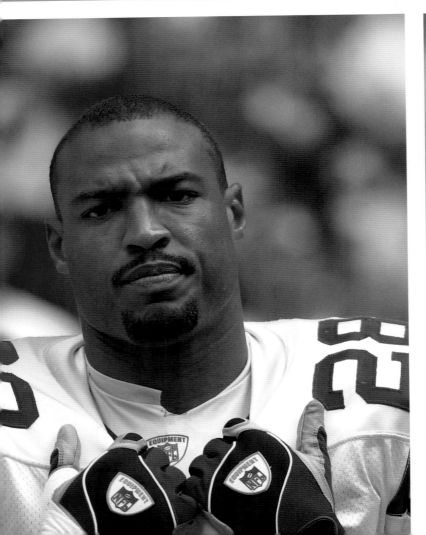
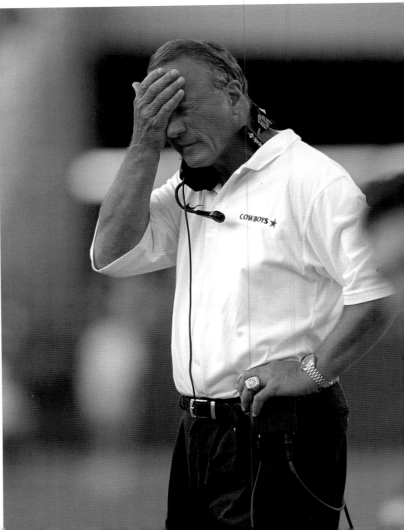

SOMETHING'S WRONG

Looks can be deceiving.

The two-time-defending Super Bowl champion Cowboys entered their Christmas eve regular season finale versus New York with a 12–3 record. Under new head coach Barry Switzer, they'd broken from the gate quickly, rolling to eleven victories in thirteen outings. By Game 13 they had clinched the NFC East by whipping Philadelphia, 31–19.

At first glance everything looked fine.

It wasn't.

Troy Aikman: "I'll be honest with you. I was concerned about that team very early in the season. Under Jimmy (Johnson) we paid attention to a lot of detail and little things. And a lot of those things were beginning to slide."

Special teams coach Joe Avezzano: "We were rockin' along still winning, but we weren't as efficient. We just weren't as dominant."

Daryl Johnston: "Usually, we peaked at the end of the season. This time we were on the sled going the other way."

The record books support Johnston's observations. Fast finishes had become a trademark of Jimmy Johnson's Cowboys.

★ 1990: Finished 4–2 to reach 7–9 for the year.

★ 1991: Ran off five straight to close at 11–5 and then posted the Pokes first playoff win in nine.

★ 1992: Ripped off five of their last six to pile up thirteen wins, the most ever for a Cowboys club in a regular season. They then pounded three straight opponents on their way to capturing Super Bowl XXVII.

★ 1993: Roared down the stretch with five in a row and continued that momentum by steamrolling three playoff foes by an average of fifteen points per game in taking a second consecutive Super Bowl.

But those were Jimmy's teams. Switzer, who'd turned the University of Oklahoma into a college football powerhouse, sensed from the beginning he'd get blamed if the Cowboys didn't three-peat.

"I knew that when I crossed the Red River going south, that day Jerry (Jones) called me," Switzer said. "I recognized you don't bust up a staff that had been to two Super Bowls . . . I was taking over someone else's staff that I didn't know their agendas. I didn't know what type of loyalty I would have. I'm to come in and keep it going down the road and out of the ditch."

Jimmy, Jimmy, Jimmy. With every decision Switzer made or any slight hint of erosion, Barry understood fully that he'd always be compared to Johnson, who'd left a team riding higher than any other in the Cowboys proud thirty-five-year history. Barry's already-hot seat grew even hotter given the stark difference in the two's personalities and styles of coaching.

Avezzano: "The intensity and hands-on scrutiny, the psychological aspect of Jimmy Johnson was much different from the laid-back, delegate-authority approach of Barry Switzer."

Johnston: "I've always stated that Barry was in a no-win situation. If he won a Super Bowl, it was 'Jimmy's team,' and if he never won it was going to be Barry's fault."

Then there were natural questions about Switzer's capacity to adapt to coaching pro football. Questions that even resonated in the Dallas locker room.

Johnston: "Absolutely we wondered about his ability to coach. He'd been removed from the game for five years. He never coached anywhere in the NFL, and at Oklahoma he was known as a great recruiter more than a great head coach."

Switzer: "I had a tough-ass job."

"Jimmy's Team" reached this regular-season finale with that solid 12–3 record.

"Barry's Team" had problems, though. Lots of alarming signs. *Dallas Morning News* columnist Frank Luksa portrayed Dallas as "the worst 12–3 team in the NFL is getting worse."

And the troubles, be they small or large, seemed to arrive as steadily as the sun rises in the East.

★ Right tackle Erik Williams, maybe the finest offensive lineman in the entire league, crashed his Mercedes into a concrete highway wall driving home after a road game in Arizona. The "lucky-to-be-alive" Williams sustained a severe, season-ending knee injury in the "alcohol-related" smashup.

★ Dallas had fallen from being the third-best rushing club in the league in '93 to the nineteenth.

★ The defense had lost to free agency three solid players from the '93 title winner—linebacker Ken Norton Jr., defensive tackle Tony Casillas, and defensive tackle Jimmie Jones. Three valuable offensive linemen, including starting guard Kevin Gogan, also left for bigger bucks.

★ A difference of opinion between middle linebacker Robert Jones and reserve corner Dave Thomas flared up. The two had to be separated by teammates.

★ Switzer caused a big brouhaha in a press conference when he aimed criticism directly at Smith saying: "I question him in the weight room. He doesn't work in the weight room like he should." Emmitt bristled at the remarks and got even more testy the next day when he found a transcript of Switzer's remarks posted in his dressing cubicle.

"People talk about us turning it off and on, but you can't do that."

★ Controversy swirled around Switzer when a story broke that he'd skipped three Saturday night team meetings to watch his son Doug play college football.

★ Emmitt Smith and James Washington engaged in a heated argument on the team charter coming home from New Orleans. During some horseplay (a food fight, perhaps?) an object (an errant beverage can, perhaps?) struck Smith. Emmitt, already in a grumpy mood after pulling a hamstring that afternoon, threw the can back, hitting Washington. An "exchange" occurred, though no punches were thrown. Michael Irvin considered the tiff serious enough to speak to the team after the plane landed.

★ Lots of areas hurt on the body of Troy "Acheman." He'd suffered the fourth concussion of his career in Arizona. Jammed his throwing thumb against San Francisco. Injured a knee versus Washington causing him to miss two games, and he returned wearing an uncomfortable-looking knee brace that affected his footwork.

★ Twenty-three veterans were headed for free agency after the season. Twenty-three! That list included five offensive and three defensive starters. Players such as wide receiver Michael Irvin, center Mark Stepnoski, tight end Jay Novacek, wide receiver Alvin Harper, defensive end Tony Tolbert, and safety James Washington.

★ Harper, leading the league in yards per catch through twelve games, had but two receptions in Games 13 through 15 and was complaining openly. "I feel like the offense has been playing with ten guys. I'm not inconsistent. The opportunities are inconsistent."

★ Rookie defensive end Shante Carver rolled his sports utility vehicle. Harper borrowed Irvin's Benz and crashed it. Smith tore up his Lexus.

★ Hurting bodies filled Kevin O'Neill's training room. Safety Brock Marion cracked a rib. Irvin nursed a quad bruise that decreased his burst off the line and ability to cut. Harper fought knee and back problems. Almost everything on Akiman throbbed. Smith's left hamstring kept him out of that Christmas Eve finale with the Giants.

Ah, back to that last, thought-to-be-meaningless date with New York. A win would make Dallas the only team to have ever swept the NFC East without a defeat.

The day would be cold and blustery. A terrific afternoon if you owned a company that manufactured lip balm. A wind chill of thirty degrees. The Cowboys weren't so hot either.

The offense produced a paltry 83 yards and ten points. That meant Dallas' once-feared attack had produced a meager twenty-nine points over its last three games.

Smith sat out to rest his hamstring.

Aikman played just five series, hitting nine of eleven passes but for only 62 yards and three points. Only one completion to a wide receiver. Harper again was shut out. Over his last four games, the once laser-like Aikman had tossed seven interceptions and one touchdown pass. He hadn't thrown a scoring pass to a wideout in six games.

But Dallas still had a chance to win, trailing 15–10, when they punted to the Giants with 9:18 left. The Cowboys never got the ball back. Slowly but steadily New York pushed the Cowboys' defense back toward their own end zone, covering 74 yards in sixteen plays. Dallas used all its timeouts plus the two-minute warning. New York marched on. It ended with Giants quarterback Dave Brown taking a knee at the Dallas 11-yard line.

After racing to an 11–2 start, Dallas had succumbed meekly to Cleveland at home (19–14), struggled to a 26–14 win at New Orleans (aided by two touchdowns from the defense) and stumbled to this lackluster 15–10 loss to New York, which had lost to Dallas five straight times by an average score of 28–13.

The manner in which the Cowboys wobbled toward the finish line worried many.

Safety Darren Woodson: "We're not playing well on offense or defense. We can't sustain a drive and, when we need to, we can't stop a drive. People talk about us turning it off and on, but you can't do that."

Daryl Johnston offered a single-word description of the Giants' defeat: "Pathetic."

Avezzano felt for Switzer: "Yes, there was a change, but hell, you've been a winner, now go out and do what you're supposed to. Does somebody have to lead you by the hand?"

Others offered bravado and stiff-upper-lip assurances. Switzer maintained his steadfast belief in his team. That they would rally. That they had champions' hearts. Players with pride who understood the urgency of what that lay ahead. Barry contended that those final three alarming efforts didn't put wrinkles in his brow.

"I didn't see anything," Switzer said. "You look at what occurred in the game . . . a few plays that made the difference in winning and losing . . . a couple of plays that we didn't make and they did."

After all this, the Cowboys had captured the NFC East and a first-round bye. Only San Francisco at 13–3 ranked above 12–4 Dallas in the final overall NFL standings.

History, however, offered an ominous footnote. Seven previous Cowboys clubs entered the playoffs having lost their final regular-season contest. None of these seven had ever reached the Super Bowl.

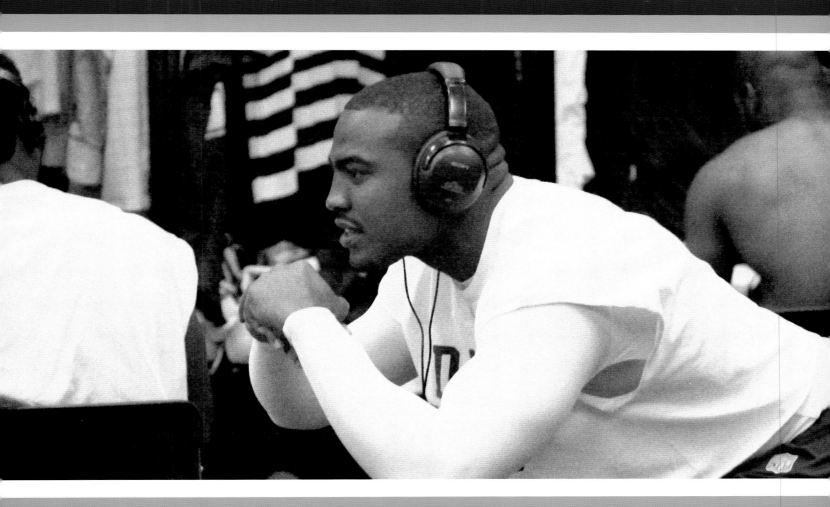

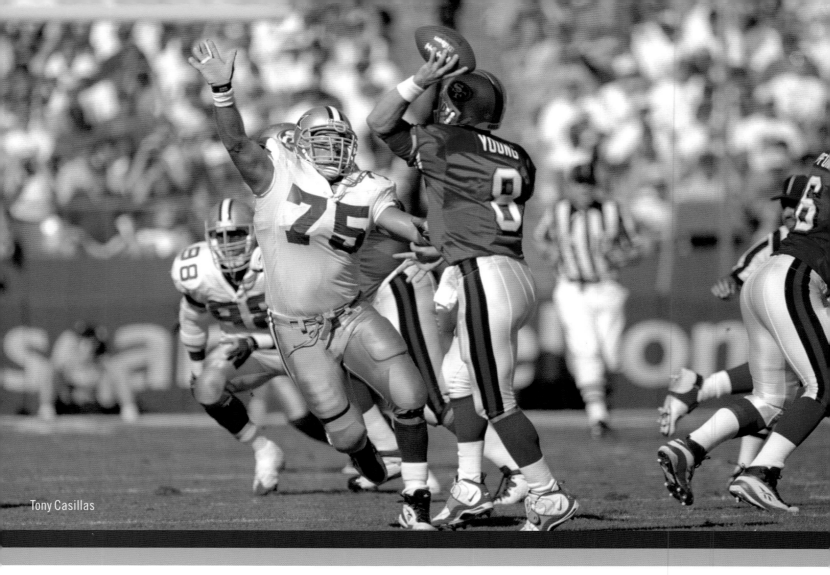

Tony Casillas

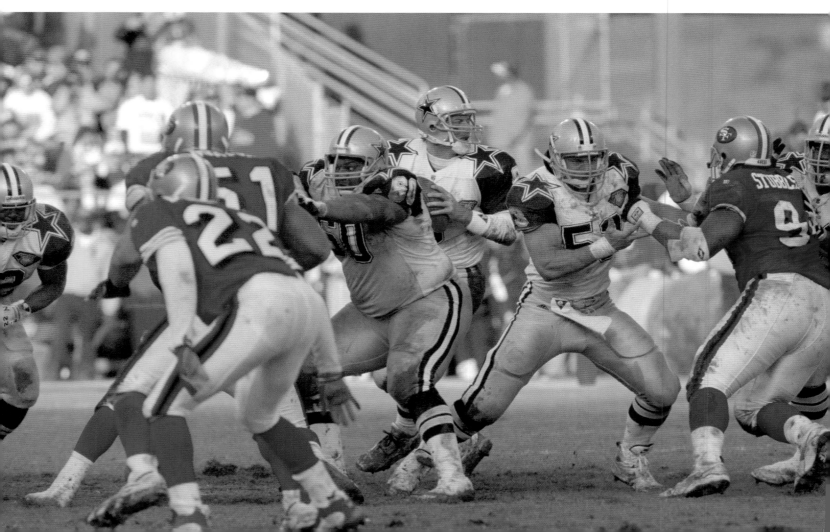

7:27 OF HELL

"The Real Super Bowl."

That's how the front cover of *Sports Illustrated* portrayed the NFC Championship Game pitting 13–4 Dallas against 14–3 San Francisco. The Niners had captured rings in '88 and '89, barely missed making it to the title game and a chance at a third consecutive crown in '90, and then had fallen to Dallas in the '92 and '93 NFC championships.

Now, it was the Cowboys who'd marched to the doorstep of history. Since the NFL-AFL merger in 1970, no franchise had ever won three straight titles. Green Bay, Miami, San Francisco, and Pittsburgh (twice) had opportunities. NFL dynasties had come and gone. There'd never been a "tri-nasty."

Dallas' attempt to "three-peat" formed the obvious storyline for the '95 season. But just beneath the surface bubbled the continuing controversy over the dismissal of Jimmy Johnson and the hiring of former Oklahoma coach Barry Switzer.

Johnson had earned the reputation of miracle worker for the way he overhauled the Cowboys almost overnight. Some players loved the discipline, focus, and direction he'd brought. Others hated his mind games, threats, and use of humiliation to motivate.

Switzer'd been out of coaching altogether for five years and had never worked a single day in the NFL. Some Cowboys loved his constant encouragement, desire to establish personal relationships, and hands-off approach. Others hated his perceived lack of discipline and attention to detail.

Every Switzer move or decision got measured by the "Johnson yardstick" Jimmy had left behind. And, though nearly ten months and seventeen games had passed, the ghost of Johnson's teams still hovered over these Cowboys.

"I don't think we'd be here at all if Jimmy were still the coach," Jones told the press. "This Jimmy-Jerry thing was not doing to die. Plus, I didn't see what I needed to see from Jimmy that would allow him to let it die."

Jones feared the ever-more-frequent disagreements between the two might ruin the '94 season. Johnson exited. Jones took his place on a very hot seat. Anything less than another Super Bowl ring, and the finger of blame would point directly at Jones.

"I accept that and live with that because, frankly, I bit that off when I bought the Cowboys," Jones said.

Switzer knew he'd taken over a "no-win job."

"I don't give a damn whether I'm considered a great pro coach," Switzer barked during the week leading up to the showdown with the Niners. "I have always championed my players and (assistant) coaches because nobody wins with just one person. It's the team, team concepts. It's never 'me' or 'I', it's 'we' and 'us' that make things happen. I'm not out to prove anything. I don't give one damn and never have."

Beneath such thick skin one got, and still gets, the impression Switzer *did* give a damn about many things and that included the way people perceived him. It's just that his hard-scrabble life growing up in the Oklahoma dust bowl would never permit anyone a peek at a softer, more vulnerable side. After all, this was the son of a bootlegger who'd held the dead body of his mother, Mary Louise, in his arms after she'd committed suicide in the backyard. Then he'd endured the murder of his father, Frank, who was shot to death by his mistress.

Though the words did not and never will pass from Switzer's lips, a Super Bowl might quiet those who questioned his NFL credentials. It might push the specter of Jimmy Johnson farther into the background—back there with Mary Louise and Frank and all the other ghosts of Switzer's past.

However much Jones still felt haunted by the collapse of his relationship with Johnson, whatever might still be lingering beneath the surface of Barry Switzer, whatever memories remained for the handful of Cowboys who'd struggled through the terrible times in '89 and '90, they all were about to spend seven minutes and twenty-seven seconds in hell.

On the game's third play Aikman fired into the right flat for Kevin Williams. The Niners' Eric

Davis anticipated the play perfectly, left the receiver he was covering (Michael Irvin), stepped in front of Williams, and was gone.

A mere 1:02 had elapsed. San Francisco led 7–0.

On the third snap of Dallas' next possession, Aikman drilled one to Irvin. A yard short of the distance needed for the first down, Irvin fought to make it to the sticks—and fumbled. Then came five straight Steve Young passes, the last to Ricky Watters, and the Niners' advantage had doubled.

With 4:19 gone, San Francisco was up, 14-0.

On the ensuing kickoff, Cowboys return man Kevin Williams raced up field, got hit, and lost the ball in front of the Cowboys' bench.

Switzer: "He (Williams) runs to the 31, right there. I'm standing there and he fumbles the SOB."

It took the opportunistic Niners seven snaps to put up another seven.

Just 7:27 gone. San Francisco 21, Dallas 0!

Switzer: "It was like a horror movie. Like I was watching *Friday the 13th* or *Halloween* or something like that. I couldn't believe it."

Troy Aikman: "Never in a million years could I anticipate that we'd get into that kind of hole to start the game."

Jones: "I was in shock."

But Dallas hadn't won a pair of Super Bowls and their "bootlegger's boy" coach hadn't risen to the heights of college football by quitting.

Switzer quickly gathered his offense together on the sidelines. "Everybody was stunned," he said. "They had that glass-eyed look and I turned to them and said 'Guys, you know what's great about being down 21–0 after seven minutes?' They all look at me like I was crazy. I said, 'Cause we got fifty-three minutes to get back in this SOB. Fifty-three minutes. Now do something about it.'"

Dallas did do something. Despite a missed 27-yard chip shot field goal by Chris Boniol, which would nag them all game long, the Cowboys had crept back to within 10 points (24–14) as the last seconds of the first half wound down.

The Forty-niners had the ball at the Dallas 28. Thirteen seconds until halftime. San Francisco had used all its timeouts. They had few play options. Perhaps a quickie toss to the sidelines to pick up a few yards, stop the clock, and shorten Doug Brien's field-goal try. Or—take a shot at the end zone.

Somehow the Niners got future Hall-of-Famer Jerry Rice matched up one-on-one with cornerback Larry Brown. Touchdown Niners. With just eight seconds left. For all the

Cowboys' comeback efforts they still trailed, 31–14, at the half. Despite the seventeen-point gap, however, high drama still lay ahead in this battle of the titans.

Dallas wouldn't quit. The Niners dug in their heels. That is, if digging one's heels remained a possibility on the Candlestick "turf" which, in some places, looked like a pig's wallow and in others seemed more like green kitty litter. Dallas scored. San Francisco replied. The fourth quarter arrived with the Forty-niners still in command by 21.

Irvin raised his arms. Sanders extended an arm across Irvin's before the ball arrived.

At first glance, it appeared Sanders had interfered. Replays confirmed it. But no yellow penalty flag flew. Switzer flew into a rage. "I threw my hip into him (the official) and said 'You mean this isn't interfering?' Then, they yellowed me."

A 15-yard walk-off for unsportsmanlike conduct left the Cowboys with a third and 25. Two more plays and Dallas'

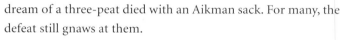

"It was like a horror movie."

A grinding fourteen-play, 89-yard Dallas drive chopped the lead to 38–28. The Cowboys defense held and Dallas had the ball back with 7:18 left and two timeouts available. On second and 10 from the Niners' 43, Aikman pump faked and lofted a pass deep down the left sideline. Star San Francisco corner Deion "Prime Time" Sanders ran stride for stride with Michael "the Playmaker" Irvin. But Irvin appeared to have him by a half step as the pass descended dead on target at the Niners' 10.

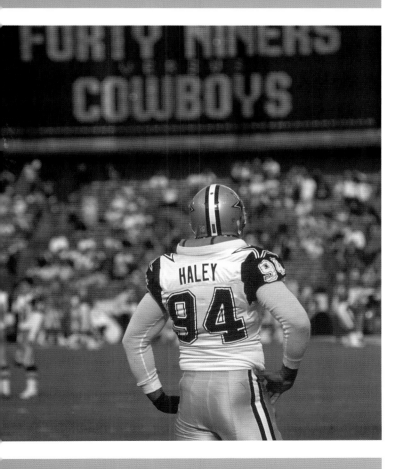

dream of a three-peat died with an Aikman sack. For many, the defeat still gnaws at them.

Larry Brown: "I was so depressed. It really, really hurts, you know, the NFC championship, and you played probably your worst game of your career."

Charles Haley: "I remember it like it was just yesterday. I thought we went into a hornet's nest. We tried to fight back, but it's hard to get momentum back."

But Aikman offers a completely different perspective: "All people had ever really seen of us was Dallas enjoying great success. It was the first they'd seen us struggle. But that game illustrated the type of team we were, how we continued to fight. I used a picture from that game on my Hall of Fame invitations. It's a shot of me full of mud. People that recognize it are surprised that I'd pick a picture from a game we lost. But it's the game I'm most proud of; we showed America what we were made of."

Switzer's post-game comments contained a mixture of anger, shedding a few tears, defiance, humor, and acceptance of guilt for protesting too vehemently the non-interference call that led to the damaging penalty.

More than a dozen seasons later, Switzer made a stunning admission about his often turbulent four-year period coaching the Cowboys.

"In that total era, that's the only game I'm ever embarrassed about," Switzer said. "We played poorly and didn't give ourselves the chance to win. If we could've won—we did win the next year—that would have been four in a row. That's the only one that ever embarrassed me."

The pain of that defeat, however, might remain sharpest in Jerry Jones.

"After the game I went out and sat in the car by myself crying," he said. "It was that emotional for me, that sad to me. I mean, I don't think I'll ever again get that close to winning three straight Super Bowls. That's asking too much of life. How many times will you have an opportunity like that, three in a row?"

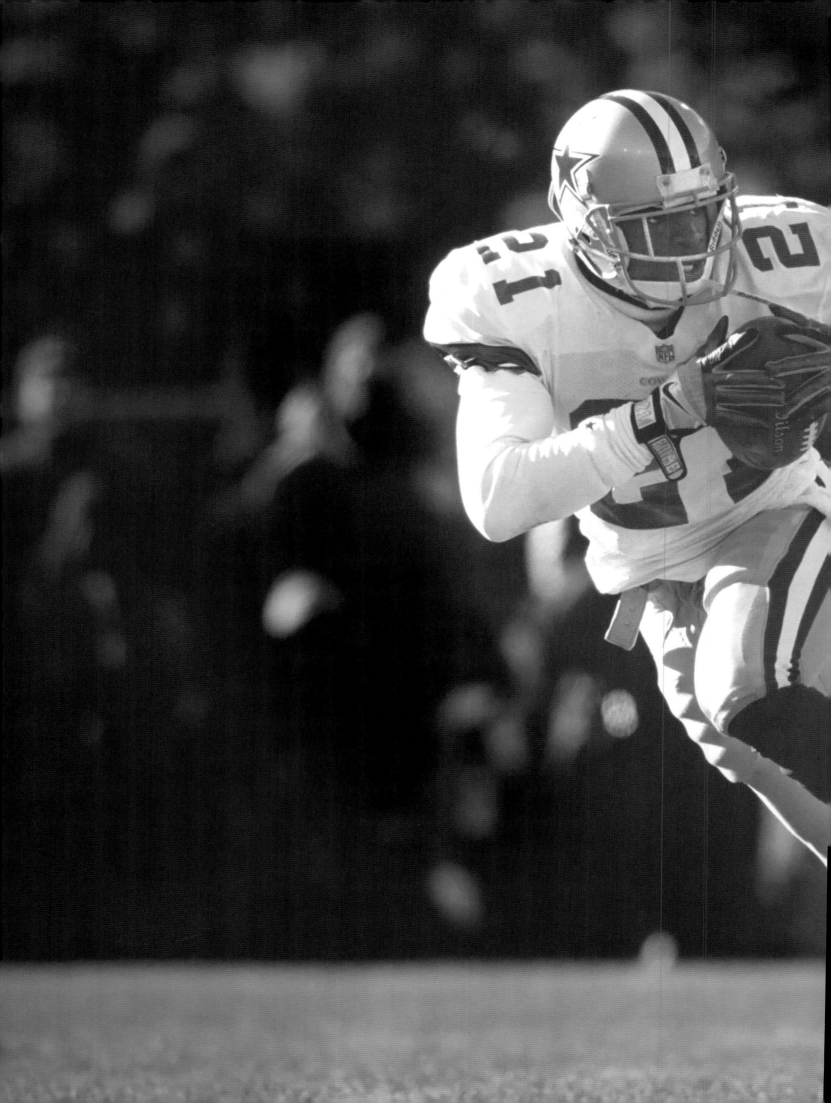

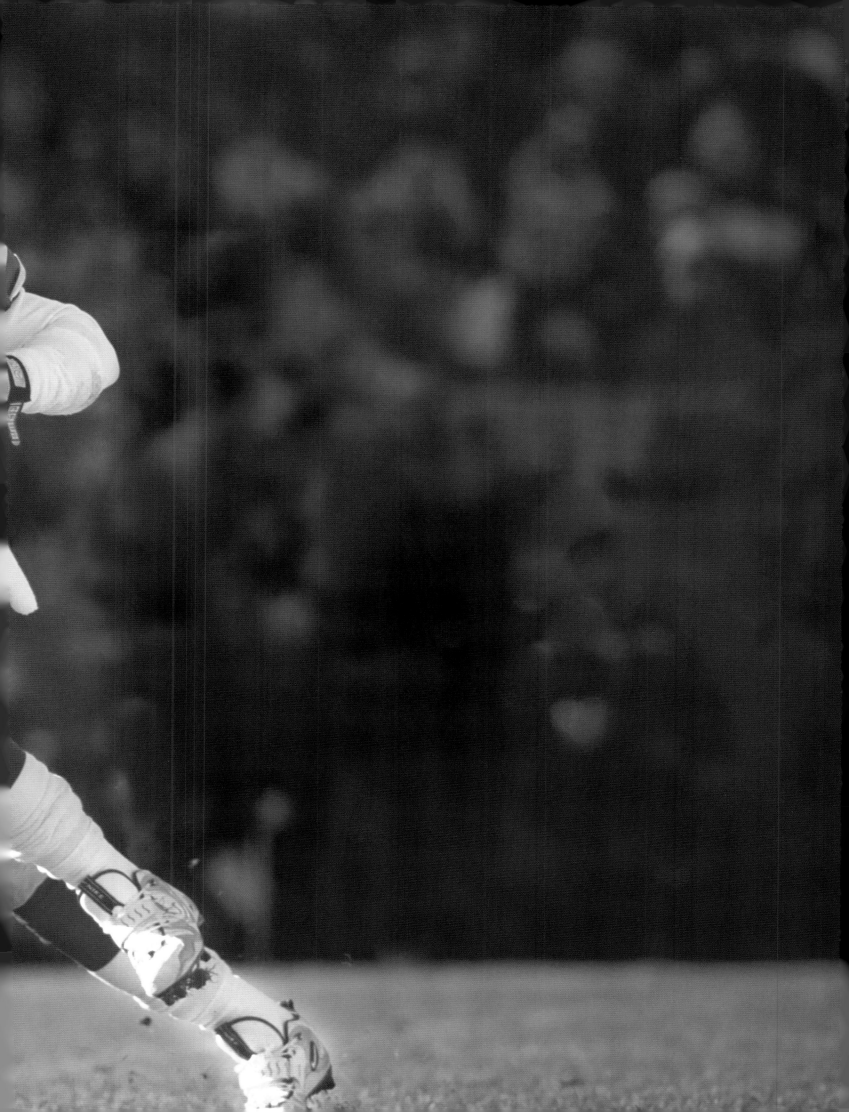

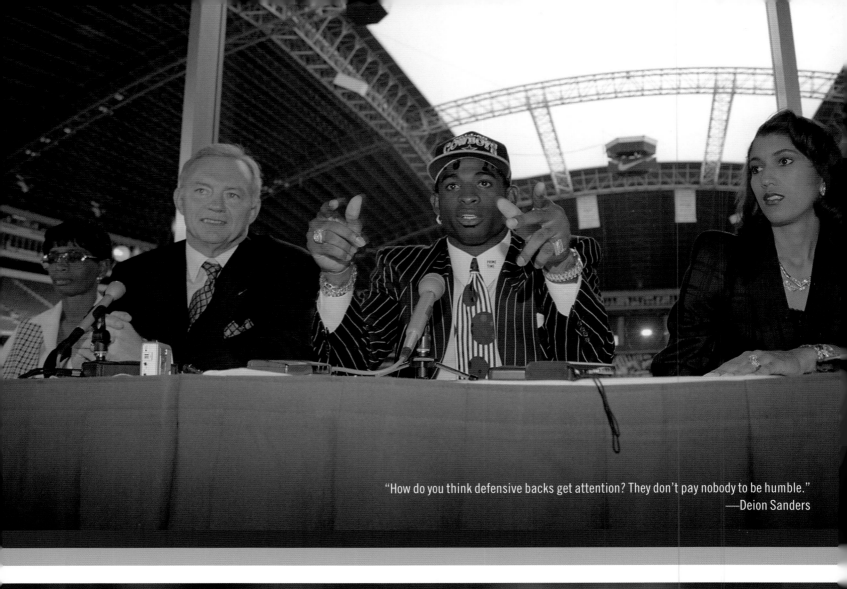

"How do you think defensive backs get attention? They don't pay nobody to be humble."
—Deion Sanders

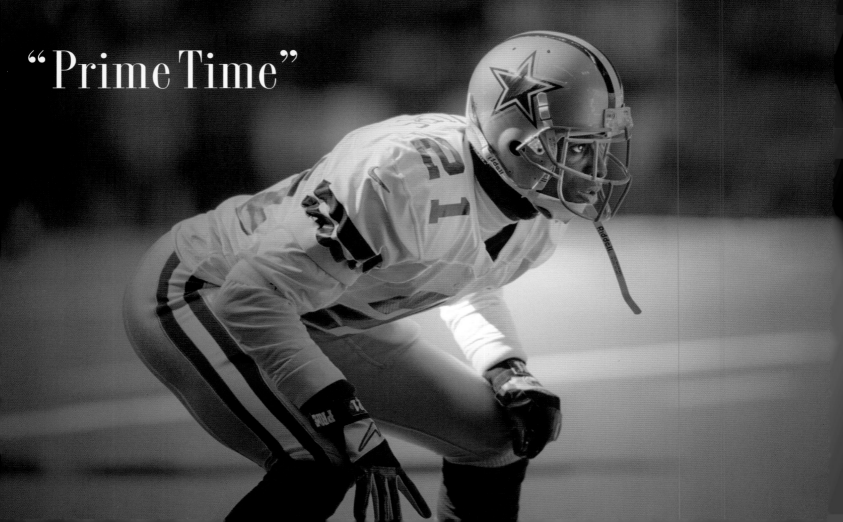

"Prime Time"

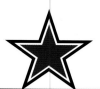

FAMILY FEUD

It's nearly midnight. Eugene Parker, the agent for mega-star cornerback Deion Sanders, waits patiently in a suite at the ritzy Mansion Hotel. But in the adjoining room voices grow steadily louder. The tone suggests this dispute's well past the simple disagreement level. The volume reaches yelling proportions. Screaming's not far away.

On the other side of that closed door Stephen Jones stands in his father Jerry's path blocking him from rejoining Parker. Stephen's neck is bowed, his jaw set, one fist clenched. Jerry, a few inches shorter, maybe thirty pounds lighter and twenty-two years older than his son, who started at linebacker for Arkansas in the '87 Orange Bowl, had also reached the "bring-it-on" stage.

"What are you fixin' to do?" Jerry hollers. "Are you gonna hit me?"

Parker'd flown to Dallas this Wednesday evening on Jones's private jet to negotiate a boxcar-sized contract. But, was his role about to change abruptly from agent to peacemaker? Family counselor? Or, maybe even referee?

Weren't the Joneses supposed to be haggling with Parker? How'd this evening become so twisted? So ugly?

Let's backtrack. Dallas' excruciating loss to San Francisco in the NFC title game eight months before still stuck in the elder Jones's craw. The Forty-niners had gone on to win the championship, denying Dallas an unprecedented third consecutive Super Bowl. Critics blamed Jones, feeling he'd run Jimmy Johnson out of Big D. Much of the super momentum that existed after consecutive Super Bowl victories had disappeared like rain on sand.

Then, more trouble in the '95 season-opening, 35–0 destruction of New York. There'd actually been two blowouts in that Monday nighter—the one of the Giants and the Achilles tendon of superb Cowboys cornerback Kevin Smith. That injury served to multiply Jones's lust to sign Sanders, who'd played a pivotal role for those '94 Forty-niner champions. Not only would signing "Neon Deion" gore the ox of their archrivals, but Jones would also be adding the only athlete who had ever:

★ Played in a World Series *and* a Super Bowl.

★ Hit a major league home run and scored an NFL touchdown in the same week.

★ Scored pro football touchdownss by rushing, pass reception, punt return, kickoff return, and fumble return.

The Cowboys had courted Sanders for weeks.

"Jerry told me he'd been writing checks with his mouth for years and then racing to cover his fanny," Parker said. "He told me Deion would be a Dallas Cowboy."

Sanders, despite bids from San Francisco, Miami, Detroit, and Denver, also knew the precise zip code of where he wanted his next fat check to come from.

"Eugene kept saying 'I don't know if it's going to get done,'" Sanders told an interviewer. "I said, 'Eugene, just get it done. I want to be a Dallas Cowboy.'"

That brings the story back to that hotel suite.

Negotiations had begun after dinner about 10 PM Jones and Parker conferred one-on-one. Stephen, who had total responsibility for managing the Cowboys' salary cap, set up shop in the next room.

"Lots of cap scenarios existed. Remember the league was just getting going under the cap [with] lots of different question marks about what you could and couldn't do," the younger Jones points out.

"At the time our roster was very front-end loaded, you know, five or six guys getting most of the money. So I was trying to figure out just how the [Sanders] deal would fit. I thought Jerry was going to come back and forth [between rooms] and say, 'Here's where we are, what can we do?'"

That assumption proved dead wrong and would be the firestarter between farther and son. Unbeknownst to Stephen, there'd be no "back and forth." Parker had done his homework and had designed the parameters of an agreement understanding full well how Jones craved "Prime Time." (Another of Deion's nicknames.)

An hour and a half passed. Jerry Jones, the owner and general manager, had yet to consult Stephen, his capologist. When he finally did, all negotiating was over. Jones had agreed to a deal and he had one angry son.

"I said, 'What do you mean you're through,'" Stephen recalled. "I just said, 'If I'd have known, I'd have gotten you more information about why to do this or why not to before you got yourself committed.'"

And, about that deal? As Gomer Pyle would say— Shazam!!! Sanders's bonus would be $12,999,999. Why not a nice, round $13 million?

Stephen: "To avoid 13, unlucky 13. We just decided we shouldn't do 13."

That gigantic check highlighted a whopping seven-year, $35 million pact. Well, that's the way the contract got announced. But, both Sanders and Dallas understood the arrangement would in reality be *five years* and *$25 million*. If you're now lost inside this maze of fuzzy math, don't feel alone. So was the NFL, and they were hopping mad.

Dallas submitted the deal as a seven-year pact enabling the Cowboys to spread that $13 million

Deal done. Mission accomplished. And that's where, according to Stephen, things got "really emotional, really heated."

Jerry (perhaps feeling giddy?): "Stephen said, 'Let's talk about this.' And I said, 'Well, you can come in here and negotiate all you want, but we've done this deal.' I was upset because I wasn't getting the approval rating that I wanted."

Stephen (perhaps feeling minimized?): "My point was, so what are you going to do if all of a sudden Troy and Michael and Emmitt see the size of this contract and want to rework. Let's *talk*!"

Jerry: "Is there anything you can see on the face of it (the terms of the contract) that's wrong?"

Stephen: "No.'"

Jerry: "Well then, get out of my way. I'm gonna go shake hands with him (Parker)."

That's when the son barred the door with clenched fist. So, when father asked, "Are you gonna hit me?" could it have happened?

"Are you gonna hit me?"

bonus over seven years, thus lowering the cap impact. At the same time Sanders would earn as his base salary only the minimum NFL wage ($178,000) each of the next three years. So, for three seasons the Cowboys owned the best corner in the league at the bargain basement price of roughly $2 million against the cap (prorated signing bonus plus base salary).

Both sides knew Sanders would be cut or the contract renegotiated before the final two years of accord ever arrived. A new term had been invented—"voidable years." All the ticked-off league cared about was that the spirit of the salary cap had been circumvented. But Jones and Parker couldn't care less how much the NFL vented.

Deion had his cash.

Jerry had his superstar.

Stephen still had his anger.

Forget the wisdom or lack thereof in offering such a pot of gold. Stephen knew how doggedly Jerry had pursued Sanders and that a contract would happen that night. But Jones the son felt his father had forgotten the painful, extended recent negotiations with "the Triplets," in which the Cowboys had convinced Emmitt Smith, Michael Irvin, and Troy Aikman to all accept somewhat less-than-market-value contracts for the good of the team and its salary cap.

Stephen worried about the impact on team chemistry. Jerry'd already erased his biggest worry.

Jerry: "I don't think he would have hit me, but he sure was getting in position to do a little bumping around there."

Sanity suddenly returned. Tempers cooled. Stephen stepped aside. Jerry and Parker shook hands. Jerry returned to the adjoining room, and father and son hugged and "we told each other that we loved each other."

Soon the threesome sat in the bar celebrating a night's work well done. Over Thursday and Friday the Joneses met with Aikman, Irvin, and Smith. All were "cool" with Deion's deal. On Saturday, September 9, Sanders officially wore the star.

Long afterward both father and son reflected on the respect they had for the stance each had taken that evening. However, in retrospect, what might Jerry have done had Stephen not stepped away?

"I quit wrestling with him when he was about sixteen," Jerry said of Stephen. He got me in a headlock, and I was clever enough to ease out of it without letting him know he had me. But I knew that I'd quit throwing him down and wrestling with him."

And, was that the maddest Stephen's ever gotten at Jerry in their years of leading the organization?

"No," Stephen confessed. "I once threw the chair at the door after he left. But that's another story."

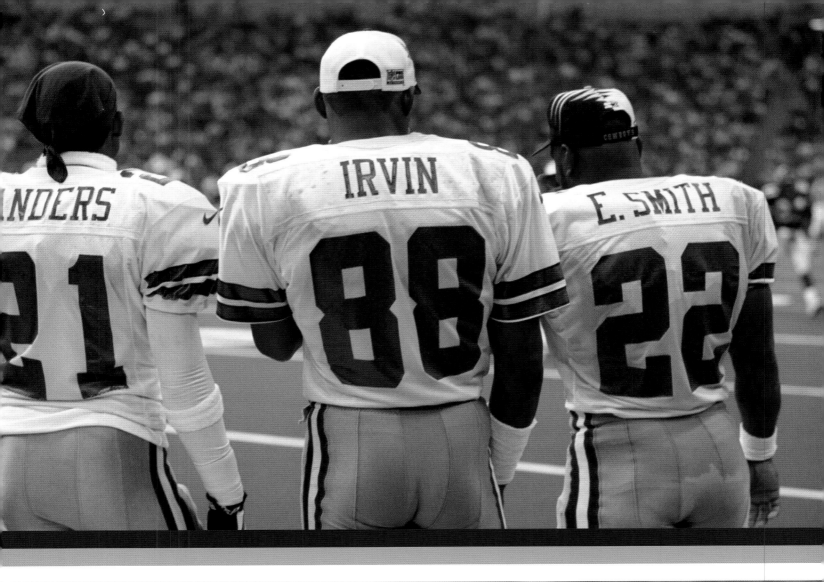

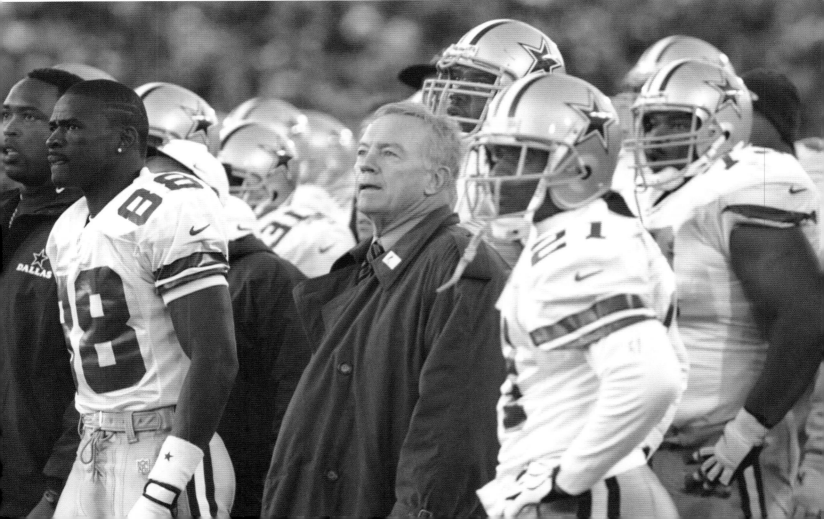

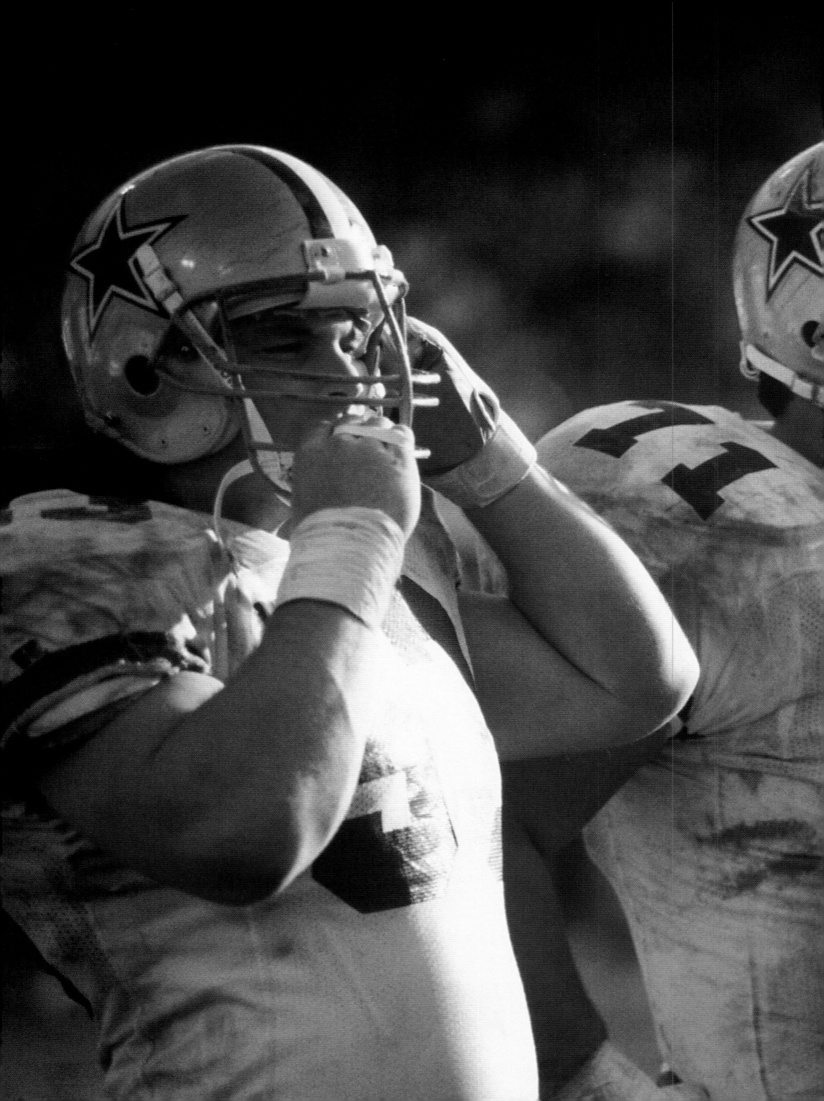

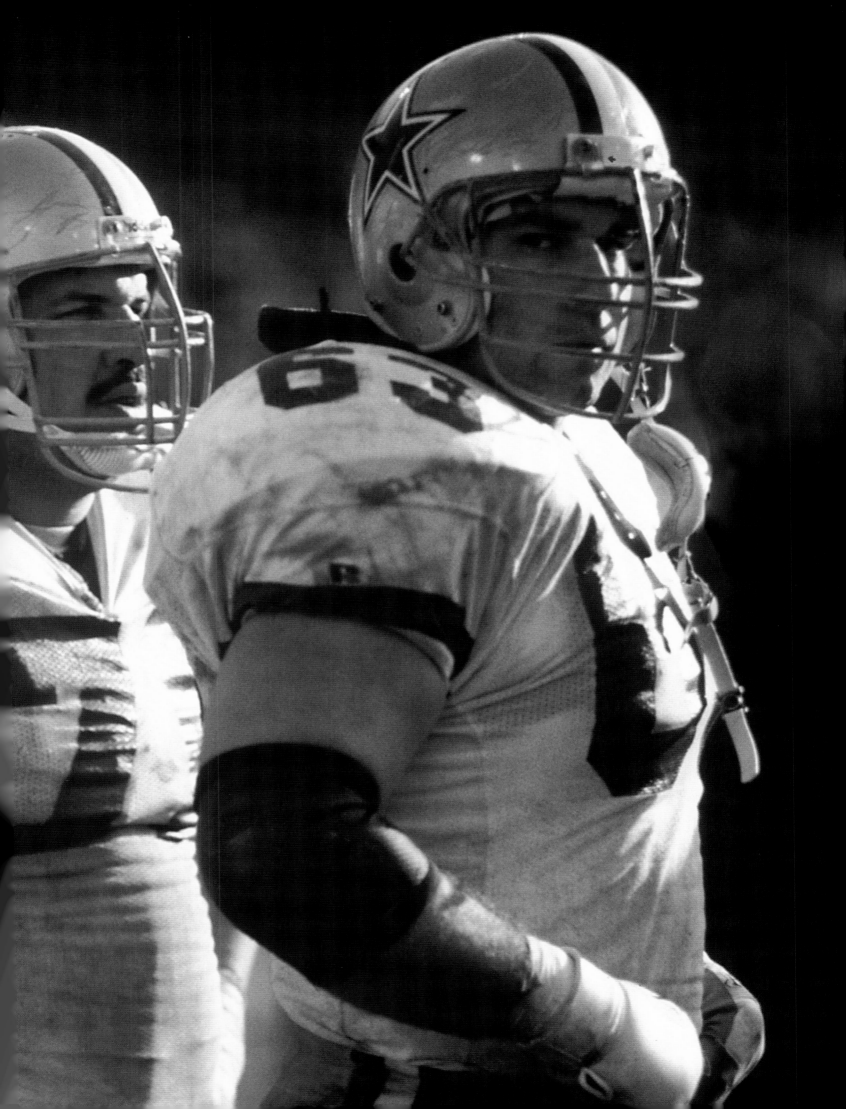

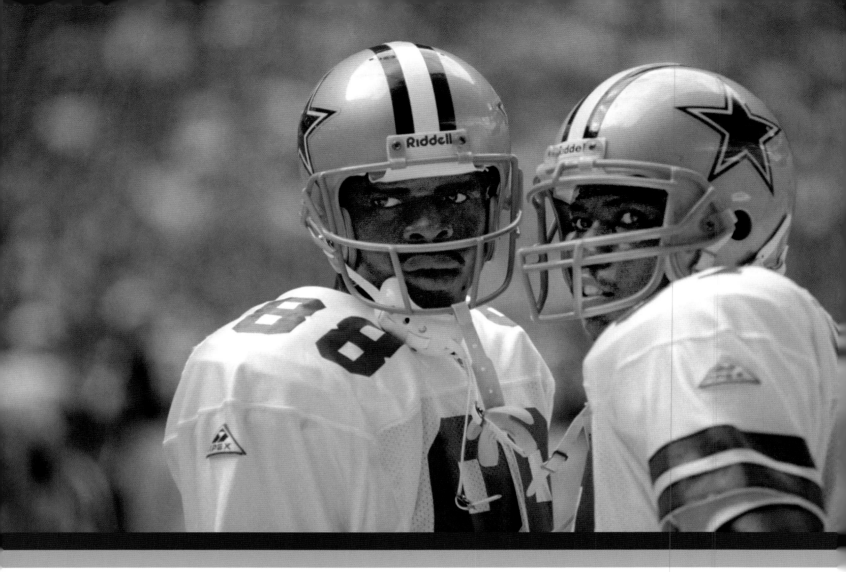
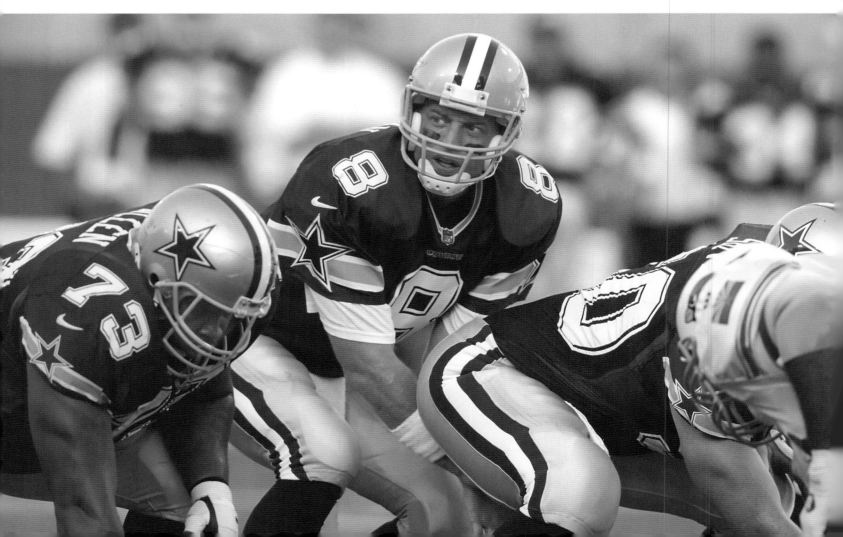

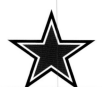
"LOAD LEFT"

Often a game, sometimes an entire season, occasionally a team's sense of worth and, once in a blue moon, the perception of a coach's competence can hinge on the outcome of a single play.

On this blustery, cold-all-the-way-down-to-your-soul afternoon at "the Vet" in Philadelphia, the Cowboys and Barry Switzer reached such a moment.

Dallas, needing a win desperately to clinch the NFC East and stay a game ahead of the Forty-niners in the battle for playoff home-field advantage, reached fourth down with a foot to go at their own 29-yard line. Game tied at 17-17. Fourth quarter. The clock ticking toward the two-minute warning. What would Dallas do? Punt or go for it?

Forget everything that had happened in the game so far. Forget the way the Cowboys dominated the contest in the first half, leading 17–3 at one point. Forget Philly's gritty 64-yard drive in the last fifty-eight seconds of the half culminating in a field goal and giving the Eagles desperately needed momentum as they headed into the locker room. Forget Philly's crucial two-point conversion after a touchdown late in the third quarter that narrowed Dallas' margin to 17–14. Forget that, just as the Cowboys appeared on the verge of putting the game out of reach, Emmitt Smith, who earlier in the season had stretched his incredible string of carries and receptions without a fumble to an astonishing 761, suddenly coughed up the ball at the Eagles' five.

Forget all of that. As time leaked away Barry Switzer had a choice—gamble or punt.

As for the season to this point, stow away memories of the mounting criticism of Switzer by fans and media. Complaints had become so pronounced that Jerry Jones felt compelled to announce, during the season, that win or lose he would not change head coaches. Put aside the public rift between quarterback Troy Aikman and Switzer over the team's level of discipline (or lack thereof). Inside the Cowboys nation, pain lingered from their agonizing loss to San Francisco in the NFC championship battle eleven months earlier. Most still blamed Switzer and Jones for the defeat that wiped out Dallas' shot at an unprecedented third consecutive Super Bowl triumph. The blown-out Achilles tendon of star cornerback Kevin Smith in the first game of the season; the substance abuse suspensions of defensive tackle Leon Lett and defensive back Clayton Holmes; the back injury that threatened the career of pass rusher Charles Haley—all of it, everything, was now simply background.

As the clock ticked toward two minutes, the time for Switzer's choice drew near.

In the few seconds that followed the third-and-10 Aikman pass to Cory Fleming that left the Cowboys oh so close to a first down, the head coach and his staff had to weigh the pluses and minuses for both options—to punt or to gamble.

The "punt people" called for booting it away and playing defense, thus hoping to hold the Eagles and force overtime.

On two previous kicks into the fierce (approximately twenty miles per hour) wind, Dallas had netted about 25 yards of difference in field position. A similar punt would leave Philly around their 45-yard line at the two-minute warning. The Eagles would need to gain one first down and about 20 yards to put Gary Anderson in long field goal range.

The Birds' offense had managed a first down and an advance of at least 20 yards only once in three possessions with the wind at their backs in the quarter, so far.

This conservative approach called for Dallas to rely on its highly acclaimed defense. Besides, "the punt people" reasoned, look at the terrible consequences of going for it and *failing*. That would immediately leave the Eagles easily within range of a winning field goal. And, even if Dallas picked up the first down on the fourth and a foot, the Cowboys had no intentions of trying to hurry into field goal position themselves. They'd only try to kill the rest of regulation time.

Finally, they ominously pointed out, the Eagles that afternoon had already stuffed Dallas in four previous third- or fourth- and short-yardage situations. Their

"Everyone of them was for going for it. Every damn one of them."

argument could be summed up easily—was the moderate reward worth the enormous risk?

The case presented by the "let's go for it people" can be summarized much more succinctly by Switzer himself. "I wanted to make a foot to control the ball because if we kick into the wind they're going to come back and kick the field goal to win anyway."

Barry Switzer it turned out, would be a member of the "let's go for it" group. Switzer made the above statement during the Cowboys' post-game press conference. In the broadcast booth TV analyst John Madden "first guessed" the decision. "Punt! That's the play you have to make. The score is tied. It's the fourth quarter. I don't think there is any other play."

Dallas decided to gamble and go for the foot needed by executing their best short-yardage play—"load left." The play sent MVP runner Emmitt Smith behind Pro Bowl blocking fullback Daryl Johnston at a hoped-for hole in the left side of the line created by Pro Bowl left guard Nate Newton and Pro Bowl left tackle Mark Tuinei. Later, running backs coach Joe Brodsky revealed that in Smith's six seasons as a Dallas star, "load left" had succeeded 94 percent of the time.

Aikman took the snap, handed the ball to Emmitt Smith and SPLAT! An Eagle avalanche landed on Smith. Load left had failed.

But wait! Whistles sounded. Like a governor's last-minute phone call staying the execution of a condemned

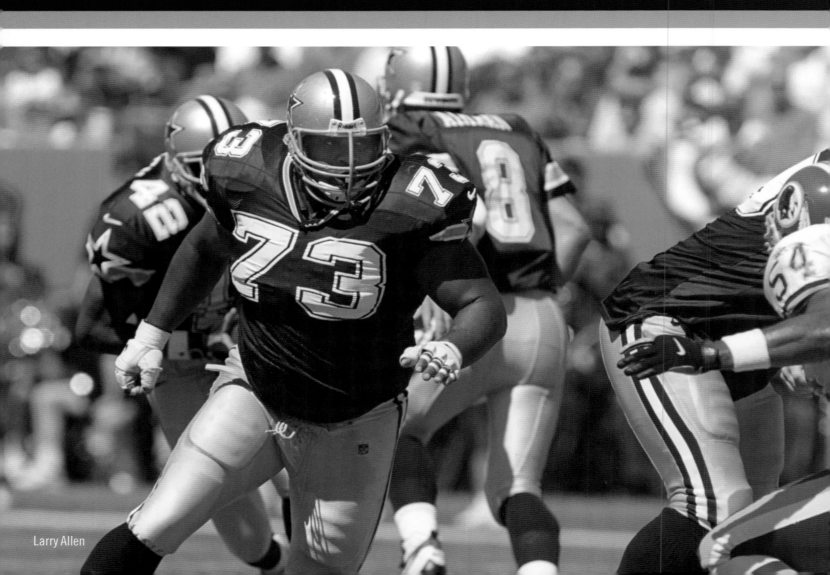

Larry Allen

man, the clock gave Dallas a reprieve. Referee Ed Hochuli ruled the Cowboys' snap had taken place a fraction of a second *after* the automatic stoppage of play for the two-minute warning.

The Cowboys now had two, maybe three, minutes to reconsider any possible error of their ways. While the network telecast sold beer, cars, and insurance, Dallas had ample time to revisit the "punt or gamble" question.

Switzer: "Every one of them was for going for it. Every damn one of them . . . I wish it would have been fourth and one because I'd have punted. But it was fourth and *inches*. Well, after you go for it the first time and don't make it, do I turn to my team and say 'Well, I don't have any confidence in you?' That's what you're saying to them if you punted it then. Hell, they still wanted to go for it so—we go for it."

After the game, to a man, the Cowboys verified Switzer's account. Everyone wanted to gamble again. About that there is, even today, still a kind of team unity.

Aikman: "I know Barry got killed on that deal but I still think it was the right call. I was for going for it."

But now, about that play selection. Switzer settled on the SAME call! "Load left"—take two. That's where the second guessers emerged.

Johnston: "I'm going, 'Don't do this.' Not the same play. They had seven guys at the point of attack and we're doing the same thing?"

Newton: "Troy's calling the play, and I kinda peeked back behind me. The Eagles, they ain't even in their huddle. They kinda know where we're gonna line up. It's like four friggin' Eagles are already standing in the hole."

Johnston: "You're just hoping Troy is gonna say, 'This isn't right.' Call a time out. Explain your point. Hey, we'll do this, but give us a different play."

Newton: "All we had to do was just fake load left and toss it to the tight end on the right side. He'd been wide open for a TD."

Should Aikman have changed the play at the line of scrimmage? Could he have? Did he have the freedom to audible into a different call?

Switzer: "No, we never did anything like that. This was the play we were going with—period!"

Philly safety Greg Jackson: "I saw them come out and I told the guys, 'Watch out. They're trying to draw us offsides.' Then I see the tight end go in motion and I say to myself 'I don't believe it. They're actually gonna run this play.'"

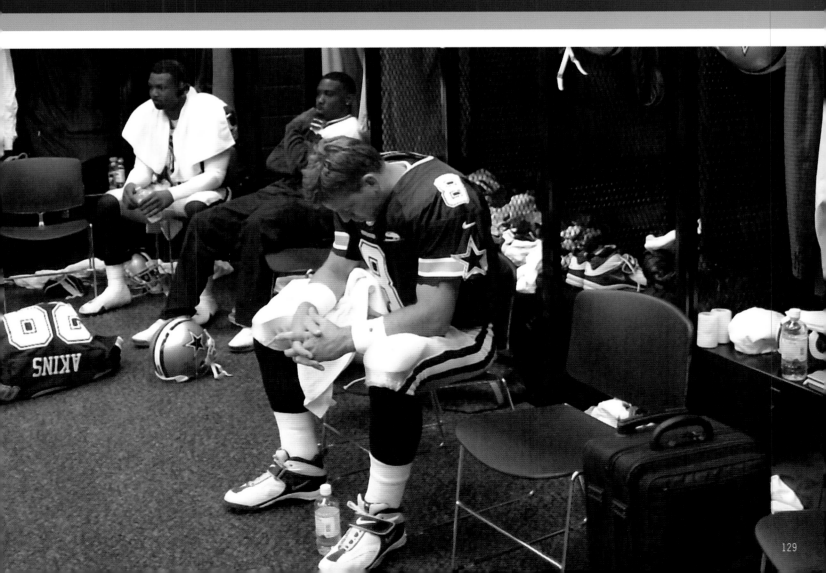

On center Derek Kennard's snap, Eagles linebacker Bill Romanowski stuffed the hole countering Johnston's lead block. The Philly defense converged on Smith. Defensive tackle Andy Harmon, middle linebacker Kurt Gouveia, Smith, and several other bodies formed a huge pile. The ball never got back to the line of scrimmage much less the required foot beyond it.

Philadelphia nudged the ball four yards forward on three running plays before kicker Anderson nailed the 41-yarder. Dallas still had 1:26 left, but their drive and the game ended on a sack of Aikman at the Dallas 45.

"They deserve to lose," was analyst Madden's blunt summary. A coast-to-coast cascade of criticism descended on Switzer.

The *New York Post* headline screamed: "Bozo the Coach."

Newsday: "It's a No-Brainer"

Philadelphia Daily News: "Thank You Barry Much"

Former coach turned analyst Mike Ditka: "It was a sequel to *Dumb and Dumber*."

Fox TV's Terry Bradshaw: "I wouldn't be surprised if Barry Switzer is fired after this season."

Bill Lyon's column in the *Philadelphia Inquirer* began thusly: "So little Barry Switzer is in school and he goes to the blackboard and writes 2+2=5. And the teacher says, 'No, Barry, that's wrong. Here's the eraser.' And Barry says, 'No, it's right, I'll show you again.'"

Even the host of the home finance show that followed the post-game programming on KRLD, the Cowboys' flagship station, implored callers still angry at Switzer to stop calling *his* show.

Meanwhile, back in a locker room Johnston described as "the quietest I've ever heard," Switzer explained and re-explained his decision while Jones and several players defended the coach. There was, however, no mistaking the mood of a Cowboys team that had now lost three of five and had surrendered the precious rights to home-field advantage in post-season.

Emmitt Smith, at times close to tears: "The morale is low. I don't know what to say. I'm not sure about a lot of things. I'm sorry. I wasted your time. I don't know nothin'."

Tuinei: "Nobody can pinpoint the problem. It's more a dumbfounded look. Like 'What's happened to us?'"

Johnston: "I think we all realized that we were in trouble."

Deion Sanders: "It's not Barry's fault. We need an *inch*. If we can't get a damn inch, we've got a problem."

Switzer tried to rally his army: "Right now it's more important than at any time that we've ever been together that we understand that it's us against everybody outside this room."

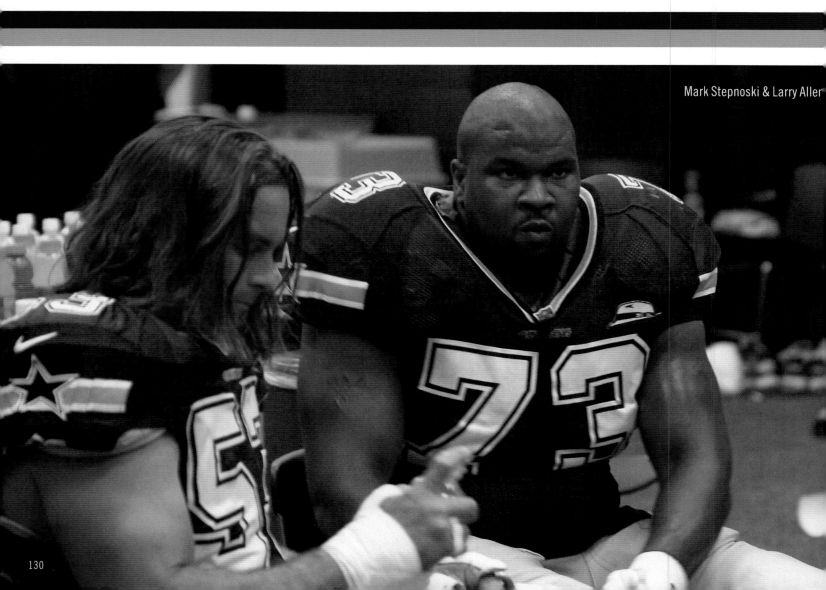

Mark Stepnoski & Larry Allen

"Right now it's more important than at any time that we've ever been together that we understand that it's us against everybody outside this room."

So many years have slipped away since "Coach Bozo's" pair of failed "load left" calls. Time for Barry Switzer to do what he always seems ready to do—to laugh at himself and all's that's happened to him. To this day people still ask about that downer of an afternoon in the City of Brotherly Love.

"I look at them and start grinning when they bring it up," Switzer chuckles. "And I say, 'Hey, by the way, who won the Super Bowl that year?'"

But how could that self-doubting Dallas team, seemingly in turmoil after flopping in Philly, have ever foreseen that? How could they have ever dreamed that they would never lose again for the rest of that season?

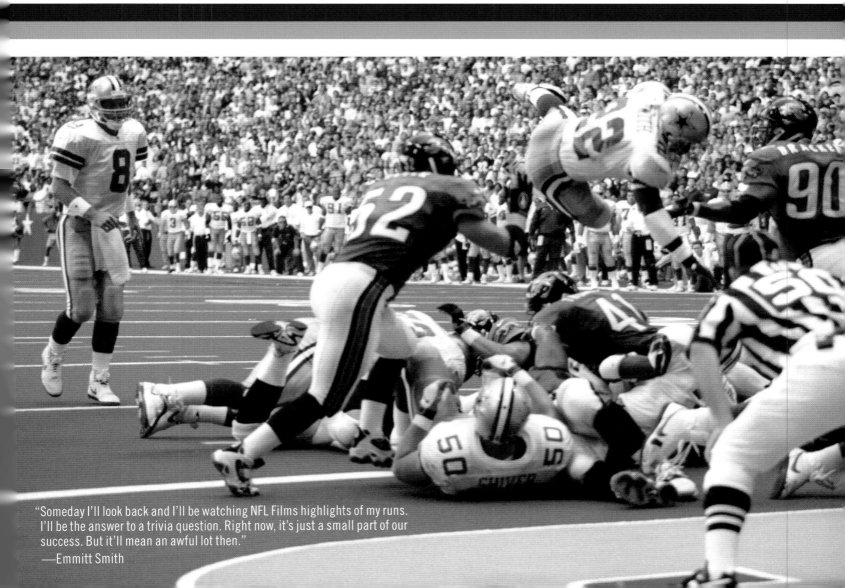

"Someday I'll look back and I'll be watching NFL Films highlights of my runs. I'll be the answer to a trivia question. Right now, it's just a small part of our success. But it'll mean an awful lot then."
—Emmitt Smith

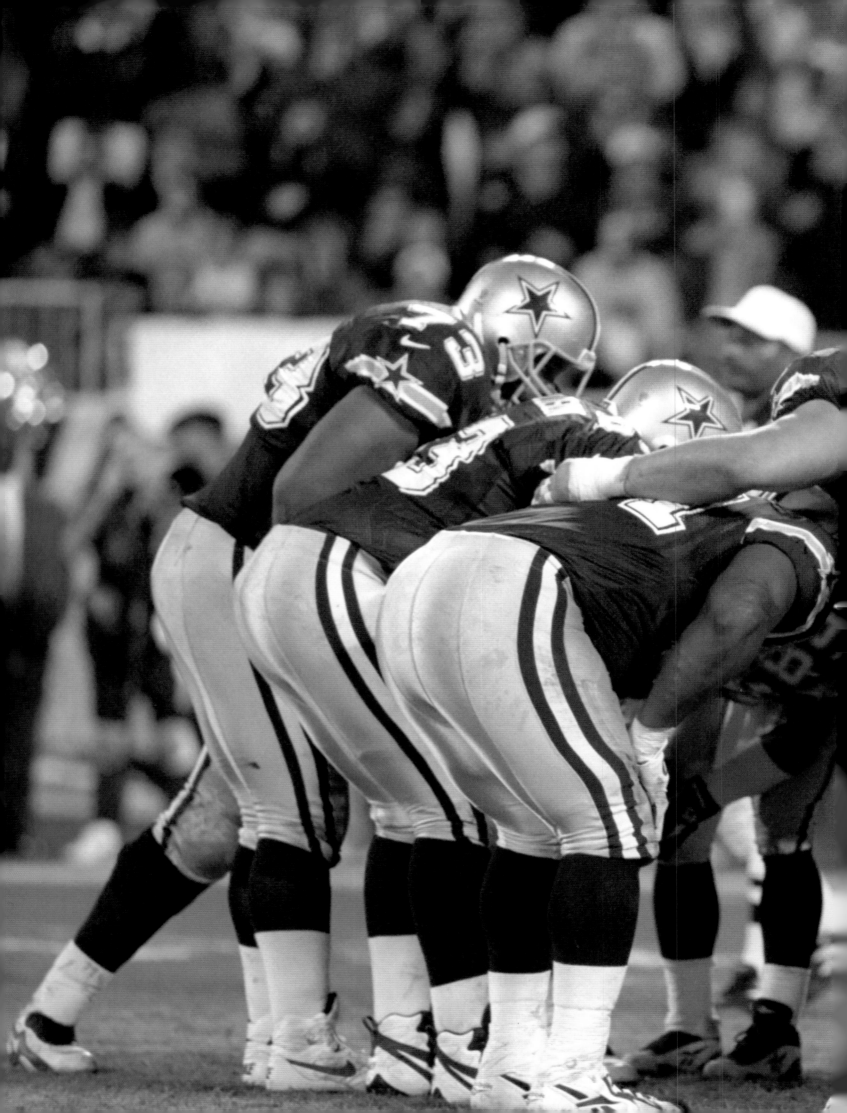

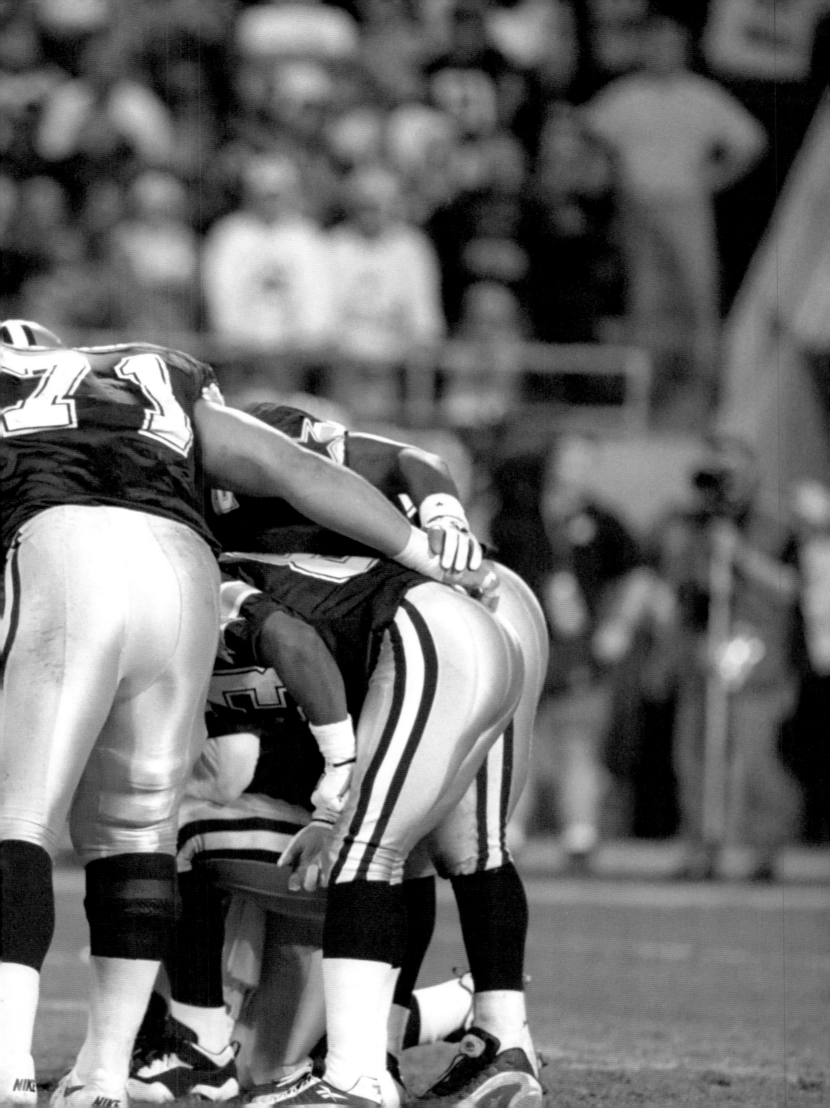

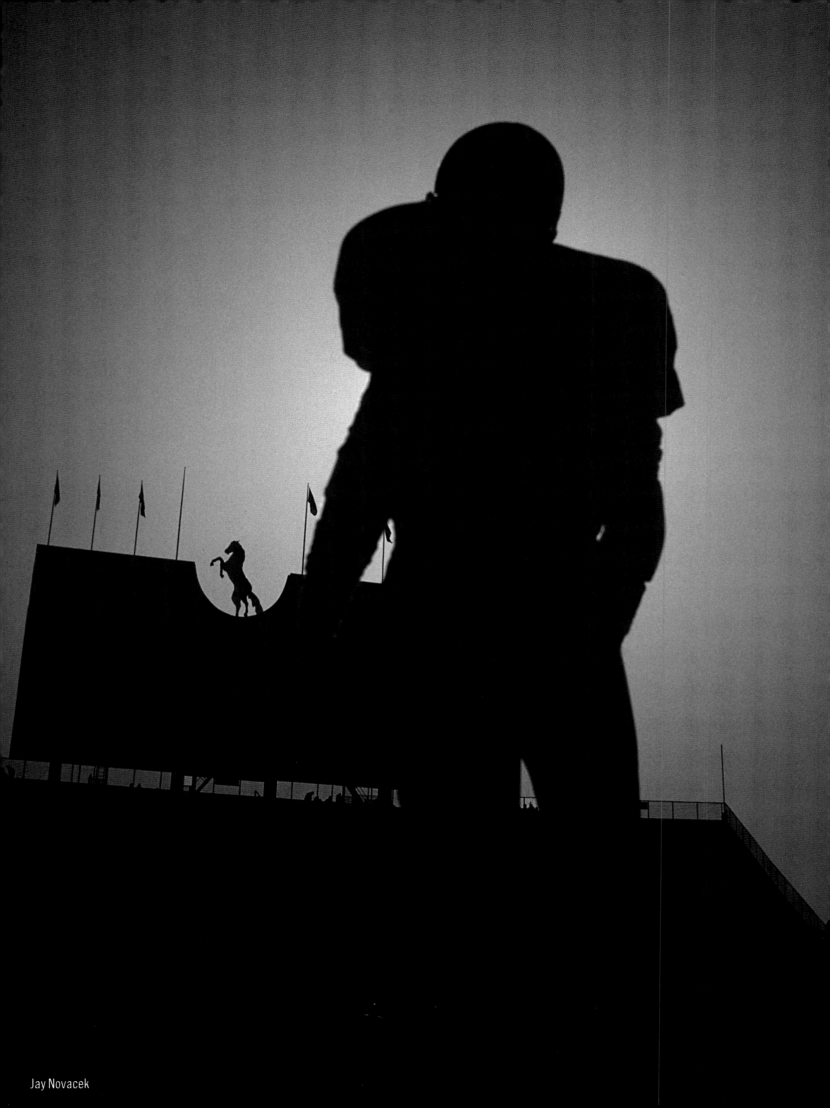

Jay Novacek

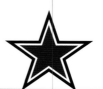

BARRY BARES HIS SOUL

For three days Barry Switzer had lived in the eye of a hurricane of controversy and criticism for his twice-failed "load left" play calls late in the fourth quarter of a costly 20–17 defeat in Philadelphia the previous Sunday.

In coaching "America's Team" Switzer had naturally become "America's Dummy"—a punchline for late-night TV talk-show jokes. They called him a "hood ornament" and described his questionable play selection as "Switzercide." One national commentary on the game began thusly:

"Admittedly, there may have been worse decisions made in the annals of time. The Edsel. The leisure suit. Adam biting the apple."

Even the governor of Texas and future president of the United States zinged Switzer. During a news conference with reporters discussing his views on Medicaid, someone asked George W. Bush for his quickie opinion: "I'd have punted, of course," "W" replied.

Success has an endless number of fathers. Failure is a bastard child. The court of public opinion placed all the blame for bungling in Philly on Switzer.

While the constant and savage level of the bombardment amazed many observers, Switzer appeared to weather the storm reasonably well. After all, he'd survived days far more troubled than these. Like this excerpt from page 57 of Switzer's autobiography *Bootlegger's Boy*:

Mother came in and sat on the bed. I didn't totally understand the hell she was living through . . . she loved me and she needed my love so much, but, as I looked at her sitting there on the bed kind of glassy and smiling, loaded on prescription drugs and booze, something broke inside of me and I said things I will always regret.

I said, "Mother, I would rather not ever see you again and know that you are safe, than to see you like this all the time."

She leaned over to kiss me.

I turned my head away.

She looked at me and got up, went to the closet and took out a pistol. I don't know why I didn't jump up and take the gun from her. She walked out of the room and started toward the back porch. I don't know why I didn't call out for her to come back.

I heard the shot.

I leaped out of bed, ran down the hall, and saw her body on the back porch. I picked her up, carried her into the house, and laid her in bed.

I have carried this guilt with me the rest of my life. Professional people, psychiatrists, have told me I was not to blame, that she had made up her mind to do it and the right time had presented itself, but still I've never been able to forget turning my face away."

Switzer had experienced, and will always be hounded by, regrets far greater than some shaky decision in some football game. But for Barry the time had come to convey that sense of context to a really good Cowboys team that seemed to be foundering in a sea of doubt. A doubt in themselves and particularly in him.

On Wednesday, the beleaguered coach gathered his players before practice for an impassioned speech delivered Switzer style: "I've always been animated. I've been emotional. I don't prepare notes . . . maybe three or four points and then I go with it. I think you come across so much more genuine and sincere. That's the way I try to communicate."

Switzer began with memories of his Arkansas childhood. Of "driving my mother to the Cummins unit of the state penitentiary to see my daddy every other Sunday." Of growing up "with a tremendous inferiority complex." Of that day his mother Mary Louise killed herself. Memories of the death of his father, Frank, when the black women he was living with caught him with another woman and shot him.

"What the hell is losing a football game and the BS the media has given me!" Switzer roared. "Do you think this means anything to me? Hell no. I had things to prove all my life. That's where I come from. What they say about me now, it's nothing in comparison."

Switzer sought no sympathy. He desired only that his players hear one clear message.

"I wanted them to know I believed in them because I made that call," he said. "And I didn't give up on them, that's why I made it again. I believed in them and I wanted them

Even Troy Aikman, who'd crossed swords often with Switzer about a variety of matters, agrees the speech made an impact. That Switzer had read the mood of the team correctly. That, without that speech, who knows what might have become of that season.

"I think that's a fair assessment. We knew that this was a tough guy and regardless of whatever happens to this team or whatever happens to Barry, he's going to survive."

Once the meeting broke up, players spilled into the training room and to their

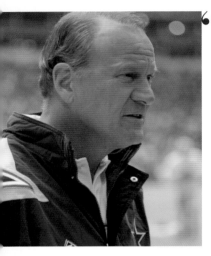

"Put it on me. I'm tough enough to handle it and if you don't think that, you don't know me."

to believe in me. I didn't turn on them, and I didn't want them to turn on me . . . 'Coaches make dumb mistakes, along with players who make dumb mistakes, but we win or lose together,' I told them. 'Don't let people outside this room, the media, affect where we are because we're still going to arrive where we want to arrive.'"

The words resonated with many Cowboys. Cornerback Larry Brown summed up the feelings of that group.

"I'm just paraphrasing here, but, when Barry said 'Put it on me. I'm tough enough to handle it and if you don't think that, you don't know me. Let me take the heat. Send the doubters to me.' I think the team needed that speech. It was heartfelt, on the spot. 'I love you guys. I care about you. I still believe in you.' I think that's when a lot of people (in that locker room) started believing in him."

individual cubicles. At that point Deion Sanders spoke up—loudly, so as to be heard in every corner. "Hey, coach, don't pay any attention to all that damn media out there. We lost with you. We had enough chances to win that ballgame. You didn't lose it, we lost it, and we want you to know that."

Eventually that day, Switzer wandered back to his office, where a clear block of crystal sat on his desk with these words inscribed on it: "There is no limit to what can be done if it doesn't matter who gets the credit."

Seven weeks later a Dallas team that had not lost since that "load left" debacle in Philadelphia would win Super Bowl XXX. And there would be plenty of credit to go around for everyone.

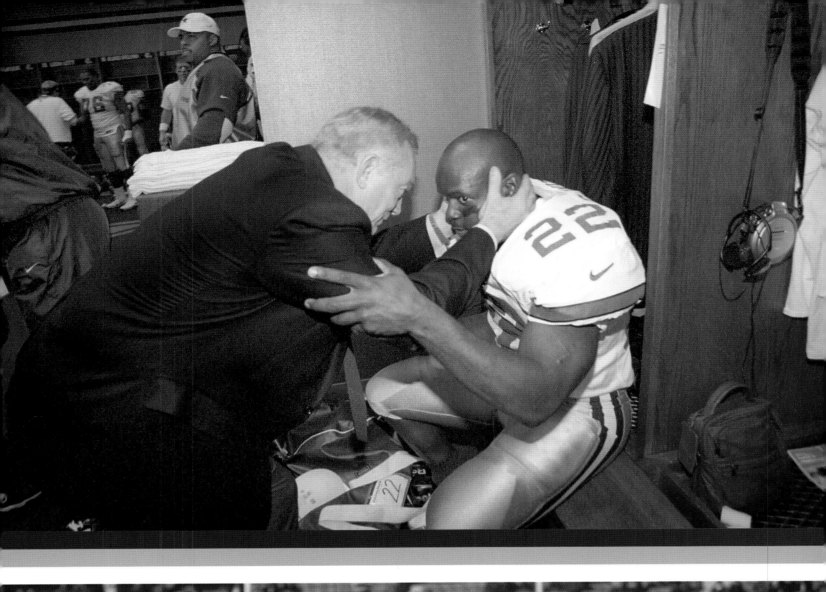
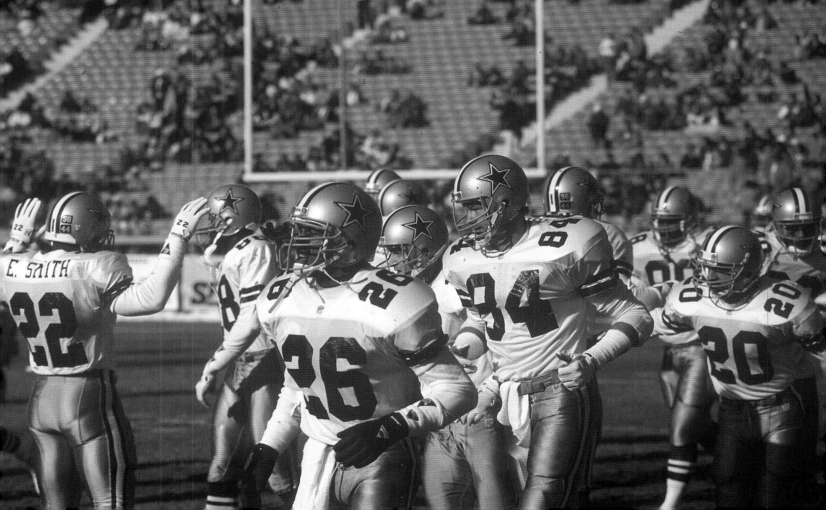

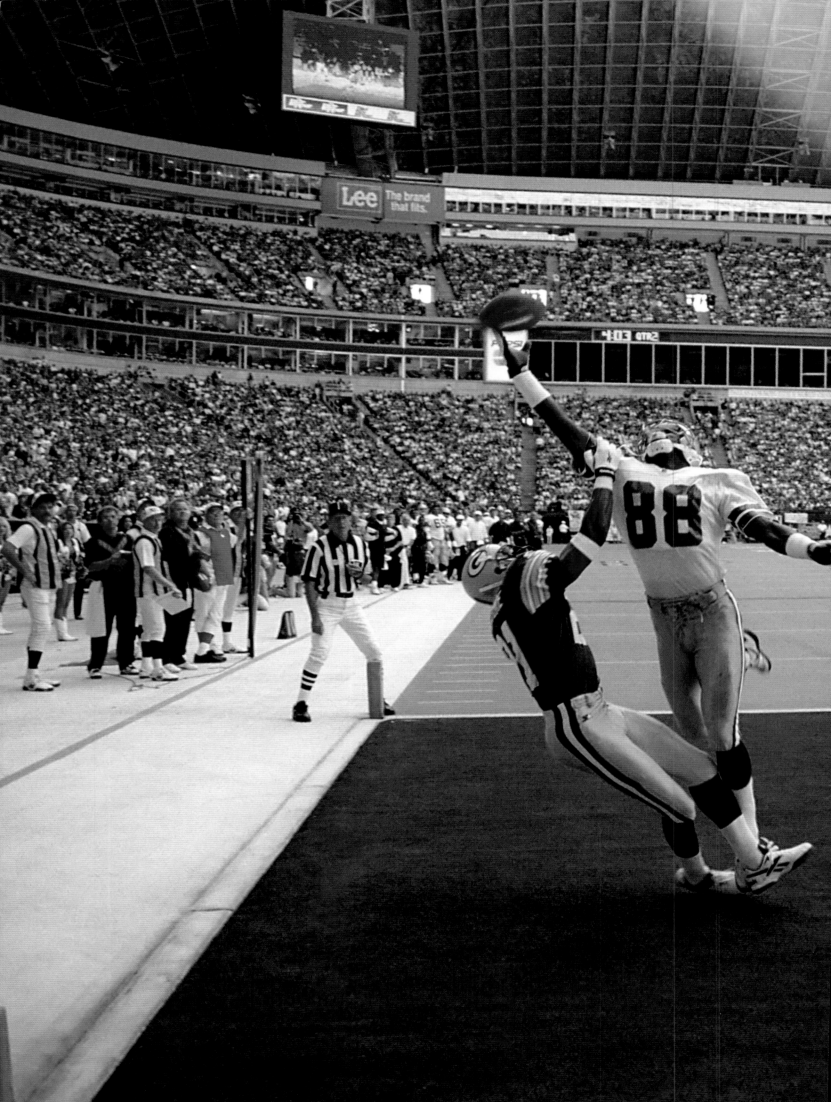

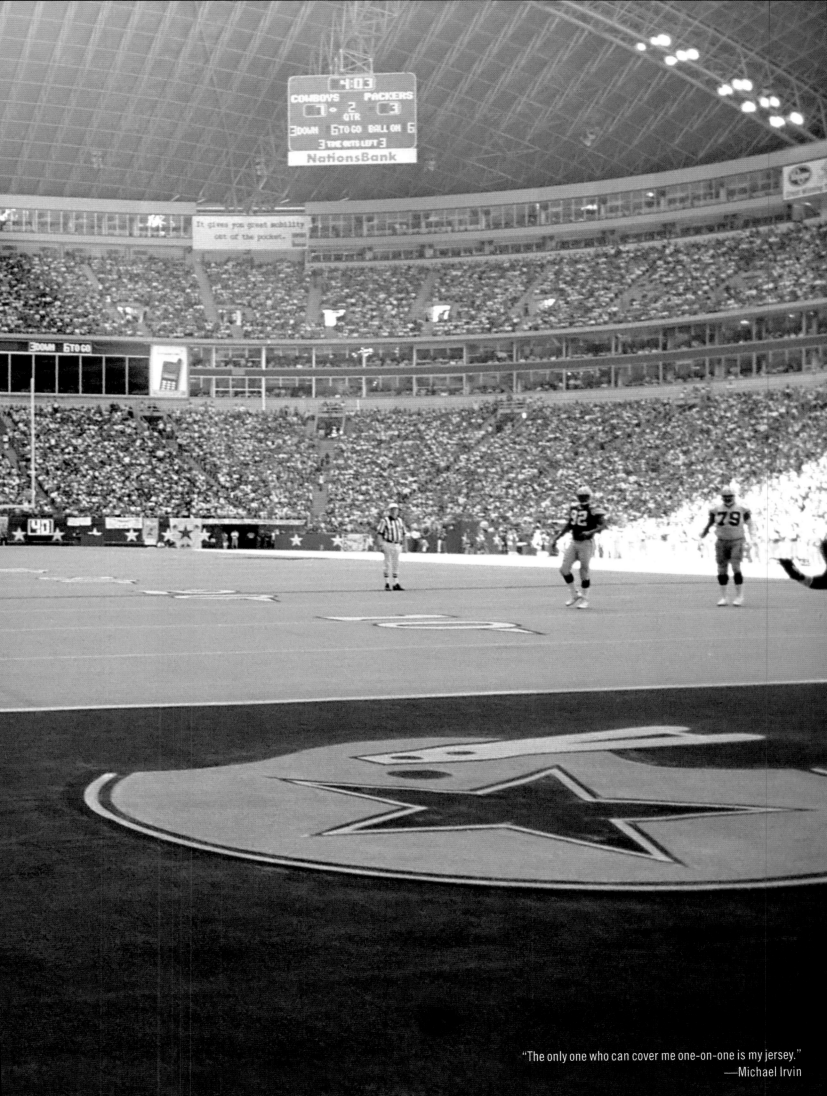

"The only one who can cover me one-on-one is my jersey."
—Michael Irvin

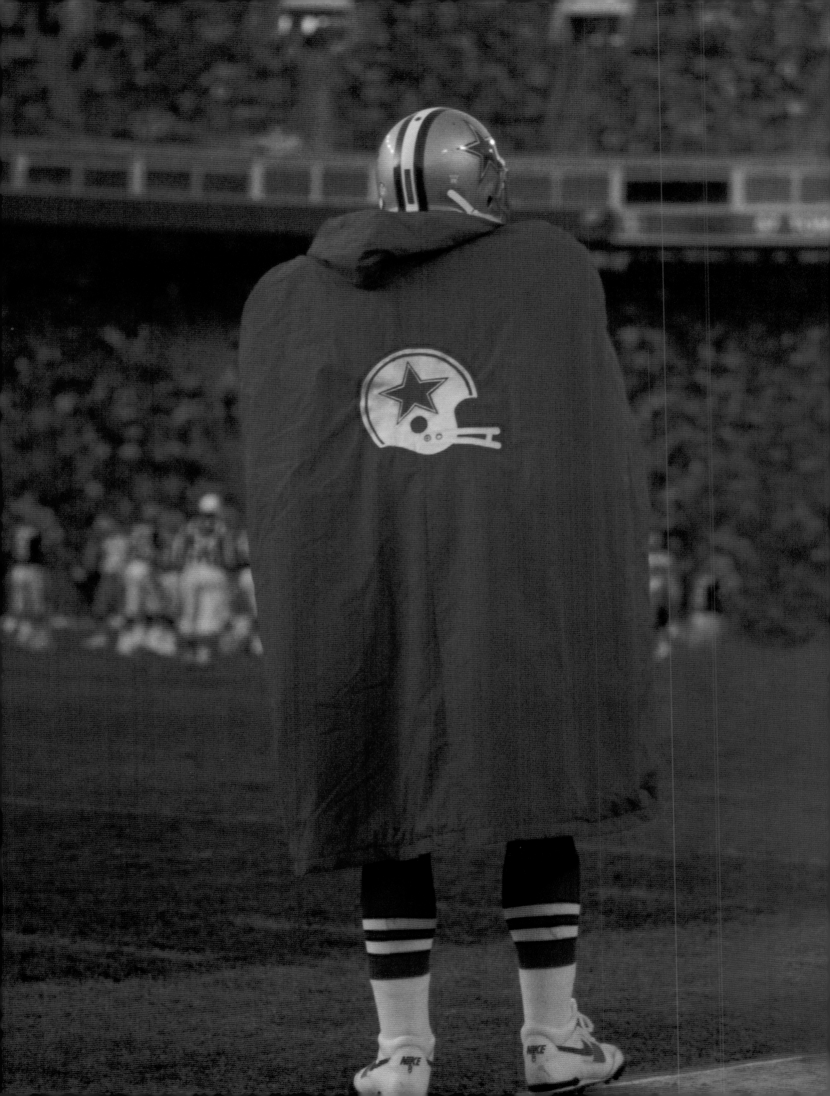

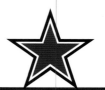

THE LOST 'BOYS

"No one felt good about anything."

Troy Aikman's simple statement summarized the somber mood of a Cowboys team boarding its Sunday afternoon charter flight for Arizona.

Dallas, at 11–4, appeared to have nothing to gain in their Monday Night Football clash with the Cardinals, the final game of the '95 regular season. They'd sewn up a fourth consecutive NFC East crown. Such a streak had been accomplished only once before in the history of the conference, and that was by the '76–'79 Cowboys.

Even if Dallas were to beat Arizona, the Niners would still wrap up homefield advantage throughout the playoffs if they could finish off Atlanta. San Francisco looked awesome. They'd blown Dallas away 38–20 at Texas Stadium six weeks ago. San Francisco had but one order of business left—whip an inferior Falcons team that Sunday afternoon and the road to Super Bowl XXX would go through San Francisco. Several starters—Aikman, Smith, et al—weren't certain they'd even suit up against 'Zona because a victory looked like it would do nothing to improve their playoff position.

That Cowboys team also brought aboard their team charter the baggage from another tumultuous season.

★ The rift between QB Aikman and Coach Switzer spilled out onto sports pages everywhere. Whispers suggested a disheartened Aikman felt Switzer had reneged on a promise to discipline the team more. In what amounted to a public threat, Aikman never specifically mentioned the coach, but his finger pointed directly at Switzer. "What I've always believed is that we all need to be committed to reaching our potential. For sixty minutes I get to do what I enjoy," Aikman said. "But this has not been an enjoyable year for me in regards to things off the field. If I ever feel there is not a commitment in this organization to win and do right, then I don't want to be a part of it."

★ Starting linebacker Darrin Smith refused to accept a Cowboys' contract offer. The team wouldn't budge. Half the season drained away before an unhappy Smith reported for duty.

★ The NFL sued Jerry Jones for $300 million, contending his Texas Stadium sponsorships with Pepsi and Nike conflicted with existing NFL deals.

★ Defensive end Charles Haley blasted Switzer for not starting him in two straight games, vowing to not play again after the season ended. A day later, Haley apologized and promised to honor his contract.

★ Switzer publicly ripped three defensive linemen—Haley, Tony Tolbert, and Leon Lett—for playing poor technique in a loss to Washington. A short time later, Switzer issued a public apology.

★ Cornerback Larry Brown's infant son, Kristopher, born several months premature, died in mid-November.

★ The NFL suspended cornerback Clayton Holmes for one year and defensive tackle Lett four games for violating the league's substance-abuse program.

★ Haley sustained another herniated disc in his back and announced his retirement. A day later, he changed his mind.

This was a distracted Cowboys team, 3–3 in its last six games and scoring just twenty-one points per game in that stretch. It was a beaten-up club that left four key starters behind in Dallas with injuries (Haley, middle linebacker Robert Jones, defensive tackle Russell Maryland and tight end Jay Novacek).

In mid-flight, at thirty thousand feet, their season turned around 180 degrees. The flight captain came on the intercom and announced that the ten-point underdog Atlanta Falcons had stunned the 49ers 28–27. That moment remains frozen in Aikman's mind. "We didn't think there was any way in hell the Falcons would win. I mean, the Falcons weren't all that good at the time," Aikman said. "All of a sudden the pilot comes on, and it was like a switch had gone off (or on) and all of a sudden the whole plane was excited, enthused. Now we were going to Arizona for a reason."

Switzer on his first thoughts: "We're coming home now! We got a chance to get 'em in *our* house! That made all the difference in the world to us."

Fullback "Moose" Johnston: "I've never seen a team get on a plane in one frame of mind and get off with such a different attitude. We got off knowing that if we win this game, we've got homefield advantage back, that, hey, we can still pull this thing out if we can win this game."

The Cardinals never got the license plate of the truck that hit them.

Six snaps into the game, all Aikman throws, Dallas forged ahead 7–0. Three plays later, Brock Marion intercepted a Dave Kreig pass and scooted 32 yards untouched. That made it 14–0. Dallas' banged-up defense forced a three-and-out. The offense drove 52 yards for a Chris Boniol field goal. Twelve eighteen gone. Dallas 17–Arizona 0.

Whatever the mystical something Dallas had lost, wherever their train had run off the tracks, the Cowboys had rediscovered themselves. Whatever *it* was—Dallas had *it* back.

Some team and NFL record-breaking was all that remained on the Cowboys' things-to-do list. Midway through the fourth quarter Emmitt Smith finished off an 82-yard drive by ramming in from three yards out. Smith's twenty-sixth touchdown of the year:

★ Broke the all-time NFL record for touchdowns in a single season.

★ Tied his Cowboys mark of eleven consecutive games with a score.

★ Tied the legendary Jim Brown as the fastest player to reach one hundred touchdowns in a career—ninety-three games.

★ Earlier that night, Smith had also shattered his single-season Cowboys rushing record with 1,773 yards.

Sunday, on that exuberant ride from the Arizona airport to the team hotel, two joyful, excited men, Jerry Jones and Barry Switzer, sat next to each other at the front of the bus. In thirty-

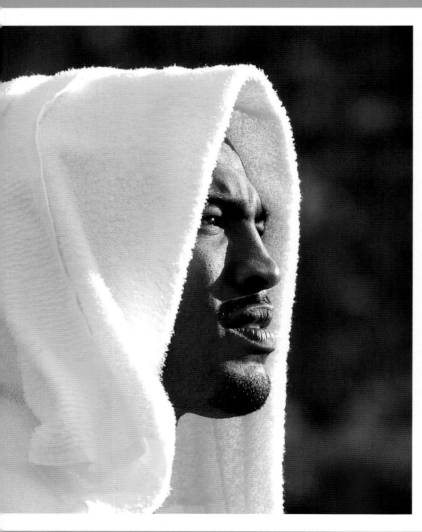
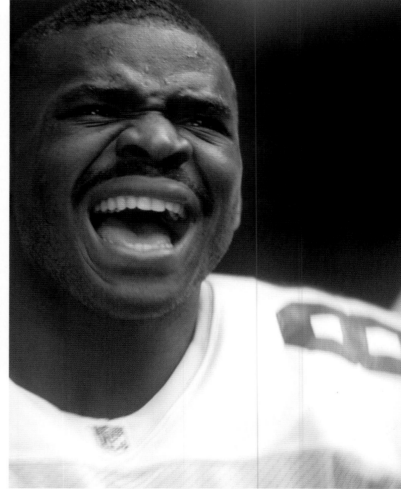

"We're coming home now! We got a chance to get 'em in our house! That made all the difference in the world to us."

five days, Arizona's Sun Devil Stadium would be the site of Super Bowl XXX.

"We pull out of the airport and we're drivin' along and we spotted this nice looking little place to have a cold beer," Jones recalls. "And we both looked at each other and said, 'When we get back here for the Super Bowl, we're gonna go to that place right there and have a cold beer.'

Less than five weeks later, Jones and Switzer had that cold beer.

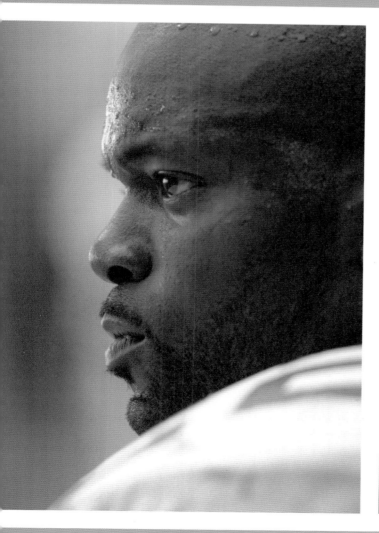

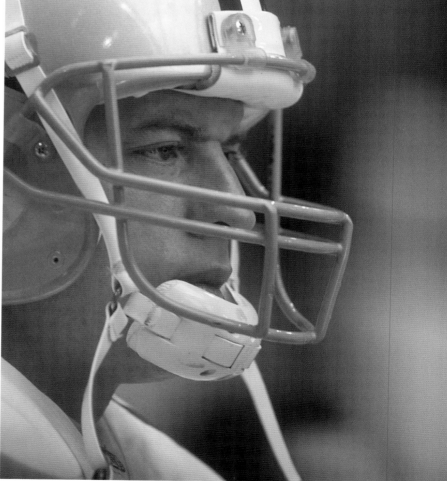

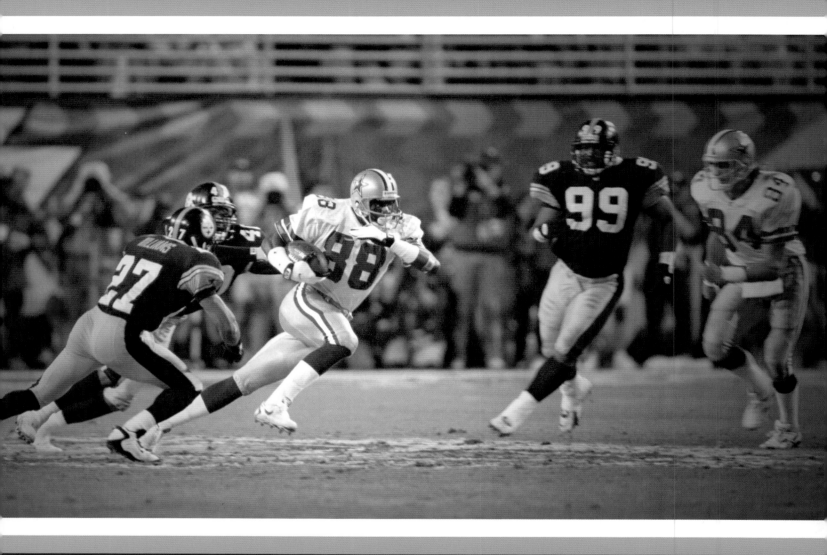

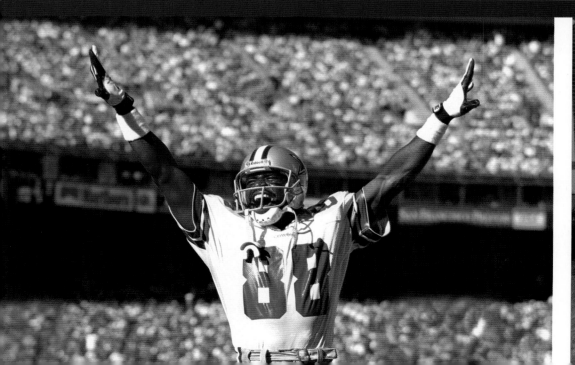

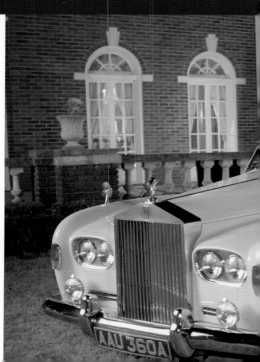

MICHAEL IRVIN

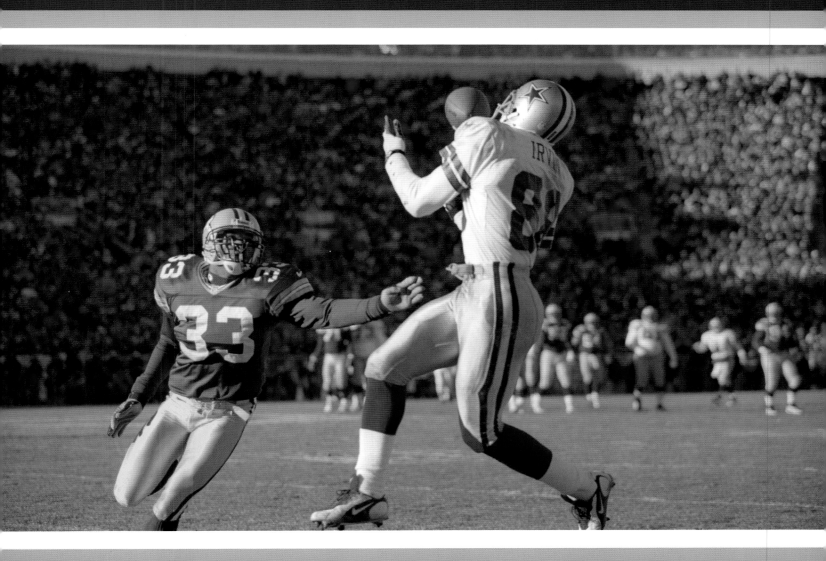

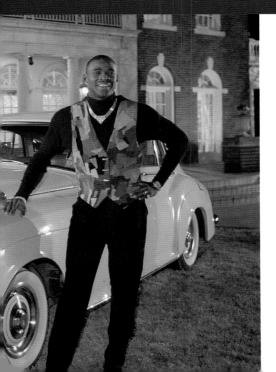

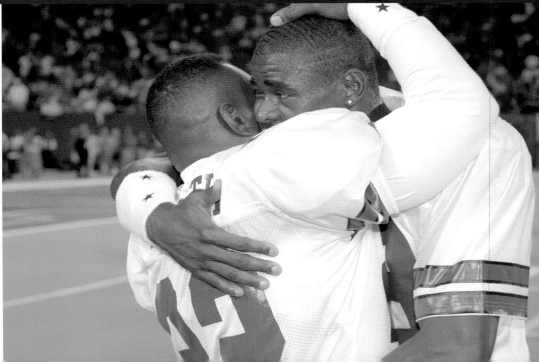

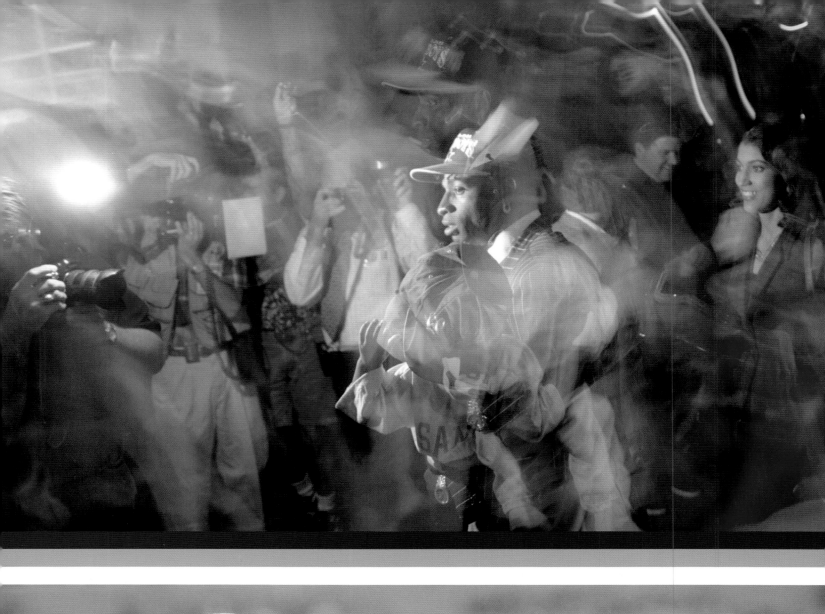
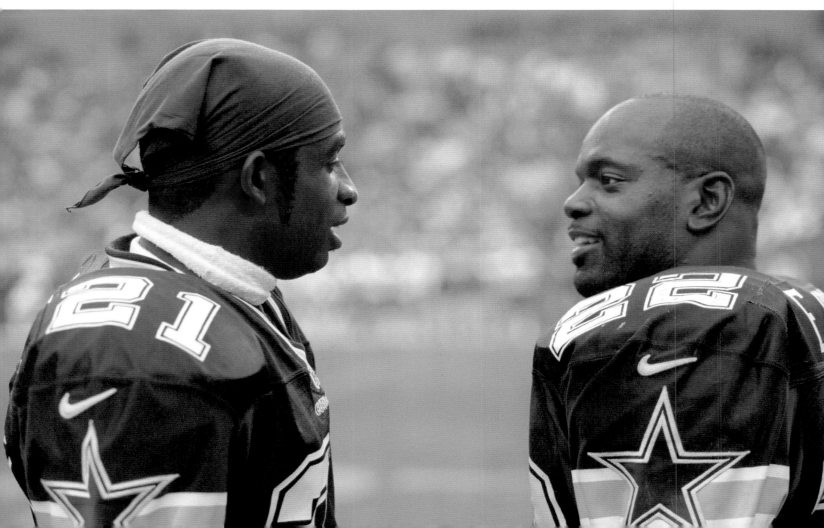

PRIME TIME

The week of the Dallas vs. Philadelphia NFC semifinal battle began with all eyes on Cowboys Coach Barry Switzer. It ended with all those eyes on Deion Sanders.

Just twenty-eight days earlier Switzer'd become a kind of NFLJ—National Football League Joke. In Philly, with two minutes left in the game, the score tied at 17-17, Switzer had opted to go for it on fourth and a foot at his own 29 rather than punt. The play—Load Left—failed. But the Gods of football smiled on Dallas and Switzer, allowing them a do over. The Cowboys' snap had come a fraction of a second after the two-minute warning whistle. The Pokes, with minutes during the timeout to mull over their options, decided to go for it again and with the very same play call—Load Left. The Eagles stuffed the Emmitt Smith run again. Philly took over already in field goal range and won 20-17.

"Bozo the Clown" . . . "Dumb and Dumber" the national headlines cried. Cowboys fans called for Switzer's head and even more sensitive body parts. Now four weeks later, Dallas and Switzer got a do-over. In the week prior to this Eagles-Cowboys playoff show-down, "load left" was getting replayed hundreds of times. Every TV report, newspaper story and radio talk show unloaded on the "load left" decision. In the eye of this storm, Switzer tried to shrug off that nightmare and focus on the Sunday ahead: "It's a different game. A different story. A different situation."

Much truth lay in Switzer's observation. This Sunday Philly would stand toe-to-toe with a rejuvenated Cowboys team. Their season-ending destruction of Arizona, coupled with San Francisco's upset loss to Atlanta, meant Dallas owned homefield advantage throughout the playoffs. The bye week gave time to heal key injured starters such as Jay Novacek, Robert Jones, and Russell Maryland.

Sunday dawned with frigid Philly-like weather. It was bitterly cold. Twenty-six degrees. A fourteen-mile-an-hour wind. Wind chill of two. It was then and still remains the coldest Cowboys home game ever.

The miserable conditions made passing difficult and field goal kicking iffy, and sitting in the stands was way beyond uncomfortable. A three-dog *day*, if you will.

The archrivals were tied 3-3 early in the second quarter. The Eagles, however, had lost starting quarterback Rodney Peete, who the season before had been Troy Aikman's backup in Dallas. Peete, diving to reach the first down sticks deep in Cowboys territory, got KO'ed by a thunderous but very clean collision with Darren Woodson.

Peete's lunge fell inches short. Fourth down and very short. Eagles Coach Ray Rhodes, perhaps mindful of Dallas' "load left" debacle of a month earlier, opted to not gamble and settled for the field goal that made it 3-3. A chance for Philly momentum had been lost. Within minutes all Eagles hopes would crater.

The moment arrived for the Cowboys $35 million man to shine. "Neon Deion" . . . "Prime Time."

Deion Sanders had joined the lineup in late October as the Cowboys "shutdown" corner. He'd also been used sparingly on offense. In '96 Sanders would become the first NFL player in thirty-four years to start regularly on both offense (wide receiver) and defense (cornerback). But, here, four minutes deep into the second quarter, Dallas fans, Cowboys bashers, critics of owner Jerry Jones, the entire NFL nation witnessed why a desperate Jones had showered Sanders with all that cash.

Dallas drove to a first down at the Philly 21. Sanders trotted out to join the offensive huddle and lined up in the right slot. The Dallas sidelines relayed the play call to Aikman—Fake Tailback Jab Right Z Reverse Left. Aikman faked a handoff to Smith up the middle. Sanders hesitated a fraction of a second then sprinted left taking the Aikman handoff. At this point a real problem popped up for Dallas. Their trickery had fooled *nobody*. The be-alert-for-Sanders Eagles recognized the play immediately. Left defensive end Mike Mamula darted up field and had Sanders dead-to-rights deep behind the line of scrimmage. But the time for "Prime Time" was upon us.

Sanders slammed on the brakes and juked the Philly defender. Mamula tackled air. Sanders reversed field. Smith threw a downfield block. Michael Irvin cleared out cornerback Bobby Taylor at the three. Sanders flew into the right corner of the end zone. With the TOUCHDOWN, "Prime Time" became the first, and, still, only, NFL player to ever score touchdowns six different ways—by rushing, pass receiving, punt return, kickoff return, fumble return and interception return. Sanders chicken danced to celebrate.

Less than seven minutes later, Smith plunged in from the one. The Cowboys headed to their locker room with a 17-3 halftime lead after playing perhaps their best half of football all season. In the opening thirty minutes, Dallas outgained the Eagles 158–87. The Cowboys had no interceptions, fumbles, blocked kicks, or sacks allowed. One penalty. One incomplete pass. It had been an "almost perfect" half.

had dogged him for four weeks. "That was a different situation. We kicked their butts today," Switzer said. "If we had played like that the last time, it wouldn't have come down to fourth and a foot. Let's bury that."

Switzer, however, had become yesterday's news. The spotlight now shined brightly on "Prime Time."

"It felt great to finally have a large impact on a game and to be fully utilized the way I want to," Sanders beamed. Then he fired back at naysayers who'd criticized his huge contract and the moderate contributions he'd made since his arrival. "Big guys have to come up in the big game. If we don't, you guys are damn sure going to let us know we're overpaid. All year supposedly I haven't earned a dime. But big guys have to set the tone in big games."

"Big guys have to come up in the big game."

Sanders tacked on a fourth quarter interception, a couple of punt returns, a 13-yard pass reception, three tackles, and one pass breakup before calling it a day.

One more flashback remained for that frigid afternoon for Switzer, however. Early in the third quarter, still up 17–3, Dallas drove to Philly's one-yard line. Fourth and one. Switzer had to make a choice. Go for it? Run "load left" again just to throw everything back into the faces of his legions of critics? Nope.

"We wanted the points—it's critical that the football team scores in that situation," Switzer explained.

Chris Boniol kicked the chip-shot field goal. Later in the quarter, he booted an outrageous (given the weather) 51-yarder, extending his Cowboys record streak to twenty-eight consecutive successful attempts.

Final score: 30-11.
Nothing to second guess.
No controversy.
No sweat.

Somewhere in the midst of the celebration, Switzer escaped the "load left" failure that

After the questions ended and the camera lights went dark, Sanders slipped into his green silk boxer shorts with dollar signs all over them. Pulled on his brown silk socks. Buttoned up his chocolate custom-made shirt with "Prime Time" embroidered on the cuff. Donned his mustard and brown plaid three-piece suit. Tied his alligator and suede shoes. Attached two gold and diamond encrusted earrings. Slipped on his gold and diamond watch as well as a thick gold necklace. Then, carrying his Louis Vuitton travel bag and flanked by bodyguards, he slipped out of the stadium to a waiting silver stretch limo and was gone.

That afternoon Green Bay bushwacked San Francisco in the other NFC semifinal. There would not be a fourth consecutive NFC championship war with the Niners.

Dallas had won at least one playoff game for a fifth consecutive season. No team in the nearly eighty-year history of pro football had ever accomplished that.

The 'Boys were back.

"Prime Time" arrived in Texas.

Switzer had *left* that four-week-old *load* behind him.

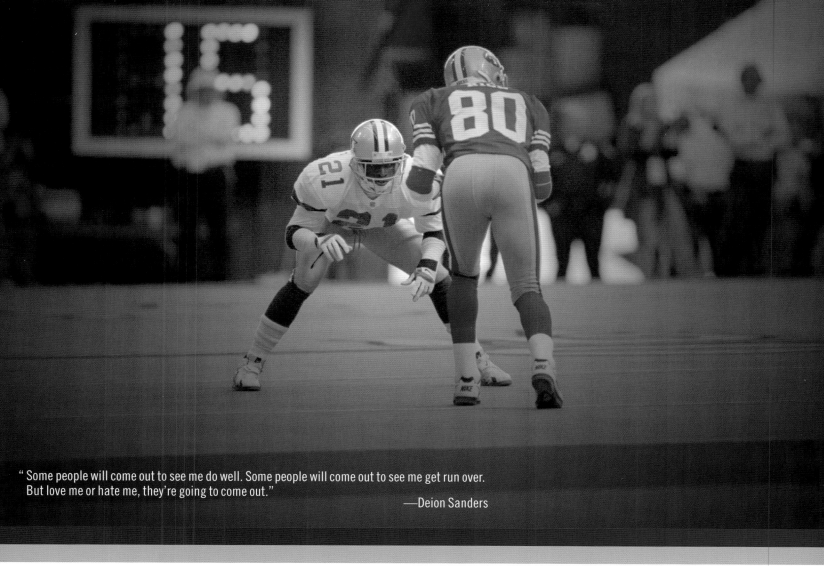

" Some people will come out to see me do well. Some people will come out to see me get run over.
But love me or hate me, they're going to come out."

—Deion Sanders

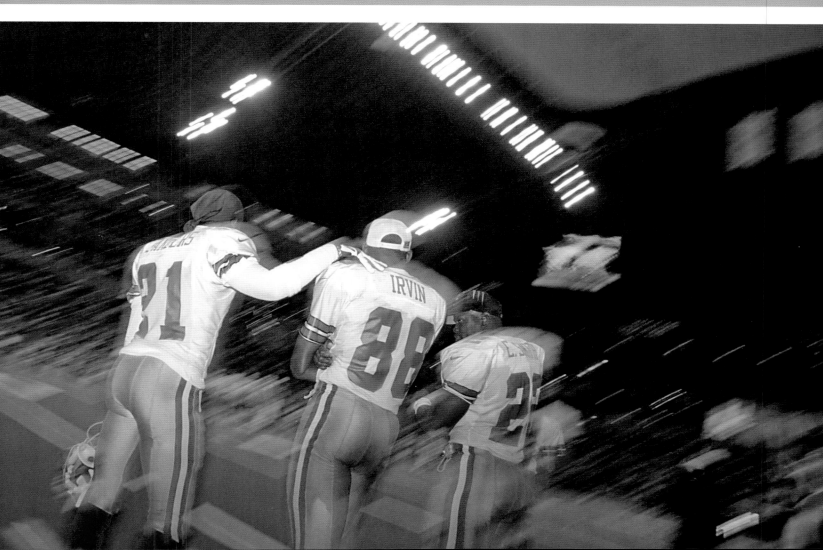

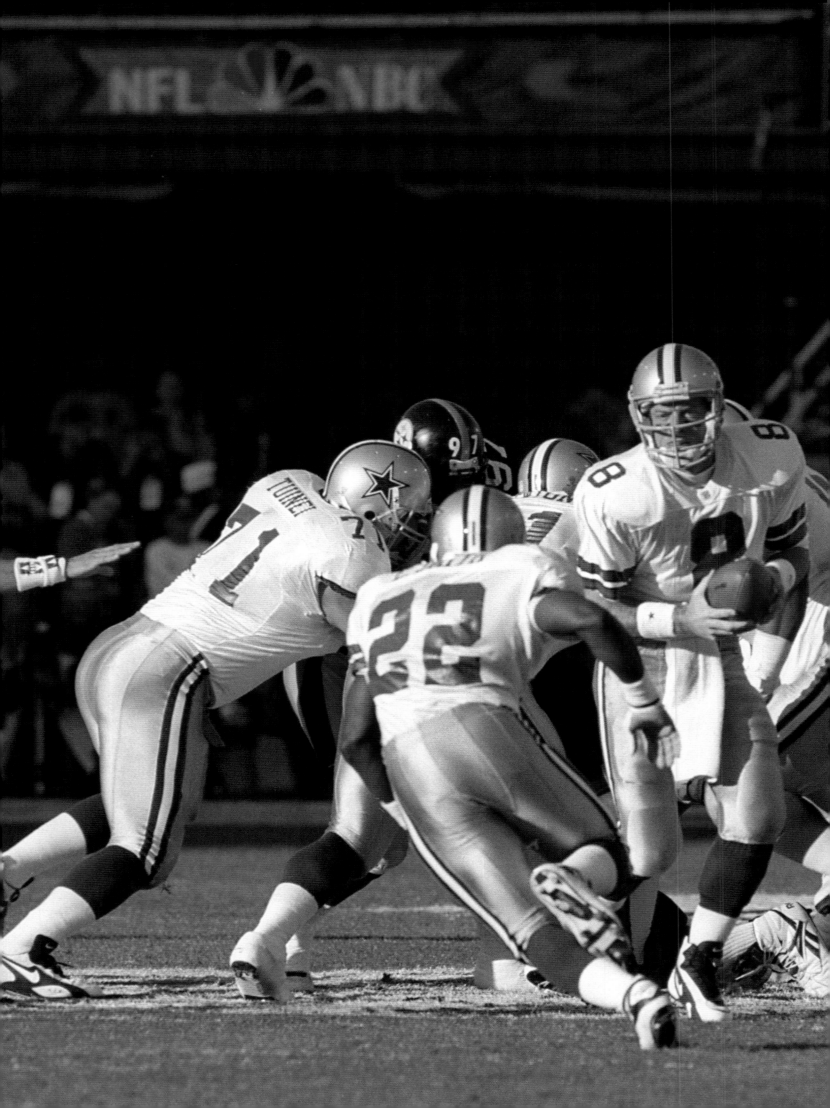

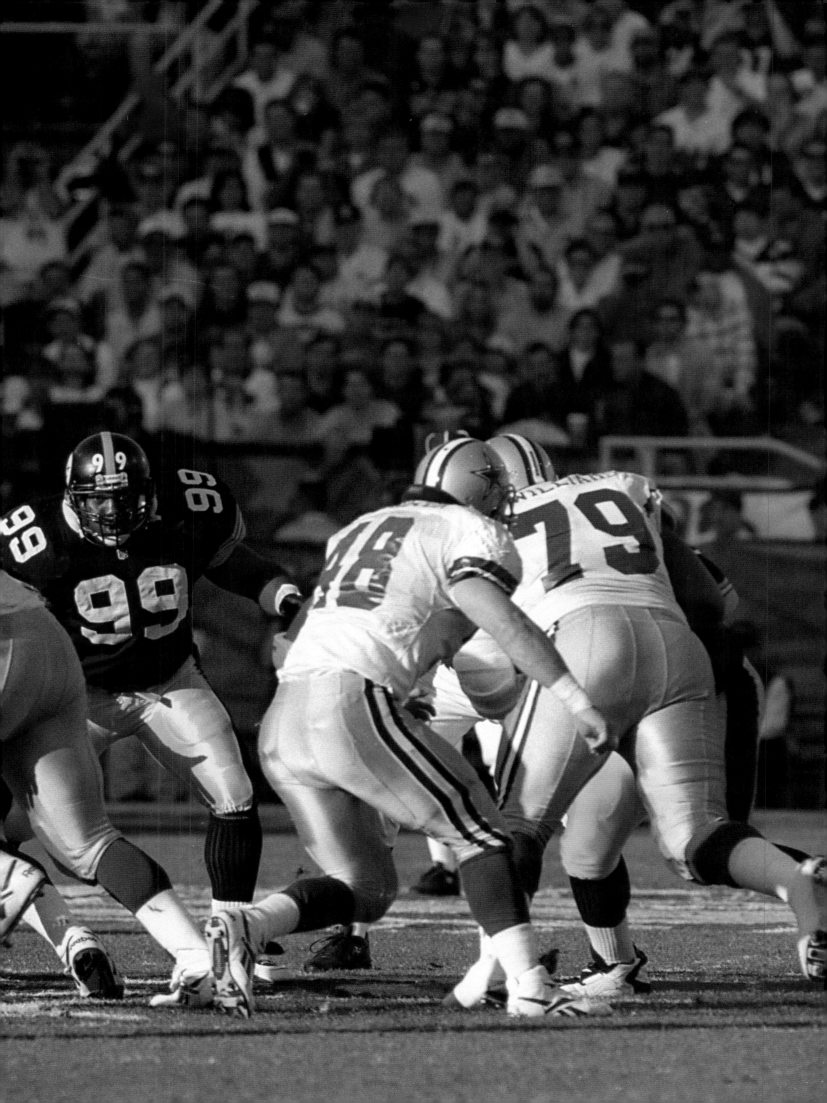

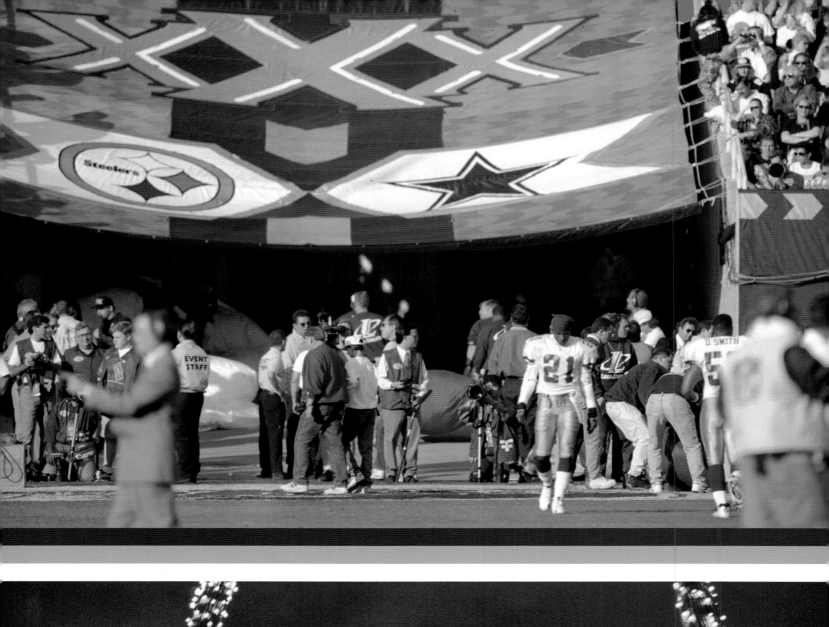

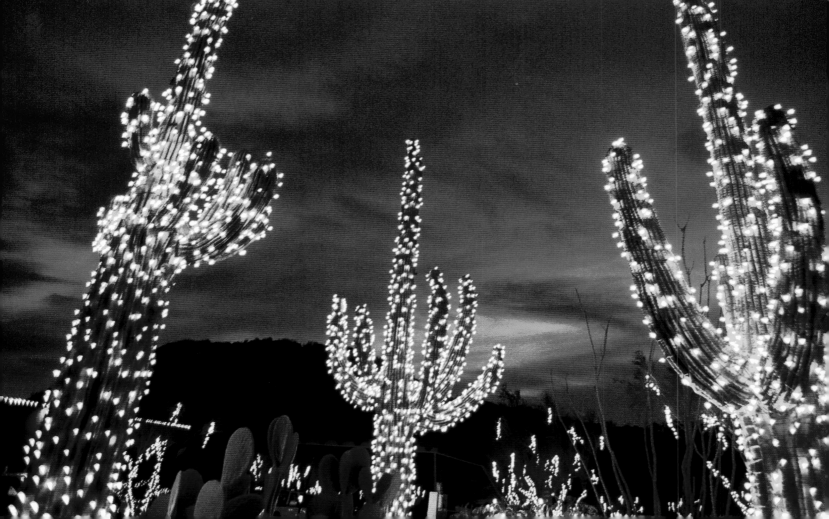

#320 BECOMES #1

Tempe—and in fact no other city that had ever hosted a Super Bowl—had ever seen anything like these party-hearty Dallas Cowboys. Champagne. Limos. Rock star lifestyles. Cockiness. Curfews? Yeah, right! Weren't celebrations supposed to happen *after* the game? Not this year. Not these Cowboys.

Less than two months earlier the bottom had fallen out of this team. They'd lost three of five. Controversy raged all around them. Then, almost magically, everything started breaking right. A season-ending trampling of the Arizona Cardinals, in the very stadium that would be the site of Super Bowl XXX, coupled with Atlanta's upset of San Francisco had given Dallas homefield advantage throughout the post-season. That 'Zona victory gave Dallas twelve for the season making them the first, and still only, NFL franchise to ever win at least a dozen games (regular season plus playoffs) in five consecutive seasons. The Cowboys smacked around Philly (36–11) to begin the playoffs and eliminated Green Bay (38–27) thanks to a late, game-sealing interception by Larry Brown.

Dallas had its swagger back. As for Tempe—the 'Boys were back in town!

★ A fleet of eleven limos convoyed from Dallas to the desert, hired by Cowboys players who felt "more comfortable" with drivers they knew. Strangers, after all, couldn't be trusted to keep secrets.

★ Owner Jerry Jones arranged for his own special ride. A six-bed luxury party bus, which once belonged to singer Whitney Houston, ferried Jones's guests to and from an almost-unending stream of bashes and blowouts.

★ "The Buttes," a swank mountaintop resort, served as Cowboys headquarters for the week. Pittsburgh stayed at the excellent but notice-ably less posh Doubletree, causing notoriously grumpy Steelers linebacker Greg Lloyd to comment about the club's "cheap" accommodations. Coach Bill Cowher, overhearing the complaint, said to Lloyd: "Greg, I'd like to introduce you to the hotel general manager who's standing right next to you."

★ "Cheap" couldn't be further from the truth when it came to Jones's personal accommodations—a 3,500-square-foot suite complete with marble floors, a full bar, three bedrooms, and its own private elevator.

★ Several players, including Deion Sanders, flew in their own personal valets, bodyguards, or "business manager" as "Prime Time" called his.

★ An enormous stretch Lincoln chauffeured Nate Newton, Erik Williams, Leon Lett, and Michael Irvin to *practice*.

★ And, speaking of Irvin. He'd taken the unofficial wardrobe championship of this "I can wear something more hip and outlandish than you" week with a canary (think phone book yellow) outfit complete with matching derby.

★ "The Tempe police gave us a list of places to not go," Newton said, laughing, "and that's where I went. I like wicked, dude."

★ Jones allowed every Cowboy to purchase up to thirty game tickets and then pressed the state of Arizona to waive its 1:00 AM "last call" law so everyone could properly party after the Sunday night game.

★ Switzer invited twenty-one people to Arizona including his ex-wife Kay *and* his girlfriend Becky Buwich. The lack of available room space ("You media guys took them all," Switzer quipped.) forced him to have six rollaway beds brought into his suite, meaning his girlfriend *and* his ex slept somewhere in the same room.

★ A Tempe radio station fittingly capped off the bizarre weeklong buildup with an outlandish Dumb-Human-Tricks contest. One Fred Flores blew away the competition and captured the prize of a pair of tickets to the game by covering himself in peanut butter and feathers, accenting the outfit with giant stuffed chicken feet, and then diving head first into a two-thousand-pound pile of cow manure.

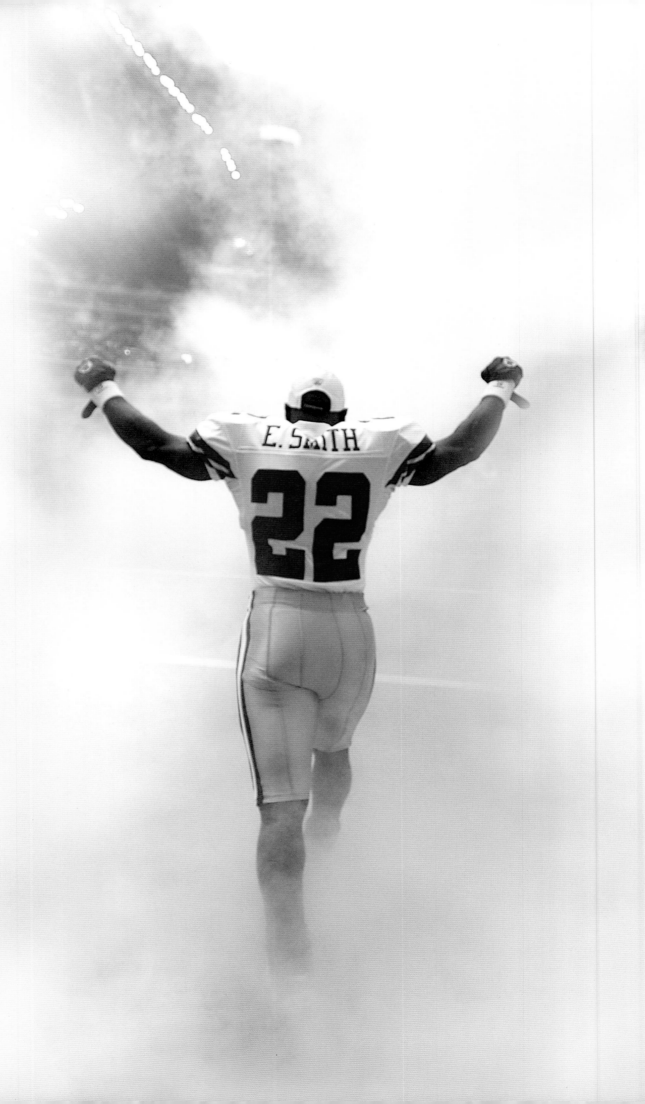

"... an exhausting, confusing, heart-breaking and hellish journey."

For one Dallas player, however, the festivities had a hollowness about them. The last five months in the life of Larry Brown had been an exhausting, confusing, heart-breaking, and hellish journey.

During a late August exhibition in San Antonio, just one week prior to the season opener, officials signaled Brown off the field and rushed him back to Dallas on Jerry Jones's private jet so he could be at the bedside of his wife Cheryl. Because of complications during her pregnancy, doctors couldn't assure the Browns the baby would survive even if Cheryl made it to term. Now, she'd gone into labor three months early. Kristopher weighed one pound and six ounces at birth. Ventilators breathed for him. Doctors told the parents the awful truth, words still etched in Brown's memory.

"They said he had brain damage," Brown recalled. "Obviously, they did everything they could but that, basically, he would have to be on a machine, brain-dead his whole life and we had to make a decision, you know, when to end it."

The weeks and months that followed would be a blurry nightmare for Brown, who'd been selected in the twelfth and last round of the 1991 draft. Pick No. 320. The NFL draft doesn't even have twelve rounds anymore. No player will ever again be able to claim he was #320.

Despite this modest pedigree, however, Brown became a starter almost instantly. Teammates had even chosen him as the club's Defensive MVP one season.

On several occasions Brown left practice to be at Kristopher's side, slept at the hospital, and then went directly back to the club's training facility.

Said Brown: "You're going through a depression, you're not eating well, not sleeping much. I wasn't even at practice for about a two-week period. I mean, literally, not even on the field, nothing, no conditioning, because, when you have to make a decision to end your child's life . . . "

Kristopher died November 16, three days before Dallas would play the Oakland Raiders, whom Brown had grown up rooting for. He strongly considered not playing the rest of the season. The organization and his teammates assured him they'd support whatever choice he made.

Kristopher's funeral took place on Saturday. Brown's grieving wife Cheryl encouraged him to play that Sunday, feeling it could prove therapeutic. Jones's jet had him in Oakland before midnight Saturday. The next afternoon, with decals memorializing Kristopher on their helmets, Dallas beat Oakland 34–21.

Super Bowl Sunday, ten weeks plus one day removed from the day of the funeral, Brown started against the Steelers.

Through nearly thirty minutes, the game looked like a laugher. Dallas scored the first three times they had the ball and bounced out to a 13–0 advantage. Everything seemed under control. Chill the champagne, rev up those limo engines, the party would begin shortly. Then Pittsburgh scored seventeen seconds before halftime. Almost thirty minutes of Dallas domination had produced a mere six-point lead (13–7).

Who could have ever imagined, though, what dramatic turns lay just ahead on Larry Brown's roller-coaster of a life? With Dallas clinging tenaciously to that lead early in the third quarter and Pittsburgh on the move hoping for a touchdown that would put them up 14–13, fate was about to make Brown the star of stars.

The Steelers lined up with five wide receivers. Quarterback Neil O'Donnell had Ernie Mills open on a middle route. "If Ernie got the ball he's still running," Steelers offensive coordinator Ron Erhardt said in hindsight. But Mills never touched it. O'Donnell's back foot got swept from under him as he threw. The replay's still crystal clear in Brown's mind:

"We were in a zone and I was looking for inside passing routes," he said. "Neil tried to hit one and the pass slipped. It didn't have much velocity. It came right to me."

Brown raced the interception back 44 yards. Two plays later Emmitt Smith leaped over right tackle to score. Dallas had breathing room, up 20–7.

155

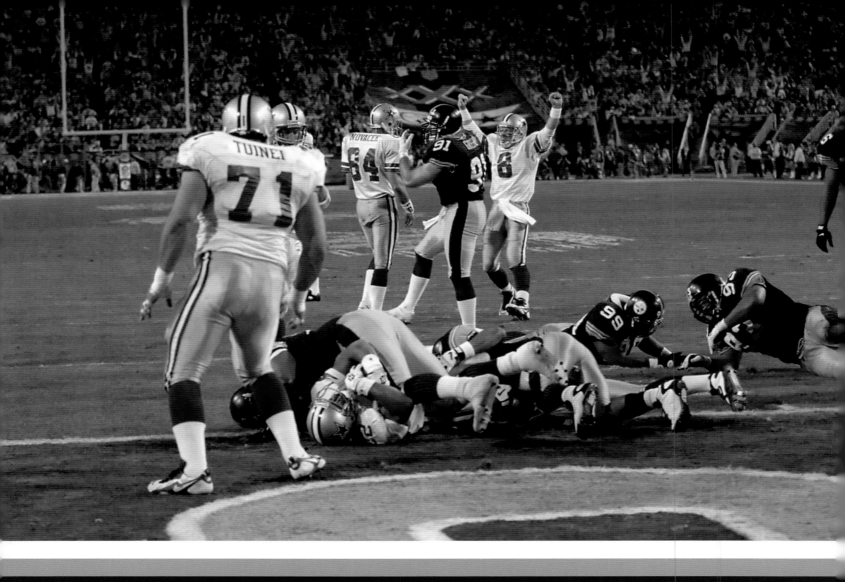

The Steelers, and O'Donnell in particular, however, simply wouldn't cave in. A field goal narrowed the Cowboys' lead to 20–10. Pitt Coach Bill Cowher then gambled on an onside kick. The Men of Steel recovered and marched 52 yards. The red hot O'Donnell had now completed fourteen of his last fifteen. Pitt trailed the 13½-point-favorite Cowboys just 20–17. The Steeler D held and the underdogs had the ball back, down by only three with 4:15 left.

Defensively Dallas decided to blitz, attack, hopefully disrupt the Steelers' offense. O'Donnell read the blitz and changed the play at the line of scrimmage. Slot receiver Andre Hastings became the "hot" receiver. At this point, the Steelers would experience what a character in the movie *Cool Hand Luke* called "a failure to communicate."

Pitt offensive coordinator Erhardt: "We had a mix-up. We ran a hitch instead of turning out. Neil just missed a read we had been very, very good on all year."

Brown: "When the ball was snapped, I peeked into the backfield and saw O'Donnell's shoulders. The way they were turned I could tell he was not going to throw the stop (inside). I came out of my backpedal real slow—then boom—I went and got the ball.

Brown's interception return took the ball all the way back to the Steelers' six. Again, in a kind of perfect symmetry, two plays later it was Smith again slamming in for the clinching score.

Brown became the first cornerback ever awarded the MVP of the Super Bowl. His 77 yards of interception returns set a new single-game Super Bowl mark.

As for the Cowboys:

- They'd become only the second team in thirty years to capture the title despite being out-gained in the game.
- The 27–17 victory gave them eleven in the post-season from '91 through '95. That's still an NFL record for a five-year period.
- Every winning margin in their last ten post-season triumphs had been by ten points or more, a streak unparalleled in league history.
- The Super Bowl title gave the Cowboys seventy-one victories from '91–'95, a total unmatched before or since.

An ecstatic Jerry Jones gave Barry Switzer a hug and the Vince Lombardi Trophy to hold aloft.

"We did it our way, BAY-BEE," Switzer screamed from the mini-stage erected in the winners' locker room. "We did it! We did it. We did it."

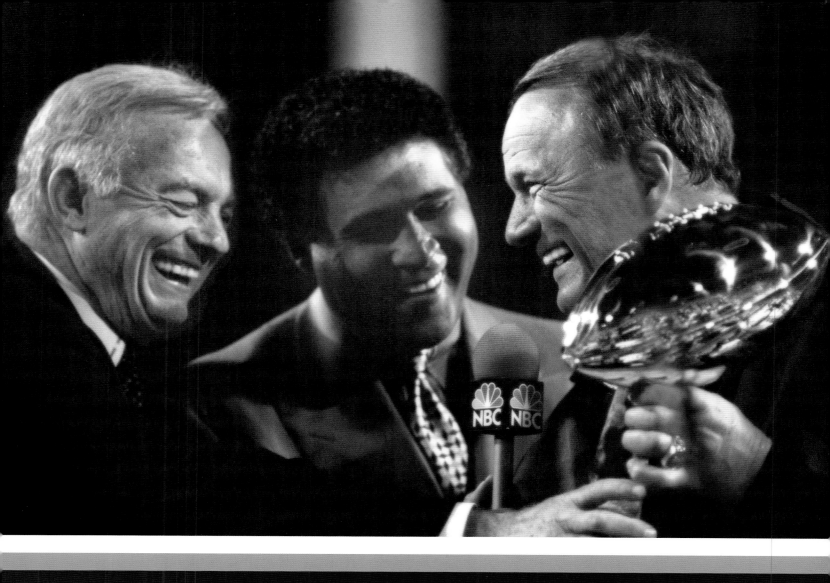

"We did it! We did it. We did it."

Earlier, Jones had become so emotional that he'd embraced his son Stephen and both had begun crying after the national anthem and prior to kickoff. "There's so much more at stake (what with) letting Jimmy go, bringing Barry in, not getting to the Super Bowl last year, the money I've spent and the criticism I've gotten," Jerry admitted. "I'm absolutely gone."

Now Jones felt more pure relief than pure joy. "I had that 'at peace' feeling," he said. "This one gave me a whole sense of closure with the Jerry-Jimmy thing."

Switzer remembers being happier for Jones than for himself.

"Whatever joy I had inside me it wasn't as great as what Jerry had inside of him. Jerry just fired a coach and went back to the Super Bowl. Think about that; his joy had to be greater. Am I not right?"

Finally, what of Larry Brown? The terrible season of turmoil and suffering had now finished on a remarkably high note—another Super Bowl ring and the incredible improbability of an MVP award also. A 320th draft choice now honored as the number one player in football's biggest game. Is it possible that this crowning moment was somehow, in some way, *meant* to be?

Switzer ponders the possibility for a moment.

"Well, I never thought about it from that aspect," he said. "Maybe things happen that way. I just don't know . . . It's almost too big a thing for me to envision."

But then, one could have almost identical thoughts about the journey the Dallas Cowboys had taken the last five seasons.

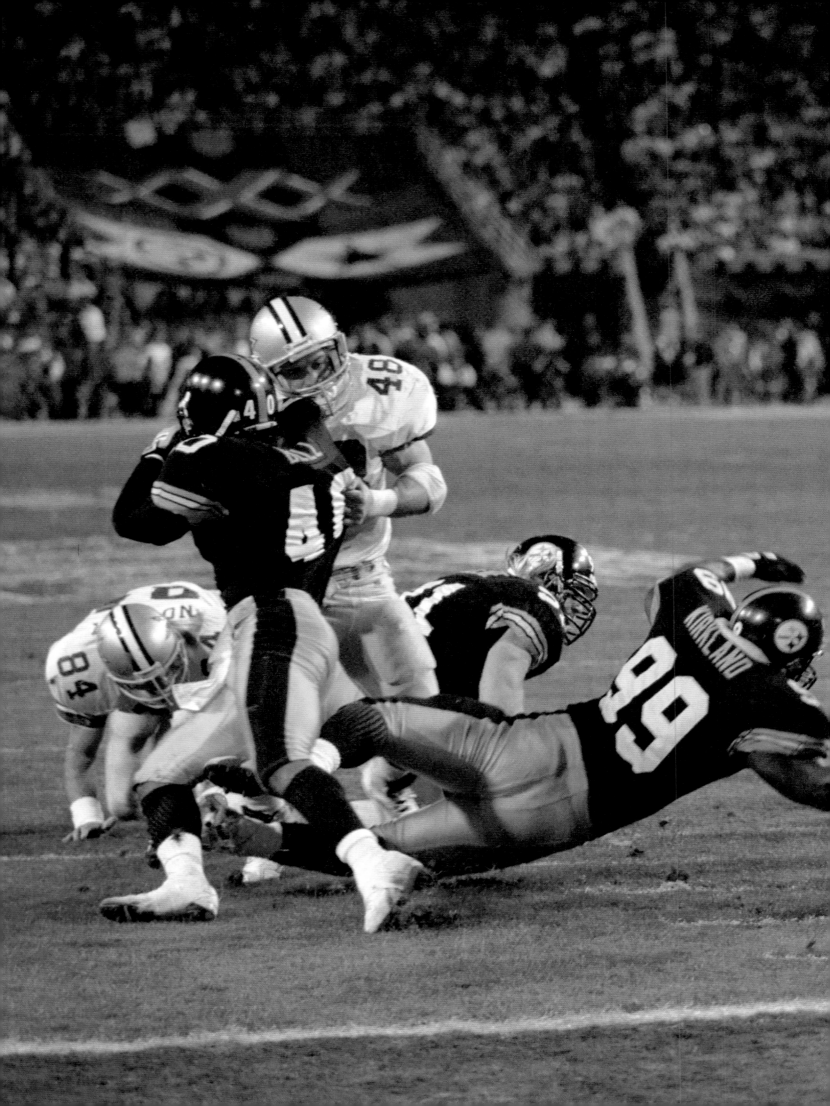

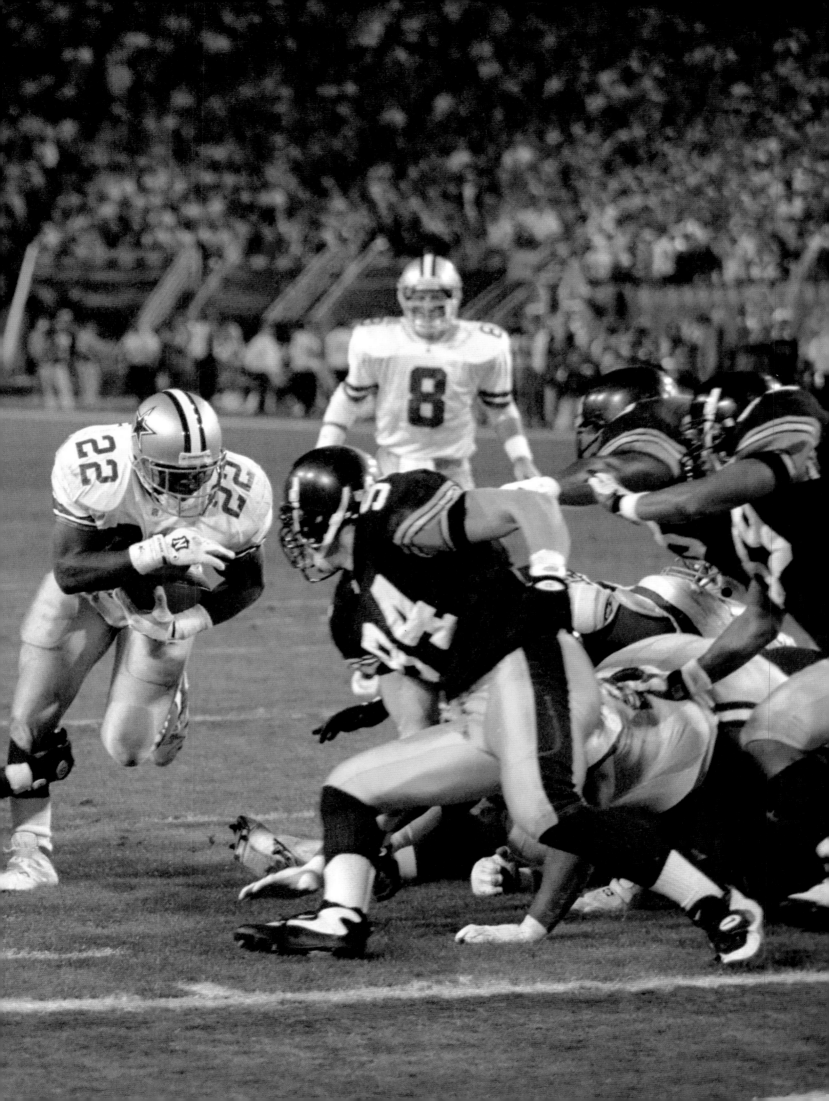

AFTERWORD

BY ROGER STAUBACH

Over the years a few extraordinary NFL teams have worn the "dynasty" label. Football fans and media hailed the Packers of the '60s, the Steelers, Dolphins, and our Cowboys in the '70s, the 49ers of the late '80s, Dallas in the early '90s, and the Patriots of 2001–05 as dynasties because of multiple championships. Excellence spread out over a number of seasons. But prior to the '90s, the NFL system actually fostered such extended dominance. With no salary cap and limited player movement, the pre-'90s NFL made it relatively simple to keep teams together. Thus, once talent was assembled, players could develop, grow, and excel together over a number of years.

The Steelers and Cowboys of the '70s perhaps best illustrate this point. If you examine the number of players who spent virtually their entire careers with those teams, it's easy to understand why these teams had such prolonged success. Joe Greene, Terry Bradshaw, Lynn Swann, John Stallworth, Mike Webster, LC Greenwood, Dwight White, Jack Lambert, Jack Ham, Mel Blount, and Franco Harris were constants in the gold and black. Randy White, Harvey Martin, Drew Pearson, Tony Dorsett, Cliff Harris, Charlie Waters, Ed Jones, Lee Roy Jordan, Chuck Howley, John Niland, Rayfield Wright, Bob Breunig, and I bled silver and blue. With rosters so stable, Pittsburgh and Dallas could fine-tune, not rebuild.

With the onset of free agency and then the salary cap in the '90s, franchises had to deal with significant annual roster upheaval. In fact, statistics now tell us nearly 33 percent of NFL rosters change yearly. The days of stability have vanished. To be successful in the new NFL you must adapt on the fly, make correct choices in both the draft and free agency and fit that talent into a capped salary structure. You must have excellent personnel evaluators, a good "capologist" and an owner willing to spend a lot of money. The '90s Cowboys had all three.

Jimmy Johnson, his assistant coaches, and the scouts shrewdly evaluated talent. Stephen Jones managed the cap. Jerry wrote the checks. Lots and lots of checks. This enabled the Cowboys to assemble an incredibly deep team. Remember that solid players like Dixon Edwards, Ken Norton, Jim Jeffcoat, Leon Lett, Chad Hennings, and Darren Woodson were all reserves when these Cowboys won the first of three Super Bowls. All eventually started on future Cowboy championship teams. But the system eventually ate away at that depth, and Dallas dealt with the losses of several key players. Center Mark Stepnoski, guard Kevin Gogan, defensive tackle Tony Casillas, linebacker Ken Norton, wide receiver Alvin Harper, linebacker Dixon Edwards, and linebacker Darrin Smith left for greener pastures. So did James Washington, cornerback Larry Brown, and defensive line stalwarts Jim Jeffcoat and Russell Maryland. The front office knew the cap wouldn't permit keeping everyone so Dallas focused on retaining its incredible core: Aikman, Smith, Irvin, Novacek, Johnston, Newton, Williams, Woodson, Haley, and Tuinei. The Cowboys constantly managed,

manipulated, and massaged the cap. While the players around them changed often, the core did not.

Yes, the Cowboys had all that fabulous talent, but I believe their most important asset was accountability. Jimmy Johnson preached it, and the best players not only bought into it; they required it of each player who wore the star. No player demanded accountability more than Troy Aikman. He exhibited professionalism, work ethic, and consistency and expected the same from every one else. Jerry Jones often said that Jimmy Johnson became a better coach, he became a better owner, and the Cowboys became a contender when Troy Aikman began to excel. That process was neither immediate nor easy. But Aikman endured and, in doing so, stepped forward as the face of the most recognized franchise in the NFL.

For a few years, I was blessed to be the Dallas quarterback. Like it or not, that position regularly calls on you to be the club spokesman. When something big happens around Dallas' Valley Ranch home, the press gathers at the quarterback's locker to measure the pulse of the team. So often, Troy had to comment on a negative or controversial situation. He did it again and again and again in a consistent manner that mirrored his play on the field. I admired him for that. I also admired how statistics always took a back seat to winning. Had Troy been called on to throw forty plus times a game like so many of his contemporaries his numbers would have been staggering. But Troy knew that, with a runner like Emmitt Smith and a dominant line, offensive balance best served the Cowboys. Aikmen was rarely flashy, just steady, driven and tough. In an era of instability, Aikman provided the guiding force. He raised the bar for the future quarterbacks in Dallas, and I loved watching him do it.

Like all Cowboys fans, the period from 1980 through 1990 was hard to bear. When I retired in 1979, I didn't emotionally detach from the team—I became a huge fan. But rooting during that era was tough. You knew deep down they just weren't talented enough to compete. Losses piled up. The star lost its shine. Coach Landry had identified a few pieces in the puzzle—Ken Norton, Jr., Mark Tuinei, Jim Jeffcoat, Nate Newton, and Michael Irvin. But they simply didn't have enough to compete at a high level. When Jimmy Johnson began to sign, draft, and trade for players in 1989, the plan began taking shape. You could see something special being built, piece by piece. I loved it. It brought back memories of our late '60s and early '70s teams. The excitement rose as those talented players began to mesh into a team that would dominate pro football for half a decade.

I had the opportunity to serve as the honorary team captain at the NFC championship game in San Francisco in January 1993. As we went out for the coin toss, I think I was more nervous than the players. Most of them were so young, and I didn't think they truly understood what was at stake for the franchise. It had been thirteen years since the Cowboys last Super Bowl appearance. I saw how far the team had come in such a short time and how special it would be if they could take the next step. I could also appreciate how difficult that step would be in the hostile environment of Candlestick Park. They did it though, and began their reign at the top of the NFL mountain.

What a wonderful five-year period for Cowboys fans! The passing game was both precise and explosive. The running game? Overpowering! A constantly underrated, unrecognized defense. And the special teams were . . . *special.* Not only did they have the chance to win every Sunday, you came to expect a victory every week. And win they did, falling just short of capturing four consecutive World Championships. What I personally loved most about those '90s Cowboys is that they beat the Steelers in the Super Bowl—something our '70s teams couldn't accomplish.

People often ask me who would have won if our '70s teams were to play the '90s Cowboys. Of course, with an admitted significant bias, I'd take my team. But how fortunate I was to play for such a fabulous team and then cheer for perhaps the finest the game has ever seen.

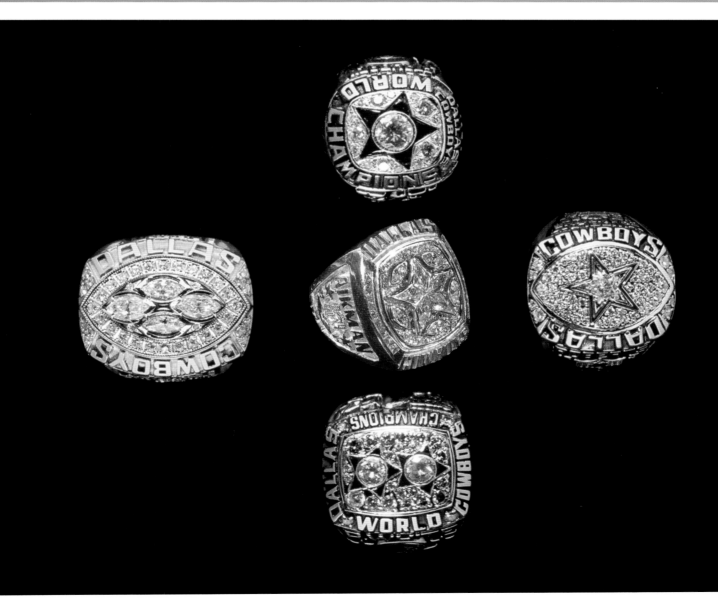

NFL STANDINGS

AFC

East
	W	L
Buffalo	13	3
Miami	8	8
New York	8	8
New England	6	10
Indianapolis	1	15

Central
	W	L
Houston	11	5
Pittsburgh	7	9
Cleveland	6	10
Cincinnati	3	13

West
	W	L
Denver	12	4
Kansas City	10	6
Los Angeles	9	7
Seattle	7	9
San Diego	4	12

NFC

East
	W	L
Washington	14	2
Dallas	11	5
Philadelphia	10	6
New York	8	8
Phoenix	4	12

Central
	W	L
Detroit	12	4
Chicago	11	5
Minnesota	8	8
Green Bay	4	12
Tampa Bay	3	13

West
	W	L
New Orleans	11	5
Atlanta	10	6
San Francisco	10	6
Los Angeles	3	13

POSTSEASON

AFC

Kansas City	10
Los Angeles	6

Houston	17
New York	10

Denver	26
Houston	24

Buffalo	37
Kansas City	14

Buffalo	10
Denver	7

NFC

Atlanta	27
New Orleans	20

Dallas	17
Chicago	13

Washington	24
Atlanta	7

Detroit	38
Dallas	6

Washington	41
Detroit	10

SUPER BOWL

Washington	37
Buffalo	24

1991

Second place, NFC East
Head Coach: Jimmy Johnson

PRESEASON (2-2)
Date	W/L	Score	Opponent	Att.
8/3	W	24-14	@ Kansas City	56,038
8/12	L	12-17	L.A. Raiders	55,981
8/18	L	20-30	@ Houston	53,314
8/23	W	20-17	Atlanta (OT)	53,689

REGULAR SEASON (11-5)
Date	W/L	Score	Opponent	Att.
9/1	W	26-14	@ Cleveland	78,860
9/9	L	31-33	WASHINGTON	63,025
9/15	L	0-24	PHILADELPHIA	62,656
9/22	W	17-9	@ Phoenix	68,814
9/29	W	21-16	N.Y. GIANTS	64,010
10/6	W	20-17	@ Green Bay	53,695
10/13	W	35-23	CINCINNATI	63,275
10/20				– Bye –
10/27	L	10-34	@ Detroit	74,906
11/3	W	27-7	PHOENIX	61,190
11/10	L	23-26	@ Houston (OT)	63,001
11/17	L	9-22	@ N.Y. Giants	76,410
11/24	W	24-21	@ Washington	55,561
11/28	W	20-10	PITTSBURGH	62,253
12/8	W	23-14	NEW ORLEANS	64,530
12/15	W	25-13	@ Philadelphia	65,854
12/22	W	31-27	ATLANTA	60,962

1991 WILD CARD GAME
Date	W/L	Score	Opponent	Att.
12/29	W	17-13	@ Chicago	62,594

1991 DIVISIONAL PLAYOFFS
Date	W/L	Score	Opponent	Att.
1/5/92	L	6-38	@ Detroit	78,290

TEAM STATISTICS	DALLAS	OPP
FIRST DOWNS	304	299
Rushing	89	103
Passing	191	180
Penalty	24	16
Third Down-Made/Att	74/196	76/194
Third Down Efficiency	37.8	39.2
Fourth Down-Made/Att	6/14	7/17
TOTAL NET YARDS	5,101	5,066
Avg. Per Game	318.8	316.6
Total Plays	971	963
Avg. Per Play	5.3	5.3
NET YARDS RUSHING	1,711	1,571
Avg. Per Game	106.9	98.2
Total Rushes	433	400
Avg. Per Rush	4.0	3.9
NET YARDS PASSING	3,390	3,495
Sacked/Yards Lost	38/273	23/151
Gross Yards	3,663	3,646
Attempts/Completions	500/305	540/320
Pct. of Completions	61.0	59.3
Had Intercepted	12	12
PUNTS/AVERAGE	57/42.6	61/38.8
Net Punting Average	36.8	32.4
PUNT RET./AVG.	29/10.7	28/8.3
KICKOFF RET./AVG.	52/21.7	69/16.9
INT./AVG. RET.	12/13.9	12/20.3
PENALTIES/YARDS	74/610	97/801
FUMBLES/BALL LOST	23/12	23/11
TOUCHDOWNS	37	32
Rushing	15	11
Passing	16	17
Returns	6	4
EXTRA POINTS/ATTEMPTS	37/37	31/32
FIELD GOALS/ATTEMPTS	27/39	29/39
AVG TIME OF POSSESSION	30:06	29:54

RUSHING	ATT	YDS	AVG	LG	TD
E. Smith	365	1,563	4.3	75t	12
Blake	15	80	5.3	30t	1
Johnston	17	54	3.2	10t	0
Agee	9	20	2.2	8t	1
Aikman	16	5	0.3	9t	1
Richards	2	4	2.0	3t	0
Wright	2	-1	-0.5	3t	0
Beuerlein	7	-14	-2.0	-1t	0
COWBOYS	433	1,711	4.0	75t	15
Opponents	400	1,571	3.9	75t	11

RECEIVING	ATT	YDS	AVG	LG	TD
Irvin	93	1,523	16.4	66t	8
Novacek	59	664	11.3	49t	4
E. Smith	49	258	5.3	14t	1
Johnston	28	244	8.7	22t	1
Harper	20	326	16.3	39t	1
Martin	16	243	15.2	27t	0
Roberts	16	136	8.5	21t	1
Wright	10	170	17.0	53t	0
Agee	7	43	6.1	9t	0
Awalt	5	57	11.4	20t	0
Blake	1	5	5.0	5t	0
Aikman	1	-6	-6.0	-6t	0
COWBOYS	305	3,663	12.0	66t	16
Opponents	320	3,646	11.4	67t	17

INTERCEPTIONS	NO	YDS	AVG	LG	TD
Holt	4	2	0.5	2t	0
Brown	2	31	15.5	20t	0
Washington	2	9	4.5	9t	0
Edwards	1	36	36.0	36t	1
Gant	1	0	0.0	0t	0
Horton	1	65	65.0	65t	1
Williams	1	24	24.0	24t	0
COWBOYS	12	167	13.9	65t	2
Opponents	12	244	20.3	96t	2

PUNTING	NO	YDS	AVG	TB	IN20	LG	BL	NET
Saxon	57	2,426	42.6	5	16	64	0	36.8
COWBOYS	57	2,426	42.6	5	16	64	0	36.8
Opp.	61	2,364	38.8	4	14	77	3	32.4

PUNT RETURNS	NO	FC	YDS	AVG	LG	TD
Martin	21	8	244	11.6	85t	1
Shepard	6	3	57	9.5	14t	0
Horton	1	0	8	8.0	8t	0
Brownlow	1	0	0	0.0	0t	0
Wright	0	1	0	0.0	0t	0
COWBOYS	29	12	309	10.7	85t	1
Opponents	28	10	231	8.3	34t	0

KICKOFF RETURNS	NO	YDS	AVG	LG	TD
Wright	21	514	24.5	102t	1
Dixon	18	398	22.1	39t	0
Gant	6	114	19.0	26t	0
Shepard	3	54	18.0	21t	0
Martin	3	47	15.7	25t	0
Horton	1	0	0.0	0t	0
COWBOYS	52	1,127	21.7	102t	1
Opponents	69	1,169	16.9	82t	1

SCORE BY QUARTERS	1	2	3	4	OT	T
COWBOYS	91	105	35	111	0	342
Opponents	61	89	66	91	3	310

FIELD GOALS	11-19	20-29	30-39	40-49	50+
Willis	2-2	6-6	9-11	6-13	4-7
COWBOYS	2-2	6-6	9-11	6-13	4-7
Opponents	1-1	11-11	5-5	9-14	3-8

Willis: (38,25,22,54),(51),(),(48M,52M,45M,41),(), (40M,23,39),(),(47B,35),(36,27),(35,37,45), (22,31,18),(51B,32M,42),(45M,18,47B,38,43),(50,41,40), (50,55M,32,37),(20,45M)

Opponents: (45M),(53,52,45,46),(42,55M),(49M, 32,32,29),(43,52M,29,25),(42),(45,24,26),(44,32),(),(52,19,22,41M,23),(27,37,22),(),(42, 51M),(54M),(37,51M, 47),(49M,25,29,49M)

SCORING	TDR	TDP	TDRt	FG	PAT	S	TP
Willis	0	0	0	27/39	37/3	0	118
E. Smith	12	1	0	0/0	0/0	0	78
Irvin	0	8	0	0/0	0/0	0	48
Novacek	0	4	0	0/0	0/0	0	24
Horton	0	0	2a	0/0	0/0	0	12
Agee	1	0	0	0/0	0/0	0	6
Aikman	1	0	0	0/0	0/0	0	6
Blake	1	0	0	0/0	0/0	0	6
Edwards	0	0	1b	0/0	0/0	0	6
Harper	0	1	0	0/0	0/0	0	6
Johnston	0	1	0	0/0	0/0	0	6
Martin	0	0	1c	0/0	0/0	0	6
Roberts	0	1	0	0/0	0/0	0	6
R. Williams	0	0	1d	0/0	0/0	0	6
Wright	0	0	1e	0/0	0/0	0	6
Hendrix	0	0	0	0/0	0/0	1#	2
COWBOYS	15	16	6	27/39	37/37	1	342
Opponents	11	17	4*	29/39	31/32	0	310

a 20 fumble return vs. N.Y. Giants (9/29)
   65 interception return vs. Green Bay (10/6)
b 36 interception return vs. Cincinnati (10/13)
c 85 punt return vs. Philadelphia (12/15)
d 18 blocked punt return vs. Houston (11/10)
e 102 kickoff return vs. Atlanta (12/22)
tackled Booty in end zone vs. Philadelphia (12/25)
* Wilson 82 kickoff return vs. Green Bay (10/6)
   White 55 blocked FG return vs. Detroit (10/27)
   Crockett 96 interception return vs. Detroit (10/27)
   Mayhew 31 interception return vs. Washington (11/24)

USUAL STARTERS

WR	Alvin Harper (5)	LE	Tony Tolbert
	Alfredo Roberts (5)	LT	Tony Casillas
	Alexander Wright (5)	RT	Russell Maryland (7)
LT	Mark Tuinei (12)		Jimmie Jones (6)
	Alan Veingrad (3)		Danny Noonan (3)
LG	Kevin Gogan	RE	Jim Jeffcoat
C	Mark Stepnoski	LLB	Ken Norton
RG	John Gesek	MLB	Jack Del Rio
RT	Nate Newton	RLB	Vinson Smith
TE	Jay Novacek (12)	LCB	Isaac Holt
	Alfredo Roberts (4)	RCB	Larry Brown (13)
WR	Michael Irvin		Manny Hendrix (3)
QB	Troy Aikman (12)	SS	James Washington
	Steve Beuerlein (4)	FS	Ray Horton
RB	Emmitt Smith		
FB	Daryl Johnston		

PASSING	ATT	COMP	YDS	PCT	AVG ATT	TD	PCT TD	PCT INT	INT	LG	SKS/YDS	RATING
Aikman	363	237	2,754	65.3	7.59	11	3.0	2.8	10	61t	32/224	86.7
Beuerlein	137	68	909	49.6	6.64	5	3.6	1.5	2	66t	6/49	77.2
COWBOYS	500	305	3,663	61.0	7.33	16	3.2	2.4	12	66t	38/273	84.1
Opponents	540	320	3,646	59.3	6.75	17	3.1	2.2	12	67t	23/151	80.8

NFL STANDINGS

AFC

East
	W	L
Miami	11	5
Buffalo	11	5
Indianapolis	9	7
New York	4	12
New England	2	14

Central
	W	L
Houston	10	6
Pittsburgh	11	5
Cleveland	7	9
Cincinnati	5	11

West
	W	L
San Diego	11	5
Kansas City	10	6
Denver	8	8
Los Angeles	7	9
Seattle	2	14

NFC

East
	W	L
Dallas	13	3
Philadelphia	11	5
Washington	9	7
New York	6	10
Phoenix	4	12

Central
	W	L
Minnesota	11	5
Green Bay	9	7
Chicago	5	11
Detroit	5	11
Tampa Bay	5	11

West
	W	L
San Francisco	14	2
New Orleans	12	4
Los Angeles	6	10
Atlanta	6	10

POSTSEASON

AFC

San Diego	17
Kansas City	0

Buffalo	41
Houston	38

Buffalo	24
Pittsburgh	3

Miami	31
San Diego	0

Buffalo	29
Miami	10

NFC

Philadelphia	36
New Orleans	20

Washingto	24
Minnesota	7

Dallas	34
Philadelphia	10

San Francisco	20
Washington	13

Dallas	30
San Francisco	20

SUPER BOWL

Dallas	52
Buffalo	17

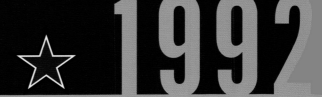

1992

First place, NFC East
Head Coach: Jimmy Johnson

PRESEASON (2-3)
Date	W/L	Score	Opponent	Att.
8/2	L	23-34	Houston @ Tokyo	51,058
8/7	W	27-24	@ Miami	50,803
8/15	L	16-17	Houston	61,334
8/22	W	17- 3	Denver	61,485
8/28	L	13-20	Chicago	60,218

REGULAR SEASON (13-3)
Date	W/L	Score	Opponent	Att.
9/7	W	23-10	WASHINGTON	63,538
9/13	W	34-28	@N.Y. Giants	76,430
9/20	W	31-20	PHOENIX	62,575
9/27			– Bye –	
10/5	L	7-31	@ Philadelphia	66,572
10/11	W	27-0	SEATTLE	62,311
10/18	W	17-10	KANSAS CITY	64,115
10/25	W	28-13	@ L.A. Raiders	91,505
11/1	W	20-10	PHILADELPHIA	65,012
11/8	W	37-3	@ Detroit	74,816
11/15	L	23-27	L.A. RAMS	63,690
11/22	W	16-10	@ Phoenix	72,439
11/26	W	30-3	N.Y. GIANTS	62,416
12/6	W	31-27	@ Denver	74,946
12/13	L	17-20	@ Washington	56,437
12/21	W	41-17	@ Atlanta	67,036
12/27	W	27-14	CHICAGO	63,101

1992 DIVISIONAL PLAYOFFS
Date	W/L	Score	Opponent	Att.
1/10/93	W	34-10	PHILADELPHIA	63,721

1992 NFC CHAMPIONSHIP GAME
Date	W/L	Score	Opponent	Att.
1/17/93	W	30-20	@ San Francisco	64,920

SUPER BOWL XXVII (Pasadena)
Date	W/L	Score	Opponent	Att.
1/31/93	W	52-17	Buffalo	98,374

TEAM STATISTICS	DALLAS	OPP
FIRST DOWNS	324	241
Rushing	119	68
Passing	183	147
Penalty	22	26
Third Down-Made/Att	87/208	50/184
Third Down Efficiency	41.8	27.2
Fourth Down-Made/Att	8/12	7/15
TOTAL NET YARDS	5,606	3,933
Avg. Per Game	350.4	245.8
Total Plays	1,014	873
Avg. Per Play	5.5	4.5
NET YARDS RUSHING	2,121	1,244
Avg. Per Game	132.6	77.8
Total Rushes	500	345
Avg. Per Rush	4.2	3.6
NET YARDS PASSING	3,485	2,689
Sacked/Yards Lost	23/112	44/347
Gross Yards	3,597	3,036
Attempts/Completions	491/314	484/263
Pct. of Completions	64.0	54.3
Had Intercepted	15	17
PUNTS/AVERAGE	61/43.0	87/42.1
Net Punting Average	33.5	35.1
PUNT RET./AVG.	44/12.5	34/11.7
KICKOFF RET./AVG.	37/18.9	60/20.3
INT./AVG. RET.	17/9.3	15/20.0
PENALTIES/YARDS	91/650	94/727
FUMBLES/BALL LOST	16/9	25/14
TOUCHDOWNS	48	29
Rushing	20	11
Passing	23	16
Returns	5	2
EXTRA POINTS/ATTEMPTS	47/48	27/29
FIELD GOALS/ATTEMPTS	24/35	14/17
AVG TIME OF POSSESSION	33:57	26:03

RUSHING	ATT	YDS	AVG	LG	TD
E. Smith	373	1,713	4.6	68t	18
Richards	49	176	3.6	15t	1
Aikman	37	105	2.8	19t	1
Johnston	17	61	3.6	14t	0
Agee	16	54	3.4	10t	0
Harper	1	15	15.0	15t	0
Martin	2	13	6.5	8t	0
Beuerlein	4	-7	-1.8	-1t	0
Irvin	1	-9	-9.0	-9t	0
COWBOYS	500	2,121	4.2	68t	20
Opponents	345	1,244	3.6	28t	11

RECEIVING	ATT	YDS	AVG	LG	TD
Irvin	78	1,396	17.9	87t	7
Novacek	68	630	9.3	34t	6
E. Smith	59	335	5.7	26t	1
Harper	35	562	16.1	52t	4
Martin	32	359	11.2	27t	3
Johnston	32	249	7.8	18t	2
Roberts	3	36	12.0	18t	0
Agee	3	18	6.0	8t	0
Richards	3	8	2.7	6t	0
Gesek	1	4	4.0	4t	0
COWBOYS	314	3,597	11.5	87t	23
Opponents	263	3,036	11.5	81t	16

INTERCEPTIONS	NO	YDS	AVG	LG	TD
Washington	3	31	10.3	16t	0
Gant	3	19	6.3	11t	0
Everett	2	28	14.0	17t	0
Horton	2	15	7.5	15t	1
Holt	2	11	5.5	8t	0
K. Smith	2	10	5.0	7t	0
Brown	1	30	30.0	30t	0
Myles	1	13	13.0	13t	0
Harper	1	1	1.0	1t	0
COWBOYS	17	158	9.3	30t	1
Opponents	15	300	20.0	59t	0

PUNTING	NO	YDS	AVG	TB	IN20	LG	BL	NET
Saxon	61	2,620	43.0	9	19	58	0	33.5
COWBOYS	61	2,620	43.0	9	19	58	0	33.5
Opp.	87	3,660	42.1	3	17	73	2	35.1

PUNT RETURNS	NO	FC	YDS	AVG	LG	TD
Martin	42	18	532	12.7	79t	2
K. Smith	1	0	17	17.0	17t	0
Horton	1	0	1	1.0	1t	0
COWBOYS	44	18	550	12.5	79t	2
Opponents	34	6	397	11.7	65t	0

KICKOFF RETURNS	NO	YDS	AVG	LG	TD
Martin	24	503	21.0	59	0
Wright	8	117	14.6	21	0
Holmes	3	70	23.3	28	0
K. Smith	1	9	9.0	9	0
Edwards	1	0	0.0	0	0
COWBOYS	37	699	18.9	59	0
Opponents	60	1,217	20.3	42	0

SCORE BY QUARTERS	1	2	3	4	OT	T
COWBOYS	108	116	134	51	0	409
Opponents	54	53	51	85	0	243

FIELD GOALS	11-19	20-29	30-39	40-49	50+
WElliot	0-0	6-7	10-14	5-10	3-4
COWBOYS	0-0	6-7	10-14	5-10	3-4
Opponents	1-1	4-4	4-5	5-7	0-0

Elliot: (32M),(39,35),(33B,29),(48M),(31,51,42M), (51M,39),(48M),(42 M,38M,35,48),(25,42, 30),(37,42,36),(28),(45,33,53),(53,32M), (23),(47,22,46M),(28M,21,34)

Opponents: (49),(),(22,42),(40),(40M),(32),(),(18), (36),(33,44),(20),(35 M,42,44M),(),(32,22),(27)

SCORING	TDR	TDP	TDRt	FG	PAT	S	TP
Elliot	0	0	0	24/35	47/48	0	119
E. Smith	18	1	0	0/0	0/0	0	114
Irvin	0	7	0	0/0	0/0	0	42
Novacek	0	6	0	0/0	0/0	0	36
Martin	0	3	2a	0/0	0/0	0	30
Harper	0	4	0	0/0	0/0	0	24
Johnston	0	2	0	0/0	0/0	0	12
Aikman	1	0	0	0/0	0/0	0	6
Horton	0	0	1b	0/0	0/0	0	6
Maryland	0	0	1c	0/0	0/0	0	6
Richards	1	0	0	0/0	0/0	0	6
R. Williams	0	0	1d	0/0	0/0	0	6
Holt	0	0	0	0/0	0/0	1#	2
COWBOYS	20	23	5	24/35	47/48	1	409
Opponents	11	16	2*	14/17	27/29	0	243

a   79 punt return vs. Washington (9/7)
    74 punt return vs. L.A. Rams (11/15)
b   15 interception return vs. Seattle (10/11)
c   26 fumble return vs. Chicago (12/27)
d   3 block punt return vs. N.Y. Giants (9/13)
Blocked punt out of end zone vs. Washington (9/7)
*   Copeland fumble recovery in end zone vs. Washington (12/13)
    Zorich 42 fumble return vs. Chicago (12/27)

USUAL STARTERS

WR	Alvin Harper	LE	Tony Tolbert
LT	Mark Tuinei	LT	Tony Casillas
LG	Nate Newton	RT	Russell Maryland
C	Mark Stepnoski	RE	Charles Haley (13)
RG	John Gesek		Jim Jeffcoat (3)
RT	Erik Williams	LLB	Vinson Smith (13)
TE	Jay Novacek		Kenneth Gant (3)
WR	Michael Irvin	MLB	Robert Jones (13)
QB	Troy Aikman		Ken Norton (3)
RB	Emmitt Smith	RLB	Ken Norton
FB	Daryl Johnston	LCB	Issiac Holt (11)
			Kevin Smith (5)
		RCB	Larry Brown
		SS	Thomas Everett (9)
			James Washington (6)
		FS	James Washington (9)
			Ray Horton (7)

PASSING	ATT	COMP	YDS	PCT	AVG ATT	TD	PCT TD	PCT INT	INT	LG	SKS/YDS	RATING
Aikman	473	302	3,445	63.8	7.28	23	4.9	3.0	14	87t	23/112	89.5
Beuerlein	18	12	152	66.7	8.44	0	0.0	5.6	1	27t	0/0	69.7
COWBOYS	491	314	3,597	64.0	7.33	23	4.7	3.1	15	87t	23/112	88.8
Opponents	484	263	3,036	54.3	6.27	16	3.3	3.5	17	67t	44/347	69.9

NFL STANDINGS

AFC

East
East	W	L
Buffalo	12	4
Miami	9	7
New York	8	8
New England	5	11
Indianapolis	4	12

Central
Central	W	L
Houston	12	4
Pittsburgh	9	7
Cleveland	7	9
Cincinnati	3	13

West
West	W	L
Kansas City	11	5
Los Angeles	10	6
Denver	9	7
San Diego	8	8
Seattle	6	10

NFC

East
East	W	L
Dallas	12	4
New York	11	5
Philadelphia	8	8
Phoenix	7	9
Washington	4	12

Central
Central	W	L
Detroit	10	6
Minnesota	9	7
Green Bay	9	7
Chicago	7	9
Tampa Bay	5	11

West
West	W	L
San Francisco	10	6
New Orleans	8	8
Atlanta	6	10
Los Angeles	5	11

POSTSEASON

AFC
Los Angeles	42			
Denver	24			
Kansas City	27			
Pittsburgh	24			
Buffalo	29			
Los Angeles	23			
Kansas City	28			
Houston	20			
Buffalo	30			
Kansas City	13			

NFC
Green Bay	28
Detroit	24
New York	17
Minnesota	10
Dallas	27
Green Bay	17
San Francisco	44
New York	3
Dallas	38
San Francisco	21

SUPER BOWL

Dallas	30
Buffalo	13

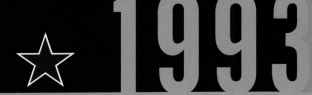

1993

First place, NFC East
Head Coach: Jimmy Johnson

PRESEASON (1-3-1)
Date	W/L	Score	Opponent	Att.
8/1	L	7-13	Minnesota	60,010
8/8	T	13-13	Det. @ London (OT)	43,522
8/14	W	13-7	L.A. Raiders	60,411
8/21	L	20-23	Houston @ San Ant.	63,285
8/27	L	21-23	@ Chicago	56,181

REGULAR SEASON (12-4)
Date	W/L	Score	Opponent	Att.
9/6	L	16-35	@ Washington	56,345
9/12	L	10-13	BUFFALO	63,226
9/19	W	17-10	@ Phoenix	73,025
9/26			– Bye –	
10/3	W	36-14	GREEN BAY	63,568
10/10	W	27-3	@ Indianapolis	60,453
10/17	W	26-17	SAN FRANCISCO	65,099
10/24			– Bye –	
10/31	W	23-10	@ Philadelphia	61,912
11/7	W	31-9	N.Y. GIANTS	64,735
11/14	W	20-15	PHOENIX	64,224
11/21	L	14-27	@ Atlanta	67,337
11/25	L	14-16	MIAMI	60,198
12/6	W	23-17	PHILADELPHIA	64,521
12/12	W	37-20	@ Minnesota	63,321
12/18	W	28-7	@ New York Jets	73,233
12/26	W	38-3	WASHINGTON	64,497
1/2/94	W	16-13	@ N.Y. Giants (OT)	77,356

DIVISIONAL PLAYOFF
Date	W/L	Score	Opponent	Att.
1/16/94	W	27-17	Green Bay	64,790

NFC CHAMPIONSHIP GAME
Date	W/L	Score	Opponent	Att.
1/23/94	W	38-21	San Francisco	64,902

SUPER BOWL XXVIII (Atlanta)
Date	W/L	Score	Opponent	Att.
1/30/94	W	30-13	Buffalo	72,817

TEAM STATISTICS	DALLAS	OPP
FIRST DOWNS	322	297
Rushing	120	94
Passing	172	176
Penalty	30	27
Third Down-Made/Att.	83/198	87/219
Third Down Efficiency	41.9	39.7
Fourth Down-Made/Att.	7/12	6/17
TOTAL NET YARDS	5,615	4,767
Avg. Per Game	350.9	297.9
Total Plays	994	1012
Avg. Per Play	5.6	4.7
NET YARDS RUSHING	2,161	1,651
Avg. Per Game	135.1	103.2
Total Rushes	490	423
Avg. Per Rush	4.4	3.9
NET YARDS PASSING	3,454	3,116
Avg. Per Game	215.9	194.8
Sacks/Yards Lost	29/163	34/231
Gross Yards	3,617	3,347
Attempts/Completions	475/317	555/334
Pct. of Completions	66.7	60.2
Had Intercepted	6	14
PUNTS/AVERAGE	56/41.8	78/41.3
Net Punting Average	37.7	34.8
PUNT RET./AVG.	37/10.3	32/5.3
KICKOFF RET./AVG.	36/21.1	66/18.6
INT./AVG. RET.	14/12.2	6/7.8
PENALTIES/YARDS	94/744	87/653
FUMBLES/BALL LOST	33/16	22/14
TOUCHDOWNS	41	23
Rushing	20	7
Passing	18	14
Returns	3	2
EXTRA POINTS/ATTEMPTS	40/41	23/23
FIELD GOALS/ATTEMPTS	30/37	22/27
AVG TIME OF POSSESSION	30:56	29:04

RUSHING	ATT	YDS	AVG	LG	TD
E. Smith	283	1,486	5.3	62t	9
Lassic	75	269	3.6	15t	3
Coleman	34	132	3.9	16t	2
Aikman	32	125	3.9	20t	0
Johnston	24	74	3.1	11t	3
Gainer	9	29	3.2	8t	0
K. Williams	7	26	3.7	12t	2
Agee	6	13	2.2	6t	0
Kosar	9	7	0.8	4t	0
Irvin	2	6	3.0	9t	0
Novacek	1	2	2.0	2t	1
J. Garret	8	-8	-1.0	0t	0
COWBOYS	490	2,161	4.4	62t	20
Opponents	423	1,651	3.9	77t	7

RECEIVING	ATT	YDS	AVG	LG	TD
Irvin	88	1,330	15.1	61t	7
E. Smith	57	414	7.3	86t	1
Johnston	50	372	7.4	20t	1
Novacek	44	445	10.1	30t	1
Harper	36	777	21.6	80t	5
K. Williams	20	151	7.6	33t	2
Lassic	9	37	4.1	9t	0
Gainer	6	37	6.3	8t	0
Coleman	4	24	6.0	10t	0
T. Williams	1	25	25.0	25t	0
Price	1	4	4.0	4t	0
Galbraith	1	1	1.0	1t	1
COWBOYS	317	3,617	11.4	86t	18
Opponents	334	3,347	10.0	70t	14

INTERCEPTIONS	NO	YDS	AVG	LG	TD
K. Smith	6	56	9.3	32t	1
Bates	2	25	12.5	22t	0
Everett	2	25	12.5	17t	0
Washington	1	38	38.0	24t	0
Norton	1	25	25.0	25t	0
Marion	1	2	2.0	2t	0
Gant	1	0	0.0	0t	0
COWBOYS	14	171	12.2	32t	1
Opponents	6	47	7.8	26t	0

PUNTING	NO	YDS	AVG	TB	IN20	LG	BL	NET
Jett	56	2,342	41.8	3	22	59	0	37.7
COWBOYS	56	2,342	41.8	3	22	59	0	37.7
Opp.	78	3,219	41.3	6	21	60	0	34.8

PUNT RETURNS	NO	FC	YDS	AVG	LG	TD
K. Williams	36	14	381	10.6	64t	2
Washington	1	0	0	0.0	0t	0
COWBOYS	37	14	381	10.3	64t	2
Opponents	32	12	169	5.3	20t	0

KICKOFF RETURNS	NO	YDS	AVG	LG	TD
K. Williams	31	689	22.2	49t	0
K. Smith	1	33	33.0	33t	0
Gant	1	18	18.0	18t	0
R. Jones	1	12	12.0	12t	0
Hennings	1	7	7.0	7t	0
Novacek	1	-1	-1.0	-1t	0
Vanderbeek	0	0	0.0	0t	0
COWBOYS	36	758	21.1	49t	0
Opponents	66	1,225	18.6	95t	1

SCORE BY QUARTERS	1	2	3	4	OT	T
COWBOYS	76	124	86	87	3	376
Opponents	43	46	79	61	0	229

FIELD GOALS	11-19	20-29	30-39	40-49	50+
Murray	4-4	4-4	9-12	8-8	3-5
Elliott	0-0	1-1	0-1	1-2	0-0
COWBOYS	4-4	5-5	9-13	9-10	3-5
Opponents	3-3	11-11	5-6	3-7	0-0

Murray: (),(),23,50M),(33,19,19,50,48),(30,32), (48,39,29,35M,18),(3 5,23,40),(34,54M), (44,43),(-),(32M),(23,19,47),(51,52,46), (),(39M,38),(32,38,41)

Elliott: (22),(49M,43,30M)

Opponents: (32M),(48,35),(20),(42M),(27),(25), (33),(21,45,29),(19,4 7),(26,24),(44M, 20,31,41B,19),(25,44M),(19,21),(), (32), (29,31)

SCORING	TDR	TDP	TDRt	FG	PAT	S	TP
E. Murray	0	0	0	28/33	38/38	0	122
E. Smith	9	1	0	0/0	0/0	0	60
Irvin	0	7	0	0/0	0/0	0	42
K. Williams	2	2	2a	0/0	0/0	0	36
Harper	0	5	0	0/0	0/0	0	30
Johnston	3	1	0	0/0	0/0	0	24
Lassic	3	0	0	0/0	0/0	0	18
Coleman	0	2	0	0/0	0/0	0	12
Novacek	1	1	0	0/0	0/0	0	12
Elliott	0	0	0	2/4	2/3	0	8
Galbraith	0	1	0	0/0	0/0	0	6
K. Smith	0	0	1b	0/0	0/0	0	6
COWBOYS	20	18	3	30/37	4014	0	376
Opponents	7	14	2*	22/27	23/23	1#	229

a 64 yd. punt return, vs. Miami (11/25)
  62 yd. punt return, vs. Washington (I12/26)
b 32 yd. interception return, @ N.Y. Jets (I2/18)
* 95 yd.kickoff ret., R Brooks, vs. G.Bay (10/3)
  47 yd. fum. ret, E. Davis, vs. S.F. (10/17)
Kosar intentional grounding in end zone vs. Phoenix (11/14)

USUAL STARTERS

WR	Alvin Harper		LE	Tony Tolbert
LT	Mark Tuinei		LT	Tony Casillas
LG	Nate Newton		RT	Russell Maryland (12)
C	Mark Stepnoski (13)			Leon Lett (4)
	Frank Cornish (3)		RE	Charles Haley (11)
RG	Kevin Gogan			Jim Jeffcoat (3)
RT	Erik Williams		LLB	Dixon Edwards
TE	Jay Novacek		MLB	Ken Norton (13)
WR	Michael Irvin			Robert Jones (3)
QB	Troy Aikman		RLB	Darrin Smith (12)
RB	Emmitt Smith (13)			Ken Norton (3)
	Derrick Lassic (3)		LCB	Kevin Smith
FB	Daryl Johnston		RCB	Larry Brown
			SS	Darren Woodson
			FS	Thomas Everett

PASSING	ATT	COMP	YDS	PCT	AVG ATT	TD	PCT TD	PCT INT	INT	LG	SKS/YDS	RATING
Aikman	392	271	3,100	69.1	7.91	15	3.8	1.5	6	80t	26/153	99.0
Kosar	63	36	410	57.1	6.51	3	4.8	0.0	0	86t	2/4	92.7
J. Garrett	19	9	61	47.4	3.21	0	0.0	0.0	0	16t	1/6	54.9
Harper	1	1	46	100.0	46.00	0	0.0	0.0	0	46t	0/0	118.8
COWBOYS	475	317	3,617	66.7	7.61	18	3.8	1.3	6	86t	29/163	96.8
Opponents	555	334	3,347	60.2	6.03	14	2.5	2.5	14	70t	34/231	75.3

NFL STANDINGS

AFC

East
East	W	L
Miami	10	6
New England	10	6
Indianapolis	8	8
Buffalo	7	9
New York	6	10

Central
Central	W	L
Pittsburgh	12	4
Cleveland	11	5
Cincinnati	3	13
Houston	2	14

West
West	W	L
San Diego	11	5
Los Angeles	9	7
Kansas City	9	7
Denver	7	9
Seattle	6	10

NFC

East
East	W	L
Dallas	12	4
New York	9	7
Arizona	8	8
Philadelphia	7	9
Washington	3	13

Central
Central	W	L
Minnesota	10	6
Green Bay	9	7
Chicago	9	7
Detroit	9	7
Tampa Bay	6	10

West
West	W	L
San Francisco	13	3
New Orleans	7	9
Atlanta	7	9
Los Angeles	4	12

POSTSEASON

AFC
Miami	27
Kansas City	17
Cleveland	20
New England	13
Pittsburgh	29
Cleveland	9
San Diego	22
Miami	21
San Diego	17
Pittsburgh	13

NFC
Chicago	35
Minnesota	18
Green Bay	16
Detroit	12
San Francisco	44
Chicago	15
Dallas	35
Green Bay	9
San Francisco	38
Dallas	28

SUPER BOWL
San Francisco	49
San Diego	26

1994

First place, NFC East
Head Coach: Barry Switzer

PRESEASON (2-3)
Date	W/L	Score	Opponent	Att.
7/31	W	17-9	Minnesota	59,062
8/7	L	19-27	L.A. Raiders	61,932
8/15	L	0-6	Hous. @ Mex. City	112,376
8/21	W	34-10	Denver	63,923
8/25	L	10-28	@ New Orleans	57,281

REGULAR SEASON (12-4)
Date	W/L	Score	Opponent	Att.
9/4	W	26-9	@ Pittsburgh	60,156
9/11	W	20-17	HOUSTON	64,402
9/19	L	17-20	DETROIT (OT)	64,102
9/25			– Bye –	
10/2	W	34-7	@ Washington	55,394
10/9	W	38-3	ARIZONA	64,518
10/16	W	24-13	PHILADELPHIA	64,703
10/23	W	28-21	@ Arizona	71,023
10/30	W	23-20	@ Cincinnati	57,096
11/7	W	38-10	N.Y. GIANTS	64,836
11/13	L	14-21	@ San Francisco	69,014
11/20	W	31-7	WASHINGTON	64,644
11/24	W	42-31	GREEN BAY	64,597
12/4	W	31-19	@ Philadelphia	65,947
12/10	L	14-19	CLEVELAND	64,826
12/19	W	24-16	@ New Orleans	67,323
12/24	L	10-15	@ N.Y. Giants	66,943

DIVISIONAL PLAYOFF
Date	W/L	Score	Opponent	Att.
1/8/95	W	35-9	GREEN BAY	64,475

NFC CHAMPIONSHIP GAME
Date	W/L	Score	Opponent	Att.
1/15/95	L	28-38	@ San Francisco	69,125

TEAM STATISTICS	DALLAS	OPP
FIRST DOWNS	322	273
Rushing	136	86
Passing	160	157
Penalty	26	30
Third Down-Made/Att.	93/209	91/229
Third Down Efficiency	44.5	39.7
Fourth Down-Made/Att.	6/7	8/17
TOTAL NET YARDS	5,321	4,313
Avg. Per Game	332.6	269.6
Total Plays	1,018	1,006
Avg. Per Play	5.2	4.3
NET YARDS RUSHING	1,953	1,561
Avg. Per Game	122.1	97.6
Total Rushes	550	437
Avg. Per Rush	3.6	3.6
NET YARDS PASSING	3,368	2,752
Avg. Per Game	210.5	172.0
Sackes/Yards Lost	20/93	47/299
Gross Yards	3,461	3,051
Attempts/Completions	4i8/282	522/269
Pct. of Completions	62.9	51.5
Had Intercepted	14	22
PUNTS/AVERAGE	70/41.9	84/43.3
Net Punting Average	35.4	36.8
PUNT RET./AVG.	44/9.2	36/10.5
KICKOFF RET./AVG.	50/25.7	82/20.8
INT./AVG. RET.	22/13.5	14/12.9
PENALTIES/YARDS	100/895	102/826
FUMBLES/BALL LOST	22/10	15/9
TOUCHDOWNS	50	27
Rushing	26	8
Passing	19	19
Returns	5	0
EXTRA POINT/ATTEMPTS	48/50	24/27
Kicking Made-Attempts	48/48	24/24
Passing Made-Attempts	0/0	0/2
Rushing Made-Attempts	0/2	0/1
FIELD GOALS/ATTEMPTS	22/29	20/25
AVG. TIME OF POSSESSION	31:35	28:25

RUSHING	ATT	YDS	AVG	LG	TD
E. Smith	368	1,484	4.0	46	21
Coleman	64	180	2.8	13	1
Johnston	40	138	3.5	9	2
B. Thomas	24	70	2.9	11	1
Aikman	30	62	2.1	13	1
K. Williams	6	20	3.3	8	0
Agee	5	4	0.8	3	0
Wilson	1	-1	-1.0	-1	0
Garrett	3	-2	-0.7	0	0
Peete	9	-2	-0.2	2	0
COWBOYS	550	1,953	3.6	46	26
Opponents	437	1,561	3.6	40	8

RECEIVING	ATT	YDS	AVG	LG	TD
Irvin	79	1,241	15.7	65t	6
E. Smith	50	341	6.8	68t	1
Novacek	47	475	10.1	27t	2
Johnston	44	325	7.4	24t	2
Harper	33	821	24.9	90t	8
K. Williams	13	181	13.9	29t	0
Coleman	8	46	5.8	14t	0
Galbraith	4	31	7.8	15t	0
B. Thomas	2	1	0.5	5t	0
Agee	1	2	2.0	2t	0
Kennard	1	-3	-3.0	-3t	0
COWBOYS	282	3,461	12.3	90t	19
Opponents	269	3,051	11.3	67t	19

INTERCEPTIONS	NO	YDS	AVG	LG	TD
Woodson	5	140	28.0	94t	1
Washington	5	43	8.6	25t	0
Brown	4	21	5.3	14t	0
D. Smith	2	13	6.5	13t	1
K. Smith	2	11	5.5	11t	0
Tolbert	1	54	54.0	54t	1
Marion	1	11	11.0	11t	0
Haley	1	1	1.0	1t	0
Gant	1	0	0.0	0t	0
Holmes	0	3	3.0	3t	0
COWBOYS	22	297	13.5	94t	3
Opponents	14	180	12.9	56t	0

PUNTING	NO	YDS	AVG	TB	IN20	LG	BL	NET
S. Jett	70	2,935	41.9	4	26	58	0	35.4
COWBOYS	70	2,935	41.9	4	26	58	0	35.4
Opp.	84	3,637	43.3	7	31	80	0	36.8

PUNT RETURNS	NO	FC	YDS	AVG	LG	TD
K. Williams	39	13	349	8.9	83t	1
Holmes	5	1	55	11.0	19t	0
COWBOYS	44	14	404	9.2	83t	1
Opponents	36	14	378	10.5	58t	0

KICKOFF RETURNS	NO	YDS	AVG	LG	TD
K. Williams	43	1,148	26.7	87t	1
Holmes	4	89	22.3	32t	0
Marion	2	39	19.5	21t	0
R. Jones	1	8	8.0	8t	0
COWBOYS	50	1,284	25.7	87t	1
Opponents	82	1,709	20.8	67t	0

SCORE BY QUARTERS	1	2	3	4	OT	T
COWBOYS	100	122	104	88	0	414
Opponents	34	93	46	72	3	248

FIELD GOALS	11-19	20-29	30-39	40-49	50+
Boniol	3-3	3-4	10-12	6-9	0-1
COWBOYS	3-3	3-4	10-12	6-9	0-1
Opponents	1-1	6-6	8-8	5-6	0-4

Boniol: (40,31,21,32),(45,29),(19),(28,47),(41M, 19),(37),(43B),(38M, 37,43,38),(45),(43M),(32,51M),(41,37,35),(19),(),(30,20B), (37, 37M)

Opponents: (41),(41),(32,51M,57B,51B,44),(),(42), (),(),(22,33),(23), (53M),(28),(22,19),(34,32,43,32),(40M, 21,32,29),(38,30)

SCORING	TDR	TDP	TDRt	FG	PAT	S	TP
E. Smith	21	1	0	0/0	0/0	0	132
Boniol	0	0	0	22/29	48/48	0	114
Harper	0	8	0	0/0	0/0	0	48
Irvin	0	6	0	0/0	0/0	0	36
Johnston	2	2	0	0/0	0/0	0	24
Novacek	0	2	0	0/0	0/0	0	12
K. Williams	0	0	2a	0/0	0/0	0	12
Aikman	1	0	0	0/0	0/0	0	6
Coleman	1	0	0	0/0	0/0	0	6
D. Smith	0	0	1b	0/0	0/0	0	6
B. Thomas	1	0	0	0/0	0/0	0	6
Tolbert	0	0	1c	0/0	0/0	0	6
Woodson	0	0	1d	0/0	0/0	0	6
COWBOYS	26	19	5	22/29	48/48	0	414
Opponents	8	19	0	20/25	24/24	1*	248

2-Pt Conversions: Team 0-2, Opponents 0-3

a 87 yd. kickoff return vs. Arizona (10/9)
   83 yd. punt return vs. Washington (11/20)
b 13 yd. interception return @ New Orleans (12/19)
c 54 yd. interception return, @ New Orleans (12/19)
d 94 yd. interception return @ Philadelphia (12/4)
* R Peete fumble out of end zone, @ NY Giants (12/24)

USUAL STARTERS

WR	Alvin Harper	LE	Tony Tolbert
LT	Mark Tuinei	LT	Russell Maryland
LG	Nate Newton	RT	Leon Lett
C	Mark Stepnoski	RE	Charles Haley
RG	Derrek Kennard	LLB	Dixon Edwards
RT	Larry Allen (9)	MLB	Robert Jones
	Erik Williams (7)	RLB	Darrin Smith
TE	Jay Novacek	LCB	Kevin Smith
WR	Michael Irvin	RCB	Larry Brown
QB	Troy Aikman	SS	Darren Woodson
RB	Emmitt Smith	FS	James Washington
FB	Daryl Johnston		

PASSING	ATT	COMP	YDS	PCT	AVG ATT	TD	PCT TD	PCT INT	INT	LG	SKS/YDS	RATING
Aikman	361	233	2,676	64.5	7.41	13	3.6	12	3.3	90t	14/59	84.9
Peete	56	33	470	58.9	8.39	4	7.1	1	1.8	65t	7/21	102.5
Garrett	31	16	315	51.6	10.16	2	6.5	1	3.2	68t	2/13	95.5
COWBOYS	448	282	3,461	62.9	7.73	19	4.2	14	3.1	90t	20/93	87.8
Opponents	522	269	3,051	51.5	5.84	19	3.6	22	4.2	67t	47/299	64.0

NFL STANDINGS

AFC

East
East	W	L
Buffalo	10	6
Miami	9	7
Indianapolis	9	7
New England	6	10
New York	3	13

Central
Central	W	L
Pittsburgh	11	5
Houston	7	9
Cincinnati	7	9
Cleveland	5	11
Jacksonville	4	12

West
West	W	L
Kansas City	13	3
San Diego	9	7
Seattle	8	8
Denver	8	8
Oakland	8	8

NFC

East
East	W	L
Dallas	12	4
Philadelphia	10	6
Washington	6	10
New York	5	11
Arizona	4	12

Central
Central	W	L
Green Bay	11	5
Detroit	10	6
Chicago	9	7
Minnesota	8	8
Tampa Bay	7	9

West
West	W	L
San Francisco	11	5
Atlanta	9	7
Carolina	7	9
St. Louis	7	9
New Orleans	7	9

POSTSEASON

AFC
Indianapolis	35		
San Diego	20		
Buffalo	37		
Miami	22		
Pittsburgh	40		
Buffalo	21		
Indianapolis	10		
Kansas City	7		
Pittsburgh	20		
Indianapolis	16		

NFC
Green Bay	37
Atlanta	20
Philadelphia	58
Detroit	37
Green Bay	27
San Francisco	17
Dallas	30
Philadelphia	11
Dallas	38
Pittsburgh	17

SUPER BOWL

Dallas	27
Pittsburgh	17

1995

First place, NFC East
Head Coach: Barry Switzer

PRESEASON (2-3)
Date	W/L	Score	Opponent	Att.
7/29	W	21-15	Buffalo	62,752
8/5	L	14-27	Oakland	62,031
8/12	L	7-9	Buffalo @ Toronto	55,799
8/21	L	17-20	@ Denver	72,451
8/26	W	10-0	Houston @ San Ant.	52,512

REGULAR SEASON (12-4)
Date	W/L	Score	Opponent	Att.
9/4	W	35-0	@ N.Y. Giants	77,454
9/10	W	31-21	DENVER	64,578
9/17	W	23-17	@ Minnesota (OT)	60,088
9/24	W	34-20	ARIZONA	64,560
10/1	L	23-27	@ Washington	55,489
10/8	W	34-24	GREEN BAY	64,806
10/15	W	23-9	@ San Diego	62,664
10/22			– Bye –	
10/29	W	28-13	@ Atlanta	70,089
11/6	W	34-12	PHILADELPHIA	64,876
11/12	L	20-38	SAN FRANCISCO	65,180
11/19	W	34-21	@ Oakland	54,092
11/23	W	24-12	KANSAS CITY	64,901
12/3	L	17-24	WASHINGTON	64,866
12/10	L	17-20	@ Philadelphia	66,198
12/17	W	21-20	N.Y. GIANTS	64,400
12/25	W	37-13	@ Arizona	72,394

DIVISIONAL PLAYOFF
Date	W/L	Score	Opponent	Att.
1/7/96	W	30-11	PHILADELPHIA	64,372

NFC CHAMPIONSHIP GAME
Date	W/L	Score	Opponent	Att.
1/14/96	W	38-27	GREEN BAY	65,135

SUPER BOWL XXX (Phoenix)
Date	W/L	Score	Opponent	Att.
1/28/96	W	27-17	Pittsburgh	76,347

TEAM STATISTICS	DALLAS	OPP
FIRST DOWNS	364	303
Rushing	141	113
Passing	195	165
Penalty	28	25
Third Down-Made/Att.	83/186	97/216
Third Down Efficiency	44.6	44.9
Fourth Down-Made/Att.	8/13	8/19
TOTAL NET YARDS	5,824	5,044
Avg. Per Game	364.0	315.3
Total Plays	1,007	1,001
Avg. Per Play	5.8	5.0
NET YARDS RUSHING	2,201	1,772
Avg. Per Game	137.6	110.8
Total Rushes	495	442
Avg. Per Rush	4.4	4.0
NET YARDS PASSING	3,623	3,272
Avg. Per Game	226.4	204.5
Sacked/Yards Lost	18/118	36/219
Gross Yards	3,741	3,491
Attempts/Completions	494/322	523/293
Pct. of Completions	65.2	56.0
Had Intercepted	10	19
PUNTS/AVERAGE	55/40.8	65/42.7
Net Punting Average	34.7	37.8
PUNT RET./AVG.	23/11.1	22/9.8
KICKOFF RET./AVG.	58/22.0	85/19.5
INT./AVG. RET.	19/13.7	10/15.5
PENALTIES/YARDS	90/695	112/913
FUMBLES/BALL LOST	24/13	16/6
TOUCHDOWNS	51	32
Rushing	29	13
Passing	18	17
Returns	4	2
EXTRA POINT/ATTEMPTS	47/50	30/32
Kicking Made-Attempts	46/48	29/29
Passing Made-Attempts	1/2	1/3
Rushing Made-Attempts	0/0	0/0
FIELD GOALS/ATTEMPTS	27/28	22/27
AVG. TIME OF POSSESSION	31:15	28:45

RUSHING	ATT	YDS	AVG	LG	TD
E. Smith	377	1,773	4.7	60t	25
S. Williams	48	205	4.3	44t	1
Johnston	25	111	4.4	18t	2
K. Williams	10	53	5.3	14t	0
Aikman	21	32	1.5	12t	1
Wilson	10	12	1.2	11t	0
Sanders	2	9	4.5	8t	0
Lang	1	7	7.0	7t	0
Garrett	1	-1	1.0	-1t	0
COWBOYS	495	2,201	4.4	60t	29
Opponents	442	1,772	4.0	48t	1

RECEIVING	ATT	YDS	AVG	LG	TD
Irvin	111	1,603	14.4	50t	10
Novacek	62	705	11.4	33t	5
E. Smith	62	375	6.0	40t	0
K. Williams	38	613	16.1	48t	2
Johnston	30	248	8.3	24t	1
Bjornson	7	53	7.6	16t	0
Fleming	6	83	13.8	16t	0
S. Williams	3	28	9.3	24t	0
Sanders	2	25	12.5	19t	0
Watkins	1	8	8.0	8t	0
COWBOYS	322	3,741	11.6	50t	18
Opponents	293	3,491	11.9	81t	17

INTERCEPTIONS	NO	YDS	AVG	LG	TD
Brown	6	124	20.7	65t	2
Marion	6	40	6.7	32t	1
Woodson	2	46	23.0	37t	1
Sanders	2	34	17.0	34t	0
Myles	1	15	15.0	15t	0
Brice	1	2	2.0	2t	0
Holmes	1	0	0.0	0t	0
COWBOYS	19	261	13.7	65t	4
Opponents	10	155	15.5	48t	1

PUNTING	NO	YDS	AVG	TB	IN20	LG	BL	NET
Jett	53	2,166	40.9	6	17	58	0	34.5
Boniol	2	77	38.5	0	2	56	0	38.5
COWBOYS	55	2,243	40.8	6	19	58	0	34.7
Opp.	65	2,775	42.7	3	22	60	0	37.8

PUNT RETURNS	NO	FC	YDS	AVG	LG	TD
K. Williams	18	15	166	9.2	30	0
Holmes	4	1	35	8.8	13	0
Sanders	1	1	54	54.0	43	0
COWBOYS	23	17	255	11.1	43	0
Opponents	22	10	216	9.8	21	0

KICKOFF RETURNS	NO	YDS	AVG	LG	TD
K. Williams	49	1,108	22.6	43	0
Holmes	5	134	26.8	46	0
Marion	1	16	16.0	16	0
Sanders	1	15	15.0	15	0
Schwantz	1	9	9.0	9	0
Watkins	1	-6	-6.0	-6	0
COWBOYS	58	1,276	22.0	46	0
Opponents	85	1,661	19.5	59	0

SCORE BY QUARTERS	1	2	3	4	OT	T
COWBOYS	102	133	83	111	6	435
Opponents	38	104	78	71	0	291

FIELD GOALS	11-19	20-29	30-39	40-49	50+
Boniol	0-0	11-12	13-13	3-3	0-0
COWBOYS	0-0	11-12	13-13	3-3	0-0
Opponents	1-1	7-7	7-8	7-10	0-1

Boniol: (),(45),(39,20M),(25,30),(32,34,23),(24, 35),(30),(),(42,37),(26, 37),(26,38),(20), (37),(21),(27,32,23,45,35),(39,23,24)

Opponents: (42B),(),(42,48M),(54M,31,19),(38, 46),(42),(),(21,40), (36,37),(26),(31M), (34,37),(47),(42,27,38,42),(40M,20, 27),(21,23)

SCORING	TDR	TDP	TDRt	2Pt	FG	PAT	S	TP
E. Smith	25	0	0	0	0/0	0/0	0	150
Boniol	0	0	0	0	27/28	46/48	0	127
Irvin	0	10	0	0	0/0	0/0	0	60
Novacek	0	5	0	1	0/0	0/0	0	32
Johnston	2	1	0	0	0/0	0/0	0	18
Brown	0	0	2a	0	0/0	0/0	0	12
K. Williams	0	2	0	0	0/0	0/0	0	12
Aikman	1	0	0	0	0/0	0/0	0	6
Marion	0	0	1b	0	0/0	0/0	0	6
S. Williams	1	0	0	0	0/0	0/0	0	6
Woodson	0	0	1c	0	0/0	0/0	0	6
COWBOYS	29	18	4	1	27/28	46/48	0	435
Opponents	13	17	2*	1	22/27	29/29	1+	291

2-Pt Conversions: Team 1-2, Opponents 1-3

a 20 yd. interception return vs Philadelphia (11/6)
   65 yd. interception return @ Philadelphia (12/10)
b 32 yd. interception return @ Arizona (IV25)
c 37yd. interception return~Washington(10/1)
* Hanks 38 yd. fumble return vs San Francisco (11/12)
   A. Williams 48 yd. int. return @ Arizona (12/25)
+ Aikman sacked in end zone @ San Diego (10/15)

USUAL STARTERS

WR	Kevin Williams	LE	Tony Tolbert
LT	Mark Tuinei	LT	Russell Maryland
LG	Nate Newton	RT	Leon Lett (10)
C	Ray Donaldson (12)		Chad Hennings (6)
	Derrek Kennard (4)	RE	Charles Haley (11)
RG	Larry Allen		Shante Carver (3)
RT	Erik Williams	LLB	Dixon Edwards
TE	Jay Novacek	MLB	Robert Jones (12)
WR	Michael Irvin		Godfrey Myles (4)
QB	Troy Aikman	RLB	Darrin Smith (9)
RB	Emmit Smith		Godfrey Myles (7)
FB	Daryl Johnston	LCB	Deion Sanders (9)
			Clayton Holmes (6)
		RCB	Larry Brown
		SS	Darren Woodson
		FS	Brock Marion

PASSING	ATT	COMP	YDS	PCT	AVG ATT	TD	PCT TD	PCT INT	INT	LG	SKS/YDS	RATING
Aikman	432	280	3,304	64.8	7.65	16	3.7	1.6	7	50	14/89	93.6
Wilson	57	38	391	66.7	6.86	1	1.8	5.3	3	38	4/29	70.1
Garrett	5	4	46	80.0	9.20	1	20.0	0.0	0	24	0/0	144.6
COWBOYS	494	322	3,741	65.2	7.57	18	3.6	2.0	10	50	18/118	91.7
Opponents	523	293	3,491	56.0	6.67	17	3.3	3.6	19	81t	36/219	72.3

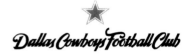

Dallas Cowboys Football Club

March 9, 1989

Mr. Ron St. Angelo
Ron St. Angelo Photography
Sammons Center for the Arts
3630 Harry Hines Blvd.
Dallas, TX 75219

Dear Ron:

Many thanks for sending a copy of the press release from your Taiwan
trip.

I would imagine that the invitation to teach in Taiwan was a great
honor and we are both happy for you and proud of your accomplishments.

Your work for the Dallas Cowboys and the Cheerleaders has always been
of the highest quality, and we look forward to the continuation of our
longtime relationship.

Best regards,

[signature]

Texas E. Schramm
President and General Manager

TES/cm

Tom Landry   July 8, 1989

Dear Ron,

Thank you for the
excellent portraits you did
for Tex and me.
I have written Danny,
Tim and Michael for
their contribution.
My continued best
wishes to you.

Sincerely

Tom Landry

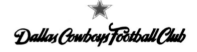

Dallas Cowboys Football Club

July 14, 1993

JIMMY JOHNSON
Head Coach

To Whom It May Concern:

Ron St. Angelo has done photography for the Dallas
Cowboys for a number of years, and we find his work
to be of the highest quality. Because of this, Ron
enjoys an excellent reputation with the Dallas Cowboys and many of the corporate sponsors he has
worked with on our behalf.

His recent work from the Super Bowl Season has been
acclaimed locally and nationally. I highly recommend him for any of your photographic needs.

Sincerely yours,

Jimmy Johnson

Jimmy Johnson

JJ:bg

Ron, Thanks for my print also.
I have it framed & it is
awesome.
Barbara

Ron St. Angelo
Ron St. Angelo Photography
3630 Harry Hines Boulevard
Dallas TX 75219

          October 9, 1995

Dear Ron:

Thank you for the spectacular framed photograph shot during
the NFC Championship game in January of this year. It is
really outstanding. You are a master of your art. The
colors are so vivid.

It will be great in my new home, and it will bring back many
memories. Thanks for capturing a special moment for me,
not to mention the great players and the superb action.

Appreciate your thoughtfulness with the special gift.

Sincerely,

[signature]

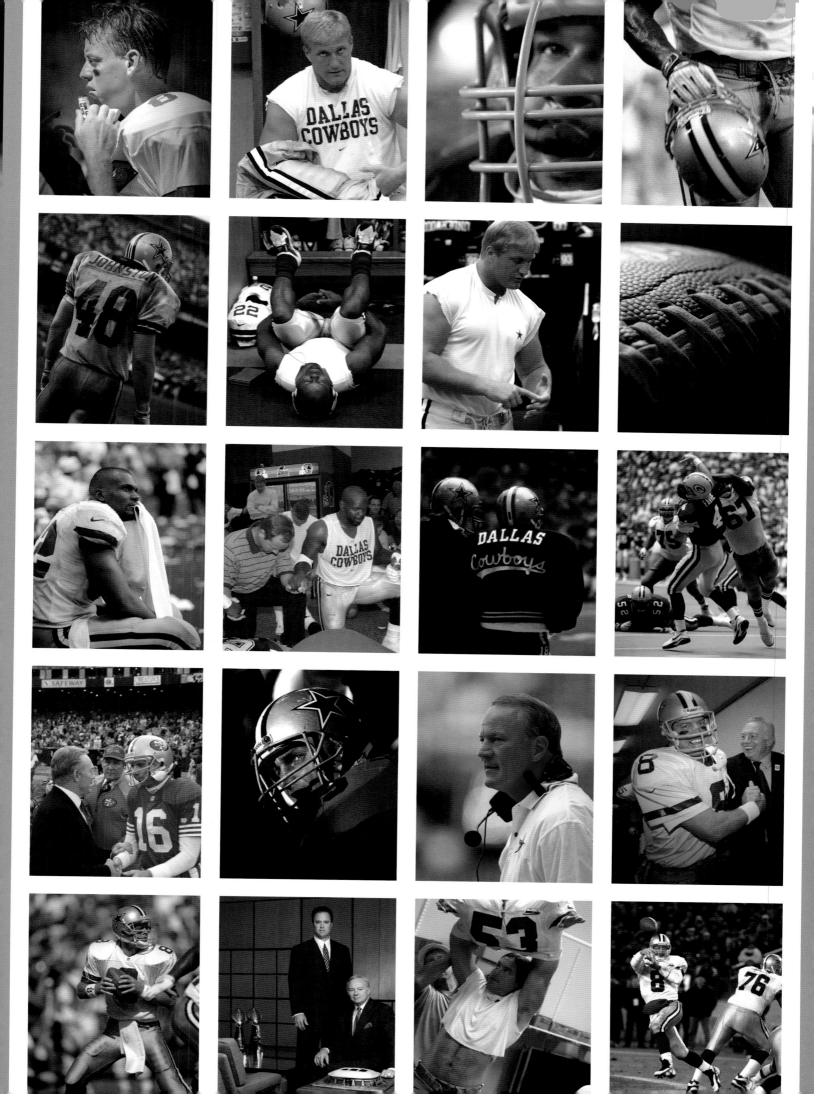

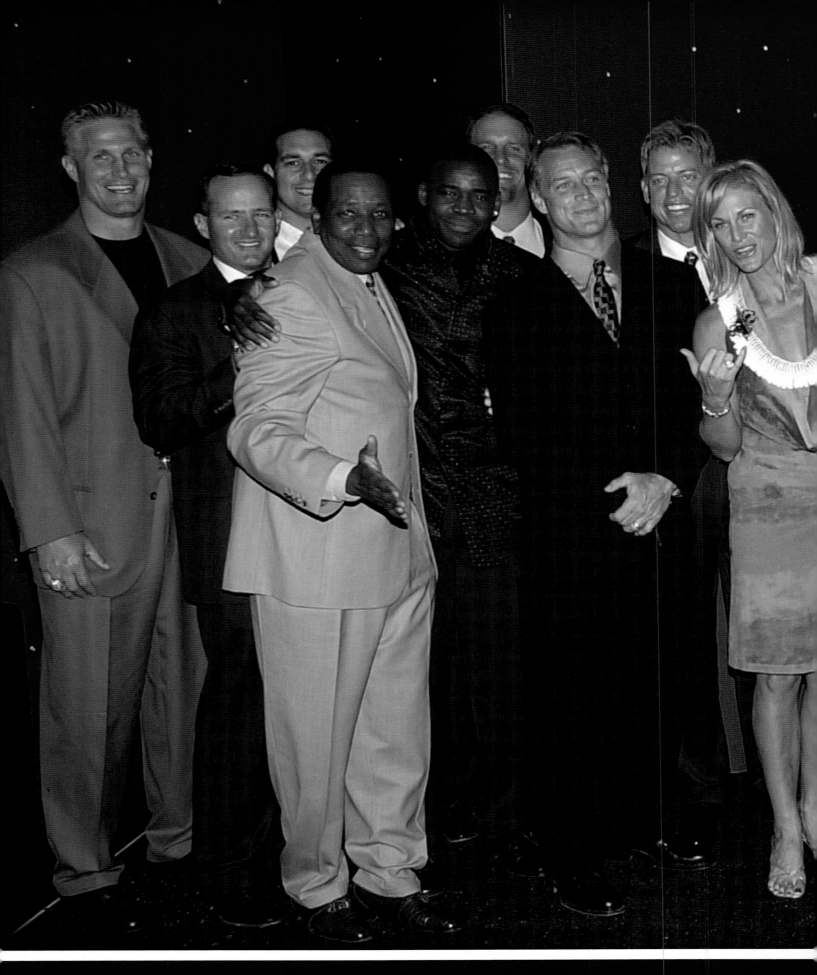

Dallas Cowboys Reunion

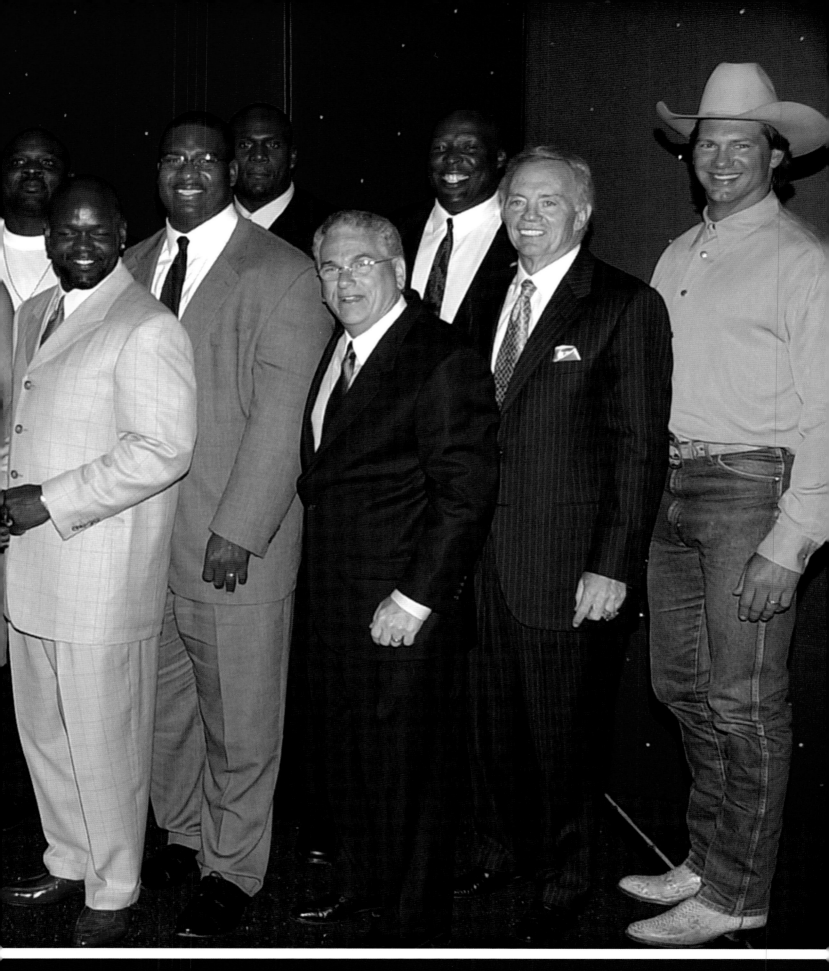

Texas Stadium / June 2001

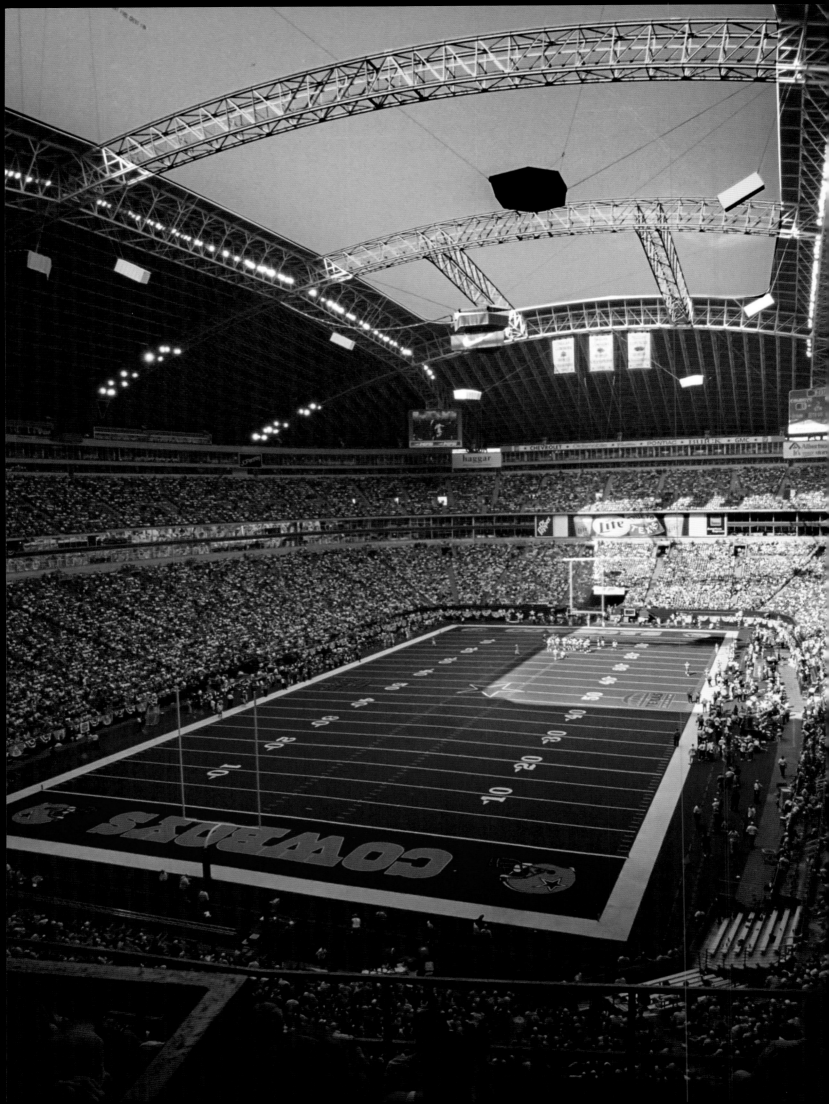

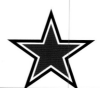

CLOSING THE HOLE IN THE ROOF

It was the spring of 1972. Just months before the Dallas Cowboys had unveiled the NFL's newest and finest pigskin palace. The debut of Texas Stadium, with its distinctive outer ring of giant concrete buttresses and trademark two-and-a-half-acre hole in the roof, had dazzled the world of sports. The eventual cost of beyond $30 million dwarfed the $6.1 million New England spent just the year before on its new football-only venue, Schaefer Stadium.

On this bright April morning, my parents took the grand tour of the sparkling showplace. Neither had ever traveled more than one hundred miles from their places of birth in western New York state before making this journey to the Southwest. And they'd never seen anything quite like Texas Stadium. Adjectives such as "beautiful," "clean," "huge," and "wonderful" dotted their comments. After one last drive on the road encircling the stadium, we paused to take in a final distant overview. After several seconds of silence, my 4'10", Polish mom asked very seriously—"When are they going to finish it?"

Now, after thirty-seven success-filled seasons, Texas Stadium itself is finished. The Cowboys and city of Arlington have built an awesome facility set to open for the 2009 NFL campaign. The price of Dallas's new digs may eventually reach *forty* times what Texas Stadium cost.

Now, if only the level of winning in their next house can equal that which Dallas enjoyed playing under their hole-in-the roof.

In the autumn of 1971, when Dallas christened the stadium, the world looked far different from now. The war in Vietnam raged on. A first-class postage stamp cost eight cents. *All in the Family* debuted on CBS, stunning television audiences with its willingness to joke about previously taboo topics such as race, sex, and antigovernment opinions. *Patton* captured the Academy Award for best picture. The U.S. thought of Iran as a trusted ally. A gallon of regular gasoline had jumped to 36 cents. Pro-football fan Richard Nixon neared the end of his first term as president. The Watergate was just another very nice hotel in Washington,

D.C. The Dow Jones had reached 950. The average home sold for $28,300.

And the Dallas Cowboys hadn't yet won anything.

The franchise had, in fact, only been in existence eleven years. But the Pokes had already picked up a generally accepted national nickname. No, not "America's Team." That tag wouldn't become commonplace until the late '70s. The Dallas team that moved into Texas Stadium was mockingly referred to as "Next Year's Champions."

Owner Clint Murchison's expansion franchise staggered through five losing seasons before starting to show signs of breaking through. But they never *broke* through. They dropped their first postseason game in '65. They lost the championship game in '66 to Green Bay. They fell again to the Packers in the celebrated 1967 "Ice Bowl." Another first-round playoff exit in '68. Again in '69. The misery reached its zenith in '70. Dallas won their way into Super Bowl V only to fritter the game away with a hailstorm of mistakes. Baltimore triumphed 16–13 in a contest

> The biggest crowd to ever witness a single event in the stadium was not there for football. Carmen, a religious singer who preached through his music, drew 71,132 for an anti–gang violence concert.

"The price of Dallas's new digs may eventually reach *forty* times what Texas Stadium cost."

so poorly played that it has forever carried the label of "the Blooper Bowl."

The eleven seasons playing in the Cotton Bowl at Fair Park had produced mounting frustration and that increasingly burdensome nickname—"Next Year's Champions." And owner Murchison tired of that home field pretty quickly.

"By 1964," Murchison once said, "it had become obvious that the Cotton Bowl, a grand lady in her day, suffered from terminal illness."

Murchison originally wanted his Cowboys to stay in downtown Dallas. He'd found what he considered a perfect location. Lots of parking. Plenty of adjacent land for the city to build museums and a music hall. Civic leaders loved it. Convention promoters jumped on board. The Dallas Citizens Council liked the idea so much that they proposed expanding the concept. Both major newspapers offered enthusiastic endorsements. Only one man hated it—Dallas mayor Erik Jonsson.

Dallas entered their final season playing at Texas Stadium with a huge "lead." In the 305 combined regular-season and playoff home games, the Cowboys have outscored their opponents 7,279 to 5,395. That's a whopping 1,884-point advantage.

The stadium proposal died. The Cowboys wound up in the suburb of Irving, on a site that had been nothing but a landfill.

Bonds necessary to finance the construction passed. Groundbreaking took place January 25, 1969, with hopes that a "dress rehearsal" North Texas State college football game could be played in December of 1970, followed by a full season of Cowboy football accompanied by all the appropriate pomp-and-circumstance. But just like Cowboys teams on the field, new problems kept cropping up with their field.

The bricklayers union struck for three weeks. Then the plumbers walked off the job. Two months of torrential rains meant sump pumps worked overtime while cranes stood idly by. Paving the parking lot became a posterior pain. At one point a local reporter asked an Irving police captain what he thought of the ability to park thousands of cars in the lots. His reply? "If you walked out there now, you'd sink up to your ankles."

Then came the almost comical haggling over alcohol.

The stadium site was in a "dry" area of Irving—no sales of spirits allowed. But who could ever imagine NFL games without any alcohol? The politicians eventually struck an interesting compromise. They decreed the stadium's 170 posh and private Circle Suites to be a "wet area" while regular seats remained "dry."

All the difficulties eventually resulted in "delay of games."

Forget that late '70 college game. Not even close. The new target date became the Cowboys' August 14, 1971, pre-season opener. But as that date neared, completion of the project still lagged. The Cowboys opted to move a three-pack of exhibitions back to the Cotton Bowl. That still wouldn't be enough leeway. The club shifted a pair of early October regular seasons back to its old home too.

Ironically, by the time the Cowboys actually played in Texas Stadium, that contest would be the fourth event held there. A ten-day Billy Graham Crusade and a pair of college games preceded the

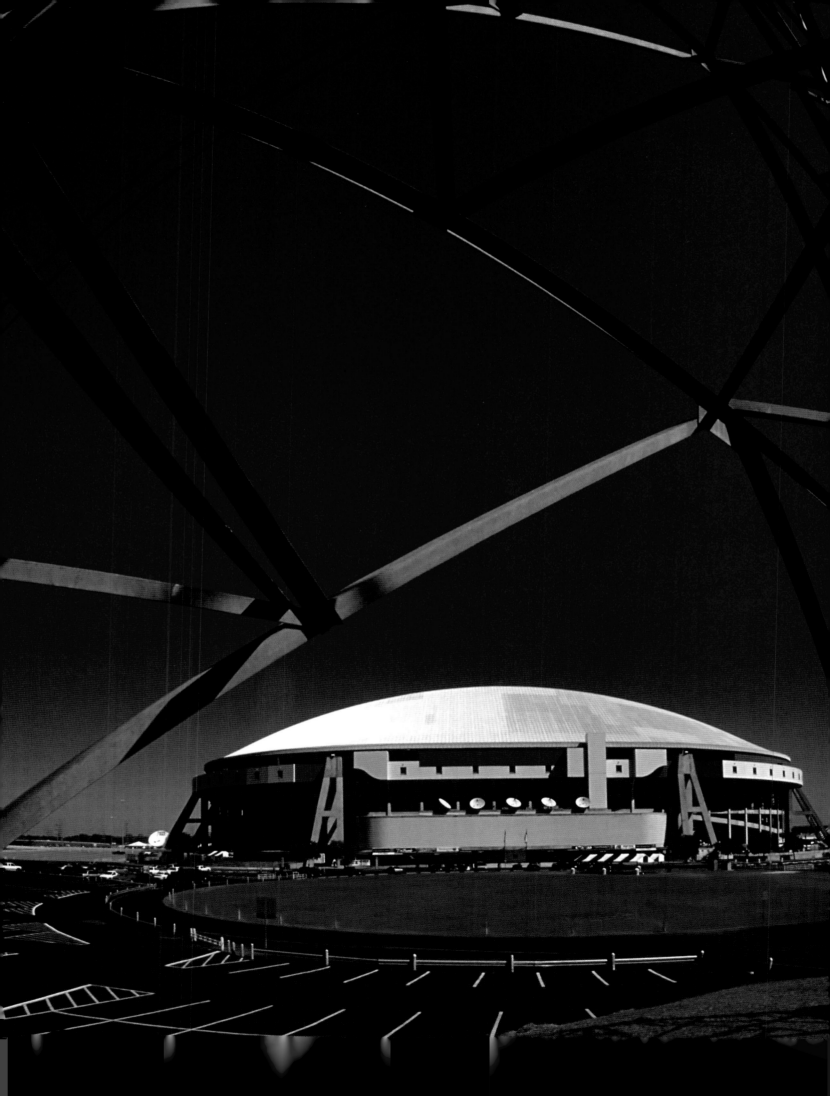

Pokes' October 24, 1971, extravaganza of an opening. Graham had said, "I hope the crusade will somehow sanctify the stadium and help the Cowboys win the Super Bowl."

How prophetic that would be!

Dallas roared into their new facility, drilling the Patriots 44–21. Roger Staubach hit Bob Hayes with a pair of touchdown passes. Dallas's "Doomsday Defense" harassed Pats QB Jim Plunkett all day. Former president Lyndon Johnson made the rounds in the victorious locker room, shaking hands and posing for photo ops.

Other than the as-expected traffic delays and the usual array of minor first-day problems, critics hailed Texas Stadium as a smashing success. The finished product resembled some European soccer venues in that the roof completely covered the seating areas but not the playing field. What made the concept of the stadium unique was the fact that builders had erected two buildings—the stadium itself and then the roof, which was a totally independent structure. Some had worried that the design could create severe noise problems as had happened with Houston's Astrodome. But in actual game conditions, much of that noise exited through the hole in the roof.

Ah, that hole in the roof. A few years later linebacker D. D. Lewis made his famous quip that builders had left the hole "so that God could watch His team play."

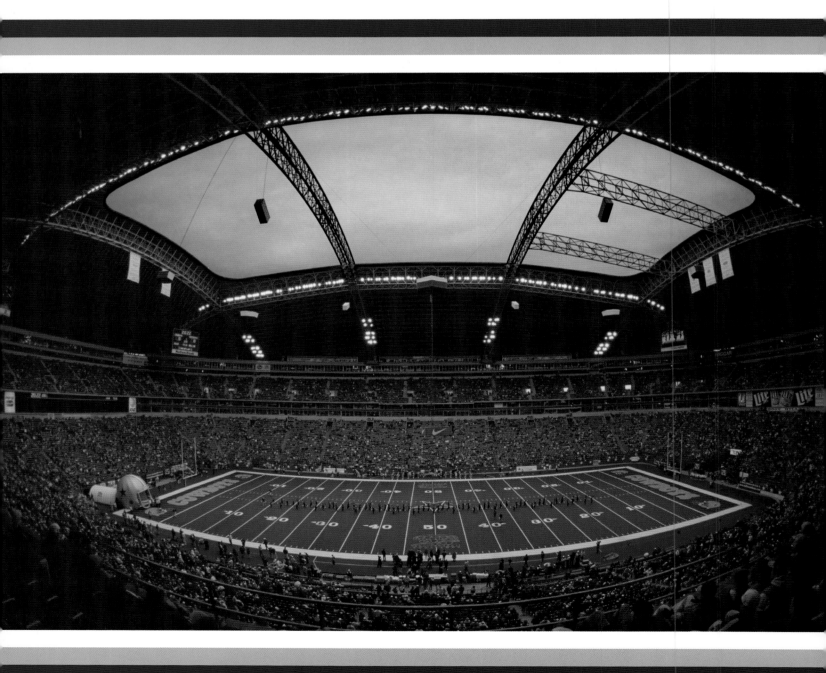

In the project's infancy, Murchison actually wanted to eventually make the stadium "whole" by covering the "hole."

"We hope to design a movable or plastic roof on the stadium" Murchison offered. "If we had started from scratch, there would be no question we could design such a roof. Whether we can do it now with the roof already built, I'm not sure."

The most magical of all Texas Stadium happenings, however, had to be the immediate elevation of the Dallas Cowboys. Following that opening-night destruction of New England, Dallas never lost at home in the entire '71 season. In fact, they only lost once more anywhere that year! The Cowboys reeled off seven consecutive victories to close out the regular season, whipped San Francisco 14–3 in their

Linebacker D. D. Lewis made his famous quip that builders had left the hole "so that God could watch His team play."

The plan never got off the ground. The topic arose again when Jerry Jones bought the team and stadium eighteen years later. But by then any such renovation had become cost prohibitive.

Over the years Texas Stadium's hosted a diverse array of high-profile events—Promise Keepers, pro soccer, high school football championships, wrestling extravaganzas, more Billy Graham Crusades, Supercross, and Cinco de Mayo celebrations. The concert calendar regularly included megastars, such as Paul McCartney, Garth Brooks, Genesis, Michael Jackson, George Strait, and Metallica.

Bruce Hardy, general manager of the Stadium for the last quarter of a century, remembers some of these acts in particular.

Madonna—"She wasn't the friendliest lady in the world . . . I'm not used to ladies using rough language."

'N Sync—"We had to get all sorts of video games in their dressing room. They got here six hours early and just played video games."

Axl Rose of Guns and Roses—"It got to be 8:30 and no Axl. Fans started chanting. I was thinking the stadium was gonna be torn up. He pulled down the tunnel at 9:10, the car door opened, and he couldn't walk. I don't know what they did, but twenty minutes later he was on stage and performed for two hours."

McCartney—"We couldn't wear leather shoes. He didn't like the idea that you killed animals to make leather shoes, so all of us, our security people, wore tennis shoes."

oh-so-comfy house for the NFC title, and "Next Year's Champions" became this year's champion with a 24–3 thumping of Miami in Super Bowl VI. Dallas jammed all that winning into just eighty-four days from stadium debut to world champs.

In its lifetime Texas Stadium's been the home of five Cowboy Super Bowl winners. No other NFL venue since the 1967 AFL-NFL merger can match that. Over the years Dallas has won an astounding 68 percent of all regular-season and playoff games there. Ten members of the organization from those years have been honored with induction into the Hall of Fame. The final scheduled regular-season game on December 20, 2008, will extend the string of consecutive sellouts to 153.

The excitement of Dallas Cowboy football will then switch to Arlington. Texas Stadium, now showing the signs of nearly four decades of use, will fall silent. But those experiencing Dallas's awesome new house may still at times be reminded of those glorious years in Irving. On lovely days, when the retractable roof's been rolled back so that anyone "above" can watch the game, fans in the Cowboys' grand, new place will see a hole-in-the-roof eerily similar in shape to that of their longtime home at Texas Stadium.

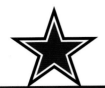

AUGUST 22, 1992

A TEXAS STADIUM MOMENT

Dallas had spent three seasons building something special—a team the Cowboys and their fans hoped would return the franchise to the glory years of the '70s.

Something else, however, had also grown during that same period—a sense of uneasiness in quarterback Troy Aikman. Simply put, heading into the exhibition season before the '92 season and even after three years together, Aikman sensed that coach Jimmy Johnson might still not think of him as the man he wanted to lead these emerging Cowboys.

"Our relationship was still very much strained at that point," Aikman remembers.

The strain, however, was about to disappear in part because a Texas Stadium halftime celebration honoring those legendary '70s Cowboys would run long.

But how, after three seasons, could the relationship between head coach and emerging quarterback still be so distant? The roots of that answer begin much farther back than that 1989 draft in which Johnson selected Aikman number one.

Coming out of high school, Aikman spurned Johnson's scholarship offer from Oklahoma State to sign with coach Barry Switzer's rival, Oklahoma. A couple of years later, after Aikman had broken a leg and decided to transfer, he again said no to Johnson, who'd moved on to Miami and wanted Aikman to join his Hurricanes. Aikman opted for UCLA instead.

One would think, though, that once Johnson grabbed Aikman in the '89 draft, there'd be little question who the Cowboys believed in as their quarterback of the future. Au contraire. Just a few weeks after that draft, Johnson used Dallas's supplemental #1 choice to take Miami of Florida All-American QB Steve Walsh, who'd quarterbacked Johnson's Hurricanes to the college national championship. Despite Johnson's claims that he chose Walsh only because using that pick represented good value, whispers began that Johnson actually preferred Walsh to be "his guy."

When an injury sidelined Aikman two-thirds of the way through his rookie season, Walsh came in and played creditably, actually posting a better quarterback rating. But Aikman seemed to have cemented the job by starting all sixteen games of the '90 season. Johnson dealt Walsh to New Orleans for first-second-and third-round draft choices (he did get good value), and all quarterback questions seemed settled in Dallas. Then

Johnson picked up accomplished veteran QB Steve Beuerlein.

In 1991, as the 6–5 Cowboys began what they hoped would be their drive to a first playoff berth in six years, Aikman suffered a serious knee injury at Washington five plays into the second half. Beuerlein entered, finished off that win, and led Dallas to four consecutive season-ending victories, an 11–5 record, and a wild card berth.

The way Aikman saw it, the backup shouldn't have even started the season finale.

"I felt I could play in the last game against the Falcons, and Jimmy came up to me before the game and said, I want to work you in some and get you some playing time."

But Aikman didn't play. Johnson told him the rain had made the artificial turf damp and that Dallas didn't want to take any chances. That was OK with Aikman.

"So, I said fine and just assumed I was starting against Chicago [in the playoffs]."

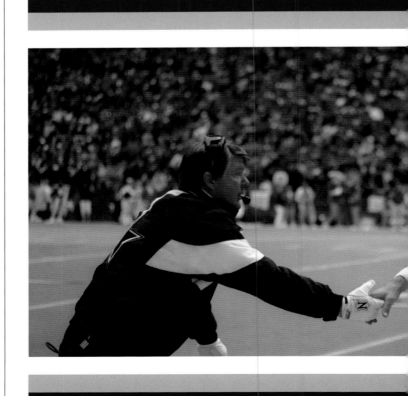

Wrong again. But it was the way Aikman found out he wasn't the starter against the Bears that truly angered him.

"I got a call from one of the beat writers saying Jimmy just announced Beuerlein was going to start. I was pretty upset and I met with Jimmy the first thing the next morning and let him know how unhappy I was with the way it was handled. He told me he didn't want me to be a distraction to the team, and I assured him I wouldn't be one."

Beuerlein quarterbacked the entire 17–13 win at Chicago and then started the week after at Detroit. He and the rest of the Cowboys played miserably that day, losing to the Lions 38–6. Aikman, the supposed "quarterback of the future," got in for mop-up duty only.

Training camp began for the '92 season with Aikman facing what he believed to be one cold, hard reality.

"Even though I don't know if it was ever publicly announced that the job was open, I realized that even if I did start the opener, I was going to be on a pretty short leash."

Which brings us to this sultry August night and halftime of this next-to-last exhibition game of the summer against Denver. The Cowboys filed out of their locker room and down the tunnel for the start of the second half, only to find on-field festivities still hadn't finished. Dallas had chosen this game to honor the twentieth anniversary of the Cowboy team that had won the club's first Super Bowl in January 1972. Convertibles containing coach Tom Landry and the stars of that team, such as Roger Staubach, Rayfield Wright, Mel Renfro, Bob Lilly, and many, many others slowly made their way around the field, accepting the adoration of the more than 61,000 fans at Texas Stadium.

As the present-day Cowboys waited for the ceremonies to conclude, Aikman walked up to Johnson and said: "Just think, coach, one of these years, after we're long out of being a part of this thing, that's going to be you and me going around in one of those cars."

Just an innocent observation. An off-the-cuff remark just to kill a little time. Johnson said nothing. But something had struck home inside this coach never known for being fond of such warm and fuzzy feelings. Aikman, however, wouldn't realize his words had connected for three more weeks.

The '92 season began two weeks later with a 23–10 thumping of the defending Super Bowl champion Redskins. Then Dallas journeyed to New York, which had won the title the season before that, and held off a late Giants rally to win 34–28.

On the jubilant flight home, Aikman took his usual seat toward the rear of the plane and passed the time having some beers and "yukking it up with a few of the guys."

Then came the moment that transformed the often-strained relationship between QB and coach.

"We were about halfway through the flight, and Jimmy came to the back of the plane, which he rarely did. He grabbed me and said, 'You'll never know how much what you said to me in the tunnel during the preseason meant to me!' And it was at that moment that I felt—OK we're starting to connect here."

Connect indeed! In the two remaining seasons, Aikman and Johnson spent together, the Cowboys went go 31-7 and won back-to-back Super Bowls.

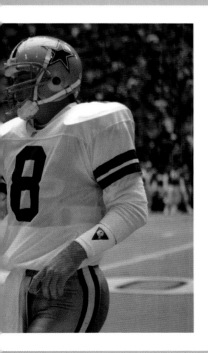
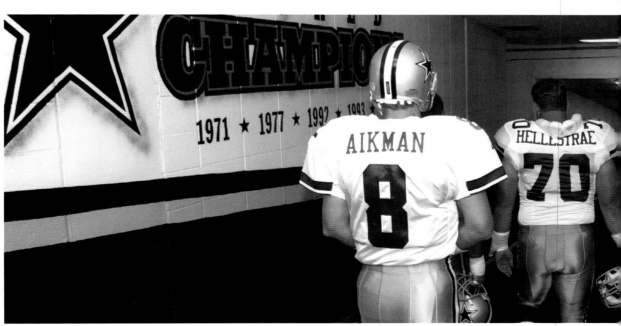

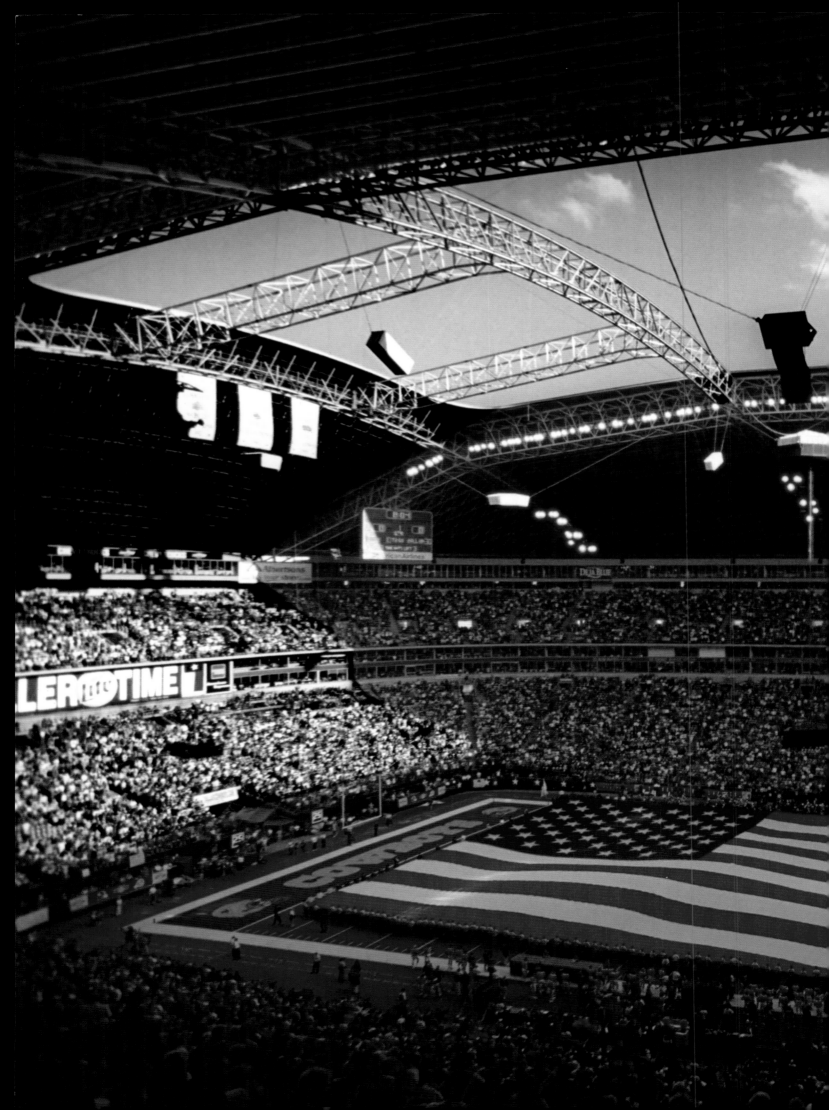

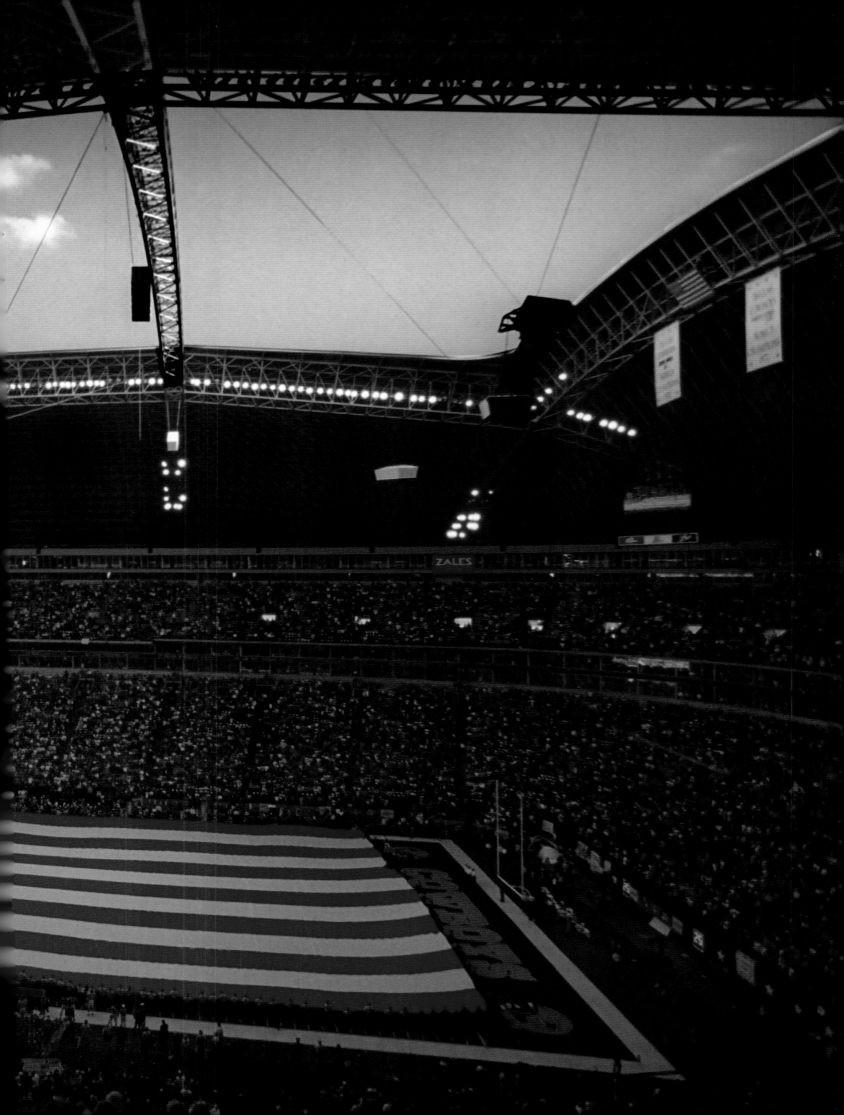

TEXAS STADIUM

25th

ANNIVERSARY

1971 • 1996

OH, THE JOYS OF TEAM OWNERSHIP
DECEMBER 24, 1989

A TEXAS STADIUM MOMENT

The phone at Jerry Jones's home rang before dawn on this Christmas Eve. The call had nothing to do with Santa Claus.

"Just when I thought things couldn't get any worse," Jones remembers, "they did."

Uncommonly cold weather struck north Texas the day before. Temperatures had fallen to an arctic, 6 degrees. Overnight, all the pipes at Texas Stadium had frozen. None of the bathrooms worked. Some upper-level pipes had burst, flooding some of the private suites. Kickoff for the last game of the season against Green Bay was just a few hours away.

How perfectly appropriate!

This Dallas season, the first of Jones's ownership, had gone in the toilet from the very beginning. Now, Texas Stadium faithful couldn't even flush those toilets. Jones himself had become a lightning rod for the unhappiness of Cowboy fans.

The clumsy firing of legendary coach Tom Landry, Jones's often controversial statements about how he intended to run the team, and the Cowboys' continued descent into obscurity on the field had worked Cowboy fans into a lather. When it came to criticism, many simply couldn't hold it in anymore. But on this day at Texas Stadium, it looked as though all those in attendance would literally have to hold it in.

General Manager Bruce Hardy and his crew sprang into action.

"We found a few hundred port-o-potties and scattered 'em all over the place. Then, as best we could, we mopped up the floor."

A few hours later, Green Bay mopped the floor with the Cowboys, beating Dallas 20–10. The season ended with seven consecutive defeats, a 1–15 record (most losses ever in a single Cowboy season) and the only year in which Dallas went winless at home (0-8).

"Yes," Jones recalls, "there were a few moments back then that I wondered what I'd gotten myself into."

> Both the hottest (109 degrees on September 3, 2000) and the coldest (26 degrees on January 7, 1996) stadium home games ever came against the same team—Philadelphia.

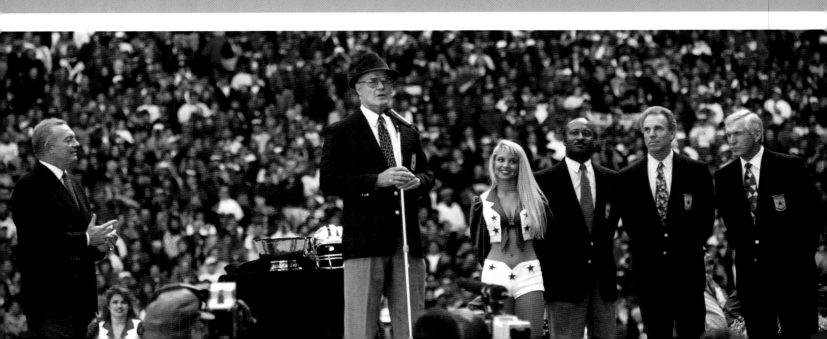

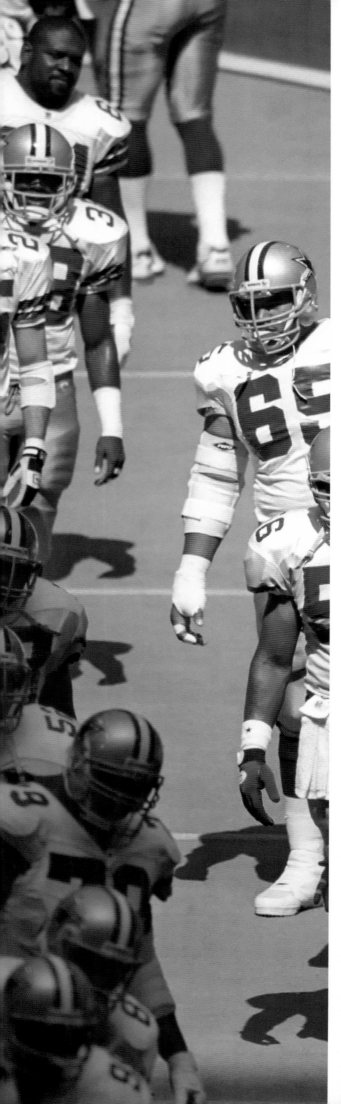
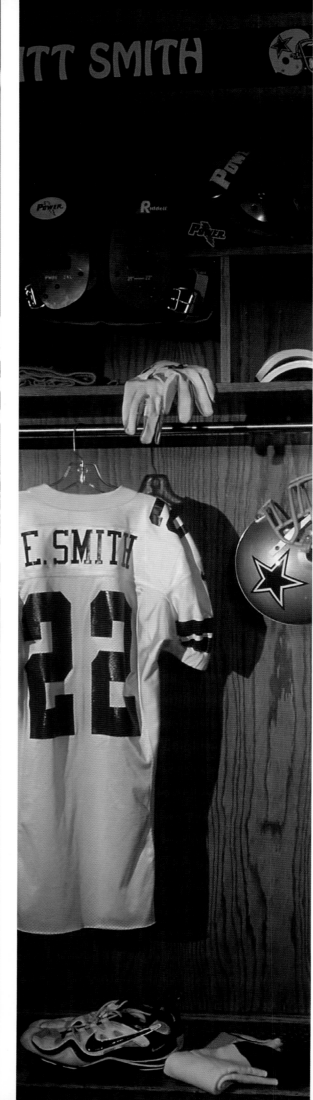
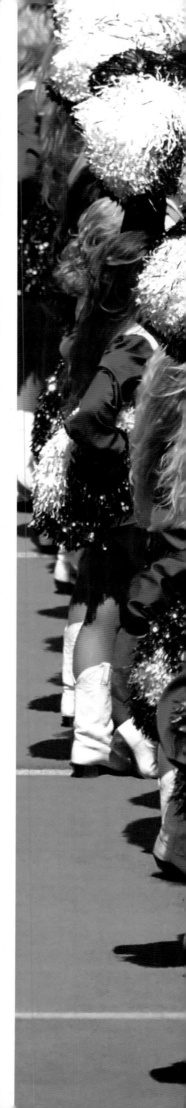

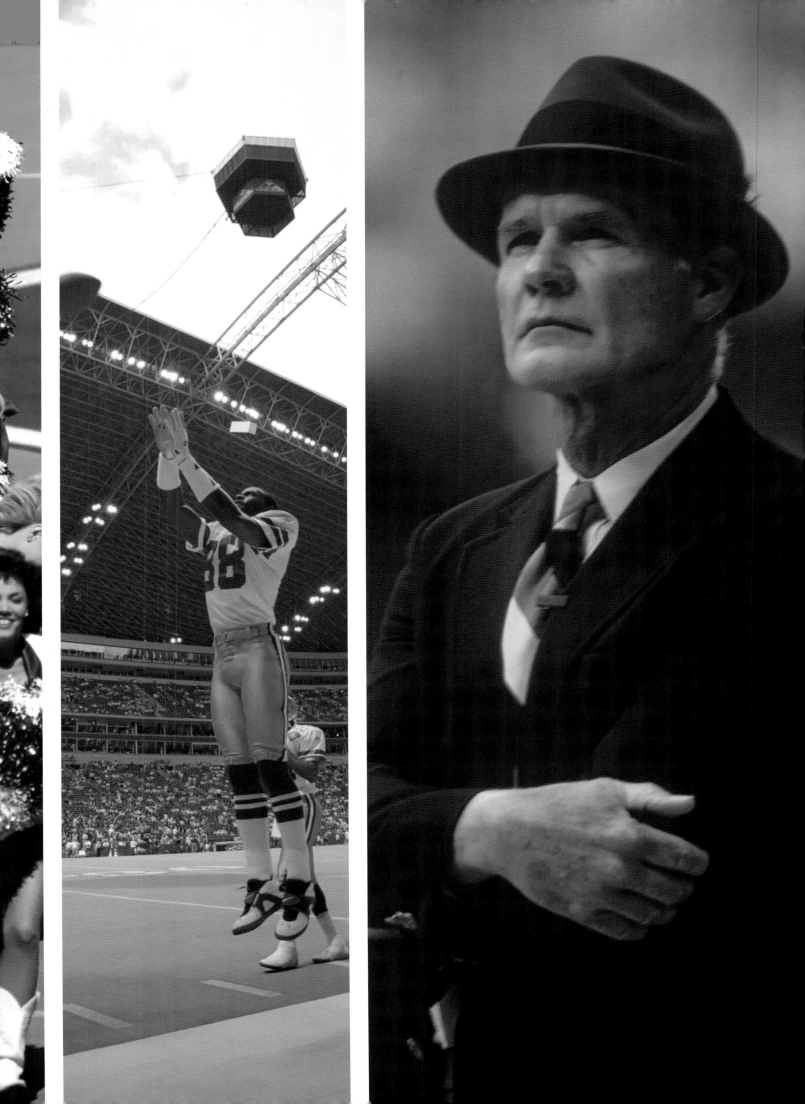

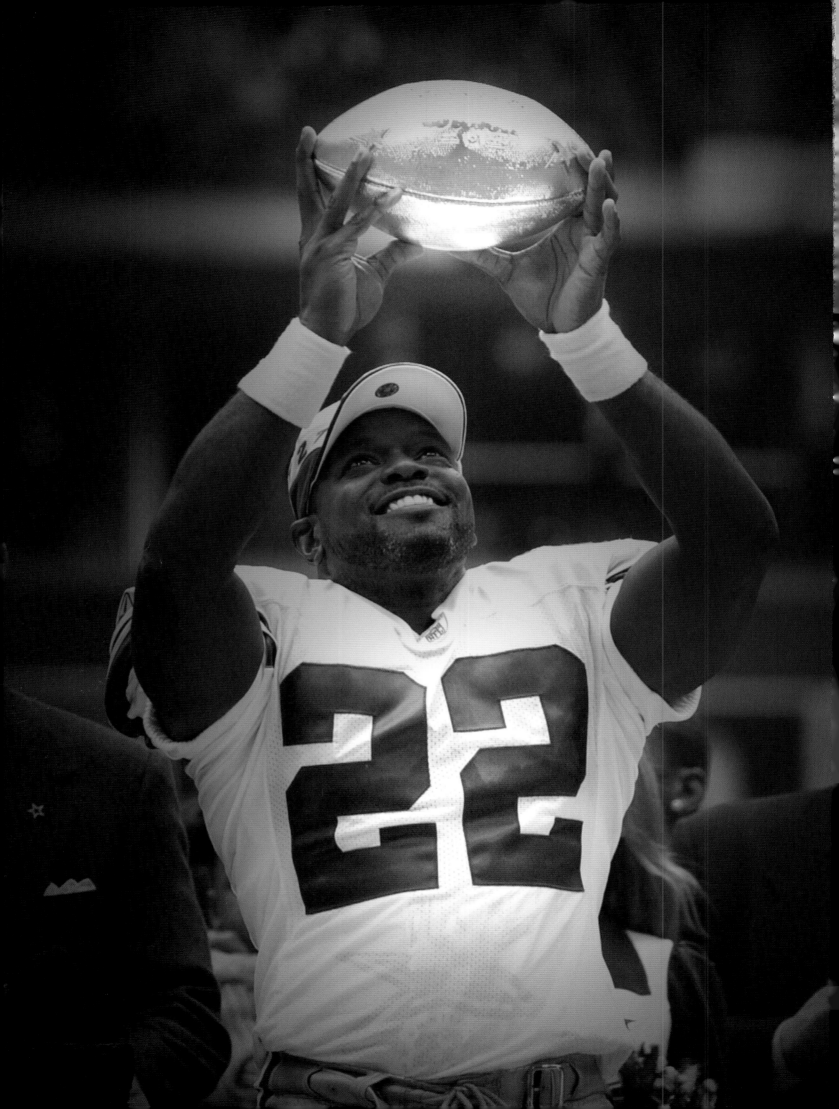